HARRISON'S
Gastroenterology and Hepatology

Editors

Dan L. Longo, MD
Scientific Director, National Institute on Aging,
National Institutes of Health, Bethesda and Baltimore

Anthony S. Fauci, MD
Chief, Laboratory of Immunoregulation;
Director, National Institute of Allergy and Infectious Diseases,
National Institutes of Health, Bethesda

Associate Editor

Carol A. Langford, MD, MHS
Associate Professor of Medicine
Cleveland Clinic, Cleveland

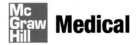 Medical

New York   Chicago   San Francisco   Lisbon   London   Madrid   Mexico City
Milan   New Delhi   San Juan   Seoul   Singapore   Sydney   Toronto

Harrison's Gastroenterology and Hepatology

2 3 4 5 6 7 8 9 0   CTP/CTP   14 13 12 11

ISBN 978-0-07-166333-5
MHID 0-07-166333-9

This book was set in Bembo by Glyph International. The editors were James Shanahan and Kim J. Davis. The production supervisor was Catherine H. Saggese. Project management was provided by Arushi Chawla of Glyph International. The cover design was by Thomas DePierro. Cover, section, and chapter opener illustrations © MedicalRF.com. All rights reserved.

China Translation & Printing Services Ltd. was the printer and binder.

Library of Congress Cataloging-in-Publication Data

Harrison's gastroenterology and hepatology / editors Dan L. Longo, Anthony S. Fauci.
      p. ; cm.
   This book is aimed at bringing together the chapters of Harrison's principles of internal medicine, 17th ed.
      ISBN-13: 978-0-07-166333-5 (pbk. : alk. paper)
      ISBN-10: 0-07-166333-9 (pbk. : alk. paper)
      1. Gastroenterology—Textbooks.   2. Hepatology—Textbooks.   3. Gastrointestinal system—Diseases—Textbooks.   4. Liver—Diseases—Textbooks.   I. Longo, Dan L. (Dan Louis), 1949-II. Fauci, Anthony S., 1940-III. Harrison, Tinsley Randolph, 1900-1978. IV. Harrison's principles of internal medicine.   V. Title: Gastroenterology and hepatology.
      [DNLM: 1. Gastrointestinal Diseases.   2. Liver Diseases. WI 140 H323 2010]
   RC801.H33 2010
   616.3'3—dc22

                                                                            2009035665

McGraw-Hill books are available at special quantity discounts to use as premiums and sales promotions, or for use in corporate training programs. To contact a representative please e-mail us at bulksales@mcgraw-hill.com.

CONTENTS

CONTRIBUTORS

Numbers in brackets refer to the chapter(s) written or co-written by the contributor.

JOHN C. ATHERTON, MD
Professor of Gastroenterology; Director, Wolfson Digestive
Diseases Centre, University of Nottingham, United Kingdom [25]

JANE C. ATKINSON, DDS
Program Director, Clinical Trials Program, Center for Clinical
Research, National Institute of Dental and Craniofacial Research,
National Institutes of Health, Bethesda [3]

BRUCE R. BACON, MD
James F. King Endowed Chair in Gastroenterology; Professor of
Internal Medicine, Division of Gastroenterology & Hepatology,
St. Louis [41, 42]

MIRIAM J. BARON, MD
Instructor in Medicine, Harvard Medical School, Boston [24]

JEAN BERGOUNIOUX, MD
Medical Doctor of Pediatrics, Unité de Pathogénie Microbienne
Moléculaire, Paris [27]

HENRY J. BINDER, MD
Professor of Medicine; Professor of Cellular & Molecular Physiology,
Yale University, New Haven [15]

BRUCE R. BISTRIAN, MD, PhD
Chief, Clinical Nutrition, Beth Israel Deaconess Medical Center;
Professor of Medicine, Harvard Medical School, Boston [54]

MARTIN J. BLASER, MD
Frederick H. King Professor of Internal Medicine; Chair,
Department of Medicine; Professor of Microbiology, New York
University School of Medicine, New York [25, 28]

GERALD BLOOMFIELD, MD, MPH
Department of Internal Medicine, The Johns Hopkins University
School of Medicine, Baltimore [Review and Self-Assessment]

RICHARD S. BLUMBERG, MD
Professor of Medicine, Harvard Medical School; Chief, Division
of Gastroenterology, Hepatology and Endoscopy, Brigham and
Women's Hospital, Boston [16]

CYNTHIA D. BROWN, MD
Department of Internal Medicine, The Johns Hopkins University
School of Medicine, Baltimore [Review and Self-Assessment]

JOAN R. BUTTERTON, MD
Assistant Clinical Professor of Medicine, Harvard Medical School;
Clinical Associate in Medicine, Massachusetts General Hospital,
Boston [22]

STEPHEN B. CALDERWOOD, MD
Morton N. Swartz, MD Academy Professor of Medicine
(Microbiology and Molecular Genetics), Harvard Medical School;
Chief, Division of Infectious Diseases, Massachusetts General
Hospital, Boston [22]

MICHAEL CAMILLERI, MD
Atherton and Winifred W. Bean Professor; Professor of Medicine
and Physiology, Mayo Clinic College of Medicine, Rochester [6]

BRIAN I. CARR, MD, PhD
Professor of Medicine, Thomas Jefferson University; Director of the
Liver Tumor Program, Kimmel Cancer Center, Philadelphia [48]

YU JO CHUA, MBBS
Research Fellow (Medical Oncology), Royal Marsden Hospital,
London [49]

RAYMOND T. CHUNG, MD
Associate Professor of Medicine, Harvard Medical School; Director
of Hepatology, Massachusetts General Hospital; Medical Director,
Liver Transplant Program, Massachusetts General Hospital,
Boston [44]

DAVID CUNNINGHAM, MD
Professor of Cancer Medicine, Institute of Cancer Research;
Consultant Medical Oncologist, Head of Gastrointestinal Unit,
Royal Marsden Hospital, London [49]

JOHN DEL VALLE, MD
Professor and Senior Associate Chair of Graduate Medical Education,
Department of Internal Medicine, Division of Gastroenterology,
University of Michigan Health System, Ann Arbor [14]

JULES L. DIENSTAG, MD
Carl W. Walter Professor of Medicine and Dean for Medical
Education, Harvard Medical School; Physician, Gastrointestinal Unit,
Massachusetts General Hospital, Boston [37–39, 44]

DAVID F. DRISCOLL, PhD
Assistant Professor of Medicine, Harvard Medical School, Boston [54]

SAMUEL C. DURSO, MD, MBA
Associate Professor of Medicine, Clinical Director, Division of
Geriatric Medicine and Gerontology, The Johns Hopkins University
School of Medicine, Baltimore [2, 3]

JOHANNA DWYER, DSc, RD
Professor of Medicine and Community Health, Tufts University
School of Medicine and Friedman School of Nutrition Science and
Policy; Senior Scientist Jean Mayer Human Nutrition Research
Center on Aging at Tufts; Director of the Frances Stern Nutrition
Center, Tufts–New England Medical Center Hospital, Boston [51]

ROBERT H. ECKEL, MD
Professor of Medicine, Division of Endocrinology, Metabolism and
Diabetes, Division of Cardiology; Professor of Physiology and
Biophysics; Charles A. Boettcher II Chair in Atherosclerosis; Program
Director, Adult General Clinical Research Center, University of
Colorado at Denver and Health Sciences Center; Director Lipid
Clinic, University Hospital, Aurora [58]

DANIEL J. FINK,[†] MD, MPH
Associate Professor of Clinical Pathology, College of Physicians
and Surgeons, Columbia University, New York [Appendix]

JEFFREY S. FLIER, MD
Caroline Shields Walker Professor of Medicine, Harvard Medical
School; Dean of the Faculty of Medicine, Harvard School of
Medicine, Boston [55]

[†]Deceased.

SONIA FRIEDMAN, MD
Assistant Professor of Medicine, Harvard Medical School; Associate Physician, Brigham and Women's Hospital, Boston [16]

SUSAN L. GEARHART, MD
Assistant Professor of Colorectal Surgery and Oncology, The Johns Hopkins University School of Medicine, Baltimore [18–21]

DALE N. GERDING, MD
Assistant Chief of Staff for Research, Hines VA Hospital, Hines; Professor, Stritch School of Medicine, Loyola University, Maywood [23]

MARC GHANY, MD
Staff Physician, Liver Diseases Branch, National Institute of Diabetes and Digestive and Kidney Diseases, National Institutes of Health, Bethesda [34]

ROGER I. GLASS, MD, PhD
Director, Fogarty International Center; Associate Director for International Research, National Institutes of Health, Bethesda [30]

ROBERT M. GLICKMAN, MD
Professor of Medicine, New York University School of Medicine, New York [10]

RAJ K. GOYAL, MD
Mallinckrodt Professor of Medicine, Harvard Medical School, Boston; Physician, VA Boston Healthcare and Beth Israel Deaconess Medical Center, West Roxbury [4, 13]

NORTON J. GREENBERGER, MD
Clinical Professor of Medicine, Harvard Medical School; Senior Physician, Brigham and Women's Hospital, Boston [43, 45, 46]

WILLIAM L. HASLER, MD
Professor of Medicine, Division of Gastroenterology, University of Michigan Health System, Ann Arbor [5, 11]

DOUGLAS C. HEIMBURGER, MD, MS
Professor of Nutrition Sciences; Professor of Medicine; Director, Clinical Nutrition Fellowship Program, University of Alabama at Birmingham, Birmingham [53]

JAY H. HOOFNAGLE, MD
Director, Liver Diseases Research Branch, Division of Digestive Diseases and Nutrition, National Institute of Diabetes and Digestive and Kidney Diseases, National Institutes of Health, Bethesda [34]

ROBERT T. JENSEN, MD
Chief, Digestive Diseases Branch, National Institute of Diabetes, Digestive and Kidney Diseases, National Institutes of Health, Bethesda [50]

STUART JOHNSON, MD
Associate Professor, Stritch School of Medicine, Loyola University, Maywood; Staff Physician, Hines VA Hospital, Hines [23]

MARSHALL M. KAPLAN, MD
Professor of Medicine, Tufts University School of Medicine; Chief Emeritus, Division of Gastroenterology, Tufts-New England Medical Center, Boston [9, 35]

DENNIS L. KASPER, MD, MA (Hon)
William Ellery Channing Professor of Medicine, Professor of Microbiology and Molecular Genetics, Harvard Medical School; Director, Channing Laboratory, Department of Medicine, Brigham and Women's Hospital, Boston [24]

GERALD T. KEUSCH, MD
Associate Provost and Associate Dean for Global Health, Boston University School of Medicine, Boston [29]

ALEXANDER KRATZ, MD, PhD, MPH
Assistant Professor of Clinical Pathology, Columbia University College of Physicians and Surgeons; Associate Director, Core Laboratory, Columbia University Medical Center, New York-Presbyterian Hospital; Director, Allen Pavilion Laboratory, New York [Appendix]

ROBERT F. KUSHNER, MD
Professor of Medicine, Northwestern University Feinberg School of Medicine, Chicago [56]

LOREN LAINE, MD
Professor of Medicine, Keck School of Medicine, University of Southern California, Los Angeles [8]

MARK E. MALLIARD, MD
Associate Professor and Chief, Division of Gastroenterology and Hepatology, Omaha [40]

ELEFTHERIA MARATOS-FLIER, MD
Associate Professor of Medicine, Harvard Medical School; Chief, Obesity Section, Joslin Diabetes Center, Boston [55]

ROBERT J. MAYER, MD
Stephen B. Kay Family Professor of Medicine, Harvard Medical School, Dana- Farber Cancer Institute, Boston [47]

SAMUEL I. MILLER, MD
Professor of Genome Sciences, Medicine, and Microbiology, University of Washington, Seattle [26]

JOSEPH A. MURRAY, MD
Professor of Medicine, Division of Gastroenterology and Hepatology, The Mayo Clinic, Rochester [6]

THOMAS B. NUTMAN, MD
Head, Helminth Immunology Section; Head, Clinical Parasitology Unit; Laboratory of Parasitic Diseases, National Institute of Allergy and Infectious Diseases, National Insitutes of Health, Bethesda [33]

CHUNG OWYANG, MD
Professor of Internal Medicine, H. Marvin Pollard Collegiate Professor; Chief, Division of Gastroenterology, University of Michigan Health System, Ann Arbor [11, 17]

UMESH D. PARASHAR, MBBS, MPH
Lead, Enteric and Respiratory Viruses Team, Epidemiology Branch, Division of Viral Diseases, National Center for Immunization and Respiratory Diseases, Centers for Disease Control and Prevention, Atlanta [30]

GUSTAV PAUMGARTNER, MD
Professor of Medicine, University of Munich, Munich, Germany [43]

DAVID A. PEGUES, MD
Professor of Medicine, Division of Infectious Diseases, David Geffen School of Medicine at UCLA, Los Angeles [26]

MICHAEL A. PESCE, PhD
Clinical Professor of Pathology, Columbia University College of Physicians and Surgeons; Director of Specialty Laboratory, New York Presbyterian Hospital, Columbia University Medical Center, New York [Appendix]

DANIEL S. PRATT, MD
Assistant Professor of Medicine, Harvard Medical School; Director, Liver- Billary-Pancreas Center, Massachusetts General Hospital, Boston [9, 35]

ROSHINI RAJAPAKSA, MD, BA
Assistant Professor, Department of Medicine, Gastroenterology, New York University Medical Center School of Medicine and Hospitals Center, New York [10]

SHARON L. REED, MD
Professor of Pathology and Medicine; Director, Microbiology and Virology Laboratories, University of California, San Diego Medical Center, San Diego [31]

CAROL M. REIFE, MD
Clinical Associate Professor of Medicine, Jefferson Medical College, Philadelphia [7]

ROBERT M. RUSSELL, MD
Director, Jean Mayer USDA Human Nutrition Research Center on Aging at Tufts University; Professor of Medicine and Nutrition, Tufts University, Boston [52]

PHILIPPE SANSONETTI
Professeur á l'Institut Pasteur, Paris, France [27]

JOSHUA SCHIFFER, MD
Department of Internal Medicine, The Johns Hopkins University School of Medicine, Baltimore [Review and Self-Assessment]

WILLIAM SILEN, MD
Johnson and Johnson Distinguished Professor of Surgery, Emeritus, Harvard Medical School, Boston [1, 20, 21]

MICHAEL F. SORRELL, MD
Robert L. Grissom Professor of Medicine, University of Nebraska Medical Center, Omaha [40]

ADAM SPIVAK, MD
Department of Internal Medicine, The Johns Hopkins University School of Medicine, Baltimore [Review and Self-Assessment]

PAOLO M. SUTER, MD, MS
Professor of Medicine, Medical Policlinic, Zurich, Switzerland [52]

MARK TOPAZIAN, MD
Associate Professor of Medicine, Mayo College of Medicine, Rochester [12]

PHILLIP P. TOSKES, MD
Professor of Medicine, Division of Gastroenterology, Hepatology and Nutrition, University of Florida College of Medicine, Gainesville [45, 46]

MATTHEW K. WALDOR, MD, PhD
Professor of Medicine (Microbiology and Molecular Genetics), Channing Laboratory, Brigham and Women's Hospital, Harvard Medical School, Boston [29]

B. TIMOTHY WALSH, MD
Professor of Psychiatry, College of Physicians & Surgeons, Columbia University; Director, Eating Disorders Research Unit, New York Psychiatric Institute, New York [57]

PETER F. WELLER, MD
Professor of Medicine, Harvard Medical School; Co-Chief, Infectious Diseases Division; Chief, Allergy and Inflammation Division; Vice-Chair for Research, Department of Medicine, Beth Israel Deaconess Medical Center, Boston [32, 33]

CHARLES WIENER, MD
Professor of Medicine and Physiology; Vice Chair, Department of Medicine; Director, Osler Medical Training Program, The Johns Hopkins University School of Medicine, Baltimore [Review and Self-Assessment]

ALLAN W. WOLKOFF, MD
Professor of Medicine and Anatomy and Structural Biology; Director, Belfer Institute for Advanced Biomedical Studies; Associate Chair of Medicine for Research; Chief, Division of Hepatology, Albert Einstein College of Medicine, Bronx [36]

LOUIS MICHEL WONG-KEE-SONG, MD
Assistant Professor of Medicine, Division of Gastroenterology and Hepatology, Mayo College of Medicine, Rochester [12]

JANET A. YELLOWITZ, DMD, MPH
Associate Professor; Director, Geriatric Dentistry, The Johns Hopkins University School of Medicine, Baltimore [3]

PREFACE

Harrison's Principles of Internal Medicine (HPIM) has long been a major source of information related to the practice of medicine for many practitioners and trainees. Yet in its aim to cover the broad spectrum of medicine, the book has become nearly 3000 pages in length and is pushing the envelope of "portability." *HPIM* has spawned several offspring tailored to diverse uses for sources of medical information. The entire book plus a large cache of supplemental visual and textual information is available as *Harrison's Online*, a component of McGraw-Hill's *Access Medicine* offering. A condensed version of *HPIM*, called *Harrison's Manual of Medicine*, has been published in print format suitable for carrying in a white coat pocket and in several electronic formats (PDA, Blackberry, iPhone). A companion to *HPIM* that serves as a study guide for standardized tests in medicine, *HPIM Self-Assessment and Board Review*, is an effective teaching tool that highlights important areas of medicine discussed in *HPIM*. *Harrison's Practice* is another electronic information source, organized by medical topic or diagnosis with information presented in a consistent structured format for ease of finding specific information to facilitate clinical care and decision-making at the bedside. All of these products retain the broad spectrum of topics presented in the *HPIM* "mother book" in variable degrees of depth.

In 2006, for the first time, the Editors of *HPIM* experimented with extracting portions of *HPIM* that were focused on a specific subspecialty of internal medicine. The products of that effort, *Harrison's Endocrinology, Harrison's Rheumatology,* and *Harrison's Neurology in Clinical Medicine*, were very well-received by audiences keenly interested in the respective subspecialities of internal medicine. Accordingly, we are expanding the effort to include books focused on other specialties.

According to a report from the National Institute of Diabetes and Digestive and Kidney Diseases, for every 100 residents of the United States, there were 35 ambulatory care contacts and 5 overnight hospital stays at which a digestive disease diagnosis was noted. In 2004, digestive diseases accounted for more than 236,000 deaths. Thus, training in the disciplines of gastroenterology and hepatology is essential to any primary care physician or general internist and even to practitioners of other internal medicine subspecialties.

This book is aimed at bringing together the chapters of *HPIM* related to gastroenterology and hepatology in a conveniently sized book for a focused study of this medical subspecialty. The book is organized into 58 chapters and 11 sections: (I) Cardinal Manifestations of Gastrointestinal Disease; (II) Evaluation of the Patient with Alimentary Tract Symptoms; (III) Disorders of the Alimentary Tract; (IV) Infections of the Alimentary Tract; (V) Evaluation of the Patient with Liver Disease; (VI) Disorders of the Liver and Biliary Tree; (VII) Liver Transplantation; (VIII) Disorders of the Pancreas; (IX) Neoplastic Diseases of the Gastrointestinal System; (X) Nutrition; and (XI) Obesity and Eating Disorders.

The information presented here is contributed by physician/authors who have personally made notable advances in the fields of their expertise. The chapters reflect authoritative analyses by individuals who have been active participants in the amazing surge of new information on genetics, cell biology, pathophysiology, and treatment that has characterized all of medicine in the last 20 years. In addition to the didactic value of the chapters, a section of test questions, answers, and an explanation of the correct answers is provided to facilitate learning and assist the reader in preparing for standardized examinations.

Gastroenterology and hepatology, like many other areas of medicine, are changing rapidly. Novel technologies of imaging, development of new drugs, and the application of molecular pathogenesis information to detect disease early and prevent disease in people at risk are just a few of the advances that have made an impact on the practice of gastroenterology. Physicians are now applying endoscopic techniques in ways that were once unimaginable including performing operations successfully without an incision; operations that once required major surgery with attendant morbidity and expense. The pace of discovery demands that physicians undertake nearly continuous self-education. It is our hope that this book will help physicians in this process.

We are grateful to Kim Davis and James Shanahan at McGraw-Hill for their help in producing this book.

Dan L. Longo, MD
Anthony S. Fauci, MD

Review and self-assessment questions and answers were taken from Wiener C, Fauci AS, Braunwald E, Kasper DL, Hauser SL, Longo DL, Jameson JL, Loscalzo J (editors) Bloomfield G, Brown CD, Schiffer J, Spivak A (contributing editors). *Harrison's Principles of Internal Medicine Self-Assessment and Board Review*, 17th ed. New York, McGraw-Hill, 2008, ISBN 978-0-07-149619-3.

 The global icons call greater attention to key epidemiologic and clinical differences in the practice of medicine throughout the world.

 The genetic icons identify a clinical issue with an explicit genetic relationship.

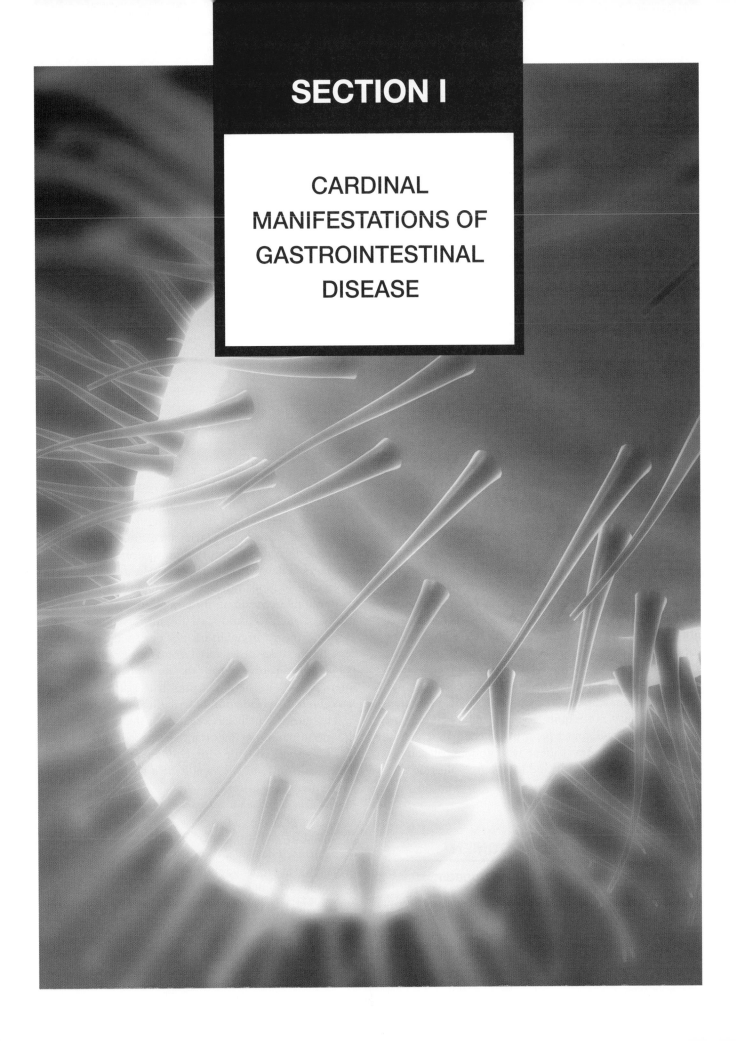

SECTION I

CARDINAL MANIFESTATIONS OF GASTROINTESTINAL DISEASE

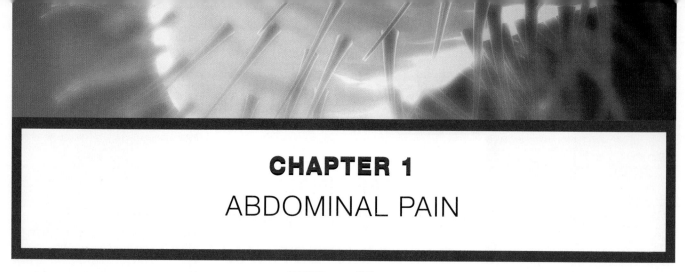

CHAPTER 1
ABDOMINAL PAIN

William Silen

The correct interpretation of acute abdominal pain is challenging. Since proper therapy may require urgent action, the unhurried approach suitable for the study of other conditions is sometimes denied. Few other clinical situations demand greater judgment, because the most catastrophic of events may be forecast by the subtlest of symptoms and signs. A meticulously executed, detailed history and physical examination are of great importance. The etiologic classification in **Table 1-1**, although not complete, forms a useful basis for the evaluation of patients with abdominal pain.

The diagnosis of "acute or surgical abdomen" is not an acceptable one because of its often misleading and erroneous connotation. The most obvious of "acute abdomens" may not require operative intervention, and the mildest of abdominal pains may herald an urgently correctable lesion. Any patient with abdominal pain of recent onset requires early and thorough evaluation and accurate diagnosis.

SOME MECHANISMS OF PAIN ORIGINATING IN THE ABDOMEN

Inflammation of the Parietal Peritoneum

The pain of parietal peritoneal inflammation is steady and aching in character and is located directly over the inflamed area, its exact reference being possible because it is transmitted by somatic nerves supplying the parietal peritoneum. The intensity of the pain is dependent on the type and amount of material to which the peritoneal surfaces are exposed in a given time period. For example, the sudden release into the peritoneal cavity of a small quantity of *sterile* acid gastric juice causes much more pain than the same amount of grossly contaminated neutral feces. Enzymatically active pancreatic juice incites more pain and inflammation than does the same amount of sterile bile containing no potent enzymes. Blood and urine are often so bland as to go undetected if their contact with the peritoneum has not been sudden and massive. In the case of bacterial contamination, such as in pelvic inflammatory disease, the pain is frequently of low intensity early in the illness until bacterial multiplication has caused the elaboration of irritating substances.

The rate at which the irritating material is applied to the peritoneum is important. Perforated peptic ulcer may be associated with entirely different clinical pictures dependent only on the rapidity with which the gastric juice enters the peritoneal cavity.

The pain of peritoneal inflammation is invariably accentuated by pressure or changes in tension of the peritoneum, whether produced by palpation or by movement, as in coughing or sneezing. The patient with peritonitis lies quietly in bed, preferring to avoid motion, in contrast to the patient with colic, who may writhe incessantly.

Another characteristic feature of peritoneal irritation is tonic reflex spasm of the abdominal musculature, localized to the involved body segment. The intensity of the tonic muscle spasm accompanying peritoneal inflammation is dependent on the location of the inflammatory

TABLE 1-1

SOME IMPORTANT CAUSES OF ABDOMINAL PAIN

PAIN ORIGINATING IN THE ABDOMEN

Parietal peritoneal inflammation
  Bacterial contamination
    Perforated appendix or other perforated
      viscus
    Pelvic inflammatory disease
  Chemical irritation
    Perforated ulcer
    Pancreatitis
    Mittelschmerz
Mechanical obstruction of hollow viscera
  Obstruction of the small or large
    intestine
  Obstruction of the biliary tree
  Obstruction of the ureter

Vascular disturbances
  Embolism or thrombosis
  Vascular rupture
  Pressure or torsional occlusion
  Sickle cell anemia
Abdominal wall
  Distortion or traction of mesentery
  Trauma or infection of muscles
Distension of visceral surfaces, e.g., by hemorrhage
  Hepatic or renal capsules
Inflammation of a viscus
  Appendicitis
  Typhoid fever
  Typhlitis

PAIN REFERRED FROM EXTRAABDOMINAL SOURCE

Cardiothoracic
  Acute myocardial infarction
  Myocarditis, endocarditis, pericarditis
  Congestive heart failure
  Pneumonia
  Pulmonary embolus
  Pleurodynia

Pneumothorax
Empyema
Esophageal disease, spasm, rupture, inflammation
Genitalia
  Torsion of the testis

METABOLIC CAUSES

Diabetes
Uremia
Hyperlipidemia
Hyperparathyroidism
Acute adrenal insufficiency

Familial Mediterranean fever
Porphyria
C1-esterase inhibitor deficiency (angioneurotic edema)

NEUROLOGIC/PSYCHIATRIC CAUSES

Herpes zoster
Tabes dorsalis
Causalgia
Radiculitis from infection or arthritis

Spinal cord or nerve root compression
Functional disorders
Psychiatric disorders

TOXIC CAUSES

Lead poisoning
Insect or animal envenomations

Black widow spiders
Snake bites

UNCERTAIN MECHANISMS

Narcotic withdrawal

Heat stroke

process, the rate at which it develops, and the integrity of the nervous system. Spasm over a perforated retrocecal appendix or perforated ulcer into the lesser peritoneal sac may be minimal or absent because of the protective effect of overlying viscera. A slowly developing process often greatly attenuates the degree of muscle spasm. Catastrophic abdominal emergencies such as a perforated ulcer may be associated with minimal or no detectable pain or muscle spasm in obtunded, seriously ill, debilitated elderly patients or in psychotic patients.

Obstruction of Hollow Viscera

The pain of obstruction of hollow abdominal viscera is classically described as intermittent, or colicky. Yet the lack of a truly cramping character should not be misleading, because distention of a hollow viscus may produce steady pain with only very occasional exacerbations. It is not nearly as well localized as the pain of parietal peritoneal inflammation.

The colicky pain of obstruction of the small intestine is usually periumbilical or supraumbilical and is poorly localized. As the intestine becomes progressively dilated with loss of muscular tone, the colicky nature of the pain may diminish. With superimposed strangulating obstruction, pain may spread to the lower lumbar region if there is traction on the root of the mesentery. The colicky pain of colonic obstruction is of lesser intensity than that of the small intestine and is often located in the infraumbilical area. Lumbar radiation of pain is common in colonic obstruction.

Sudden distention of the biliary tree produces a steady rather than colicky type of pain; hence the term *biliary colic* is misleading. Acute distention of the gallbladder usually causes pain in the right upper quadrant with radiation to the right posterior region of the thorax or to the tip of the right scapula, and distention of the common bile duct is often associated with pain in the epigastrium radiating to the upper part of the lumbar region. Considerable variation is common, however, so that differentiation between these may be impossible. The typical subscapular pain or lumbar radiation is frequently absent. Gradual dilatation of the biliary tree, as in carcinoma of the head of the pancreas, may cause no pain or only a mild aching sensation in the epigastrium or right upper quadrant. The pain of distention of the pancreatic ducts is similar to that described for distention of the common bile duct but, in addition, is very frequently accentuated by recumbency and relieved by the upright position.

Obstruction of the urinary bladder results in dull suprapubic pain, usually low in intensity. Restlessness without specific complaint of pain may be the only sign of a distended bladder in an obtunded patient. In contrast, acute obstruction of the intravesicular portion of the ureter is characterized by severe suprapubic and flank pain that radiates to the penis, scrotum, or inner aspect of the upper thigh. Obstruction of the ureteropelvic junction is felt as pain in the costovertebral angle, whereas obstruction of the remainder of the ureter is associated with flank pain that often extends into the same side of the abdomen.

Vascular Disturbances

A frequent misconception, despite abundant experience to the contrary, is that pain associated with intraabdominal vascular disturbances is sudden and catastrophic in nature. The pain of embolism or thrombosis of the superior mesenteric artery, or that of impending rupture of an abdominal aortic aneurysm, certainly may be severe and diffuse. Yet just as frequently, the patient with occlusion of the superior mesenteric artery has only mild continuous diffuse pain for 2 or 3 days before vascular collapse or findings of peritoneal inflammation appear. The early, seemingly insignificant discomfort is caused by hyperperistalsis rather than peritoneal inflammation. Indeed, absence of tenderness and rigidity in the presence of continuous, diffuse pain in a patient likely to have vascular disease is quite characteristic of occlusion of the superior mesenteric artery. Abdominal pain with radiation to the sacral region, flank, or genitalia should always signal the possible presence of a rupturing abdominal aortic aneurysm. This pain may persist over a period of several days before rupture and collapse occur.

Abdominal Wall

Pain arising from the abdominal wall is usually constant and aching. Movement, prolonged standing, and pressure accentuate the discomfort and muscle spasm. In the case of hematoma of the rectus sheath, now most frequently encountered in association with anticoagulant therapy, a mass may be present in the lower quadrants of the abdomen. Simultaneous involvement of muscles in other parts of the body usually serves to differentiate myositis of the abdominal wall from an intraabdominal process that might cause pain in the same region.

REFERRED PAIN IN ABDOMINAL DISEASES

Pain referred to the abdomen from the thorax, spine, or genitalia may prove a vexing diagnostic problem, because diseases of the upper part of the abdominal cavity such as acute cholecystitis or perforated ulcer are frequently associated with intrathoracic complications. A most important, yet often forgotten, dictum is that the possibility of intrathoracic disease must be considered in every patient with abdominal pain, especially if the pain is in the upper part of the abdomen. Systematic questioning and examination directed toward detecting myocardial or pulmonary infarction, pneumonia, pericarditis, or esophageal disease (the intrathoracic diseases that most often masquerade as abdominal emergencies) will often provide sufficient clues to establish the proper diagnosis. Diaphragmatic pleuritis resulting from pneumonia or pulmonary infarction may cause pain in the right upper quadrant and pain in the supraclavicular area, the latter radiation to be distinguished from the referred subscapular pain caused by acute distention of the extrahepatic biliary tree. The ultimate decision as to the origin of abdominal pain may require deliberate and planned observation over a period of several hours, during which repeated questioning and examination will provide the diagnosis or suggest the appropriate studies.

Referred pain of thoracic origin is often accompanied by splinting of the involved hemithorax with respiratory lag and decrease in excursion more marked than that seen in the presence of intraabdominal disease. In addition, apparent abdominal muscle spasm caused by referred pain will diminish during the inspiratory phase of respiration, whereas it is persistent throughout both respiratory phases if it is of abdominal origin. Palpation over the area of referred pain in the abdomen also does not usually accentuate the pain and in many instances actually seems to relieve it. Thoracic disease and abdominal disease frequently coexist and may be difficult or impossible to differentiate. For example, the patient with known biliary tract disease often has epigastric pain during myocardial infarction, or biliary colic may be referred to the precordium or left shoulder in a patient who has suffered previously from angina pectoris.

Referred pain from the spine, which usually involves compression or irritation of nerve roots, is characteristically intensified by certain motions such as cough, sneeze, or strain, and is associated with hyperesthesia over the involved dermatomes. Pain referred to the abdomen from the testes or seminal vesicles is generally accentuated by the slightest pressure on either of these organs. The abdominal discomfort is of dull aching character and is poorly localized.

METABOLIC ABDOMINAL CRISES

Pain of metabolic origin may simulate almost any other type of intraabdominal disease. Several mechanisms may be at work. In certain instances, such as hyperlipidemia, the metabolic disease itself may be accompanied by an intraabdominal process such as pancreatitis, which can lead to unnecessary laparotomy unless recognized. C1-esterase deficiency associated with angioneurotic edema is often associated with episodes of severe abdominal pain. Whenever the cause of abdominal pain is obscure, a metabolic origin always must be considered. Abdominal pain is also the hallmark of familial Mediterranean fever.

The problem of differential diagnosis is often not readily resolved. The pain of porphyria and of lead colic is usually difficult to distinguish from that of intestinal obstruction, because severe hyperperistalsis is a prominent feature of both. The pain of uremia or diabetes is nonspecific, and the pain and tenderness frequently shift in location and intensity. Diabetic acidosis may be precipitated by acute appendicitis or intestinal obstruction, so if prompt resolution of the abdominal pain does not result from correction of the metabolic abnormalities, an underlying organic problem should be suspected. Black widow spider bites produce intense pain and rigidity of the abdominal muscles and back, an area infrequently involved in intraabdominal disease.

NEUROGENIC CAUSES

Causalgic pain may occur in diseases that injure sensory nerves. It has a burning character and is usually limited to the distribution of a given peripheral nerve. Normal stimuli such as touch or change in temperature may be transformed into this type of pain, which is frequently present in a patient at rest. The demonstration of irregularly spaced cutaneous pain spots may be the only indication of an old nerve lesion underlying causalgic pain. Even though the pain may be precipitated by gentle palpation, rigidity of the abdominal muscles is absent, and the respirations are not disturbed. Distention of the abdomen is uncommon, and the pain has no relationship to the intake of food.

Pain arising from spinal nerves or roots comes and goes suddenly and is of a lancinating type. It may be caused by herpes zoster, impingement by arthritis, tumors, herniated nucleus pulposus, diabetes, or syphilis. It is not associated with food intake, abdominal distention, or changes in respiration. Severe muscle spasm, as in the gastric crises of tabes dorsalis, is common but is either relieved or is not accentuated by abdominal palpation. The pain is made worse by movement of the spine and is usually confined to a few dermatomes. Hyperesthesia is very common.

Pain due to functional causes conforms to none of the aforementioned patterns. The mechanism is hard to define. Irritable bowel syndrome (IBS) is a functional gastrointestinal disorder characterized by abdominal pain and altered bowel habits. The diagnosis is made on the basis of clinical criteria (Chap. 17) and after exclusion of demonstrable structural abnormalities. The episodes of abdominal pain are often brought on by stress, and the pain varies considerably in type and location. Nausea and vomiting are rare. Localized tenderness and muscle spasm are inconsistent or absent. The causes of IBS or related functional disorders are not known.

Approach to the Patient:
ABDOMINAL PAIN

Few abdominal conditions require such urgent operative intervention that an orderly approach need be abandoned, no matter how ill the patient. Only those patients with exsanguinating intraabdominal hemorrhage (e.g., ruptured aneurysm) must be rushed to the operating room immediately, but in such instances only a few minutes are required to assess the critical nature of the problem. Under these circumstances, all obstacles must be swept aside, adequate venous access for fluid replacement obtained, and the operation begun. Many patients of this type have died in the radiology department or the emergency room while awaiting such unnecessary examinations as electrocardiograms or abdominal films. *There are no contraindications to operation when massive intraabdominal hemorrhage is present.* Fortunately, this situation is relatively rare. These comments do not pertain to gastrointestinal hemorrhage, which can often be managed by other means (Chap. 8).

Nothing will supplant an orderly, painstakingly *detailed history*, which is far more valuable than any laboratory or radiographic examination. This kind of history is laborious and time-consuming, making it not especially popular, even though a reasonably accurate diagnosis can be made on the basis of the history alone in the majority of cases. Computer-aided diagnosis of abdominal pain provides no advantage over clinical assessment alone. In cases of *acute* abdominal pain, a diagnosis is readily established in most instances, whereas success is not so frequent in patients with *chronic* pain. IBS is one of the most common causes of abdominal pain and must always be kept in mind (Chap. 17). The location of the pain can assist in narrowing the differential diagnosis (see Table 1-2); however, the *chronological sequence of events* in the patient's history is often more important than emphasis on the location of pain. If the examiner is sufficiently open-minded and unhurried, asks the proper questions, and listens, the patient will usually provide the diagnosis. Careful attention should be paid to the extraabdominal regions that may be responsible for abdominal pain. An accurate menstrual history in a female patient is essential. Narcotics or analgesics should *not* be withheld until a definitive diagnosis or a definitive plan has been formulated; obfuscation of the diagnosis by adequate analgesia is unlikely.

In the examination, simple critical inspection of the patient, e.g., of facies, position in bed, and respiratory activity, may provide valuable clues. The amount of information to be gleaned is directly proportional to the *gentleness* and thoroughness of the examiner. Once a patient with peritoneal inflammation has been examined brusquely, accurate assessment by the next examiner becomes almost impossible. Eliciting rebound tenderness by sudden release of a deeply palpating hand in a patient with suspected peritonitis is cruel and unnecessary. The same information can be obtained by gentle percussion of the abdomen (rebound tenderness on a miniature scale), a maneuver that can be far more precise and localizing. Asking the patient to cough will elicit true rebound tenderness without the need for placing a hand on the abdomen. Furthermore, the forceful demonstration of rebound tenderness will startle and induce protective spasm in a nervous or worried patient in whom true rebound tenderness is not present. A palpable gallbladder will be missed if palpation is so brúsque that voluntary muscle spasm becomes superimposed on involuntary muscular rigidity.

TABLE 1-2

DIFFERENTIAL DIAGNOSES OF ABDOMINAL PAIN BY LOCATION

RIGHT UPPER QUADRANT	EPIGASTRIC	LEFT UPPER QUADRANT
Cholecystitis	Peptic ulcer disease	Splenic infarct
Cholangitis	Gastritis	Splenic rupture
Pancreatitis	GERD	Splenic abscess
Pneumonia/empyema	Pancreatitis	Gastritis
Pleurisy/pleurodynia	Myocardial infarction	Gastric ulcer
Subdiaphragmatic abscess	Pericarditis	Pancreatitis
Hepatitis	Ruptured aortic aneurysm	Subdiaphragmatic abscess
Budd-Chiari syndrome	Esophagitis	

RIGHT LOWER QUADRANT	PERIUMBILICAL	LEFT LOWER QUADRANT
Appendicitis	Early appendicitis	Diverticulitis
Salpingitis	Gastroenteritis	Salpingitis
Inguinal hernia	Bowel obstruction	Inguinal hernia
Ectopic pregnancy	Ruptured aortic aneurysm	Ectopic pregnancy
Nephrolithiasis		Nephrolithiasis
Inflammatory bowel disease		Irritable bowel syndrome
Mesenteric lymphadenitis		Inflammatory bowel disease
Typhlitis		

DIFFUSE NONLOCALIZED PAIN	
Gastroenteritis	Diabetes
Mesenteric ischemia	Malaria
Bowel obstruction	Familial Mediterranean fever
Irritable bowel syndrome	Metabolic diseases
Peritonitis	Psychiatric disease

As in history taking, sufficient time should be spent in the examination. Abdominal signs may be minimal but nevertheless, if accompanied by consistent symptoms, may be exceptionally meaningful. Abdominal signs may be virtually or totally absent in cases of pelvic peritonitis, so careful *pelvic and rectal examinations are mandatory in every patient with abdominal pain.* Tenderness on pelvic or rectal examination in the absence of other abdominal signs can be caused by operative indications such as perforated appendicitis, diverticulitis, twisted ovarian cyst, and many others.

Much attention has been paid to the presence or absence of peristaltic sounds, their quality, and their frequency. Auscultation of the abdomen is one of the least revealing aspects of the physical examination of a patient with abdominal pain. Catastrophes such as strangulating small intestinal obstruction or perforated appendicitis may occur in the presence of normal peristaltic sounds. Conversely, when the proximal part of the intestine above an obstruction becomes markedly distended and edematous, peristaltic sounds may lose the characteristics of borborygmi and become weak or absent, even when peritonitis is not present. It is usually the severe chemical peritonitis of sudden onset that is associated with the truly silent abdomen. Assessment of the patient's state of hydration is important.

Laboratory examinations may be of great value in assessment of the patient with abdominal pain, yet with few exceptions they rarely establish a diagnosis. Leukocytosis should never be the single deciding factor as to whether or not operation is indicated. A white blood cell count >20,000/μL may be observed with perforation of a viscus, but pancreatitis, acute cholecystitis, pelvic inflammatory disease, and intestinal infarction may be associated with marked leukocytosis. A normal white blood cell count is not rare in cases of perforation of abdominal viscera. The diagnosis of anemia may be more helpful than the white blood cell count, especially when combined with the history.

The urinalysis may reveal the state of hydration or rule out severe renal disease, diabetes, or urinary infection. Blood urea nitrogen, glucose, and serum bilirubin levels may be helpful. Serum amylase levels may be increased by many diseases other than pancreatitis, e.g., perforated ulcer, strangulating intestinal obstruction, and acute cholecystitis; thus, elevations of serum amylase do not rule out the need for an operation. The determination of the serum lipase may have greater accuracy than that of the serum amylase.

Plain and upright or lateral decubitus radiographs of the abdomen may be of value in cases of intestinal obstruction, perforated ulcer, and a variety of other conditions. They are usually unnecessary in patients with acute appendicitis or strangulated external hernias.

In rare instances, barium or water-soluble contrast study of the upper part of the gastrointestinal tract may demonstrate partial intestinal obstruction that may elude diagnosis by other means. If there is any question of obstruction of the colon, oral administration of barium sulfate should be avoided. On the other hand, in cases of suspected colonic obstruction (without perforation), contrast enema may be diagnostic.

In the absence of trauma, peritoneal lavage has been replaced as a diagnostic tool by ultrasound, CT, and laparoscopy. Ultrasonography has proved to be useful in detecting an enlarged gallbladder or pancreas, the presence of gallstones, an enlarged ovary, or a tubal pregnancy. Laparoscopy is especially helpful in diagnosing pelvic conditions, such as ovarian cysts, tubal pregnancies, salpingitis, and acute appendicitis. Radioisotopic scans (HIDA) may help differentiate acute cholecystitis from acute pancreatitis. A CT scan may demonstrate an enlarged pancreas, ruptured spleen, or thickened colonic or appendiceal wall and streaking of the mesocolon or mesoappendix characteristic of diverticulitis or appendicitis.

Sometimes, even under the best circumstances with all available aids and with the greatest of clinical skill, a definitive diagnosis cannot be established at the time of the initial examination. Nevertheless, despite lack of a clear anatomic diagnosis, it may be abundantly clear to an experienced and thoughtful physician and surgeon that on clinical grounds alone operation is indicated. Should that decision be questionable, watchful waiting with repeated questioning and examination will often elucidate the true nature of the illness and indicate the proper course of action.

FURTHER READINGS

ASSAR AN, ZARINS CK: Ruptured abdominal aortic aneurysm: A surgical emergency with many clinical presentations. Postgrad Med J 85:268, 2009

CERVERO F, LAIRD JM: Visceral pain. Lancet 353:2145, 1999

FORD AC et al: Yield of diagnostic tests for celiac disease in individuals with symptoms suggestive of irritable bowel syndrome: Systematic review and meta-analysis. Arch Intern Med 169:651, 2009

JAMES AW et al: Portomesenteric venous thrombosis after laparoscopic surgery: A systematic literature review. Arch Surg 144:520, 2009

JONES PF: Suspected acute appendicitis: Trends in management over 30 years. Br J Surg 88:1570, 2001

LYON C, CLARK DC: Diagnosis of acute abdominal pain in older patients. Am Fam Physician 74:1537, 2006

RICHARDSON WS et al: The role of diagnostic laparoscopy for chronic abdominal conditions: An evidence-based review. Surg Endosc 23:2073, 2009

SILEN W: *Cope's Early Diagnosis of the Acute Abdomen,* 21st ed. New York and Oxford: Oxford University Press, 2005

SMITH JE, HALL EJ: The use of plain abdominal x-rays in the emergency department. Emerg Med J 26:160, 2009

TAIT IS et al: Do patients with abdominal pain wait unduly long for analgesia? J R Coll Surg Edinb 44:181, 1999

CHAPTER 2
ORAL MANIFESTATIONS OF DISEASE

Samuel C. Durso

As primary care physicians and consultants, internists are often asked to evaluate patients with disease of the oral soft tissues, teeth, and pharynx. Knowledge of the oral milieu and its unique structures is necessary to guide preventive services and recognize oral manifestations of local or systemic disease (Chap. 3). Furthermore, internists frequently collaborate with dentists in the care of patients who have a variety of medical conditions that affect oral health or who undergo dental procedures that increase their risk of medical complications.

DISEASES OF THE TEETH AND PERIODONTAL STRUCTURES

TOOTH AND PERIODONTAL STRUCTURE

Tooth formation begins during the sixth week of embryonic life and continues through the first 17 years of age. Tooth development begins in utero and continues until after the tooth erupts. Normally all 20 deciduous teeth have erupted by age 3 and have been shed by age 13. Permanent teeth, eventually totaling 32, begin to erupt by age 6 and have completely erupted by age 14, though third molars (wisdom teeth) may erupt later.

The erupted tooth consists of the visible crown covered with enamel and the root submerged below the gum line and covered with bonelike cementum. *Dentin*, a material that is denser than bone and exquisitely sensitive to pain, forms the majority of the tooth substance. Dentin surrounds a core of myxomatous *pulp* containing the vascular and nerve supply. The tooth is held firmly in the alveolar socket by the *periodontium*, supporting structures that consist of the gingivae, alveolar bone, cementum, and periodontal ligament. The periodontal ligament tenaciously binds the tooth's cementum to the alveolar bone. Above this ligament is a collar of attached gingiva just below the crown. A few millimeters of unattached or free gingiva (1–3 mm) overlap the base of the crown, forming a shallow sulcus along the gum–tooth margin.

Dental Caries, Pulpal and Periapical Disease, and Complications

Dental caries begin asymptomatically as a destructive process of the hard surface of the tooth. *Streptococcus mutans*, principally, along with other bacteria colonize the organic buffering film on the tooth surface to produce *plaque*. If not removed by brushing or the natural cleaning action of saliva and oral soft tissues, bacterial acids demineralize the enamel. Fissures and pits on the occlusion surfaces are the most frequent sites of decay. Surfaces adjacent to tooth restorations and exposed roots are also vulnerable, particularly as teeth are retained in an aging population. Over time, dental caries extend to the underlying dentin, leading to cavitation of the enamel and ultimately penetration to the tooth pulp, producing *acute pulpitis*. At this early stage, when the pulp infection is limited, the tooth becomes sensitive to percussion and hot or cold, and pain resolves immediately when the irritating stimulus is removed. Should the infection spread throughout the pulp, *irreversible pulpitis* occurs, leading to pulp necrosis. At this late stage pain is severe and has a sharp or throbbing visceral quality that may be worse when the patient lies down. Once pulp necrosis is complete, pain may be constant or intermittent, but cold sensitivity is lost.

Treatment of caries involves removal of the softened and infected hard tissue; sealing the exposed dentin; and restoration of the tooth structure with silver amalgam, composite plastic, gold, or porcelain. Once irreversible pulpitis occurs, root canal therapy is necessary, and the contents of the pulp chamber and root canals are removed, followed by thorough cleaning, antisepsis, and filling with an inert material. Alternatively, the tooth may be extracted.

Pulpal infection, if it does not egress through the decayed enamel, leads to *periapical abscess* formation, which produces pain on chewing. If the infection is mild and chronic, a *periapical granuloma* or eventually a *periapical cyst* forms, either of which produces radiolucency at the root apex. When unchecked, a periapical abscess can erode into the alveolar bone, producing osteomyelitis; penetrate and drain through the gingivae (parulis or gumboil); or track along deep fascial planes, producing a virulent cellulitis (Ludwig's angina) involving the submandibular space and floor of the mouth. Elderly patients, those with diabetes mellitus, and patients taking glucocorticoids may experience little or no pain and fever as these complications develop.

Periodontal Disease

Periodontal disease accounts for more tooth loss than caries, particularly in the elderly. Like dental caries, chronic infection of the gingiva and anchoring structures of the tooth begins with formation of bacterial plaque. The process begins invisibly above the gum line and in the gingival sulcus. Plaque, including mineralized plaque (calculus), is preventable by appropriate dental hygiene, including periodic professional cleaning. Left undisturbed, chronic inflammation ensues and produces a painless hyperemia of the free and attached gingivae (*gingivitis*) that typically bleeds with brushing. If ignored, severe *periodontitis* occurs, leading to deepening of the physiologic sulcus and destruction of the periodontal ligament. Pockets develop around the teeth and become filled with pus and debris. As the periodontium is destroyed, teeth loosen and exfoliate. Eventually there is

resorption of the alveolar bone. A role for the chronic inflammation resulting from chronic periodontal disease in promoting coronary heart disease and stroke has been proposed. Epidemiologic studies demonstrate a moderate but significant association between chronic periodontal inflammation and atherogenesis, though a causal role remains unproven.

Acute and aggressive forms of periodontal disease are less common than the chronic forms described above. However, if the host is stressed or exposed to a new pathogen, rapidly progressive and destructive disease of the periodontal tissue can occur. A virulent example is *acute necrotizing ulcerative gingivitis* (ANUG), or *Vincent's infection*, characterized as "trench mouth" during World War I. Stress, poor oral hygiene, and tobacco and alcohol use are risk factors. The presentation includes sudden gingival inflammation, ulceration, bleeding, interdental gingival necrosis, and fetid halitosis. *Localized juvenile periodontitis*, seen in adolescents, is particularly destructive and appears to be associated with impaired neutrophil chemotaxis. *AIDS-related periodontitis* resembles ANUG in some patients or a more destructive form of adult chronic periodontitis in others. It may also produce a gangrene-like destructive process of the oral soft tissues and bone that resembles *noma*, seen in severely malnourished children in developing nations.

Prevention of Tooth Decay and Periodontal Infection

Despite the reduced prevalence of dental caries and periodontal disease in the United States, due in large part to water fluoridation and improved dental care, respectively, both diseases constitute a major public health problem worldwide and for certain groups. The internist should promote preventive dental care and hygiene as part of health maintenance. Special populations at high risk for dental caries and periodontal disease include those with xerostomia, diabetics, alcoholics, tobacco users, those with Down's syndrome, and those with gingival hyperplasia. Furthermore, patients lacking dental care access (low socioeconomic status) and those with reduced ability to provide self-care (e.g., nursing home residents, those with dementia or upper extremity disability) suffer at a disproportionate rate. It is important to provide counseling regarding regular dental hygiene and professional cleaning, use of fluoride-containing toothpaste, professional fluoride treatments, and use of electric toothbrushes for patients with limited dexterity, and to give instruction to caregivers for those unable to perform self-care. Internists caring for international students studying in the United States should be aware of the high prevalence of dental decay in this population. Cost, fear of dental care, and language and cultural differences may create barriers that prevent some from seeking preventive dental services.

Developmental and Systemic Disease Affecting the Teeth and Periodontium

Malocclusion is the most common developmental problem, which, in addition to a problem with cosmesis, can interfere with mastication unless corrected through orthodontic techniques. Impacted third molars are common and occasionally become infected. Acquired prognathism due to *acromegaly* may also lead to malocclusion, as may deformity of the maxilla and mandible due to *Paget's disease* of the bone. Delayed tooth eruption, receding chin, and a protruding tongue are occasional features of *cretinism* and *hypopituitarism*. Congenital syphilis produces tapering, notched (Hutchinson's) incisors and finely nodular (mulberry) molar crowns.

Enamel hypoplasia results in crown defects ranging from pits to deep fissures of primary or permanent teeth. Intrauterine infection (syphilis, rubella), vitamin deficiency (A, C, or D), disorders of calcium metabolism (malabsorption, vitamin D–resistant rickets, hypoparathyroidism), prematurity, high fever, or rare inherited defects (*amelogenesis imperfecta*) are all causes. Tetracycline, given in sufficiently high doses during the first 8 years, may produce enamel hypoplasia and discoloration. Exposure to endogenous pigments can discolor developing teeth: *erythroblastosis fetalis* (green or bluish-black), congenital liver disease (green or yellow-brown), and porphyria (red or brown that fluoresces with ultraviolet light). *Mottled enamel* occurs if excessive fluoride is ingested during development. Worn enamel is seen with age, bruxism, or excessive acid exposure (e.g., chronic gastric reflux or bulimia).

Premature tooth loss resulting from periodontitis is seen with cyclic neutropenia, Papillon-Lefèvre syndrome, Chédiak-Higashi syndrome, and leukemia. Rapid focal tooth loosening is most often due to infection, but rarer causes include histiocytosis X, Ewing's sarcoma, osteosarcoma, or Burkitt's lymphoma. Early loss of primary teeth is a feature of *hypophosphatasia*, a rare inborn error of metabolism.

Pregnancy may produce severe gingivitis and localized *pyogenic granulomas*. Severe periodontal disease occurs with Down's syndrome and diabetes mellitus. *Gingival hyperplasia* may be caused by phenytoin, calcium channel blockers (e.g., nifedipine), and cyclosporine. *Idiopathic familial gingival fibromatosis* and several syndrome-related disorders appear similar. Removal of the medication often reverses the drug-induced form, though surgery may be needed to control both. *Linear gingival erythema* is variably seen in patients with advanced HIV infection and probably represents immune deficiency and decreased neutrophil activity. Diffuse or focal gingival swelling may be a feature of early or late acute myelomonocytic leukemia (AML) as well as of other lymphoproliferative disorders. A rare, but pathognomonic, sign of Wegener's granulomatosis is a red-purplish, granular gingivitis (strawberry gums).

DISEASES OF THE ORAL MUCOSA

Infection

Most oral mucosal diseases involve microorganisms (**Table 2–1**).

Pigmented Lesions

See **Table 2–2**.

Dermatologic Diseases

See Tables 2–1, 2–2, and **2–3**.

Diseases of the Tongue

See **Table 2–4**.

HIV Disease and AIDS

See Tables 2–1, 2–2, 2–3, and **2–5**.

Ulcers

Ulceration is the most common oral mucosal lesion. Although there are many causes, the host and pattern of lesions, including the presence of systemic features, narrow the differential diagnosis (Table 2–1). Most acute ulcers are painful and self-limited. Recurrent aphthous ulcers and herpes simplex infection constitute the majority. Persistent and deep aphthous ulcers can be idiopathic or seen with HIV/AIDS. Aphthous lesions are often the presenting symptom in *Behçet's syndrome*. Similar-appearing, though less painful, lesions may occur with Reiter's syndrome, and aphthous ulcers are occasionally present during phases of discoid or *systemic lupus erythematosus*. Aphthous-like ulcers are seen in Crohn's disease (Chap. 16), but unlike the common aphthous variety, they may exhibit granulomatous inflammation histologically. Recurrent aphthae in some patients with *celiac disease* have been reported to remit with elimination of gluten.

Of major concern are chronic, relatively painless ulcers and mixed red/white patches (erythroplakia and leukoplakia) of more than 2 weeks' duration. Squamous cell carcinoma and premalignant dysplasia should be considered early and a diagnostic biopsy obtained. The importance is underscored because early-stage malignancy is vastly more treatable than late-stage disease. High-risk sites include the lower lip, floor of the mouth, ventral and lateral tongue, and soft palate–tonsillar pillar complex. Significant risk factors for oral cancer in Western countries include sun exposure (lower lip) and tobacco and alcohol use. In India and some other Asian countries, smokeless tobacco mixed with betel nut, slaked lime, and spices is a common cause of oral cancer.

TABLE 2-1

11

CHAPTER 2

Oral Manifestations of Disease

VESICULAR, BULLOUS, OR ULCERATIVE LESIONS OF THE ORAL MUCOSA

CONDITION	USUAL LOCATION	CLINICAL FEATURES	COURSE
Viral Diseases			
Primary acute herpetic gingivostomatitis [herpes simplex virus (HSV) type 1, rarely type 2]	Lip and oral mucosa (buccal, gingival, lingual mucosa)	Labial vesicles that rupture and crust, and intraoral vesicles that quickly ulcerate; extremely painful; acute gingivitis, fever, malaise, foul odor, and cervical lymphadenopathy; occurs primarily in infants, children, and young adults	Heals spontaneously in 10–14 days. Unless secondarily infected, lesions lasting >3 weeks are not due to primary HSV infection
Recurrent herpes labialis	Mucocutaneous junction of lip, perioral skin	Eruption of groups of vesicles that may coalesce, then rupture and crust; painful to pressure or spicy foods	Lasts about 1 week, but condition may be pro-longed if secondarily infected. If severe, topical or oral antiviral may reduce healing time
Recurrent intraoral herpes simplex	Palate and gingiva	Small vesicles on keratinized epithelium that rupture and coalesce; painful	Heals spontaneously in about 1 week. If severe, topical or oral antiviral may reduce healing time
Chickenpox (varicella-zoster virus)	Gingiva and oral mucosa	Skin lesions may be accompanied by small vesicles on oral mucosa that rupture to form shallow ulcers; may coalesce to form large bullous lesions that ulcerate; mucosa may have generalized erythema	Lesions heal spontaneously within 2 weeks
Herpes zoster (reactivation of varicella-zoster virus)	Cheek, tongue, gingiva, or palate	Unilateral vesicular eruptions and ulceration in linear pattern following sensory distribution of trigeminal nerve or one of its branches	Gradual healing without scarring unless secondarily infected; postherpetic neuralgia is common. Oral acyclovir, famciclovir, or valacyclovir reduce healing time and postherpetic neuralgia
Infectious mononucleosis (Epstein-Barr virus)	Oral mucosa	Fatigue, sore throat, malaise, fever, and cervical lymphadenopathy; numerous small ulcers usually appear several days before lymphadenopathy; gingival bleeding and multiple petechiae at junction of hard and soft palates	Oral lesions disappear during convalescence; no treatment though gluco-corticoids indicated if tonsillar swelling compromises airway
Herpangina (coxsack-ievirus A; also possi-bly coxsackie B and echovirus)	Oral mucosa, pharynx, tongue	Sudden onset of fever, sore throat, and oropharyngeal vesicles, usually in children under 4 years, during summer months; diffuse pharyngeal congestion and vesicles (1–2 mm), grayish-white surrounded by red areola; vesicles enlarge and ulcerate	Incubation period 2–9 days; fever for 1–4 days; recovery uneventful
Hand, foot, and mouth disease (coxsack-ievirus A16 most common)	Oral mucosa, pharynx, palms, and soles	Fever, malaise, headache with oropharyngeal vesicles that become painful, shallow ulcers; highly infectious; usually affects children under age 10	Incubation period 2–18 days; lesions heal sponta-neously in 2–4 weeks
Primary HIV infection	Gingiva, palate, and pharynx	Acute gingivitis and oropharyngeal ulceration, associated with febrile illness resembling mononucleosis and including lymphadenopathy	Followed by HIV serocon-version, asymptomatic HIV infection, and usually ultimately by HIV disease

(Continued)

TABLE 2-1 (CONTINUED)

VESICULAR, BULLOUS, OR ULCERATIVE LESIONS OF THE ORAL MUCOSA

CONDITION	USUAL LOCATION	CLINICAL FEATURES	COURSE
Bacterial or Fungal Diseases			
Acute necrotizing ulcerative gingivitis ("trench mouth," Vincent's infection)	Gingiva	Painful, bleeding gingiva characterized by necrosis and ulceration of gingival papillae and margins plus lymphadenopathy and foul odor	Debridement and diluted (1:3) peroxide lavage provide relief within 24 h; antibiotics in acutely ill patients; relapse may occur
Prenatal (congenital) syphilis	Palate, jaws, tongue, and teeth	Gummatous involvement of palate, jaws, and facial bones; Hutchinson's incisors, mulberry molars, glossitis, mucous patches, and fissures on corner of mouth	Tooth deformities in permanent dentition irreversible
Primary syphilis (chancre)	Lesion appears where organism enters body; may occur on lips, tongue, or tonsillar area	Small papule developing rapidly into a large, painless ulcer with indurated border; unilateral lymphadenopathy; chancre and lymph nodes containing spirochetes; serologic tests positive by third to fourth weeks	Healing of chancre in 1–2 months, followed by secondary syphilis in 6–8 weeks
Secondary syphilis	Oral mucosa frequently involved with mucous patches, primarily on palate, also at commissures of mouth	Maculopapular lesions of oral mucosa, 5–10 mm in diameter with central ulceration covered by grayish membrane; eruptions occurring on various mucosal surfaces and skin accompanied by fever, malaise, and sore throat	Lesions may persist from several weeks to a year
Tertiary syphilis	Palate and tongue	Gummatous infiltration of palate or tongue followed by ulceration and fibrosis; atrophy of tongue papillae produces characteristic bald tongue and glossitis	Gumma may destroy palate, causing complete perforation
Gonorrhea	Lesions may occur in mouth at site of inoculation or secondarily by hematogenous spread from a primary focus elsewhere	Most pharyngeal infection is asymptomatic; may produce burning or itching sensation; oropharynx and tonsils may be ulcerated and erythematous; saliva viscous and fetid	More difficult to eradicate than urogenital infection, though pharyngitis usually resolves with appropriate antimicrobial treatment
Tuberculosis	Tongue, tonsillar area, soft palate	A painless, solitary, 1–5 cm, irregular ulcer covered with a persistent exudate; ulcer has a firm undermined border	Autoinoculation from pulmonary infection usual; lesions resolve with appropriate antimicrobial therapy
Cervicofacial actinomycosis	Swellings in region of face, neck, and floor of mouth	Infection may be associated with an extraction, jaw fracture, or eruption of molar tooth; in acute form resembles an acute pyogenic abscess, but contains yellow "sulfur granules" (gram-positive mycelia and their hyphae)	Typically swelling is hard and grows painlessly; multiple abscesses with draining tracks develop; penicillin first choice; surgery usually necessary
Histoplasmosis	Any area of the mouth, particularly tongue, gingiva, or palate	Nodular, verrucous, or granulomatous lesions; ulcers are indurated and painful; usual source hematogenous or pulmonary, but may be primary	Systemic antifungal therapy necessary to treat
Candidiasis (Table 2-3)			

(Continued)

TABLE 2-1 (*CONTINUED*)

13

CHAPTER 2

Oral Manifestations of Disease

VESICULAR, BULLOUS, OR ULCERATIVE LESIONS OF THE ORAL MUCOSA

CONDITION	USUAL LOCATION	CLINICAL FEATURES	COURSE
Dermatologic Diseases			
Mucous membrane pemphigoid	Typically produces marked gingival erythema and ulceration; other areas of oral cavity, esophagus, and vagina may be affected	Painful, grayish-white collapsed vesicles or bullae of full-thickness epithelium with peripheral erythematous zone; gingival lesions desquamate, leaving ulcerated area	Protracted course with remissions and exacerbations; involvement of different sites occurs slowly; glucocorticoids may temporarily reduce symptoms but do not control the disease
Erythema multiforme minor and major (Stevens-Johnson syndrome)	Primarily the oral mucosa and the skin of hands and feet	Intraoral ruptured bullae surrounded by an inflammatory area; lips may show hemorrhagic crusts; the "iris," or "target," lesion on the skin is pathognomonic; patient may have severe signs of toxicity	Onset very rapid; usually idiopathic, but may be associated with trigger such as drug reaction; condition may last 3–6 weeks; mortality with EM major 5–15% if untreated
Pemphigus vulgaris	Oral mucosa and skin; sites of mechanical trauma (soft/hard palate, frenulum, lips, buccal mucosa)	Usually (>70%) presents with oral lesions; fragile, ruptured bullae and ulcerated oral areas; mostly in older adults	With repeated occurrence of bullae, toxicity may lead to cachexia, infection, and death within 2 years; often controllable with oral glucocorticoids
Lichen planus	Oral mucosa and skin	White striae in mouth; purplish nodules on skin at sites of friction; occasionally causes oral mucosal ulcers and erosive gingivitis	White striae alone usually asymptomatic; erosive lesions often difficult to treat, but may respond to glucocorticoids
Other Conditions			
Recurrent aphthous ulcers	Usually on nonkeratinized oral mucosa (buccal and labial mucosa, floor of mouth, soft palate, lateral and ventral tongue)	Single or clusters of painful ulcers with surrounding erythematous border; lesions may be 1–2 mm in diameter in crops (herpetiform), 1–5 mm (minor), or 5–15 mm (major)	Lesions heal in 1–2 weeks but may recur monthly or several times a year; protective barrier with orabase and topical steroids give symptomatic relief; systemic glucocorticoids may be needed in severe cases
Behçet's syndrome	Oral mucosa, eyes, genitalia, gut, and CNS	Multiple aphthous ulcers in mouth; inflammatory ocular changes, ulcerative lesions on genitalia; inflammatory bowel disease and CNS disease	Oral lesions often first manifestation; persist several weeks and heal without scarring
Traumatic ulcers	Anywhere on oral mucosa; dentures frequently responsible for ulcers in vestibule	Localized, discrete ulcerated lesions with red border; produced by accidental biting of mucosa, penetration by a foreign object, or chronic irritation by a denture	Lesions usually heal in 7–10 days when irritant is removed, unless secondarily infected
Squamous cell carcinoma	Any area in the mouth, most commonly on lower lip, tongue, and floor of mouth	Ulcer with elevated, indurated border; failure to heal, pain not prominent; lesions tend to arise in areas of erythro/leukoplakia or in smooth atrophic tongue	Invades and destroys underlying tissues; frequently metastasizes to regional lymph nodes
Acute myeloid leukemia (usually monocytic)	Gingiva	Gingival swelling and superficial ulceration followed by hyperplasia of gingiva with extensive necrosis and hemorrhage; deep ulcers may occur elsewhere on the mucosa complicated by secondary infection	Usually responds to systemic treatment of leukemia; occasionally requires local radiation therapy
Lymphoma	Gingiva, tongue, palate and tonsillar area	Elevated, ulcerated area that may proliferate rapidly, giving the appearance of traumatic inflammation	Fatal if untreated; may indicate underlying HIV infection
Chemical or thermal burns	Any area in mouth	White slough due to contact with corrosive agents (e.g., aspirin, hot cheese) applied locally; removal of slough leaves raw, painful surface	Lesion heals in several weeks if not secondarily infected

Note: CNS, central nervous system.

TABLE 2-2

PIGMENTED LESIONS OF THE ORAL MUCOSA

CONDITION	USUAL LOCATION	CLINICAL FEATURES	COURSE
Oral melanotic macule	Any area of the mouth	Discrete or diffuse localized, brown to black macule	Remains indefinitely; no growth
Diffuse melanin pigmentation	Any area of the mouth	Diffuse pale to dark-brown pigmentation; may be physiologic ("racial") or due to smoking	Remains indefinitely
Nevi	Any area of the mouth	Discrete, localized, brown to black pigmentation	Remains indefinitely
Malignant melanoma	Any area of the mouth	Can be flat and diffuse, painless, brown to black, or can be raised and nodular	Expands and invades early; metastasis leads to death
Addison's disease	Any area of the mouth, but mostly buccal mucosa	Blotches or spots of bluish-black to dark-brown pigmentation occurring early in the disease, accompanied by diffuse pigmentation of skin; other symptoms of adrenal insufficiency	Condition controlled by adrenal steroid replacement
Peutz-Jeghers syndrome	Any area of the mouth	Dark-brown spots on lips, buccal mucosa, with characteristic distribution of pigment around lips, nose, eyes, and on hands; concomitant intestinal polyposis	Oral pigmented lesions remain indefinitely; gastrointestinal polyps may become malignant
Drug ingestion (neuroleptics, oral contraceptives, minocycline, zidovudine, quinine derivatives)	Any area of the mouth	Brown, black, or gray areas of pigmentation	Gradually disappears following cessation of drug
Amalgam tattoo	Gingiva and alveolar mucosa	Small blue-black pigmented areas associated with embedded amalgam particles in soft tissues; these may show up on radiographs as radiopaque particles in some cases	Remains indefinitely
Heavy metal pigmentation (bismuth, mercury, lead)	Gingival margin	Thin blue-black pigmented line along gingival margin; rarely seen except for children exposed to lead-based paint	Indicative of systemic absorption; no significance for oral health
Black hairy tongue	Dorsum of tongue	Elongation of filiform papillae of tongue, which become stained by coffee, tea, tobacco, or pigmented bacteria	Improves within 1–2 weeks with gentle brushing of tongue or discontinuation of antibiotic if due to bacterial overgrowth
Fordyce "spots"	Buccal and labial mucosa	Numerous small yellowish spots just beneath mucosal surface; no symptoms; due to hyperplasia of sebaceous glands	Benign; remains without apparent change
Kaposi's sarcoma	Palate most common, but may occur in any other site	Red or blue plaques of variable size and shape; often enlarge, become nodular and may ulcerate	Usually indicative of HIV infection or non-Hodgkin's lymphoma; rarely fatal, but may require treatment for comfort or cosmesis
Mucous retention cysts	Buccal and labial mucosa	Bluish-clear fluid-filled cyst due to extravasated mucous from injured minor salivary gland	Benign; painless unless traumatized; may be removed surgically

TABLE 2-3

15

CHAPTER 2

Oral Manifestations of Disease

WHITE LESIONS OF ORAL MUCOSA

CONDITION	USUAL LOCATION	CLINICAL FEATURES	COURSE
Lichen planus	Buccal mucosa, tongue, gingiva, and lips; skin	Striae, white plaques, red areas, ulcers in mouth; purplish papules on skin; may be asymptomatic, sore, or painful; lichenoid drug reactions may look similar	Protracted; responds to topical glucocorticoids
White sponge nevus	Oral mucosa, vagina, anal mucosa	Painless white thickening of epithelium; adolescent/early adult onset; familial	Benign and permanent
Smoker's leukoplakia and smokeless tobacco lesions	Any area of oral mucosa, sometimes related to location of habit	White patch that may become firm, rough, or red-fissured and ulcerated; may become sore and painful but usually painless	May or may not resolve with cessation of habit; 2% develop squamous cell carcinoma; early biopsy essential
Erythroplakia with or without white patches	Floor of mouth common in men; tongue and buccal mucosa in women	Velvety, reddish plaque; occasionally mixed with white patches or smooth red areas	High risk of squamous cell cancer; early biopsy essential
Candidiasis	Any area in mouth	*Pseudomembranous type* ("thrush"): creamy white curdlike patches that reveal a raw, bleeding surface when scraped; found in sick infants, debilitated elderly patients receiving high doses of glucocorticoids or broad-spectrum antibiotics, or in patients with AIDS	Responds favorably to antifungal therapy and correction of predisposing causes where possible
		Erythematous type: flat, red, sometimes sore areas in same groups of patients	Course same as for pseudomembranous type
		Candidal leukoplakia: nonremovable white thickening of epithelium due to *Candida*	Responds to prolonged antifungal therapy
		Angular cheilitis: sore fissures at corner of mouth	Responds to topical antifungal therapy
Hairy leukoplakia	Usually lateral tongue, rarely elsewhere on oral mucosa	White areas ranging from small and flat to extensive accentuation of vertical folds; found in HIV carriers in all risk groups for AIDS	Due to EBV; responds to high dose acyclovir but recurs; rarely causes discomfort unless secondarily infected with *Candida*
Warts (papillomavirus)	Anywhere on skin and oral mucosa	Single or multiple papillary lesions, with thick, white keratinized surfaces containing many pointed projections; cauliflower lesions covered with normal-colored mucosa or multiple pink or pale bumps (focal epithelial hyperplasia)	Lesions grow rapidly and spread; consider squamous cell carcinoma and rule out with biopsy; excision or laser therapy; may regress in HIV infected patients on antiretroviral therapy

Note: EBV, Epstein-Barr virus.

TABLE 2-4

ALTERATIONS OF THE TONGUE

TYPE OF CHANGE	CLINICAL FEATURES
Size or Morphology Changes	
Macroglossia	Enlarged tongue that may be part of a syndrome found in developmental conditions such as Down syndrome, Simpson-Golabi-Behmel syndrome, or Beckwith-Wiedemann syndrome may be due to tumor (hemangioma or lymphangioma), metabolic disease (such as primary amyloidosis), or endocrine disturbance (such as acromegaly or cretinism)
Fissured ("scrotal") tongue	Dorsal surface and sides of tongue covered by painless shallow or deep fissures that may collect debris and become irritated
Median rhomboid glossitis	Congenital abnormality of tongue with ovoid, denuded area in median posterior portion of the tongue; may be associated with candidiasis and may respond to antifungals
Color Changes	
"Geographic" tongue (benign migratory glossitis)	Asymptomatic inflammatory condition of the tongue, with rapid loss and regrowth of filiform papillae, leading to appearance of denuded red patches "wandering" across the surface of the tongue
Hairy tongue	Elongation of filiform papillae of the medial dorsal surface area due to failure of keratin layer of the papillae to desquamate normally; brownish-black coloration may be due to staining by tobacco, food, or chromogenic organisms
"Strawberry" and "raspberry" tongue	Appearance of tongue during scarlet fever due to the hypertrophy of fungiform papillae plus changes in the filiform papillae
"Bald" tongue	Atrophy may be associated with xerostomia, pernicious anemia, iron-deficiency anemia, pellagra, or syphilis; may be accompanied by painful burning sensation; may be an expression of erythematous candidiasis and respond to antifungals

TABLE 2-5

ORAL LESIONS ASSOCIATED WITH HIV INFECTION

LESION MORPHOLOGY	ETIOLOGIES
Papules, nodules, plaques	Candidiasis (hyperplastic and pseudomembranous)[a]
	Condyloma acuminatum (human papillomavirus infection)
	Squamous cell carcinoma (preinvasive and invasive)
	Non-Hodgkin's lymphoma[a]
	Hairy leukoplakia[a]
Ulcers	Recurrent aphthous ulcers[a]
	Angular cheilitis
	Squamous cell carcinoma
	Acute necrotizing ulcerative gingivitis[a]
	Necrotizing ulcerative periodontitis[a]
	Necrotizing ulcerative stomatitis
	Non-Hodgkin's lymphoma[a]
	Viral infection (herpes simplex, herpes zoster, cytomegalovirus)
	Mycobacterium tuberculosis, Mycobacterium avium-intracellulare
	Fungal infection (histoplasmosis, cryptococcosis, candidiasis, geotrichosis, aspergillosis)
	Bacterial infection (*Escherichia coli, Enterobacter cloacae, Klebsiella pneumoniae, Pseudomonas aeruginosa*)
	Drug reactions (single or multiple ulcers)
Pigmented lesions	Kaposi's sarcoma[a]
	Bacillary angiomatosis (skin and visceral lesions more common than oral)
	Zidovudine pigmentation (skin, nails, and occasionally oral mucosa)
	Addison's disease
Miscellaneous	Linear gingival erythema[a]

[a]Strongly associated with HIV infection.

Less common etiologies include syphilis and Plummer-Vinson syndrome (iron deficiency).

Rarer causes of chronic oral ulcer such as tuberculosis, fungal infection, Wegener's granulomatosis, and midline granuloma may look identical to carcinoma. Making the correct diagnosis depends on recognizing other clinical features and biopsy of the lesion. The syphilitic chancre is typically painless and therefore easily missed. Regional lymphadenopathy is invariably present. Confirmation is achieved using appropriate bacterial and serologic tests.

Disorders of mucosal fragility often produce painful oral ulcers that fail to heal within 2 weeks. *Mucous membrane pemphigoid* and *pemphigus vulgaris* are the major acquired disorders. While clinical features are often distinctive, immunohistochemical examination should be performed for diagnosis and to distinguish these entities from *lichen planus* and drug reactions.

Hematologic and Nutritional Disease

Internists are more likely to encounter patients with acquired, rather than congenital, bleeding disorders. Bleeding after minor trauma should stop after 15 min and within an hour of tooth extraction if local pressure is applied. More prolonged bleeding, if not due to continued injury or rupture of a large vessel, should lead to investigation for a clotting abnormality. In addition to bleeding, petechiae and ecchymoses are prone to occur at the line of vibration between the soft and hard palates in patients with platelet dysfunction or thrombocytopenia.

All forms of leukemia, but particularly acute myelomonocytic leukemia, can produce gingival bleeding, ulcers, and gingival enlargement. Oral ulcers are a feature of agranulocytosis, and ulcers and mucositis are often severe complications of chemotherapy and radiation therapy for hematologic and other malignancies. Plummer-Vinson syndrome (iron deficiency, angular stomatitis, glossitis, and dysphagia) raises the risk of oral squamous cell cancer and esophageal cancer at the postcricoidal tissue web. Atrophic papillae and a red, burning tongue may occur with pernicious anemia. B-group vitamin deficiencies produce many of these same symptoms as well as oral ulceration and cheilosis. Cheilosis may also be seen in iron deficiency. Swollen, bleeding gums, ulcers, and loosening of the teeth are a consequence of scurvy.

NONDENTAL CAUSES OF ORAL PAIN

Most but not all oral pain emanates from inflamed or injured tooth pulp or periodontal tissues. Nonodontogenic causes may be overlooked. In most instances toothache is predictable and proportional to the stimulus applied, and an identifiable condition (e.g., caries, abscess) is found. Local anesthesia eliminates pain originating from dental or periodontal structures, but not referred pain. The most common nondental origin is myofascial pain referred from muscles of mastication, which become tender and ache with increased use. Many sufferers exhibit bruxism (the grinding of teeth, often during sleep) that is secondary to stress and anxiety. *Temporomandibular disorder* is closely related. It predominantly affects females ages 15–45. Features include pain, limited mandibular movement, and temporomandibular joint sounds. The etiologies are complex, and malocclusion does not play the primary role once attributed to it. *Osteoarthritis* is a common cause of masticatory pain. Anti-inflammatory medication, jaw rest, soft foods, and heat provide relief. The temporomandibular joint is involved in 50% of patients with *rheumatoid arthritis* and is usually a late feature of severe disease. Bilateral preauricular pain, particularly in the morning, limits range of motion.

Migrainous neuralgia may be localized to the mouth. Episodes of pain and remission without identifiable cause and absence of relief with local anesthesia are important clues. *Trigeminal neuralgia* (*tic douloureux*) may involve the entire branch or part of the mandibular or maxillary branches of the fifth cranial nerve and produce pain in one or a few teeth. Pain may occur spontaneously or may be triggered by touching the lip or gingiva, brushing the teeth, or chewing. *Glossopharyngeal neuralgia* produces similar acute neuropathic symptoms in the distribution of the ninth cranial nerve. Swallowing, sneezing, coughing, or pressure on the tragus of the ear triggers pain that is felt in the base of the tongue, pharynx, and soft palate and may be referred to the temporomandibular joint. *Neuritis* involving the maxillary and mandibular divisions of the trigeminal nerve (e.g., maxillary sinusitis, neuroma, and leukemic infiltrate) is distinguished from ordinary toothache by the neuropathic quality of the pain. Occasionally *phantom pain* follows tooth extraction. Often the earliest symptom of Bell's palsy in the day or so before facial weakness develops is pain and hyperalgesia behind the ear and side of the face. Likewise, similar symptoms may precede visible lesions of herpes zoster infecting the seventh nerve (Ramsey-Hunt syndrome) or trigeminal nerve. *Postherpetic neuralgia* may follow either condition. *Coronary ischemia* may produce pain exclusively in the face and jaw and, like typical angina pectoris, is usually reproducible with increased myocardial demand. Aching in several upper molar or premolar teeth that is unrelieved by anesthetizing the teeth may point to *maxillary sinusitis*.

Giant cell arteritis is notorious for producing headache, but it may also produce facial pain or sore throat without headache. Jaw and tongue claudication with chewing or talking is relatively common. Tongue infarction is rare. Patients with subacute thyroiditis often experience pain referred to the face or jaw before the tender thyroid gland and transient hyperthyroidism are appreciated.

Burning mouth syndrome (glossodynia) is present in the absence of an identifiable cause (e.g., vitamin B_{12} deficiency, iron deficiency, Plummer-Vinson syndrome, diabetes mellitus, low-grade *Candida* infection, food sensitivity, or subtle xerostomia) and predominantly affects postmenopausal women. The etiology may be neuropathic. Clonazepam, alpha-lipoic acid, and cognitive behavioral therapy have benefited some.

DISEASES OF THE SALIVARY GLANDS

Saliva is essential to oral health. Its major components, water and mucin, serve as a cleansing solvent and lubricating fluid. In addition, it contains antimicrobial factors (e.g., lysozyme, lactoperoxidase, secretory IgA), epidermal growth factor, minerals, and buffering systems. The major salivary glands secrete intermittently in response to autonomic stimulation, which is high during a meal but low otherwise. Hundreds of minor glands in the lips and cheeks secrete mucus continuously. Consequently, oral function becomes impaired when salivary function is reduced. Dry mouth (*xerostomia*) is perceived when salivary flow is reduced by 50%. The most common etiology is medication, especially drugs with anticholinergic properties, but also alpha and beta blockers, calcium channel blockers, and diuretics. Other causes include Sjögren's syndrome, chronic parotitis, salivary duct obstruction, diabetes mellitus, HIV/AIDS, and irradiation for head and neck cancer. Management involves eliminating or limiting drying medications, preventive dental care, and supplementing oral liquid. Sugarless mints or chewing gum may stimulate salivary secretion if dysfunction is mild. When sufficient exocrine tissue remains, pilocarpine or cevimeline has been shown to increase secretions. Commercial saliva substitutes or gels relieve dryness but must be supplemented with fluoride applications to prevent caries.

Sialolithiasis presents most often as painful swelling but in some instances as just swelling or pain. The obstructing stone produces spasm upon eating. Conservative therapy consists of local heat, massage, and hydration. Promotion of salivary secretion with mints or lemon drops may flush out small stones. Antibiotic treatment is necessary when bacterial infection in suspected. In adults, *acute bacterial parotitis* is typically unilateral and most commonly affects postoperative patients within the first 2 weeks of surgery. *Staphylococcus aureus* is the most common bacterial agent. Dehydration, advanced age, and chronic debilitating disease are major risks. Chronic bacterial sialadenitis results from lowered salivary secretion and recurrent bacterial infection. When suspected bacterial infection is not responsive to therapy, the differential diagnosis should be expanded to include benign and malignant neoplasms, lymphoproliferative

disorders, Sjögren's syndrome, sarcoidosis, tuberculosis, lymphadenitis, actinomycosis, and Wegener's granulomatosis. Bilateral nontender parotid enlargement occurs with diabetes mellitus, cirrhosis, bulimia, HIV/AIDS, and drugs (e.g., iodide, propylthiouracil).

Pleomorphic adenoma comprises two-thirds of all salivary neoplasms. The parotid is the principal salivary gland affected, and the tumor presents as a firm, slow-growing mass. Though benign, recurrence is common if resection is incomplete. Malignant tumors such as mucoepidermoid carcinoma, adenoid cystic carcinoma, and adenocarcinoma tend to grow relatively fast, depending upon grade. They may ulcerate and invade nerves, producing numbness and facial paralysis. Neutron-beam radiation therapy is an effective treatment; 5-year survival is about 68% for malignant salivary gland tumors.

DENTAL CARE OF MEDICALLY COMPLEX PATIENTS

Routine dental care (e.g., extraction, scaling and cleaning, tooth restoration, and root canal) is remarkably safe. The most common concerns regarding care of dental patients with medical disease are fear of excessive bleeding for patients on anticoagulants, infection of the heart valves and prosthetic devices from hematogenous seeding of oral flora, and cardiovascular complications resulting from vasopressors used with local anesthetics during dental treatment. Experience confirms that the risks of any of these complications are very low.

Patients undergoing tooth extraction or alveolar and gingival surgery rarely experience uncontrolled bleeding when warfarin anticoagulation is maintained within the therapeutic range currently recommended for prevention of venous thrombosis, atrial fibrillation, or mechanical heart valve. Embolic complications and death, however, have been reported during subtherapeutic anticoagulation. Therapeutic anticoagulation should be confirmed before and continued through the procedure. Likewise, low-dose aspirin (e.g., 81–325 mg) can be safely continued.

Patients at high or moderate risk for bacterial endocarditis should maintain optimal oral hygiene, including flossing, and have regular professional cleaning. Prophylactic antibiotics are recommended for all at-risk patients who undergo dental and oral procedures likely to cause significant bleeding and bacteremia. Should unexpected bleeding occur, antibiotics given within 2 h following the procedure provide effective prophylaxis.

Hematogenous bacterial seeding from oral infection can undoubtedly produce late prosthetic joint infection and therefore requires removal of the infected tissue (e.g., drainage, extraction, root canal) and appropriate antibiotic therapy. However, evidence that late prosthetic joint infection occurs following routine dental procedures is lacking. For this reason, antibiotic prophylaxis is not recommended before dental surgery in patients with orthopedic pins, screws, and plates. It is, however, advised within the first 2 years after joint replacement for patients who have inflammatory arthropathies, immunosuppression, type 1 diabetes mellitus, previous prosthetic joint infection, hemophilia, or malnourishment.

Concern often arises regarding the use of vasoconstrictors in patients with hypertension and heart disease. Vasoconstrictors enhance the depth and duration of local anesthesia, thus reducing the anesthetic dose and potential toxicity. If intravascular injection is avoided, 2% lidocaine with 1:100,000 epinephrine (limited to a total of 0.036 mg epinephrine) can be used safely in those with controlled hypertension and stable coronary heart disease, arrhythmia, or congestive heart failure. Precaution should be taken with patients taking tricyclic antidepressants and nonselective beta blockers as these drugs may potentiate the effect of epinephrine.

Elective dental treatments should be postponed for at least 1 month after myocardial infarction, after which the risk of reinfarction is low provided the patient is medically stable (e.g., stable rhythm, stable angina, and free of heart failure). Patients who have suffered a stroke should have elective dental care deferred for 6 months. In both situations, effective stress reduction requires good pain control, including the use of the minimal amount of vasoconstrictor necessary to provide good hemostasis and local anesthesia.

Bisphosphonate therapy can be associated with *osteonecrosis* of the jaw. Most patients affected have received high-dose aminobisphosphonate therapy for multiple myeloma or metastatic breast cancer and have undergone tooth extraction or dental surgery. Intra-oral lesions appear as exposed yellow-white hard bone involving the mandible or maxilla. Two-thirds are painful. Patients about to receive aminobisphosphonate therapy should receive preventive dental care that reduces the risk of infection and need for future dentoalveolar surgery.

HALITOSIS

Halitosis typically emanates from the oral cavity or nasal passages. Volatile sulfur compounds resulting from bacterial decay of food and cellular debris account for the malodor. Periodontal disease, caries, acute forms of gingivitis, poorly fitting dentures, oral abscess, and tongue coating are usual causes. Treatment includes correcting poor hygiene, treating infection, and tongue brushing. Xerostomia can produce and exacerbate halitosis. Pockets of decay in the tonsillar crypts, esophageal diverticulum, esophageal stasis (e.g., achalasia, stricture), sinusitis, and lung abscess account for some instances. A few systemic diseases produce distinctive odors: renal failure (ammoniacal), hepatic (fishy), and ketoacidosis (fruity).

Helicobacter pylori gastritis can also produce ammoniac breath. If no odor is detectable, then pseudohalitosis or even halitophobia must be considered. These conditions represent varying degrees of psychiatric illness.

AGING AND ORAL HEALTH

While tooth loss and dental disease are not normal consequences of aging, a complex array of structural and functional changes occurs with age that can affect oral health. Subtle changes in tooth structure (e.g., diminished pulp space and volume, sclerosis of dentinal tubules, altered proportions of nerve and vascular pulp content) result in diminished or altered pain sensitivity, reduced reparative capacity, and increased tooth brittleness. In addition, age-associated fatty replacement of salivary acini may reduce physiologic reserve, thus increasing the risk of xerostomia.

Poor oral hygiene often results when vision fails or when patients lose manual dexterity and upper extremity flexibility. This is particularly common for nursing home residents and must be emphasized, since regular oral cleaning and dental care have been shown to reduce the incidence of pneumonia. Other risks for dental decay include limited lifetime fluoride exposure and preference by some older adults for intensely sweet foods when taste and olfaction wane. These factors occur in an increasing proportion of persons over age 75 who retain teeth that have extensive restorations and exposed roots. Without assiduous care, decay can become quite advanced yet remain asymptomatic. Consequently, much or all of the tooth can be destroyed before the process is detected.

Periodontal disease, a leading cause of tooth loss, is indicated by loss of alveolar bone height. Over 90% of Americans have some degree of periodontal disease by age 50. Healthy adults who have not experienced significant alveolar bone loss by the sixth decade do not typically develop significant worsening with advancing age.

Complete edentulousness with advanced age, though less common than in previous decades, is still present in approximately 50% of Americans age ≥85. Speech, mastication, and facial contours are dramatically affected. Edentulousness may also worsen obstructive sleep apnea, particularly in those without symptoms while wearing dentures. Dentures can improve speech articulation and restore diminished facial contours. Mastication is restored less predictably, and those expecting dentures to improve oral intake are often disappointed. Dentures require periodic adjustment to accommodate inevitable remodeling that leads to a diminished volume of the alveolar ridge. Pain can result from friction or traumatic lesions produced by loose dentures. Poor fit and poor oral hygiene may permit candidiasis to develop. This may be asymptomatic or painful and is indicated by erythematous smooth or granular tissue conforming to an area covered by the appliance.

ACKNOWLEDGMENT

The author acknowledges the contribution to this chapter by the previous author, Dr. John S. Greenspan.

FURTHER READINGS

BAUM BJ et al: Aquaporin-1 gene transfer to correct radiation-induced salivary hypofunction. Handb Exp Pharmacol 190:403, 2009

DURSO SC: Interaction with other health team members in caring for elderly patients. Dent Clin North Am 49:377, 2005

GONSALVES WC et al: Common oral conditions in older persons. Am Fam Physician 78:845, 2008

GUEIROS LA et al: Impact of ageing and drug consumption on oral health. Gerodontology 26:297, 2009

LITTLE JW et al (eds): *Dental Management of the Medically Compromised Patient*, 6th ed. St. Louis, Mosby, 2002

REGEZI JA, SCIUBBA JJ: *Oral Pathology: Clinical Pathologic Correlations*, 4th ed. Philadelphia, Saunders, 2002

SPAHR A et al: Periodontal infection and coronary heart disease. Role of periodontal bacteria and importance of total pathogen burden in the coronary event and periodontal disease (CORODONT) study. Arch Intern Med 166:554, 2006

WOO SB et al: Systematic review: Bisphosphonates and osteonecrosis of the jaws. Ann Intern Med 144:753, 2006

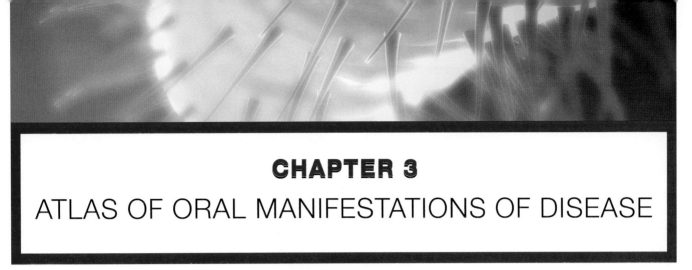

CHAPTER 3
ATLAS OF ORAL MANIFESTATIONS OF DISEASE

Samuel C. Durso ■ Janet A. Yellowitz ■ Jane C. Atkinson

The health status of the oral cavity is linked to cardiovascular disease, diabetes, and other systemic illnesses. Thus, there is significant clinical value in examining the oral cavity for signs of disease. This chapter presents numerous outstanding clinical photographs illustrating many of the conditions discussed in Chap. 2, Oral Manifestations of Disease. Conditions affecting the teeth, periodontal tissues, and oral mucosa are all represented.

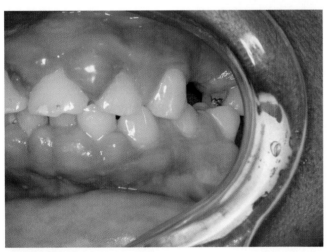

FIGURE 3-1
Gingival overgrowth secondary to calcium channel blocker use.

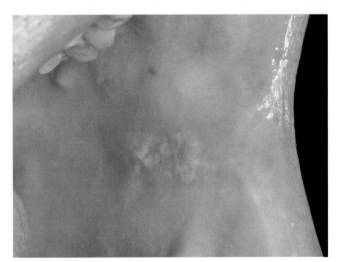

FIGURE 3-2
Oral lichen planus.

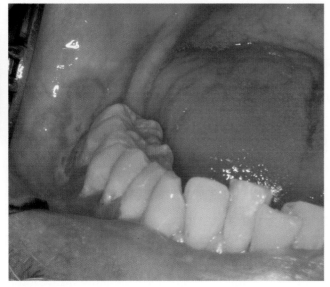

FIGURE 3-3
Erosive lichen planus.

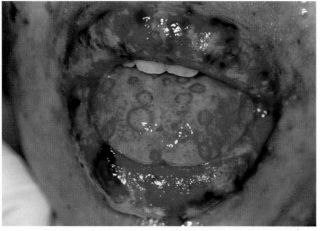

FIGURE 3-4
Stevens-Johnson syndrome—reaction to nevirapine.

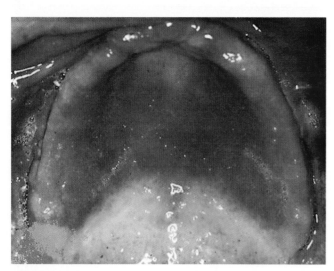

FIGURE 3-5
Inflamed palate.

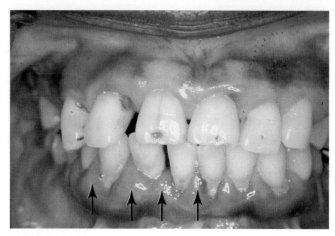

FIGURE 3-6
Severe periodontitis.

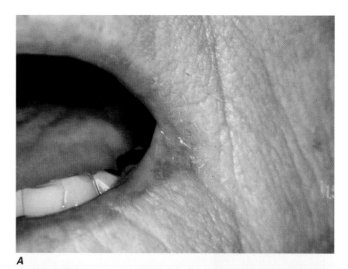

A

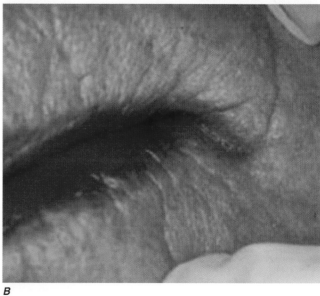

B

FIGURE 3-7
Angular cheilitis.

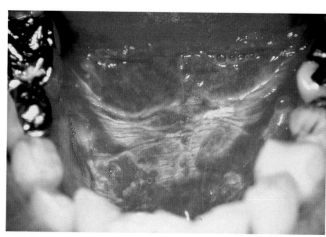

FIGURE 3-8
Sublingual leukoplakia.

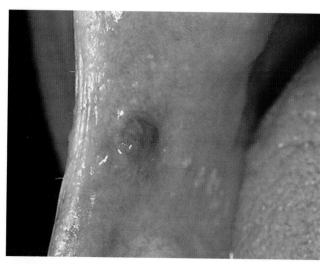

FIGURE 3-10
Traumatic lesion inside of cheek.

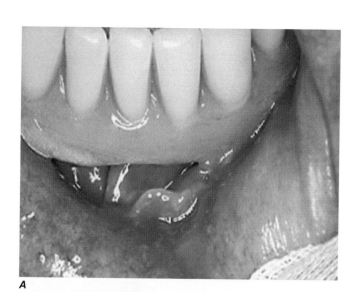

A

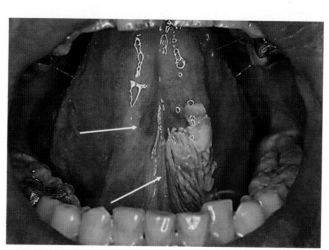

FIGURE 3-11
Sublingual keratosis.

FIGURE 3-9

A. Epulis (gingival hypertrophy) under denture. *B.* Epulis fissuratum.

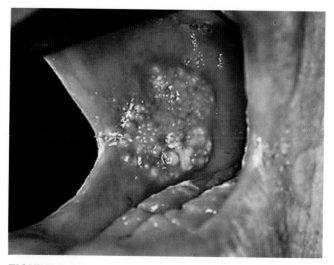

FIGURE 3-12
Oral carcinoma.

B

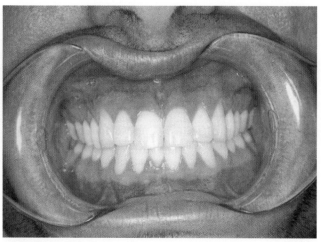

FIGURE 3-13
Healthy mouth.

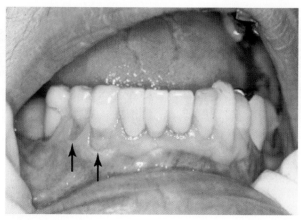

FIGURE 3-16
Gingival recession.

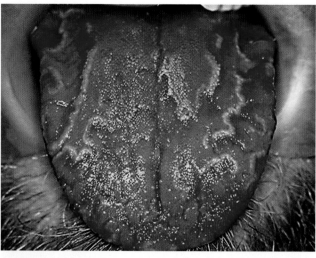

FIGURE 3-14
Geographic tongue.

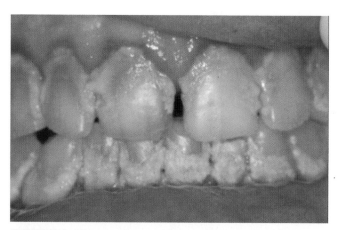

FIGURE 3-17
Heavy calculus and gingival inflammation.

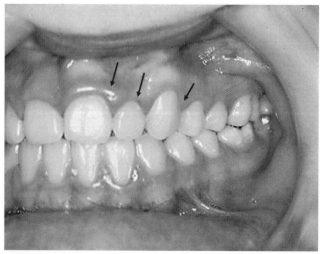

FIGURE 3-15
Moderate gingivitis.

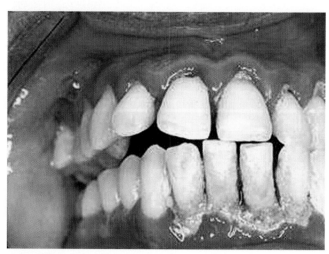

FIGURE 3-18
Severe gingival inflammation and heavy calculus.

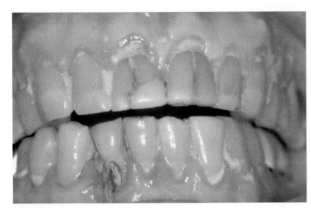

FIGURE 3-19
Heavy plaque and gingival inflammation.

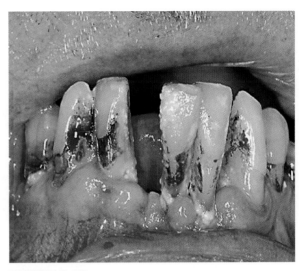

FIGURE 3-22
Severe periodontal disease, missing tooth, very mobile teeth.

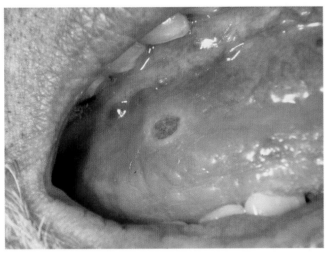

FIGURE 3-20
Ulcer on lateral border of tongue—potential carcinoma.

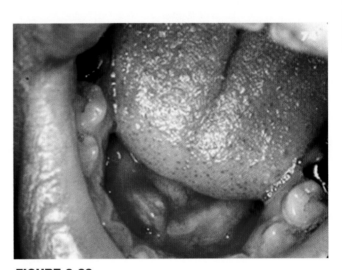

FIGURE 3-23
Salivary stone.

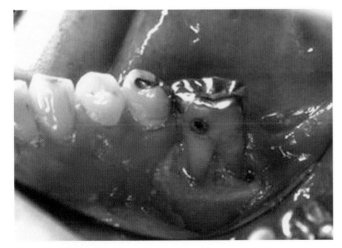

FIGURE 3-21
Osteonecrosis.

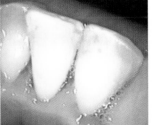

A *B*

FIGURE 3-24
A. Calculus. *B.* Teeth cleaned.

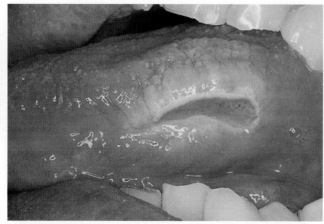

FIGURE 3-25
Traumatic ulcer.

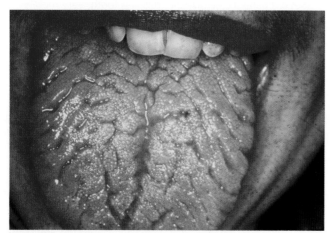

FIGURE 3-26
Fissured tongue.

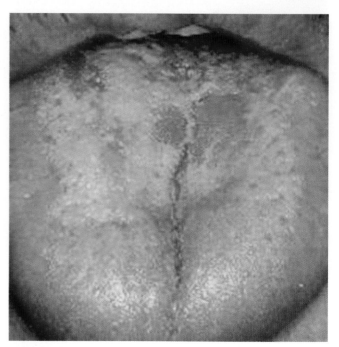

FIGURE 3-27
White coated tongue—likely candidiasis.

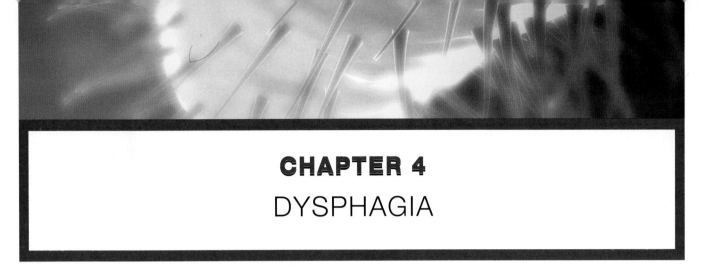

CHAPTER 4
DYSPHAGIA

Raj K. Goyal

Dysphagia is defined as a sensation of "sticking" or obstruction of the passage of food through the mouth, pharynx, or esophagus. However, it is often used as an umbrella term to include other symptoms related to swallowing difficulty. *Aphagia* signifies complete esophageal obstruction, which is usually due to bolus impaction and represents a medical emergency. *Difficulty in initiating a swallow* occurs in disorders of the voluntary phase of swallowing. However, once initiated, swallowing is completed normally. *Odynophagia* means painful swallowing. Frequently, odynophagia and dysphagia occur together. *Globus pharyngeus* is the sensation of a lump lodged in the throat. However, no difficulty is encountered when swallowing is performed. *Misdirection of food*, resulting in nasal regurgitation and laryngeal and pulmonary aspiration during swallowing, is characteristic of oropharyngeal dysphagia. *Phagophobia*, meaning fear of swallowing, and *refusal to swallow* may occur in hysteria, rabies, tetanus, and pharyngeal paralysis due to fear of aspiration. Painful inflammatory lesions that cause odynophagia may also cause refusal to swallow. Some patients may feel the food as it goes down the esophagus. This esophageal sensitivity is not associated with either food sticking or obstruction.

PHYSIOLOGY OF SWALLOWING

The process of swallowing begins with a voluntary (oral) phase that includes a preparatory phase during which a food bolus suitable for swallowing is prepared and a transfer phase during which the bolus is pushed into the pharynx by contraction of the tongue. The bolus then activates oropharyngeal sensory receptors that initiate the deglutition reflex. The deglutition reflex is centrally mediated and involves a complex series of events. It serves both to propel food through the pharynx and the esophagus and to prevent its entry into the airway. When the bolus is propelled backward by the tongue, the larynx moves forward and the upper esophageal sphincter (UES) opens. As the bolus moves into the pharynx, contraction of the superior pharyngeal constrictor against the contracted soft palate initiates a peristaltic contraction that proceeds rapidly downward to move the bolus through the pharynx and the esophagus. The lower esophageal sphincter (LES) opens as the food enters the esophagus and remains open until the peristaltic contraction has swept the bolus into the stomach. Peristaltic contraction in response to a swallow is called *primary peristalsis*. It involves inhibition followed by sequential contraction of muscles along the entire swallowing passage. The inhibition that precedes the peristaltic contraction is called *deglutitive inhibition*. Local distention of the esophagus from residual food activates *secondary peristalsis*.

Muscles of the oral cavity, pharynx, UES, and cervical esophagus are striated and are directly innervated by the lower motor neurons carried in the cranial nerves. Oral cavity muscles are innervated by the Vth and the VIIth cranial nerves and the tongue muscles by the XIIth cranial nerve. Pharyngeal muscles are innervated by the IXth and the Xth cranial nerves.

The UES consists of constrictor and dilator muscles. The constrictor muscles include the cricopharyngeus

27

and inferior pharyngeal constrictor muscles. The dilator muscles include a number of suprahyoid muscles including the geniohyoid muscle. The constrictor muscles are innervated by the Xth cranial nerve and the dilator muscles are innervated by the XIIth and also the Vth and the VIIth cranial nerves. The UES remains closed owing to the elastic properties of its wall and to neurogenic tonic contraction of the cricopharyngeus muscle. Inhibition of the vagal excitatory activity in the central nervous system relaxes the cricopharyngeus, and contraction of the dilator muscles opens the UES by causing upward and forward displacement of the larynx.

The neuromuscular apparatus for peristalsis is different in cervical and thoracic parts of the esophagus. The cervical esophagus, like the pharyngeal muscles, is composed of striated muscles and is innervated by lower motor neurons in the vagus (Xth cranial) nerve. Peristalsis in the cervical esophagus is due to sequential activation of the vagal motor neurons in the nucleus ambiguus.

In contrast, the thoracic esophagus and LES are composed of smooth-muscle fibers and are innervated by excitatory and inhibitory neurons within the esophageal myenteric plexus. Neurotransmitters of the excitatory nerves are acetylcholine and substance P, and of the inhibitory nerves are vasoactive intestinal peptide (VIP) and nitric oxide. Separate groups of parasympathetic preganglionic nerve fibers in the Xth cranial nerve arising from its dorsal motor nucleus project onto the inhibitory and excitatory postganglionic myenteric neurons. Patterned activation of inhibitory followed by excitatory vagal pathways is responsible for peristalsis, which consists of a sequence of inhibition (deglutitive inhibition) followed by contraction. The LES relaxes, with deglutitive inhibition, at the onset of esophageal peristalsis.

The LES is closed at rest because of its intrinsic myogenic tone, influenced by excitatory and inhibitory nerves. The function of the LES is supplemented by the striated muscle of the diaphragmatic crura, which surrounds the LES and acts as an external LES.

PATHOPHYSIOLOGY OF DYSPHAGIA

Based on anatomic site of involvement, dysphagia may be divided into oral, pharyngeal, and esophageal dysphagia. Normal transport of an ingested bolus through the swallowing passage depends on the size of the ingested bolus and size of the lumen, the force of peristaltic contraction, and deglutitive inhibition, including normal relaxation of UES and LES during swallowing. Dysphagia caused by a large bolus or a narrow lumen is called *mechanical dysphagia*, whereas dysphagia due to weakness of peristaltic contractions or to impaired deglutitive inhibition causing nonperistaltic contractions and impaired sphincter relaxation is called *motor dysphagia*.

Oral and Pharyngeal (Oropharyngeal) Dysphagia

Oral-phase dysphagia is associated with poor bolus formation and control, so that food may either drool out of the mouth or overstay in the mouth or the patient may experience difficulty in initiating the swallowing reflex. Poor bolus control may also lead to premature spillage of food into the pharynx and aspiration into the unguarded larynx and/or nasal cavity. Pharyngeal-phase dysphagia is associated with stasis of food in the pharynx due to poor pharyngeal propulsion and obstruction at the UES. Pharyngeal stasis leads to nasal regurgitation and laryngeal aspiration during or after a swallow. Nasal regurgitation and laryngeal aspiration during the process of swallowing are hallmarks of oropharyngeal dysphagia.

Oropharyngeal dysphagia may be due to mechanical causes, including a variety of developmental abnormalities, head and neck tumors, radiation therapy, and inflammatory processes (Table 4-1).

Oropharyngeal motor dysphagia results from impairment of the voluntary effort required in bolus preparation or neuromuscular disorders affecting bolus preparation, initiation of the swallowing reflex, timely passage of food through the pharynx, and prevention of entry of food into the nasal and the laryngeal opening. Paralysis of the suprahyoid muscles leads to loss of opening of the UES and severe dysphagia. Because each side of the pharynx is innervated by ipsilateral nerves, a unilateral lesion of motor neurons leads to unilateral pharyngeal paralysis.

Neuromuscular disorders causing dysphagia are listed in Table 4-1. They include a variety of cortical and suprabulbar disorders, lesions of the cranial nerves in their nuclei in the brainstem or their course to the muscles, defects of neurotransmission at the motor end plates, and muscular diseases. Some of these disorders also involve laryngeal muscles and vocal cords, causing hoarseness.

Since the oropharyngeal phase of swallowing lasts no more than a second, rapid-sequence videofluoroscopy is necessary to permit detection and analysis of abnormalities of oral and pharyngeal function. However, such studies can only be performed in a fully conscious and cooperative patient. A videofluoroscopic swallowing study (VFSS) using barium of different consistencies may reveal difficulties in the oral phase of swallowing. The pharynx is examined to detect stasis of barium in the valleculae and pyriform sinuses and regurgitation of barium into the nose and tracheobronchial tree. Pharyngeal contraction waves and opening of UES with a swallow are carefully monitored. Manometric studies may demonstrate reduced amplitude of pharyngeal contractions and reduced UES pressure without further fall in pressure on swallowing (see Fig. 13-3). General treatment consists of maneuvers to reduce pharyngeal stasis and to enhance airway protection under the direction of

TABLE 4-1

OROPHARYNGEAL DYSPHAGIA

OROPHARYNGEAL MECHANICAL DYSPHAGIA

I. Wall defects
  A. Congenital
    1. Cleft lip, cleft palate
    2. Laryngeal clefts
  B. Post surgical
II. Intrinsic narrowing
  A. Inflammatory
    1. Viral (herpes simplex, varicella-zoster, cytomegalovirus)
    2. Bacterial (peritonsillar abscess)
    3. Fungal (Candida)
    4. Mucocutaneous bullous diseases
    5. Caustic, chemical, thermal injury
  B. Web
    1. Plummer-Vinson syndrome
  C. Strictures
    1. Congenital micrognathia
    2. Caustic ingestion
    3. Post-radiation
  D. Tumors
    1. Benign
    2. Malignant
III. Extrinsic compression
  A. Retropharyngeal abscess, mass
  B. Zenker's diverticulum
  C. Thyroid disorders
  D. Vertebral osteophytes

OROPHARYNGEAL MOTOR DYSPHAGIA

I. Diseases of cerebral cortex and brainstem
  A. With altered consciousness or dementia
    1. Dementias including Alzheimer's disease
    2. Altered consciousness, metabolic encephalopathy, encephalitis, meningitis, cerebrovascular accident, brain injury
  B. With normal cognitive functions
    1. Brain injury
    2. Cerebral palsy
    3. Rabies, tetanus, neurosyphilis
    4. Cerebrovascular disease
    5. Parkinson's disease and other extrapyramidal lesions
    6. Multiple sclerosis (bulbar and pseudobulbar palsy)
    7. Amyotrophic lateral sclerosis (motor neuron disease)
    8. Poliomyelitis and post-poliomyelitis syndrome
II. Diseases of cranial nerves (V, VII, IX, X, XII)
  A. Basilar meningitis (chronic inflammatory, neoplastic)
  B. Nerve injury
  C. Neuropathy (Guillain-Barré syndrome, familial dysautonomia, sarcoid, diabetic and other causes)
III. Neuromuscular
  A. Myasthenia gravis
  B. Eaton-Lambert syndrome
  C. Botulinum toxin
  D. Aminoglycoside and other drugs
IV. Muscle disorders
  A. Myositis (polymyositis, dermatomyositis, sarcoidosis)
  B. Metabolic myopathy (mitochondrial myopathy, thyroid myopathy)
  C. Primary myopathies (myotonic dystrophy, oculopharyngeal myopathy)

a trained swallow therapist. Feeding by a nasogastric tube or an endoscopically placed gastrostomy tube may be necessary for nutritional support; however, these maneuvers do not provide protection against aspiration of salivary secretions. Gastrostomy tube feeding may actually increase gastroesophageal reflux and lead to more aspiration. Jejunostomy tube feeding may lessen reflux.

Dysphagia resulting from a cerebrovascular accident usually improves with time, although often not completely. Patients with myasthenia gravis and polymyositis may respond to treatment of the primary disease. Cricopharyngeal myotomy is usually not helpful. Extensive operative procedures to prevent aspiration are rarely needed. Death is often due to pulmonary complications.

A cricopharyngeal bar results from failure of the cricopharyngeus to relax but with normal activity of the suprahyoid muscles on swallowing. Barium swallow shows a prominent projection on the posterior wall of the pharynx at the level of the lower part of the cricoid cartilage (see Fig. 13-1). A transient cricopharyngeal bar is seen in up to 5% of individuals without dysphagia undergoing upper gastrointestinal studies; it can be produced in normal individuals during a Valsalva maneuver. A persistent cricopharyngeal bar may be caused by fibrosis in the cricopharyngeus. Cricopharyngeal myotomy may be helpful in severely symptomatic case with functional evidence of obstruction by the cricopharyngeus muscle, but is contraindicated in the presence of gastroesophageal reflux because it may lead to pharyngeal and pulmonary aspiration. Globus pharyngeus mainly occurs in individuals with emotional disorders, particularly in women. Results of barium studies and manometry are normal. Treatment consists primarily of reassurance. Some patients with globus pharyngeus have associated reflux esophagitis, and they may respond to treatment of the esophagitis.

Esophageal Dysphagia

In an adult, the esophageal lumen can distend up to 4 cm in diameter. When the esophagus cannot dilate beyond 2.5 cm in diameter, dysphagia to normal solid food can occur. Dysphagia is always present when the esophagus cannot distend beyond 1.3 cm. Circumferential lesions produce dysphagia more consistently than do lesions that involve only a portion of circumferences of the esophageal wall, as uninvolved segments retain their distensibility. The esophageal causes of mechanical dysphagia are listed in Table 4-2. Common causes include carcinoma, peptic and other benign strictures, and lower esophageal ring. Esophageal motor dysphagia may result from abnormalities in peristalsis and deglutitive inhibition due to diseases of the esophageal striated or smooth muscle.

Diseases of the striated muscle often also involve the cervical part of the esophagus, in addition to affecting

TABLE 4-2

ESOPHAGEAL DYSPHAGIA

ESOPHAGEAL MECHANICAL DYSPHAGIA

I. Wall defects
  A. Congenital
  B. Tracheoesophageal fistula
II. Intrinsic narrowing
  A. Inflammatory esophagitis
    1. Viral (herpes simplex, varicella-zoster, cytomegalovirus)
    2. Bacterial
    3. Fungal (Candida)
    4. Mucocutaneous bullous diseases
    5. Caustic, chemical, thermal injury
    6. Eosinophilic esophagitis
  B. Webs and rings
    1. Esophageal (congenital, inflammatory)
    2. Lower esophageal mucosal ring (Schatzki's ring)
    3. Eosinophilic esophagitis
    4. Host-versus-graft disease, mucocutaneous disorders
  C. Benign strictures
    1. Peptic
    2. Caustic

  3. Pill-induced
  4. Inflammatory (Crohn's disease, Candida, mucocutaneous lesions)
  5. Ischemic
  6. Postoperative
  7. Post-radiation
  8. Congenital
  D. Tumors
    1. Benign
    2. Malignant
III. Extrinsic compression
  A. Vascular compression (dysphagia lusoria, aberrant right subclavian artery, right-sided aorta, left atrial enlargement, aortic aneurysm)
  B. Posterior mediastinal mass
  C. Postvagotomy hematoma and fibrosis

ESOPHAGEAL MOTOR DYSPHAGIA

I. Disorders of cervical esophagus (see oropharyngeal motor dysphagia, Table 4-1)
II. Disorders of thoracic esophagus
  A. Diseases of smooth muscle or excitatory nerves
    1. Weak muscle contraction or LES tone
      a. Idiopathic
      b. Scleroderma and related collagen vascular diseases
      c. Hollow visceral myopathy
      d. Myotonic dystrophy
      e. Metabolic neuromyopathy (amyloid, alcohol?, diabetes?)
      f. Drugs: anticholinergics, smooth muscle relaxants

    2. Enhanced muscle contraction
      a. Hypertensive peristalsis (nutcracker esophagus)
      b. Hypertensive LES, hypercontracting LES
  B. Disorders of inhibitory innervation
    1. Diffuse esophageal spasm
    2. Achalasia
      a. Primary
      b. Secondary (Chagas' disease, carcinoma, lymphoma, neuropathic intestinal pseudo-obstruction syndrome)
    3. Contractile (muscular) lower esophageal ring

Note: LES, lower esophageal sphincter.

the oropharyngeal muscles. Clinical manifestations of the cervical esophageal involvement are usually overshadowed by those of the oropharyngeal dysphagia.

Diseases of the smooth-muscle segment involve the thoracic part of the esophagus and the LES. Dysphagia occurs when the peristaltic contractions are weak or absent or when the contractions are nonperistaltic. Loss of peristalsis may be associated with failure of LES relaxation. Weakness of contractile power occurs due to muscle weakness, as in scleroderma or impaired cholinergic effect. Nonperistaltic contractions and failure of LES relaxation occur due to impaired inhibitory innervation. In diffuse esophageal spasm (DES), inhibitory innervation only to the esophageal body is impaired, whereas in achalasia inhibitory innervation to both the esophageal body and LES is impaired. Dysphagia due to esophageal muscle

weakness is often associated with symptoms of gastroesophageal reflux disease (GERD). Dysphagia due to loss of the inhibitory innervation is typically not associated with GERD but may be associated with chest pain.

The causes of esophageal motor dysphagia are also listed in Table 4-2; they include scleroderma of the esophagus, achalasia, DES, and other motor disorders.

Approach to the Patient:
DYSPHAGIA

Figure 4-1 shows an algorithm of approach to a patient with dysphagia.

HISTORY The history can provide a presumptive diagnosis in >80% of patients. The site of dysphagia

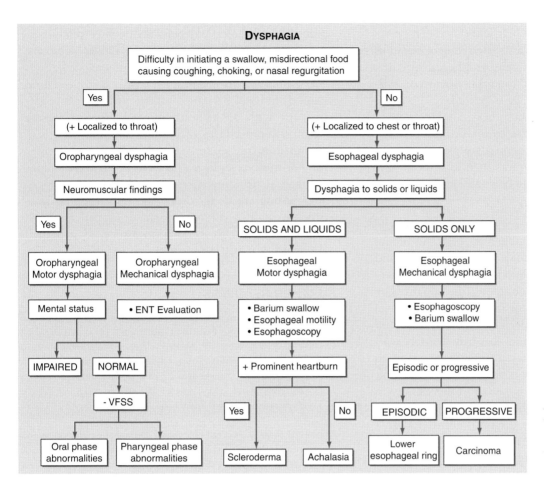

DYSPHAGIA

FIGURE 4-1
Approach to the patient with dysphagia. ENT, ear, nose, and throat; VFSS, videofluoroscopic swallowing study.

described by the patient helps to determine the site of esophageal obstruction; the lesion is at or below the perceived location of dysphagia.

Associated symptoms provide important diagnostic clues. Nasal regurgitation and tracheobronchial aspiration with swallowing are hallmarks of pharyngeal paralysis or a tracheoesophageal fistula. Tracheobronchial aspiration unrelated to swallowing may be due to achalasia, Zenker's diverticulum, or gastroesophageal reflux.

Association of laryngeal symptoms and dysphagia occurs in various neuromuscular disorders. The presence of hoarseness may be an important diagnostic clue. When hoarseness precedes dysphagia, the primary lesion is usually in the larynx; hoarseness following dysphagia may suggest involvement of the recurrent laryngeal nerve by extension of esophageal carcinoma. Sometimes hoarseness may be due to laryngitis secondary to gastroesophageal reflux. Hiccups may rarely occur with a lesion in the distal portion of the esophagus. Unilateral wheezing with dysphagia may indicate a mediastinal mass involving the esophagus and a large bronchus.

The type of food causing dysphagia provides useful information. Difficulty only with solids implies

mechanical dysphagia with a lumen that is not severely narrowed. In advanced obstruction, dysphagia occurs with liquids as well as solids. In contrast, motor dysphagia due to achalasia and DES is equally affected by solids and liquids from the very onset. Patients with scleroderma have dysphagia to solids that is unrelated to posture and to liquids while recumbent but not upright. When peptic stricture develops in patients with scleroderma, dysphagia becomes more persistent.

The duration and course of dysphagia are helpful in diagnosis. Transient dysphagia may be due to an inflammatory process. Progressive dysphagia lasting a few weeks to a few months is suggestive of carcinoma of the esophagus. Episodic dysphagia to solids lasting several years indicates a benign disease characteristic of a lower esophageal ring.

Severe weight loss that is out of proportion to the degree of dysphagia is highly suggestive of carcinoma.

Chest pain with dysphagia occurs in DES and related motor disorders. Chest pain resembling DES may occur in esophageal obstruction due to a large bolus. A prolonged history of heartburn and reflux preceding dysphagia indicates peptic stricture. A history of prolonged nasogastric intubation, ingestion of caustic agents, ingestion of pills without water, previous radiation therapy, or associated mucocutaneous diseases may provide the cause of esophageal stricture. If odynophagia is present, candidal, herpes, or pill-induced esophagitis should be suspected.

In patients with AIDS or other immunocompromised states, esophagitis due to opportunistic infections such as *Candida*, herpes simplex virus, or cytomegalovirus and to tumors such as Kaposi's sarcoma and lymphoma should be considered.

PHYSICAL EXAMINATION Physical examination is important in oral and pharyngeal motor dysphagia. Signs of bulbar or pseudobulbar palsy, including dysarthria, dysphonia, ptosis, tongue atrophy, and hyperactive jaw jerk, in addition to evidence of generalized neuromuscular disease, should be sought. The neck should be examined for thyromegaly or a spinal abnormality. A careful inspection of the mouth and pharynx should disclose lesions that may interfere with passage of food. Pulmonary complications such as acute or chronic aspiration pneumonia may be present.

Physical examination is often unrevealing in esophageal dysphagia. Changes in the skin and extremities may suggest a diagnosis of scleroderma and other collagen vascular diseases or mucocutaneous diseases such as pemphigoid or epidermolysis bullosa, which may involve the esophagus. Cancer spread to lymph nodes and liver may be evident.

DIAGNOSTIC PROCEDURES Dysphagia is usually a symptom of organic disease rather than a functional complaint. If oral or pharyngeal dysphagia is suspected, VFSS by both a radiologist and a swallow therapist is the procedure of choice. Videoendoscopy is currently performed only in specialized centers. Otolaryngoscopic and neurologic evaluation are also usually required.

If esophageal mechanical dysphagia is suspected on clinical history, barium swallow and esophagogastroscopy with or without mucosal biopsies are the diagnostic procedures of choice. In some cases, CT examination and endoscopic ultrasound may be useful. For motor esophageal dysphagia, barium swallow, esophageal manometry, esophageal pH, and impedance testing are useful diagnostic tests. Esophagogastroscopy is also often performed in patients with motor dysphagia to exclude an associated structural abnormality (Chap. 13).

FURTHER READINGS

ATKINS D et al: Eosinophilic esophagitis: the newest esophageal inflammatory disease. Nat Rev Gastroenterol Hepatol 6:267, 2009

BELHOCINE K, GALMICHE JP: Epidemiology of the complications of gastroesophageal reflux disease. Dig Dis 27:7, 2009

BHARDWAJ A et al: A meta-analysis of the diagnostic accuracy of esophageal capsule endoscopy for Barrett's esophagus in patients with gastroesophageal reflux disease. Am J Gastroenterol 104:1533, 2009

MASSEY B, SHAKER R: Oral pharyngeal and upper esophageal sphincter motility disorders. *http://www.nature.com/gimo/index.html; doi:10.1038/gimo19,* 2006

MCCULLOUGH TM, JAFFE D: Head and neck disorders causing dysphagia. *www.GI motilityonline.com; doi:10.1038/gimo36,* 2006

PATERSON WG et al: Esophageal motility disorders. *www.GImotility online.com; doi:10.1038/gimo20,* 2006

VELA MF: Non-acid reflux: detection by multichannel intraluminal impedance and pH, clinical significance, and management. Am J Gastroenterol 104:277, 2009

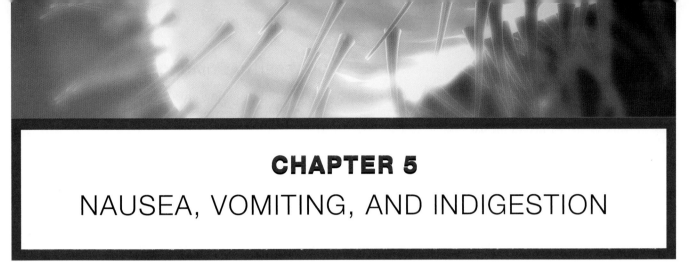

CHAPTER 5
NAUSEA, VOMITING, AND INDIGESTION

William L. Hasler

Nausea is the subjective feeling of a need to vomit. *Vomiting* (emesis) is the oral expulsion of gastrointestinal contents resulting from contractions of gut and thoracoabdominal wall musculature. Vomiting is contrasted with *regurgitation*, the effortless passage of gastric contents into the mouth. *Rumination* is the repeated regurgitation of stomach contents, which may be rechewed and reswallowed. In contrast to vomiting, these phenomena often exhibit volitional control. *Indigestion* is a nonspecific term that encompasses a variety of upper abdominal complaints including nausea, vomiting, heartburn, regurgitation, and dyspepsia (the presence of symptoms thought to originate in the gastroduodenal region). Some individuals with dyspepsia report predominantly epigastric burning, gnawing discomfort, or pain. Others with dyspepsia experience a constellation of symptoms including postprandial fullness, early satiety (an inability to complete a meal due to premature fullness), bloating, eructation (belching), and anorexia.

NAUSEA AND VOMITING

MECHANISMS

Vomiting is coordinated by the brainstem and is effected by neuromuscular responses in the gut, pharynx, and thoracoabdominal wall. The mechanisms underlying nausea are poorly understood but likely involve the cerebral cortex, as nausea requires conscious perception.

This is supported by electroencephalographic studies showing activation of temporofrontal cortical regions during nausea.

Coordination of Emesis

Several brainstem nuclei—including the nucleus tractus solitarius, dorsal vagal and phrenic nuclei, medullary nuclei that regulate respiration, and nuclei that control pharyngeal, facial, and tongue movements—coordinate the initiation of emesis. Neurotransmitters involved in this coordination are uncertain; however, roles for neurokinin NK_1, serotonin 5-HT_3, and vasopressin pathways are postulated.

Somatic and visceral muscles exhibit stereotypic responses during emesis. Inspiratory thoracic and abdominal wall muscles contract, producing high intrathoracic and intraabdominal pressures that facilitate expulsion of gastric contents. The gastric cardia herniates across the diaphragm and the larynx moves upward to promote oral propulsion of the vomitus. Under normal conditions, distally migrating gut contractions are regulated by an electrical phenomenon, the slow wave, which cycles at 3 cycles/min in the stomach and 11 cycles/min in the duodenum. With emesis, there is slow-wave abolition and initiation of orally propagating spike activity, which evokes retrograde contractions that assist in oral expulsion of intestinal contents.

Emetic stimuli act at several sites. Emesis provoked by unpleasant thoughts or smells originates in the cerebral cortex, whereas cranial nerves mediate vomiting after gag reflex activation. Motion sickness and inner ear disorders act on the labyrinthine apparatus, whereas gastric irritants and cytotoxic agents such as cisplatin stimulate gastroduodenal vagal afferent nerves. Nongastric visceral afferents are activated by intestinal and colonic obstruction and mesenteric ischemia. The area postrema, a medullary nucleus, responds to bloodborne emetic stimuli and is termed the *chemoreceptor trigger zone*. Many emetogenic drugs act on the area postrema, as do bacterial toxins and metabolic factors produced during uremia, hypoxia, and ketoacidosis.

Neurotransmitters that mediate induction of vomiting are selective for these anatomic sites. Labyrinthine disorders stimulate vestibular cholinergic muscarinic M_1 and histaminergic H_1 receptors, whereas gastroduodenal vagal afferent stimuli activate serotonin 5-HT$_3$ receptors. The area postrema is richly served by nerve fibers acting on 5-HT$_3$, M_1, H_1, and dopamine D_2 receptor subtypes. Transmitter mediators in the cerebral cortex are poorly understood, although cortical cannabinoid CB_1 pathways have been characterized. Optimal pharmacologic management of vomiting requires understanding of these pathways.

DIFFERENTIAL DIAGNOSIS

Nausea and vomiting are caused by conditions within and outside the gut as well as by drugs and circulating toxins (**Table 5-1**).

Intraperitoneal Disorders

Visceral obstruction and inflammation of hollow and solid viscera may produce vomiting as the main symptom. Gastric obstruction results from ulcer disease and malignancy, while small-bowel and colonic obstruction occur because of adhesions, benign or malignant tumors, volvulus, intussusception, or inflammatory diseases such as Crohn's disease. The superior mesenteric artery syndrome, occurring after weight loss or prolonged bed rest, results when the duodenum is compressed by the overlying superior mesenteric artery. Abdominal irradiation impairs intestinal contractile function and induces strictures. Biliary colic causes nausea via action on visceral afferent nerves. Vomiting with pancreatitis, cholecystitis, and appendicitis is due to localized visceral irritation and induction of ileus. Enteric infections with viruses or bacteria such as *Staphylococcus aureus* and *Bacillus cereus* are common causes of acute vomiting, especially in children. Opportunistic infections such as cytomegalovirus or herpes

TABLE 5-1

CAUSES OF NAUSEA AND VOMITING

INTRAPERITONEAL	EXTRAPERITONEAL	MEDICATIONS/METABOLIC DISORDERS
Obstructing disorders	Cardiopulmonary disease	Drugs
Pyloric obstruction	Cardiomyopathy	Cancer chemotherapy
Small bowel obstruction	Myocardial infarction	Antibiotics
Colonic obstruction	Labyrinthine disease	Cardiac antiarrhythmics
Superior mesenteric artery syndrome	Motion sickness	Digoxin
Enteric infections	Labyrinthitis	Oral hypoglycemics
Viral	Malignancy	Oral contraceptives
Bacterial	Intracerebral disorders	Endocrine/metabolic disease
Inflammatory diseases	Malignancy	Pregnancy
Cholecystitis	Hemorrhage	Uremia
Pancreatitis	Abscess	Ketoacidosis
Appendicitis	Hydrocephalus	Thyroid and parathyroid disease
Hepatitis	Psychiatric illness	Adrenal insufficiency
Altered sensorimotor function	Anorexia and bulimia nervosa	Toxins
Gastroparesis	Depression	Liver failure
Intestinal pseudoobstruction	Postoperative vomiting	Ethanol
Functional dyspepsia		
Gastroesophageal reflux		
Chronic idiopathic nausea		
Functional vomiting		
Cyclic vomiting syndrome		
Biliary colic		
Abdominal irradiation		

simplex virus induce emesis in immunocompromised individuals.

Disordered gut sensorimotor function also commonly causes nausea and vomiting. *Gastroparesis* is defined as a delay in emptying of food from the stomach and occurs after vagotomy, with pancreatic adenocarcinoma, with mesenteric vascular insufficiency, or in systemic diseases such as diabetes, scleroderma, and amyloidosis. Idiopathic gastroparesis occurring in the absence of systemic illness may follow a viral prodrome, suggesting an infectious etiology. Intestinal pseudoobstruction is characterized by disrupted intestinal and colonic motor activity and leads to retention of food residue and secretions, bacterial overgrowth, nutrient malabsorption, and symptoms of nausea, vomiting, bloating, pain, and altered defecation. *Intestinal pseudoobstruction* may be idiopathic or inherited as a familial visceral myopathy or neuropathy, or it may result from systemic disease or as a paraneoplastic complication of a malignancy such as small cell lung carcinoma. Patients with gastroesophageal reflux may report nausea and vomiting, as do some individuals with functional dyspepsia and irritable bowel syndrome.

Three other functional disorders without organic abnormalities have been characterized in adults. *Chronic idiopathic nausea* is defined as nausea without vomiting occurring several times weekly, whereas *functional vomiting* is defined as one or more vomiting episodes weekly in the absence of an eating disorder or psychiatric disease. *Cyclic vomiting syndrome* is a rare disorder of unknown etiology that produces periodic discrete episodes of relentless nausea and vomiting. The syndrome shows a strong association with migraine headaches, suggesting that some cases may be migraine variants. Cyclic vomiting is most common in children, although adult cases have been described in association with rapid gastric emptying and with chronic cannabis use.

Extraperitoneal Disorders

Myocardial infarction and congestive heart failure are cardiac causes of nausea and vomiting. Postoperative emesis occurs after 25% of surgeries, most commonly laparotomy and orthopedic surgery, and is more prevalent in women. Increased intracranial pressure from tumors, bleeding, abscess, or obstruction to cerebrospinal fluid outflow produces prominent vomiting with or without nausea. Motion sickness, labyrinthitis, and Ménière's disease evoke symptoms via labyrinthine pathways. Patients with psychiatric illnesses including anorexia nervosa, bulimia nervosa, anxiety, and depression may report significant nausea that may be associated with delayed gastric emptying.

Drugs evoke vomiting by action on the stomach (analgesics, erythromycin) or area postrema (digoxin, opiates, anti-Parkinsonian drugs). Emetogenic agents include antibiotics, cardiac antiarrhythmics, antihypertensives, oral hypoglycemics, and contraceptives. Cancer chemotherapy causes vomiting that is acute (within hours of administration), delayed (after 1 or more days), or anticipatory. Acute emesis resulting from highly emetogenic agents such as cisplatin is mediated by 5-HT$_3$ pathways, whereas delayed emesis is 5-HT$_3$-independent. Anticipatory nausea often responds better to anxiolytic therapy than to antiemetics.

Several metabolic disorders elicit nausea and vomiting. Pregnancy is the most prevalent endocrinologic cause of nausea, occurring in 70% of women in the first trimester. Hyperemesis gravidarum is a severe form of nausea of pregnancy that can produce significant fluid loss and electrolyte disturbances. Uremia, ketoacidosis, and adrenal insufficiency, as well as parathyroid and thyroid disease, are other metabolic causes of emesis.

Circulating toxins evoke symptoms via effects on the area postrema. Endogenous toxins are generated in fulminant liver failure, whereas exogenous enterotoxins may be produced by enteric bacterial infection. Ethanol intoxication is a common toxic etiology of nausea and vomiting.

Approach to the Patient:
NAUSEA AND VOMITING

HISTORY AND PHYSICAL EXAMINATION The history helps define the etiology of unexplained nausea and vomiting. Drugs, toxins, and gastrointestinal infections commonly cause acute symptoms, whereas established illnesses evoke chronic complaints. Pyloric obstruction and gastroparesis produce vomiting within 1 h of eating, whereas emesis from intestinal obstruction occurs later. In severe cases of gastroparesis, the vomitus may contain food residue ingested hours or days previously. Hematemesis raises suspicion of an ulcer, malignancy, or Mallory-Weiss tear, whereas feculent emesis is noted with distal intestinal or colonic obstruction. Bilious vomiting excludes gastric obstruction, while emesis of undigested food is consistent with a Zenker's diverticulum or achalasia. Relief of abdominal pain by emesis characterizes small-bowel obstruction, whereas vomiting has no effect on pancreatitis or cholecystitis pain. Pronounced weight loss raises concern about malignancy or obstruction. Fevers suggest inflammation; an intracranial source is considered if there are headaches or visual field changes. Vertigo or tinnitus indicates labyrinthine disease.

The physical examination complements information obtained in the history. Demonstration of orthostatic hypotension and reduced skin turgor indicate intravascular fluid loss. Pulmonary abnormalities raise concern for aspiration of vomitus. Abdominal auscultation may reveal absent bowel sounds with ileus. High-pitched rushes suggest bowel obstruction, while a succussion splash upon abrupt lateral movement of the patient is found with gastroparesis or pyloric obstruction. Tenderness or involuntary guarding raises suspicion of inflammation, whereas fecal blood suggests mucosal injury from ulcer, ischemia, or tumor. Neurologic etiologies present with papilledema, visual field loss, or focal neural abnormalities. Neoplasm is suggested by palpation of masses or adenopathy.

DIAGNOSTIC TESTING   For intractable symptoms or an elusive diagnosis, selected diagnostic tests can direct clinical management. Electrolyte replenishment is indicated for hypokalemia or metabolic alkalosis. Detection of iron-deficiency anemia mandates a search for mucosal injury. Pancreaticobiliary disease is indicated by abnormal pancreatic enzymes or liver biochemistries, whereas endocrinologic, rheumatologic, or paraneoplastic etiologies are suggested by specific hormone or serologic testing. If luminal obstruction is suspected, supine and upright abdominal radiographs may show intestinal air-fluid levels with reduced colonic air. Ileus is characterized by diffusely dilated air-filled bowel loops.

Anatomic studies may be indicated if initial testing is nondiagnostic. Upper endoscopy detects ulcers or malignancy, while small-bowel barium radiography diagnoses partial small-bowel obstruction. Colonoscopy or contrast enema radiography can detect colonic obstruction. Abdominal ultrasound or computed tomography (CT) defines intraperitoneal inflammatory processes, while CT or magnetic resonance imaging (MRI) of the head can delineate intracranial disease. Mesenteric angiography or MRI is useful when ischemia is considered.

Gastrointestinal motility testing may detect a motor disorder that contributes to symptoms when anatomic abnormalities are absent. Gastroparesis commonly is diagnosed using gastric scintigraphy, by which emptying of a radiolabeled meal is measured. Isotopic breath tests and telemetry capsule methods also have been validated. Electrogastrography, a noninvasive test of gastric slow-wave activity using cutaneous electrodes placed over the stomach, has been proposed as an alternate means of diagnosing gastroparesis. The diagnosis of intestinal pseudoobstruction often is suggested by abnormal barium transit and luminal dilation on small-bowel contrast radiography. Small-intestinal manometry can confirm the diagnosis and further characterize the motor abnormality as neuropathic or myopathic based on contractile patterns. Such investigation can obviate the need for open intestinal biopsy to evaluate for smooth muscle or neuronal degeneration.

℞ **Treatment:**
NAUSEA AND VOMITING

GENERAL PRINCIPLES   Therapy of vomiting is tailored to correction of medically or surgically remediable abnormalities if possible. Hospitalization is considered for severe dehydration especially if oral fluid replenishment cannot be sustained. Once oral intake is tolerated, nutrients are restarted with liquids that are low in fat, as lipids delay gastric emptying. Foods high in indigestible residues are avoided as these also prolong gastric retention.

ANTIEMETIC MEDICATIONS   The most commonly used antiemetic agents act on sites within the central nervous system (**Table 5-2**). Antihistamines such as meclizine and dimenhydrinate and anticholinergic drugs like scopolamine act on labyrinthine-activated pathways and are useful in motion sickness and inner ear disorders. Dopamine D_2 antagonists treat emesis evoked by area postrema stimuli and are useful for medication, toxic, and metabolic etiologies. Dopamine antagonists freely cross the blood-brain barrier and cause anxiety, dystonic reactions, hyperprolactinemic effects (galactorrhea and sexual dysfunction), and irreversible tardive dyskinesia.

Other drug classes exhibit antiemetic properties. Serotonin $5\text{-}HT_3$ antagonists such as ondansetron and granisetron exhibit utility in postoperative vomiting, after radiation therapy, and in the prevention of cancer chemotherapy–induced emesis. The usefulness of $5\text{-}HT_3$ antagonists for other causes of emesis is less well established. Low-dose tricyclic antidepressant agents provide symptomatic benefit in patients with chronic idiopathic nausea and functional vomiting as well as in diabetic patients with nausea and vomiting whose disease is long standing.

GASTROINTESTINAL MOTOR STIMULANTS
Drugs that stimulate gastric emptying are indicated for gastroparesis (Table 5-2). Metoclopramide, a combined $5\text{-}HT_4$ agonist and D_2 antagonist, exhibits efficacy in gastroparesis, but antidopaminergic side effects limit its use in 25% of patients. Erythromycin, a macrolide antibiotic, increases gastroduodenal motility by action on receptors for motilin, an endogenous stimulant of fasting motor activity. Intravenous erythromycin is useful for inpatients with refractory gastroparesis; however, oral forms also have some utility. Domperidone, a D_2 antagonist not available in the United States, exhibits prokinetic and antiemetic effects but does not cross into

TABLE 5-2

37

TREATMENT OF NAUSEA AND VOMITING

TREATMENT	MECHANISM	EXAMPLES	CLINICAL INDICATIONS
Antiemetic agents	Antihistaminergic	Dimenhydrinate, meclizine	Motion sickness, inner ear disease
	Anticholinergic	Scopolamine	Motion sickness, inner ear disease
	Antidopaminergic	Prochlorperazine, thiethylperazine	Medication-, toxin-, or metabolic-induced emesis
	5-HT$_3$ antagonist	Ondansetron, granisetron	Chemotherapy- and radiation-induced emesis, postoperative emesis
	NK$_1$ antagonist	Aprepitant	Chemotherapy-induced nausea and vomiting
	Tricyclic antidepressant	Amitriptyline, nortriptyline	Chronic idiopathic nausea, functional vomiting, cyclic vomiting syndrome
Prokinetic agents	5-HT$_4$ agonist and antidopaminergic	Metoclopramide	Gastroparesis
	Motilin agonist	Erythromycin	Gastroparesis, ?intestinal pseudoobstruction
	Peripheral antidopaminergic	Domperidone	Gastroparesis
	5-HT$_4$ agonist	Tegaserod	?Gastroparesis, ?intestinal pseudoobstruction
	Somatostatin analogue	Octreotide	Intestinal pseudoobstruction
Special settings	Benzodiazepines	Lorazepam	Anticipatory nausea and vomiting with chemotherapy
	Glucocorticoids	Methylprednisolone, dexamethasone	Chemotherapy-induced emesis
	Cannabinoids	Tetrahydrocannabinol	?Chemotherapy-induced emesis

most other brain regions; thus, anxiety and dystonic reactions are rare. The main side effects of domperidone relate to induction of hyperprolactinemia via effects on pituitary regions served by a porous blood-brain barrier. The 5-HT$_4$ agonist tegaserod potently stimulates gastric emptying in patients with gastroparesis; however, its effects on symptoms of gastric retention are unproven.

Patients with refractory upper gut motility disorders pose significant challenges. Liquid suspensions of prokinetic drugs may be beneficial, as liquids empty from the stomach more rapidly than pills. Metoclopramide can be administered subcutaneously in patients unresponsive to oral drugs. Intestinal pseudoobstruction may respond to the somatostatin analogue octreotide, which induces propagative small intestinal motor complexes. Pyloric injections of botulinum toxin are reported in uncontrolled studies to benefit patients with gastroparesis. Placement of a feeding jejunostomy reduces hospitalizations and improves overall health in some patients with gastroparesis who do not respond to drug therapy. Surgical options are limited for refractory cases, but postvagotomy gastroparesis may improve with near-total resection of the stomach. Implanted gastric electrical stimulators may reduce symptoms, enhance nutrition, improve quality of life, and decrease health care expenditures in patients with medication-refractory gastroparesis.

SELECTED CLINICAL SETTINGS Cancer chemotherapeutic agents such as cisplatin are intensely emetogenic. Given prophylactically, 5-HT$_3$ antagonists prevent chemotherapy-induced acute vomiting in most cases (Table 5-2). Optimal antiemetic effects often are obtained with a 5-HT$_3$ antagonist combined with a glucocorticoid. High-dose metoclopramide also exhibits efficacy in chemotherapy-evoked emesis, while benzodiazepines such as lorazepam are useful in reducing anticipatory nausea and vomiting. Therapy of delayed emesis 1–5 days after chemotherapy is less successful. Neurokinin NK$_1$ antagonists (e.g., aprepitant) exhibit antiemetic and antinausea effects during both the acute and delayed periods after chemotherapy. Cannabinoids such as tetrahydrocannabinol, long advocated for cancer-associated emesis, produce significant side effects and exhibit no more efficacy than antidopaminergic agents. Most current drug regimens produce greater reductions in vomiting than in nausea.

The clinician should exercise caution in managing the pregnant patient with nausea. Studies of the teratogenic effects of available antiemetic agents provide conflicting results. Few controlled trials have been performed in nausea of pregnancy, although antihistamines such as meclizine and antidopaminergics such as prochlorperazine demonstrate efficacy greater than placebo. Some obstetricians offer alternative therapies such as pyridoxine, acupressure, or ginger.

Controlling emesis in cyclic vomiting syndrome is a challenge. In many individuals, prophylactic treatment with tricyclic antidepressants, cyproheptadine, or β-adrenoceptor antagonists can reduce the frequency of attacks. Intravenous 5-HT$_3$ antagonists combined with the sedating effects of a benzodiazepine such as lorazepam are a mainstay of treatment of acute symptom flares. Small studies report benefits with antimigraine therapies, including the serotonin 5-HT$_1$ agonist sumatriptan as well as certain newer anticonvulsant drugs.

INDIGESTION

MECHANISMS

The most common causes of indigestion are gastroesophageal acid reflux and functional dyspepsia. Other cases are a consequence of a more serious organic illness.

Gastroesophageal Acid Reflux

Acid reflux can result from a variety of physiologic defects. Reduced lower esophageal sphincter (LES) tone is an important cause of reflux in scleroderma and pregnancy; it may also be a factor in patients without other systemic conditions. Many individuals exhibit frequent transient LES relaxations during which acid bathes the esophagus. Overeating and aerophagia can transiently override the barrier function of the LES, whereas impaired esophageal body motility and reduced salivary secretion prolong acid exposure. The role of hiatal hernias is controversial—although most reflux patients exhibit hiatal hernias, most individuals with hiatal hernias do not have excess heartburn.

Gastric Motor Dysfunction

Disturbed gastric motility is purported to cause acid reflux in some cases of indigestion. Delayed gastric emptying is also found in 25–50% of functional dyspeptics. The relation of these defects to symptom induction is uncertain; many studies show poor correlation between symptom severity and the degree of motor dysfunction. Impaired gastric fundus relaxation after eating may underlie selected dyspeptic symptoms like bloating, nausea, and early satiety.

Visceral Afferent Hypersensitivity

Disturbed gastric sensory function is proposed as a pathogenic factor in functional dyspepsia. Visceral afferent hypersensitivity was first demonstrated in patients with irritable bowel syndrome who had heightened perception of rectal balloon inflation without changes in rectal compliance. Similarly, dyspeptic patients experience discomfort with fundic distention to lower pressures than healthy controls. Some patients with heartburn exhibit normal esophageal acid exposure. These individuals with

functional heartburn are believed to have heightened perception of normal esophageal pH.

Other Factors

Helicobacter pylori has a clear etiologic role in peptic ulcer disease, but ulcers cause a minority of cases of dyspepsia. Infection with *H. pylori* is considered to be a minor factor in the genesis of functional dyspepsia. In contrast, functional dyspepsia is associated with a reduced sense of physical and mental well-being and is exacerbated by stress, suggesting an important role for psychological factors. Analgesics cause dyspepsia, while nitrates, calcium channel blockers, theophylline, and progesterone promote acid reflux. Other exogenous stimuli that induce acid reflux include ethanol, tobacco, and caffeine via LES relaxation. Genetic factors may contribute to development of acid reflux.

DIFFERENTIAL DIAGNOSIS

Gastroesophageal Reflux Disease

Gastroesophageal reflux disease (GERD) is prevalent in Western society. Heartburn is reported once monthly by 40% of Americans and daily by 7–10%. Most cases of heartburn occur because of excess acid reflux; however, approximately 10% of patients with functional heartburn exhibit normal degrees of esophageal acid exposure.

Functional Dyspepsia

Nearly 25% of the populace has dyspeptic symptoms at least six times yearly, but only 10–20% of these individuals present to physicians. Functional dyspepsia, the cause of symptoms in 60% of dyspeptic patients, is defined as ≥3 months of bothersome postprandial fullness, early satiety, epigastric pain, or epigastric burning with symptom onset at least 6 months before diagnosis in the absence of organic cause. Most patients follow a benign course, but a small number with *H. pylori* infection or on nonsteroidal anti-inflammatory drugs (NSAIDs) progress to ulcer formation. As with idiopathic gastroparesis, some cases of functional dyspepsia result from prior gastrointestinal infection.

Ulcer Disease

In most cases of GERD, there is no destruction of the esophagus. However, 5% of patients develop esophageal ulcers, and some form strictures. Symptoms do not reliably distinguish nonerosive from erosive or ulcerative esophagitis. Some 15–25% of cases of dyspepsia stem from ulcers of the stomach or duodenum. The most common causes of ulcer disease are gastric infection with *H. pylori* and use of NSAIDs. Other rare causes of gastroduodenal ulcer include Crohn's disease (Chap. 16) and Zollinger-Ellison syndrome (Chap. 14), a condition resulting from gastrin overproduction by an endocrine tumor.

Malignancy

Dyspeptic patients often seek care because of fear of cancer. However, <2% of cases result from gastroesophageal malignancy. Esophageal squamous cell carcinoma occurs most often in those with histories of tobacco or ethanol intake. Other risk factors include prior caustic ingestion, achalasia, and the hereditary disorder tylosis. Esophageal adenocarcinoma usually complicates long-standing acid reflux. Between 8 and 20% of GERD patients exhibit intestinal metaplasia of the esophagus, termed *Barrett's metaplasia*. This condition predisposes to esophageal adenocarcinoma (Chap. 47). Gastric malignancies include adenocarcinoma, which is prevalent in certain Asian societies, and lymphoma.

Other Causes

Alkaline reflux esophagitis produces GERD-like symptoms in patients who have had surgery for peptic ulcer disease. Opportunistic fungal or viral esophageal infections may produce heartburn or chest discomfort but more often cause odynophagia. Other causes of esophageal inflammation include eosinophilic esophagitis and pill esophagitis. Biliary colic is in the differential diagnosis of dyspepsia, but most patients with true biliary colic report discrete episodes of right upper quadrant or epigastric pain rather than chronic burning discomfort, nausea, and bloating. Intestinal lactase deficiency produces gas, bloating, discomfort, and diarrhea after lactose ingestion. Lactase deficiency occurs in 15–25% of Caucasians of northern European descent but is more common in African Americans and Asians. Intolerance of other carbohydrates (e.g., fructose, sorbitol) produces similar symptoms. Small-intestinal bacterial overgrowth may produce dyspepsia, often with bowel dysfunction, distention, and malabsorption. Pancreatic disease (chronic pancreatitis and malignancy), hepatocellular carcinoma, celiac disease, Ménétrier's disease, infiltrative diseases (sarcoidosis and eosinophilic gastroenteritis), mesenteric ischemia, thyroid and parathyroid disease, and abdominal wall strain cause dyspepsia. Extraperitoneal etiologies of indigestion include congestive heart failure and tuberculosis.

Approach to the Patient:
INDIGESTION

HISTORY AND PHYSICAL EXAMINATION Care of the patient with indigestion requires a thorough interview. GERD classically produces heartburn, a substernal warmth in the epigastrium that moves toward the neck. Heartburn often is exacerbated by meals and may awaken the patient. Associated symptoms include regurgitation of acid and water brash, the reflex release of salty salivary secretions into the mouth. Atypical symptoms include pharyngitis, asthma, cough, bronchitis, hoarseness, and chest pain that mimics angina. Some patients with acid reflux on esophageal pH testing do not report heartburn and note abdominal pain or other symptoms.

Some individuals with dyspepsia report a predominance of epigastric pain or burning that is intermittent and not generalized or localized to other regions. Others experience a postprandial distress syndrome characterized by fullness occurring after normal-sized meals and early satiety that prevents completion of regular meals several times weekly, with associated bloating, belching, or nausea. Functional dyspepsia overlaps with other functional bowel disorders such as irritable bowel syndrome.

The physical exam with GERD and functional dyspepsia usually is normal. In atypical GERD, pharyngeal erythema and wheezing may be noted. Poor dentition may be seen with prolonged acid regurgitation. Functional dyspeptics may exhibit epigastric tenderness or abdominal distention.

Discrimination between functional and organic causes of indigestion mandates exclusion of selected historic and examination features. Odynophagia suggests esophageal infection, while dysphagia is worrisome for a benign or malignant esophageal blockage. Other alarming features include unexplained weight loss, recurrent vomiting, occult or gross gastrointestinal bleeding, jaundice, a palpable mass or adenopathy, and a family history of gastrointestinal malignancy.

DIAGNOSTIC TESTING As indigestion is prevalent and because most cases result from GERD or functional dyspepsia, a general principle is to perform only limited and directed diagnostic testing of selected individuals.

Once alarm factors are excluded (Table 5-3), patients with typical GERD do not need further evaluation and are treated empirically. Upper endoscopy is indicated to exclude mucosal injury in cases with atypical symptoms, symptoms unresponsive to acid-suppressing drugs, or alarm factors. For heartburn >5 years in duration, especially in patients >50 years old, endoscopy is recommended to screen for Barrett's metaplasia. However, the clinical benefits and cost-effectiveness of this approach have not been validated in controlled studies. Ambulatory esophageal pH testing using a catheter method or an implanted esophageal capsule device is considered for drug-refractory symptoms and atypical symptoms like unexplained chest pain. Esophageal manometry most commonly is ordered when surgical treatment of GERD is considered. A low LES pressure may predict

TABLE 5-3

ALARM SYMPTOMS IN GERD
Odynophagia
Unexplained weight loss
Recurrent vomiting
Occult or gross gastrointestinal bleeding
Jaundice
Palpable mass or adenopathy
Family history of gastrointestinal malignancy

failure of drug therapy and helps select patients who may require surgery. Demonstration of disordered esophageal body peristalsis may affect the decision to operate or modify the type of operation chosen. Manometry with provocative testing may clarify the diagnosis in patients with atypical symptoms. Blind perfusion of saline and then acid into the esophagus, known as the *Bernstein test*, can delineate whether unexplained chest discomfort results from acid reflux.

Upper endoscopy is performed as the initial diagnostic test in patients with unexplained dyspepsia who are >55 years old or have alarm factors because of the elevated risks of malignancy and ulcer in these groups. The management approach to patients <55 years old without alarm factors is dependent on the prevalence of *H. pylori* infection in the local population. For individuals who reside in regions with low *H. pylori* prevalence (<10%), a 4–week trial of a potent acid–suppressing medication such as a proton pump inhibitor is recommended. If this fails, a "test and treat" approach is most commonly applied. *H. pylori* status is determined with urea breath testing, stool antigen measurement, or blood serology testing. Those who are *H. pylori* positive are given therapy to eradicate the infection. If symptoms resolve on either of these regimens, no further intervention is required. For patients in areas with high *H. pylori* prevalence (>10%), an initial test and treat approach is advocated, with a subsequent trial of an acid–suppressing regimen offered for those who fail *H. pylori* treatment or for those who are negative for the infection. In each of these patient subsets, upper endoscopy is reserved for those who fail to respond to therapy.

Further testing is indicated if other factors are present. If bleeding is reported, a blood count is obtained to exclude anemia. Thyroid chemistries or calcium levels screen for metabolic disease, whereas specific serologies may suggest celiac disease. For suspected pancreaticobiliary causes, pancreatic and liver chemistries are obtained. If abnormalities are found, abdominal ultrasound or CT may give important information. Gastric emptying scintigraphy is considered to exclude

gastroparesis in patients whose dyspeptic symptoms resemble postprandial distress when drug treatment fails. Gastric scintigraphy also assesses for gastroparesis in patients with GERD, especially if surgical intervention is being considered. Breath testing after carbohydrate ingestion may detect lactase deficiency, intolerance to other dietary carbohydrates, or small-intestinal bacterial overgrowth.

℞ **Treatment:**
INDIGESTION

GENERAL PRINCIPLES For mild indigestion, reassurance that a careful evaluation revealed no serious organic disease may be the only intervention needed. Drugs that cause acid reflux or dyspepsia should be stopped if possible. Patients with GERD should limit ethanol, caffeine, chocolate, and tobacco use because of their effects on the LES. Other measures in GERD include ingesting a low-fat diet, avoiding snacks before bedtime, and elevating the head of the bed.

Specific therapies for organic disease should be offered when possible. Surgery is appropriate in disorders like biliary colic, while diet changes are indicated for lactase deficiency or celiac disease. Some illnesses such as peptic ulcer disease may be cured by specific medical regimens. However, as most indigestion is caused by GERD or functional dyspepsia, medications that reduce gastric acid, stimulate motility, or blunt gastric sensitivity are indicated.

ACID-SUPPRESSING OR NEUTRALIZING MEDICATIONS Drugs that reduce or neutralize gastric acid are most often prescribed for GERD. Histamine H_2 antagonists such as cimetidine, ranitidine, famotidine, and nizatidine are useful in mild to moderate GERD. For severe symptoms or many cases of erosive or ulcerative esophagitis, proton pump inhibitors such as omeprazole, lansoprazole, rabeprazole, pantoprazole, or esomeprazole are needed. These drugs, which inhibit gastric H^+-, K^+-ATPase activity, are more potent than H_2 antagonists. Acid suppressants may be taken continuously or on demand depending on symptom severity. Many patients initially started on a proton pump inhibitor can be stepped down to an H_2 antagonist. Combination therapy with a proton pump inhibitor and an H_2 antagonist has been proposed for some refractory cases.

Acid-suppressing drugs are also effective in appropriately selected patients with functional dyspepsia. Meta-analysis of eight controlled trials calculated a risk ratio of 0.86, with a 95% confidence interval of 0.78–0.95, favoring proton pump inhibitor therapy over placebo. The benefits of less potent acid-reducing therapies such as H_2 antagonists are unproven.

Liquid antacids are useful for short-term control of mild GERD but are less effective for severe disease unless given at high doses that elicit side effects (diarrhea and constipation with magnesium- and aluminum-containing agents, respectively). Alginic acid in combination with antacids may form a floating barrier to acid reflux in individuals with upright symptoms. Sucralfate is a salt of aluminum hydroxide and sucrose octasulfate that buffers acid and binds pepsin and bile salts. Its efficacy in GERD is felt to be comparable to that of H_2 antagonists.

HELICOBACTER PYLORI ERADICATION

H. pylori eradication is clearly indicated only for peptic ulcer and mucosa-associated lymphoid tissue gastric lymphoma. The utility of eradication therapy in functional dyspepsia is less well established, but <15% of cases relate to this infection. Meta-analysis of 13 controlled trials calculated a risk ratio of 0.91, with a 95% confidence interval of 0.87–0.96, favoring *H. pylori* eradication therapy over placebo. Several drug combinations show efficacy in eliminating the infection (Chap. 14); most include 10–14 days of a proton pump inhibitor or bismuth subsalicylate in concert with two antibiotics. *H. pylori* infection is associated with reduced prevalence of GERD, especially in the elderly. However, eradication of the infection does not worsen GERD symptoms. To date, no consensus recommendations regarding *H. pylori* eradication in GERD patients have been offered.

GASTROINTESTINAL MOTOR STIMULANTS

Motor stimulants (also known as prokinetics) such as metoclopramide, erythromycin, domperidone, and tegaserod have limited utility in GERD. The γ-aminobutyric acid B (GABA-B) agonist baclofen reduces esophageal acid exposure by inhibiting transient LES relaxations; the clinical benefits of this drug are yet to be defined in large trials. Several studies have evaluated the effectiveness of motor-stimulating drugs in functional dyspepsia; however, convincing evidence of their benefits has not been found. Some clinicians suggest that patients with symptoms resembling postprandial distress may respond preferentially to prokinetic drugs.

OTHER OPTIONS

Antireflux surgery (fundoplication) is offered to GERD patients who are young and may require lifelong therapy, have typical heartburn and regurgitation, and are responsive to proton pump inhibitors. Individuals who may respond less well to operative therapy include those with atypical symptoms, those with poor response to proton pump inhibitors, and those who have esophageal motor disturbances. Fundoplications are performed laparoscopically when possible and include the Nissen and Toupet procedures in which the proximal stomach is partly or completely wrapped around the distal esophagus to increase LES pressure. Dysphagia, gas-bloat syndrome, and gastroparesis may be long-term complications of these procedures. Endoscopic therapies for increasing the barrier function of the gastroesophageal junction, including radiofrequency energy delivery, suturing, biopolymer implantation, and gastroplication, have been investigated in patients with refractory GERD with variable results and some adverse consequences.

Some patients with functional heartburn and functional dyspepsia refractory to standard therapies may respond to low-dose tricyclic antidepressants. Their mechanism of action is unknown but may involve blunting of visceral pain processing in the brain. Gas and bloating are among the most troubling symptoms in some patients with indigestion and can be difficult to treat. Dietary exclusion of gas-producing foods such as legumes and use of simethicone or activated charcoal provide symptom benefits in some patients. Therapies that modify gut flora, including antibiotics and probiotic preparations containing active bacterial cultures, are useful for cases of bacterial overgrowth and functional lower gastrointestinal disorders, but their utility in functional dyspepsia is unproven. Psychological treatments may be offered for refractory functional dyspepsia, but no convincing data suggest their efficacy.

FURTHER READINGS

ABELL TL et al: Treatment of gastroparesis: A multidisciplinary clinical review. Neurogastroenterol Motil 18:263, 2006

DEVAULT KR, CASTELL DO: American College of Gastroenterology. Updated guidelines for the diagnosis and treatment of gastroesophageal reflux disease. Am J Gastroenterol 100:190, 2005

GALMICHE JP et al: Functional esophageal disorders. Gastroenterology 130:1459, 2006

HASLER WL: Management of gastroparesis. Expert Rev Gastroenterol Hepatol 2:411, 2008

HASLER WL, CHEY WD: Nausea and vomiting. Gastroenterology 125:1860, 2003

KAHRILAS PJ, LEE TJ: Pathophysiology of gastroesophageal reflux disease. Thorac Surg Clin 15:323, 2005

PARKMAN HP et al: American Gastroenterological Association technical review on the diagnosis and treatment of gastroparesis. Gastroenterology 127:1592, 2004

REDDYMASU SC, MCCALLUM RW: Pharmacotherapy of gastroparesis. Expert Opin Pharmacother 10:469, 2009

SCHWARTZBERG LS: Chemotherapy-induced nausea and vomiting: Clinician and patient perspectives. J Support Oncol 5(suppl 1):5, 2007

SZARKA LA, CAMILLERI M: Methods for measurement of gastric motility. Am J Physiol Liver Physiol 296:G461, 2009

TACK J et al: Functional gastroduodenal disorders. Gastroenterology 130:1466, 2006

TALLEY NJ: Green light from the FDA for new drug development in irritable bowel syndrome and functional dyspepsia. Am J Gastroenterol 104:1339, 2009

TALLEY NJ et al: American Gastroenterological Association technical review on the evaluation of dyspepsia. Gastroenterology 129:1756, 2005

TALLEY NJ et al: Guidelines for the management of dyspepsia. Am J Gastroenterol 100:2324, 2005

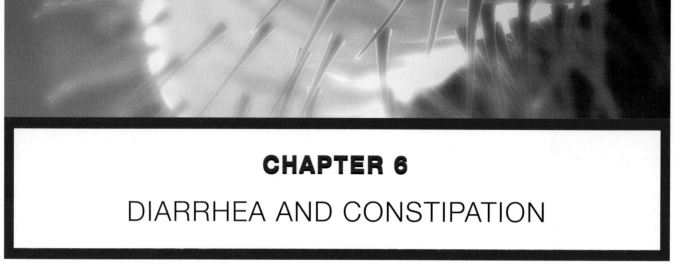

CHAPTER 6

DIARRHEA AND CONSTIPATION

Michael Camilleri ■ Joseph A. Murray

Diarrhea and constipation are exceedingly common and together exact an enormous toll in terms of mortality, morbidity, social inconvenience, loss of work productivity, and consumption of medical resources. Worldwide, >1 billion individuals suffer one or more episodes of acute diarrhea each year. Among the 100 million persons affected annually by acute diarrhea in the United States, nearly half must restrict activities, 10% consult physicians, ~250,000 require hospitalization, and ~5000 die (primarily the elderly). The annual economic burden to society may exceed $20 billion. Acute infectious diarrhea remains one of the most common causes of mortality in developing countries, particularly among children, accounting for 2–3 million deaths per year. Constipation, by contrast, is rarely associated with mortality and is exceedingly common in developed countries, leading to frequent self-medication and, in a third of those, to medical consultation. Population statistics on chronic diarrhea and constipation are more uncertain, perhaps due to variable definitions and reporting, but the frequency of these conditions is also high. United States population surveys put prevalence rates for chronic diarrhea at 2–7% and for chronic constipation at 12–19%, with women being affected twice as often as men. Diarrhea and constipation are among the most common patient complaints faced by internists and primary care physicians, and they account for nearly 50% of referrals to gastroenterologists.

Although diarrhea and constipation may present as mere nuisance symptoms at one extreme, they can be severe or life-threatening at the other. Even mild symptoms may signal a serious underlying gastrointestinal lesion, such as colorectal cancer, or systemic disorder, such as thyroid disease. Given the heterogeneous causes and potential severity of these common complaints, it is imperative for clinicians to appreciate the pathophysiology, etiologic classification, diagnostic strategies, and principles of management of diarrhea and constipation, so that rational and cost-effective care can be delivered.

NORMAL PHYSIOLOGY

While the primary function of the small intestine is the digestion and assimilation of nutrients from food, the small intestine and colon together perform important functions that regulate the secretion and absorption of water and electrolytes, the storage and subsequent transport of intraluminal contents aborally, and the salvage of some nutrients after bacterial metabolism of carbohydrate that are not absorbed in the small intestine. The main motor functions are summarized in **Table 6-1**.

TABLE 6-1

NORMAL GASTROINTESTINAL MOTILITY: FUNCTIONS AT DIFFERENT ANATOMIC LEVELS
Stomach and Small Bowel
Synchronized MMCs in fasting
Accommodation, trituration, mixing, transit
Stomach ~3 h
Small bowel ~3 h
Ileal reservoir empties boluses
Colon: Irregular Mixing, Fermentation, Absorption, Transit
Ascending, transverse: reservoirs
Descending: conduit
Sigmoid/rectum: volitional reservoir

Note: MMC, migrating motor complex.

Alterations in fluid and electrolyte handling contribute significantly to diarrhea. Alterations in motor and sensory functions of the colon result in highly prevalent syndromes such as irritable bowel syndrome (IBS), chronic diarrhea, and chronic constipation.

NEURAL CONTROL

The small intestine and colon have intrinsic and extrinsic innervation. The *intrinsic innervation*, also called the enteric nervous system, comprises myenteric, submucosal, and mucosal neuronal layers. The function of these layers is modulated by interneurons through the actions of neurotransmitter amines or peptides, including acetylcholine, vasoactive intestinal peptide (VIP), opioids, norepinephrine, serotonin, ATP, and nitric oxide. The myenteric plexus regulates smooth-muscle function, and the submucosal plexus affects secretion, absorption, and mucosal blood flow.

The *extrinsic innervations* of the small intestine and colon are part of the autonomic nervous system and also modulate motor and secretory functions. The parasympathetic nerves convey visceral sensory and excitatory pathways to the colon. Parasympathetic fibers via the vagus nerve reach the small intestine and proximal colon along the branches of the superior mesenteric artery. The distal colon is supplied by sacral parasympathetic nerves (S_{2-4}) via the pelvic plexus; these fibers course through the wall of the colon as ascending intracolonic fibers as far as, and in some instances including, the proximal colon. The chief excitatory neurotransmitters controlling motor function are acetylcholine and the tachykinins, such as substance P. The sympathetic nerve supply modulates motor functions and reaches the small intestine and colon alongside their arterial vessels. Sympathetic input to the gut is generally excitatory to sphincters and inhibitory to nonsphincteric muscle. Visceral afferents convey sensation from the gut to the central nervous system; initially, they course along

sympathetic fibers, but as they approach the spinal cord they separate, have cell bodies in the dorsal root ganglion, and enter the dorsal horn of the spinal cord. Afferent signals are conveyed to the brain along the lateral spinothalamic tract and the nociceptive dorsal column pathway and are then projected beyond the thalamus and brainstem to the insula and cerebral cortex to be perceived. Other afferent fibers synapse in the prevertebral ganglia and reflexly modulate intestinal motility.

INTESTINAL FLUID ABSORPTION AND SECRETION

On an average day, 9 L of fluid enter the gastrointestinal (GI) tract; ~1 L of residual fluid reaches the colon; the stool excretion of fluid constitutes about 0.2 L/d. The colon has a large capacitance and functional reserve and may recover up to four times its usual volume of 0.8 L/d, provided the rate of flow permits reabsorption to occur. Thus, the colon can partially compensate for excess fluid delivery to the colon because of intestinal absorptive or secretory disorders.

In the colon, sodium absorption is predominantly electrogenic, and uptake takes place at the apical membrane; it is compensated for by the export functions of the basolateral sodium pump. A variety of neural and non-neural mediators regulate colonic fluid and electrolyte balance, including cholinergic, adrenergic, and serotonergic mediators. Angiotensin and aldosterone also influence colonic absorption, reflecting the common embryologic development of the distal colonic epithelium and the renal tubules.

SMALL-INTESTINAL MOTILITY

During fasting, the motility of the small intestine is characterized by a cyclical event called the migrating motor complex (MMC), which serves to clear nondigestible residue from the small intestine (the intestinal "housekeeper"). This organized, propagated series of contractions lasts on average 4 min, occurs every 60–90 min, and usually involves the entire small intestine. After food ingestion, the small intestine produces irregular, mixing contractions of relatively low amplitude, except in the distal ileum where more powerful contractions occur intermittently and empty the ileum by bolus transfers.

ILEOCOLONIC STORAGE AND SALVAGE

The distal ileum acts as a reservoir, emptying intermittently by bolus movements. This action allows time for salvage of fluids, electrolytes, and nutrients. Segmentation by haustra compartmentalizes the colon and facilitates mixing, retention of residue, and formation of solid stools. There is increased appreciation of the intimate interaction between the colonic function and the luminal ecology.

The resident bacteria in the colon are necessary for the digestion of unabsorbed carbohydrates that reach the colon even in health, thereby providing a vital source of nutrients to the mucosa. Normal colonic flora also keeps pathogens at bay by a variety of mechanisms. In health, the ascending and transverse regions of colon function as reservoirs (average transit, 15 h), and the descending colon acts as a conduit (average transit, 3 h). The colon is efficient at conserving sodium and water, a function that is particularly important in sodium-depleted patients in whom the small intestine alone is unable to maintain sodium balance. Diarrhea or constipation may result from alteration in the reservoir function of the proximal colon or the propulsive function of the left colon. Constipation may also result from disturbances of the rectal or sigmoid reservoir, typically as a result of dysfunction of the pelvic floor or the coordination of defecation.

COLONIC MOTILITY AND TONE

The small intestinal MMC only rarely continues into the colon. However, short duration or phasic contractions mix colonic contents, and high-amplitude (>75 mmHg) propagated contractions (HAPCs) are sometimes associated with mass movements through the colon and normally occur approximately five times per day, usually on awakening in the morning and postprandially. Increased frequency of HAPCs may result in diarrhea or urgency. The predominant phasic contractions in the colon are irregular and nonpropagated and serve a "mixing" function.

Colonic tone refers to the background contractility upon which phasic contractile activity (typically contractions lasting <15 s) is superimposed. It is an important cofactor in the colon's capacitance (volume accommodation) and sensation.

COLONIC MOTILITY AFTER MEAL INGESTION

After meal ingestion, colonic phasic and tonic contractility increase for a period of ~2 h. The initial phase (~10 min) is mediated by the vagus nerve in response to mechanical distention of the stomach. The subsequent response of the colon requires caloric stimulation and is mediated at least in part by hormones, e.g., gastrin and serotonin.

DEFECATION

Tonic contraction of the puborectalis muscle, which forms a sling around the rectoanal junction, is important to maintain continence; during defecation, sacral parasympathetic nerves relax this muscle, facilitating the straightening of the rectoanal angle (Fig. 6-1). Distention of the rectum results in transient relaxation of the internal anal sphincter via intrinsic and reflex sympathetic innervation. As sigmoid and rectal contractions increase the pressure within the rectum, the rectosigmoid angle opens by >15°. Voluntary relaxation of the external anal sphincter (striated muscle innervated by the pudendal nerve) in response to the sensation produced by distention permits the evacuation of feces; this evacuation process can be augmented by an increase in intraabdominal pressure created by the Valsalva maneuver. Defecation can also be delayed voluntarily by contraction of the external anal sphincter.

DIARRHEA

DEFINITION

Diarrhea is loosely defined as passage of abnormally liquid or unformed stools at an increased frequency. For adults on a typical Western diet, stool weight >200 g/d can

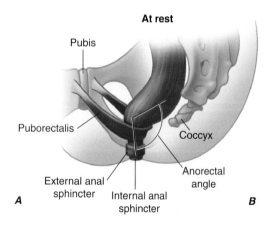
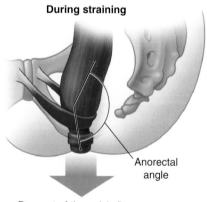

At rest — Pubis, Puborectalis, External anal sphincter, Internal anal sphincter, Coccyx, Anorectal angle

During straining — Anorectal angle, Descent of the pelvic floor

A **B**

FIGURE 6-1

Sagittal view of the anorectum (A) at rest and (B) during straining to defecate. Continence is maintained by normal rectal sensation and tonic contraction of the internal anal sphincter and the puborectalis muscle, which wraps around the anorectum, maintaining an anorectal angle between 80° and 110°. During defecation, the pelvic floor muscles (including the puborectalis) relax, allowing the anorectal angle to straighten by at least 15°, and the perineum descends by 1.0–3.5 cm. The external anal sphincter also relaxes and reduces pressure on the anal canal. *(Reproduced with permission from Lembo and Camilleri.)*

generally be considered diarrheal. Diarrhea may be further defined as *acute* if <2 weeks, *persistent* if 2–4 weeks, and *chronic* if >4 weeks in duration.

Two common conditions, usually associated with the passage of stool totaling <200 g/d, must be distinguished from diarrhea, as diagnostic and therapeutic algorithms differ. *Pseudodiarrhea*, or the frequent passage of small volumes of stool, is often associated with rectal urgency and accompanies IBS or proctitis. *Fecal incontinence* is the involuntary discharge of rectal contents and is most often caused by neuromuscular disorders or structural anorectal problems. Diarrhea and urgency, especially if severe, may aggravate or cause incontinence. Pseudodiarrhea and fecal incontinence occur at prevalence rates comparable to or higher than that of chronic diarrhea and should always be considered in patients complaining of "diarrhea." Overflow diarrhea may occur in nursing home patients due to fecal impaction that is readily detectable by rectal examination. A careful history and physical examination generally allow these conditions to be discriminated from true diarrhea.

ACUTE DIARRHEA

More than 90% of cases of acute diarrhea are caused by infectious agents; these cases are often accompanied by vomiting, fever, and abdominal pain. The remaining 10% or so are caused by medications, toxic ingestions, ischemia, and other conditions.

Infectious Agents

Most infectious diarrheas are acquired by fecal-oral transmission or, more commonly, via ingestion of food or water contaminated with pathogens from human or animal feces. In the immunocompetent person, the resident fecal microflora, containing >500 taxonomically distinct species, are rarely the source of diarrhea and may actually play a role in suppressing the growth of ingested pathogens. Disturbances of flora by antibiotics can lead to diarrhea by reducing the digestive function or by allowing the overgrowth of pathogens, such as *Clostridium difficile* (Chap. 23). Acute infection or injury occurs when the ingested agent overwhelms the host's mucosal immune and nonimmune (gastric acid, digestive enzymes, mucus secretion, peristalsis, and suppressive resident flora) defenses. Established clinical associations with specific enteropathogens may offer diagnostic clues.

In the United States, five high-risk groups are recognized:

1. *Travelers.* Nearly 40% of tourists to endemic regions of Latin America, Africa, and Asia develop so-called traveler's diarrhea, most commonly due to enterotoxigenic or enteroaggregative *Escherichia coli* as well as to *Campylobacter, Shigella, Aeromonas*, norovirus, *Coronavirus*, and *Salmonella*. Visitors to Russia (especially St. Petersburg) may have increased risk of *Giardia*-associated diarrhea; visitors to Nepal may acquire *Cyclospora*. Campers, backpackers, and swimmers in wilderness areas may become infected with *Giardia*. Cruise ships may be affected by outbreaks of gastroenteritis caused by agents such as Norwalk virus.

2. *Consumers of certain foods.* Diarrhea closely following food consumption at a picnic, banquet, or restaurant may suggest infection with *Salmonella, Campylobacter,* or *Shigella* from chicken; enterohemorrhagic *E. coli* (O157:H7) from undercooked hamburger; *Bacillus cereus* from fried rice; *Staphylococcus aureus* or *Salmonella* from mayonnaise or creams; *Salmonella* from eggs; and *Vibrio* species, *Salmonella*, or acute hepatitis A from seafood, especially if raw.

3. *Immunodeficient persons.* Individuals at risk for diarrhea include those with either primary immunodeficiency (e.g., IgA deficiency, common variable hypogammaglobulinemia, chronic granulomatous disease) or the much more common secondary immunodeficiency states (e.g., AIDS, senescence, pharmacologic suppression). Common enteric pathogens often cause a more severe and protracted diarrheal illness, and, particularly in persons with AIDS, opportunistic infections, such as by *Mycobacterium* species, certain viruses (cytomegalovirus, adenovirus, and herpes simplex), and protozoa (*Cryptosporidium, Isospora belli*, Microsporida, and *Blastocystis hominis*) may also play a role. In patients with AIDS, agents transmitted venereally per rectum (e.g., *Neisseria gonorrhoeae, Treponema pallidum, Chlamydia*) may contribute to proctocolitis. Persons with hemochromatosis are especially prone to invasive, even fatal, enteric infections with *Vibrio* species and *Yersinia* infections and should avoid raw fish.

4. *Daycare attendees and their family members.* Infections with *Shigella, Giardia, Cryptosporidium*, rotavirus, and other agents are very common and should be considered.

5. *Institutionalized persons.* Infectious diarrhea is one of the most frequent categories of nosocomial infections in many hospitals and long-term care facilities; the causes are a variety of microorganisms but most commonly *C. difficile.*

The pathophysiology underlying acute diarrhea by infectious agents produces specific clinical features that may also be helpful in diagnosis (Table 6-2). Profuse watery diarrhea secondary to small bowel hypersecretion occurs with ingestion of preformed bacterial toxins, enterotoxin-producing bacteria, and enteroadherent pathogens. Diarrhea associated with marked vomiting and minimal or no fever may occur abruptly within a few hours after ingestion of the former two types; vomiting is usually less, and abdominal cramping or bloating is greater; fever is higher with the latter. Cytotoxin-producing and invasive microorganisms all cause high fever

TABLE 6-2

ASSOCIATION BETWEEN PATHOBIOLOGY OF CAUSATIVE AGENTS AND CLINICAL FEATURES IN ACUTE INFECTIOUS DIARRHEA

PATHOBIOLOGY/AGENTS	INCUBATION PERIOD	VOMITING	ABDOMINAL PAIN	FEVER	DIARRHEA
Toxin producers					
Preformed toxin					
Bacillus cereus, Staphylococcus aureus,	1–8 h	3–4+	1–2+	0–1+	3–4+, watery
Clostridium perfringens	8–24 h				
Enterotoxin					
Vibrio cholerae, enterotoxigenic *Escherichia coli, Klebsiella pneumoniae, Aeromonas* species	8–72 h	2–4+	1–2+	0–1+	3–4+, watery
Enteroadherent					
Enteropathogenic and enteroadherent *E. coli, Giardia* organisms, cryptosporidiosis, helminths	1–8 d	0–1+	1–3+	0–2+	1–2+, watery, mushy
Cytotoxin-producers					
Clostridium difficile	1–3 d	0–1+	3–4+	1–2+	1–3+, usually watery, occasionally bloody
Hemorrhagic *E. coli*	12–72 h	0–1+	3–4+	1–2+	1–3+, initially watery, quickly bloody
Invasive organisms					
Minimal inflammation					
Rotavirus and Norwalk agent	1–3 d	1–3+	2–3+	3–4+	1–3+, watery
Variable inflammation					
Salmonella, Campylobacter, and *Aeromonas* species, *Vibrio parahaemolyticus, Yersinia*	12 h–11 d	0–3+	2–4+	3–4+	1–4+, watery or bloody
Severe inflammation					
Shigella species, enteroinvasive *E. coli, Entamoeba histolytica*	12 h–8 d	0–1+	3–4+	3–4+	1–2+, bloody

Source: Adapted from DW Powell, in T Yamada (ed): *Textbook of Gastroenterology and Hepatology,* 4th ed. Philadelphia, Lippincott Williams & Wilkins, 2003; and DR Syndman, in SL Gorbach (ed): *Infectious Diarrhea.* London, Blackwell, 1986.

and abdominal pain. Invasive bacteria and *Entamoeba histolytica* often cause bloody diarrhea (referred to as *dysentery*). *Yersinia* invades the terminal ileal and proximal colon mucosa and may cause especially severe abdominal pain with tenderness mimicking acute appendicitis.

Finally, infectious diarrhea may be associated with systemic manifestations. Reiter's syndrome (arthritis, urethritis, and conjunctivitis) may accompany or follow infections by *Salmonella, Campylobacter, Shigella,* and *Yersinia.* Yersiniosis may also lead to an autoimmune-type thyroiditis, pericarditis, and glomerulonephritis. Both enterohemorrhagic *E. coli* (O157:H7) and *Shigella* can lead to the *hemolytic-uremic syndrome* with an attendant

high mortality rate. The syndrome of postinfectious IBS has now been recognized as a complication of infectious diarrhea. Acute diarrhea can also be a major symptom of several systemic infections including *viral hepatitis, listeriosis, legionellosis,* and *toxic shock syndrome.*

Other Causes

Side effects from medications are probably the most common noninfectious cause of acute diarrhea, and etiology may be suggested by a temporal association between use and symptom onset. Although innumerable medications may produce diarrhea, some of the more frequently incriminated include antibiotics, cardiac antidysrhythmics, antihypertensives, nonsteroidal anti-inflammatory drugs (NSAIDs), certain antidepressants, chemotherapeutic agents, bronchodilators, antacids, and laxatives. Occlusive or nonocclusive *ischemic colitis* typically occurs in persons >50 years; often presents as acute lower abdominal pain preceding watery, then bloody diarrhea; and generally results in acute inflammatory changes in the sigmoid or left colon while sparing the rectum. Acute diarrhea may accompany colonic *diverticulitis* and *graft-versus-host disease*. Acute diarrhea, often associated with systemic compromise, can follow ingestion of toxins including organophosphate insecticides, amanita and other mushrooms, arsenic, and preformed environmental toxins in seafood, such as ciguatera and scombroid. Conditions causing chronic diarrhea can also be confused with acute diarrhea early in their course. This confusion may occur with inflammatory bowel disease (IBD) and some of the other inflammatory chronic diarrheas that may have an abrupt rather than insidious onset and exhibit features that mimic infection.

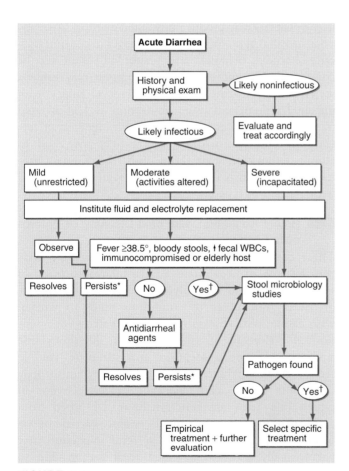

FIGURE 6-2

Algorithm for the management of acute diarrhea. Consider empirical Rx before evaluation with (*) metronidazole and with (†) quinolone. WBCs, white blood cells.

Approach to the Patient:
ACUTE DIARRHEA

The decision to evaluate acute diarrhea depends on its severity and duration and on various host factors (**Fig. 6-2**). Most episodes of acute diarrhea are mild and self-limited and do not justify the cost and potential morbidity of diagnostic or pharmacologic interventions. Indications for evaluation include profuse diarrhea with dehydration, grossly bloody stools, fever ≥38.5°C, duration >48 h without improvement, recent antibiotic use, new community outbreaks, associated severe abdominal pain in patients >50 years, and elderly (≥70 years) or immunocompromised patients. In some cases of moderately severe febrile diarrhea associated with fecal leukocytes (or increased fecal levels of the leukocyte proteins) or with gross blood, a diagnostic evaluation might be avoided in favor of an empirical antibiotic trial (see below).

The cornerstone of diagnosis in those suspected of severe acute infectious diarrhea is microbiologic analysis of the stool. Workup includes cultures for bacterial and viral pathogens, direct inspection for ova and parasites, and immunoassays for certain bacterial toxins (*C. difficile*), viral antigens (rotavirus), and protozoal antigens (*Giardia, E. histolytica*). The aforementioned clinical and epidemiologic associations may assist in focusing the evaluation. If a particular pathogen or set of possible pathogens is so implicated, then either the whole panel of routine studies may not be necessary or, in some instances, special cultures may be appropriate as for enterohemorrhagic and other types of *E. coli*, *Vibrio* species, and *Yersinia*. Molecular diagnosis of pathogens in stool can be made by identification of unique DNA sequences; and evolving microarray technologies could lead to a more rapid, sensitive, specific, and cost-effective diagnostic approach in the future.

Persistent diarrhea is commonly due to *Giardia* (Chap. 31), but additional causative organisms that should be considered include *C. difficile* (especially if antibiotics had been administered), *E. histolytica*, *Cryptosporidium*, *Campylobacter*, and others. If stool studies are unrevealing, then flexible sigmoidoscopy with biopsies and upper endoscopy with duodenal aspirates and biopsies may be indicated. Brainerd diarrhea is an increasingly recognized entity characterized by an abrupt-onset diarrhea that persists for at least 4 weeks, but may last 1–3 years, and is thought to be of infectious origin. It may be associated with subtle inflammation of the distal small intestine or proximal colon.

Structural examination by sigmoidoscopy, colonoscopy, or abdominal CT scanning (or other imaging approaches) may be appropriate in patients with uncharacterized persistent diarrhea to exclude IBD, or as an initial approach in patients with suspected noninfectious acute diarrhea such as might be caused by ischemic colitis, diverticulitis, or partial bowel obstruction.

℞ **Treatment:**
ACUTE DIARRHEA

Fluid and electrolyte replacement are of central importance to all forms of acute diarrhea. Fluid replacement alone may suffice for mild cases. Oral sugar-electrolyte solutions (sport drinks or designed formulations) should be instituted promptly with severe diarrhea to limit dehydration, which is the major cause of death. Profoundly dehydrated patients, especially infants and the elderly, require IV rehydration.

In moderately severe nonfebrile and nonbloody diarrhea, antimotility and antisecretory agents such as loperamide can be useful adjuncts to control symptoms. Such agents should be avoided with febrile dysentery, which may be exacerbated or prolonged by them. Bismuth subsalicylate may reduce symptoms of vomiting and diarrhea but should not be used to treat immunocompromised patients or those with renal impairment because of the risk of bismuth encephalopathy.

Judicious use of antibiotics is appropriate in selected instances of acute diarrhea and may reduce its severity and duration (Fig. 6-2). Many physicians treat moderately to severely ill patients with febrile dysentery empirically without diagnostic evaluation using a quinolone, such as ciprofloxacin (500 mg bid for 3–5 d). Empirical treatment can also be considered for suspected giardiasis with metronidazole (250 mg qid for 7 d). Selection of antibiotics and dosage regimens are otherwise dictated by specific pathogens, geographic patterns of resistance, and conditions found (Chaps. 22 and 26-29). Antibiotic coverage is indicated whether or not a causative organism is discovered in patients who are immunocompromised, have mechanical heart valves or recent vascular grafts, or are elderly. Antibiotic prophylaxis is indicated for certain patients traveling to high-risk countries in whom the likelihood or seriousness of acquired diarrhea would be especially high, including those with immunocompromise, IBD, hemochromatosis, or gastric achlorhydria. Use of trimethoprim/sulfamethoxazole, ciprofloxacin, or rifaximin may reduce bacterial diarrhea in such travelers by 90%, though rifaximin may not be suitable for invasive disease. Finally, physicians should be vigilant to identify if an outbreak of diarrheal illness is occurring and to alert the public health authorities promptly. This may reduce the ultimate size of the affected population.

CHRONIC DIARRHEA

Diarrhea lasting >4 weeks warrants evaluation to exclude serious underlying pathology. In contrast to acute diarrhea, most of the causes of chronic diarrhea are noninfectious. The classification of chronic diarrhea by pathophysiologic mechanism facilitates a rational approach to management, though many diseases cause diarrhea by more than one mechanism (Table 6-3).

Secretory Causes

Secretory diarrheas are due to derangements in fluid and electrolyte transport across the enterocolonic mucosa. They are characterized clinically by watery, large-volume fecal outputs that are typically painless and persist with fasting. Because there is no malabsorbed solute, stool osmolality is accounted for by normal endogenous electrolytes with no fecal osmotic gap.

Medications
Side effects from regular ingestion of drugs and toxins are the most common secretory causes of chronic diarrhea. Hundreds of prescription and over-the-counter medications (see "Other Causes" under "Acute Diarrhea" earlier in the chapter) may produce unwanted diarrhea. Surreptitious or habitual use of stimulant laxatives [e.g., senna, cascara, bisacodyl, ricinoleic acid (castor oil)] must also be considered. Chronic ethanol consumption may cause a secretory-type diarrhea due to enterocyte injury with impaired sodium and water absorption as well as rapid transit and other alterations. Inadvertent ingestion of certain environmental toxins (e.g., arsenic) may lead to chronic rather than acute forms of diarrhea. Certain bacterial infections may occasionally persist and be associated with a secretory-type diarrhea.

Bowel Resection, Mucosal Disease, or Enterocolic Fistula
These conditions may result in a secretory-type diarrhea because of inadequate surface for reabsorption of secreted fluids and electrolytes. Unlike other secretory diarrheas, this subset of conditions tends to worsen with eating. With disease (e.g., Crohn's ileitis) or resection of <100 cm of terminal ileum, dihydroxy bile acids may escape absorption and stimulate colonic secretion (cholorrheic diarrhea). This mechanism may contribute to so-called *idiopathic secretory diarrhea*, in which bile acids are functionally malabsorbed from a normal-appearing terminal ileum. Partial bowel obstruction, ostomy stricture, or fecal impaction may paradoxically lead to increased fecal output due to fluid hypersecretion.

Hormones
Although uncommon, the classic examples of secretory diarrhea are those mediated by hormones. *Metastatic*

TABLE 6-3   49

MAJOR CAUSES OF CHRONIC DIARRHEA ACCORDING TO PREDOMINANT PATHOPHYSIOLOGIC MECHANISM

Secretory causes
Exogenous stimulant laxatives
Chronic ethanol ingestion
Other drugs and toxins
Endogenous laxatives (dihydroxy bile acids)
Idiopathic secretory diarrhea
Certain bacterial infections
Bowel resection, disease, or fistula ($\downarrow$ absorption)
Partial bowel obstruction or fecal impaction
Hormone-producing tumors (carcinoid, VIPoma, medullary
  cancer of thyroid, mastocytosis, gastrinoma, colorectal
  villous adenoma)
Addison's disease
Congenital electrolyte absorption defects

Osmotic causes
Osmotic laxatives (Mg^{2+}, PO_4^{-3}, SO_4^{-2})
Lactase and other disaccharide
  deficiencies
Nonabsorbable carbohydrates (sorbitol, lactulose,
  polyethylene glycol)

Steatorrheal causes
Intraluminal maldigestion (pancreatic exocrine insufficiency,
  bacterial overgrowth, bariatric surgery, liver disease)
Mucosal malabsorption (celiac sprue, Whipple's disease,
  infections, abetalipoproteinemia, ischemia)
Post-mucosal obstruction (1° or 2° lymphatic obstruction)

Inflammatory causes
Idiopathic inflammatory bowel disease (Crohn's, chronic
  ulcerative colitis)
Lymphocytic and collagenous colitis
  Immune-related mucosal disease (1° or 2°
  immunodeficiencies, food allergy, eosinophilic
  gastroenteritis, graft-vs-host disease)
Infections (invasive bacteria, viruses, and parasites,
  Brainerd diarrhea)
Radiation injury
Gastrointestinal malignancies

Dysmotile causes
Irritable bowel syndrome (including post-infectious IBS)
Visceral neuromyopathies
Hyperthyroidism
Drugs (prokinetic agents)
Postvagotomy

Factitial causes
Munchausen
Eating disorders

Iatrogenic causes
Cholecystectomy
Ileal resection
Bariatric surgery
Vagotomy, fundoplication

---

gastrointestinal carcinoid tumors or, rarely, *primary bronchial carcinoids* may produce watery diarrhea alone or as part of the carcinoid syndrome that comprises episodic flushing, wheezing, dyspnea, and right-sided valvular heart disease. Diarrhea is due to the release into the circulation of potent intestinal secretagogues including serotonin, histamine, prostaglandins, and various kinins. Pellagra-like skin lesions may rarely occur as the result of serotonin overproduction with niacin depletion. *Gastrinoma*, one of the most common neuroendocrine tumors, most typically presents with refractory peptic ulcers, but diarrhea occurs in up to one-third of cases and may be the only clinical manifestation in 10%. While other secretagogues released with gastrin may play a role, the diarrhea most often results from fat maldigestion owing to pancreatic enzyme inactivation by low intraduodenal pH. The watery diarrhea hypokalemia achlorhydria syndrome, also called *pancreatic cholera*, is due to a non-β cell pancreatic adenoma, referred to as a *VIPoma*, that secretes VIP and a host of other peptide hormones including pancreatic polypeptide, secretin, gastrin, gastrin-inhibitory polypeptide (also called glucose-dependent insulinotropic peptide), neurotensin, calcitonin, and prostaglandins. The secretory diarrhea is often massive with stool volumes >3 L/d; daily volumes as high as 20 L have been reported.

Life-threatening dehydration; neuromuscular dysfunction from associated hypokalemia, hypomagnesemia, or hypercalcemia; flushing; and hyperglycemia may accompany a VIPoma. *Medullary carcinoma of the thyroid* may present with watery diarrhea caused by calcitonin, other secretory peptides, or prostaglandins. This tumor occurs sporadically or, in 25–50% of cases, as a feature of multiple endocrine neoplasia type 2a with pheochromocytomas and hyperparathyroidism. Prominent diarrhea is often associated with metastatic disease and poor prognosis. *Systemic mastocytosis*, which may be associated with the skin lesion urticaria pigmentosa, may cause diarrhea that is either secretory and mediated by histamine, or inflammatory due to intestinal infiltration by mast cells. Large *colorectal villous adenomas* may rarely be associated with a secretory diarrhea that may cause hypokalemia, can be inhibited by NSAIDs, and is apparently mediated by prostaglandins.

Congenital Defects in Ion Absorption

Rarely, defects in specific carriers associated with ion absorption cause watery diarrhea from birth, and these disorders include defective Cl^-/HCO_3^- exchange (*congenital chloridorrhea*) with alkalosis and defective Na^+/H^+ exchange with acidosis. Some hormone deficiencies may be associated with watery diarrhea, such as occurs with adrenocortical insufficiency (Addison's disease) that may be accompanied by skin hyperpigmentation.

Osmotic Causes

Osmotic diarrhea occurs when ingested, poorly absorbable, osmotically active solutes draw enough fluid into the lumen to exceed the reabsorptive capacity of the colon. Fecal water output increases in proportion to such a solute load. Osmotic diarrhea characteristically ceases with fasting or with discontinuation of the causative agent.

▇▇ Osmotic Laxatives

Ingestion of magnesium-containing antacids, health supplements, or laxatives may induce osmotic diarrhea typified by a stool osmotic gap (>50 mosmol/L): serum osmolarity (typically 290 mosmol/kg)[2 × (fecal sodium + potassium concentration)]. Measurement of fecal osmolarity is no longer recommended since, even when measured immediately after evacuation, it may be erroneous, as carbohydrates are metabolized by colonic bacteria, causing an increase in osmolarity.

▇▇ Carbohydrate Malabsorption

Carbohydrate malabsorption due to acquired or congenital defects in brush-border disaccharidases and other enzymes leads to osmotic diarrhea with a low pH. One of the most common causes of chronic diarrhea in adults is *lactase deficiency*, which affects three-fourths of non-Caucasians worldwide and 5–30% of persons in the United States; the total lactose load at any one time influences the symptoms experienced. Most patients learn to avoid milk products without requiring treatment with enzyme supplements. Some sugars, such as sorbitol, lactulose, or fructose, are frequently malabsorbed, and diarrhea ensues with ingestion of medications, gum, or candies sweetened with these poorly or incompletely absorbed sugars.

Steatorrheal Causes

Fat malabsorption may lead to greasy, foul-smelling, difficult-to-flush diarrhea often associated with weight loss and nutritional deficiencies due to concomitant malabsorption of amino acids and vitamins. Increased fecal output is caused by the osmotic effects of fatty acids, especially after bacterial hydroxylation, and, to a lesser extent, by the neutral fat. Quantitatively, steatorrhea is defined as stool fat exceeding the normal 7 g/d; rapid-transit diarrhea may result in fecal fat up to 14 g/d; daily fecal fat averages 15–25 g with small intestinal diseases and is often >32 g with pancreatic exocrine insufficiency. Intraluminal maldigestion, mucosal malabsorption, or lymphatic obstruction may produce steatorrhea.

▇▇ Intraluminal Maldigestion

This condition most commonly results from pancreatic exocrine insufficiency, which occurs when >90% of pancreatic secretory function is lost. *Chronic pancreatitis*, usually a sequel of ethanol abuse, most frequently causes pancreatic insufficiency. Other causes include *cystic fibrosis*, *pancreatic duct obstruction*, and rarely, *somatostatinoma*. Bacterial overgrowth in the small intestine may deconjugate bile acids and alter micelle formation, impairing fat digestion; it occurs with stasis from a blind-loop, small bowel diverticulum or dysmotility and is especially likely in the elderly. Finally, cirrhosis or biliary obstruction may lead to mild steatorrhea due to deficient intraluminal bile acid concentration.

▇▇ Mucosal Malabsorption

Mucosal malabsorption occurs from a variety of enteropathies, but most commonly from *celiac disease*. This gluten-sensitive enteropathy affects all ages and is characterized by villous atrophy and crypt hyperplasia in the proximal small bowel and can present with fatty diarrhea associated with multiple nutritional deficiencies of varying severity. Celiac disease is much more frequent than previously thought; it affects ~1% of the population, frequently presents without steatorrhea, can mimic IBS, and has many other GI and extraintestinal manifestations. *Tropical sprue* may produce a similar histologic and clinical syndrome but occurs in residents of or travelers to tropical climates; abrupt onset and response to antibiotics suggest an infectious etiology. *Whipple's disease*, due to the bacillus *Tropheryma whipplei* and histiocytic infiltration of the small-bowel mucosa, is a less common cause of steatorrhea that most typically occurs in young or middle-aged men; it is frequently associated with arthralgias, fever, lymphadenopathy, and extreme fatigue and may affect the central nervous system and endocardium. A similar clinical and histologic picture results from *Mycobacterium avium-intracellulare* infection in patients with AIDS. *Abetalipoproteinemia* is a rare defect of chylomicron formation and fat malabsorption in children, associated with acanthocytic erythrocytes, ataxia, and retinitis pigmentosa. Several other conditions may cause mucosal malabsorption including infections, especially with protozoa such as *Giardia*, numerous medications (e.g., colchicine, cholestyramine, neomycin), and chronic ischemia.

▇▇ Postmucosal Lymphatic Obstruction

The pathophysiology of this condition, which is due to the rare *congenital intestinal lymphangiectasia* or to *acquired lymphatic obstruction* secondary to trauma, tumor, or infection, leads to the unique constellation of fat malabsorption with enteric losses of protein (often causing edema) and lymphocytopenia. Carbohydrate and amino acid absorption are preserved.

Inflammatory Causes

Inflammatory diarrheas are generally accompanied by pain, fever, bleeding, or other manifestations of inflammation. The mechanism of diarrhea may not only be exudation but, depending on lesion site, may include fat malabsorption, disrupted fluid/electrolyte absorption, and hypersecretion or hypermotility from release of cytokines and other inflammatory mediators. The unifying feature on stool analysis is the presence of leukocytes or leukocyte-derived proteins such as calprotectin. With severe inflammation, exudative protein loss can lead to anasarca (generalized edema). Any middle-aged or older person with chronic inflammatory-type diarrhea, especially with blood, should be carefully evaluated to exclude a colorectal tumor.

Idiopathic Inflammatory Bowel Disease

The illnesses in this category, which include *Crohn's disease* and *chronic ulcerative colitis*, are among the most common organic causes of chronic diarrhea in adults and range in severity from mild to fulminant and life-threatening. They may be associated with uveitis, polyarthralgias, cholestatic liver disease (primary sclerosing cholangitis), and skin lesions (erythema nodosum, pyoderma gangrenosum). *Microscopic colitis*, including both lymphocytic and *collagenous colitis*, is an increasingly recognized cause of chronic watery diarrhea, especially in middle-aged women and those on NSAIDS; biopsy of a normal-appearing colon is required for histologic diagnosis. It may coexist with symptoms suggesting IBS or with celiac sprue. It typically responds well to anti-inflammatory drugs (e.g., bismuth), to the opioid agonist loperamide, or to budesonide.

Primary or Secondary Forms of Immunodeficiency

Immunodeficiency may lead to prolonged infectious diarrhea. With common variable *hypogammaglobulinemia*, diarrhea is particularly prevalent and often the result of giardiasis.

Eosinophilic Gastroenteritis

Eosinophil infiltration of the mucosa, muscularis, or serosa at any level of the GI tract may cause diarrhea, pain, vomiting, or ascites. Affected patients often have an atopic history, Charcot-Leyden crystals due to extruded eosinophil contents may be seen on microscopic inspection of stool, and peripheral eosinophilia is present in 50–75% of patients. While hypersensitivity to certain foods occurs in adults, true food allergy causing chronic diarrhea is rare.

Other Causes

Chronic inflammatory diarrhea may be caused by *radiation enterocolitis*, *chronic graft-versus-host disease*, *Behçet's syndrome*, and *Cronkite-Canada syndrome*, among others.

Dysmotility Causes

Rapid transit may accompany many diarrheas as a secondary or contributing phenomenon, but primary dysmotility is an unusual etiology of true diarrhea. Stool features often suggest a secretory diarrhea, but mild steatorrhea of up to 14 g of fat per day can be produced by maldigestion from rapid transit alone. *Hyperthyroidism*, *carcinoid syndrome*, and certain drugs (e.g., prostaglandins, prokinetic agents) may produce hypermotility with resultant diarrhea. Primary visceral neuromyopathies or idiopathic acquired intestinal pseudoobstruction may lead to stasis with secondary bacterial overgrowth causing diarrhea. *Diabetic diarrhea*, often accompanied by peripheral and generalized autonomic neuropathies, may occur in part because of intestinal dysmotility.

The exceedingly common *irritable bowel syndrome* (10% point prevalence, 1–2% per year incidence) is characterized by disturbed intestinal and colonic motor and sensory responses to various stimuli. Symptoms of stool frequency typically cease at night, alternate with periods of constipation, are accompanied by abdominal pain relieved with defecation, and rarely result in weight loss or true diarrhea.

Factitial Causes

Factitial diarrhea accounts for up to 15% of unexplained diarrheas referred to tertiary care centers. Either as a form of *Munchausen syndrome* (deception or self-injury for secondary gain) or *eating disorders*, some patients covertly self-administer laxatives alone or in combination with other medications (e.g., diuretics) or surreptitiously add water or urine to stool sent for analysis. Such patients are more often female than male, often with histories of psychiatric illness, and disproportionately from careers in health care. Hypotension and hypokalemia are common co-presenting features. The evaluation of such patients may be difficult: contamination of the stool with water or urine is suggested by very low or high stool osmolarity, respectively. Such patients often deny this possibility when confronted, but they do benefit from psychiatric counseling when they acknowledge their behavior.

Approach to the Patient:
CHRONIC DIARRHEA

The laboratory tools available to evaluate the very common problem of chronic diarrhea are extensive, and many are costly and invasive. As such, the diagnostic evaluation must be rationally directed by a careful history and physical examination (Fig. 6-3A). When this strategy is unrevealing, simple triage tests are often warranted to direct the choice of more complex investigations (Fig. 6-3B). The history, physical examination

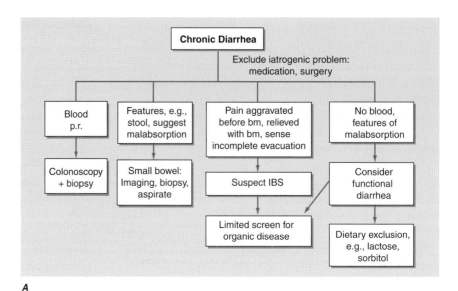

A

FIGURE 6-3

Chronic diarrhea. *A.* Initial management based on accompanying symptoms or features. ***B.*** Evaluation based on findings from a limited age appropriate screen for organic disease. p.r., per rectum; bm, bowel movement; IBS, irritable bowel syndrome; Hb, hemoglobin; Alb, albumin; MCV, mean corpuscular volume; MCH, mean corpuscular hemoglobin; OSM, osmolality. *(Reprinted from M Camilleri: Clin Gastroenterol Hepatol. 2:198, 2004.)*

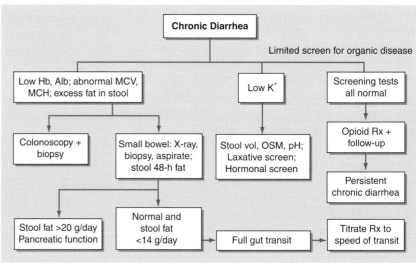

B

(Table 6-4), and routine blood studies should attempt to characterize the mechanism of diarrhea, identify diagnostically helpful associations, and assess the patient's fluid/electrolyte and nutritional status. Patients should be questioned about the onset, duration, pattern, aggravating (especially diet) and relieving factors, and stool characteristics of their diarrhea. The presence or absence of fecal incontinence, fever, weight loss, pain, certain exposures (travel, medications, contacts with diarrhea), and common extraintestinal manifestations (skin changes, arthralgias, oral aphthous ulcers) should be noted. A family history of IBD or sprue may indicate those possibilities. Physical findings may offer clues such as a thyroid mass, wheezing, heart murmurs, edema, hepatomegaly, abdominal masses, lymphadenopathy, mucocutaneous abnormalities, perianal fistulae, or anal sphincter laxity. Peripheral blood leukocytosis, elevated sedimentation rate, or C-reactive protein suggests inflammation; anemia reflects blood loss or nutritional deficiencies; or eosinophilia may occur with parasitoses, neoplasia, collagen-vascular disease, allergy, or

eosinophilic gastroenteritis. Blood chemistries may demonstrate electrolyte, hepatic, or other metabolic disturbances. Measuring tissue transglutaminase antibodies may help detect celiac disease.

TABLE 6-4

PHYSICAL EXAMINATION IN PATIENTS WITH CHRONIC DIARRHEA

1. Are there general features to suggest malabsorption or inflammatory bowel disease (IBD) such as anemia, dermatitis herpetiformis, edema, or clubbing?
2. Are there features to suggest underlying autonomic neuropathy or collagen-vascular disease in the pupils, orthostasis, skin, hands, or joints?
3. Is there an abdominal mass or tenderness?
4. Are there any abnormalities of rectal mucosa, rectal defects, or altered anal sphincter functions?
5. Are there any mucocutaneous manifestations of systemic disease such as dermatitis herpetiformis (celiac disease), erythema nodosum (ulcerative colitis), flushing (carcinoid), or oral ulcers for IBD or celiac disease?

A therapeutic trial is often appropriate, definitive, and highly cost effective when a specific diagnosis is suggested on the initial physician encounter. For example, chronic watery diarrhea, which ceases with fasting in an otherwise healthy young adult, may justify a trial of a lactose-restricted diet; bloating and diarrhea persisting since a mountain backpacking trip may warrant a trial of metronidazole for likely giardiasis; and postprandial diarrhea persisting since an ileal resection might be due to bile acid malabsorption and be treated with cholestyramine before further evaluation. Persistent symptoms require additional investigation.

Certain diagnoses may be suggested on the initial encounter, e.g., idiopathic IBD; however, additional focused evaluations may be necessary to confirm the diagnosis and characterize the severity or extent of disease so that treatment can be best guided. Patients suspected of having IBS should be initially evaluated with flexible sigmoidoscopy with colorectal biopsies; those with normal findings might be reassured and, as indicated, treated empirically with antispasmodics, antidiarrheals, bulk agents, anxiolytics, or antidepressants. Any patient who presents with chronic diarrhea and hematochezia should be evaluated with stool microbiologic studies and colonoscopy.

In an estimated two-thirds of cases, the cause for chronic diarrhea remains unclear after the initial encounter, and further testing is required. Quantitative stool collection and analyses can yield important objective data that may establish a diagnosis or characterize the type of diarrhea as a triage for focused additional studies (Fig. 6-3B). If stool weight is >200 g/d, additional stool analyses should be performed that might include electrolyte concentration, pH, occult blood testing, leukocyte inspection (or leukocyte protein assay), fat quantitation, and laxative screens.

For secretory diarrheas (watery, normal osmotic gap), possible medication-related side effects or surreptitious laxative use should be reconsidered. Microbiologic studies should be done including fecal bacterial cultures (including media for *Aeromonas* and *Plesiomonas*), inspection for ova and parasites, and *Giardia* antigen assay (the most sensitive test for giardiasis). Small-bowel bacterial overgrowth can be excluded by intestinal aspirates with quantitative cultures or with glucose or lactulose breath tests involving measurement of breath hydrogen, methane, or other metabolite (e.g., $^{14}CO_2$). However, interpretation of these breath tests may be confounded by disturbances of intestinal transit. When suggested by history or other findings, screens for peptide hormones should be pursued (e.g., serum gastrin, VIP, calcitonin, and thyroid hormone/thyroid-stimulating hormone, or urinary 5-hydroxyindolacetic acid and histamine). Upper endoscopy and colonoscopy with biopsies and small-bowel barium x-rays are helpful to rule out structural or occult inflammatory disease.

Further evaluation of osmotic diarrhea should include tests for lactose intolerance and magnesium ingestion, the two most common causes. Low fecal pH suggests carbohydrate malabsorption; lactose malabsorption can be confirmed by lactose breath testing or by a therapeutic trial with lactose exclusion and observation of the effect of lactose challenge (e.g., a liter of milk). Lactase determination on small-bowel biopsy is generally not available. If fecal magnesium or laxative levels are elevated, then inadvertent or surreptitious ingestion should be considered and psychiatric help should be sought.

For those with proven fatty diarrhea, endoscopy with small-bowel biopsy (including aspiration for *Giardia* and quantitative cultures) should be performed; if this procedure is unrevealing, a small-bowel radiograph is often an appropriate next step. If small-bowel studies are negative or if pancreatic disease is suspected, pancreatic exocrine insufficiency should be excluded with direct tests, such as the secretin-cholecystokinin stimulation test or a variation that could be performed endoscopically. In general, indirect tests such as assay of fecal chymotrypsin activity or a bentiromide test have fallen out of favor because of low sensitivity and specificity.

Chronic inflammatory-type diarrheas should be suspected by the presence of blood or leukocytes in the stool. Such findings warrant stool cultures, inspection for ova and parasites, *C. difficile* toxin assay, colonoscopy with biopsies, and, if indicated, small-bowel contrast studies.

℞ Treatment:
CHRONIC DIARRHEA

Treatment of chronic diarrhea depends on the specific etiology and may be curative, suppressive, or empirical. If the cause can be eradicated, treatment is curative as with resection of a colorectal cancer, antibiotic administration for Whipple's disease, or discontinuation of a drug. For many chronic conditions, diarrhea can be controlled by suppression of the underlying mechanism. Examples include elimination of dietary lactose for lactase deficiency or gluten for celiac sprue, use of glucocorticoids or other anti-inflammatory agents for idiopathic IBDs, adsorptive agents such as cholestyramine for ileal bile acid malabsorption, proton pump inhibitors such as omeprazole for the gastric hypersecretion of gastrinomas, somatostatin analogues such as octreotide for malignant carcinoid syndrome, prostaglandin inhibitors such as indomethacin for medullary carcinoma of the thyroid, and pancreatic enzyme replacement for pancreatic insufficiency. When the specific cause or mechanism of chronic diarrhea evades diagnosis, empirical therapy may be beneficial. Mild opiates, such as diphenoxylate or loperamide, are often helpful in mild or moderate watery diarrhea. For those with more severe diarrhea, codeine or tincture of opium may be beneficial. Such antimotility agents should be avoided with IBD, as toxic megacolon may be precipitated. Clonidine, an α_2-adrenergic agonist, may allow control of diabetic diarrhea. For all patients with chronic diarrhea, fluid and electrolyte repletion is an important component of management (see "Acute Diarrhea," earlier in the chapter). Replacement of fat-soluble vitamins may also be necessary in patients with chronic steatorrhea.

CONSTIPATION

DEFINITION

Constipation is a common complaint in clinical practice and usually refers to persistent, difficult, infrequent, or seemingly incomplete defecation. Because of the wide range of normal bowel habits, constipation is difficult to define precisely. Most persons have at least three bowel movements per week; however, low stool frequency alone is not the sole criterion for the diagnosis of constipation. Many constipated patients have a normal frequency of defecation but complain of excessive straining, hard stools, lower abdominal fullness, or a sense of incomplete evacuation. The individual patient's symptoms must be analyzed in detail to ascertain what is meant by "constipation" or "difficulty" with defecation.

Stool form and consistency are well correlated with the time elapsed from the preceding defecation. Hard, pellety stools occur with slow transit, while loose watery stools are associated with rapid transit. Both small pellety or very large stools are more difficult to expel than normal stools.

The perception of hard stools or excessive straining is more difficult to assess objectively, and the need for enemas or digital disimpaction is a clinically useful way to corroborate the patient's perceptions of difficult defecation.

Psychosocial or cultural factors may also be important. A person whose parents attached great importance to daily defecation will become greatly concerned when he or she misses a daily bowel movement; some children withhold stool to gain attention or because of fear of pain from anal irritation; and some adults habitually ignore or delay the call to have a bowel movement.

CAUSES

Pathophysiologically, chronic constipation generally results from inadequate fiber or fluid intake or from disordered colonic transit or anorectal function. These result from

TABLE 6-5

CAUSES OF CONSTIPATION IN ADULTS

TYPES OF CONSTIPATION AND CAUSES	EXAMPLES
Recent Onset	
Colonic obstruction	Neoplasm; stricture: ischemic, diverticular, inflammatory
Anal sphincter spasm Medications	Anal fissure, painful hemorrhoids
Chronic	
Irritable bowel syndrome	Constipation-predominant, alternating
Medications	Ca^{2+} blockers, antidepressants
Colonic pseudo-obstruction	Slow-transit constipation, megacolon (rare Hirschsprung's, Chagas)
Disorders of rectal evacuation	Pelvic floor dysfunction; anismus; descending perineum syndrome; rectal mucosal prolapse; rectocele
Endocrinopathies	Hypothyroidism, hypercalcemia, pregnancy
Psychiatric disorders	Depression, eating disorders, drugs
Neurologic disease	Parkinsonism, multiple sclerosis, spinal cord injury
Generalized muscle disease	Progressive systemic sclerosis

neurogastroenterologic disturbance, certain drugs, advancing age, or in association with a large number of systemic diseases that affect the gastrointestinal tract (Table 6-5). Constipation of recent onset may be a symptom of significant organic disease such as tumor or stricture. In *idiopathic constipation*, a subset of patients exhibit delayed emptying of the ascending and transverse colon with prolongation of transit (often in the proximal colon) and a reduced frequency of propulsive HAPCs. *Outlet obstruction to defecation* (also called *evacuation disorders*) may cause delayed colonic transit, which is usually corrected by biofeedback retraining of the disordered defecation. Constipation of any cause may be exacerbated by hospitalization or chronic illnesses that lead to physical or mental impairment and result in inactivity or physical immobility.

Approach to the Patient:
CONSTIPATION

A careful history should explore the patient's symptoms and confirm whether he or she is indeed constipated based on frequency (e.g., fewer than three bowel movements per week), consistency (lumpy/hard), excessive straining, prolonged defecation time, or need to support the perineum or digitate the anorectum. In the vast majority of cases (probably >90%), there is no underlying cause (e.g., cancer, depression, or hypothyroidism), and constipation responds to ample hydration, exercise, and supplementation of dietary fiber (15–25 g/d). A good diet and medication history and attention to psychosocial issues are key. Physical examination and, particularly, a rectal examination should exclude fecal impaction and most of the important diseases that present with constipation and possibly indicate features suggesting an evacuation disorder (e.g., high anal sphincter tone).

The presence of weight loss, rectal bleeding, or anemia with constipation mandates either flexible sigmoidoscopy plus barium enema or colonoscopy alone, particularly in patients >40 years, to exclude structural diseases such as cancer or strictures. Colonoscopy alone is most cost effective in this setting since it provides an opportunity to biopsy mucosal lesions, perform polypectomy, or dilate strictures. Barium enema has advantages over colonoscopy in the patient with isolated constipation, since it is less costly and identifies colonic dilatation and all significant mucosal lesions or strictures that are likely to present with constipation. Melanosis coli, or pigmentation of the colon mucosa, indicates the use of anthraquinone laxatives such as cascara or senna; however, this is usually apparent from a careful history. An unexpected disorder such as megacolon or cathartic colon may also be detected by colonic radiographs. Measurement of serum calcium, potassium, and thyroid-stimulating hormone levels will identify rare patients with metabolic disorders.

Patients with more troublesome constipation may not respond to fiber alone and may be helped by a bowel training regimen: taking an osmotic laxative (lactulose, sorbitol, polyethylene glycol) and evacuating with enema or glycerine suppository as needed. After breakfast, a distraction-free 15–20 min on the toilet without straining is encouraged. Excessive straining may lead to development of hemorrhoids, and, if there is weakness of the pelvic floor or injury to the pudendal nerve, may result in obstructed defecation from descending perineum syndrome several years later. Those few who do not benefit from the simple measures delineated above or require long-term treatment with potent laxatives with the attendant risk of developing laxative abuse syndrome are assumed to have severe or intractable constipation and should have further investigation (Fig. 6-4). Novel agents that induce secretion (e.g., lubiprostone, a chloride channel activator) are also available.

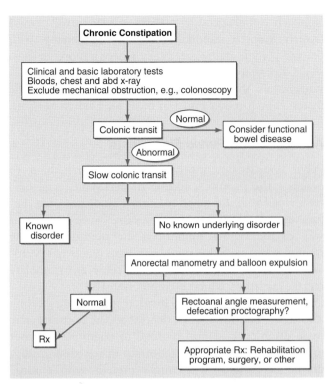

FIGURE 6-4
Algorithm for the management of constipation.

INVESTIGATION OF SEVERE CONSTIPATION

A small minority (probably <5%) of patients have severe or "intractable" constipation. These are the patients most likely to be seen by gastroenterologists or in referral centers. Further observation of the patient may occasionally reveal a previously unrecognized cause, such as an evacuation disorder, laxative abuse, malingering, or psychological disorder. In these patients, evaluations of the physiologic function of the colon and pelvic floor and of psychological status aid in the rational choice of treatment. Even among these highly selected patients with severe constipation, a cause can be identified in only about two-thirds of tertiary referral patients (see later).

Measurement of Colonic Transit

Radiopaque marker transit tests are easy, repeatable, generally safe, inexpensive, reliable, and highly applicable in evaluating constipated patients in clinical practice. Several validated methods are very simple. For example, radiopaque markers are ingested; an abdominal flat film taken 5 days later should indicate passage of 80% of the markers out of the colon without the use of laxatives or enemas. This test does not provide useful information about the transit profile of the stomach and small bowel.

Radioscintigraphy with a delayed-release capsule containing radiolabeled particles has been used to noninvasively characterize normal, accelerated, or delayed colonic function over 24–48 h with low radiation exposure. This approach simultaneously assesses gastric, small bowel (which may be important in ~20% of patients with delayed colonic transit since they reflect a more generalized GI motility disorder), and colonic transit. The disadvantages are the greater cost and the need for specific materials prepared in a nuclear medicine laboratory.

Anorectal and Pelvic Floor Tests

Pelvic floor dysfunction is suggested by the inability to evacuate the rectum, a feeling of persistent rectal fullness, rectal pain, the need to extract stool from the rectum digitally, application of pressure on the posterior wall of the vagina, support of the perineum during straining, and excessive straining. These significant symptoms should be contrasted with the sense of incomplete rectal evacuation, which is common in IBS.

Formal psychological evaluation may identify eating disorders, "control issues," depression, or posttraumatic stress disorders that may respond to cognitive or other intervention and may be important in restoring quality of life to patients who might present with chronic constipation.

A simple clinical test in the office to document a nonrelaxing puborectalis muscle is to have the patient strain to expel the index finger during a digital rectal examination. Motion of the puborectalis posteriorly during straining indicates proper coordination of the pelvic floor muscles.

Measurement of perineal descent is relatively easy to gauge clinically by placing the patient in the left decubitus position and watching the perineum to detect inadequate descent (<1.5 cm, a sign of pelvic floor dysfunction) or perineal ballooning during straining relative to bony landmarks (>4 cm, suggesting excessive perineal descent).

A useful overall test of evacuation is the balloon expulsion test. A balloon-tipped urinary catheter is placed and inflated with 50 mL of water. Normally, a patient can expel it while seated on a toilet or in the left lateral decubitus position. In the lateral position, the weight needed to facilitate expulsion of the balloon is determined; normally expulsion occurs with <200 g added.

Anorectal manometry when used in the evaluation of patients with severe constipation may find an excessively high resting (>80 mmHg) or squeeze anal sphincter tone, suggesting anismus (anal sphincter spasm). This test also identifies rare syndromes, such as adult Hirschsprung's disease, by the absence of the rectoanal inhibitory reflex.

Defecography (a dynamic barium enema including lateral views obtained during barium expulsion) reveals "soft abnormalities" in many patients; the most relevant findings are the measured changes in rectoanal angle, anatomic defects of the rectum such as internal mucosal prolapse, and enteroceles or rectoceles. Surgically remediable conditions are identified in only a few patients. These include severe, whole-thickness intussusception

with complete outlet obstruction due to funnel-shaped plugging at the anal canal or an extremely large rectocele that fills preferentially during attempts at defecation instead of expulsion of the barium through the anus. In summary, defecography requires an interested and experienced radiologist, and abnormalities are not pathognomonic for pelvic floor dysfunction. The most common cause of outlet obstruction is failure of the puborectalis muscle to relax; this is not identified by defecography but requires a dynamic study such as proctography. MRI is being developed as an alternative and provides more information about the structure and function of the pelvic floor, distal colorectum, and anal sphincters.

Dynamic imaging studies such as proctography during defecation or scintigraphic expulsion of artificial stool help measure perineal descent and the rectoanal angle during rest, squeezing, and straining, and scintigraphic expulsion quantitates the amount of "artificial stool" emptied. Lack of straightening of the rectoanal angle by at least 15° during defecation confirms pelvic floor dysfunction.

Neurologic testing (electromyography) is more helpful in the evaluation of patients with incontinence than of those with symptoms suggesting obstructed defecation. The absence of neurologic signs in the lower extremities suggests that any documented denervation of the puborectalis results from pelvic (e.g., obstetric) injury or from stretching of the pudendal nerve by chronic, longstanding straining. Constipation is common among patients with spinal cord injuries, neurologic diseases such as Parkinson's disease, multiple sclerosis, and diabetic neuropathy.

Spinal-evoked responses during electrical rectal stimulation or stimulation of external anal sphincter contraction by applying magnetic stimulation over the lumbosacral cord identify patients with limited sacral neuropathies with sufficient residual nerve conduction to attempt biofeedback training.

In summary, a balloon expulsion test is an important screening test for anorectal dysfunction. If positive, an anatomic evaluation of the rectum or anal sphincters and an assessment of pelvic floor relaxation are the tools for evaluating patients in whom obstructed defecation is suspected.

℞ **Treatment:**
CONSTIPATION

After the cause of constipation is characterized, a treatment decision can be made. Slow-transit constipation requires aggressive medical or surgical treatment; anismus or pelvic floor dysfunction usually responds to biofeedback management (Fig. 6-4). However, only ~60% of patients with severe constipation are found to have such a physiologic disorder (half with colonic transit delay and half with evacuation disorder). Patients with spinal cord injuries or other neurologic disorders require a dedicated bowel regime that often includes rectal stimulation, enema therapy, and carefully timed laxative therapy.

Patients with slow-transit constipation are treated with bulk, osmotic, prokinetic, secretory, and stimulant laxatives including fiber, psyllium, milk of magnesia, lactulose, polyethylene glycol (colonic lavage solution), lubiprostone, and bisacodyl. Newer treatment aimed at enhancing motility and secretion may have application in circumstances such as constipation-predominant IBS in females or severe constipation. If a 3- to 6-month trial of medical therapy fails and patients continue to have documented slow-transit constipation unassociated with obstructed defecation, the patients should be considered for laparoscopic colectomy with ileorectostomy; however, this should not be undertaken if there is continued evidence of an evacuation disorder or a generalized GI dysmotility. Referral to a specialized center for further tests of colonic motor function is warranted. The decision to resort to surgery is facilitated in the presence of megacolon and megarectum. The complications after surgery include small-bowel obstruction (11%) and fecal soiling, particularly at night during the first postoperative year. Frequency of defecation is 3–8 per day during the first year, dropping to 1–3 per day from the second year after surgery.

Patients who have a combined (evacuation and transit/motility) disorder should pursue pelvic floor retraining (biofeedback and muscle relaxation), psychological counseling, and dietetic advice first, followed by colectomy and ileorectostomy if colonic transit studies do not normalize and symptoms are intractable despite biofeedback and optimized medical therapy. In patients with pelvic floor dysfunction alone, biofeedback training has a 70–80% success rate, measured by the acquisition of comfortable stool habits. Attempts to manage pelvic floor dysfunction with operations (internal anal sphincter or puborectalis muscle division) have achieved only mediocre success and have been largely abandoned.

FURTHER READINGS

ATIA AN, BUCHMAN AL: Oral rehydration solutions in non-cholera diarrhea: A review. Am J Gastroenterol 2009 epub ahead of print

BARTLETT JG: Narrative review: The new epidemic of *Clostridium difficile*-associated enteric disease. Ann Intern Med 145:758, 2006

CAMILLERI M: Chronic diarrhea: A review on pathophysiology and management for the clinical gastroenterologist. Clin Gastroenterol Hepatol 2:198, 2004

CAMILLERI M: Serotonin in the gastrointestinal tract. Curr Opin Endocrinol Diabetes Obes 16:53, 2009

FARRELL RJ, KELLY CP: Celiac sprue. N Engl J Med 346:180, 2002

GADEWAR S, FASANO A: Current concepts in the evaluation, diagnosis and management of acute infectious diarrhea. Curr Opin Pharmacol 5:559, 2005

LEMBO A, CAMILLERI M: Chronic constipation. N Engl J Med 349:1360, 2003

McCALLUM IJ et al: Chronic constipation in adults. BMJ 338:b831, 2009

MENNIGEN R, BRUEWER M: Effect of probiotics on intestinal barrier function. Ann NY Acad Sci 1165:183, 2009

MUSHER DM, MUSHER BL: Contagious acute gastrointestinal infections. N Engl J Med 351:2417, 2004

WALD A: Clinical practice. Fecal incontinence in adults. N Engl J Med 356:1648, 2007

————: Constipation in the primary care setting: Current concepts and misconceptions. Am J Med 119:736, 2006

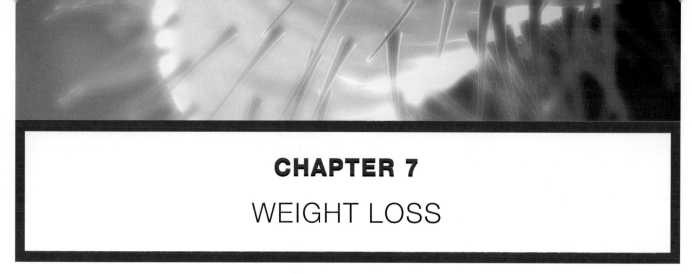

CHAPTER 7
WEIGHT LOSS

Carol M. Reife

Significant unintentional weight loss in a previously healthy individual is often a harbinger of underlying systemic disease. During the routine medical examination, changes in weight should always be assessed; loss of 5% of body weight over 6–12 months should prompt further evaluation.

PHYSIOLOGY OF WEIGHT REGULATION

The normal individual maintains body weight at a remarkably stable "set point," given the wide variation in daily caloric intake and level of activity. Because of the physiologic importance of maintaining energy stores, voluntary weight loss is difficult to achieve and sustain.

Appetite and metabolism are regulated by an intricate network of neural and hormonal factors. The hypothalamic feeding and satiety centers play a central role in these processes (Chap. 55). Neuropeptides such as corticotropin-releasing hormone (CRH), α-melanocyte-stimulating hormone (α-MSH), and cocaine- and amphetamine-related transcript (CART) induce anorexia by acting centrally on satiety centers. The gastrointestinal peptides ghrelin, glucagon, somatostatin, and cholecystokinin signal satiety and thus decrease food intake. Hypoglycemia suppresses insulin, reducing glucose utilization and inhibiting the satiety center.

Leptin is produced by adipose tissue, and it plays a central role in the long-term maintenance of weight homeostasis by acting on the hypothalamus to decrease food intake and increase energy expenditure (Chap. 55). Leptin suppresses expression of hypothalamic neuropeptide Y, a potent appetite stimulatory peptide, and it increases the expression of α-MSH, which acts through the MC4R melanocortin receptor to decrease appetite. Thus, leptin activates a series of downstream neural pathways that alter food-seeking behavior and metabolism. Leptin deficiency, which occurs in conjunction with the loss of adipose tissue, stimulates appetite and induces adaptive responses including inhibition of hypothalamic thyrotropin-releasing hormone (TRH) and gonadotropin-releasing hormone (GnRH).

A variety of cytokines, including tumor necrosis factor α (TNF-α), interleukin (IL) 6 (IL-6), IL-1, interferon γ (IFN-γ), ciliary neurotrophic factor (CNTF), and leukemia inhibitory factor (LIF), can induce cachexia. In addition to causing anorexia, these factors may stimulate fever, depress myocardial function, modulate immune and inflammatory responses, and induce a variety of specific metabolic alterations. TNF-α, for example, preferentially mobilizes fat but spares skeletal muscle. Levels of these cytokines may be increased in patients with cancer, sepsis, chronic inflammatory conditions, AIDS, or congestive heart failure.

Weight loss occurs when energy expenditure exceeds calories available for energy utilization (Chap. 53). In most individuals, approximately half of food energy is utilized for basal processes such as maintenance of body temperature. In a 70-kg person, basal activity consumes ~1800 kcal/d. About 40% of caloric intake is used for physical activity, although athletes may use >50% during vigorous exercise. About 10% of caloric intake is used for dietary thermogenesis, the energy

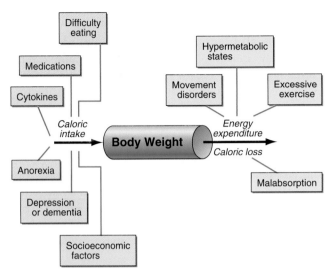

FIGURE 7-1
Energy balance and pathophysiology of weight loss.

expended for digestion, absorption, and metabolism of food.

Mechanisms of weight loss include decreased food intake, malabsorption, loss of calories, and increased energy requirements (Fig. 7-1). Changes in weight may involve loss of tissue mass or body fluid content. A deficit of 3500 kcal generally correlates with the loss of 0.45 kg (1 lb) of body fat, but one must also consider water weight [1 kg/L (2.2 lb/L)] gained or lost. Weight loss that persists over weeks to months reflects the loss of tissue mass.

Food intake may be influenced by a wide variety of visual, olfactory, and gustatory stimuli as well as by genetic, psychological, and social factors. Absorption may be impaired because of pancreatic insufficiency, cholestasis, celiac sprue, intestinal tumors, radiation injury, inflammatory bowel disease, infection, or medication effect. These disease processes may be manifest as changes in stool frequency and consistency. Calories may also be lost due to vomiting or diarrhea, glucosuria in diabetes mellitus, or fistulous drainage. Resting energy expenditure decreases with age and can be affected by thyroid status. Beginning at about age 60, body weight declines by an average of 0.5% per year. Body composition is also affected by aging; adipose tissue increases and lean muscle mass decreases with age.

SIGNIFICANCE OF WEIGHT LOSS

Unintentional weight loss, especially in the elderly, is relatively common and is associated with increased morbidity and mortality rates, even after comorbid conditions have been taken into account. Prospective studies indicate that significant involuntary weight loss is associated with a mortality rate of 25% over the next 18 months.

Retrospective studies of significant weight loss in the elderly document mortality rates of 9–38% over a 2- to 3-year period.

Cancer patients with weight loss have decreased performance status, impaired responses to chemotherapy, and reduced median survival. Marked weight loss also predisposes to infection. Patients undergoing elective surgery, who have lost >4.5 kg (>10 lb) in 6 months, have higher surgical mortality rates. Vitamin and nutrient deficiencies may also accompany significant weight loss (Chap. 52).

CAUSES OF WEIGHT LOSS

The list of possible causes of weight loss is extensive (Table 7-1). In the elderly, the most common causes of weight loss are depression, cancer, and benign gastrointestinal disease. Lung and gastrointestinal cancer are the

TABLE 7-1

CAUSES OF WEIGHT LOSS	
Cancer	Medications
Endocrine and	Antibiotics
metabolic	Nonsteroidal anti-
Hyperthyroidism	inflammatory
Diabetes mellitus	drugs
Pheochromocytoma	Serotonin reuptake
Adrenal	inhibitors
insufficiency	Metformin
Gastrointestinal	Levodopa
disorders	ACE inhibitors
Malabsorption	Other drugs
Obstruction	Disorders of the mouth
Pernicious anemia	and teeth
Cardiac disorders	Age-related factors
Chronic ischemia	Physiologic changes
Chronic congestive	Decreased taste and
heart failure	smell
Respiratory disorders	Functional disabilities
Emphysema	Neurologic
Chronic obstructive	Stroke
pulmonary	Parkinson's disease
disease	Neuromuscular
Renal insufficiency	disorders
Rheumatologic disease	Dementia
Infections	Social
HIV	Isolation
Tuberculosis	Economic hardship
Parasitic infection	Psychiatric and
Subacute bacterial	behavioral
endocarditis	Depression
	Anxiety
	Bereavement
	Alcoholism
	Eating disorders
	Increased activity
	or exercise
	Idiopathic

most common malignancies in patients presenting with weight loss. In younger individuals, diabetes mellitus, hyperthyroidism, psychiatric disturbances including eating disorders, and infection, especially with HIV, should be considered.

The cause of involuntary weight loss is rarely occult. Careful history and physical examination, in association with directed diagnostic testing, will identify the cause of weight loss in 75% of patients. The etiology of weight loss may not be found in the remaining patients, despite extensive testing. Patients with negative evaluations tend to have lower mortality rates than those found to have organic disease.

Patients with medical causes of weight loss usually have signs or symptoms that suggest involvement of a particular organ system. Gastrointestinal tumors, including those of the pancreas and liver, may affect food intake early in the course of illness, causing weight loss before other symptoms are apparent. Lung cancer may present with post-obstructive pneumonia, dyspnea, or cough and hemoptysis; however, it may be silent and should be considered even in those without a history of cigarette smoking. Depression and isolation can cause profound weight loss, especially in the elderly. Chronic pulmonary disease and congestive heart failure can produce anorexia, and they also increase resting energy expenditure. Weight loss may be the presenting sign of infectious diseases such as HIV infection, tuberculosis, endocarditis, and fungal or parasitic infections. Hyperthyroidism or pheochromocytoma increases metabolism. Elderly patients with apathetic hyperthyroidism may present with weight loss and weakness, with few other manifestations of thyrotoxicosis. New-onset diabetes mellitus is often accompanied by weight loss, reflecting glucosuria and loss of the anabolic actions of insulin. Adrenal insufficiency may be suggested by increased pigmentation, hyponatremia, and hyperkalemia.

The review of systems should focus on signs or symptoms that are associated with disorders that commonly cause weight loss. These include fever, pain, shortness of breath or cough, palpitations, and evidence of neurologic disease. Gastrointestinal disturbances, including difficulty eating, dysphagia, anorexia, nausea, and change in bowel habits, should be sought. Travel history, use of cigarettes and alcohol, and all medications should be reviewed, and patients should be questioned about previous illness or surgery as well as diseases in family members. Risk factors for HIV infection should be assessed. Signs of depression, evidence of dementia, and social factors, including financial issues that might affect food intake, should be considered.

Physical examination should begin with weight determination and documentation of vital signs. The skin should be examined for pallor, jaundice, turgor, scars from prior surgery, and stigmata of systemic disease. The search for oral thrush or dental disease, thyroid gland enlargement, adenopathy, and respiratory or cardiac abnormalities and a detailed examination of the abdomen often lead to clues for further evaluation. Rectal examination, including prostate examination, should be performed in men; and all women should have a pelvic examination, even if they have had a hysterectomy. Neurologic examination should include mental status assessment and screening for depression.

Laboratory testing should confirm or exclude possible diagnoses elicited from the history and physical examination (Table 7-2). An initial phase of testing should include a complete blood count with differential, serum chemistry tests including glucose, electrolytes, renal and liver tests, calcium, thyroid-stimulating hormone (TSH), urinalysis, and chest x-ray. Patients at risk for HIV infection should have HIV antibody testing. In all cases, recommended cancer screening tests appropriate for the

Approach to the Patient:
WEIGHT LOSS

Before extensive evaluation is undertaken, it is important to confirm weight loss and to determine the time interval over which it has occurred. Almost half of patients who claim significant weight loss have no actual change when body weight is measured objectively. In the absence of documentation, changes in belt notch position or the fit of clothing may be confirmatory. Not infrequently, patients who have actually sustained significant weight loss are unaware that it has occurred. Routine documentation of weight during office visits is therefore important.

TABLE 7-2

SCREENING TESTS FOR EVALUATION OF INVOLUNTARY WEIGHT LOSS	
Initial testing	Additional testing
CBC	HIV test
Electrolytes, calcium, glucose	Upper and/or lower gastrointestinal
Renal and liver function tests	endoscopy
Urinalysis	Abdominal CT scan or MRI
TSH	Chest CT sca
Chest x-ray	
Recommended cancer screening	

gender and age group, such as mammograms and colonoscopies, should be updated. If gastrointestinal signs or symptoms are present, upper and/or lower endoscopy and abdominal imaging with either CT or MRI have a relatively high yield, consistent with the high prevalence of gastrointestinal disorders in patients with weight loss. If an etiology of weight loss is not found, careful clinical follow-up, rather than persistent undirected testing, is reasonable.

FURTHER READINGS

ALIBHAI S: An approach to the management of unintentional weight loss in elderly people. CMAJ 172:773, 2005

BOURAS EP, LANGE SM: Rational approach to patients with unintentional weight loss. Mayo Clinic Proc 76:923, 2001

HARRINGTON M et al: A review and meta-analysis of the effect of weight loss on all-cause mortality risk. Nutr Res Rev 22:93, 2009

HERNANDEZ JL, MATORRAS JA: Involuntary weight loss without specific symptoms: A clinical prediction score for malignant neoplasm. Q J Med 96: 649, 2003

INUI A: Cancer anorexia-cachexia syndrome: Current issues in research and management. Cancer J Clinicians 52:72, 2002

NORA E, RAMAN A: Hypermetabolism, cachexia and wasting. Curr Opin Endocrinol Diabetes 12:326, 2005

SCHWARTZ MW: Brain pathways controlling food intake and body weight. Exp Biol Med 226:978, 2001

STRASSER F, BRUERA ED: Update on anorexia and cachexia. Hematol Oncol Clin North Am 16:589, 2002

TISDALE MJ: Mechanisms of cancer cachexia. Physiol Rev 89:381, 2009

WALLACE JI: Involuntary weight loss in elderly outpatients: Recognition, etiologies, and treatment. Clin Geriatr Med 13:717, 1997

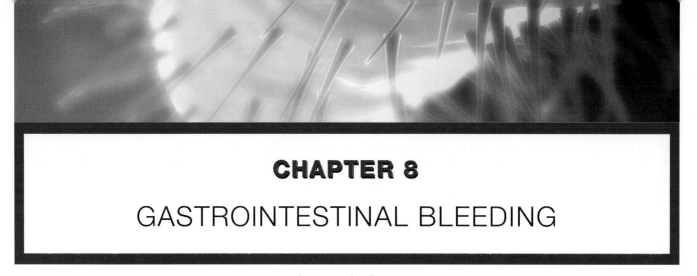

CHAPTER 8

GASTROINTESTINAL BLEEDING

Loren Laine

Bleeding from the gastrointestinal (GI) tract may present in five ways. *Hematemesis* is vomitus of red blood or "coffee-grounds" material. *Melena* is black, tarry, foul-smelling stool. *Hematochezia* is the passage of bright red or maroon blood from the rectum. *Occult GI bleeding* (GIB) may be identified in the absence of overt bleeding by a fecal occult blood test or the presence of iron deficiency. Finally, patients may present only with *symptoms of blood loss or anemia* such as lightheadedness, syncope, angina, or dyspnea.

SOURCES OF GASTROINTESTINAL BLEEDING

Upper Gastrointestinal Sources of Bleeding

(Table 8-1) The annual incidence of hospital admissions for upper GIB (UGIB) in the United States and Europe is ~0.1%, with a mortality rate of ~5–10%. Patients rarely die from exsanguination; rather, they die due to decompensation from other underlying illnesses. The mortality rate for patients <60 years in the absence of major concurrent illness is <1%. Independent predictors of rebleeding and death in patients hospitalized with UGIB include increasing age, comorbidities, and hemodynamic compromise (tachycardia or hypotension).

Peptic ulcers are the most common cause of UGIB, accounting for up to ~50% of cases; an increasing proportion is due to nonsteroidal anti-inflammatory drugs (NSAIDs), with the prevalence of *Helicobacter pylori* decreasing. Mallory-Weiss tears account for ~5–10 or 15% of cases. The proportion of patients bleeding from varices varies widely from ~5 to 30%, depending on the population. Hemorrhagic or erosive gastropathy (e.g., due to NSAIDs or alcohol) and erosive esophagitis often cause mild UGIB, but major bleeding is rare.

Peptic Ulcers

In addition to clinical features, characteristics of an ulcer at endoscopy provide important prognostic information. One-third of patients with active bleeding or a non-bleeding visible vessel have further bleeding that requires urgent surgery if they are treated conservatively. These patients clearly benefit from endoscopic therapy with bipolar electrocoagulation, heater probe, injection therapy (e.g., absolute alcohol, 1:10,000 epinephrine), and/or clips with reductions in bleeding, hospital stay, mortality rate, and costs. In contrast, patients with clean-based ulcers have rates of recurrent bleeding approaching zero. If there is no other reason for hospitalization, such

TABLE 8-1

SOURCES OF BLEEDING IN PATIENTS HOSPITALIZED FOR UPPER GI BLEEDING IN YEARS 2000–2002	
SOURCES OF BLEEDING	**PROPORTION OF PATIENTS, %**
Ulcers	31–59
Varices	7–20
Mallory-Weiss tears	4–8
Gastroduodenal erosions	2–7
Erosive esophagitis	1–13
Neoplasm	2–7
Vascular ectasias	0–6
No source identified	8–14

Source: Data from M Van Leerdam et al: Am J Gastroenterol 98:1494, 2003; DM Jensen et al: Gastrointest Endosc 57:AB147, 2003; KC Thomopoulos et al: Eur J Gastroenterol Hepatol 16:177, 2004; F Di Fiore et al: Eur J Gastroenterol Hepatol 17:641, 2005.

patients may be discharged on the first hospital day, following stabilization. Patients without clean-based ulcers should usually remain in the hospital for 3 days, as most episodes of recurrent bleeding occur within 3 days.

Randomized controlled trials document that a high-dose constant-infusion IV proton pump inhibitor (PPI) (e.g., omeprazole 80-mg bolus and 8-mg/h infusion), designed to sustain intragastric pH >6 and enhance clot stability, decreases further bleeding (but not mortality), in patients with high-risk ulcers (active bleeding, nonbleeding visible vessel, adherent clot), even after appropriate endoscopic therapy. Institution of therapy at presentation in all patients with UGIB does not significantly improve outcomes such as further bleeding, transfusions, or mortality as compared to initiating therapy only when high-risk ulcers are identified at the time of endoscopy.

One-third of patients with a bleeding ulcer will rebleed within the next 1–2 years. Prevention of recurrent bleeding focuses on the three main factors in ulcer pathogenesis, *H. pylori*, NSAIDs, and acid. Eradication of *H. pylori* in patients with bleeding ulcers decreases rates of rebleeding to <5%. If a bleeding ulcer develops in a patient taking NSAIDs, the NSAIDs should be discontinued, if possible. If NSAIDs must be continued, initial treatment should be with a PPI. Long-term preventive strategies to decrease NSAID-associated ulcers include use of a cyclooxygenase 2 (COX-2) selective inhibitor (coxib) or addition of GI co-therapy to a traditional NSAID. PPIs and misoprostol are effective co-therapies, but PPIs are more commonly used due to less frequent dosing (once daily) and fewer side effects (e.g., diarrhea). However, either PPI co-therapy alone or use of a coxib alone is associated with an annual rebleeding rate of ~10% in high-risk patients (i.e., a recent bleeding ulcer). Combination of a coxib and PPI provides a further significant decrease in ulcers and recurrent bleeding and should be employed in very high-risk patients. Patients with bleeding ulcers unrelated to *H. pylori* or NSAIDs should remain on full-dose antisecretory therapy indefinitely. Peptic ulcers are discussed in Chap. 14.

Mallory-Weiss Tears

The classic history is vomiting, retching, or coughing preceding hematemesis, especially in an alcoholic patient. Bleeding from these tears, which are usually on the gastric side of the gastroesophageal junction, stops spontaneously in 80–90% of patients and recurs in only 0–7%. Endoscopic therapy is indicated for actively bleeding Mallory-Weiss tears. Angiographic therapy with embolization and operative therapy with oversewing of the tear are rarely required. Mallory-Weiss tears are discussed in Chap. 13.

Esophageal Varices

Patients with variceal hemorrhage have poorer outcomes than patients with other sources of UGIB. Endoscopic therapy for acute bleeding and repeated sessions of endoscopic therapy to eradicate esophageal varices significantly reduce rebleeding and mortality. Ligation is the endoscopic therapy of choice for esophageal varices because it has less rebleeding, a lower mortality rate, fewer local complications, and requires fewer treatment sessions to achieve variceal eradication than sclerotherapy.

Octreotide (50-μg bolus and 50-μg/h IV infusion for 2–5 days) further helps in the control of acute bleeding when used in combination with endoscopic therapy. Other vasoactive agents such as somatostatin and terlipressin, available outside the United States, are also effective. Antibiotic therapy (e.g., quinolones) is also recommended for patients with cirrhosis presenting with UGIB, as antibiotics decrease bacterial infections and mortality in this population. Over the long term, treatment with nonselective beta blockers decreases recurrent bleeding from esophageal varices. Chronic therapy with beta blockers plus endoscopic ligation is recommended for prevention of recurrent esophageal variceal bleeding.

In patients who have persistent or recurrent bleeding despite endoscopic and medical therapy, more invasive therapy is warranted. Transjugular intrahepatic portosystemic shunt (TIPS) decreases rebleeding more effectively than endoscopic therapy, although hepatic encephalopathy is more common and the mortality rates are comparable. Most patients with TIPS have shunt stenosis within 1–2 years and require reintervention to maintain shunt patency, although the use of coated stents appears to markedly decrease shunt dysfunction, at least in the first year. A randomized comparison of TIPS and distal splenorenal shunt in Child-Pugh class A or B cirrhotic patients with refractory variceal bleeding revealed no significant difference in rebleeding, encephalopathy, or survival, but a much higher rate of reintervention with TIPS (82% vs 11%). Therefore, TIPS is most appropriate in patients with more severe liver disease and those in whom transplant is anticipated. Patients with milder, well-compensated cirrhosis should require fewer re-interventions with decompressive surgery, although the higher initial risks of surgery must also be considered.

Portal hypertension is also responsible for bleeding from gastric varices, varices in the small and large intestine, and portal hypertensive gastropathy and enterocolopathy.

Hemorrhagic and Erosive Gastropathy ("Gastritis")

Hemorrhagic and erosive gastropathy, often labeled gastritis, refers to endoscopically visualized subepithelial hemorrhages and erosions. These are mucosal lesions and thus do not cause major bleeding. They develop in various clinical settings, the most important of which are NSAID use, alcohol intake, and stress. Half of patients who chronically ingest NSAIDs have erosions (15–30% have ulcers), while up to 20% of actively drinking alcoholic patients with symptoms of UGIB have evidence of subepithelial hemorrhages or erosions.

Stress-related gastric mucosal injury occurs only in extremely sick patients: those who have experienced serious trauma, major surgery, burns covering more than one-third of the body surface area, major intracranial disease, or severe medical illness (i.e., ventilator dependence, coagulopathy). Significant bleeding probably does not develop unless ulceration occurs. The mortality rate in these patients is quite high because of their serious underlying illnesses.

The incidence of bleeding from stress-related gastric mucosal injury or ulceration has decreased dramatically in recent years, most likely due to better care of critically ill patients. Pharmacologic prophylaxis for bleeding may be considered in the high-risk patients mentioned above. Multiple trials document the efficacy of intravenous H_2-receptor antagonist therapy, which is more effective than sucralfate but not superior to a PPI immediate-release suspension given via nasogastric tube. Prophylactic therapy decreases bleeding but does not lower the mortality rate.

Other Causes

Other, less frequent causes of UGIB include erosive duodenitis, neoplasms, aortoenteric fistulas, vascular lesions [including hereditary hemorrhagic telangiectasias (Osler-Weber-Rendu) and gastric antral vascular ectasia ("watermelon stomach")], Dieulafoy's lesion (in which an aberrant vessel in the mucosa bleeds from a pinpoint mucosal defect), prolapse gastropathy (prolapse of proximal stomach into esophagus with retching, especially in alcoholics), and hemobilia and hemosuccus pancreaticus (bleeding from the bile duct or pancreatic duct).

Small-Intestinal Sources of Bleeding

Small-intestinal sources of bleeding (bleeding from sites beyond the reach of the standard upper endoscope) are difficult to diagnose and are responsible for the majority of cases of obscure GIB. Fortunately, small-intestinal bleeding is uncommon. The most common causes are vascular ectasias and tumors (e.g., adenocarcinoma, leiomyoma, lymphoma, benign polyps, carcinoid, metastases, and lipoma). Other less common causes include Crohn's disease, infection, ischemia, vasculitis, small-bowel varices, diverticula, Meckel's diverticulum, duplication cysts, and intussusception. NSAIDs induce small-intestinal erosions and ulcers and may be a relatively common cause of chronic, obscure GIB; coxibs induce less small-intestinal injury than traditional NSAIDs.

Meckel's diverticulum is the most common cause of significant lower GIB (LGIB) in children, decreasing in frequency as a cause of bleeding with age. In adults <40–50 years, small-bowel tumors often account for obscure GIB; in patients >50–60 years, vascular ectasias are usually responsible.

Vascular ectasias should be treated with endoscopic therapy if possible. Surgical therapy can be used for vascular ectasias isolated to a segment of the small intestine when endoscopic therapy is unsuccessful. Although estrogen/progesterone compounds have been used for vascular ectasias, a double-blind trial found no benefit in prevention of recurrent bleeding. Isolated lesions, such as tumors, diverticula, or duplications, are generally treated with surgical resection.

Colonic Sources of Bleeding

The incidence of hospitalizations for LGIB is about one-fifth that for UGIB. Hemorrhoids are probably the most common cause of LGIB; anal fissures also cause minor bleeding and pain. If these local anal processes, which rarely require hospitalization, are excluded, the most common causes of LGIB in adults are diverticula, vascular ectasias (especially in the proximal colon of patients >70 years), neoplasms (primarily adenocarcinoma), and colitis—most commonly infectious or idiopathic inflammatory bowel disease, but occasionally ischemic or radiation-induced. Uncommon causes include post-polypectomy bleeding, solitary rectal ulcer syndrome, NSAID-induced ulcers or colitis, trauma, varices (most commonly rectal), lymphoid nodular hyperplasia, vasculitis, and aortocolic fistulas. In children and adolescents, the most common colonic causes of significant GIB are inflammatory bowel disease and juvenile polyps.

Diverticular bleeding is abrupt in onset, usually painless, sometimes massive, and often from the right colon; minor and occult bleeding is not characteristic. Clinical reports suggest that bleeding colonic diverticula stop bleeding spontaneously in ~80% of patients and rebleed in about 20–25% of patients. Intraarterial vasopressin or embolization by superselective technique should stop bleeding in a majority of patients. If bleeding persists or recurs, segmental surgical resection is indicated.

Bleeding from right colonic vascular ectasias in the elderly may be overt or occult; it tends to be chronic and only occasionally is hemodynamically significant. Endoscopic hemostatic therapy may be useful in the treatment of vascular ectasias, as well as discrete bleeding ulcers and post-polypectomy bleeding, while endoscopic polypectomy, if possible, is used for bleeding colonic polyps. Surgical therapy is generally required for major, persistent, or recurrent bleeding from the wide variety of colonic sources of GIB that cannot be treated medically, angiographically, or endoscopically.

Approach to the Patient:
GASTROINTESTINAL BLEEDING

Measurement of the heart rate and blood pressure is the best way to assess a patient with GIB. Clinically significant bleeding leads to postural changes in heart rate or blood pressure, tachycardia, and, finally, recumbent hypotension. In contrast, the hemoglobin does not fall immediately with acute GIB, due to proportionate reductions in plasma and red cell volumes (i.e., "people bleed whole blood"). Thus, hemoglobin may be normal or only minimally decreased at the initial presentation of a severe bleeding episode. As extravascular fluid enters the vascular space to restore volume, the hemoglobin falls, but this process may take up to 72 h. Patients with slow, chronic GIB may have very low hemoglobin values despite normal blood pressure and heart rate. With the development of iron-deficiency anemia, the mean corpuscular volume will be low and red blood cell distribution width will be increased.

DIFFERENTIATION OF UPPER FROM LOWER GIB

Hematemesis an upper GI source of bleeding (above the ligament of Treitz). Melena indicates that blood has been present in the GI tract for at least 14 h. Thus, the more proximal the bleeding site, the more likely melena will occur. Hematochezia usually represents a lower GI source of bleeding, although an upper GI lesion may bleed so briskly that blood does not remain in the bowel long enough for melena to develop. When hematochezia is the presenting symptom of UGIB, it is associated with hemodynamic instability and dropping hemoglobin. Bleeding lesions of the small bowel may present as melena or hematochezia. Other clues to UGIB include hyperactive bowel sounds and an elevated blood urea nitrogen level (due to volume depletion and blood proteins absorbed in the small intestine).

A nonbloody nasogastric aspirate may be seen in up to 18% of patients with UGIB—usually from a duodenal source. Even a bile-stained appearance does not exclude a bleeding postpyloric lesion since reports of bile in the aspirate are incorrect in ~50% of cases. Testing of aspirates that are not grossly bloody for occult blood is not useful.

DIAGNOSTIC EVALUATION OF THE PATIENT WITH GIB

Upper GIB (Fig. 8-1) History and physical examination are not usually diagnostic of the source of GIB. Upper endoscopy is the test of choice in patients with UGIB and should be performed urgently in patients with hemodynamic instability (hypotension, tachycardia, or postural changes in heart rate or blood pressure). Early endoscopy is also beneficial in cases of milder bleeding for management decisions. Patients with major bleeding and high-risk endoscopic findings (e.g., varices, ulcers with active bleeding or a visible vessel) benefit from endoscopic hemostatic therapy, while patients with low-risk lesions (e.g., clean-based ulcers, nonbleeding Mallory-Weiss tears, erosive or hemorrhagic gastropathy) who have stable vital signs and hemoglobin, and no other medical problems, can be discharged home.

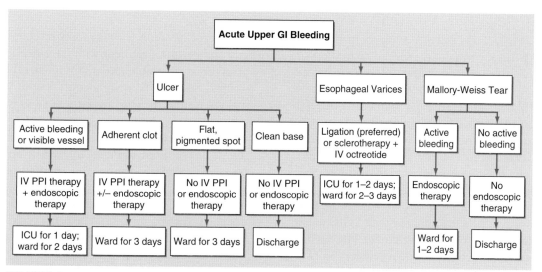

FIGURE 8-1

Suggested algorithm for patients with acute upper gastrointestinal bleeding. Recommendations on level of care and time of discharge assume patient is stabilized without further bleeding or other concomitant medical problems. PPI, proton pump inhibitor; ICU, intensive care unit.

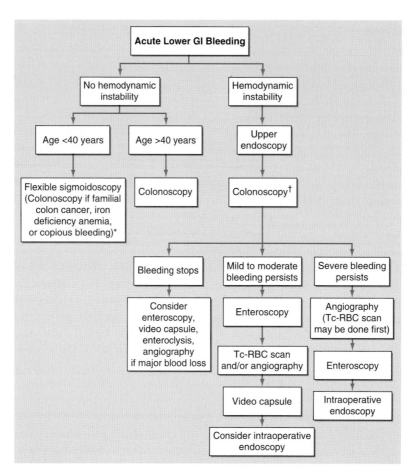

FIGURE 8-2

Suggested algorithm for patients with acute lower gastrointestinal bleeding. Sequential recommendations under "Hemodynamic instability" assume a test is found to be nondiagnostic before next test is performed. *Some suggest colonoscopy for any degree of rectal bleeding in patients <40 years as well. †If massive bleeding does not allow time for colonic lavage, proceed to angiography. Tc-RBC, ^{99m}technetium-labeled red blood cell.

Lower GIB (Fig. 8-2) Patients with hematochezia and hemodynamic instability should have upper endoscopy to rule out an upper GI source before evaluation of the lower GI tract. Patients with presumed LGIB may undergo early sigmoidoscopy for the detection of obvious, low-lying lesions. However, the procedure is difficult with brisk bleeding, and it is usually not possible to identify the area of bleeding. Sigmoidoscopy is useful primarily in patients <40 years with minor bleeding.

Colonoscopy after an oral lavage solution is the procedure of choice in patients admitted with LGIB unless bleeding is too massive or unless sigmoidoscopy has disclosed an obvious actively bleeding lesion. ^{99m}Tc-labeled red cell scan allows repeated imaging for up to 24 h and may identify the general location of bleeding. However, radionuclide scans should be interpreted with caution because results, especially from later images, are highly variable. In active LGIB, angiography can detect the site of bleeding (extravasation of contrast into the gut) and permits treatment with intraarterial infusion of vasopressin or embolization. Even after bleeding has stopped, angiography may identify lesions with abnormal vasculature, such as vascular ectasias or tumors.

GIB of Obscure Origin Obscure GIB is defined as persistent or recurrent bleeding for which no source has been identified by routine endoscopic and contrast x-ray studies; it may be overt (e.g., melena, hematochezia) or occult. Push enteroscopy, with a specially designed enteroscope or a pediatric colonoscope to inspect the entire duodenum and part of the jejunum, is generally the next step. Push enteroscopy may identify probable bleeding sites in 20–40% of patients with obscure GIB. Video capsule endoscopy, which allows endoscopic examination of the entire small intestine, increases diagnostic yield in obscure GIB: a systematic review of 14 trials comparing push enteroscopy to capsule revealed "clinically significant findings" in 26% and 56% of patients, respectively. However, lack of control of the capsule prevents its manipulation and full visualization of the intestine; in addition, tissue cannot be sampled and therapy cannot be applied. A new endoscopic technique, double-balloon enteroscopy, allows the endoscopist to potentially examine and provide therapy to much or all of the small intestine. If enteroscopy and video capsule endoscopy are negative or unavailable, a specialized radiographic examination of the small bowel (e.g., enteroclysis) should be performed. Newer imaging techniques being investigated include CT and MR enterography.

Patients with continued obscure GIB who require transfusions or repeated hospitalizations warrant further investigations. ^{99m}Tc-labeled red blood cell scintigraphy should be employed. Angiography is useful even if bleeding has subsided, since it may disclose vascular anomalies or tumor vessels. ^{99m}Tc-pertechnetate scintigraphy for diagnosis of Meckel's diverticulum should be done, especially in the evaluation of young patients. When all tests are unrevealing, intraoperative endoscopy is indicated in patients with severe recurrent or persistent bleeding requiring repeated transfusions.

Occult GIB Occult GIB is manifested by a positive test for fecal occult blood or iron-deficiency anemia. Evaluation of a positive test for fecal occult blood generally should begin with colonoscopy, particularly in patients >40 years. If evaluation of the colon is negative, many perform upper endoscopy only if iron-deficiency anemia or upper GI symptoms are present, while others recommend upper endoscopy in all patients since up to 25–40% of these patients may have some abnormality noted on upper endoscopy. If standard endoscopic tests are unrevealing, enteroscopy, video capsule endoscopy, and/or enteroclysis may be considered in patients with iron-deficiency anemia.

FURTHER READINGS

CHAN FK et al: Proton pump inhibitor plus a COX-2 inhibitor for the prevention of recurrent ulcer bleeding in patients with arthritis: A double blinded, randomized trial. Gastroenterology 130:A-105, 2006

CHIU PW, NG EK: Predicting poor outcome from acute upper gastrointestinal hemorrhage. Gastroenterol Clin North Am 38:215, 2009

CIPOLLETTA L et al: Outpatient management for low-risk nonvariceal upper GI bleeding: A randomized controlled trial. Gastrointest Endosc 55:1, 2002

CONRAD SA et al: Randomized, double-blind comparison of immediate-release omeprazole oral suspension versus intravenous cimetidine for the prevention of upper gastrointestinal bleeding in critically ill patients. Crit Care Med 33:760, 2005

D'AMICO G et al: Pharmacological treatment of portal hypertension: An evidence-based approach. Semin Liver Dis 19:475, 1999

ELMUNZER BJ et al: Systematic review of the predictors of recurrent hemorrhage after endoscopic hemostatic therapy for bleeding peptic ulcers. Am J Gastroenterol 103:2625, 2008

HENDERSON JM et al: Distal splenorenal shunt versus transjugular intrahepatic portal systematic shunt for variceal bleeding: A randomized trial. Gastroenterology 130:1643, 2006

LAINE L, COOK D: Endoscopic ligation compared with sclerotherapy for treatment of esophageal variceal bleeding: A meta-analysis. Ann Intern Med 123:280, 1995

LAU JYW et al: Effect of intravenous omeprazole on recurrent bleeding after endoscopic treatment of bleeding peptic ulcers. N Engl J Med 343:310, 2000

LEONTIADIS GI, HOWDEN CW: The role of proton pump inhibitors in the management of upper gastrointestinal bleeding. Gastroenterol Clin North Am 38:199, 2009

MARMO R et al: Dual therapy versus monotherapy in endoscopic treatment of high-risk bleeding ulcers: A meta-analysis of controlled trials. Am J Gastroenterol 102:279, 2007

ROCKALL TA et al: Risk assessment after acute upper gastrointestinal haemorrhage. Gut 38:316, 1996

SASS DA, CHOPRA KB: Portal hypertension and variceal hemorrhage. Med Clin North Am 93:837, 2009

TRIESTER SL et al: A meta-analysis of the yield of capsule endoscopy compared to other diagnostic modalities in patients with obscure gastrointestinal bleeding. Am J Gastroenterol 100:2407, 2005

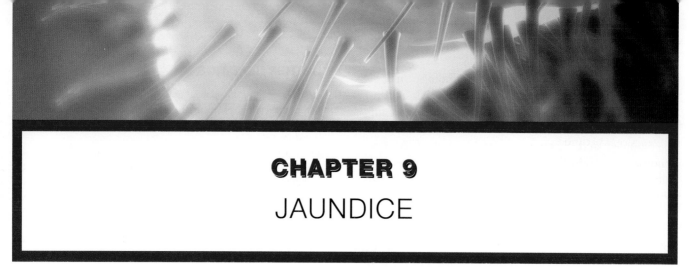

CHAPTER 9
JAUNDICE

Daniel S. Pratt ■ Marshall M. Kaplan

Jaundice, or icterus, is a yellowish discoloration of tissue resulting from the deposition of bilirubin. Tissue deposition of bilirubin occurs only in the presence of serum hyperbilirubinemia and is a sign of either liver disease or, less often, a hemolytic disorder. The degree of serum bilirubin elevation can be estimated by physical examination. Slight increases in serum bilirubin are best detected by examining the sclerae, which have a particular affinity for bilirubin due to their high elastin content. The presence of scleral icterus indicates a serum bilirubin of at least 51 μmol/L (3.0 mg/dL). The ability to detect scleral icterus is made more difficult if the examining room has fluorescent lighting. If the examiner suspects scleral icterus, a second place to examine is underneath the tongue. As serum bilirubin levels rise, the skin will eventually become yellow in light-skinned patients and even green if the process is long-standing; the green color is produced by oxidation of bilirubin to biliverdin.

The differential diagnosis for yellowing of the skin is limited. In addition to jaundice, it includes carotenoderma, the use of the drug quinacrine, and excessive exposure to phenols. Carotenoderma is the yellow color imparted to the skin by the presence of carotene; it occurs in healthy individuals who ingest excessive amounts of vegetables and fruits that contain carotene, such as carrots, leafy vegetables, squash, peaches, and oranges. Unlike jaundice, where the yellow coloration of the skin is uniformly distributed over the body, in carotenoderma the pigment is concentrated on the palms, soles, forehead, and nasolabial folds. Carotenoderma can be distinguished from jaundice by the sparing of the sclerae. Quinacrine causes a yellow discoloration of the skin in 4–37% of patients treated with it. Unlike carotene, quinacrine can cause discoloration of the sclerae.

Another sensitive indicator of increased serum bilirubin is darkening of the urine, which is due to the renal excretion of conjugated bilirubin. Patients often describe their urine as tea or cola colored. Bilirubinuria indicates an elevation of the direct serum bilirubin fraction and therefore the presence of liver disease.

Increased serum bilirubin levels occur when an imbalance exists between bilirubin production and clearance. A logical evaluation of the patient who is jaundiced requires an understanding of bilirubin production and metabolism.

PRODUCTION AND METABOLISM OF BILIRUBIN

(See also Chap. 36) Bilirubin, a tetrapyrrole pigment, is a breakdown product of heme (ferroprotoporphyrin IX). About 70–80% of the 250–300 mg of bilirubin produced each day is derived from the breakdown of hemoglobin in senescent red blood cells. The remainder comes from prematurely destroyed erythroid cells in bone marrow and from the turnover of hemoproteins such as myoglobin and cytochromes found in tissues throughout the body.

The formation of bilirubin occurs in reticuloendothelial cells, primarily in the spleen and liver. The first reaction, catalyzed by the microsomal enzyme heme oxygenase, oxidatively cleaves the α bridge of the porphyrin group and opens the heme ring. The end products of this reaction are biliverdin, carbon monoxide, and iron. The second reaction, catalyzed by the cytosolic enzyme biliverdin reductase, reduces the central methylene bridge of biliverdin and converts it to bilirubin. Bilirubin formed in the reticuloendothelial cells is virtually insoluble in water. This is due to tight internal hydrogen bonding between the water-soluble moieties of bilirubin, propionic acid carboxyl groups of one dipyrrolic half of the molecule with the imino and lactam groups of the opposite half. This configuration blocks solvent access to the polar residues of bilirubin and places the hydrophobic residues on the outside. To be transported in blood, bilirubin must be solubilized. This is accomplished by its reversible, noncovalent binding to albumin. Unconjugated bilirubin bound to albumin is transported to the liver, where it, but not the albumin, is taken up by hepatocytes via a process that at least partly involves carrier-mediated membrane transport. No specific bilirubin transporter has yet been identified (Chap. 36, Fig. 36-1).

After entering the hepatocyte, unconjugated bilirubin is bound to the cytosolic protein ligandin, or glutathione S-transferase B. Whereas ligandin was initially thought to be a transport protein, responsible for delivering unconjugated bilirubin from the plasma membrane to the endoplasmic reticulum, it now appears that its role may in fact be to reduce bilirubin efflux back into the plasma. Studies suggest that unconjugated bilirubin may well rapidly diffuse unaided through the aqueous cytosol between membranes. In the endoplasmic reticulum, bilirubin is solubilized by conjugation to glucuronic acid, a process that disrupts the internal hydrogen bonds and yields bilirubin monoglucuronide and diglucuronide. The conjugation of glucuronic acid to bilirubin is catalyzed by bilirubin uridine diphosphate-glucuronosyl transferase (UDPGT). The now hydrophilic bilirubin conjugates diffuse from the endoplasmic reticulum to the canalicular membrane, where bilirubin monoglucuronide and diglucuronide are actively transported into canalicular bile by an energy-dependent mechanism involving the multiple drug resistance protein 2.

The conjugated bilirubin excreted into bile drains into the duodenum and passes unchanged through the proximal small bowel. Conjugated bilirubin is not taken up by the intestinal mucosa. When the conjugated bilirubin reaches the distal ileum and colon, it is hydrolyzed to unconjugated bilirubin by bacterial β-glucuronidases. The unconjugated bilirubin is reduced by normal gut bacteria to form a group of colorless tetrapyrroles called urobilinogens. About 80–90% of these products are excreted in feces, either unchanged or oxidized to orange derivatives called urobilins. The remaining 10–20% of the urobilinogens are passively absorbed, enter the portal venous blood, and are reexcreted by the liver. A small fraction (usually <3 mg/dL) escapes hepatic uptake, filters across the renal glomerulus, and is excreted in urine.

MEASUREMENT OF SERUM BILIRUBIN

The terms direct- and indirect-reacting bilirubin are based on the original van den Bergh reaction. This assay, or a variation of it, is still used in most clinical chemistry laboratories to determine the serum bilirubin level. In this assay, bilirubin is exposed to diazotized sulfanilic acid, splitting into two relatively stable dipyrrylmethene azopigments that absorb maximally at 540 nm, allowing for photometric analysis. The direct fraction is that which reacts with diazotized sulfanilic acid in the absence of an accelerator substance such as alcohol. The direct fraction provides an approximate determination of the conjugated bilirubin in serum. The total serum bilirubin is the amount that reacts after the addition of alcohol. The indirect fraction is the difference between the total and the direct bilirubin and provides an estimate of the unconjugated bilirubin in serum.

With the van den Bergh method, the normal serum bilirubin concentration usually is 17 μmol/L (<1 mg/dL). Up to 30%, or 5.1 μmol/L (0.3 mg/dL), of the total may be direct-reacting (conjugated) bilirubin. Total serum bilirubin concentrations are between 3.4 and 15.4 μmol/L (0.2 and 0.9 mg/dL) in 95% of a normal population.

Several new techniques, although less convenient to perform, have added considerably to our understanding of bilirubin metabolism. First, they demonstrate that in normal persons or those with Gilbert's syndrome, almost 100% of the serum bilirubin is unconjugated; <3% is monoconjugated bilirubin. Second, in jaundiced patients with hepatobiliary disease, the total serum bilirubin concentration measured by these new, more accurate methods is lower than the values found with diazo methods. This suggests that there are diazo-positive compounds distinct from bilirubin in the serum of patients with hepatobiliary disease. Third, these studies indicate that in jaundiced patients with hepatobiliary disease, monoglucuronides of bilirubin predominate over the diglucuronides. Fourth, part of the direct-reacting bilirubin fraction includes conjugated bilirubin that is covalently linked to albumin. This albumin-linked bilirubin fraction (*delta fraction,* or *biliprotein*) represents an important fraction of total serum bilirubin in patients with cholestasis and hepatobiliary disorders. Albumin-bound conjugated bilirubin is formed in serum when hepatic excretion of bilirubin glucuronides is impaired and the glucuronides are present in serum in increasing amounts. By virtue of its tight binding to albumin, the clearance rate of albumin-bound bilirubin from serum approximates the half-life of albumin, 12–14 days, rather than the short half-life of bilirubin, about 4 h.

The prolonged half-life of albumin-bound conjugated bilirubin explains two previously unexplained enigmas in jaundiced patients with liver disease: (1) that some patients with conjugated hyperbilirubinemia do not exhibit bilirubinuria during the recovery phase of their disease because the bilirubin is covalently bound to albumin and therefore not filtered by the renal glomeruli, and (2) that the elevated serum bilirubin level declines more slowly than expected in some patients who otherwise appear to be recovering satisfactorily. Late in the recovery phase of hepatobiliary disorders, all the conjugated bilirubin may be in the albumin-linked form. Its value in serum falls slowly because of the long half-life of albumin.

MEASUREMENT OF URINE BILIRUBIN

Unconjugated bilirubin is always bound to albumin in the serum, is not filtered by the kidney, and is not found in the urine. Conjugated bilirubin is filtered at the glomerulus and the majority is reabsorbed by the proximal tubules; a small fraction is excreted in the urine. Any bilirubin found in the urine is conjugated bilirubin. The presence of bilirubinuria implies the presence of liver disease. A urine dipstick test (Ictotest) gives the same information as fractionation of the serum bilirubin. This test is very accurate. A false-negative test is possible in patients with prolonged cholestasis due to the predominance of conjugated bilirubin covalently bound to albumin.

Approach to the Patient:
BILIRUBIN

The bilirubin present in serum represents a balance between input from production of bilirubin and hepatic/biliary removal of the pigment. Hyperbilirubinemia may result from (1) overproduction of bilirubin; (2) impaired uptake, conjugation, or excretion of bilirubin; or (3) regurgitation of unconjugated or conjugated bilirubin from damaged hepatocytes or bile ducts. An increase in unconjugated bilirubin in serum results from either overproduction, impairment of uptake, or conjugation of bilirubin. An increase in conjugated bilirubin is due to decreased excretion into the bile ductules or backward leakage of the pigment. The initial steps in evaluating the patient with jaundice are to determine (1) whether the hyperbilirubinemia is predominantly conjugated or unconjugated in nature, and (2) whether other biochemical liver tests are abnormal. The thoughtful interpretation of limited data will allow for a rational evaluation of the patient (Fig. 9-1). This discussion will focus solely on the evaluation of the adult patient with jaundice.

ISOLATED ELEVATION OF SERUM BILIRUBIN

Unconjugated Hyperbilirubinemia The differential diagnosis of an isolated unconjugated hyperbilirubinemia is limited (Table 9-1). The critical determination is whether the patient is suffering from a hemolytic process resulting in an overproduction of bilirubin (hemolytic disorders and ineffective erythropoiesis) or from impaired hepatic uptake/conjugation of bilirubin (drug effect or genetic disorders).

Hemolytic disorders that cause excessive heme production may be either inherited or acquired. Inherited disorders include spherocytosis, sickle cell anemia, thalassemia, and deficiency of red cell enzymes such as pyruvate kinase and glucose-6-phosphate dehydrogenase. In these conditions, the serum bilirubin rarely exceeds 86 μmol/L (5 mg/dL). Higher levels may occur when there is coexistent renal or hepatocellular dysfunction or in acute hemolysis such as a sickle cell crisis. In evaluating jaundice in patients with chronic hemolysis, it is important to remember the high incidence of pigmented (calcium bilirubinate) gallstones found in these patients, which increases the likelihood of choledocholithiasis as an alternative explanation for hyperbilirubinemia.

Acquired hemolytic disorders include microangiopathic hemolytic anemia (e.g., hemolytic-uremic syndrome), paroxysmal nocturnal hemoglobinuria, spur cell anemia, and immune hemolysis. Ineffective erythropoiesis occurs in cobalamin, folate, and iron deficiencies.

In the absence of hemolysis, the physician should consider a problem with the hepatic uptake or conjugation of bilirubin. Certain drugs, including rifampicin and probenecid, may cause unconjugated hyperbilirubinemia by diminishing hepatic uptake of bilirubin. Impaired bilirubin conjugation occurs in three genetic conditions: Crigler-Najjar syndrome, types I and II, and Gilbert's syndrome. *Crigler-Najjar type I* is an exceptionally rare condition found in neonates and characterized by severe jaundice [bilirubin > 342 μmol/L (>20 mg/dL)] and neurologic impairment due to kernicterus, frequently leading to death in infancy or childhood. These patients have a complete absence of bilirubin UDPGT activity, usually due to mutations in the critical 3′ domain of the *UDPGT* gene, and are totally unable to conjugate, hence cannot excrete bilirubin. The only effective treatment is orthotopic liver transplantation. Use of gene therapy and allogeneic hepatocyte infusion are experimental approaches of future promise for this devastating disease.

Crigler-Najjar type II is somewhat more common than type I. Patients live into adulthood with serum bilirubin levels that range from 103–428 μmol/L (6–25 mg/dL). In these patients, mutations in the

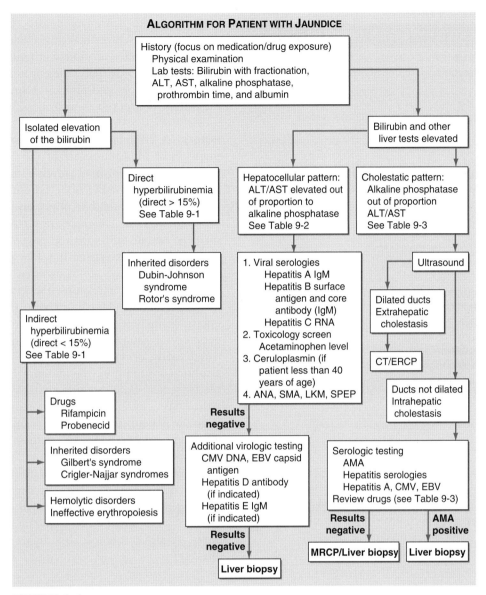

FIGURE 9-1

Evaluation of the patient with jaundice. MRCP, magnetic resonance cholangiopancreatography; ALT, alanine aminotransferase; AST, aspartate aminotransferase; SMA, smooth-muscle antibody; AMA, antimitochondrial antibody; LKM, liver-kidney microsomal antibody; SPEP, serum protein electrophoresis; CMV, cytomegalovirus; EBV, Epstein-Barr virus.

bilirubin *UDPGT* gene cause reduced but not completely absent activity of the enzyme. Bilirubin *UDPGT* activity can be induced by the administration of phenobarbital, which can reduce serum bilirubin levels in these patients. Despite marked jaundice, these patients usually survive into adulthood, although they may be susceptible to kernicterus under the stress of intercurrent illness or surgery.

Gilbert's syndrome is also marked by the impaired conjugation of bilirubin due to reduced bilirubin UDPGT activity. Patients with Gilbert's syndrome have a mild

unconjugated hyperbilirubinemia with serum levels almost always <103 μmol/L (6 mg/dL). The serum levels may fluctuate, and jaundice is often identified only during periods of fasting. One molecular defect that has been identified in patients with Gilbert's syndrome is in the TATAA element in the 5′ promoter region of the bilirubin *UDPGT* gene upstream of exon 1. This defect alone is not necessarily sufficient for producing the clinical syndrome of Gilbert's as there are patients who are homozygous for this defect yet do not have the levels of hyperbilirubinemia typically seen in

CAUSES OF ISOLATED HYPERBILIRUBINEMIA

I. Indirect hyperbilirubinemia
  A. Hemolytic disorders
    1. Inherited
      a. Spherocytosis, elliptocytosis
        Glucose-6-phosphate dehydrogenase
        and pyruvate kinase deficiencies
      b. Sickle cell anemia
    2. Acquired
      a. Microangiopathic hemolytic anemias
      b. Paroxysmal nocturnal hemoglobinuria
      c. Spur cell anemia
      d. Immune hemolysis
  B. Ineffective erythropoiesis
    1. Cobalamin, folate, thalassemia, and
      severe iron deficiencies
  C. Drugs
    1. Rifampicin, probenecid, ribavirin
  D. Inherited conditions
    1. Crigler-Najjar types I and II
    2. Gilbert's syndrome
II. Direct hyperbilirubinemia
  A. Inherited conditions
    1. Dubin-Johnson syndrome
    2. Rotor's syndrome

Gilbert's syndrome. An enhancer polymorphism that lowers transcriptional activity has recently been identified. The decrease in transcription caused by both mutations together may be critical for producing the syndrome. Unlike both Crigler-Najjar syndromes, Gilbert's syndrome is very common. The reported incidence is 3–7% of the population with males predominating over females by a ratio of 2–7:1.

Conjugated Hyperbilirubinemia Elevated conjugated hyperbilirubinemia is found in two rare inherited conditions: *Dubin-Johnson syndrome* and *Rotor's syndrome* (Table 9-1). Patients with both conditions present with asymptomatic jaundice, typically in the second generation of life. The defects in Dubin-Johnson syndrome are mutations in the gene for multiple drug resistance protein 2. These patients have altered excretion of bilirubin into the bile ducts. Rotor's syndrome seems to be a problem with the hepatic storage of bilirubin. Differentiating between these syndromes is possible, but clinically unnecessary, due to their benign nature.

ELEVATION OF SERUM BILIRUBIN WITH OTHER LIVER TEST ABNORMALITIES

The remainder of this chapter will focus on the evaluation of the patient with a conjugated hyperbilirubinemia in the setting of other liver test abnormalities. This group of patients can be divided into those with a primary hepatocellular process and those with intra- or extrahepatic cholestasis. Being able to make this differentiation will guide the physician's evaluation (Fig. 9-1). This differentiation is made on the basis of the history and physical examination as well as the pattern of liver test abnormalities.

History A complete medical history is perhaps the single most important part of the evaluation of the patient with unexplained jaundice. Important considerations include the use of or exposure to any chemical or medication, either physician-prescribed, over-the-counter, complementary or alternative medicines such as herbal and vitamin preparations, or other drugs such as anabolic steroids. The patient should be carefully questioned about possible parenteral exposures, including transfusions, IV and intranasal drug use, tattoos, and sexual activity. Other important questions include recent travel history, exposure to people with jaundice, exposure to possibly contaminated foods, occupational exposure to hepatotoxins, alcohol consumption, the duration of jaundice, and the presence of any accompanying symptoms such as arthralgias, myalgias, rash, anorexia, weight loss, abdominal pain, fever, pruritus, and changes in the urine and stool. While none of these latter symptoms are specific for any one condition, they can suggest a particular diagnosis. A history of arthralgias and myalgias predating jaundice suggests hepatitis, either viral or drug-related. Jaundice associated with the sudden onset of severe right upper quadrant pain and shaking chills suggests choledocholithiasis and ascending cholangitis.

Physical Examination The general assessment should include assessment of the patient's nutritional status. Temporal and proximal muscle wasting suggests long-standing diseases such as pancreatic cancer or cirrhosis. Stigmata of chronic liver disease, including spider nevi, palmar erythema, gynecomastia, caput medusae, Dupuytren's contractures, parotid gland enlargement, and testicular atrophy are commonly seen in advanced alcoholic (Laennec's) cirrhosis and occasionally in other types of cirrhosis. An enlarged left supraclavicular node (Virchow's node) or periumbilical nodule (Sister Mary Joseph's nodule) suggests an abdominal malignancy. Jugular venous distention, a sign of right-sided heart failure, suggests hepatic congestion. Right pleural effusion, in the absence of clinically apparent ascites, may be seen in advanced cirrhosis.

The abdominal examination should focus on the size and consistency of the liver, whether the spleen is palpable and hence enlarged, and whether there is ascites present. Patients with cirrhosis may have an enlarged left lobe of the liver, which is felt below the xiphoid, and an enlarged spleen. A grossly enlarged nodular liver or an obvious abdominal mass suggests malignancy. An enlarged tender liver could be viral or alcoholic hepatitis, an infiltrative process such as amyloid, or, less often, an acutely congested liver secondary to right-sided heart failure. Severe right upper quadrant tenderness with respiratory arrest on inspiration (Murphy's sign) suggests cholecystitis or, occasionally, ascending cholangitis. Ascites in the presence of jaundice suggests either cirrhosis or malignancy with peritoneal spread.

Laboratory Tests When the physician encounters a patient with unexplained jaundice, there is a battery of tests that are helpful in the initial evaluation. These include total and direct serum bilirubin with fractionation, aminotransferases, alkaline phosphatase, albumin, and prothrombin time tests. Enzyme tests [alanine aminotransferase (ALT), aspartate aminotransferase (AST), and alkaline phosphatase] are helpful in differentiating between a hepatocellular process and a cholestatic process (Table 35-1; Fig. 9-1), a critical step in determining what additional workup is indicated. Patients with a hepatocellular process generally have a disproportionate rise in the aminotransferases compared to the alkaline phosphatase. Patients with a cholestatic process have a disproportionate rise in the alkaline phosphatase compared to the aminotransferases. The bilirubin can be prominently elevated in both hepatocellular and cholestatic conditions and therefore is not necessarily helpful in differentiating between the two.

In addition to the enzyme tests, all jaundiced patients should have additional blood tests, specifically an albumin level and a prothrombin time, to assess liver function. A low albumin suggests a chronic process such as cirrhosis or cancer. A normal albumin is suggestive of a more acute process such as viral hepatitis or choledocholithiasis. An elevated prothrombin time indicates either vitamin K deficiency due to prolonged jaundice and malabsorption of vitamin K or significant hepatocellular dysfunction. The failure of the prothrombin time to correct with parenteral administration of vitamin K indicates severe hepatocellular injury.

The results of the bilirubin, enzyme tests, albumin, and prothrombin time tests will usually indicate whether a jaundiced patient has a hepatocellular or a cholestatic disease, as well as some indication of the duration and severity of the disease. The causes and evaluation of hepatocellular and cholestatic diseases are quite different.

Hepatocellular Conditions Hepatocellular diseases that can cause jaundice include viral hepatitis, drug or environmental toxicity, alcohol, and end-stage cirrhosis from

any cause (Table 9-2). Wilson's disease, once believed to occur primarily in young adults, should be considered in all adults if no other cause of jaundice is found. Autoimmune hepatitis is typically seen in young to middle-aged women but may affect men and women of any age. Alcoholic hepatitis can be differentiated from viral and toxin-related hepatitis by the pattern of the aminotransferases. Patients with alcoholic hepatitis typically have an AST:ALT ratio of at least 2:1. The AST rarely exceeds 300 U/L. Patients with acute viral hepatitis and toxin-related injury severe enough to produce jaundice typically have aminotransferases >500 U/L, with the ALT greater than or equal to the AST. The degree of aminotransferase elevation can occasionally help in differentiating between hepatocellular and cholestatic processes. While ALT and AST values less than 8 times normal may be seen in either hepatocellular or cholestatic liver disease, values 25 times normal or higher are seen primarily in acute hepatocellular diseases. Patients with jaundice from cirrhosis can have normal or only slight elevations of the aminotransferases.

When the physician determines that the patient has a hepatocellular disease, appropriate testing for acute viral hepatitis includes a hepatitis A IgM antibody, a hepatitis B surface antigen and core IgM antibody, and a hepatitis C viral RNA test. It can take many weeks for the hepatitis C antibody to become detectable, making it an unreliable test if acute hepatitis C is suspected. Depending on circumstances, studies for hepatitis D, E, Epstein-Barr virus (EBV), and cytomegalovirus (CMV) may be indicated. Ceruloplasmin is the initial screening test for Wilson's disease.

TABLE 9-2

HEPATOCELLULAR CONDITIONS THAT MAY PRODUCE JAUNDICE

Viral hepatitis
  Hepatitis A, B, C, D, and E
  Epstein-Barr virus
  Cytomegalovirus
  Herpes simplex
Alcohol
Drug toxicity
  Predictable, dose-dependent, e.g., acetaminophen
  Unpredictable, idiosyncratic, e.g., isoniazid
Environmental toxins
  Vinyl chloride
  Jamaica bush tea—pyrrolizidine alkaloids
  Kava Kava
  Wild mushrooms—*Amanita phalloides* or *A. verna*
Wilson's disease
Autoimmune hepatitis

Testing for autoimmune hepatitis usually includes an antinuclear antibody and measurement of specific immunoglobulins.

Drug-induced hepatocellular injury can be classified either as predictable or unpredictable. Predictable drug reactions are dose-dependent and affect all patients who ingest a toxic dose of the drug in question. The classic example is acetaminophen hepatotoxicity. Unpredictable or idiosyncratic drug reactions are not dose-dependent and occur in a minority of patients. A great number of drugs can cause idiosyncratic hepatic injury. Environmental toxins are also an important cause of hepatocellular injury. Examples include industrial chemicals such as vinyl chloride, herbal preparations containing pyrrolizidine alkaloids (Jamaica bush tea) and Kava Kava, and the mushrooms *Amanita phalloides* or *A. verna* that contain highly hepatotoxic amatoxins.

Cholestatic Conditions   When the pattern of the liver tests suggests a cholestatic disorder, the next step is to determine whether it is intra- or extrahepatic cholestasis (Fig. 9-1). Distinguishing intrahepatic from extrahepatic cholestasis may be difficult. History, physical examination, and laboratory tests are often not helpful. The next appropriate test is an ultrasound. The ultrasound is inexpensive, does not expose the patient to ionizing radiation, and can detect dilation of the intra- and extrahepatic biliary tree with a high degree of sensitivity and specificity. The absence of biliary dilatation suggests intrahepatic cholestasis, while the presence of biliary dilatation indicates extrahepatic cholestasis. False-negative results occur in patients with partial obstruction of the common bile duct or in patients with cirrhosis or primary sclerosing cholangitis (PSC) where scarring prevents the intrahepatic ducts from dilating.

Although ultrasonography may indicate extrahepatic cholestasis, it rarely identifies the site or cause of obstruction. The distal common bile duct is a particularly difficult area to visualize by ultrasound because of overlying bowel gas. Appropriate next tests include CT, magnetic resonance cholangiography (MRCP), and endoscopic retrograde cholangiopancreatography (ERCP). CT scanning and MRCP are better than ultrasonography for assessing the head of the pancreas and for identifying choledocholithiasis in the distal common bile duct, particularly when the ducts are not dilated. ERCP is the "gold standard" for identifying choledocholithiasis. It is performed by introducing a side-viewing endoscope perorally into the duodenum. The ampulla of Vater is visualized and a catheter is advanced through the ampulla. Injection of dye allows for the visualization of the common bile duct and the pancreatic duct. The success rate for cannulation of the

common bile duct ranges from 80–95%, depending on the operator's experience. Beyond its diagnostic capabilities, ERCP allows for therapeutic interventions, including the removal of common bile duct stones and the placement of stents. In patients in whom ERCP is unsuccessful and there is a high likelihood of the need for a therapeutic intervention, transhepatic cholangiography can provide the same information and allow for intervention. MRCP is a now widely available, noninvasive technique for imaging the bile and pancreatic ducts; it has replaced ERCP as the initial diagnostic test in cases where the need for intervention is felt to be small.

In patients with apparent *intrahepatic cholestasis*, the diagnosis is often made by serologic testing in combination with percutaneous liver biopsy. The list of possible causes of intrahepatic cholestasis is long and varied (Table 9–3). A number of conditions that typically cause a hepatocellular pattern of injury can also present as a cholestatic variant. Both hepatitis B and C can cause a cholestatic hepatitis (fibrosing cholestatic hepatitis). This disease variant has been reported in patients who have undergone solid organ transplantation. Hepatitis A, alcoholic hepatitis, EBV, and CMV may also present as cholestatic liver disease.

Drugs may cause intrahepatic cholestasis, a variant of drug-induced hepatitis. Drug-induced cholestasis is usually reversible after eliminating the offending drug, although it may take many months for cholestasis to resolve. Drugs most commonly associated with cholestasis are the anabolic and contraceptive steroids. Cholestatic hepatitis has been reported with chlorpromazine, imipramine, tolbutamide, sulindac, cimetidine, and erythromycin estolate. It also occurs in patients taking trimethoprim, sulfamethoxazole, and penicillin-based antibiotics such as ampicillin, dicloxacillin, and clavulanic acid. Rarely, cholestasis may be chronic and associated with progressive fibrosis despite early discontinuation of the drug. Chronic cholestasis has been associated with chlorpromazine and prochlorperazine.

Primary biliary cirrhosis is an autoimmune disease predominantly of middle-aged women in which there is a progressive destruction of interlobular bile ducts. The diagnosis is made by the presence of the antimitochondrial antibody that is found in 95% of patients. *Primary sclerosing cholangitis* is characterized by the destruction and fibrosis of larger bile ducts. The disease may involve only the intrahepatic ducts and present as intrahepatic cholestasis. However, in 95% of patients with PSC, both intra- and extrahepatic ducts are involved. The diagnosis of PSC is made by imaging the biliary tree. The pathognomonic findings are multiple strictures of bile ducts with dilatations proximal to the strictures. Approximately 75% of patients with PSC have inflammatory bowel disease.

TABLE 9-3

CHOLESTATIC CONDITIONS THAT MAY PRODUCE JAUNDICE

I. Intrahepatic
   A. Viral hepatitis
      1. Fibrosing cholestatic hepatitis—hepatitis B and C
      2. Hepatitis A, Epstein-Barr virus, cytomegalovirus
   B. Alcoholic hepatitis
   C. Drug toxicity
      1. Pure cholestasis—anabolic and contraceptive steroids
      2. Cholestatic hepatitis—chlorpromazine, erythromycin estolate
      3. Chronic cholestasis—chlorpromazine and prochlorperazine
   D. Primary biliary cirrhosis
   E. Primary sclerosing cholangitis
   F. Vanishing bile duct syndrome
      1. Chronic rejection of liver transplants
      2. Sarcoidosis
      3. Drugs
   G. Inherited
      1. Progressive familial intrahepatic cholestasis
      2. Benign recurrent cholestasis
   H. Cholestasis of pregnancy
   I. Total parenteral nutrition
   J. Nonhepatobiliary sepsis
   K. Benign postoperative cholestasis
   L. Paraneoplastic syndrome
   M. Venoocclusive disease
   N. Graft-versus-host disease
   O. Infiltrative disease
      1. TB
      2. Lymphoma
      3. Amyloid
II. Extrahepatic
   A. Malignant
      1. Cholangiocarcinoma
      2. Pancreatic cancer
      3. Gallbladder cancer
      4. Ampullary cancer
      5. Malignant involvement of the porta hepatis lymph nodes
   B. Benign
      1. Choledocholithiasis
      2. Postoperative biliary strictures
      3. Primary sclerosing cholangitis
      4. Chronic pancreatitis
      5. AIDS cholangiopathy
      6. Mirizzi syndrome
      7. Parasitic disease (ascariasis)

The *vanishing bile duct syndrome* and *adult bile ductopenia* are rare conditions in which there are a decreased number of bile ducts seen in liver biopsy specimens. The histologic picture is similar to that found in primary biliary cirrhosis. This picture is seen in patients who develop chronic rejection after liver transplantation and in those who develop graft-versus-host disease after bone marrow transplantation. Vanishing bile duct syndrome also occurs in rare cases of sarcoidosis, in patients taking certain drugs including chlorpromazine, and idiopathically.

There are also familial forms of intrahepatic cholestasis. The familial intrahepatic cholestatic syndromes include *progressive familial intrahepatic cholestasis* (PFIC) *types 1–3,* and *benign recurrent cholestasis* (BRC). PFIC1 and BRC are autosomal recessive diseases that result from mutations in the *ATP8B1* gene that encodes a protein belonging to the subfamily of P-type ATPases; the exact function of this protein remains poorly defined. While PFIC1 is a progressive condition that manifests in childhood, BRC presents later than PFIC1 and is marked by recurrent episodes of jaundice and pruritus; the episodes are self-limited but can be debilitating. PFIC2 is caused by mutations in the *ABCB11* gene, which encodes the bile salt export pump, and PFIC3 is caused by mutations in the multidrug-resistant P-glycoprotein 3. *Cholestasis of pregnancy* occurs in the second and third trimesters and resolves after delivery. Its cause is unknown, but the condition is probably inherited and cholestasis can be triggered by estrogen administration.

Other causes of intrahepatic cholestasis include total parenteral nutrition (TPN), nonhepatobiliary sepsis, benign postoperative cholestasis, and a paraneoplastic syndrome associated with a number of different malignancies, including Hodgkin's disease, medullary thyroid cancer, renal cell cancer, renal sarcoma, T cell lymphoma, prostate cancer, and several gastrointestinal malignancies. The term *Stauffer's syndrome* has been used for intrahepatic cholestasis specifically associated with renal cell cancer. In patients developing cholestasis in the intensive care unit, the major considerations should be sepsis, shock liver, and TPN jaundice. Jaundice occurring after bone marrow transplantation is most likely due to venoocclusive disease or graft-versus-host disease.

Causes of *extrahepatic cholestasis* can be split into malignant and benign (Table 9-3). Malignant causes include pancreatic, gallbladder, ampullary, and cholangiocarcinoma. The latter is most commonly associated with PSC and is exceptionally difficult to diagnose because its appearance is often identical to that of PSC. Pancreatic and gallbladder tumors, as well as cholangiocarcinoma, are rarely resectable and have poor prognoses. Ampullary carcinoma has the highest surgical cure rate of all the tumors that present as painless jaundice. Hilar lymphadenopathy due to metastases from other cancers may cause obstruction of the extrahepatic biliary tree.

Choledocholithiasis is the most common cause of extrahepatic cholestasis. The clinical presentation can range from mild right upper quadrant discomfort with only minimal elevations of the enzyme tests to ascending cholangitis with jaundice, sepsis, and circulatory collapse. PSC may occur with clinically important strictures limited to the extrahepatic biliary tree. In cases where there is a dominant stricture, patients can be effectively managed with serial endoscopic dilatations. Chronic pancreatitis rarely causes strictures of the distal common bile duct, where it passes through the head of the pancreas. AIDS cholangiopathy is a condition, usually due to infection of the bile duct epithelium with CMV or cryptosporidia, which has a cholangiographic appearance similar to that of PSC. These patients usually present with greatly elevated serum alkaline phosphatase levels (mean, 800 IU/L), but the bilirubin is often near normal. These patients do not typically present with jaundice.

SUMMARY

The goal of this chapter is not to provide an encyclopedic review of all of the conditions that can cause jaundice. Rather, it is intended to provide a framework that helps a physician to evaluate the patient with jaundice in a logical way (Fig. 9-1).

Simply stated, the initial step is to obtain appropriate blood tests to determine if the patient has an isolated elevation of serum bilirubin. If so, is the bilirubin elevation due to an increased unconjugated or conjugated fraction? If the hyperbilirubinemia is accompanied by other liver test abnormalities, is the disorder hepatocellular or cholestatic? If cholestatic, is it intra- or extrahepatic? All of these questions can be answered with a thoughtful history, physical examination, and interpretation of laboratory and radiologic tests and procedures.

FURTHER READINGS

BOSMA PJ: Inherited disorders of bilirubin metabolism. J Hepatol 38:107, 2003

FERENCI P: Wilson's disease. Clin Gastroenterol Hepatol 3:726, 2005

FOX IJ et al: Treatment of the Crigler-Najjar syndrome type I with hepatocyte transplantation. N Engl J Med 338:1422, 1998

GLASOVA H, BEUERS U: Extrahepatic manifestations of cholestasis. J Gastroenterol Hepatol 9:938, 2002

PRATT DS, KAPLAN MM: Laboratory tests, in Schiff's Diseases of the Liver, 9th ed, ER Schiff et al (eds). Philadelphia, Lippincott Williams & Wilkins, 2003

TRAUNER M et al: Molecular pathogenesis of cholestasis. N Engl J Med 339:1217, 1998

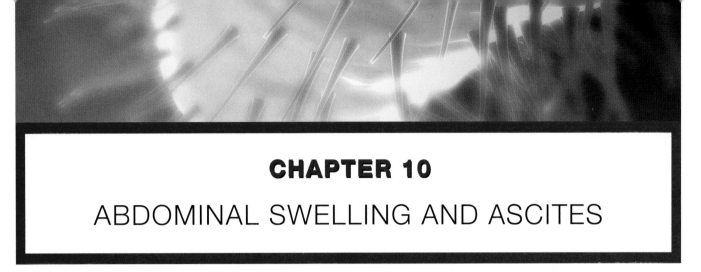

CHAPTER 10
ABDOMINAL SWELLING AND ASCITES

Robert M. Glickman ■ Roshini Rajapaksa

ABDOMINAL SWELLING

Abdominal swelling or distention is a common problem in clinical medicine and may be the initial manifestation of a systemic disease or of otherwise unsuspected abdominal disease. *Subjective* abdominal enlargement, often described as a sensation of fullness or bloating, is usually transient and is often related to a functional gastrointestinal disorder when it is not accompanied by objective physical findings of increased abdominal girth or local swelling. *Obesity* and lumbar lordosis, which may be associated with prominence of the abdomen, may usually be distinguished from true increases in the volume of the peritoneal cavity by history and careful physical examination.

CLINICAL HISTORY

Abdominal swelling may first be noticed by the patient because of a progressive increase in belt or clothing size, the appearance of abdominal or inguinal hernias, or the development of a localized swelling. Often, considerable abdominal enlargement has gone unnoticed for weeks or months, either because of coexistent obesity or because the ascites formation has been insidious, without pain or localizing symptoms. Progressive abdominal distention may be associated with a sensation of "pulling" or "stretching" of the flanks or groins and vague low back pain. Localized pain usually results from involvement of an abdominal organ (e.g., a passively congested liver, large spleen, or colonic tumor). Pain is

uncommon in cirrhosis with ascites, and when it is present, pancreatitis, hepatocellular carcinoma, or peritonitis should be considered. Tense ascites or abdominal tumors may produce increased intraabdominal pressure, resulting in indigestion and heartburn due to gastroesophageal reflux or dyspnea, abdominal wall hernias (inguinal and umbilical), orthopnea, and tachypnea from elevation of the diaphragm. A coexistent pleural effusion, more commonly on the right, presumably due to leakage of ascitic fluid through lymphatic channels in the diaphragm, may also contribute to respiratory embarrassment. A large pleural effusion, obscuring most of the lung, is known as a *hepatic hydrothorax*. The patient with diffuse abdominal swelling should be questioned about increased alcohol intake, a prior episode of jaundice or hematuria, or a change in bowel habits. Such historic information may provide the clues that will lead one to suspect an occult cirrhosis, a colonic tumor with peritoneal seeding, congestive heart failure, or nephrosis.

PHYSICAL EXAMINATION

A carefully executed general physical examination can yield valuable clues concerning the etiology of abdominal swelling. Thus palmar erythema and spider angiomas suggest an underlying cirrhosis, while supraclavicular adenopathy (Virchow's node) should raise the question of an underlying gastrointestinal malignancy.

Inspection of the abdomen is important. By noting the abdominal contour, one may be able to distinguish localized from generalized swelling. The tensely distended abdomen with tightly stretched skin, bulging flanks, and everted umbilicus is characteristic of ascites. A prominent abdominal venous pattern with the direction of flow away from the umbilicus is often a reflection of portal hypertension; venous collaterals with flow from the lower part of the abdomen toward the umbilicus suggest obstruction of the inferior vena cava; flow downward toward the umbilicus suggests superior vena cava obstruction. "Doming" of the abdomen with visible ridges from underlying intestinal loops is usually due to intestinal obstruction or distention. An epigastric mass, with evident peristalsis proceeding from left to right, usually indicates underlying pyloric obstruction. A liver with metastatic deposits may be visible as a nodular right upper quadrant mass moving with respiration.

Auscultation may reveal the high-pitched, rushing sounds of early intestinal obstruction or a succussion sound due to increased fluid and gas in a dilated hollow viscus. Careful auscultation over an enlarged liver occasionally reveals a harsh bruit signifying a vascular tumor (especially a hepatocellular carcinoma) or alcoholic hepatitis, or the leathery friction rub of a surface nodule. A venous hum at the umbilicus may signify portal hypertension and an increased collateral blood flow around the liver. A fluid wave and flank dullness that shifts with change in position of the patient are important signs that indicate the presence of peritoneal fluid, although a minimum of 1500 mL of fluid is usually required to produce these findings. In obese patients, small amounts of fluid may be difficult to demonstrate and often can only be detected by ultrasound examination of the abdomen, which can detect as little as 100 mL of fluid. Careful percussion should serve to distinguish generalized abdominal enlargement from localized swelling due to an enlarged uterus, ovarian cyst, or distended bladder. Percussion can also outline an abnormally small or large liver. Loss of normal liver dullness may result from massive hepatic necrosis; it also may be a clue to free gas in the peritoneal cavity, as from perforation of a hollow viscus.

Palpation is often difficult with massive ascites, and ballottement of overlying fluid may be the only method of palpating the liver or spleen. A slightly enlarged spleen in association with ascites may be the only evidence of an occult cirrhosis. When there is evidence of portal hypertension, a soft liver suggests that obstruction to portal flow is extrahepatic; a firm liver suggests cirrhosis as the likely cause of the portal hypertension. A very hard or nodular liver is a clue that the liver is infiltrated with tumor, and when accompanied by ascites, it suggests that the latter is due to peritoneal seeding. The presence of a hard periumbilical nodule (Sister Mary Joseph's nodule) suggests metastatic disease from a pelvic or gastrointestinal primary tumor. A pulsatile liver and ascites may be found in tricuspid insufficiency.

An attempt should be made to determine whether a mass is solid or cystic, smooth or irregular, and whether it moves with respiration. The liver, spleen, and gallbladder should descend with respiration unless they are fixed by adhesions or extension of tumor beyond the organ. A fixed mass not descending with respiration may indicate that it is retroperitoneal. Tenderness, especially if localized, may indicate an inflammatory process such as an abscess; it also may be due to stretching of the visceral peritoneum or tumor necrosis. Rectal and pelvic examinations are mandatory; they may reveal otherwise undetected masses due to tumor or infection.

Radiographic and laboratory examinations are essential for confirming or extending the impressions gained on physical examination. Upright and recumbent films of the abdomen may demonstrate the dilated loops of intestine with fluid levels characteristic of intestinal obstruction or the diffuse abdominal haziness and loss of psoas margins suggestive of ascites. Ultrasonography is often of value in detecting ascites, determining the presence of a mass, or evaluating the size of the liver and spleen. CT scanning provides similar information and is often necessary to visualize the retroperitoneum, pancreas, and lymph nodes. A plain film of the abdomen may reveal the distended colon of otherwise unsuspected ulcerative colitis and give valuable information as to the size of the liver and spleen. An irregular and elevated right side of the diaphragm may be a clue to a liver abscess or hepatocellular carcinoma. Studies of the gastrointestinal tract with barium or other contrast media are usually necessary in the search for a primary tumor.

Laboratory abnormalities that are highly suggestive of cirrhosis as the cause of ascites include unexplained thrombocytopenia, decreased albumin, and a prolonged prothrombin time.

ASCITES

The evaluation of a patient with ascites requires that the cause of the ascites be established. In most cases ascites appears as part of a well-recognized illness, i.e., cirrhosis, congestive heart failure, nephrosis, or disseminated carcinomatosis. In these situations, the physician should determine that the development of ascites is indeed a consequence of the basic underlying disease and not due to the presence of a separate or related disease process. This distinction is necessary even when the cause of ascites seems obvious. For example, when the patient with compensated cirrhosis and minimal ascites develops progressive ascites that is increasingly difficult to control with sodium restriction or diuretics, the temptation is to attribute the worsening of the clinical picture to progressive liver disease. However, an occult hepatocellular carcinoma, portal vein thrombosis, spontaneous bacterial peritonitis, alcoholic hepatitis, viral infection, or even tuberculosis may be responsible for the decompensation. The disappointingly low success in diagnosing tuberculous peritonitis or hepatocellular carcinoma in the patient with cirrhosis and ascites reflects the too-low index of suspicion for the development of such superimposed conditions. Similarly, the patient with congestive heart failure may develop ascites from a disseminated carcinoma with peritoneal seeding. It is important to note, however, that while there are many different causes of ascites, in the United States >80% of cases are due to cirrhosis. Risk factors for the development of cirrhosis include alcoholism, viral hepatitis, nonalcoholic steatohepatitis, and a family history of liver disease.

Diagnostic paracentesis (50–100 mL) should be part of the routine evaluation of the patient with ascites, and does not routinely require the prior administration of platelets or fresh-frozen plasma unless disseminated intravascular coagulation is suspected. The fluid should be examined for its gross appearance; protein content, albumin level, cell

count, and differential cell count should be determined; and Gram's and acid-fast stains and culture should be performed. Cytologic and cell-block examination may disclose an otherwise unsuspected carcinoma. A serum ascites–albumin gradient (SAAG) should be calculated to determine if the fluid has the features of a transudate or an exudate. The gradient correlates directly with portal pressure. A gradient >1.1 g/dL (high gradient) is characteristic of uncomplicated cirrhotic ascites and differentiates ascites due to portal hypertension from ascites not due to portal hypertension >97% of the time. Other etiologies of high-gradient ascites include alcoholic hepatitis, congestive heart failure, hepatic metastases, constrictive pericarditis, and Budd-Chiari syndrome. A gradient <1.1 g/dL (low gradient) suggests that the ascites is not due to portal hypertension with >97% accuracy and mandates a search for other causes such as peritoneal carcinomatosis, tuberculous peritonitis, pancreatitis, serositis, pyogenic peritonitis, and nephrotic syndrome (Table 10-1). Table 10-1

TABLE 10-1

CHARACTERISTICS OF ASCITIC FLUID IN VARIOUS DISEASE STATES

CONDITION	GROSS APPEARANCE	PROTEIN, g/L	SERUM-ASCITES ALBUMIN GRADIENT, g/dL	CELL COUNT RED BLOOD CELLS, >10,000/µL	WHITE BLOOD CELLS, PER µL	OTHER TESTS
Cirrhosis	Straw-colored or bile-stained	<25 (95%)	>1.1	1%	<250 (90%)[a]; predominantly mesothelial	
Neoplasm	Straw-colored, hemorrhagic, mucinous, or chylous	>25 (75%)	<1.1	20%	>1000 (50%); variable cell types	Cytology, cell block, peritoneal biopsy
Tuberculous peritonitis	Clear, turbid, hemorrhagic, chylous	>25 (50%)	<1.1	7%	>1000 (70%); usually >70% lymphocytes	Peritoneal biopsy, stain and culture for acid-fast bacilli
Pyogenic peritonitis	Turbid or purulent	If purulent, >25	<1.1	Unusual	Predominantly polymorphonuclear leukocytes	Positive Gram's stain, culture
Congestive heart failure	Straw-colored	Variable, 15–53	>1.1	10%	<1000 (90%); usually mesothelial, mononuclear	
Nephrosis	Straw-colored or chylous	<25 (100%)	<1.1	Unusual	<250; mesothelial, mononuclear	If chylous, ether extraction, Sudan staining
Pancreatic ascites (pancreatitis, pseudocyst)	Turbid, hemorrhagic, or chylous	Variable, often >25	<1.1	Variable, may be blood-stained	Variable	Increased amylase in ascitic fluid and serum

[a]Because the conditions of examining fluid and selecting patients were not identical in each series, the percentage figures (in parentheses) should be taken as an indication of the order of magnitude rather than as the precise incidence of any abnormal finding.

presents some of the disease states that produce high-SAAG and low-SAAG ascites. Although there is variability of the ascitic fluid in any given disease state, some features are sufficiently characteristic to suggest certain diagnostic possibilities. For example, blood-stained fluid with >25 g/L protein is unusual in uncomplicated cirrhosis but is consistent with tuberculous peritonitis or neoplasm. Cloudy fluid with a predominance of polymorphonuclear cells (>250/μL) and a positive Gram's stain are characteristic of bacterial peritonitis, which requires antibiotic therapy; if most cells are lymphocytes, tuberculosis should be suspected. The complete examination of each fluid is most important, for occasionally only one finding may be abnormal. For example, if the fluid is a typical transudate but contains >250 white blood cells per microliter, the finding should be recognized as atypical for cirrhosis and should warrant a search for tumor or infection. This is especially true in the evaluation of cirrhotic ascites where occult peritoneal infection may be present with only minor elevations in the white blood cell count of the peritoneal fluid (300–500/μL). Since Gram's stain of the fluid may be negative in a high proportion of such cases, careful culture of the peritoneal fluid is mandatory. Bedside inoculation of blood culture flasks with ascitic fluid results in a dramatically increased incidence of positive cultures when bacterial infection is present (90 vs 40% positivity with conventional cultures done by the laboratory). Direct visualization of the peritoneum (laparoscopy) may disclose peritoneal deposits of tumor, tuberculosis, or metastatic disease of the liver. Biopsies are taken under direct vision, often adding to the diagnostic accuracy of the procedure.

Chylous ascites refers to a turbid, milky, or creamy peritoneal fluid due to the presence of thoracic or intestinal lymph. Such a fluid shows Sudan-staining fat globules microscopically and an increased triglyceride content by chemical examination. Opaque milky fluid usually has a triglyceride concentration of >11.3 mmol/L (>1000 mg/dL), but a triglyceride concentration of >2.3 mmol/L (>200 mg/dL) is sufficient for the diagnosis. A turbid fluid due to leukocytes or tumor cells may be confused with chylous fluid (pseudochylous), and it is often helpful to carry out alkalinization and ether extraction of the specimen. Alkali tend to dissolve cellular proteins and thereby reduce turbidity; ether extraction leads to clearing if the turbidity of the fluid is due to lipid. Chylous ascites is most often the result of lymphatic disruption or obstruction from cirrhosis, tumor, trauma, tuberculosis, filariasis, or congenital abnormalities. It may also be seen in the nephrotic syndrome.

Rarely, ascitic fluid may be *mucinous* in character, suggesting either pseudomyxoma peritonei (Chap. 18) or rarely a colloid carcinoma of the stomach or colon with peritoneal implants.

On occasion, ascites may develop as a seemingly isolated finding in the absence of a clinically evident underlying disease. Then, a careful analysis of ascitic fluid may indicate the direction the evaluation should take. A useful framework for the workup starts with an analysis of whether the fluid is classified as a high (transudate) or low (exudate) gradient fluid. *High-gradient (transudative) ascites* of unclear etiology is most often due to occult cirrhosis, right-sided venous hypertension raising hepatic sinusoidal pressure, Budd–Chiari syndrome, or massive hepatic metastases. Cirrhosis with well-preserved liver function (normal albumin) resulting in ascites is invariably associated with significant portal hypertension (Chap. 40). Evaluation should include liver function tests and a hepatic imaging procedure (i.e., CT or ultrasound) to detect nodular changes in the liver suggesting portal hypertension. On occasion, a wedged hepatic venous pressure can be useful to document portal hypertension. Finally, if clinically indicated, a liver biopsy will confirm the diagnosis of cirrhosis and perhaps suggest its etiology. Other etiologies may result in hepatic venous congestion and resultant ascites. Right-sided cardiac valvular disease and particularly constrictive pericarditis should raise a high index of suspicion and may require cardiac imaging and cardiac catheterization for definitive diagnosis. Hepatic vein thrombosis is evaluated by visualizing the hepatic veins with imaging techniques (Doppler ultrasound, angiography, CT scans, MRI) to demonstrate obliteration, thrombosis, or obstruction by tumor. Uncommonly, transudative ascites may be associated with benign tumors of the ovary, particularly fibroma (Meigs' syndrome) with ascites and hydrothorax.

Low-gradient (exudative) ascites should initiate an evaluation for primary peritoneal processes, most importantly infection and tumor. Tuberculous peritonitis (Table 10-1) is best diagnosed by peritoneal biopsy, either percutaneously or via laparoscopy. Histologic examination invariably shows granulomata that may contain acid-fast bacilli. Since cultures of peritoneal fluid and biopsies for tuberculosis may require 6 weeks, characteristic histology with appropriate stains allows antituberculosis therapy to be started promptly. Similarly, the diagnosis of peritoneal seeding by tumor can usually be made by cytologic analysis of peritoneal fluid or by peritoneal biopsy if cytology is negative. Appropriate diagnostic studies can then be undertaken to determine the nature and site of the primary tumor. Pancreatic ascites (Table 10-1) is invariably associated with an extravasation of pancreatic fluid from the pancreatic ductal system, most commonly from a leaking pseudocyst. Ultrasound or CT examination of the pancreas followed by visualization of the pancreatic duct by direct cannulation [viz., endoscopic retrograde cholangiopancreatography (ERCP)] usually discloses the site of leakage and permits resective surgery to be carried out.

An analysis of the physiologic and metabolic factors involved in the production of ascites (detailed in Chap. 40), coupled with a complete evaluation of the nature of the ascitic fluid, invariably discloses the etiology of the ascites and permits appropriate therapy to be instituted.

ACKNOWLEDGMENT

Dr. Kurt J. Isselbacher was the co-author of this chapter in previous editions.

FURTHER READINGS

LIPSKY MS, STERNBACH MR: Evaluation and initial management of patients with ascites. Am Fam Physician 54:1327, 1996

McHUTCHISON JG: Differential diagnosis of ascites. Semin Liver Dis 17:191, 1997

PARSONS SL et al: Malignant ascites. Br J Surg 83:6, 1996

PINTO PC et al: Large volume paracentesis in nonedematous patients with tense ascites: Its effect on intravascular volume. Hepatology 8:207, 1988

RUNYON BA: Management of adult patients with ascites due to cirrhosis. Hepatology 39:841, 2004

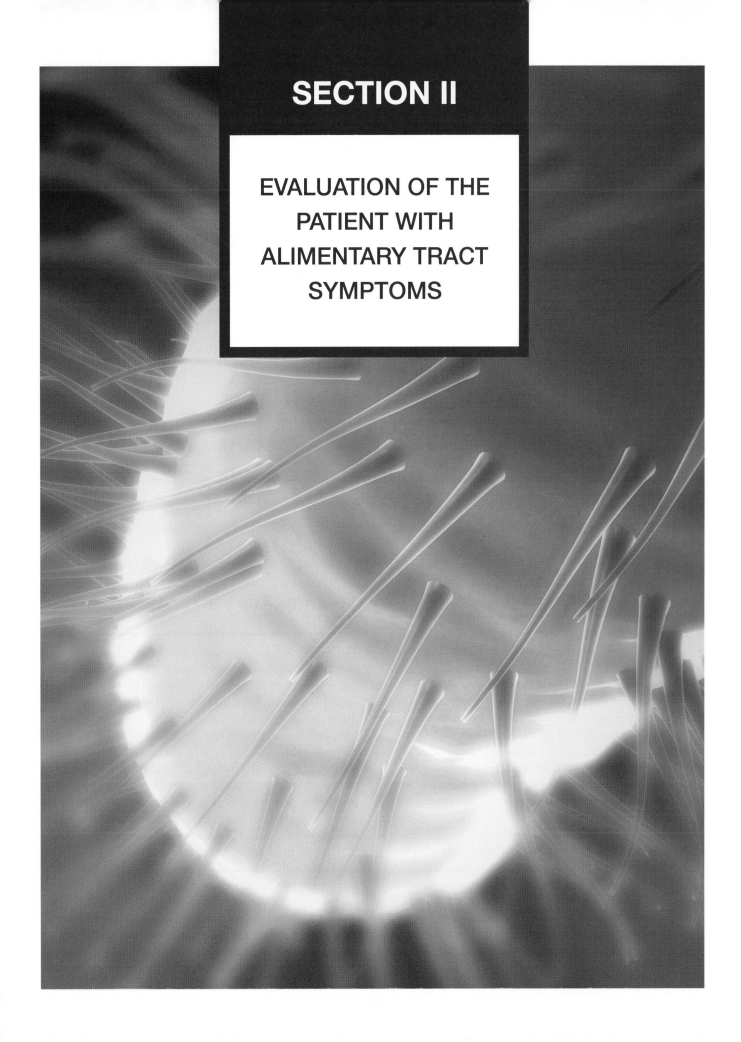

SECTION II

EVALUATION OF THE PATIENT WITH ALIMENTARY TRACT SYMPTOMS

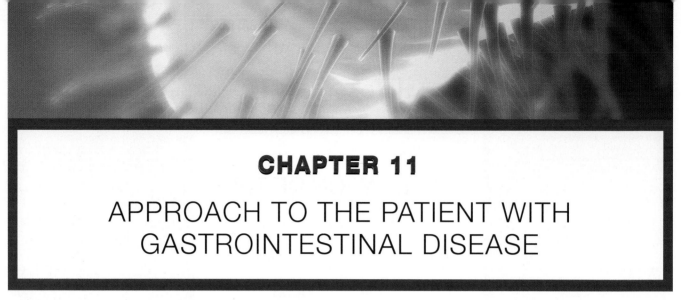

CHAPTER 11

APPROACH TO THE PATIENT WITH GASTROINTESTINAL DISEASE

William L. Hasler ■ Chung Owyang

ANATOMIC CONSIDERATIONS

The gastrointestinal (GI) tract extends from the mouth to the anus and comprises several organs with distinct functions. Separating the organs are specialized independently controlled thickened sphincters that assist in gut compartmentalization. The gut wall is organized into well-defined layers that contribute to the functional activities in each region. The mucosa serves as a barrier to luminal contents or as a site for transfer of fluids or nutrients. Gut smooth muscle mediates propulsion from one region to the next. Many GI organs possess a serosal layer that provides a supportive foundation but that also permits external input.

Interactions with other organ systems serve the needs both of the gut and the body. Pancreaticobiliary conduits deliver bile and enzymes into the duodenum. A rich vascular supply is modulated by GI tract activity. Lymphatic channels assist in gut immune activities. Intrinsic gut wall nerves provide the basic controls for propulsion and fluid regulation. Extrinsic neural input provides volitional or involuntary control to degrees that are specific for each gut region.

FUNCTIONS OF THE GASTROINTESTINAL TRACT

The GI tract serves two main functions—assimilation of nutrients and elimination of waste. The gut anatomy is organized to serve these functions. In the mouth, food is processed, mixed with salivary amylase, and delivered to the luminal GI tract. The esophagus propels the bolus into the stomach, and the lower esophageal sphincter prevents oral reflux of gastric contents. The esophageal mucosa has a protective squamous histology that does not permit significant diffusion or absorption. The propulsive activities of the esophagus are exclusively aboral and are coordinated with relaxation of the upper and lower esophageal sphincters upon swallowing.

The stomach furthers food preparation by triturating and mixing the bolus with pepsin and acid. Gastric acid also sterilizes the upper gut. Gastric motor activities exhibit regional variability. The proximal stomach serves a storage function by relaxing to accommodate the meal. The distal stomach exhibits phasic contractions that propel solid food residue against the pylorus where it is repeatedly propelled proximally for further mixing before

84

it is emptied into the duodenum. Finally, the stomach secretes intrinsic factor for vitamin B_{12} absorption.

The small intestine serves most of the nutrient absorptive function of the gut. The intestinal mucosa exhibits villous architecture to provide maximal surface area for absorption and is endowed with specialized enzymes and transporters. Triturated food from the stomach is mixed with pancreatic juice and bile in the proximal duodenum to facilitate digestion. Pancreatic juice contains the main enzymes for carbohydrate, protein, and fat digestion as well as bicarbonate to optimize the pH for activation of these enzymes. Bile secreted by the liver and stored in the gallbladder is essential for intestinal lipid digestion. The proximal intestine is optimized for rapid absorption of nutrient breakdown products and most minerals, while the ileum is better suited for absorption of vitamin B_{12} and bile acids. The small intestine also aids in waste elimination. Bile contains byproducts of erythrocyte degradation, toxins, metabolized and unaltered medications, and cholesterol. Motor function of the small intestine delivers indigestible food residue and sloughed enterocytes into the colon for further processing. The small intestine terminates in the ileocecal junction, a sphincteric structure that prevents coloileal reflux and maintains small-intestinal sterility.

The colon prepares the waste material for controlled evacuation. The colonic mucosa dehydrates the stool, decreasing daily fecal volumes from 1000–1500 mL delivered from the ileum to 100–200 mL expelled from the rectum. The colonic lumen possesses a dense bacterial colonization that ferments undigested carbohydrates and short-chain fatty acids. Whereas transit times in the esophagus are on the order of seconds and times in the stomach and small intestine range from minutes to a few hours, propagation through the colon takes >1 day in most individuals. Colonic motor patterns exhibit a to-and-fro character that facilitates slow fecal desiccation. The proximal colon serves to mix and absorb fluid, while the distal colon exhibits peristaltic contractions and mass actions that function to expel the stool. The colon terminates in the anus, a structure with volitional and involuntary controls to permit retention of the fecal bolus until it can be released in a socially convenient setting.

EXTRINSIC MODULATION OF GUT FUNCTION

GI function is modified by influences outside of the gut. Unlike other organ systems, the gut is in physical continuity with the outside environment. Thus, protective mechanisms are vigilant against the deleterious effects of consumed foods, medications, toxins, and infectious organisms. Mucosal immune mechanisms include an indwelling lymphocyte and plasma cell population in the epithelial layer and lamina propria backed up by

lymph node chains to prevent noxious agents from entering the circulation. All substances absorbed into the bloodstream are filtered through the liver via the portal venous circulation. In the liver, many drugs and toxins are detoxified by a variety of mechanisms. Although intrinsic nerves control most basic gut activities, extrinsic neural input affects a number of functions. The two activities under voluntary control are swallowing and defecation. Many normal GI reflexes involve extrinsic vagus or splanchnic nerve pathways. An active brain gut axis further alters function in regions not under volitional regulation. As an example, stress has potent effects on gut motor, secretory, and sensory function.

OVERVIEW OF GASTROINTESTINAL DISEASES

GI diseases develop as a consequence of abnormalities within or outside of the gut and range in severity from those that produce mild symptoms and no long-term morbidity to those with intractable symptoms or an adverse outcome. Diseases may be localized to a single organ or exhibit diffuse involvement at a number of sites.

CLASSIFICATION OF GI DISEASES

GI diseases are manifestations of alterations in nutrient assimilation or waste evacuation or in the activities supporting these main functions.

Impaired Digestion and Absorption

Diseases of the stomach, intestine, biliary tree, and pancreas can disrupt nutrient digestion and absorption. Gastric hypersecretory conditions such as Zollinger-Ellison syndrome damage the intestinal mucosa, impair pancreatic enzyme activation, and accelerate transit due to excess gastric acid. The most common intestinal maldigestion syndrome, lactase deficiency, produces gas and diarrhea after consumption of dairy products and has no adverse effect on survival. Other intestinal enzyme deficiencies produce similar symptoms with ingestion of other simple sugars. Conversely, celiac disease, bacterial overgrowth, infectious enteritis, Crohn's ileitis, and radiation damage, which affect digestion and/or absorption more diffusely, produce anemia, dehydration, electrolyte disorders, or malnutrition. Biliary obstruction from stricture or neoplasm may impair fat digestion. Impaired release of pancreatic enzymes in chronic pancreatitis or pancreatic cancer decreases intraluminal digestion and can lead to profound malnutrition.

Altered Secretion

Selected GI diseases result from dysregulation of gut secretion. Gastric acid hypersecretion occurs in Zollinger-Ellison syndrome, G cell hyperplasia, retained antrum syndrome, and some individuals with duodenal ulcer disease. Conversely, patients with atrophic gastritis or pernicious anemia release little or no gastric acid. Inflammatory and infectious small-intestinal and colonic diseases produce fluid loss through impaired absorption or enhanced secretion, but usually do not cause malnutrition. Common intestinal and colonic hypersecretory conditions cause diarrhea and these include acute bacterial or viral infection, chronic *Giardia* or *Cryptosporidia* infections, small-intestinal bacterial overgrowth, bile salt diarrhea, microscopic colitis, diabetic diarrhea, and abuse of certain laxatives. Less common causes include large colonic villous adenomas and endocrine neoplasias with tumor overproduction of secretagogue transmitters such as vasoactive intestinal polypeptide.

Altered Gut Transit

Alterations in gut transit may be due to mechanical obstruction. Esophageal occlusion often results from acid-induced stricture or neoplasm. Gastric outlet obstruction develops from peptic ulcer disease or gastric cancer. Small-intestinal obstruction most commonly results from adhesions but may also occur with Crohn's disease, radiation- or drug-induced strictures, and less likely malignancy. The most common cause of colonic obstruction is colon cancer, although inflammatory strictures develop in patients with inflammatory bowel disease, after certain infections, or with some drugs.

Retardation of propulsion also develops from disordered gut motor function. *Achalasia* is characterized by impaired esophageal body peristalsis and incomplete lower esophageal sphincter relaxation. *Gastroparesis* is the symptomatic delay in gastric emptying of solid or liquid meals secondary to impaired gastric motility. Intestinal pseudoobstruction causes marked delays in small-bowel transit due to injury to enteric nerves or intestinal smooth muscle. Slow-transit constipation is produced by diffusely impaired colonic propulsion. Constipation is also produced by outlet abnormalities such as rectal prolapse, intussusception, or failure of anal relaxation upon attempted defecation.

Disorders of rapid propulsion are less common than those with delayed transit. Rapid gastric emptying occurs in postvagotomy dumping syndrome, with gastric hypersecretion, and in some cases of functional dyspepsia and cyclic vomiting syndrome. Exaggerated intestinal or colonic motor patterns may be responsible for diarrhea in irritable bowel syndrome. Accelerated transit with hyperdefecation is noted in hyperthyroidism.

Immune Dysregulation

Many inflammatory GI conditions are consequences of altered gut immune function. The mucosal inflammation of celiac disease results from dietary ingestion of gluten-containing grains. Some patients with food allergy also exhibit altered immune populations. Eosinophilic esophagitis and eosinophilic gastroenteritis are inflammatory disorders with prominent mucosal eosinophils. Ulcerative colitis and Crohn's disease are disorders of uncertain etiology that produce mucosal injury primarily in the lower gut. The microscopic colitides, lymphocytic and collagenous colitis, exhibit colonic subepithelial infiltrates without visible mucosal damage. Bacterial, viral, and protozoal organisms may produce ileitis or colitis in selected patient populations.

Impaired Gut Blood Flow

Different GI regions are at variable risk for ischemic damage from impaired blood flow. Rare cases of gastroparesis result from blockage of the celiac and superior mesenteric arteries. More commonly encountered are intestinal and colonic ischemia, which are consequences of arterial embolus, arterial thrombosis, venous thrombosis, or hypoperfusion from dehydration, sepsis, hemorrhage, or reduced cardiac output. These may produce mucosal injury, hemorrhage, or even perforation. Some cases of radiation enterocolitis exhibit reduced mucosal blood flow.

Neoplastic Degeneration

All GI regions are susceptible to malignant degeneration to varying degrees. In the United States, colorectal cancer is most common and typically presents after age 50. Worldwide, gastric cancer is prevalent, especially in certain Asian regions. Esophageal cancer develops with chronic acid reflux or in those with an extensive alcohol or tobacco use history. Small-intestinal neoplasms are rare and occur with underlying inflammatory disease. Anal cancers may arise with prior anal infection or inflammation. Pancreatic and biliary cancers elicit severe pain, weight loss, and jaundice and have poor prognoses. Hepatocellular carcinoma usually arises in the setting of chronic viral hepatitis or cirrhosis secondary to other causes. Most GI cancers are carcinomas, but lymphomas and tumors of other cell types also are observed.

Disorders without Obvious Organic Abnormalities

The most common GI disorders show no abnormalities on biochemical or structural testing and include irritable bowel syndrome (IBS), functional dyspepsia, non-cardiac chest pain, and functional heartburn. These functional bowel disorders exhibit altered gut motor function; however, the pathogenic relevance of these abnormalities is uncertain. Exaggerated visceral sensory responses to noxious stimulation may cause discomfort in these disorders. Symptoms in other patients result from altered processing of visceral pain sensations in the central nervous system. Functional bowel patients with severe symptoms may exhibit significant emotional disturbances on psychometric testing.

Genetic Influences

Although many GI diseases result from environmental factors, others exhibit hereditary components. Family members of inflammatory bowel disease (IBD) patients show a genetic predisposition to disease development themselves. Colonic and esophageal malignancies arise in certain inherited disorders. Rare genetic dysmotility syndromes are described. Familial clustering is even observed in the functional bowel disorders, although this may be learned familial illness behavior rather than a true hereditary factor.

SYMPTOMS OF GASTROINTESTINAL DISEASE

The most common GI symptoms are abdominal pain, heartburn, nausea and vomiting, altered bowel habits, GI bleeding, and jaundice (Table 11-1). Others are dysphagia, anorexia, weight loss, fatigue, and extraintestinal symptoms.

Abdominal Pain

Abdominal pain results from GI disease and extraintestinal conditions involving the genitourinary tract, abdominal wall, thorax, or spine. Visceral pain generally is midline in location and vague in character, while parietal pain is localized and precisely described. Common inflammatory diseases with pain include peptic ulcer, appendicitis, diverticulitis, IBD, and infectious enterocolitis. Other intraabdominal causes of pain include gallstone disease and pancreatitis. Noninflammatory visceral sources include mesenteric ischemia and neoplasia. The most common causes of abdominal pain are IBS and functional dyspepsia.

Heartburn

Heartburn, a burning substernal sensation, is reported intermittently by at least 40% of the population. Classically, heartburn is felt to result from excess gastroesophageal reflux of acid. However, some cases exhibit normal esophageal acid exposure and may result from heightened sensitivity of esophageal mucosal nerves.

Nausea and Vomiting

Nausea and vomiting are caused by GI diseases, medications, toxins, acute and chronic infection, endocrine disorders, labyrinthine conditions, and central nervous system disease. The best-characterized GI etiologies relate to mechanical obstruction of the upper gut; however, disorders of propulsion including gastroparesis and intestinal pseudoobstruction also elicit prominent symptoms. Nausea and vomiting also are commonly reported by patients with IBS and functional disorders of the upper gut (including chronic idiopathic nausea and functional vomiting).

Altered Bowel Habits

Altered bowel habits are common complaints of patients with GI disease. Constipation is reported as infrequent defecation, straining with defecation, passage of hard stools, or a sense of incomplete fecal evacuation. Causes of constipation include obstruction, motor disorders of the colon, medications, and endocrine diseases such as

TABLE 11-1

COMMON CAUSES OF COMMON GI SYMPTOMS

ABDOMINAL PAIN	NAUSEA AND VOMITING	DIARRHEA	GI BLEEDING	OBSTRUCTIVE JAUNDICE
Appendicitis	Medications	Infection	Ulcer disease	Bile duct stones
Gallstone disease	GI obstruction	Poorly absorbed sugars	Esophagitis	Cholangiocar cinoma
Pancreatitis	Motor disorders	Inflammatory bowel disease	Varices	Cholangitis
Diverticulitis	Functional bowel disorder	Microscopic colitis	Vascular lesions	Sclerosing cholangitis
Ulcer disease	Enteric infection	Functional bowel disorder	Neoplasm	Ampullary stenosis
Esophagitis	Pregnancy	Celiac disease	Diverticula	Ampullary carcinoma
GI obstruction	Endocrine disease	Pancreatic insufficiency	Hemorrhoids	Pancreatitis
Inflammatory bowel disease	Motion sickness	Hyperthyroidism	Fissures	Pancreatic tumor
Functional bowel disorder	Central nervous system disease	Ischemia	Inflammatory bowel disease	
Vascular disease		Endocrine tumor	Infectious colitis	
Gynecologic causes				
Renal stone				

hypothyroidism and hyperparathyroidism. Diarrhea is reported as frequent defecation, passage of loose or watery stools, fecal urgency, or a similar sense of incomplete evacuation. The differential diagnosis of diarrhea is broad and includes infections, inflammatory causes, malabsorption, and medications. IBS produces constipation, diarrhea, or an alternating bowel pattern. Fecal mucus is common in IBS, while pus characterizes inflammatory disease. Steatorrhea develops with malabsorption.

GI Bleeding

Hemorrhage may develop from any gut organ. Most commonly, upper GI bleeding presents with melena or hematemesis, whereas lower GI bleeding produces passage of bright red or maroon stools. However, briskly bleeding upper sites can elicit voluminous red rectal bleeding, while slowly bleeding ascending colon sites may produce melena. Chronic slow GI bleeding may present with iron-deficiency anemia. The most common upper GI causes of bleeding are ulcer disease, gastroduodenitis, and esophagitis. Other etiologies include portal hypertension, malignancy, tears across the gastroesophageal junction, and vascular lesions. The most prevalent lower GI sources of hemorrhage include hemorrhoids, anal fissures, diverticula, ischemic colitis, and arteriovenous malformations. Other causes include neoplasm, IBD, infectious colitis, drug-induced colitis, and other vascular lesions.

Jaundice

Jaundice results from prehepatic, intrahepatic, or posthepatic disease. Posthepatic causes of jaundice include biliary diseases such as choledocholithiasis, cholangitis, stricture, and neoplasm and pancreatic disorders such as acute and chronic pancreatitis, stricture, and malignancy.

Other Symptoms

Other symptoms may be manifestations of GI disease. Dysphagia, odynophagia, and unexplained chest pain suggest esophageal disease. A globus sensation is reported with esophagopharyngeal conditions but also occurs with functional GI disorders. Weight loss, anorexia, and fatigue are nonspecific symptoms of neoplastic, inflammatory, gut motility, pancreatic, small-bowel mucosal, and psychiatric conditions. Fever is reported with inflammatory illness, but malignancies also evoke febrile responses. GI disorders also produce extraintestinal symptoms. IBD is associated with hepatobiliary dysfunction, skin and eye lesions, and arthritis. Celiac disease may present with dermatitis herpetiformis. Jaundice can produce pruritus. Conversely, systemic diseases can have GI consequences. Systemic lupus may cause gut ischemia, presenting with pain or bleeding. Overwhelming stress or severe burns may lead to gastric ulcer formation.

EVALUATION OF THE PATIENT WITH GASTROINTESTINAL DISEASE

Evaluation of the patient with GI disease begins with a careful history and physical examination. Subsequent investigation with a variety of tools designed to test the structure or function of the gut is indicated in selected cases. Some patients exhibit normal findings on diagnostic testing. In these individuals, validated symptom profiles are employed for confident diagnosis of a functional bowel disorder.

HISTORY

The history of the patient with suspected GI disease has several components. Symptom timing can suggest specific etiologies. Symptoms of short duration commonly result from acute infection, toxin exposure, or abrupt inflammation or ischemia. Long-standing symptoms point to an underlying chronic inflammatory or neoplastic condition or a functional bowel disorder. Symptoms from mechanical obstruction, ischemia, IBD, and functional bowel disorders are worsened by meal ingestion. Conversely, ulcer symptoms may be relieved by eating or antacids. The symptom pattern and duration may suggest underlying etiologies. Ulcer pain occurs at intermittent intervals lasting weeks to months, whereas biliary colic has a sudden onset and lasts up to several hours. Pain from acute inflammation, as with acute pancreatitis, is severe and persists for days to weeks. Meals elicit diarrhea in some cases of IBD and IBS; defecation relieves discomfort in both. Functional bowel disorders are exacerbated by stress. Sudden awakening from sound sleep suggests organic disease rather than a functional bowel disorder. Diarrhea from malabsorption usually improves with fasting, while secretory diarrhea persists without oral intake.

Symptom relation to other factors narrows the list of diagnostic possibilities. Obstructive symptoms with prior abdominal surgery raise concern for adhesions, whereas loose stools after gastrectomy or gallbladder excision suggest dumping syndrome or post-cholecystectomy diarrhea. Symptom onset after travel prompts a search for enteric infection. Medications or food supplements may produce pain, altered bowel habits, or GI bleeding. Lower GI bleeding likely results from a neoplasm, diverticula, or vascular lesions in an older person and anorectal abnormalities or IBD in a younger individual. Celiac disease is prevalent in people of Irish descent, whereas IBD is more common in certain Jewish populations. A sexual history may raise concern for sexually transmitted diseases or immunodeficiency.

Over the past two decades, working groups have been convened to devise symptom criteria to improve the confident diagnosis of the functional bowel disorders and to minimize the numbers of unnecessary diagnostic tests performed. The most widely accepted symptom-based criteria are the *Rome criteria*. When tested against findings of structural investigations, the Rome criteria exhibit diagnostic specificities >90% for many of the functional bowel disorders.

PHYSICAL EXAMINATION

The physical examination complements information from the history. Abnormal vital signs provide diagnostic clues and determine the need for acute intervention. Fever suggests inflammation or neoplasm. Orthostasis is found with significant blood loss, dehydration, sepsis, or autonomic neuropathy. Skin, eye, or joint findings may point to specific diagnoses. Neck examination with swallowing assessment evaluates dysphagia. Cardiopulmonary disease may present with abdominal pain or nausea; thus, lung and cardiac examinations are important. Pelvic examination tests for a gynecologic source of abdominal pain. Rectal examination may detect blood indicating gut mucosal injury or neoplasm or a palpable inflammatory mass in appendicitis. Metabolic conditions and gut motor disorders have associated peripheral neuropathy.

Inspection of the abdomen may reveal distention from obstruction, tumor, or ascites or vascular abnormalities with liver disease. Ecchymoses develop with severe pancreatitis. Auscultation can detect bruits or friction rubs from vascular disease or hepatic tumors. Loss of bowel sounds signifies ileus, while high-pitched, hyperactive sounds characterize intestinal obstruction. Percussion assesses liver size and can detect shifting dullness from ascites. Palpation assesses for hepatosplenomegaly as well as neoplastic or inflammatory masses. Abdominal examination is helpful in evaluating unexplained pain. Intestinal ischemia elicits severe pain but little tenderness. Patients with visceral pain may exhibit generalized discomfort, while those with parietal pain or peritonitis have directed pain, often with involuntary guarding, rigidity, or rebound. Patients with musculoskeletal abdominal wall pain may note tenderness exacerbated by Valsalva or straight leg lift maneuvers.

TOOLS FOR PATIENT EVALUATION

Laboratory, radiographic, and functional tests can assist in diagnosis of suspected GI disease. The GI tract is also amenable to internal evaluation with upper and lower endoscopy and to examination of luminal contents. Histopathologic examinations of gastrointestinal tissues complement these tests.

Laboratory

Selected laboratory tests facilitate the diagnosis of GI disease. Iron-deficiency anemia suggests mucosal blood loss, whereas vitamin B_{12} deficiency results from small-intestinal, gastric, or pancreatic disease. Either can also

result from inadequate oral intake. Leukocytosis and increased sedimentation rates are found in inflammatory conditions, while leukopenia is seen in viremic illness. Severe vomiting or diarrhea elicits electrolyte disturbances, acid-base abnormalities, and elevated blood urea nitrogen. Pancreaticobiliary or liver disease is suggested by elevated pancreatic or liver chemistries. Thyroid chemistries, cortisol, and calcium levels are obtained to exclude endocrinologic causes of GI symptoms. Pregnancy testing is considered for young women with unexplained nausea. Serologies tests are available to screen for celiac disease, IBD, and rheumatologic diseases such as lupus or scleroderma. Hormone levels are obtained for suspected endocrine neoplasia. Intraabdominal malignancies produce tumor markers including the carcinoembryonic antigen CA 19-9 and α-fetoprotein. Paraneoplastic serology panels can be ordered for individuals with gut dysmotility that is believed to be a consequence of extraintestinal neoplasm. Other body fluids are sampled under certain circumstances. Ascitic fluid is analyzed for infection, malignancy, or findings of portal hypertension. Cerebrospinal fluid is obtained for suspected central nervous system causes of vomiting. Urine samples are screened for carcinoid, porphyria, and heavy metal intoxication.

Luminal Contents

Luminal contents can be examined for diagnostic clues. Stool samples are cultured for bacterial pathogens, examined for leukocytes and parasites, or tested for *Giardia* antigen. Duodenal aspirates can be examined for parasites or cultured for bacterial overgrowth. Fecal fat is quantified in possible malabsorption. Stool electrolytes can be measured in diarrheal conditions. Laxative screens are done when laxative abuse is suspected. Gastric acid is quantified to rule out Zollinger-Ellison syndrome. Esophageal pH testing is done for refractory symptoms of acid reflux, whereas newer impedance techniques assess for nonacidic reflux. Pancreatic juice is analyzed for enzyme or bicarbonate content to exclude pancreatic exocrine insufficiency.

Endoscopy

The gut is accessible with endoscopy, which can provide the diagnosis of the causes of bleeding, pain, nausea and vomiting, weight loss, altered bowel function, and fever. Table 11-2 lists the most common indications for the major endoscopic procedures. Upper endoscopy evaluates the esophagus, stomach, and duodenum, while colonoscopy assesses the colon and distal ileum. Upper endoscopy is advocated as the initial structural test performed in patients with suspected ulcer disease, esophagitis, neoplasm, malabsorption, and Barrett's metaplasia because of its ability to directly visualize as well as biopsy the abnormality. Colonoscopy is the procedure of choice

TABLE 11-2

COMMON INDICATIONS FOR ENDOSCOPY

UPPER ENDOSCOPY	COLONOSCOPY	ENDOSCOPIC RETROGRADE CHOLANGIOPANCREATOGRAPHY	ENDOSCOPIC ULTRASOUND
Dyspepsia despite treatment	Cancer screening	Jaundice	Staging of malignancy
Dyspepsia with signs of organic disease	Lower GI bleeding	Postbiliary surgery complaints	Characterize and biopsy submucosal mass
Refractory vomiting	Diarrhea	Cholangitis	Bile duct stones
Dysphagia	Polypectomy	Gallstone pancreatitis	Chronic pancreatitis
Upper GI bleeding	Obstruction	Pancreatic/biliary/am pullary tumor	Drain pseudocyst
Anemia	Biopsy radiologic abnormality	Unexplained pancreatitis	Large gastric folds
Weight loss	Cancer surveillance:	Pancreatitis with unrelenting pain	Anal continuity
Malabsorption	family history, prior	Fistulas	
Biopsy radiologic abnormality	polyp/cancer, colitis	Biopsy radiologic abnormality	
Polypectomy	Palliate neoplasm	Pancreaticobiliary drainage	
Place gastrostomy	Remove foreign body	Sample bile	
Barrett's surveillance		Sphincter of Oddi manometry	
Palliate neoplasm			
Sample duodenal tissue/fluid			
Remove foreign body			

for colon cancer screening and surveillance as well as diagnosis of colitis secondary to infection, ischemia, radiation, and IBD. Sigmoidoscopy examines the colon up to the splenic flexure and is currently used to exclude distal colonic inflammation or obstruction in young patients not at significant risk for colon cancer. For elusive GI bleeding due to arteriovenous malformations or superficial ulcers, small-intestinal examination is performed with push enteroscopy, capsule endoscopy, or the novel technique of double-balloon enteroscopy. Capsule endoscopy is also increasingly being employed to visualize small-intestinal Crohn's disease in individuals with negative barium radiography. Endoscopic retrograde cholangiopancreatography (ERCP) provides diagnoses of pancreatic and biliary disease. Endoscopic ultrasound can evaluate the extent of disease in GI malignancy as well as exclude choledocholithiasis, evaluate pancreatitis, drain pancreatic pseudocysts, and assess anal continuity.

Radiography/Nuclear Medicine

Radiographic tests evaluate diseases of the gut and extraluminal structures. Oral or rectal contrast agents such as barium provide mucosal definition from the esophagus to the rectum. Contrast radiography also assesses gut transit and pelvic floor dysfunction. Barium swallow is the initial procedure for evaluation of dysphagia to exclude subtle rings or strictures and assess for achalasia, whereas small-bowel contrast radiology reliably diagnoses intestinal tumors and Crohn's ileitis.

Contrast enemas are performed when colonoscopy is unsuccessful or contraindicated. Ultrasound and CT evaluate regions not accessible by endoscopy or contrast studies, including the liver, pancreas, gallbladder, kidneys, and retroperitoneum. These tests are useful for diagnosis of mass lesions, fluid collections, organ enlargement, and in the case of ultrasound gallstones. CT and MR colonography are being evaluated as alternatives to colonoscopy for colon cancer screening. MRI assesses the pancreaticobiliary ducts to exclude neoplasm, stones, and sclerosing cholangitis, and the liver to characterize benign and malignant tumors. Angiography excludes mesenteric ischemia and determines spread of malignancy. Angiographic techniques also access the biliary tree in obstructive jaundice. CT and MR techniques can be used to screen for mesenteric occlusion, thereby limiting exposure to angiographic dyes. Positron emission tomography is showing promise in distinguishing malignant from benign disease in several organ systems.

Scintigraphy both evaluates structural abnormalities and quantifies luminal transit. Radionuclide bleeding scans localize bleeding sites in patients with brisk hemorrhage so that therapy with endoscopy, angiography, or surgery may be directed. Radiolabeled leukocyte scans can search for intraabdominal abscesses not visualized on CT. Biliary scintigraphy is complementary to ultrasound in the assessment of cholecystitis. Scintigraphy to quantify esophageal and gastric emptying are well established, while techniques to measure small-intestinal or colonic transit are less widely used.

Histopathology

Gut mucosal biopsies obtained at endoscopy evaluate for inflammatory, infectious, and neoplastic disease. Deep rectal biopsies assist with diagnosis of Hirschsprung's disease or amyloid. Liver biopsy is indicated in cases with abnormal liver chemistries, unexplained jaundice, following liver transplant to exclude rejection, and to characterize the degree of inflammation in patients with chronic viral hepatitis before initiating antiviral therapy. Biopsies obtained during CT or ultrasound can evaluate for other intraabdominal conditions not accessible by endoscopy.

Functional Testing

Tests of gut function provide important data when structural testing is nondiagnostic. In addition to gastric acid and pancreatic function testing, functional testing of motor activity is provided by regional manometric techniques. Esophageal manometry is useful for suspected achalasia, whereas small–intestinal manometry tests for pseudoobstruction. In addition to scintigraphy, breath tests and capsule techniques are available for quantifying gastric emptying. Anorectal manometry with balloon expulsion testing is employed for unexplained incontinence or constipation from outlet dysfunction. Biliary manometry tests for sphincter of Oddi dysfunction with unexplained biliary pain. Electrogastrography measures gastric electrical activity in individuals with nausea and vomiting, whereas electromyography assesses anal function in fecal incontinence. Measurement of breath hydrogen while fasting and after oral mono- or oligosaccharide challenge can screen for carbohydrate intolerance and small-intestinal bacterial overgrowth.

℞ Treatment: GASTROINTESTINAL DISEASE

Management options for the patient with GI disease depend on the cause of symptoms. Available treatments include modifications in dietary intake, medications, interventional endoscopy or radiology techniques, surgery, and therapies directed to external influences.

NUTRITIONAL MANIPULATION Dietary modifications for GI disease include treatments that only reduce symptoms, therapies that correct pathologic defects, and measures that replace normal food intake with enteral or parenteral formulations. Changes that improve symptoms but do not reverse an organic abnormality include lactose restriction for lactase deficiency, liquid meals in gastroparesis, carbohydrate restrictions in dumping syndrome, and high-fiber diets in IBS. The gluten-free diet for celiac disease exemplifies a modification that serves as primary therapy to reduce mucosal inflammation. Enteral medium-chain triglycerides replace normal fats with short-gut syndrome or severe ileal disease. Perfusion of liquid meals through a gastrostomy is performed in those who cannot swallow safely. Enteral feeding through a jejunostomy is considered for gastric dysmotility syndromes that preclude feeding into the stomach. Intravenous hyperalimentation is employed for individuals with generalized gut malfunction who cannot tolerate or who cannot be sustained with enteral nutrition.

PHARMACOTHERAPY Several medications are available to treat GI diseases. Considerable health care resources are expended on over-the-counter remedies. Many prescription drug classes are offered as short-term or continuous therapy of GI illness. A plethora of alternative treatments have gained popularity in GI conditions for which traditional therapies provide incomplete relief.

Over-the-Counter Agents Over-the-counter agents are reserved for mild GI symptoms. Antacids and histamine H_2 antagonists decrease symptoms in gastroesophageal reflux and dyspepsia, whereas antiflatulents and adsorbents reduce gaseous symptoms. More potent acid inhibitors such as proton pump inhibitors are now available over the counter for treatment of chronic gastrointestinal reflux disease. Fiber supplements, stool softeners, enemas, and laxatives are used for constipation. Laxatives are categorized as stimulants, saline cathartics, and poorly absorbed sugars. Nonprescription antidiarrheal agents include bismuth subsalicylate, kaolin-pectin combinations, and loperamide. Supplemental enzymes include lactase pills for lactose intolerance and bacterial α-galactosidase to treat excess gas. In general, use of a nonprescription preparation for more than a short time for chronic persistent symptoms should be supervised by a health care provider.

Prescription Drugs Prescription drugs for GI diseases are a major focus of attention from pharmaceutical companies. Potent acid suppressants including drugs that inhibit the proton pump are advocated for acid reflux when over-the-counter preparations are inadequate. Cytoprotective agents sometimes are used for upper gut ulcers. Prokinetic drugs stimulate GI propulsion in gastroparesis, pseudoobstruction, and constipation as well as the functional bowel disorders. Prosecretory drugs and isotonic solutions containing polyethylene glycol are prescribed for constipation refractory to other agents. Prescription antidiarrheals include opiate drugs, anticholinergic antispasmodics, tricyclics, bile acid binders, and serotonin antagonists. Antispasmodics and tricyclic drugs are also useful for functional abdominal pain, whereas narcotics are used for pain control in organic conditions such as disseminated malignancy and chronic pancreatitis. Antiemetics in several classes reduce nausea and vomiting. Potent pancreatic enzymes decrease malabsorption and pain from pancreatic disease. Antisecretory drugs such as the somatostatin analogue octreotide treat hypersecretory states. Antibiotics treat ulcer disease secondary to *Helicobacter pylori*, infectious diarrhea, diverticulitis, intestinal bacterial overgrowth, and Crohn's disease. Anti-inflammatory and immunosuppressive drugs are used in ulcerative colitis, Crohn's disease, microscopic colitis, refractory celiac disease, and gut vasculitis. Chemotherapy with or without radiotherapy is offered for GI malignancies. Most GI carcinomas respond poorly to such therapy, whereas lymphomas may be cured with such intervention.

Alternative Therapies Alternative treatments are marketed to treat selected GI symptoms. Ginger, acupressure, and acustimulation have been advocated for nausea, while pyridoxine has been investigated for nausea of first-trimester pregnancy. Probiotics containing active bacterial cultures are used as adjuncts in some cases of refractory infectious diarrhea and are being advocated by some as primary therapy of IBS. Low-potency pancreatic enzyme preparations are sold as general digestive aids but have little evidence to support their efficacy.

ENTERIC THERAPIES/INTERVENTIONAL ENDOSCOPY AND RADIOLOGY

Simple luminal interventions are commonly performed for GI diseases. Nasogastric tube suction decompresses the upper gut in ileus or mechanical obstruction. Nasogastric lavage of saline or water in the patient with upper GI hemorrhage determines the rate of bleeding and helps evacuate blood prior to endoscopy. Enteral feedings can be initiated through a nasogastric or nasoenteric tube. Enemas relieve fecal impaction or assist in gas evacuation in acute colonic pseudoobstruction. A rectal tube can be left in place to vent the distal colon in colonic pseudoobstruction and other colonic distention disorders.

In addition to its diagnostic role, endoscopy has therapeutic capabilities in certain settings. Cautery techniques can stop hemorrhage from ulcers, vascular malformations, and tumors. Injection with vasoconstrictor substances or sclerosants is used for bleeding ulcers, vascular malformations, varices, and hemorrhoids. Endoscopic encirclement of varices and hemorrhoids with constricting bands stops hemorrhage from these sites, while endoscopically placed clips can occlude arterial bleeding sites. Endoscopy can remove polyps or debulk lumen-narrowing malignancies. Endoscopic sphincterotomy of the ampulla of Vater relieves symptoms of choledocholithiasis. Obstructions of the gut lumen and pancreaticobiliary tree are relieved by endoscopic dilation or placement of plastic or expandable metal stents. In cases of acute colonic pseudoobstruction, colonoscopy is employed to withdraw luminal gas. Finally, endoscopy is commonly used to insert feeding tubes.

Radiologic measures also are useful in GI disease. Angiographic embolization or vasoconstriction decrease bleeding from sites not amenable to endoscopic intervention. Dilation or stenting with fluoroscopic guidance relieves luminal strictures. Contrast enemas can reduce volvulus and evacuate air in acute colonic pseudoobstruction. CT and ultrasound help drain abdominal fluid collections, in many cases obviating the need for surgery. Percutaneous transhepatic cholangiography relieves biliary obstruction when ERCP is contraindicated. Lithotripsy can fragment gallstones in patients who are not candidates for surgery. In some instances, radiologic approaches offer advantages over endoscopy for gastroenterostomy placement. Finally, central venous catheters for parenteral nutrition may be placed using radiographic techniques.

SURGERY

Surgery is performed to cure GI disease, control symptoms without cure, maintain nutrition, or palliate unresectable neoplasm. Medication-unresponsive ulcerative colitis, diverticulitis, cholecystitis, appendicitis, and intraabdominal abscess are curable with surgery, whereas only symptom control without cure is possible with Crohn's disease. Surgery is mandated for ulcer complications such as bleeding, obstruction, or perforation and intestinal obstructions that do not resolve with conservative care. Fundoplication of the gastroesophageal junction is performed for presentations ranging from ulcerative esophagitis to drug-refractory symptoms of acid reflux. Achalasia responds to operations to relieve lower esophageal sphincter pressure. Novel operative therapies for motility disorders have been introduced including implanted electrical stimulators for gastroparesis and electrical devices and artificial sphincters for fecal incontinence. Surgery may be needed to place a jejunostomy for long-term enteral feedings. The threshold for performing surgery depends on the clinical setting. In all cases, the benefits of operation must be weighed against the potential for postoperative complications.

THERAPY DIRECTED TO EXTERNAL INFLUENCES

In some conditions, GI symptoms respond to treatments directed outside the gut. Psychological therapies including psychotherapy, behavior modification, hypnosis, and biofeedback have shown efficacy in functional bowel disorders. Patients with significant psychological dysfunction and those with little response to treatments targeting the gut are likely to benefit from this form of therapy.

FURTHER READINGS

AMERICAN SOCIETY FOR GASTROINTESTINAL ENDOSCOPY: Appropriate use of gastrointestinal endoscopy. Gastrointest Endosc 52:831, 2000

LONGSTRETH GF et al: Functional bowel disorders. Gastroenterology 130:1480, 2006

MANDEVILLE KL et al: Gastroenterology in developing countries: issues and advances. World J Gastroenterol 15:2839, 2009

WINAWER S et al: Colorectal cancer screening and surveillance: Clinical guidelines and rationale—Update based on new evidence. Gastroenterology 124:544, 2003

YAMADA T (ed): *Textbook of Gastroenterology and Hepatology*, 4th ed. Philadelphia, Lippincott Williams & Wilkins, 2003

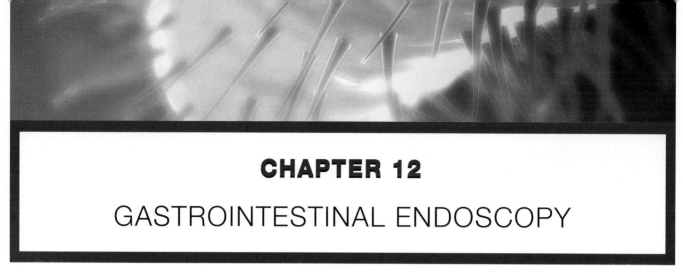

CHAPTER 12

GASTROINTESTINAL ENDOSCOPY

Louis Michel Wong-Kee-Song ■ Mark Topazian

Gastrointestinal endoscopy has been attempted for over 200 years, but the introduction of semirigid gastroscopes in the middle of the twentieth century marked the dawn of the modern endoscopic era. Since then, rapid advances in endoscopic technology have led to dramatic changes in the diagnosis and treatment of many digestive diseases. Innovative endoscopic devices and new endoscopic treatment modalities continue to expand the use of endoscopy in patient care.

Flexible endoscopes provide either an optical image (transmitted over fiberoptic bundles) or an electronic video image (generated by a charge-coupled device in the tip of the endoscope). Operator controls permit deflection of the endoscope tip; fiberoptic bundles bring light to the tip of the endoscope; and working channels allow washing, suctioning, and the passage of instruments. Progressive changes in the diameter and stiffness of endoscopes have improved the ease and patient tolerance of endoscopy.

ENDOSCOPIC PROCEDURES

UPPER ENDOSCOPY

Upper endoscopy, also referred to as esophagogastroduodenoscopy (EGD), is performed by passing a flexible endoscope through the mouth into the esophagus, stomach, bulb, and second duodenum. The procedure is the best method for examining the upper gastrointestinal mucosa. While the upper gastrointestinal radiographic series has similar accuracy for diagnosis of duodenal ulcer (Fig. 12-1), EGD is superior for detection of gastric ulcers (Fig. 12-2) and flat mucosal lesions such as Barrett's esophagus (Fig. 12-3), and it permits directed biopsy and endoscopic therapy. Intravenous conscious sedation is given to most patients in the United States to ease the anxiety and discomfort of the procedure, although in many countries EGD is routinely performed with topical pharyngeal anesthesia only. Patient tolerance of unsedated EGD is improved by the use of an ultrathin, 5-mm diameter endoscope that can be passed transorally or transnasally.

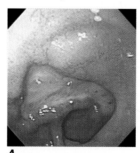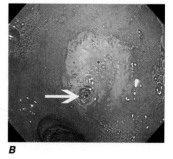

A   B

FIGURE 12-1

Duodenal ulcers. *A.* Ulcer with a clean base. ***B.*** Ulcer with a visible vessel (*arrow*) in a patient with recent hemorrhage.

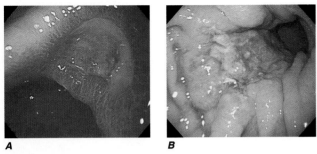

FIGURE 12-2

Gastric ulcers. *A.* Benign gastric ulcer. ***B.*** Malignant gastric ulcer involving greater curvature of stomach.

COLONOSCOPY

Colonoscopy is performed by passing a flexible colonoscope through the anal canal into the rectum and colon. The cecum is reached in >95% of cases, and the terminal ileum can often be examined. Colonoscopy is the "gold standard" for diagnosis of colonic mucosal disease. Colonoscopy has greater sensitivity than barium enema or CT for colitis (Fig. 12-4), polyps (Fig. 12-5), and cancer (Fig. 12-6). Conscious sedation is usually given before colonoscopy in the United States, although a willing patient and a skilled examiner can complete the procedure without sedation in many cases.

FLEXIBLE SIGMOIDOSCOPY

Flexible sigmoidoscopy is similar to colonoscopy but visualizes only the rectum and a variable portion of the left colon, typically to 60 cm from the anal verge. This procedure causes brief abdominal cramping and is usually performed without sedation. Flexible sigmoidoscopy is primarily used for evaluation of diarrhea and rectal outlet bleeding.

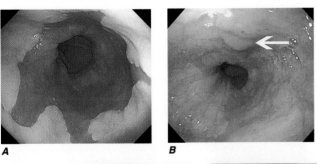

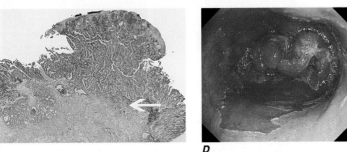

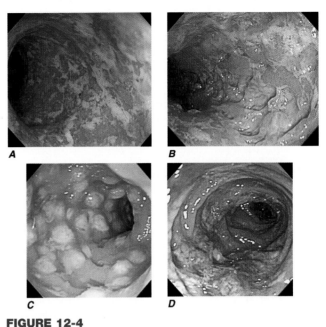

FIGURE 12-4

Causes of colitis. *A.* Chronic ulcerative colitis with diffuse ulcerations and exudates. ***B.*** Severe Crohn's colitis with deep ulcers. ***C.*** Pseudomembranous colitis with yellow, adherent pseudomembranes. ***D.*** Ischemic colitis with patchy mucosal edema, subepithelial hemorrhage, and cyanosis.

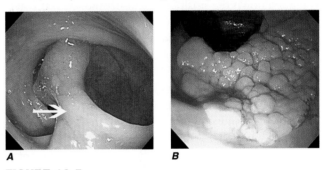

FIGURE 12-5

Colonic polyps. *A.* Pedunculated colon polyp on a thick stalk covered with normal mucosa (*arrow*). ***B.*** Sessile rectal polyp.

FIGURE 12-3

Barrett's esophagus. *A.* Pink tongues of Barrett's mucosa extending proximally from the gastro-esophageal junction. ***B.*** Barrett's esophagus with a suspicious nodule (*arrow*) identified during endoscopic surveillance. ***C.*** Histologic finding of intramucosal adenocarcinoma in the endoscopically resected nodule. Tumor extends into the esophageal submucosa (*arrow*). ***D.*** Barrett's esophagus with locally advanced adenocarcinoma.

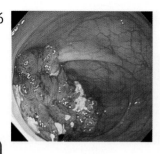

FIGURE 12-6
Colon adenocarcinoma growing into the lumen.

SMALL-BOWEL ENDOSCOPY

Three techniques are currently used to evaluate the small intestine, most often in patients presenting with presumed small-bowel bleeding. For *capsule endoscopy* the patient swallows a disposable capsule that contains a complementary metal oxide silicon (CMOS) chip camera. Color still images (Fig. 12-7) are transmitted wirelessly to an external receiver at several frames per second until the capsule's battery is exhausted or it is passed into the toilet. Although capsule endoscopy allows visualization of the jejunal and ileal mucosa beyond the reach of a conventional endoscope, it remains purely a diagnostic procedure at present.

Push enteroscopy is performed with a long endoscope similar in design to an upper endoscope. The enteroscope is pushed down the small bowel, sometimes with the help of a stiffening overtube that extends from the mouth to the small intestine. The mid-jejunum is usually reached, and the endoscope's instrument channel allows for biopsies or endoscopic therapy. In *double-balloon enteroscopy* (Fig. 12-8), a long overtube and endoscope are both equipped with balloons that, when inflated, appose the intestinal wall and allow for pleating of the small intestine over the endoscope and overtube. The double-balloon enteroscope may be passed orally or anally, and the entire small bowel can be visualized in some patients when both approaches are used. Biopsies and endoscopic therapy can be performed throughout the visualized small bowel.

ENDOSCOPIC RETROGRADE CHOLANGIOPANCREATOGRAPHY (ERCP)

During ERCP, a side-viewing endoscope is passed through the mouth to the duodenum, the ampulla of Vater is identified and cannulated with a thin plastic catheter, and radiographic contrast material is injected into the bile duct and pancreatic duct under fluoroscopic guidance. When indicated, the sphincter of Oddi can be opened using the technique of endoscopic sphincterotomy (Fig. 12-9). Stones can be retrieved from the ducts (Fig. 12-10), biopsies can be obtained,

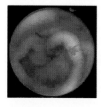

FIGURE 12-7
Capsule endoscopy image of jejunal vascular ectasia.

FIGURE 12-8
Radiograph of a double-balloon enteroscope in the small intestine. (*Image courtesy of Dr. Ananya Das; with permission.*)

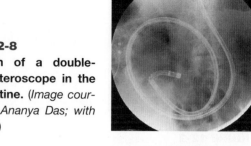

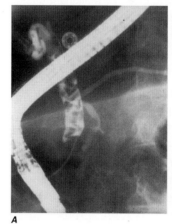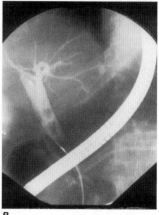

A   *B*

FIGURE 12-9
Endoscopic retrograde cholangiopancreatography (ERCP) for bile duct stones with cholangitis. *A.* Faceted bile duct stones are demonstrated in the common bile duct. ***B.*** After endoscopic sphincterotomy, the stones are extracted with a Dormia basket. A small abscess communicates with the left hepatic duct.

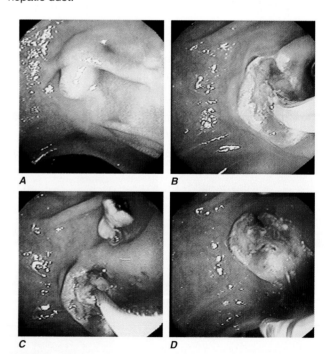

C   *D*

FIGURE 12-10
Endoscopic sphincterotomy. *A.* A normal-appearing ampulla of Vater. ***B.*** Sphincterotomy is performed with electrocautery. ***C.*** Bile duct stones are extracted with a balloon catheter. ***D.*** Final appearance of the sphincterotomy.

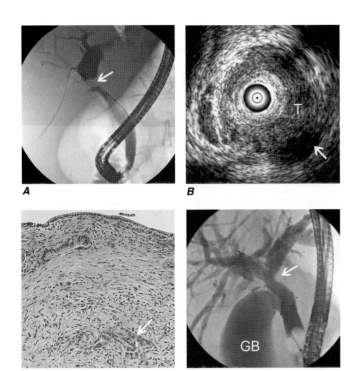

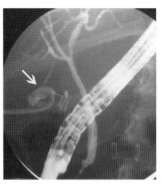

FIGURE 12-12

Bile leak (*arrow*) from a duct of Luschka after laparoscopic cholecystectomy. Contrast leaks from a small right intrahepatic duct into the gallbladder fossa, then flows into the pigtail of a percutaneous drainage catheter.

FIGURE 12-11

Endoscopic diagnosis, staging, and palliation of hilar cholangiocarcinoma. *A.* ERCP in a patient with obstructive jaundice demonstrates a malignant-appearing stricture of the biliary confluence extending into the left and right intrahepatic ducts (*arrow*). ***B.*** Intraductal ultrasound of the biliary stricture demonstrates marked bile duct wall thickening due to tumor (T) with partial encasement of the hepatic artery (*arrow*). ***C.*** Intraductal biopsy obtained during ERCP demonstrates malignant cells infiltrating the submucosa of the bile duct wall (*arrow*). ***D.*** Endoscopic placement of bilateral self-expanding metal stents (*arrow*) relieves the biliary obstruction.

and strictures (Fig. 12-11) or ductal leaks (Fig. 12-12) can be dilated and stented. ERCP is often performed for therapy but remains important in diagnosis, especially for ductal strictures and bile duct stones.

ENDOSCOPIC ULTRASOUND (EUS)

EUS utilizes high-frequency ultrasound transducers incorporated into the tip of a flexible endoscope. Ultrasound images are obtained of the gut wall and adjacent organs, vessels, and lymph nodes. By sacrificing depth of ultrasound penetration and bringing the ultrasound transducer close to the area of interest via endoscopy, very-high-resolution images are obtained. EUS provides the most accurate preoperative local staging of esophageal, pancreatic, and rectal malignancies, although it does not detect most distant metastases. Examples of EUS tumor staging are shown in Fig. 12-13. EUS is also highly sensitive for diagnosis of bile duct stones,

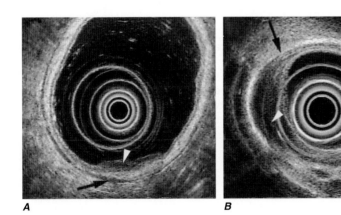

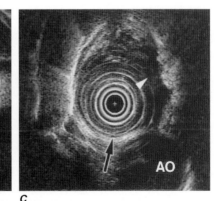

FIGURE 12-13

Local staging of gastrointestinal cancers with endoscopic ultrasound. In each example the white arrowhead marks the primary tumor and the black arrow indicates the muscularis propria (mp) of the intestinal wall. "AO" indicates aorta. ***A.*** T1 gastric cancer. The tumor does not invade the mp. ***B.*** T2 esophageal cancer. The tumor invades the mp. ***C.*** T3 esophageal cancer. The tumor extends through the mp into the surrounding tissue, and focally abuts the aorta.

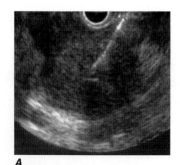
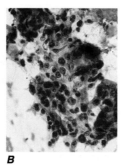

A   **B**

FIGURE 12-14

Endoscopic ultrasound (EUS)-guided fine-needle aspiration (FNA). *A.* Ultrasound image of a 22-gauge needle passed through the duodenal wall and positioned in a hypoechoic pancreatic head mass. *B.* Micrograph of aspirated malignant cells. (*Image B courtesy of Dr. Mary S. Chacho; with permission.*)

gallbladder disease, submucosal gastrointestinal lesions, and chronic pancreatitis. Fine-needle aspiration of masses and lymph nodes in the posterior mediastinum, abdomen, and pelvis can be performed under EUS guidance (**Fig. 12-14**).

RISKS OF ENDOSCOPY

All endoscopic procedures carry some risk of bleeding and gastrointestinal perforation. These risks are quite low with diagnostic upper endoscopy and colonoscopy (<1:1000 procedures), although the risk is as high as 2:100 when therapeutic procedures such as polypectomy, control of hemorrhage, or stricture dilation are performed. Bleeding and perforation are rare with flexible sigmoidoscopy. The risks for diagnostic EUS (without needle aspiration) are similar to the risks for diagnostic upper endoscopy.

Infectious complications are unusual with most endoscopic procedures. Some procedures carry a higher incidence of postprocedure bacteremia, and prophylactic antibiotics may be indicated for these procedures in some patients (**Table 12-1**).

ERCP carries additional risks. Pancreatitis occurs in about 5% of patients undergoing ERCP and in up to 25% of patients with sphincter of Oddi dysfunction. Young anicteric patients with normal ducts are at

TABLE 12-1

ANTIBIOTIC PROPHYLAXIS FOR SELECTED ENDOSCOPIC PROCEDURES

PATIENT CONDITION	PROCEDURE CONTEMPLATED	ANTIBIOTIC PROPHYLAXIS[a]
High risk: Prosthetic valve, history of endocarditis, systemic-pulmonary shunt, synthetic vascular graft <1 year old), complex cyanotic congenital heart disease	High risk[b] Low risk[c]	Recommended Optional (insufficient data)
Moderate risk: Most other congenital abnormalities, acquired valvular disfunction (rheumatic heart disease), hypertrophic cardiomyopathy, mitral valve prolapse with regurgitation or thickened leaflets	High risk Low risk	Optional (insufficient data) Not recommended[d]
Low risk: CABG, repaired septal defect or patent ductus, mitral valve prolapse without valvular regurgitation, pacemakers, implantable defibrillators	High or low risk	Not recommended
Obstructed bile duct	ERCP	Recommended
Pancreatic cystic lesion	ERCP, EUS-FNA	Recommended
Cirrhosis acute GI bleed	All endoscopic procedures	Recommended
Ascites, immunocompromised patients	High risk Low risk	No recommendation Not recommended
Prosthetic joints	All endoscopic procedures	Not recommended
All patients	Percutaneous endoscopic feed tube placement	Recommended (parenteral cephalosporin or equivalent)

[a]Cardiac prophylaxis regimens include amoxicillin, 2 g PO, 1 h before; or ampicillin, 2 g IV, 30 min before procedure. In penicillin-allergic patients, may substitute clindamycin, 600 mg PO; or cephalexin or cefadroxil, 2 g PO; or azithromycin or clarithromycin 500 mg PO; or cefazolin 1 g IV or IM; or vancomycin 1 g IV. Regimens for noncardiac indications vary.
[b]High-risk endoscopic procedures: stricture dilation, variceal sclerotherapy, ERCP/obstructed biliary tree.
[c]Low-risk endoscopic procedures: EGD and colonoscopy with or without biopsy and polyp removal, variceal ligation.
[d]Controversy exists and recommendations may vary. See, e.g., Dajani AS et al: Clin Infect Dis 25:1448, 1997.
Note: CABG, coronary artery bypass grafting; ERCP, endoscopic retrograde cholangiopancreatography; EUS, endoscopic ultrasound; FNA, fine-needle aspiration; EGD, esophagogastroduodenoscopy.
Source: Adapted from WK Hirota et al: Guidelines for antibiotic prophylaxis for GI endoscopy. Gastrointest Endosc 58(4):475, 2003; with permission.

increased risk. Post-ERCP pancreatitis is usually mild and self-limited but may rarely result in prolonged hospitalization, surgery, diabetes, or death. Bleeding occurs in 1% of endoscopic sphincterotomies. Ascending cholangitis, pseudocyst infection, retroperitoneal perforation, and abscess formation may all occur as a result of ERCP.

The conscious sedation used during endoscopy may cause respiratory depression or allergic reactions. Percutaneous gastrostomy tube placement during EGD is associated with a 10–15% incidence of complications, most often wound infections. Fasciitis, pneumonia, bleeding, and colonic injury may result from gastrostomy tube placement.

URGENT ENDOSCOPY

ACUTE GASTROINTESTINAL HEMORRHAGE

Endoscopy is an important diagnostic and therapeutic technique for patients with acute gastrointestinal hemorrhage. Although most gastrointestinal bleeding stops spontaneously, a minority of patients will have persistent or recurrent hemorrhage that may be life-threatening. Clinical predictors of rebleeding help identify patients most likely to benefit from urgent endoscopy and endoscopic, angiographic, or surgical hemostasis.

Initial Evaluation

The initial evaluation of the bleeding patient focuses on the magnitude of hemorrhage as reflected by the postural vital signs, the frequency of hematemesis or melena, and (in some cases) findings on nasogastric lavage. Decreases in hematocrit and hemoglobin lag behind the clinical course and are not reliable gauges of the magnitude of acute bleeding. This initial evaluation, completed well before the bleeding source is confidently identified, guides immediate supportive care of the patient and helps determine the timing of endoscopy. The magnitude of the initial hemorrhage is the most important indication for urgent endoscopy, since a large initial bleed increases the likelihood of ongoing or recurrent bleeding. Patients with resting hypotension, repeated hematemesis, nasogastric aspirate that does not clear with large volume lavage, or orthostatic change in vital signs, or those requiring blood transfusions, should be considered for urgent endoscopy. In addition, patients with cirrhosis, coagulopathy, or respiratory or renal failure and those over 70 years are more likely to have significant rebleeding.

Bedside evaluation also suggests an upper or lower gastrointestinal source of bleeding in most patients. Over 90% of patients with melena are bleeding proximal to the ligament of Treitz, and about 90% of patients with hematochezia are bleeding from the colon. Melena can result from bleeding in the small bowel or right colon,

especially in older patients with slow colonic transit. Conversely, some patients with massive hematochezia may be bleeding from an upper GI source, such as a gastric Dieulafoy's lesion or duodenal ulcer, with rapid intestinal transit. Early upper endoscopy should be considered in such patients.

Endoscopy should be performed after the patient has been resuscitated with intravenous fluids and transfusions as necessary. Marked coagulopathy or thrombocytopenia is usually treated before endoscopy, since correction of these abnormalities may lead to resolution of bleeding, and techniques for endoscopic hemostasis are limited in such patients. Metabolic derangements should also be addressed. Tracheal intubation for airway protection should be considered before upper endoscopy in patients with repeated recent hematemesis and suspected variceal hemorrhage.

Most patients with impressive hematochezia can undergo colonoscopy after a rapid colonic purge with a polyethylene glycol solution; the preparation fluid may be administered via a nasogastric tube. Colonoscopy has a higher diagnostic yield than bleeding scans or angiography in lower gastrointestinal bleeding, and endoscopic therapy can be applied in some cases. In a minority of patients, endoscopic assessment is hindered by poor visualization due to persistent vigorous bleeding with recurrent hemodynamic instability, and other techniques (such as bleeding scans, angiography, or emergency subtotal colectomy) must be employed. In such patients, massive bleeding originating from an upper GI source should be excluded by upper endoscopy. The anal and rectal mucosa should be visualized endoscopically early in the course of massive rectal bleeding, as bleeding lesions in or close to the anal canal may be identified that are often amenable to endoscopic or surgical transanal hemostatic techniques.

Peptic Ulcer

The endoscopic appearance of peptic ulcers provides useful prognostic information and guides the need for endoscopic therapy in patients with acute hemorrhage (Fig. 12-15). A clean-based ulcer is associated with a low 3–5% risk of rebleeding; patients with melena and a clean-based ulcer are often discharged home from the emergency room or endoscopy suite if they are young, reliable, and otherwise healthy. Flat red or purple spots in the ulcer base and large adherent clots covering the ulcer base have a 10 and 20% risk of rebleeding, respectively. Endoscopic therapy is often considered for an ulcer with an adherent clot. When a platelet plug is seen protruding from a vessel wall in the base of an ulcer (so-called sentinel clot or visible vessel), the risk of rebleeding from the ulcer is 40%. This finding generally leads to local endoscopic therapy to decrease the rebleeding rate. Occasionally, active spurting from an ulcer is seen with >90% risk of ongoing bleeding.

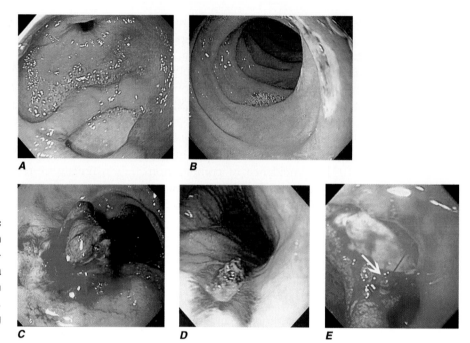

FIGURE 12-15
Stigmata of hemorrhage in peptic ulcers. *A.* Gastric antral ulcer with a clean base. *B.* Duodenal ulcer with flat pigmented spots. *C.* Duodenal ulcer with a dense adherent clot. *D.* Gastric ulcer with a pigmented protuberance/visible vessel. *E.* Duodenal ulcer with active spurting (*arrow*).

Endoscopic therapy of ulcers with high-risk stigmata typically reduces the rebleeding rate to 5–10%. Several hemostatic techniques are available, including injection of epinephrine or sclerosant into and around the vessel, "coaptive coagulation" of the vessel in the base of the ulcer using a thermal probe that is pressed against the site of bleeding, placement of hemoclips, or a combination of these modalities. Proton pump inhibitor therapy also decreases the risk of recurrent hemorrhage and should be administered in patients with endoscopic stigmata of recent bleeding.

Varices

Two complementary strategies guide therapy of bleeding varices: local treatment of the bleeding vessel and treatment of the underlying portal hypertension. Local therapies, including endoscopic sclerotherapy, endoscopic band ligation, and balloon tamponade with a Sengstaken-Blakemore tube, effectively control acute hemorrhage in most patients and are the mainstay of acute treatment, although therapies that decrease portal pressures (pharmacologic treatment, surgical shunts, or radiologically placed intrahepatic shunts) also play an important role.

When feasible, endoscopic band ligation is the preferred local therapy for control of active esophageal variceal bleeding and for subsequent eradication of esophageal varices (**Fig. 12-16**). In this technique a varix is suctioned into a cap fitted on the end of the endoscope, and a rubber band is then released from the cap, ligating the varix. Acute hemorrhage can be controlled in up to 90% of patients, and complications (such as

sepsis, symptomatic esophageal ulceration, or esophageal stenosis) are uncommon. Endoscopic sclerotherapy is another technique in which a sclerosing, thrombogenic solution is injected into or next to the esophageal varices. Sclerotherapy also controls acute hemorrhage in most patients but has a higher complication rate. Bleeding from large gastric fundic varices is best treated by cyanoacrylate ("glue") injection, since band ligation or sclerotherapy of these varices are associated with a high rebleeding rate. These techniques are used when varices are actively bleeding during endoscopy or (more commonly) when varices are the only identifiable cause of acute hemorrhage.

After treatment of the acute hemorrhage, an elective course of endoscopic therapy can be undertaken with the goal of eradicating esophageal varices and preventing rebleeding months to years later. This chronic therapy is less successful, however, preventing long-term rebleeding in ~50% of patients. Pharmacologic therapies that decrease portal pressure have similar efficacy, and the two modalities may be combined.

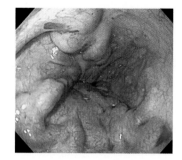

FIGURE 12-16
Esophageal varices.

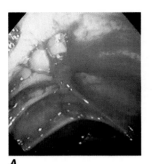
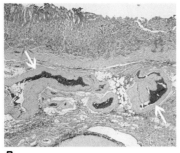

A   **B**

FIGURE 12-17
Dieulafoy's lesion. ***A.*** Actively spurting jejunal Dieulafoy's lesion. There is no underlying mucosal lesion. ***B.*** Histology of a gastric Dieulafoy's lesion. A persistent caliber artery (*arrows*) is present in the gastric submucosa, immediately beneath the mucosa.

Dieulafoy's Lesion

This lesion, also called *persistent caliber artery*, is a large-caliber arteriole that runs immediately beneath the gastrointestinal mucosa and bleeds through a pinpoint mucosal erosion (**Fig. 12-17**). Dieulafoy's lesion is seen most commonly on the lesser curvature of the proximal stomach, causes impressive arterial hemorrhage, and may be difficult to diagnose; it is often recognized only after repeated endoscopy for recurrent bleeding. Endoscopic therapy is typically effective for control of bleeding and ablation of the underlying vessel once the lesion has been identified. Angiographic embolization or surgical over-sewing is considered when endoscopic therapy has failed.

Mallory-Weiss Tear

A Mallory-Weiss tear is a linear mucosal rent near or across the gastroesophageal junction that is often associated with retching or vomiting (**Fig. 12-18**). When the tear disrupts a submucosal arteriole, brisk hemorrhage may result. Endoscopy is the best diagnostic method, and an actively bleeding tear can be treated endoscopically with epinephrine injection, coaptive coagulation, hemoclips, or band ligation. Unlike peptic ulcer, a Mallory-Weiss tear with a nonbleeding sentinel clot in its base rarely rebleeds and thus does not require endoscopic therapy.

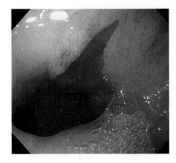

FIGURE 12-18
Mallory-Weiss tear at the gastroesophageal junction.

Vascular Ectasias

Vascular ectasias are flat mucosal vascular anomalies that are best diagnosed by endoscopy. They usually cause slow intestinal blood loss and have several characteristic distributions in the gastrointestinal tract (**Fig. 12-19**). Cecal vascular ectasias (senile lesions), gastric antral vascular ectasias ("watermelon stomach"), and radiation-induced rectal ectasias are often responsive to local endoscopic ablative therapy, such as argon plasma coagulation (APC). Patients with diffuse small-bowel vascular ectasias (associated with chronic renal failure and hereditary hemorrhagic telangiectasia) may continue to bleed despite endoscopic treatment of easily accessible lesions by conventional endoscopy. These patients may benefit from double balloon enteroscopy with endoscopic therapy, pharmacologic treatment with octreotide or estrogen/progesterone therapy, or intraoperative enteroscopy.

Colonic Diverticula

Diverticula form where nutrient arteries penetrate the muscular wall of the colon en route to the colonic mucosa. The artery found in the base or neck of a diverticulum may bleed, causing painless and impressive hematochezia. Colonoscopy is indicated in patients with hematochezia and suspected diverticular hemorrhage, since other causes of bleeding (such as vascular ectasias, colitis, and colon cancer) must be excluded. In addition, an actively bleeding diverticulum may be seen and treated during colonoscopy.

GASTROINTESTINAL OBSTRUCTION AND PSEUDOOBSTRUCTION

Endoscopy is useful for evaluation and treatment of several causes of gastrointestinal obstruction. An important exception is small-bowel obstruction due to surgical adhesions, which is generally not diagnosed or treated endoscopically. Esophageal, gastroduodenal, and colonic obstruction or pseudoobstruction can all be diagnosed and often managed endoscopically.

Acute Esophageal Obstruction

Esophageal obstruction by impacted food or an ingested foreign body is a potentially life-threatening event and represents an endoscopic emergency. Left untreated, the patient may develop esophageal ulceration, ischemia, and perforation. Patients with persistent esophageal obstruction often have hypersalivation and are usually unable to swallow water; endoscopy is generally the best initial test in such patients, since endoscopic removal of the obstructing material is usually possible, and the presence of underlying esophageal pathology can often be determined. Radiographs of the chest and neck should be considered before endoscopy in patients with fever,

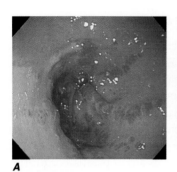 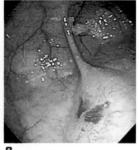 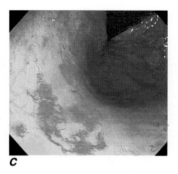

FIGURE 12-19

Gastrointestinal vascular ectasias. *A.* Gastric antral vascular ectasias, or "watermelon stomach," characterized by prominent flat or raised red angioectatic stripes radiating in a spoke-like fashion from the pylorus to the antrum. ***B.*** Cecal vascular ectasias. ***C.*** Radiation-induced vascular ectasias of the rectum in a patient previously treated for prostate cancer.

obstruction for ≥24 h, or ingestion of a sharp object such as a fishbone. Radiographic contrast studies interfere with subsequent endoscopy and are not advisable in most patients with a clinical picture of esophageal obstruction. Occasionally, sublingual nifedipine or nitrates, or intravenous glucagon, may resolve an esophageal food impaction, but in most patients an underlying web, ring, or stricture is present, and endoscopic removal of the obstructing food bolus is necessary.

Gastric Outlet Obstruction

Obstruction of the gastric outlet is commonly caused by malignancy of the prepyloric gastric antrum or chronic peptic ulceration with stenosis of the pylorus. Patients vomit partially digested food many hours after eating. Gastric decompression with a nasogastric tube and subsequent lavage for removal of retained material is the first step in treatment. The diagnosis can then be confirmed with a saline load test, if desired. Endoscopy is useful for diagnosis and treatment. Patients with benign pyloric stenosis may be treated with endoscopic balloon dilation of the pylorus, and a course of endoscopic dilation results in long-term relief of symptoms in about 50% of patients. Malignant pyloric obstruction can be palliated with endoscopically placed expandable stents in a patient with an inoperable malignancy.

Colonic Obstruction and Pseudoobstruction

These both present with abdominal distention and discomfort; tympany; and a dilated, air-filled colon on plain abdominal radiography. The radiographic appearance can be characteristic of a particular cause, such as sigmoid volvulus (**Fig. 12-20**). Both structural obstruction and pseudoobstruction may lead to colonic perforation if untreated. Acute colonic pseudoobstruction is a form of colonic ileus that is usually attributable to electrolyte disorders, narcotic and anticholinergic medications, immobility

(as after surgery), and retroperitoneal hemorrhage or mass. Multiple causative factors are often present. Either colonoscopy or a water-soluble contrast enema may be used to look for an obstructing lesion and differentiate obstruction from pseudoobstruction. One of these diagnostic studies should be strongly considered if the patient does not have clear risk factors for pseudoobstruction, if radiographs do not show air in the rectum, or if the patient fails to improve when the underlying causes of pseudoobstruction have been addressed. The risk of cecal perforation in pseudoobstruction rises when the cecal diameter exceeds 12 cm, and in such patients decompression of the colon may be achieved using intravenous neostigmine, colonoscopic decompression, or placement of a cecostomy tube. Most patients should receive a trial of conservative therapy (with correction of electrolyte disorders, removal of offending medications, and increased mobilization) before undergoing an invasive decompressive procedure for colonic pseudoobstruction.

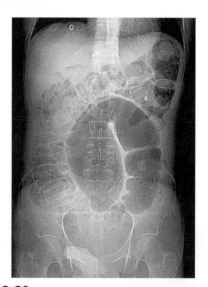

FIGURE 12-20

Sigmoid volvulus with the characteristic radiologic appearance of a "bent inner tube."

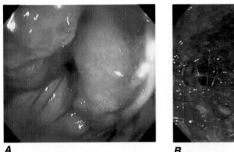
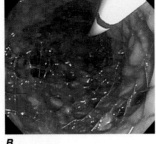
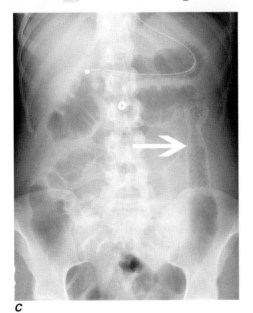

FIGURE 12-21

Obstructing colonic carcinoma. *A.* Colonic adenocarcinoma causing marked luminal narrowing of the descending colon. ***B.*** Endoscopic placement of a self-expanding metal stent. ***C.*** Radiograph of expanded stent across the obstructing tumor with a residual waist (*arrow*). (*Image A courtesy of Dr. Glenn Alexander; with permission.*)

Colonic obstruction is an indication for urgent intervention. Emergency diverting colostomy may be performed with a subsequent second operation after bowel preparation to treat the underlying cause of obstruction. Colonoscopic placement of an expandable stent is an alternative that can relieve the malignant obstruction without emergency surgery and permit bowel preparation for an elective one-stage operation (**Fig. 12–21**).

ACUTE BILIARY OBSTRUCTION

The steady, severe pain that occurs when a gallstone acutely obstructs the common bile duct often brings patients to a hospital. The diagnosis of a ductal stone is suspected when the patient is jaundiced or when serum liver tests or pancreatic enzyme levels are elevated; it is confirmed by direct cholangiography (performed endoscopically, percutaneously, or during surgery). ERCP is currently the primary means of diagnosing and treating

Bile Duct Imaging

While transabdominal ultrasound diagnoses only a minority of bile duct stones, magnetic resonance cholangiopancreatography (MRCP) and EUS are >90% accurate and have an important role in diagnosis. Examples of these modalities are shown in **Fig. 12–22**.

If the suspicion for a bile duct stone is high and urgent treatment is required (as in a patient with jaundice and biliary sepsis), ERCP is the procedure of choice, since it remains the gold standard for diagnosis and provides immediate treatment. If a persistent bile duct stone is unlikely (as in a patient with gallstone pancreatitis), ERCP may be supplanted by less-invasive, safer imaging techniques.

Ascending Cholangitis

Charcot's triad of jaundice, abdominal pain, and fever is present in about 70% of patients with ascending cholangitis and biliary sepsis. Initially, such patients are managed with fluid resuscitation and intravenous antibiotics. Abdominal ultrasound is often done to look for gallbladder stones and bile duct dilation. However, the bile duct may not be dilated early in the course of acute biliary obstruction. Medical management usually improves the patient's clinical status, providing a window of approximately 24 h during which biliary drainage should be established, typically by ERCP. Undue delay can result in recrudescence of overt sepsis and increased morbidity. In addition to Charcot's triad, the presence of shock and confusion (Reynolds' pentad) should prompt urgent attempts at restoring biliary drainage.

Gallstone Pancreatitis

Gallstones may cause acute pancreatitis as they pass through the ampulla of Vater. The occurrence of gallstone pancreatitis usually implies passage of a stone into the duodenum, and only about 20% of patients harbor a persistent stone in the ampulla or the common bile duct. Retained stones are more common in patients with jaundice, rising serum liver tests following hospitalization, severe pancreatitis, or superimposed ascending cholangitis.

Urgent ERCP decreases the morbidity of gallstone pancreatitis in some subsets of patients. It remains unclear whether the benefit of ERCP is mainly attributable to treatment and prevention of ascending cholangitis or to relief of pancreatic duct obstruction. ERCP is warranted early in the course of gallstone pancreatitis if ascending cholangitis is also suspected, especially in a jaundiced patient. Urgent ERCP also appears to benefit

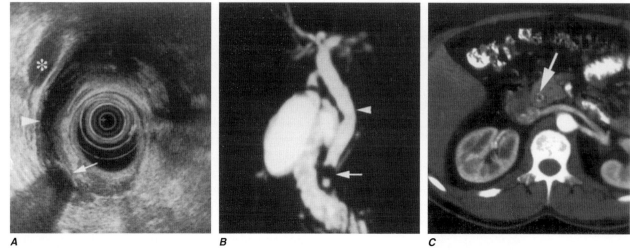

FIGURE 12-22

Methods of bile duct imaging. Arrows mark bile duct stones. Arrowheads indicate the common bile duct, and the asterisk marks the portal vein. **A.** Endoscopic ultrasound (EUS). **B.** Magnetic resonance cholangiopancreatography (MRCP). **C.** CT.

patients predicted to have severe pancreatitis using a clinical index of severity such as the Glasgow or Ranson score.

ELECTIVE ENDOSCOPY

DYSPEPSIA AND REFLUX

Dyspepsia is a chronic or recurrent burning discomfort or pain in the upper abdomen that may be caused by diverse processes such as gastroesophageal reflux, peptic ulcer disease, and "nonulcer dyspepsia," a heterogeneous category that includes disorders of motility, sensation, and somatization. Gastric and esophageal malignancies are less-common causes of dyspepsia. Careful history-taking allows accurate differential diagnosis of dyspepsia in only about half of patients. In the remainder, endoscopy can be a useful diagnostic tool, especially in those patients whose symptoms are not resolved by an empirical trial of symptomatic treatment.

GASTROESOPHAGEAL REFLUX DISEASE (GERD)

When classic symptoms of gastroesophageal reflux are present, such as water brash and substernal heartburn, presumptive diagnosis and empirical treatment are often sufficient. Although endoscopy is sensitive for diagnosis of esophagitis (Fig. 12-23), it can miss cases of nonerosive reflux disease (NERD), since some patients have symptomatic reflux without esophagitis. The most sensitive test for diagnosis of GERD is 24-h ambulatory pH monitoring. To assess the esophagus and exclude other diseases, endoscopy is indicated in patients with reflux symptoms refractory to medical therapy; in those with

alarm symptoms such as dysphagia, weight loss, or gastrointestinal bleeding; and in those with recurrent dyspepsia after treatment that is not clearly due to reflux on clinical grounds alone. Endoscopy may be indicated in patients with long-standing (≥10 years) frequent heartburn, who are at sixfold increased risk of Barrett's esophagus compared to a patient with <1 year of reflux

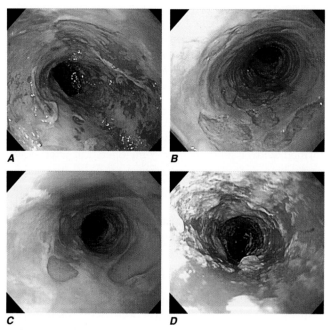

FIGURE 12-23

Causes of esophagitis. A. Severe reflux esophagitis with mucosal ulceration and friability. **B.** Cytomegalovirus esophagitis. **C.** Herpes simplex virus esophagitis with numerous shallow ulcerations. **D.** Candida esophagitis with white plaques adherent to the esophageal mucosa.

symptoms. Patients with Barrett's esophagus (Fig. 12-3) usually enter a program of periodic endoscopy with biopsies to detect dysplasia or early carcinoma. Endoscopic treatments for GERD have been developed as alternatives to pharmacologic and laparoscopic therapies, and their role in the treatment of patients is still being assessed.

PEPTIC ULCER

Peptic ulcer classically causes epigastric gnawing or burning, often occurring nocturnally and promptly relieved by food or antacids. Although endoscopy is the most sensitive diagnostic test for peptic ulcer, it is not a cost-effective strategy in young patients with ulcer-like dyspeptic symptoms unless endoscopy is available at low cost. Patients with suspected peptic ulcer should be evaluated for *Helicobacter pylori* infection. Serology (past or present infection), urea breath testing (current infection), and stool tests are less invasive and costly than endoscopy with biopsy. Patients with alarm symptoms and those with persistent symptoms despite treatment should undergo endoscopy to exclude gastric malignancy and other etiologies.

NONULCER DYSPEPSIA

Nonulcer dyspepsia may be associated with bloating and, unlike peptic ulcer, tends not to remit and recur. Most patients obtain little relief with acid-reducing, prokinetic, or anti-*Helicobacter* therapy, and they are typically referred for endoscopy to exclude a refractory ulcer and assess for other causes. Although endoscopy is useful for excluding other diagnoses, its impact on the treatment of patients with nonulcer dyspepsia is marginal.

DYSPHAGIA

About 50% of patients with difficulty swallowing have a mechanical obstruction; the remainder have a motility disorder, such as achalasia or diffuse esophageal spasm. Careful history-taking often suggests a diagnosis and leads to the appropriate use of diagnostic tests. Esophageal strictures (Fig. 12-24) typically cause progressive dysphagia, first for solids, then for liquids; motility disorders often cause inter-

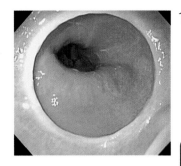

FIGURE 12-25
Schatzki's ring at the gas-troesophageal junction.

mittent dysphagia for both solids and liquids. Some underlying disorders have characteristic historic features: Schatzki's ring (Fig. 12-25) causes episodic dysphagia for solids, typically at the beginning of a meal; pharyngeal motor disorders are associated with difficulty initiating deglutition ("transfer dysphagia") and nasal reflux or coughing with swallowing; and achalasia may cause nocturnal regurgitation of undigested food.

When mechanical obstruction is suspected, endoscopy is a useful initial diagnostic test, since it permits immediate biopsy and/or dilation of strictures, masses, or rings. The presence of multiple corrugated rings throughout a narrowed esophagus should raise suspicion for eosinophilic esophagitis, an increasingly recognized cause of recurrent dysphagia and food impaction (Fig. 12-26). Blind or forceful passage of an endoscope may lead to perforation in a patient with stenosis of the cervical esophagus or a Zencker's diverticulum, but gentle passage of an endoscope under direct visual guidance is reasonably safe. Endoscopy can miss a subtle stricture or ring in some patients.

When a motility disorder is suspected, esophageal radiography and/or a video-swallow study are the best initial diagnostic tests. The pharyngeal swallowing mechanism, esophageal peristalsis, and the lower esophageal sphincter can all be assessed. In some disorders, subsequent esophageal manometry may also be important for diagnosis.

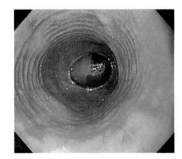

FIGURE 12-26
Eosinophilic esophagitis with multiple circular rings of the esophagus creating a corrugated appearance, and an impacted grape at the narrowed esophagogastric junction. The diagnosis requires biopsy with histologic finding of ≥20 eosinophils/high-power field.

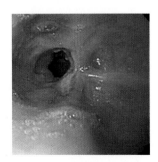

FIGURE 12-24
Peptic esophageal stricture associated with ulceration and scarring of the distal esophagus.

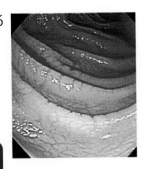

FIGURE 12-27
Scalloped duodenal folds in a patient with celiac sprue.

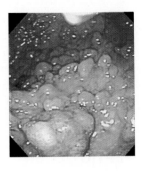

FIGURE 12-29
Innumerable colon polyps of various sizes in a patient with familial adenomatous polyposis syndrome.

ANEMIA AND OCCULT BLOOD IN THE STOOL

Iron-deficiency anemia may be attributed to poor iron absorption (as in celiac sprue) or, more commonly, chronic blood loss. Intestinal bleeding should be strongly suspected in men and postmenopausal women with iron-deficiency anemia, and colonoscopy is indicated in such patients, even in the absence of detectable occult blood in the stool. Approximately 30% of patients will have colon polyps, 10% will have colorectal cancer, and a few additional patients will have colonic vascular lesions. When a convincing source of blood loss is not found in the colon, upper gastrointestinal endoscopy should be considered; if no lesion is found, duodenal biopsies should be obtained to exclude sprue (**Fig. 12-27**). Small bowel evaluation with capsule endoscopy may be appropriate if both EGD and colonoscopy are unrevealing (**Fig. 12-28**).

Tests for occult blood in the stool detect hemoglobin or the heme moiety and are most sensitive for colonic blood loss, although they will also detect larger amounts of upper gastrointestinal bleeding. Patients over age 50 with occult blood in normal-appearing stool should undergo colonoscopy to diagnose or exclude colorectal neoplasia. The diagnostic yield is lower than in iron-deficiency anemia. Whether upper endoscopy is also indicated depends on the patient's symptoms.

The small intestine may be the source of chronic intestinal bleeding, especially if colonoscopy and upper endoscopy are not diagnostic. The utility of small-bowel evaluation varies with the clinical setting and is most important in patients in whom bleeding causes chronic

or recurrent anemia. While small-bowel radiography is usually of low diagnostic yield, capsule endoscopy provides a specific diagnosis in about 50% of such patients (Fig. 12-28). The most common finding is mucosal vascular ectasias.

COLORECTAL CANCER SCREENING

The majority of colon cancers develop from preexisting colonic adenomas, and colorectal cancer can be largely prevented by the detection and removal of adenomatous polyps. The choice of screening strategy for an asymptomatic person depends on his or her personal and family history. Individuals with inflammatory bowel disease, a history of colorectal polyps, family members with adenomatous polyps or cancer, or certain familial syndromes (**Fig. 12-29**) are at increased risk for colon cancer. An individual without these factors is generally considered at average risk.

Screening strategies are summarized in **Table 12-2**. While stool tests for occult blood have been shown to decrease mortality from colorectal cancer, they do not detect some cancers and many polyps, and direct visualization of the colon is a more effective screening strategy. Either sigmoidoscopy or colonoscopy may be used for cancer screening in asymptomatic average-risk patients. The use of sigmoidoscopy was based on the historic finding that the majority of colorectal cancers occurred in the rectum and left colon and that patients with right-sided colon cancers had left-sided polyps. Over the past several decades, however, the distribution of colon cancers has changed, with proportionally fewer rectal and left-sided cancers than in the past. Large studies of colonoscopy for screening of average-risk individuals show that cancers are roughly equally distributed between left and right colon, and half of patients with right-sided lesions have no polyps in the left colon. Visualization of the entire colon thus appears to be the optimal strategy for colorectal cancer screening and prevention.

Virtual colonoscopy (VC) is a radiologic technique that images the colon with CT following rectal insufflation of the colonic lumen. Computer rendering of CT images generates an electronic display of a virtual "flight" along the colonic lumen, simulating colonoscopy (**Fig. 12-30**).

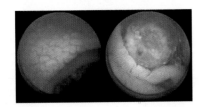

FIGURE 12-28
Capsule endoscopy images of a mildly scalloped jejunal fold (*left*) and an ileal tumor (*right*) in a patient with celiac sprue. (*Images courtesy of Dr. Elizabeth Rajan; with permission.*)

TABLE 12-2

107

COLORECTAL CANCER SCREENING STRATEGIES

	RECOMMENDATION	COMMENTS
Average-Risk Patients		
Asymptomatic individuals ≥50 years of age	Annual fecal occult blood testing, two samples from each of three consecutive stools	Fails to detect many polyps and some cancers
	Flexible sigmoidoscopy every 5 years *or*	Fails to detect some polyps and cancers
	Colonoscopy every 10 years	CT colonography may become a reasonable alternative (see text)
	Double-contrast barium enema every 5 years	Less sensitivity than colonoscopy for polyps and cancer
High-Risk Patients		
Personal history: colon cancer	Evaluate entire colon around the time of resection, then colonoscopy in 3 years	
Personal history: advanced, large, or fewer than three adenomas, completely removed	Repeat colonoscopy in 3 years	
One or two small tubular adenomas	Repeat colonoscopy in 5 years	
Personal history: long-standing (>8 years) extensive ulcerative colitis or Chrohn's colitis, or left-sided ulcerative colitis >15 years' duration	Colonoscopy with biopsies every 1–3 years	
Family history: first-degree relative with colorectal cancer or adenomatous polyp at age ≥60 years, or two second-degree relatives with a history of colorectal cancer	Same as average risk, but start at age 40	
Family history: fewer than two first-degree relatives with colon cancer, or a single first-degree relative with colon cancer or adenomatous polyps diagnosed at an age <60 years	Colonoscopy every 5 years beginning at age 40 or 10 years younger than the earliest diagnosis in the family, whichever comes first	
Family history: one second-degree or third-degree relative with colorectal cancer	Same as average risk	
Family history: familial adenomatous polyposis	Sigmoidoscopy annually, beginning at age 10–12 years	Consider genetic counseling and testing
Family history: hereditary nonpolyposis colorectal cancer (HNPCC)	Colonoscopy every 1–2 years, beginning at age 20–25 years or 10 years younger than the earliest case in the family, whichever comes first	Consider genetic counseling and testing

Source: Adapted from S Winawer et al: Colonorectal cancer screening and surveillance: clinical guidelines and rationale-update based on new evidence. Gastroenterology 124:544, 2003; with permission from the American Gastroenterological Association.

Most comparative studies of VC and conventional colonoscopy have shown that VC lacks adequate sensitivity for polyps, but technical refinements have improved its performance characteristics, and in one study it detected more polyps than conventional colonoscopy. VC may become more widely used for colorectal cancer screening, particularly at institutions with demonstrated skill with this technique. Findings detected during VC often require subsequent conventional colonoscopy for confirmation and treatment.

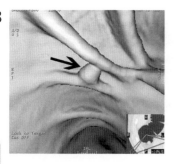

FIGURE 12-30
Virtual colonoscopy image of a colon polyp (*arrow*). *(Image courtesy of Dr. Jeff Fidler; with permission.)*

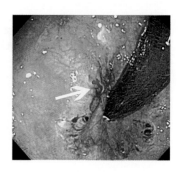

FIGURE 12-31
Internal hemorrhoids with bleeding (*arrow*) as seen on a retroflexed view of the rectum.

DIARRHEA

Most cases of diarrhea are acute, self-limited, and due to infections or medication. Chronic diarrhea (lasting >6 weeks) is more often due to a primary inflammatory, malabsorptive, or motility disorder; is less likely to resolve spontaneously; and generally requires diagnostic evaluation. Patients with chronic diarrhea or severe, unexplained acute diarrhea often undergo endoscopy if stool tests for pathogens are unrevealing. The choice of endoscopic testing depends on the clinical setting.

Patients with colonic symptoms and findings such as bloody diarrhea, tenesmus, fever, or stool leukocytes generally undergo sigmoidoscopy or colonoscopy to search for colitis (Fig. 12-4). Sigmoidoscopy is often adequate and is the best initial test in most of these patients. On the other hand, patients with symptoms and findings suggestive of small-bowel disease, such as large-volume watery stools, substantial weight loss, and malabsorption of iron, calcium, or fat, may undergo upper endoscopy with duodenal biopsies and aspirates.

Many patients with chronic diarrhea do not fit either of these patterns. In the setting of a long-standing history of alternating constipation and diarrhea dating to early adulthood, without findings such as blood in the stool or anemia, a diagnosis of irritable bowel syndrome may be made without direct visualization of the bowel. Steatorrhea and upper abdominal pain may prompt evaluation of the pancreas rather than the gut. Patients whose chronic diarrhea is not easily categorized often undergo initial colonoscopy to examine the entire colon and terminal ileum for inflammatory or neoplastic disease.

MINOR HEMATOCHEZIA

Bright red blood passed with or on formed brown stool usually has a rectal, anal, or distal sigmoid source (**Fig. 12-31**). Patients with even trivial amounts of hematochezia should be investigated with flexible sigmoidoscopy and anoscopy to exclude large polyps or cancers in the distal bowel. Patients reporting red blood on the toilet tissue only, without blood in the toilet or on the stool, are generally bleeding from a lesion in the anal canal. Careful external inspection, digital examination, and anoscopy are sufficient for diagnosis in most cases.

PANCREATITIS

Approximately 20% of patients with pancreatitis have no identifiable cause after routine clinical investigation (including a review of medication and alcohol use, measurement of serum triglyceride and calcium levels, abdominal ultrasonography, and CT). Endoscopic techniques lead to a specific diagnosis in the majority of such patients, often altering clinical management. Endoscopic investigation is particularly appropriate if the patient has had more than one episode of pancreatitis.

Microlithiasis, or the presence of microscopic crystals in bile, is a leading cause of previously unexplained acute pancreatitis and is sometimes seen during abdominal ultrasonography as layering sludge or flecks of floating, echogenic material in the gallbladder. Gallbladder bile can be obtained for microscopic analysis by administering a cholecystokinin analogue during endoscopy, causing contraction of the gallbladder. Bile is suctioned from the duodenum as it drains from the papilla, and the darkest fraction is examined for cholesterol crystals or bilirubinate granules. Combined EUS of the gallbladder and bile microscopy is probably the most sensitive means of diagnosing microlithiasis.

Previously undetected chronic pancreatitis, pancreatic malignancy, or pancreas divisum may be diagnosed by either ERCP or EUS. Sphincter of Oddi dysfunction probably causes some cases of pancreatitis and can be diagnosed by manometric studies performed during ERCP.

Severe pancreatitis often results in pancreatic fluid collections. Both pseudocysts and areas of organized pancreatic necrosis can be drained into the stomach or duodenum endoscopically, using transpapillary and transmural endoscopic techniques.

CANCER STAGING

Local staging of esophageal, gastric, pancreatic, bile duct, and rectal cancers can be obtained with EUS (Fig. 12-13). EUS with fine-needle aspiration (Fig. 12-14) currently provides the most accurate preoperative assessment of local tumor and nodal staging, but it does not detect most distant metastases. Details of the local tumor stage can guide treatment decisions including resectability and need for neoadjuvant therapy. EUS with transesophageal needle biopsy may also be used to assess the presence of non-small cell lung cancer in mediastinal nodes.

OPEN-ACCESS ENDOSCOPY

Direct scheduling of endoscopic procedures by primary care physicians without preceding gastroenterology consultation, or *open-access endoscopy*, is an increasingly common practice. When the indications for endoscopy are clear-cut and appropriate, the procedural risks are low, and the patient understands what to expect, open-access endoscopy streamlines patient care and decreases costs.

Patients referred for open-access endoscopy should have a recent history, physical examination, and medication review. A copy of such an evaluation should be available when the patient comes to the endoscopy suite. Patients with unstable cardiovascular or respiratory conditions should not be referred directly for open-access endoscopy. Patients with selected cardiac conditions undergoing certain procedures should be prescribed prophylactic antibiotics prior to endoscopy (Table 12-1). In addition, patients on anticoagulants and antiplatelet drugs may require adjustment of these agents before endoscopy (Table 12-3). Most evidence suggests that, in the absence of a preexisting bleeding disorder, it is safe to perform endoscopic procedures in patients taking aspirin and nonsteroidal anti-inflammatory drugs. Little data are available regarding the risks of hemorrhage in patients receiving clopidogrel who undergo endoscopic biopsy or therapy, but current guidelines advise discontinuation of this agent at least 5 days before elective endoscopic procedures.

Common indications for open-access EGD include dyspepsia resistant to a trial of appropriate therapy, gastrointestinal bleeding, and persistent anorexia or early satiety. Open-access colonoscopy is often requested in men or postmenopausal women with iron-deficiency anemia, in patients over age 50 with occult blood in the stool, in patients with a previous history of colorectal adenomatous polyps or cancer, and for colorectal cancer screening. Flexible sigmoidoscopy is commonly performed as an open-access procedure.

When patients are referred for open-access colonoscopy, the primary care provider may need to choose a colonic preparation. Commonly used oral preparations include polyethylene glycol lavage solution and oral sodium phosphate. Sodium phosphate may cause fluid and electrolyte abnormalities, especially in patients with renal failure or congestive heart failure and those over 70 years of age.

FURTHER READINGS

BARON TH: Expandable metal stents for the treatment of cancerous obstruction of the gastrointestinal tract. N Engl J Med 344:1681, 2001

BHAT YM et al: Transluminal endosurgery: novel use of endoscopic tacks for the closure of access sites in natural orifice transluminal endoscopic surgery. Gastrointest Endosc 69:1161, 2009

TABLE 12-3

MANAGEMENT OF ANTICOAGULANTS AND ANTIPLATELET DRUGS BEFORE ENDOSCOPIC PROCEDURES

DRUG	PROCEDURAL RISK OF BLEEDING[a,b]	HIGH PATIENT RISK OF THROMBOEMBOLISM[c]	LOW PATIENT RISK OF THROMBOEMBOLISM[d]
Warfarin	High	Stop warfarin 3–5 days before the procedure; consider heparin while INR is below the therapeutic range	Stop warfarin 3–5 days before the procedure; restart warfarin after the procedure
	Low	No change in anticoagulation; elective procedures should be delayed while INR is in the supratherapeutic range	
Low molecular weight heparin	High	Consider discontinuation at least 8 h before procedure	
	Low	No change in therapy	
Clopidogrel or ticlopidine	High	Consider discontinuation 5–10 days before procedure	
	Low	No change in therapy	
Aspirin	High or Low	No change in therapy	

[a]High-risk procedures: Polypectomy, stricture dilation, treatment of varices, gastrostomy tube placement, biliary sphincterotomy, endoscopic ultrasound (EUS) with fine-needle aspiration (FNA), laser ablation and coagulation.
[b]Low-risk procedures: Diagnostic upper endoscopy, colonoscopy, or sigmoidoscopy, with or without biopsy; endoscopic retrograde cholangiopancreatography (ERCP) without endoscopic sphincterotomy; EUS without FNA.
[c]High-risk conditions: Atrial fibrillation associated with valvular heart disease, mechanical valve in the mitral position, mechanical valve and prior thromboembolic event.
[d]Low-risk conditions: Uncomplicated or paroxysmal nonvalvular atrial fibrillation, mechanical valve in the aortic position, bioprosthetic valve, deep vein thrombosis.
Note: INR, international normalized ratio.
Source: Adapted from G Eisen et al: Guideline on the management of anticoagulation and antiplatelet therapy for endoscopic procedures. Gastrointest Endosc 55:775, 2002; and from M Zuckerman et al: ASGE guideline: The management of low molecular weight heparin and nonaspirin antiplatelet agents for endoscopic procedures. Gastrointest Endosc 61:189, 2005; with permission.

110 Hu WH et al: Comparison between empirical prokinetics, helicobacter test-and-treat and empirical endoscopy in primary-care patients presenting with dyspepsia: A one-year study. World J Gastroenterol 12:5010, 2006

Imperiale TF et al: Risk of advanced proximal neoplasms in asymptomatic adults according to the distal colorectal findings. N Engl J Med 343:169, 2000

Jensen DM et al: Urgent colonoscopy for the diagnosis and treatment of severe diverticular hemorrhage. N Engl J Med 342:78, 2000

Lin S, Rockey DC: Obscure gastrointestinal bleeding. Gastroenterol Clin North Am 34:679–98, 2005

Pennazio M: Enteroscopy in the diagnosis and management of obscure gastrointestinal bleeding. Gastrointest Endosc Clin N Am 19:409, 2009

Respici A et al: Endoscopic mucosal resection for early colorectal neoplasia: pathologic basis, procedures, and outcome. Dis Colon Rectum 52:1502, 2009

Rosman AS, Horsten MA: Meta-analysis comparing CT colonography, air contrast barium enema, and colonoscopy. Am J Med 120:203, 2007

Semrad CE: Small bowel enteroscopy: territory conquered, future horizons. Curr Opin Gastroenterol 25:110, 2009

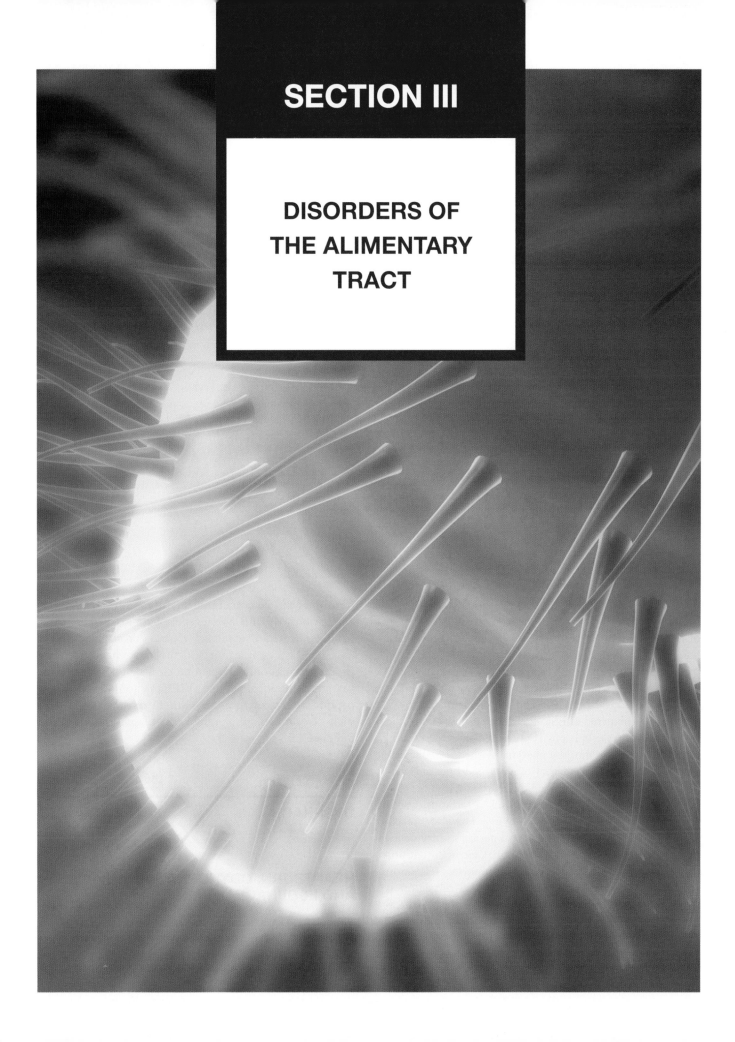

SECTION III

DISORDERS OF THE ALIMENTARY TRACT

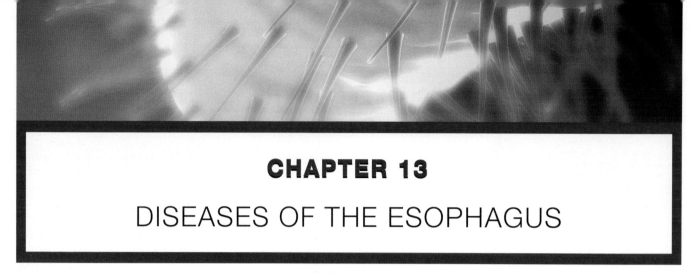

CHAPTER 13

DISEASES OF THE ESOPHAGUS

Raj K. Goyal

Two major functions of the esophagus are transport of food bolus from the mouth to the stomach and prevention of retrograde flow of gastrointestinal contents. Esophageal transport function begins with the transfer of food from the mouth and pharynx through the opened upper esophageal sphincter (UES) into the esophagus, and it involves esophageal peristalsis and relaxation of the lower esophageal sphincter (LES). Retrograde flow from the stomach into the esophagus is prevented by the LES and from the esophagus into the pharynx by the UES. Physiology of swallowing, esophageal motility, and oral and pharyngeal dysphagia are described in Chap. 4.

Normally, the LES relaxes in association with esophageal peristalsis with swallowing. However, relaxation of the LES without esophageal peristalsis may occur during belching and gastric distention. Gastric distention-evoked transient lower esophageal sphincter relaxation (tLESR) is a vagovagal reflex. Reflex LES relaxation is augmented by phosphodiesterase-5 inhibitors such as sildenafil that increase cyclic guanosine monophosphate (cGMP) in the sphincter muscle, and it is inhibited by GABA-B agonists such as baclofen. Fatty meals, smoking, and beverages with high xanthine content (tea, coffee, cola) also cause a reduction in sphincter pressure. Many

hormones and neurotransmitters can modify LES pressure. Muscarinic M_2 and M_3 receptor agonists, α-adrenergic agonists, gastrin, substance P, and prostaglandin $F_2\alpha$ all cause LES contraction. On the other hand, nicotine, β-adrenergic agonists, dopamine, cholecystokinin, secretin, vasoactive intestinal peptide (VIP), calcitonin gene-related peptide, adenosine, prostaglandin E, nitric oxide donors such as nitrates, and inhibitors of phosphodiesterase 5 reduce LES pressure.

SYMPTOMS

DYSPHAGIA

See Chap. 4.

HEARTBURN, ODYNOPHAGIA, AND ESOPHAGEAL PAIN

Heartburn, or pyrosis, is characterized by burning retrosternal discomfort that may move up and down the chest like a wave. When severe, it may radiate to the sides of the chest, the neck, and the angles of the jaw. Heartburn is a characteristic symptom of *reflux esophagitis* and may be associated with regurgitation or a feeling of warm fluid climbing up the throat. It is aggravated by bending forward, straining, or lying recumbent and is worse after meals. It is relieved by an upright posture, by the swallowing of saliva or water, and, more reliably, by antacids. Heartburn is produced by heightened mucosal sensitivity and can be reproduced by infusion of dilute (0.1 N) hydrochloric acid (Bernstein test) or neutral hyperosmolar solutions into the esophagus.

Odynophagia, or painful swallowing, is characteristic of nonreflux esophagitis (particularly monilial), herpes, and pill-induced esophagitis. Odynophagia may occur with peptic ulcer of the esophagus (Barrett's ulcer), carcinoma with periesophageal involvement, caustic damage of the esophagus, and esophageal perforation. Odynophagia is unusual in uncomplicated reflux esophagitis. Crampy chest pain associated with a food bolus impaction should be distinguished from odynophagia.

Esophageal chest pain resembling cardiac pain is called *noncardiac chest pain* or *atypical chest pain*. Such pain is different from heartburn or odynophagia, and it may occur in gastroesophageal reflux disease (GERD) or esophageal motility disorders such as diffuse esophageal spasm (DES). Chest pain due to periesophageal involvement with carcinoma or peptic ulcer may be constant and agonizing. Sometimes different types of esophageal pains exist concomitantly in the same patient, and frequently patients are not able to describe the pain accurately enough to allow its classification. Coronary artery disease should always be excluded before the esophagus is considered as the origin of atypical chest pain. The most frequent esophageal cause of chest pain is reflux esophagitis. Therefore, studies to investigate GERD should be performed. A trial of proton pump inhibitors (PPIs) is usual; an esophageal motility study may be useful in these cases. A few patients with atypical chest pain are found to have DES or achalasia. However, achalasia usually has associated dysphagia. Some patients have nonspecific esophageal motor abnormalities of uncertain significance. Smooth-muscle relaxants may be tried in selected cases. However, a large number of these patients are thought to have esophageal hypersensitivity syndrome, which can be revealed by a low threshold of pain production by esophageal balloon distension. A low-dose antidepressant treatment may be helpful in these cases. Many of these patients also have behavioral and psychosomatic disorders such as depression, anxiety, or panic reactions.

REGURGITATION

Regurgitation is the effortless appearance of gastric or esophageal contents in the mouth. In distal esophageal obstruction and stasis, as in achalasia or the presence of a large diverticulum, the regurgitated material consists of tasteless mucoid fluid or undigested food. Regurgitation of sour or bitter-tasting material occurs in severe gastroesophageal reflux and is associated with incompetence of both the UES and the LES. Regurgitation may result in chronic cough, laryngitis, and laryngeal aspiration, with spells of coughing and choking that may awaken the patient from sleep. It may also result in aspiration pneumonia. In some patients, regurgitation and rumination may be a behavioral problem. Water brash is reflex salivary hypersecretion that occurs in response to peptic esophagitis and should not be confused with regurgitation.

DIAGNOSTIC TESTS

RADIOLOGIC STUDIES

Barium swallow with fluoroscopy and an esophagogram is often used to evaluate both structural and motor disorders and is the initial test of choice in the motility disorders. Videofluoroscopic swallow study focuses on oral and pharyngeal phases of swallowing (Chap. 4). A finding of spontaneous reflux of barium from the stomach into the esophagus as an indicator of gastroesophageal reflux is unreliable. Esophageal peristalsis is best studied in the recumbent position, because in the upright position barium passage occurs largely by gravity alone. A double-contrast esophagogram, obtained by coating the esophageal mucosa with barium and distending the esophageal lumen with air using effervescent granules, is particularly useful in demonstrating mucosal ulcers and early cancers. A barium-soaked piece of bread or a 13-mm barium tablet is sometimes used to demonstrate an obstructive lesion. **Figures 13-1** and **13-2** illustrate the radiographic appearance of some structural and motor disorders of the esophagus. CT examination of the chest may be helpful in assessing the esophageal wall and the structures surrounding the esophagus.

ESOPHAGOSCOPY

Esophagoscopy is the direct method of establishing the cause of mechanical dysphagia. It can identify mucosal lesions that may not be revealed by the usual barium swallow. Ultrathin endoscopes have been used when the lumen is markedly narrowed; on occasion, a stricture must be dilated before the examination can be completed. Endoscopy is usually performed under sedation. Unsedated esophagoscopy using an ultrathin endoscope is an alternative approach in patients without known stricture. Endoscopic biopsies are useful in diagnosing carcinoma, esophagitis, and other mucosal diseases such as eosinophilic esophagitis. Cells obtained by a cytology balloon or by brushing the mucosa can be evaluated for carcinoma. Endoscopic ultrasonography permits evaluation of intramural and periesophageal masses and staging of esophageal cancer.

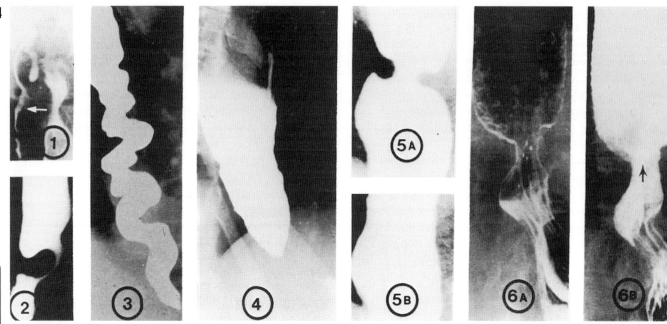

FIGURE 13-1

Radiographic appearance of some motor disorders of the esophagus. *(1)* Pharyngeal paralysis with tracheal aspiration (*arrow*). *(2)* Cricopharyngeal achalasia. Note the prominent cricopharyngeus, which is recognized by its smoothness and location in the posterior wall. *(3)* Diffuse esophageal spasm. Note the typical corkscrew appearance of the lower part of the esophagus. *(4)* Achalasia, showing a dilated esophageal body with an air-fluid level and a closed lower esophageal sphincter. *(5)* Muscular (contractile) lower esophageal ring. The asymmetric contraction visible in *(5A)* has disappeared in *(5B)*, obtained during the same examination. *(6)* Scleroderma esophagus showing dilated esophagus with a stricture *(6A)* and reflux of barium from the stomach into the esophagus *(6B)*.

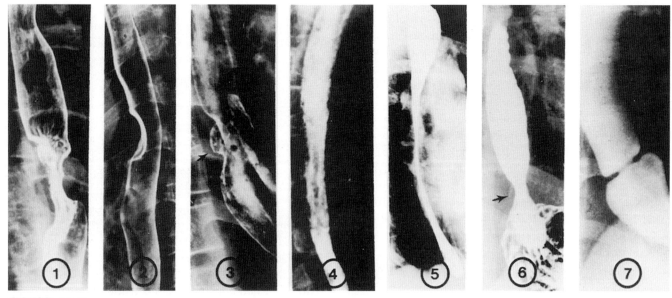

FIGURE 13-2

Selected structural lesions of the esophagus. *(1)* Carcinoma of the esophagus, with typical annular narrowing with overhanging margins and destruction of the mucosa. *(2)* Leiomyoma of the esophagus, with a smooth filling defect and right angles of origin from the esophageal wall. *(3)* Esophageal ulcer in columnar cell–lined esophagus (Barrett's esophagus). *(4)* Monilial esophagitis, with irregular plaquelike filling defects. *(5)* Long stricture secondary to lye ingestion. *(6)* Peptic stricture, short and tubular, with associated hiatal hernia. *(7)* Lower esophageal mucosal (Schatzki) ring. A thin, weblike annular constriction at the esophagogastric junction is associated with a small hiatal hernia.

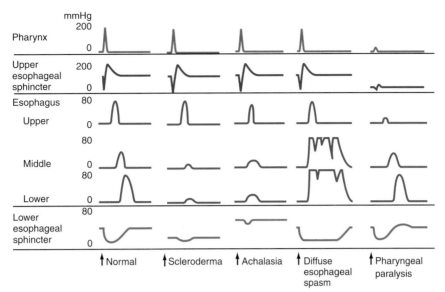

FIGURE 13-3

Motility patterns in selected esophageal and pharyngeal disorders. In normal individuals, the upper and lower esophageal sphincters (UES and LES) appear as zones of high pressure. With a swallow (indicated by ↑), pressure in the sphincters falls and a contraction wave starts in the pharynx and progresses down the esophagus. In scleroderma, the thoracic esophagus (smooth muscle) shows reduced amplitude of contractions, which may be peristaltic or simultaneous in onset, and hypotension of the LES. In achalasia, the lower part of the esophagus shows contractions that are reduced in amplitude and simultaneous in onset. In contrast to scleroderma, the LES in achalasia is hypertensive and fails to relax in response to a swallow. In diffuse esophageal spasm, the lower part of the esophagus shows simultaneous-onset, large-amplitude, prolonged, repetitive contractions. In contrast, in motor disorders of the cervical esophagus, the cervical esophagus shows poor contractions while contractions in the thoracic esophagus are normal. Moreover, these cases also show poor pharyngeal contractions and a hypotensive UES that fails to fully relax on swallowing.

ESOPHAGEAL MOTILITY

The study of esophageal motility entails simultaneous recording of pressures from different sites in the esophageal lumen with an assembly of pressure sensors positioned 5 cm apart. The UES and LES appear as zones of high pressure that relax on swallowing. The esophagus normally shows peristaltic waves with each swallow.

Esophageal motility studies are helpful in the diagnosis of esophageal motor disorders (achalasia, spasm, and scleroderma) (**Fig. 13-3**) but are of little value in the differential diagnosis of mechanical dysphagia. In patients with reflux esophagitis, esophageal manometry is useful in quantifying LES competence and providing information on the status of the esophageal body motor activity. Manometry provides quantitative data that cannot be obtained by barium swallow or endoscopy. Esophageal impedance testing identifies the nature (fluid or gas) and the direction of movement (oral or aboral) by measuring impedance across segments using a special catheter positioned in the esophagus. It may be helpful in the study of transit of the contents, particularly nonacid gastric contents. Other tests for reflux esophagitis are described later.

MOTOR DISORDERS

CERVICAL ESOPHAGUS

Motor disorders of the cervical esophagus (striated muscle) are accompanied by oral and pharyngeal dysphagia. Their clinical manifestations are described in Chap. 4.

THORACIC AND ABDOMINAL ESOPHAGUS

Achalasia

Achalasia is a motor disorder of the esophageal smooth muscle and involves thoracic and abdominal parts of the esophagus. In achalasia, the esophageal body loses peristaltic contractions and the LES does not relax normally in response to swallowing.

Pathophysiology

The underlying abnormality is the loss of intramural neurons. Inhibitory neurons containing VIP and nitric oxide synthase are predominantly involved, but cholinergic neurons are also affected in advanced disease. Primary idiopathic achalasia accounts for most of the cases seen in the United States. Secondary achalasia may be caused by gastric carcinoma that infiltrates the esophagus, lymphoma, Chagas' disease, certain viral infections, eosinophilic gastroenteritis, and neurodegenerative disorders.

Clinical Features

Achalasia affects patients of all ages and both sexes. Dysphagia, chest pain, and regurgitation are the main symptoms. Dysphagia occurs early with both liquids and solids and is worsened by emotional stress and hurried eating. Various maneuvers designed to increase intraesophageal pressure, including the Valsalva maneuver, may aid the passage of the bolus into the stomach. Regurgitation and pulmonary aspiration occur because of retention of a large amount of saliva and ingested food in the esophagus. Patients may complain of difficulty belching. The presence of gastroesophageal reflux argues against achalasia; in patients with long-standing heartburn, cessation of heartburn and appearance of dysphagia may suggest development of achalasia, peptic stricture, or carcinoma on top of reflux esophagitis. The course is usually chronic, with progressive dysphagia and weight loss over months to years. Achalasia associated with carcinoma is characterized by severe weight loss and a rapid downhill course.

Diagnosis

A chest x-ray shows absence of the gastric air bubble and sometimes a tubular mediastinal mass beside the aorta. An air-fluid level in the mediastinum in the upright position represents retained food in the esophagus. Barium swallow shows esophageal dilation, and in advanced cases the esophagus may become sigmoid. On fluoroscopy with barium swallow, normal peristalsis is lost in the lower two-thirds of the esophagus. The terminal part of the esophagus shows a persistent beaklike narrowing representing the nonrelaxing LES (Fig. 13-1, panel 4).

Manometry shows the basal LES pressure to be normal or elevated, and swallow-induced relaxation either does not occur or is reduced in degree, duration, and consistency. The esophageal body shows an elevated resting pressure. In response to swallows, primary peristaltic waves are replaced by simultaneous contractions (Fig. 13-3). These contractions may be of poor amplitude (classic achalasia) or of large amplitude and long duration (vigorous achalasia). Cholecystokinin (CCK), which normally causes a fall in the sphincter pressure, paradoxically causes contraction of the LES (the CCK test). This paradoxical response occurs because, in achalasia, the neurally transmitted inhibitory effect of CCK is absent and the direct excitatory effect of CCK remains unopposed.

Endoscopy is helpful in excluding the secondary causes of achalasia, particularly gastric carcinoma.

℞ Treatment: ACHALASIA

Treatment with soft food, sedatives, and anticholinergics is usually unsatisfactory. Nitrates and calcium channel blockers provide short-term benefit, but their use may be limited by side effects. Nitroglycerin, 0.3–0.6 mg, is used sublingually before meals and as needed for chest pain. Isosorbide dinitrate, 2.5–5 mg sublingually or 10–20 mg orally before meals, can also be used. Nitrates are associated with headache and postural hypotension. The calcium channel blocker nifedipine, 10–20 mg orally or sublingually before meals, may be effective. Sildenafil provides symptomatic relief by increasing cGMP that may reduce LES pressure and augment swallow-induced relaxation. Botulinum toxin acts by blocking cholinergic excitatory nerves in the sphincter. Endoscopic intrasphincteric injection of botulinum toxin is effective with clinical improvement in 60% of patients at 6 months; it may be very useful in temporizing symptoms in elderly or high-risk patients. However, repeated injections may lead to fibrosis, complicating further operative therapy. Balloon dilatation reduces the basal LES pressure by tearing muscle fibers. In experienced hands, this technique is effective in ~85% of patients; perforation and bleeding are potential complications. Heller's extramucosal myotomy of the LES, in which the circular muscle layer is incised, is equally effective. Laparoscopic myotomy is currently the procedure of choice. Since reflux esophagitis and peptic stricture may follow after a successful treatment (more often with myotomy than with balloon dilatation), surgical myotomy is sometimes accompanied by partial fundoplication to lessen postoperative reflux.

Diffuse Esophageal Spasm and Hypertensive Motor Disorders

DES is characterized by nonperistaltic contractions. The contraction may have low, normal, or large amplitude. The duration of contraction may be prolonged, and repetitive contractions may be present. The hypertensive disorders include nutcracker esophagus, hypercontracting LES, and hypertensive LES. In *nutcracker esophagus*, esophageal contractions are normally peristaltic but hypertensive. In *hypercontracting LES*, the normal sphincter relaxation is followed by hypertensive contraction. In *hypertensive LES*, basal LES pressure is elevated, but sphincter relaxation and contraction are normal.

Pathophysiology

Nonperistaltic contractions are due to dysfunction of inhibitory nerves. Histopathology shows patchy neural degeneration localized to nerve processes, rather than the prominent degeneration of nerve cell bodies seen in achalasia. DES may progress to achalasia. Hypertensive peristaltic contractions and hypertensive or hypercontracting LES may represent cholinergic or myogenic hyperactivity.

Clinical Features

DES and hypertensive motor disorders may present with chest pain. Chest pain is particularly marked in patients with esophageal contractions of large amplitude with long duration. It usually occurs at rest but may be brought on by swallowing or by emotional stress. The pain is retrosternal; it may radiate to the back, the sides of the chest, both arms, or the sides of the jaw and may last from a few seconds to several minutes. Pain may be acute and severe, mimicking the pain of myocardial ischemia. Dysphagia with solids and liquids may occur with or without chest pain and is correlated with simultaneous contractions.

DES and hypertensive esophageal motor disorders must be differentiated from other causes of chest pain, particularly ischemic heart disease with atypical angina. A complete cardiac workup should be done before a noncardiac etiology is considered. The presence of dysphagia in association with pain should point to the esophagus as the origin. Esophageal motility disorders are uncommon causes of noncardiac chest pain.

Diagnosis

In DES, barium swallow shows that normal sequential peristalsis below the aortic arch is replaced by uncoordinated simultaneous contractions that produce the appearance of curling or multiple ripples in the wall, sacculations, and pseudodiverticula—the "corkscrew" esophagus (Fig. 13-1, panel 3). Sometimes an esophageal contraction obliterates the lumen, and barium is pushed away in both directions. The barium swallow may be normal.

Diffuse esophageal spasm (Fig. 13-3) is best diagnosed by manometry. Because these abnormalities may be episodic, manometry may be normal at the time of the study. Several techniques are used to provoke esophageal spasm. Cold swallows produce chest pain but do not produce spasm on manometric studies. Solid boluses and pharmacologic agents, particularly edrophonium, may induce both chest pain and motor abnormalities. However, correlation between induction of pain and manometric changes is poor. The usefulness of pharmacologic provocative tests is limited.

Treatment:
℞ DIFFUSE ESOPHAGEAL SPASM AND HYPERTENSIVE MOTOR DISORDERS

Anticholinergics are usually of limited value. Agents that relax smooth muscle, such as sublingual nitroglycerin

(0.3–0.6 mg) or longer-acting agents such as isosorbide dinitrate (10–30 mg orally before meals) or nifedipine (10–20 mg orally before meals) may be helpful. Reassurance and tranquilizers are helpful in allaying apprehension.

Scleroderma Esophagus

The esophageal lesions in systemic sclerosis consist of atrophy of smooth muscle, manifested by weakness in the lower two-thirds of the esophagus and incompetence of the LES. The esophageal wall is atrophic and thin and may exhibit areas of patchy fibrosis. Patients usually present with dysphagia to solids. Liquids may cause dysphagia when the patient is recumbent. These patients usually also complain of heartburn, regurgitation, and other symptoms of GERD. Barium swallow shows dilation and loss of peristaltic contractions in the middle and distal portions of the esophagus. The LES is patulous, and gastroesophageal reflux may occur freely (Fig. 13-1, panel 6). Mucosal changes due to esophageal ulceration and stricture may be present. Motility studies show a marked reduction in the amplitude of smooth-muscle contractions, which is usually peristaltic but may be nonperistaltic. The resting pressure of the LES is subnormal, but sphincter relaxation is normal (Fig. 13-3). Similar esophageal motor abnormalities are found in other collagen vascular diseases, including Raynaud's phenomenon. Dietary adjustments with the use of soft foods are helpful in management. GERD and its complications should be treated aggressively.

GASTROESOPHAGEAL REFLUX DISEASE

GERD is one of the most prevalent gastrointestinal disorders. Population-based studies show that up to 15% of individuals have heartburn and/or regurgitation at least once a week, and 7% have symptoms daily. Symptoms are caused by backflow of gastric acid and other gastric contents into the esophagus due to incompetent barriers at the gastroesophageal junction.

PATHOPHYSIOLOGY

The normal antireflux mechanisms consist of the LES, the crural diaphragm, and the anatomic location of the gastroesophageal junction below the diaphragmatic hiatus. Reflux occurs only when the gradient of pressure between the LES and the stomach is lost. It can be caused by a sustained or transient decrease in LES tone. A sustained hypotension of the LES may be due to muscle weakness that is often without apparent cause. Secondary causes of sustained LES incompetence include scleroderma-like diseases, myopathy associated with chronic intestinal pseudo-obstruction, pregnancy, smoking, anticholinergic drugs, smooth-muscle relaxants (β-adrenergic agents, aminophylline, nitrates, calcium channel blockers, and phosphodiesterase inhibitors), surgical damage to the LES, and esophagitis. tLESR without associated esophageal contraction is due to a vagovagal reflex in which LES relaxation is elicited by gastric distention. Increased episodes of tLESR are associated with GERD. A similar reflex operates during belching. Apart from incompetent barriers, gastric contents are most likely to reflux (1) when gastric volume is increased (after meals, in pyloric obstruction, in gastric stasis, during acid hypersecretion states), (2) when gastric contents are near the gastroesophageal junction (in recumbency, bending down, hiatal hernia), and (3) when gastric pressure is increased (obesity, pregnancy, ascites, tight clothes). Incompetence of the diaphragmatic crural muscle, which surrounds the esophageal hiatus in the diaphragm and functions as an external LES, also predisposes to GERD. Obesity is a risk factor for GERD.

Esophageal exposure to refluxed gastric contents depends on the amount of refluxed material per episode, the frequency of reflux episodes, and the rate of clearing of the esophagus by gravity and peristaltic contractions. When peristaltic contractions are impaired, esophageal clearance is impaired. Acid refluxed into the esophagus is neutralized by saliva. Thus, impaired salivary secretion also increases esophageal exposure time. If the refluxed material extends to the cervical esophagus and crosses the upper sphincter, it can enter the pharynx, larynx, and trachea.

Reflux esophagitis is a complication of reflux. It develops when mucosal defenses are unable to counteract the damage caused by acid, pepsin, and bile. *Mild esophagitis* involves microscopic changes of mucosal infiltration with granulocytes or small numbers of eosinophils, hyperplasia of basal cells, and elongation of dermal pegs. In nonerosive reflux disease (NERD), the mucosa may be normal or mildly erythematous. *Erosive esophagitis* reveals clear mucosal damage with redness, friability, superficial linear ulcers, and exudates. Histology shows polymorphonuclear or mild eosinophilic infiltrates and granulation tissue. *Peptic stricture* results from fibrosis that causes luminal constriction. These strictures occur in ~10% of patients with untreated GERD. Short strictures caused by spontaneous reflux are usually 1–3 cm long and are present in the distal esophagus near the squamocolumnar junction (Fig. 13-2, panel 6). Long, tubular peptic strictures can result from persistent vomiting or prolonged nasogastric intubation. Erosive esophagitis may heal by intestinal metaplasia (*Barrett's esophagus*), a risk factor for adenocarcinoma.

CLINICAL FEATURES

Heartburn and regurgitation of sour material into the mouth are the characteristic symptoms of GERD. Heartburn is induced by the contact of refluxed material with the sensitized or ulcerated esophageal mucosa. Angina-like or atypical chest pain occurs in some patients. Persistent dysphagia suggests development of a peptic stricture. Most patients with peptic stricture have a history of several years of heartburn preceding dysphagia. However, in one-third of patients, dysphagia is the presenting symptom. Rapidly progressive dysphagia and weight loss may indicate the development of adenocarcinoma in Barrett's esophagus. Bleeding occurs due to mucosal erosions or Barrett's ulcer. Many patients with GERD remain asymptomatic, while many symptomatic patients treat themselves and do not seek medical help until severe symptoms or complications occur.

Extraesophageal manifestations of GERD are due to reflux of gastric contents into the pharynx, larynx, tracheobronchial tree, nose, and mouth. It may cause chronic cough, laryngitis, and pharyngitis. Morning hoarseness may be noted. Recurrent pulmonary aspiration may cause or aggravate chronic bronchitis, asthma, pulmonary fibrosis, chronic obstructive pulmonary disease, or pneumonia. Chronic sinusitis and dental decay have also been ascribed to GERD.

DIAGNOSIS

The diagnosis can be made by history alone in many cases. A therapeutic trial with a PPI such as omeprazole, 40 mg bid for 1 week, provides support for the diagnosis of GERD.

Diagnostic studies are indicated in patients with persistent symptoms or symptoms while on therapy, or in those with complications. The diagnostic approach to GERD can be divided into three categories: (1) documentation of mucosal injury, (2) documentation and quantitation of reflux, and (3) definition of the pathophysiology.

Mucosal damage is documented by the use of barium swallow, esophagoscopy, and mucosal biopsy. Barium swallow is usually normal but may reveal an ulcer or a stricture. A high esophageal peptic stricture, a deep ulcer, or adenocarcinoma suggests Barrett's esophagus. Esophagoscopy may reveal the presence of erosions, ulcers, peptic strictures, or Barrett's metaplasia with or without ulcer, peptic stricture, or adenocarcinoma. A variety of in vivo imaging techniques that facilitate the identification of Barrett's mucosa, dysplasia, or carcinoma during the endoscopy are being developed. Esophagoscopy is not diagnostic of GERD; it is normal in NERD, which constitutes one-third to one-half of all cases of GERD. Mucosal biopsies and the Bernstein test may be helpful in the diagnosis of NERD. Mucosal biopsies may show early changes of esophagitis, including dilation of intracellular spaces. The mucosal biopsies should be performed at least 5 cm above the LES, as the esophageal mucosal changes of chronic esophagitis are quite frequent in the most distal esophagus in otherwise normal individuals. The Bernstein test involves the infusion of solutions of 0.1 *N* HCl or normal saline into the esophagus. In patients with symptomatic esophagitis, infusion of acid, but not of saline, reproduces the symptoms of heartburn. Infusion of acid in normal individuals usually produces no symptoms. Supraesophageal manifestations are documented by careful otolaryngologic and pulmonary examination.

Documentation and quantitation of reflux, when necessary, can be done by ambulatory long-term (24–48 h) esophageal pH recording. Long-term pH recording may be performed using a pH-sensitive capsule (BRAVO) that is anchored into the esophageal mucosa via an endoscope, rather than the traditional nasally placed pH probe. For evaluation of pharyngeal reflux, a system of recording simultaneously from pharyngeal and esophageal sites may be useful. The pH recordings are helpful only in the evaluation of acid reflux. Endoscopic esophagitis does not correlate with gastroesophageal reflux. Documentation of reflux is necessary only when the role of reflux in the symptom complex is unclear, particularly in evaluation of supraesophageal symptoms, in cases with NERD, and in cases with noncardiac chest pain. Reflux of nonacid contents may be responsible for symptoms of regurgitation and extraesophageal manifestations of GERD. Reflux of nonacid contents can be documented by the use of an impedance test.

Determination of pathophysiologic factors in GERD is sometimes indicated for management decisions such as antireflux surgery. Esophageal motility studies may provide useful quantitative information on the competence of the LES and on esophageal motor function. Determination of tLESR as a cause of GERD requires studies that are usually not available in the clinical laboratory.

℞ **Treatment:**
GASTROESOPHAGEAL REFLUX DISEASE

The goals of treatment are to provide symptom relief, heal erosive esophagitis, and prevent complications. The management of mild cases includes weight reduction, sleeping with the head of the bed elevated by about 4–6 in. with blocks, and elimination of factors that increase abdominal pressure. Patients should not smoke and should avoid consuming fatty foods, coffee, chocolate, alcohol, mint, orange juice, and certain medications (such as anticholinergic drugs, calcium channel blockers, and other smooth-muscle relaxants). They should also avoid ingesting large quantities of fluids with meals. The lifestyle change and over-the-counter antisecretory agents may be adequate. H_2 receptor blocking agents (cimetidine, 300 mg qid; ranitidine, 150 mg bid; famotidine, 20 mg bid; nizatidine, 150 mg bid) are effective in symptom relief. PPIs are more effective and more commonly used.

The PPIs are comparably effective: omeprazole (20 mg/d), lansoprazole (30 mg/d), pantoprazole (40 mg/d), esomeprazole (40 mg/d), or rabeprazole (20 mg/d) for 8 weeks can heal erosive esophagitis in up to 90% of patients. The PPI should be taken 30 min before breakfast. Refractory patients can double the dose. Since GERD is a chronic disease, long-term maintenance therapy is often required, and symptoms may relapse in up to 80% of patients within 1 year if therapy is discontinued. PPIs are most effective in preventing recurrences. The side effects of PPI therapy are generally minimal. However, aggressive acid suppression may cause hypergastrinemia but does not increase the risk for carcinoid tumors or gastrinomas. Vitamin B_{12} and calcium absorption may be compromised by the treatment. Patients on PPIs for prolonged periods have an increased incidence of hip fractures. Patients who have Barrett's esophagus with concomitant esophagitis should be treated similarly; however, acid suppression does not lead to resolution of the Barrett's metaplasia or cancer prevention. Patients who have an associated peptic stricture are treated with endoscopic dilation to relieve dysphagia, and such patients should be vigorously treated for reflux. Esophagoscopy should also be performed in patients suspected of other complications such as bleeding or development of cancer.

Antireflux surgery, in which the gastric fundus is wrapped around the esophagus (fundoplication), creates an antireflux barrier. The efficacy of the antireflux barrier depends on the type of surgery and experience of the operator. Open fundoplication has mostly been replaced by laparoscopic fundoplication, and endoscopic antireflux procedures are being vigorously tested. Laparoscopic or endoscopic antireflux procedures should be considered as alternatives in young patients who require long-term, high-dose PPIs. Ideal candidates for fundoplication are those who have classical GERD with good response to PPI therapy and in whom motility studies show poor LES pressures but normal peristaltic contractions in the esophageal body.

Symptomatic GERD patients with low or no acid or alkaline (bile) reflux are also considered candidates for antireflux operations. Nonoperative treatment of alkaline esophagitis includes general antireflux measures and neutralization of bile salts with cholestyramine, aluminum hydroxide, or sucralfate. Sucralfate is particularly useful in these cases, as it also serves as a mucosal protector.

BARRETT'S ESOPHAGUS

The metaplasia of esophageal squamous epithelium to columnar epithelium (Barrett's esophagus) is a complication of severe reflux esophagitis, and it is a risk factor for esophageal adenocarcinoma (Chap. 47). Metaplastic columnar epithelium develops during healing of erosive esophagitis with continued acid reflux because columnar epithelium is more resistant to acid-pepsin damage than is squamous epithelium. The metaplastic epithelium is a mosaic of different epithelial types, including goblet cells and columnar cells, which have features of both secretory and absorptive cells. Finding intestinal metaplasia with goblet cells in the esophagus is diagnostic of Barrett's esophagus; this type of mucosa is thought to be at risk of cancer. Barrett's esophagus is arbitrarily divided into long-segment (>2–3 cm) and short-segment (<2–3 cm) groups; long-segment disease is diagnosed in about 1.5% and short-segment disease in 10–15% of the GERD population.

The rate of cancer development is 0.5% per year in long-segment disease, a 30- to 125-fold increased risk as compared to the general population. Short-segment Barrett's esophagus may also progress to cancer, but the actual risk in these cases is unclear.

Barrett's intestinal metaplasia progresses to adenocarcinoma through dysplastic stages, including low-grade dysplasia (LGD) and high-grade dysplasia (HGD). The sequence of disease progression is variable and inconsistent. Sampling error is a major problem in monitoring progression of the disease by mucosal biopsies. Therefore, optical methods of recognizing dysplasia during the endoscopy (laser-induced fluorescence spectroscopy, optical coherence tomography) are being developed. Moreover, an intense search for molecular markers of neoplastic progression is ongoing.

Barrett's esophagus can also lead to chronic peptic ulcer of the esophagus with high (midesophageal) and long strictures. Barrett's esophagus is more common in obese white men; its incidence increases with age. Usefulness of routine endoscopic population screening for Barrett's esophagus has not been established. However, a one-time esophagoscopy is recommended in patients with persistent GERD symptoms at age 50, particularly in white males. Over 90% of patients with esophageal adenocarcinoma are diagnosed during their first visit to a physician. When Barrett's esophagus is identified for the first time, no effort should be spared to exclude the presence of concurrent dysplasia or carcinoma. This effort may require a follow-up endoscopic study after aggressive treatment of esophagitis, with multiple esophageal mucosal biopsies.

The frequency of surveillance endoscopies in patients with established Barrett's esophagus depends on the initial endoscopic findings. HGD is often associated with concurrent carcinoma and progresses to cancer in about 20% of the cases. Currently, patients with HGD can be treated with esophagectomy, endoscopic mucosal resection, or photodynamic therapy with HGD. Close endoscopic follow-up (every 3 months) is recommended in all patients with HGD. In LGD, follow-up endoscopy is recommended at 6 and 12 months initially and yearly thereafter, as long as LGD persists. Patients with Barrett's esophagus without dysplasia should have two examinations within the first year and subsequently every 3 years. Acid suppression and fundoplication are indicated when active esophagitis is also present. Established metaplasia does not regress with antisecretory treatment.

INFLAMMATORY DISORDERS

INFECTIOUS ESOPHAGITIS

Infectious esophagitis can be due to viral, bacterial, fungal, or parasitic organisms. In severely immunocompromised patients, multiple organisms may coexist.

Viral Esophagitis

Herpes simplex virus (HSV) type 1 occasionally causes esophagitis in immunocompetent individuals, but either HSV-1 or HSV-2 may afflict patients who are immunosuppressed. Patients may complain of an acute onset of chest pain, odynophagia, and dysphagia. Bleeding may occur in severe cases; tracheoesophageal fistula and food impaction have been reported. Systemic manifestations such as nausea, vomiting, fever, chills, and mild leukocytosis may be present. Herpetic vesicles on the nose and lips may provide a clue to the diagnosis. Barium swallow is inadequate to detect early lesions and cannot reliably distinguish HSV infection from other types of infections. Endoscopy shows vesicles and small, discrete, punched-out ("volcano-like") superficial ulcerations with or without a fibrinous exudate. In later stages, a diffuse erosive esophagitis develops from enlargement and coalescence of the ulcers. Mucosal cells from a biopsy sample taken at the edge of an ulcer or from a cytologic smear show ballooning degeneration, ground-glass changes in the nuclei with eosinophilic intranuclear inclusions (Cowdry type A), and giant cell formation on routine stains. Culture for HSV becomes positive within days and is helpful in diagnosis and to identify acyclovir-resistant strains. PCR assays are more sensitive than viral cultures. Spontaneous resolution may occur in 1–2 weeks. Acyclovir (400 mg PO 5 times a day for 14–21 days) causes early resolution of symptoms. Valacyclovir (1 g PO tid for 7 days) may be more convenient and have better patient adherence. In patients with severe odynophagia, intravenous acyclovir, 5 mg/kg every 8 h for 7–14 days, is used. Symptoms usually resolve in 1 week, but large ulcerations may take longer to heal. Foscarnet (90 mg/kg intravenously bid for 2–4 weeks) is used if acyclovir resistance occurs. Oral famciclovir may be considered in patients who are able to swallow.

Varicella-zoster virus (VZV) sometimes produces esophagitis in children with chickenpox and adults with herpes zoster. Esophageal VZV can also be the source of disseminated VZV infection without skin involvement. In an immunocompromised host, VZV esophagitis causes vesicles and confluent ulcers and usually resolves spontaneously, but it may cause necrotizing esophagitis in severely compromised patients. On routine histologic examination of mucosal biopsy samples or cytology specimens, VZV is difficult to distinguish from HSV, but the distinction can be made immunohistologically or by culture. Acyclovir and valacyclovir reduce duration of symptoms and may be used in combination with glucocorticoids.

Cytomegalovirus (CMV) infections occur only in immunocompromised patients. CMV is usually activated from a latent stage or may be acquired from blood product transfusions. CMV lesions initially appear as serpiginous ulcers in an otherwise normal mucosa. These may coalesce to form giant ulcers, particularly in the distal esophagus. Patients present with odynophagia, persistent and focal chest pain, nausea, vomiting, and hematemesis. Diagnosis requires endoscopy and biopsies from the ulcer base. Mucosal brushings are not useful. Routine histologic examination shows intranuclear and small intracytoplasmic inclusions in large fibroblasts and endothelial cells. Immunohistology with monoclonal antibodies to CMV and in situ hybridization tests are useful for early diagnosis. Ganciclovir, 5 mg/kg every 12 h intravenously, is the treatment of choice. Valganciclovir (900 mg bid), an oral formulation of ganciclovir, can be used. Foscarnet (90 mg/kg every 12 h intravenously) may be used in resistant cases. Therapy is continued until healing occurs, which may take 3-6 weeks.

HIV may be associated with a self-limited syndrome of acute esophageal ulceration associated with oral ulcers and a maculopapular skin rash, which occurs at the time of HIV seroconversion. Some patients with advanced disease have deep, persistent esophageal ulcers requiring treatment with oral glucocorticoids or thalidomide. Some ulcers respond to local steroid injection.

Bacterial and Fungal Esophagitis

Bacterial esophagitis is unusual, but *Lactobacillus* and β-hemolytic streptococci can cause esophagitis in immunocompromised patients. In patients with profound granulocytopenia and patients with cancer, bacterial esophagitis is often overlooked because it is commonly present with other organisms, including viruses and fungi. In patients with AIDS, infection with *Cryptosporidium* or *Pneumocystis carinii* may cause nonspecific inflammation, and *Mycobacterium tuberculosis* infection may cause deep ulcerations of the distal esophagus. Very rarely, other types of fungi may cause esophagitis.

CANDIDA ESOPHAGITIS

Candida species are normal commensals in the throat but become pathogenic and produce esophagitis in a compromised host. Candida esophagitis can occur without any predisposing factors. Patients may be asymptomatic or complain of odynophagia and dysphagia. Oral thrush or other evidence of mucocutaneous candidiasis may be absent. Rarely, Candida esophagitis is complicated by esophageal bleeding, perforation, and stricture or by systemic invasion. Barium swallow may be normal or show multiple nodular filling defects of various sizes (Fig. 13-2, panel 4). Large nodular defects may resemble grape clusters. Endoscopy shows small, yellow-white raised plaques with surrounding erythema in mild disease. Confluent linear and nodular plaques reflect extensive disease. Diagnosis is made by demonstration of yeast or hyphal forms in plaque smears and exudate stained with periodic acid–Schiff or Gomori silver stains. Histologic examination is often negative. Culture is not useful in diagnosis but may define the species and the drug sensitivities of the yeast; *Candida albicans* is most common. Oral fluconazole (200 mg on the first day, followed by 100 mg daily) for 7–14 days is the preferred treatment. Patients refractory to fluconazole often respond to itraconazole. Patients who respond poorly or cannot swallow oral medications can be treated with an intravenous echinocandin such as caspofungin (50 mg daily for 7–21 days). Amphotericin B (10–15 mg IV infusion for 6 h daily to a total dose of 300–500 mg) is used in severe cases.

OTHER TYPES OF ESOPHAGITIS

Eosinophilic Esophagitis

Eosinophilic esophagitis is characterized by eosinophilic inflammation and submucosal fibrosis. The eosinophil chemokine eotaxin-3 is involved in the pathogenesis of the disease. Clinically, eosinophilic esophagitis is more common in children and in males. Presenting symptoms vary with age. Younger children present with failure to thrive and refusal to swallow. Older children present with regurgitation, vomiting, and pain. Adolescents usually present with heartburn and dysphagia. Adults often present with intermittent dysphagia and food impaction. A history of allergic disease or mild peripheral eosinophilia is present in about half of patients. Barium esophagogram may show a small-caliber esophagus, isolated esophageal narrowing, or single or multiple esophageal rings. Esophagoscopy may reveal one or more longitudinal fissures, fixed or transient concentric rings, proximal strictures, and focal white specks (abscesses). Endoscopic ultrasound may show thickening of the esophageal wall. Differential diagnosis includes reflux esophagitis, eosinophilic gastroenteritis, and esophageal rings and strictures. Diagnosis is confirmed by esophageal mucosal biopsies that show increased eosinophils (>15) per high-power field or eosinophilic microabscesses. Treatment consists of a 12-week course of swallowed fluticasone propionate (440 μg bid) using a metered dose inhaler. Oral prednisone may also be used. Dietary management involves identification of the offending food and its elimination from the diet or a trial of elemental diet for 4 weeks. Food impaction requires endoscopic dislodging. Esophageal dilation should be performed with great care because of a high rate of esophageal perforation in these cases. Antibody to interleukin 5 is an effective therapy emerging from clinical trials.

Radiation esophagitis is a common occurrence during radiation treatment for thoracic cancers. The frequency and severity of esophagitis increase with the amount of radiation delivered and may be enhanced by radiosensitizing drugs like doxorubicin, bleomycin, cyclophosphamide, and cisplatin. Dysphagia and odynophagia may last several weeks to several months after therapy. The esophageal mucosa becomes erythematous, edematous, and friable. Superficial erosions coalesce to form larger ulcers. Submucosal fibrosis and degenerative changes in the blood vessels, muscles, and myenteric neurons may occur, and esophageal stricture may develop. The treatment aims to relieve the pain with viscous lidocaine during the acute phase; indomethacin treatment may reduce radiation damage. Esophageal stricture may need to be dilated.

Corrosive esophagitis is caused by the ingestion of caustic agents, such as strong alkali or acid. Severe corrosive injury may lead to esophageal perforation, bleeding, and death. Glucocorticoids are not useful in acute corrosive esophagitis. Healing is usually associated with stricture formation. Caustic strictures are usually long and rigid (Fig. 13-2, panel 5) and generally require dilatation with dilators passed over a guide wire through the stricture.

Pill-induced esophagitis is associated with the ingestion of certain types of pills. Antibiotics such as doxycycline, tetracycline, oxytetracycline, minocycline, penicillin, and clindamycin account for more than half the cases. Nonsteroidal anti-inflammatory agents such as aspirin, indomethacin, and ibuprofen may cause injury. Other commonly prescribed pills that cause esophageal injury include potassium chloride, ferrous sulfate or succinate, quinidine, alprenolol, theophylline, ascorbic acid, and pinaverium bromide. Bisphosphonates, particularly alendronate and pamidronate, are more common offenders. Pill-induced esophagitis can be prevented by avoiding the offending agents or taking pills in the upright position with copious amount of fluid.

Sclerotherapy for bleeding esophageal varices usually produces transient retrosternal chest pain and dysphagia; esophageal ulcer, stricture, hematoma, or perforation may occur. Variceal banding causes similar complications, but less frequently. Esophagitis associated with mucocutaneous and systemic diseases is usually associated with blister and bulla formation, epithelial desquamation, and thin, weblike, or dense esophageal strictures. Pemphigus vulgaris and bullous pemphigoid form intraepithelial and subepithelial bullae, respectively, and can be distinguished by specific immunohistology; both

are characterized by sloughing of epithelium or the presence of esophageal casts. Glucocorticoid treatment is usually effective. Cicatricial pemphigoid, Stevens-Johnson syndrome, and toxic epidermolysis bullosa can produce esophageal bullous lesions and strictures requiring gentle dilatation. Graft-versus-host disease (GVHD) occurs in patients who have received allogeneic bone marrow or cord blood transplant. If it involves the esophagus, dysphagia and odynophagia are common symptoms. Radiologic findings include mid- and upper esophageal rings or webs and strictures. Esophageal ulcers may be seen. Behçet's syndrome and eosinophilic gastroenteritis may involve the esophagus and respond to glucocorticoid therapy. An erosive lichen planus can also involve the esophagus. Crohn's disease may cause inflammatory strictures, sinus tracts, filiform polyps, and fistulas in the esophagus.

OTHER ESOPHAGEAL DISORDERS

DIVERTICULA

Diverticula are outpouchings of the esophagus wall. A *Zenker's diverticulum* appears in the natural zone of weakness in the posterior hypopharyngeal wall (Killian's triangle) and causes halitosis and regurgitation of saliva and food that may have been consumed several days earlier. When it becomes large and filled with food, it can compress the esophagus and cause dysphagia or complete obstruction. Nasogastric intubation and endoscopy should be performed with utmost care in these patients, as the diverticulum may perforate. A *midesophageal diverticulum* may be caused by traction from old adhesions or by propulsion associated with esophageal motor abnormalities. An *epiphrenic diverticulum* may be associated with achalasia. Small or medium-sized diverticula and midesophageal and epiphrenic diverticula are usually asymptomatic. *Diffuse intramural esophageal diverticulosis* is due to dilation of the deep esophageal glands and may lead to chronic candidiasis or to the development of a stricture that is usually high up in the esophagus. These patients may present with dysphagia. Symptomatic Zenker's diverticula are treated by cricopharyngeal myotomy with or without diverticulectomy. Large symptomatic esophageal diverticula are removed surgically. Diverticula associated with DES or achalasia are treated with distal myotomy. Strictures associated with diffuse intramural diverticulosis are treated with rubber dilators.

WEBS AND RINGS

Weblike constrictions of the esophagus are usually congenital or inflammatory in origin. Asymptomatic hypopharyngeal webs are demonstrated in <10% of normal individuals. When concentric, they cause intermittent dysphagia to solids. The combination of symptomatic hypopharyngeal webs and iron-deficiency anemia in middle-aged women constitutes *Plummer-Vinson syndrome*. The clinical importance of this syndrome is uncertain. Midesophageal webs are rare. Often they are inflammatory in nature and may occur in mucocutaneous disorders, GVHD, and eosinophilic esophagitis. Multiple mucosal rings (feline esophagus) are characteristic of eosinophilic esophagitis.

A *lower esophageal mucosal ring* (Schatzki ring) is a thin, weblike constriction located at the squamocolumnar mucosal junction at or near the border of the LES (Fig. 13-2, panel 7). It may result from GERD or be congenital in origin. It invariably produces dysphagia when the lumen diameter is <1.3 cm. Dysphagia to solids is the only symptom, and it is usually episodic. A lower esophageal ring is one of the common causes of dysphagia. Asymptomatic rings may be present in ~10% of normal individuals. Symptomatic rings and webs are easily treated by dilatation.

A *lower esophageal muscular ring* (contractile ring) is located proximal to the site of mucosal rings and may represent an abnormal uppermost segment of the LES. These rings can be recognized by the fact that they are not constant in size and shape. They may also cause dysphagia and should be differentiated from peptic strictures, achalasia, and lower esophageal mucosal rings. Muscular rings do not respond well to dilatation.

HIATAL HERNIA

A *hiatal hernia* is a herniation of part of the stomach into the thoracic cavity through the esophageal hiatus in the diaphragm. A *sliding hiatal hernia* is one in which the gastroesophageal junction and fundus of the stomach slide upward. A sliding hernia may result from weakening of the anchors of the gastroesophageal junction to the diaphragm, from longitudinal contraction of the esophagus, or from increased intraabdominal pressure. Small sliding hernias can be demonstrated commonly during barium studies if intraabdominal pressure is increased. Incidence increases with age; in individuals in the sixth decade of life, the prevalence of such hernias is ~60%. Small sliding hiatal hernias alone probably produce no symptoms but can contribute to reflux esophagitis. A *paraesophageal hernia* is one in which the esophagogastric junction remains fixed in its normal location and a pouch of stomach is herniated beside the gastroesophageal junction through the esophageal hiatus. A paraesophageal or mixed paraesophageal and sliding hernia may become incarcerated and strangulated, leading to acute chest pain, dysphagia, and a mediastinal mass and requiring surgery. A herniated gastric pouch may cause dysphagia, gastritis, ulceration, or chronic blood loss. Large paraesophageal hernias should be surgically repaired.

MECHANICAL TRAUMA

Esophageal rupture may be caused by (1) iatrogenic damage from instrumentation of the esophagus or external trauma, (2) increased intraesophageal pressure associated with forceful vomiting or retching (*spontaneous rupture* or *Boerhaave's syndrome*), or (3) diseases of the esophagus such as corrosive esophagitis, esophageal ulcer, and neoplasm. The site of perforation depends on the cause. Instrumental perforation usually occurs in the pharynx or lower esophagus, just above the diaphragm in the posterolateral wall. Esophageal perforation causes severe retrosternal chest pain, which may be worsened by swallowing and breathing. Free air enters the mediastinum and spreads to neighboring structures, causing palpable subcutaneous emphysema in the neck, mediastinal crackling sounds on auscultation, and pneumothorax. With time, secondary infection supervenes, and mediastinal abscess may develop. Esophageal perforation associated with vomiting usually deposits gastric contents in the mediastinum and causes severe mediastinal complications. By contrast, instrumental perforation may be clinically mild and free of severe complications. Spontaneous rupture of the esophagus may mimic myocardial infarction, pancreatitis, or rupture of an abdominal viscus. Symptoms of chest pain may be mild, particularly in the elderly. Mediastinal emphysema may develop late. An x-ray of the chest shows abnormalities in most patients, but CT of the chest is more sensitive in detecting mediastinal air. Fluid from pleural effusions may have a high content of (salivary) amylase. The diagnosis is confirmed by swallow of radiopaque contrast material. Gastrografin is used initially, and if no leak is found, a small amount of thin barium is used to confirm the diagnosis. Treatment includes esophageal and gastric suction and parenteral broad-spectrum antibiotics. Surgical drainage and repair of the laceration should be performed as soon as possible. In patients with terminal carcinoma, surgical repair may not be feasible. Endoscopic clipping or stent placement may be indicated in some cases. Patients with minor instrumental perforation can be treated conservatively. Extensive corrosive damage may require esophageal diversion and excision of the damaged portion.

Mucosal Tear (Mallory-Weiss Syndrome)

This tear is usually caused by vomiting, retching, or vigorous coughing. The tear usually involves the gastric mucosa near the squamocolumnar mucosal junction. Patients present with upper gastrointestinal bleeding, which may be severe. In most patients, bleeding ceases spontaneously; continued bleeding may respond to vasopressin therapy or angiographic embolization. Surgery is rarely needed.

Intramural Hematoma

Emetogenic injury, particularly in patients with bleeding abnormalities, can cause bleeding between the mucosal and muscle layers of the esophagus. The patients may develop sudden chest pain and dysphagia. The diagnosis is made by barium swallow and CT. Resolution is usually spontaneous.

FOREIGN BODIES AND FOOD IMPACTION

Foreign bodies may lodge in the cervical esophagus just beyond the UES, near the aortic arch, or above the LES. They usually require endoscopic removal. Impaction of food may occur when the esophageal lumen is narrowed due to stricture, carcinoma, lower esophageal ring, or eosinophilic esophagitis. Acute impaction may cause complete inability to swallow and severe chest pain. Impacted food is dislodged endoscopically. Use of a meat tenderizer to facilitate passage of a meat bolus is discouraged because of potential esophageal perforation and aspiration pneumonia. Glucagon (1.0 mg IV) is sometimes tried before endoscopic dislodgement. Esophageal dilation is needed to avoid recurrence. In eosinophilic esophagitis, esophageal dilation should be performed cautiously because of a high risk of perforation.

FURTHER READINGS

Ford CN: Evaluation and management of laryngopharyngeal reflux. JAMA 28:1534, 2005

Gill SK et al: The safety of proton pump inhibitors in pregnancy: a meta-analysis. Am J Gastroenterol 104:1541, 2009

Hirano I: Pathophysiology of achalasia and diffuse esophageal spasm. GI Motility Online, *http://www.nature.com/gimo/contents/pt1/full/gimo22.html*, 2006

Logemann JA: Medical and rehabilitative therapy of oral, pharyngeal motor disorders. GI Motility Online, *http://www.nature.com/gimo/contents/pt1/full/gimo50.html*, 2006

Lowe RC: Medical management of gastroesophageal reflux disease. GI Motility Online, *http://www.nature.com/gimo/contents/pt1/full/gimo54.html*, 2006

Ney DM et al: Senescent swallowing: impact, strategies, and interventions. Nutr Clin Pract 24:395, 2009

Nurko S, Furuta GT: Eosinophilic esophagitis. GI Motility Online, *http://www.nature.com/gimo/contents/pt1/full/gimo49.html*, 2006

Pehlivanov N, Pasricha PJ: Medical and endoscopic treatment of achalasia. GI Motility Online, *http://www.nature.com/gimo/contents/pt1/full/gimo52.html*, 2006

Peters MJ et al: Meta-analysis of randomized clinical trials comparing open and laparoscopic anti-reflux surgery. Am J Gastroenterol 104:1548, 2009

Spechler SJ: Clinical practice: Barrett's esophagus. N Engl J Med 346:836, 2002

Spechler SJ et al: Thoughts on the complex relationship between gastroesophageal reflux disease and eosinophilic esophagitis. Am J Gastroenterol 102:1301, 2007

Whitney-Miller CL et al: Eosinophilic esophagitis: a retrospective review of esophageal biopsy specimens from 1992 to 2004 at an adult academic medical center. Am J Clin Pathol 131:788, 2009

Wise JL, Murray JA: Oral, pharyngeal and esophageal motility disorders in systemic diseases Systemic diseases. GI Motility Online, *http://www.nature.com/gimo/contents/pt1/full/gimo40.html*, 2006

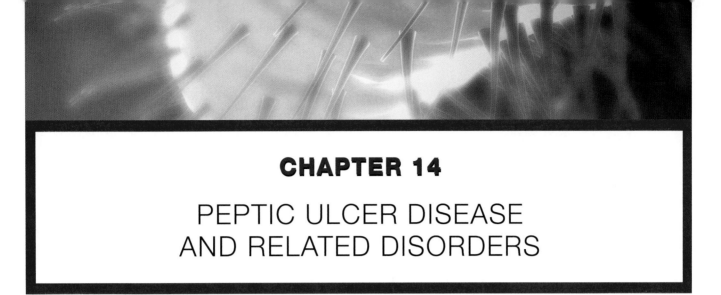

CHAPTER 14

PEPTIC ULCER DISEASE AND RELATED DISORDERS

John Del Valle

PEPTIC ULCER DISEASE

Burning epigastric pain exacerbated by fasting and improved with meals is a symptom complex associated with peptic ulcer disease (PUD). An *ulcer* is defined as disruption of the mucosal integrity of the stomach and/or duodenum leading to a local defect or excavation due to active inflammation. Ulcers occur within the stomach and/or duodenum and are often chronic in nature. Acid peptic disorders are very common in the United States, with 4 million individuals (new cases and recurrences) affected per year. Lifetime prevalence of PUD in the United States is ~12% in men and 10% in women. Moreover, an estimated 15,000 deaths per year occur as a consequence of complicated PUD. The financial impact of these common disorders has been substantial, with an estimated burden on direct and indirect health care costs of ~$10 billion per year in the United States.

GASTRIC PHYSIOLOGY

Despite the constant attack on the gastroduodenal mucosa by a host of noxious agents (acid, pepsin, bile acids, pancreatic enzymes, drugs, and bacteria), integrity is maintained by an intricate system that provides mucosal defense and repair.

Gastric Anatomy

The gastric epithelial lining consists of rugae that contain microscopic gastric pits, each branching into four or five gastric glands made up of highly specialized epithelial cells. The makeup of gastric glands varies with their anatomic location. Glands within the gastric cardia comprise <5% of the gastric gland area and contain mucous and endocrine cells. The 75% of gastric glands are found within the oxyntic mucosa and contain mucous neck, parietal, chief, endocrine, and enterochromaffin cells (**Fig. 14-1**). Pyloric glands contain mucous and endocrine cells (including gastrin cells) and are found in the antrum.

The parietal cell, also known as the oxyntic cell, is usually found in the neck, or isthmus, or in the oxyntic gland. The resting, or unstimulated, parietal cell has prominent cytoplasmic tubulovesicles and intracellular canaliculi containing short microvilli along its apical surface (**Fig. 14-2**). H^+,K^+-ATPase is expressed in the tubulovesicle membrane; upon cell stimulation, this membrane, along with apical membranes, transforms into a dense network of apical intracellular canaliculi containing long microvilli. Acid secretion, a process requiring high energy, occurs at the apical canalicular surface. Numerous mitochondria (30–40% of total cell volume) generate the energy required for secretion.

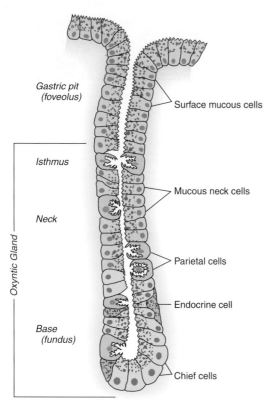

FIGURE 14-1
Diagrammatic representation of the oxyntic gastric gland.
(Adapted from S Ito, RJ Winchester: Cell Biol 16:541, 1963.)

Gastroduodenal Mucosal Defense

The gastric epithelium is under constant assault by a series of endogenous noxious factors, including HCl, pepsinogen/pepsin, and bile salts. In addition, a steady flow of exogenous substances such as medications, alcohol, and bacteria encounter the gastric mucosa. A highly intricate biologic system is in place to provide defense from mucosal injury and to repair any injury that may occur.

The mucosal defense system can be envisioned as a three-level barrier, composed of preepithelial, epithelial, and subepithelial elements (**Fig. 14-3**). The first line of

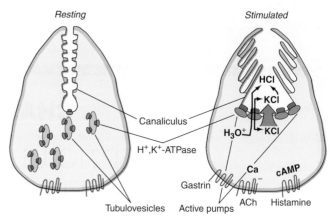

FIGURE 14-2
Gastric parietal cell undergoing transformation after secretagogue-mediated stimulation. *(Adapted from SJ Hersey, G Sachs: Physiol Rev 75:155, 1995.)*

defense is a mucus-bicarbonate layer, which serves as a physicochemical barrier to multiple molecules, including hydrogen ions. Mucus is secreted in a regulated fashion by gastroduodenal surface epithelial cells. It consists primarily of water (95%) and a mixture of lipids and glycoproteins (mucin). The mucous gel functions as a nonstirred water layer impeding diffusion of ions and molecules such as pepsin. Bicarbonate, secreted in a regulated manner by surface epithelial cells of the gastroduodenal mucosa into the mucous gel, forms a pH gradient ranging from 1 to 2 at the gastric luminal surface and reaching 6 to 7 along the epithelial cell surface.

Surface epithelial cells provide the next line of defense through several factors, including mucus production, epithelial cell ionic transporters that maintain intracellular pH and bicarbonate production, and intracellular tight junctions. If the preepithelial barrier were breached, gastric epithelial cells bordering a site of injury can migrate to restore a damaged region (*restitution*). This process occurs independent of cell division and requires uninterrupted blood flow and an alkaline pH in the surrounding environment. Several growth factors, including epidermal

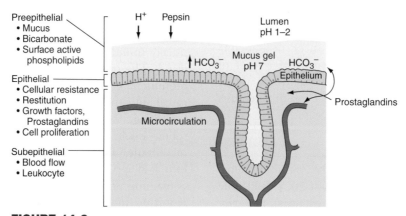

FIGURE 14-3
Components involved in providing gastroduodenal mucosal defense and repair.

growth factor (EGF), transforming growth factor (TGF)-α, and basic fibroblast growth factor (FGF), modulate the process of restitution. Larger defects that are not effectively repaired by restitution require cell proliferation. Epithelial cell regeneration is regulated by prostaglandins and growth factors such as EGF and TGF-α. In tandem with epithelial cell renewal, formation of new vessels (*angiogenesis*) within the injured microvascular bed occurs. Both FGF and vascular endothelial growth factor (VEGF) are important in regulating angiogenesis in the gastric mucosa.

An elaborate microvascular system within the gastric submucosal layer is the key component of the subepithelial defense/repair system, providing HCO_3^-, which neutralizes the acid generated by parietal cell. Moreover, this microcirculatory bed provides an adequate supply of micronutrients and oxygen while removing toxic metabolic by-products.

Prostaglandins play a central role in gastric epithelial defense/repair (Fig. 14-4). The gastric mucosa contains abundant levels of prostaglandins that regulate the release of mucosal bicarbonate and mucus, inhibit parietal cell secretion, and are important in maintaining mucosal blood flow and epithelial cell restitution. Prostaglandins are derived from esterified arachidonic acid, which is formed from phospholipids (cell membrane) by the action of phospholipase A_2. A key enzyme that controls the rate-limiting step in prostaglandin synthesis is cyclooxygenase (COX), which is present in two isoforms (COX-1, COX-2), each having distinct characteristics regarding structure, tissue distribution, and expression. COX-1 is expressed in a host of tissues, including the stomach, platelets, kidneys, and endothelial cells. This isoform is expressed in a constitutive manner and plays an important role in maintaining the integrity of renal function, platelet aggregation, and gastrointestinal mucosal integrity. In contrast, the expression of COX-2 is inducible by inflammatory stimuli, and it is expressed in macrophages, leukocytes, fibroblasts, and synovial cells. The beneficial effects of nonsteroidal anti-inflammatory drugs (NSAIDs) on tissue inflammation are due to inhibition of COX-2; the toxicity of these drugs (e.g., gastrointestinal mucosal ulceration and renal dysfunction) is related to inhibition of the COX-1 isoform. The highly COX-2–selective NSAIDs have the potential to provide the beneficial effect of decreasing tissue inflammation while minimizing toxicity in the gastrointestinal tract. Selective COX-2 inhibitors have had adverse effects on the cardiovascular system, leading to increased risk of myocardial infarction. Therefore, the FDA has removed two of these agents (valdecoxib and rofecoxib) from the market (see "Therapy of NSAID-Related Gastric or Duodenal Injury" later in the chapter).

Nitric oxide (NO) is important in the maintenance of gastric mucosal integrity. The key enzyme NO synthase is constitutively expressed in the mucosa and contributes to cytoprotection by stimulating gastric mucus, increasing mucosal blood flow and maintaining epithelial cell barrier function.

Physiology of Gastric Secretion

Hydrochloric acid and pepsinogen are the two principal gastric secretory products capable of inducing mucosal injury. Acid secretion should be viewed as occurring under basal and stimulated conditions. Basal acid production occurs in a circadian pattern, with highest levels occurring during the night and lowest levels during the morning hours. Cholinergic input via the vagus nerve and histaminergic input from local gastric sources are the principal contributors to basal acid secretion. Stimulated gastric acid secretion occurs primarily in three phases based on the site where the signal originates (cephalic, gastric, and intestinal). Sight, smell, and taste of food are the components of the cephalic phase, which stimulates gastric secretion via the vagus nerve. The gastric phase is activated once food enters the stomach. This component of secretion is driven by nutrients (amino acids and amines) that directly stimulate the G cell to release gastrin, which in turn activates the parietal cell via direct and indirect mechanisms. Distention of the stomach wall also leads to gastrin release and acid production. The last phase of gastric acid secretion is initiated as food enters the intestine and is mediated by luminal distention and nutrient assimilation. A series of pathways that inhibit gastric acid production are also set into motion during these phases. The gastrointestinal hormone somatostatin is released from endocrine cells found in the gastric mucosa (D cells) in response to HCl. Somatostatin can inhibit acid production by both direct (parietal cell) and indirect mechanisms [decreased histamine release from enterochromaffin-like (ECL) cells and gastrin release from G cells]. Additional neural

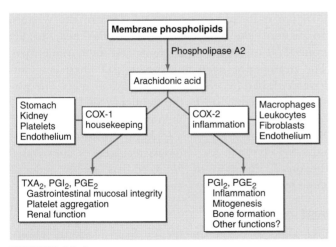

FIGURE 14-4
Schematic representation of the steps involved in synthesis of prostaglandin E$_2$ (PGE$_2$) and prostacyclin (PGI$_2$). Characteristics and distribution of the cyclooxygenase (COX) enzymes 1 and 2 are also shown. TXA$_2$, thromboxane A$_2$.

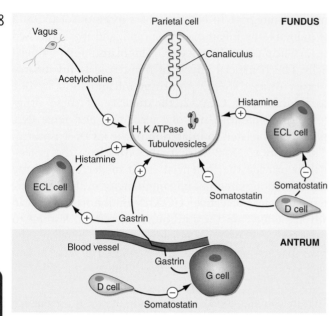

FIGURE 14-5
Regulation of gastric acid secretion at the cellular level.
ECL cell, enterochromaffin-like cell.

(central and peripheral) and hormonal (secretin, cholecystokinin) factors play a role in counterbalancing acid secretion. Under physiologic circumstances, these phases occur simultaneously.

The acid-secreting parietal cell is located in the oxyntic gland, adjacent to other cellular elements (ECL cell, D cell) important in the gastric secretory process (**Fig. 14-5**). This unique cell also secretes intrinsic factor (IF). The parietal cell expresses receptors for several stimulants of acid secretion, including histamine (H_2), gastrin (cholecystokinin B/gastrin receptor), and acetylcholine (muscarinic, M_3). Binding of histamine to the H_2 receptor leads to activation of adenylate cyclase and an increase in cyclic AMP. Activation of the gastrin and muscarinic receptors results in activation of the protein kinase C/phosphoinositide signaling pathway. Each of these signaling pathways in turn regulates a series of downstream kinase cascades, which control the acid-secreting pump, H^+,K^+-ATPase. The discovery that different ligands and their corresponding receptors lead to activation of different signaling pathways explains the potentiation of acid secretion that occurs when histamine and gastrin or acetylcholine are combined. More importantly, this observation explains why blocking one receptor type (H_2) decreases acid secretion stimulated by agents that activate a different pathway (gastrin, acetylcholine). Parietal cells also express receptors for ligands that inhibit acid production (prostaglandins, somatostatin, and EGF).

The enzyme H^+,K^+-ATPase is responsible for generating the large concentration of H^+. It is a membrane-bound protein that consists of two subunits, α and β. The active catalytic site is found within the α subunit; the function of the β subunit is unclear. This enzyme uses the chemical energy of ATP to transfer H^+ ions from parietal cell cytoplasm to the secretory canaliculi in exchange for K^+. The H^+,K^+-ATPase is located within the secretory canaliculus and in nonsecretory cytoplasmic tubulovesicles. The tubulovesicles are impermeable to K^+, which leads to an inactive pump in this location. The distribution of pumps between the nonsecretory vesicles and the secretory canaliculus varies according to parietal cell activity (Fig. 14-2). Proton pumps are recycled back to the inactive state in cytoplasmic vesicles once parietal cell activation ceases.

The chief cell, found primarily in the gastric fundus, synthesizes and secretes pepsinogen, the inactive precursor of the proteolytic enzyme pepsin. The acid environment within the stomach leads to cleavage of the inactive precursor to pepsin and provides the low pH (<2.0) required for pepsin activity. Pepsin activity is significantly diminished at a pH of 4 and irreversibly inactivated and denatured at a pH of ≥7. Many of the secretagogues that stimulate acid secretion also stimulate pepsinogen release. The precise role of pepsin in the pathogenesis of PUD remains to be established.

PATHOPHYSIOLOGIC BASIS OF PEPTIC ULCER DISEASE

PUD encompasses both gastric and duodenal ulcers. *Ulcers* are defined as breaks in the mucosal surface >5 mm in size, with depth to the submucosa. Duodenal ulcers (DUs) and gastric ulcers (GUs); share many common features in terms of pathogenesis, diagnosis, and treatment, but several factors distinguish them from one another.

Epidemiology

Duodenal Ulcers

DUs are estimated to occur in 6–15% of the Western population. The incidence of DUs declined steadily from 1960 to 1980 and has remained stable since then. The death rates, need for surgery, and physician visits have decreased by >50% over the past 30 years. The reason for the reduction in the frequency of DUs is likely related to the decreasing frequency of *Helicobacter pylori*. Before the discovery of *H. pylori*, the natural history of DUs was typified by frequent recurrences after initial therapy. Eradication of *H. pylori* has greatly reduced these recurrence rates.

Gastric Ulcers

GUs tend to occur later in life than duodenal lesions, with a peak incidence reported in the sixth decade. More than half of GUs occur in males and are less common than DUs, perhaps due to the higher likelihood of GUs being silent and presenting only after a complication develops. Autopsy studies suggest a similar incidence of DUs and GUs.

Pathology

Duodenal Ulcers

DUs occur most often in the first portion of duodenum (>95%), with ~90% located within 3 cm of the pylorus. They are usually ≤1 cm in diameter but can occasionally reach 3–6 cm (giant ulcer). Ulcers are sharply demarcated, with depth at times reaching the muscularis propria. The base of the ulcer often consists of a zone of eosinophilic necrosis with surrounding fibrosis. Malignant DUs are extremely rare.

Gastric Ulcers

In contrast to DUs, GUs can represent a malignancy. Benign GUs are most often found distal to the junction between the antrum and the acid secretory mucosa. Benign GUs are quite rare in the gastric fundus and are histologically similar to DUs. Benign GUs associated with *H. pylori* are also associated with antral gastritis. In contrast, NSAID-related GUs are not accompanied by chronic active gastritis but may instead have evidence of a chemical gastropathy, typified by foveolar hyperplasia, edema of the lamina propria and epithelial regeneration in the absence of *H. pylori*. Extension of smooth-muscle fibers into the upper portions of the mucosa, where they are not typically found, may also occur.

Pathophysiology

Duodenal Ulcers

H. pylori and NSAID-induced injury account for the majority of DUs. Many acid secretory abnormalities have been described in DU patients. Of these, average basal and nocturnal gastric acid secretion appears to be increased in DU patients as compared to controls; however, the level of overlap between DU patients and control subjects is substantial. The reason for this altered secretory process is unclear, but *H. pylori* infection may contribute. Accelerated gastric emptying of liquids has been noted in some DU patients, but its role in DU formation, if any, is unclear. Bicarbonate secretion is significantly decreased in the duodenal bulb of patients with an active DU as compared to control subjects. *H. pylori* infection may also play a role in this process (see later).

Gastric Ulcers

As in DUs, the majority of GUs can be attributed to either *H. pylori* or NSAID-induced mucosal damage. GUs that occur in the prepyloric area or those in the body associated with a DU or a duodenal scar are similar in pathogenesis to DUs. Gastric acid output (basal and stimulated) tends to be normal or decreased in GU patients. When GUs develop in the presence of minimal acid levels, impairment of mucosal defense factors may be present.

Abnormalities in resting and stimulated pyloric sphincter pressure with a concomitant increase in duodenal gastric reflux have been implicated in some GU patients. Although bile acids, lysolecithin, and pancreatic enzymes may injure gastric mucosa, a definite role for these in GU pathogenesis has not been established. Delayed gastric emptying of solids has been described in GU patients but has not been reported consistently.

H. Pylori and Acid Peptic Disorders

Gastric infection with the bacterium *H. pylori* accounts for the majority of PUD. This organism also plays a role in the development of gastric mucosal-associated lymphoid tissue (MALT) lymphoma and gastric adenocarcinoma. Although the entire genome of *H. pylori* has been sequenced, it is still not clear how this organism, which resides in the stomach, causes ulceration in the duodenum, or whether its eradication will lead to a decrease in gastric cancer.

The Bacterium

The bacterium, initially named *Campylobacter pyloridis*, is a gram-negative microaerophilic rod found most commonly in the deeper portions of the mucous gel coating the gastric mucosa or between the mucous layer and the gastric epithelium. It may attach to gastric epithelium but under normal circumstances does not appear to invade cells. It is strategically designed to live within the aggressive environment of the stomach. It is S-shaped (~0.5 × 3 μm in size) and contains multiple sheathed flagella. Initially, *H. pylori* resides in the antrum but, over time, migrates toward the more proximal segments of the stomach. The organism is capable of transforming into a coccoid form, which represents a dormant state that may facilitate survival in adverse conditions. The genome of *H. pylori* (1.65 million base pairs) encodes ~1500 proteins. Among this multitude of proteins there are factors that are essential determinants of *H. pylori*–mediated pathogenesis and colonization, such as the outer membrane protein (Hop proteins), urease, and the vacuolating cytotoxin (Vac A). Moreover, the majority of *H. pylori* strains contain a genomic fragment that encodes the cag pathogenicity island (cag-PAI). Several of the genes that make up cag-PAI encode components of a type IV secretion island that translocates Cag A into host cells. Once in the cell, Cag A activates a series of cellular events important in cell growth and cytokine production. The first step in infection by *H. pylori* is dependent on the bacteria's motility and its ability to produce urease. Urease produces ammonia from urea, an essential step in alkalinizing the surrounding pH. Additional bacterial factors include catalase, lipase, adhesins, platelet-activating factor, and pic B (induces cytokines). Multiple strains of *H. pylori* exist and are characterized by their ability to express several of these factors (Cag A, Vac A, etc.). It is possible that the different diseases related to *H. pylori* infection can be attributed to different strains of the organism with distinct pathogenic features.

Epidemiology

The prevalence of *H. pylori* varies throughout the world and depends largely on the overall standard of living in the region. In developing parts of the world, 80% of the population may be infected by the age of 20, whereas the prevalence is 20–50% in industrialized countries. In contrast, in the United States this organism is rare in childhood. The overall prevalence of *H. pylori* in the United States is ~30%, with individuals born before 1950 having a higher rate of infection than those born later. About 10% of Americans <30 years of age are colonized with the bacteria. The rate of infection with *H. pylori* in industrialized countries has decreased substantially in recent decades. The steady increase in the prevalence of *H. pylori* noted with increasing age is due primarily to a cohort effect, reflecting higher transmission during a period in which the earlier cohorts were children. It has been calculated through mathematical models that improved sanitation during the latter half of the nineteenth century dramatically decreased transmission of *H. pylori*. Moreover, with the present rate of intervention, the organism will be ultimately eliminated from the United States. Two factors that predispose to higher colonization rates include poor socioeconomic status and less education. These factors, not race, are responsible for the rate of *H. pylori* infection in blacks and Hispanic Americans being double the rate seen in whites of comparable age. Other risk factors for *H. pylori* infection are (1) birth or residence in a developing country, (2) domestic crowding, (3) unsanitary living conditions, (4) unclean food or water, and (5) exposure to gastric contents of an infected individual.

Transmission of *H. pylori* occurs from person to person, following an oral-oral or fecal-oral route. The risk of *H. pylori* infection is declining in developing countries. The rate of infection in the United States has fallen by >50% when compared to 30 years ago.

Pathophysiology

H. pylori infection is virtually always associated with a chronic active gastritis, but only 10–15% of infected individuals develop frank peptic ulceration. The basis for this difference is unknown. Initial studies suggested that >90% of all DUs were associated with *H. pylori*, but *H. pylori* is present in only 30–60% of individuals with GUs and 50–70% of patients with DUs. The pathophysiology of ulcers not associated with *H. pylori* or NSAID ingestion [or the rare Zollinger-Ellison syndrome (ZES)] is becoming more relevant as the incidence of *H. pylori* is dropping, particularly in the Western world (see below).

The particular end result of *H. pylori* infection (gastritis, PUD, gastric MALT lymphoma, gastric cancer) is

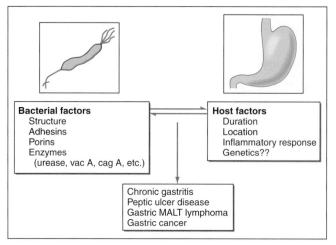

FIGURE 14-6

Outline of the bacterial and host factors important in determining *H. pylori*–induced gastrointestinal disease. MALT, mucosal-associated lymphoid tissue.

determined by a complex interplay between bacterial and host factors (**Fig. 14-6**).

1. *Bacterial factors.* *H. pylori* is able to facilitate gastric residence, induce mucosal injury, and avoid host defense. Different strains of *H. pylori* produce different virulence factors. A specific region of the bacterial genome, the pathogenicity island, encodes the virulence factors Cag A and pic B. Vac A also contributes to pathogenicity, though it is not encoded within the pathogenicity island. These virulence factors, in conjunction with additional bacterial constituents, can cause mucosal damage. Urease, which allows the bacteria to reside in the acidic stomach, generates NH_3, which can damage epithelial cells. The bacteria produce surface factors that are chemotactic for neutrophils and monocytes, which in turn contribute to epithelial cell injury (see below). *H. pylori* makes proteases and phospholipases that break down the glycoprotein lipid complex of the mucous gel, thus reducing the efficacy of this first line of mucosal defense. *H. pylori* expresses adhesins, which facilitate attachment of the bacteria to gastric epithelial cells. Although lipopolysaccharide (LPS) of gram-negative bacteria often plays an important role in the infection, *H. pylori* LPS has low immunologic activity compared to that of other organisms. It may promote a smoldering chronic inflammation.

2. *Host factors.* The inflammatory response to *H. pylori* includes recruitment of neutrophils, lymphocytes (T and B), macrophages, and plasma cells. The pathogen leads to local injury by binding to class II MHC molecules expressed on gastric epithelial cells, leading to cell death (*apoptosis*). Moreover, bacterial strains that encode cag-PAI can introduce Cag A into the host cells, leading to further cell injury and activation

of cellular pathways involved in cytokine production. Elevated concentrations of multiple cytokines are found in the gastric epithelium of *H. pylori*–infected individuals, including interleukin (IL) 1α/β, IL-2, IL-6, IL-8, tumor necrosis factor (TNF)-α, and interferon (IFN-γ). *H. pylori* infection also leads to both a mucosal and a systemic humoral response, which does not lead to eradication of the bacteria but further compounds epithelial cell injury. Additional mechanisms by which *H. pylori* may cause epithelial cell injury include (1) activated neutrophil-mediated production of reactive oxygen or nitrogen species and enhanced epithelial cell turnover and (2) apoptosis related to interaction with T cells (T helper 1, or T_H1, cells) and IFN-γ.

The reason for *H. pylori*–mediated duodenal ulceration remains unclear. One potential explanation is that gastric metaplasia in the duodenum of DU patients permits *H. pylori* to bind to it and produce local injury secondary to the host response. Another hypothesis is that *H. pylori* antral infection could lead to increased acid production, increased duodenal acid, and mucosal injury. Basal and stimulated [meal, gastrin-releasing peptide (GRP)] gastrin release are increased in *H. pylori*–infected individuals, and somatostatin-secreting D cells may be decreased. *H. pylori* infection might induce increased acid secretion through both direct and indirect actions of *H. pylori* and proinflammatory cytokines (IL-8, TNF, and IL-1) on G, D, and parietal cells (Fig. 14-7).

H. pylori infection has also been associated with decreased duodenal mucosal bicarbonate production. Data supporting and contradicting each of these interesting theories have been demonstrated. Thus, the mechanism by which *H. pylori* infection of the stomach leads to duodenal ulceration remains to be established.

In summary, the final effect of *H. pylori* on the gastrointestinal tract is variable and determined by microbial and host factors. The type and distribution of gastritis correlate with the ultimate gastric and duodenal pathology observed. Specifically, the presence of antral-predominant gastritis is associated with DU formation; gastritis involving primarily the corpus predisposes to the development of GUs, gastric atrophy, and ultimately gastric carcinoma (Fig. 14-8).

NSAID-Induced Disease
Epidemiology

NSAIDs represent a group of the most commonly used medications in the United States. More than 30 billion over-the-counter tablets and over 100 million prescriptions are sold yearly in the United States alone. In fact, after the introduction of COX-2 inhibitors in the year 2000, the number of prescriptions written for NSAIDs was >111 million at a cost of $4.8 billion. Side effects and complications due to NSAIDs are considered the most common drug-related toxicities in the United States. The spectrum of NSAID-induced morbidity ranges from nausea and dyspepsia (prevalence reported as high as 50–60%) to a serious gastrointestinal complication such as endoscopy-documented peptic ulceration (15–30% of individuals taking NSAIDs regularly) complicated by bleeding or perforation in as many as 1.5% of users per year. About 20,000 patients die each year from serious gastrointestinal complications from NSAIDs.

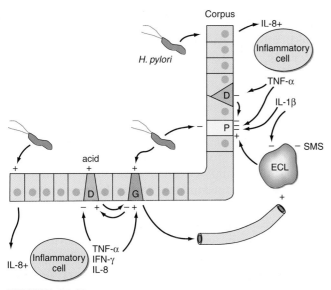

FIGURE 14-7

Summary of potential mechanisms by which *H. pylori* may lead to gastric secretory abnormalities. D, somatostatin cell; ECL, enterochromaffin-like cell; G, G cell; IFN, interferon; IL, interleukin; P, parietal cell; SMS, somatostatin; TNF, tumor necrosis factor. *(Adapted from J Calam et al: Gastroenterology 113:543, 1997.)*

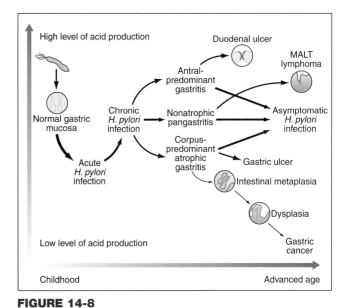

FIGURE 14-8

Natural history of *H. pylori* infection. *(Used with permission from Suerbaum and Michetti.)*

Unfortunately, dyspeptic symptoms do not correlate with NSAID-induced pathology. Over 80% of patients with serious NSAID-related complications did not have preceding dyspepsia. In view of the lack of warning signs, it is important to identify patients who are at increased risk for morbidity and mortality related to NSAID usage. Even 75 mg/d of aspirin may lead to serious gastrointestinal ulceration; thus, no dose of NSAID is completely safe. Established risk factors include advanced age, history of ulcer, concomitant use of glucocorticoids, high-dose NSAIDs, multiple NSAIDs, concomitant use of anticoagulants, and serious or multisystem disease. Possible risk factors include concomitant infection with *H. pylori*, cigarette smoking, and alcohol consumption.

Pathophysiology

Prostaglandins play a critical role in maintaining gastroduodenal mucosal integrity and repair. It therefore follows that interruption of prostaglandin synthesis can impair mucosal defense and repair, thus facilitating mucosal injury via a systemic mechanism. A summary of the pathogenetic pathways by which systemically administered NSAIDs may lead to mucosal injury is shown in **Fig. 14–9**.

Injury to the mucosa also occurs as a result of the topical encounter with NSAIDs. Aspirin and many NSAIDs are weak acids that remain in a nonionized lipophilic form when found within the acid environment of the stomach. Under these conditions, NSAIDs migrate across lipid membranes of epithelial cells, leading to cell injury once trapped intracellularly in an ionized form. Topical NSAIDs can also alter the surface mucous layer, permitting back diffusion of H^+ and pepsin, leading to further epithelial cell damage. Moreover, enteric-coated or buffered preparations are also associated with risk of peptic ulceration.

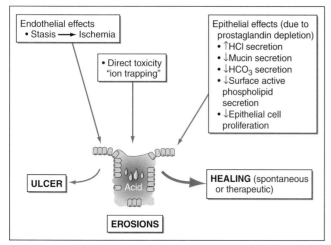

FIGURE 14-9
Mechanisms by which NSAIDs may induce mucosal injury. *(Adapted from J Scheiman et al: J Clin Outcomes Management 3:23, 1996.)*

The interplay between *H. pylori* and NSAIDs in the pathogenesis of PUD is complex. Meta-analysis supports the conclusion that each of these aggressive factors are independent and synergistic risk factors for PUD and its complications, such as gastrointestinal bleeding.

Pathogenetic Factors Unrelated to *H. Pylori* and NSAIDs in Acid Peptic Disease

Cigarette smoking has been implicated in the pathogenesis of PUD. Not only have smokers been found to have ulcers more frequently than do nonsmokers, but smoking appears to decrease healing rates, impair response to therapy, and increase ulcer-related complications such as perforation. The mechanism responsible for increased ulcer diathesis in smokers is unknown. Theories have included altered gastric emptying, decreased proximal duodenal bicarbonate production, increased risk for *H. pylori* infection, and cigarette-induced generation of noxious mucosal free radicals. Despite these interesting theories, the mechanism for the cigarette-induced peptic ulcer diathesis has not been established.

Genetic predisposition may play a role in ulcer development. First-degree relatives of DU patients are three times as likely to develop an ulcer; however, the potential role of *H. pylori* infection in contacts is a major consideration. Increased frequency of blood group O and of the nonsecretor status have also been implicated as genetic risk factors for peptic diathesis. However, *H. pylori* preferentially binds to group O antigens. The role of genetic predisposition in common PUD has not been established.

Psychological stress has been thought to contribute to PUD, but studies examining the role of psychological factors in its pathogenesis have generated conflicting results. Although PUD is associated with certain personality traits (neuroticism), these same traits are also present in individuals with nonulcer dyspepsia (NUD) and other functional and organic disorders. Although more work in this area is needed, no typical PUD personality has been found.

Diet has also been thought to play a role in peptic diseases. Certain foods can cause dyspepsia, but no convincing studies indicate an association between ulcer formation and a specific diet. This is also true for beverages containing alcohol and caffeine. Specific chronic disorders have been associated with PUD. Those with a strong association are (1) systemic mastocytosis, (2) chronic pulmonary disease, (3) chronic renal failure, (4) cirrhosis, (5) nephrolithiasis, and (6) α_1-antitrypsin deficiency. Those with a possible association are (1) hyperparathyroidism, (2) coronary artery disease, (3) polycythemia vera, and (4) chronic pancreatitis.

Multiple factors play a role in the pathogenesis of PUD. The two predominant causes are *H. pylori* infection and NSAID ingestion. PUD not related to *H. pylori* or NSAIDs is increasing. Other less common

TABLE 14-1

CAUSES OF ULCERS NOT CAUSED BY *HELICOBACTER PYLORI* AND NSAIDS

Infection

Cytomegalovirus
Herpes simplex virus
Helicobacter heilmannii

Drug/Toxin

Bisphosphonates
Chemotherapy
Clopidogrel
Crack cocaine
Glucocorticoids (when combined with NSAIDs)
Mycophenolate mofetil
Potassium chloride

Miscellaneous

Basophilia in myeloproliferative disease
Duodenal obstruction (e.g., annular pancreas)
Infiltrating disease
Ischemia
Radiation therapy
Sarcoidosis
Crohn's disease
Idiopathic hypersecretory state

Note: Hp, *Helicobacter pylori*; NSAID, nonsteroidal anti-inflammatory drug.

causes of PUD are shown in Table 14-1. These etiologic agents should be considered as the incidence of *H. pylori* is decreasing. Independent of the inciting or injurious agent, peptic ulcers develop as a result of an imbalance between mucosal protection/repair and aggressive factors. Gastric acid plays an essential role in mucosal injury.

CLINICAL FEATURES

History

Abdominal pain is common to many gastrointestinal disorders, including DU and GU, but has a poor predictive value for the presence of either DU or GU. Up to 10% of patients with NSAID-induced mucosal disease can present with a complication (bleeding, perforation, and obstruction) without antecedent symptoms. Despite this poor correlation, a careful history and physical examination are essential components of the approach to a patient suspected of having peptic ulcers.

Epigastric pain described as a burning or gnawing discomfort can be present in both DU and GU. The discomfort is also described as an ill-defined, aching sensation or as hunger pain. The typical pain pattern in DU occurs 90 min to 3 h after a meal and is frequently relieved by antacids or food. Pain that awakes the patient from sleep (between midnight and 3 A.M.) is the most discriminating symptom, with two-thirds of DU patients describing this complaint. Unfortunately, this symptom is also present in one-third of patients with NUD. The pain pattern in GU patients may be different from that in DU patients, where discomfort may actually be precipitated by food. Nausea and weight loss occur more commonly in GU patients. Endoscopy detects ulcers in <30% of patients who have dyspepsia.

The mechanism for development of abdominal pain in ulcer patients is unknown. Several possible explanations include acid-induced activation of chemical receptors in the duodenum, enhanced duodenal sensitivity to bile acids and pepsin, or altered gastroduodenal motility.

Variation in the intensity or distribution of the abdominal pain, as well as the onset of associated symptoms such as nausea and/or vomiting, may be indicative of an ulcer complication. Dyspepsia that becomes constant, is no longer relieved by food or antacids, or radiates to the back may indicate a penetrating ulcer (pancreas). Sudden onset of severe, generalized abdominal pain may indicate perforation. Pain worsening with meals, nausea, and vomiting of undigested food suggest gastric outlet obstruction. Tarry stools or coffee-ground emesis indicate bleeding.

Physical Examination

Epigastric tenderness is the most frequent finding in patients with GU or DU. Pain may be found to the right of the midline in 20% of patients. Unfortunately, the predictive value of this finding is rather low. Physical examination is critically important for discovering evidence of ulcer complication. Tachycardia and orthostasis suggest dehydration secondary to vomiting or active gastrointestinal blood loss. A severely tender, boardlike abdomen suggests a perforation. Presence of a succussion splash indicates retained fluid in the stomach, suggesting gastric outlet obstruction.

PUD-Related Complications

Gastrointestinal Bleeding

Gastrointestinal bleeding is the most common complication observed in PUD. It occurs in ~15% of patients and more often in individuals >60 years old. The higher incidence in the elderly is likely due to the increased use of NSAIDs in this group. Up to 20% of patients with ulcer-related hemorrhage bleed without any preceding warning signs or symptoms.

Perforation

The second most common ulcer-related complication is perforation, being reported in as many as 6–7% of PUD patients. As in the case of bleeding, the incidence of perforation in the elderly appears to be increasing secondary to increased use of NSAIDs. *Penetration* is a form of perforation in which the ulcer bed tunnels into an adjacent organ. DUs tend to penetrate posteriorly into the pancreas, leading to pancreatitis, whereas GUs tend to penetrate into the left hepatic lobe. Gastrocolic fistulas associated with GUs have also been described.

Gastric Outlet Obstruction

Gastric outlet obstruction is the least common ulcer-related complication, occurring in 1–2% of patients. A patient may have relative obstruction secondary to ulcer-related inflammation and edema in the peripyloric region. This process often resolves with ulcer healing. A fixed, mechanical obstruction secondary to scar formation in the peripyloric areas is also possible. The latter requires endoscopic (balloon dilation) or surgical intervention. Signs and symptoms relative to mechanical obstruction may develop insidiously. New onset of early satiety, nausea, vomiting, increase of postprandial abdominal pain, and weight loss should make gastric outlet obstruction a possible diagnosis.

Differential Diagnosis

The list of gastrointestinal and nongastrointestinal disorders that can mimic ulceration of the stomach or duodenum is quite extensive. The most commonly encountered diagnosis among patients seen for upper abdominal discomfort is NUD. NUD, also known as *functional dyspepsia* or *essential dyspepsia*, refers to a group of heterogeneous disorders typified by upper abdominal pain without the presence of an ulcer. Dyspepsia has been reported to occur in up to 30% of the U.S. population. Up to 60% of patients seeking medical care for dyspepsia have a negative diagnostic evaluation. The etiology of NUD is not established, and the potential role of *H. pylori* in NUD remains controversial.

Several additional disease processes that may present with "ulcer-like" symptoms include proximal gastrointestinal tumors, gastroesophageal reflux, vascular disease, pancreaticobiliary disease (biliary colic, chronic pancreatitis), and gastroduodenal Crohn's disease.

Diagnostic Evaluation

In view of the poor predictive value of abdominal pain for the presence of a gastroduodenal ulcer and the multiple disease processes that can mimic this disease, the clinician is often confronted with having to establish the presence of an ulcer. Documentation of an ulcer requires either a radiographic (barium study) or an endoscopic procedure. However, a large percentage of patients with symptoms suggestive of an ulcer have NUD; empirical therapy is appropriate for individuals who are otherwise healthy and <45, before embarking on a diagnostic evaluation (Chap. 5).

Barium studies of the proximal gastrointestinal tract are still commonly used as a first test for documenting an ulcer. The sensitivity of older single-contrast barium meals for detecting a DU is as high as 80%, with a double-contrast study providing detection rates as high as 90%. Sensitivity for detection is decreased in small ulcers (<0.5 cm), presence of previous scarring, or in postoperative patients. A DU appears as a well-demarcated crater, most often seen in the bulb (**Fig. 14-10***A*). A GU may represent benign or malignant disease. Typically, a benign GU also appears as a discrete crater with radiating mucosal folds originating from the ulcer margin (**Fig. 14-10***B*). Ulcers >3 cm in size or those associated with a mass are more often malignant. Unfortunately, up to 8% of GUs that appear to be benign by radiographic appearance are malignant by endoscopy or surgery.

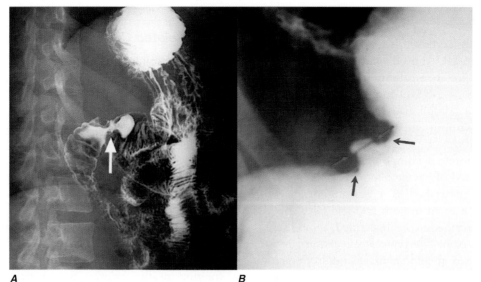

A   *B*

FIGURE 14-10
Barium study demonstrating: *A.* a benign duodenal ulcer; *B.* a benign gastric ulcer.

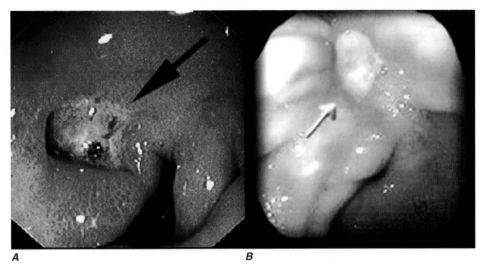

FIGURE 14-11
Endoscopy demonstrating: **A.** a benign duodenal ulcer; **B.** a benign gastric ulcer.

Radiographic studies that show a GU must be followed by endoscopy and biopsy.

Endoscopy provides the most sensitive and specific approach for examining the upper gastrointestinal tract (Fig. 14-11). In addition to permitting direct visualization of the mucosa, endoscopy facilitates photographic documentation of a mucosal defect and tissue biopsy to rule out malignancy (GU) or *H. pylori*. Endoscopic examination is particularly helpful in identifying lesions too small to detect by radiographic examination, for evaluation of atypical radiographic abnormalities, or to determine if an ulcer is a source of blood loss.

Although the methods for diagnosing *H. pylori* are outlined in Chap. 25, a brief summary will be included here (Table 14-2). Several biopsy urease tests have been developed (PyloriTek, Clotest, Hpfast, Pronto Dry) that have a sensitivity and specificity of >90–95%. Several noninvasive methods for detecting this organism have been developed. Three types of studies routinely used include serologic testing, the ^{13}C- or ^{14}C-urea breath test, and the fecal *H. pylori* (Hp) antigen test. A urinary Hp antigen test, as well as a refined monoclonal antibody stool antigen test, appears promising.

Occasionally, specialized testing such as serum gastrin and gastric acid analysis or sham feeding may be needed in individuals with complicated or refractory PUD (see "Zollinger-Ellison Syndrome" later in the chapter). Screening for aspirin or NSAIDs (blood or urine) may also be necessary in refractory *H. pylori*–negative PUD patients.

TABLE 14-2

TESTS FOR DETECTION OF *H. PYLORI*		
TEST	**SENSITIVITY/SPECIFICITY, %**	**COMMENTS**
Invasive (Endoscopy/Biopsy Required)		
Rapid urease	80–95/95–100	Simple, false negative with recent use of PPIs, antibiotics, or bismuth compounds
Histology	80–90/>95	Requires pathology processing and staining; provides histologic information
Culture	–/–	Time-consuming, expensive, dependent on experience; allows determination of antibiotic susceptibility
Non-Invasive		
Serology	>80/>90	Inexpensive, convenient; not useful for early follow-up
Urea breath test	>90/>90	Simple, rapid; useful for early follow-up; false negatives with recent therapy (see rapid urease test); exposure to low-dose radiation with ^{14}C test
Stool antigen	>90/>90	Inexpensive, convenient; not established for eradication but promising

Note: PPIs, proton pump inhibitors.

℞ **Treatment:**
PEPTIC ULCER DISEASE

Before the discovery of *H. pylori*, the therapy of PUD was centered on the old dictum by Schwartz of "no acid, no ulcer." Although acid secretion is still important in the pathogenesis of PUD, eradication of *H. pylori* and therapy/prevention of NSAID-induced disease is the mainstay of treatment. A summary of commonly used drugs for treatment of acid peptic disorders is shown in Table 14-3.

ACID NEUTRALIZING/INHIBITORY DRUGS

Antacids Before we understood the important role of histamine in stimulating parietal cell activity, neutralization of secreted acid with antacids constituted the main form of therapy for peptic ulcers. They are now rarely, if ever, used as the primary therapeutic agent but instead are often used by patients for symptomatic relief of dyspepsia. The most commonly used agents are mixtures of aluminum and magnesium hydroxide. Aluminum can produce constipation and phosphate depletion; magnesium hydroxide may cause loose stools. Many of the commonly used antacids (e.g., Maalox, Mylanta) have a combination of both aluminum and magnesium hydroxide in order to avoid these side effects. The magnesium-containing preparation should not be used in chronic renal failure patients because of possible hypermagnesemia, and aluminum may cause chronic neurotoxicity in these patients.

TABLE 14-3

DRUGS USED IN THE TREATMENT OF PEPTIC ULCER DISEASE		
DRUG TYPE/ MECHANISM	**EXAMPLES**	**DOSE**
Acid-Suppressing Drugs		
Antacids	Mylanta, Maalox, Tums, Gaviscon	100–140 meq/L 1 and 3 h after meals and hs
H₂ receptor antagonists	Cimetidine	400 mg bid
	Ranitidine	300 mg hs
	Famotidine	40 mg hs
	Nizatidine	300 mg hs
Proton pump inhibitors	Omeprazole	20 mg/d
	Lansoprazole	30 mg/d
	Rabeprazole	20 mg/d
	Pantoprazole	40 mg/d
	Esomeprazole	20 mg/d
Mucosal Protective Agents		
Sucralfate	Sucralfate	1 g qid
Prostaglandin analogue	Misoprostol	200 μg qid
Bismuth-containing compounds	Bismuth subsalicylate (BSS)	See anti-*H. pylori* regimens (Table 14-4)

Calcium carbonate and sodium bicarbonate are potent antacids with varying levels of potential problems. The long-term use of calcium carbonate (converts to calcium chloride in the stomach) can lead to milk-alkali syndrome (hypercalcemia, hyperphosphatemia with possible renal calcinosis and progression to renal insufficiency). Sodium bicarbonate may induce systemic alkalosis.

H₂ Receptor Antagonists Four of these agents are presently available (cimetidine, ranitidine, famotidine, and nizatidine), and their structures share homology with histamine. Although each has different potency, all will significantly inhibit basal and stimulated acid secretion to comparable levels when used at therapeutic doses. Moreover, similar ulcer-healing rates are achieved with each drug when used at the correct dosage. Presently, this class of drug is often used for treatment of active ulcers (4–6 weeks) in combination with antibiotics directed at eradicating *H. pylori* (see below).

Cimetidine was the first H₂ receptor antagonist used for the treatment of acid peptic disorders. The initial recommended dosing profile for cimetidine was 300 mg qid. Subsequent studies have documented the efficacy of using 800 mg at bedtime for treatment of active ulcer, with healing rates approaching 80% at 4 weeks. Cimetidine may have weak antiandrogenic side effects resulting in reversible gynecomastia and impotence, primarily in patients receiving high doses for prolonged periods of time (months to years, as in ZES). In view of cimetidine's ability to inhibit cytochrome P450, careful monitoring of drugs such as warfarin, phenytoin, and theophylline is indicated with long-term usage. Other rare reversible adverse effects reported with cimetidine include confusion and elevated levels of serum aminotransferases, creatinine, and serum prolactin. Ranitidine, famotidine, and nizatidine are more potent H₂ receptor antagonists than cimetidine. Each can be used once a day at bedtime for ulcer prevention, which was commonly done before the discovery of *H. pylori* and the development of proton pump inhibitors (PPIs). Patients may develop tolerance to H₂ blockers, a rare event with PPIs (see below). Comparable nighttime dosing regimens are ranitidine 300 mg, famotidine 40 mg, and nizatidine 300 mg.

Additional rare, reversible systemic toxicities reported with H₂ receptor antagonists include pancytopenia, neutropenia, anemia, and thrombocytopenia, with a prevalence rate varying from 0.01 to 0.2%. Cimetidine and ranitidine (to a lesser extent) can bind to hepatic cytochrome P450; famotidine and nizatidine do not.

Proton Pump (H⁺,K⁺-ATPase) Inhibitors Omeprazole, esomeprazole, lansoprazole, rabeprazole, and pantoprazole are substituted benzimidazole derivatives that covalently bind and irreversibly inhibit H⁺,K⁺-ATPase.

Esomeprazole, the newest member of this drug class, is the S-enantiomer of omeprazole, which is a racemic mixture of both S- and R-optical isomers. These are the most potent acid inhibitory agents available. Omeprazole and lansoprazole are the PPIs that have been used for the longest time. Both are acid-labile and are administered as enteric-coated granules in a sustained-release capsule that dissolves within the small intestine at a pH of 6. Lansoprazole is available in an orally disintegrating tablet that can be taken with or without water, an advantage for individuals who have significant dysphagia. Absorption kinetics are similar to the capsule. In addition, a lansoprazole-naproxen combination preparation that has been made available is targeted at decreasing NSAID-related gastrointestinal injury (see below). Omeprazole is available as non-enteric-coated granules mixed with sodium bicarbonate in a powder form which can be administered orally or via gastric tube. The sodium bicarbonate has two purposes: to protect the omeprazole from acid degradation and to promote rapid gastric alkalinization and subsequent proton pump activation, which facilitates rapid action of the PPI. Pantoprazole and rabeprazole are available as enteric-coated tablets. Pantoprazole is also available as a parenteral formulation for intravenous use. These agents are lipophilic compounds; upon entering the parietal cell, they are protonated and trapped within the acid environment of the tubulovesicular and canalicular system. These agents potently inhibit all phases of gastric acid secretion. Onset of action is rapid, with a maximum acid inhibitory effect between 2 and 6 h after administration and duration of inhibition lasting up to 72–96 h. With repeated daily dosing, progressive acid inhibitory effects are observed, with basal and secretagogue-stimulated acid production being inhibited by >95% after 1 week of therapy. The half-life of PPIs is ~18 h; thus, it can take between 2 and 5 days for gastric acid secretion to return to normal levels once these drugs have been discontinued. Because the pumps need to be activated for these agents to be effective, their efficacy is maximized if they are administered before a meal (except for the immediate-release formulation of omeprazole) (e.g., in the morning before breakfast). Mild to moderate hypergastrinemia has been observed in patients taking these drugs. Carcinoid tumors developed in some animals given the drugs preclinically; however, extensive experience has failed to demonstrate gastric carcinoid tumor development in humans. Serum gastrin levels return to normal levels within 1–2 weeks after drug cessation. Intrinsic factor (IF) production is also inhibited, but vitamin B_{12}-deficiency anemia is uncommon, probably because of the large stores of the vitamin. As with any agent that leads to significant hypochlorhydria, PPIs may interfere with absorption of drugs such as ketoconazole, ampicillin, iron, and digoxin. Hepatic cytochrome P450 can be inhibited by the earlier PPIs (omeprazole, lansoprazole). Rabeprazole, pantoprazole, and esomeprazole do not appear to interact significantly with drugs metabolized by the cytochrome P450 system. The overall clinical significance of this observation is not definitely established. Caution should be taken when using warfarin, diazepam, atazanavir, and phenytoin concomitantly with PPIs. Long-term acid suppression, especially with PPIs, has been associated with a higher incidence of community-acquired pneumonia. This observation requires confirmation but should alert the practitioner to take caution when recommending these agents for long-term use, especially in elderly patients at risk for developing pneumonia.

Two new formulations of acid inhibitory agents are being developed. Tenatoprazole is a PPI containing an imidazopyridine ring instead of a benzimidazole ring, which promotes irreversible proton pump inhibition. This agent has a longer half-life than the other PPIs and may be beneficial for inhibiting nocturnal acid secretion, which has significant relevance in gastroesophageal reflux disease (GERD). A second new class of agents is the potassium-competitive acid pump antagonists (P-CABs). These compounds inhibit gastric acid secretion via potassium competitive binding of the H^+,K^+-ATPase.

CYTOPROTECTIVE AGENTS

Sucralfate Sucralfate is a complex sucrose salt in which the hydroxyl groups have been substituted by aluminum hydroxide and sulfate. This compound is insoluble in water and becomes a viscous paste within the stomach and duodenum, binding primarily to sites of active ulceration. Sucralfate may act by several mechanisms: serving as a physicochemical barrier, promoting a trophic action by binding growth factors such as EGF, enhancing prostaglandin synthesis, stimulating mucous and bicarbonate secretion, and enhancing mucosal defense and repair. Toxicity from this drug is rare, with constipation being most common (2–3%). It should be avoided in patients with chronic renal insufficiency to prevent aluminum-induced neurotoxicity. Hypophosphatemia and gastric bezoar formation have also been reported rarely. Standard dosing of sucralfate is 1 g qid.

Bismuth-Containing Preparations Sir William Osler considered bismuth-containing compounds as the drug of choice for treating PUD. The resurgence in the use of these agents is due to their effect against *H. pylori*. Colloidal bismuth subcitrate (CBS) and bismuth subsalicylate (BSS, Pepto-Bismol) are the most widely used preparations. The mechanism by which these agents induce ulcer healing is unclear. Potential mechanisms include ulcer coating; prevention of further pepsin/HCl-induced damage; binding of pepsin; and stimulation of prostaglandins, bicarbonate, and mucous secretion.

Adverse effects with short-term usage include black stools, constipation, and darkening of the tongue. Long-term usage with high doses, especially with the avidly absorbed CBS, may lead to neurotoxicity. These compounds are commonly used as one of the agents in an anti-*H. pylori* regimen (see below).

Prostaglandin Analogues In view of their central role in maintaining mucosal integrity and repair, stable prostaglandin analogues were developed for the treatment of PUD. The mechanism by which this rapidly absorbed drug provides its therapeutic effect is through enhancement of mucosal defense and repair. Prostaglandin analogues enhance mucous bicarbonate secretion, stimulate mucosal blood flow, and decrease mucosal cell turnover. The most common toxicity noted with this drug is diarrhea (10–30% incidence). Other major toxicities include uterine bleeding and contractions; misoprostol is contraindicated in women who may be pregnant, and women of childbearing age must be made clearly aware of this potential drug toxicity. The standard therapeutic dose is 200 μg qid.

Miscellaneous Drugs A number of drugs aimed at treating acid peptic disorders have been developed over the years. In view of their limited utilization in the United States, if any, they will only be listed briefly. Anticholinergics, designed to inhibit activation of the muscarinic receptor in parietal cells, met with limited success due to their relatively weak acid-inhibiting effect and significant side effects (dry eyes, dry mouth, urinary retention). Tricyclic antidepressants have been suggested by some, but again the toxicity of these agents in comparison to the safe, effective drugs already described precludes their utility.

THERAPY OF *H. PYLORI* Extensive effort has been made into determining who of the many individuals with *H. pylori* infection should be treated. The common conclusion arrived at by multiple consensus conferences around the world is that *H. pylori* should be eradicated in patients with documented PUD. This holds true independent of time of presentation (first episode or not), severity of symptoms, presence of confounding factors such as ingestion of NSAIDs, or whether the ulcer is in remission. Some have advocated treating patients with a history of documented PUD who are found to be *H. pylori*–positive by serology or breath testing. Over half of patients with gastric MALT lymphoma experience complete remission of the tumor in response to *H. pylori* eradication. Treating patients with NUD, to prevent gastric cancer, or patients with GERD requiring long-term acid suppression, remains controversial.

Multiple drugs have been evaluated in the therapy of *H. pylori*. No single agent is effective in eradicating the organism. Combination therapy for 14 days provides the greatest efficacy. A shorter course administration (7–10 days), although attractive, has not proved as successful as the 14-day regimens. The agents used with the greatest frequency include amoxicillin, metronidazole, tetracycline, clarithromycin, and bismuth compounds.

The physician's goal in treating PUD is to provide relief of symptoms (pain or dyspepsia), promote ulcer healing, and ultimately prevent ulcer recurrence and complications. The greatest impact of understanding the role of *H. pylori* in peptic disease has been the ability to prevent recurrence. Documented eradication of *H. pylori* in patients with PUD is associated with a dramatic decrease in ulcer recurrence to <10–20% as compared to 59% in GU patients and 67% in DU patients when the organism is not eliminated. Eradication of the organism may lead to diminished recurrent ulcer bleeding. The impact of its eradication on ulcer perforation is unclear.

Suggested treatment regimens for *H. pylori* are outlined in Table 14-4. Choice of a particular regimen will be influenced by several factors, including efficacy, patient tolerance, existing antibiotic resistance, and cost of the drugs. The aim for initial eradication rates should be 85–90%. Dual therapy [PPI plus amoxicillin, PPI plus clarithromycin, ranitidine bismuth citrate (Tritec) plus clarithromycin] are not recommended in view of studies demonstrating eradication rates of <80–85%. The combination of bismuth, metronidazole, and tetracycline was the first triple regimen found effective against *H. pylori*. The combination of two antibiotics plus either a PPI, H_2 blocker, or bismuth compound has comparable

TABLE 14-4

REGIMENS RECOMMENDED FOR ERADICATION OF *H. PYLORI* INFECTION

DRUG	DOSE
Triple Therapy	
1. Bismuth subsalicylate *plus*	2 tablets qid
Metronidazole *plus*	250 mg qid
Tetracycline[a]	500 mg qid
2. Ranitidine bismuth citrate *plus*	400 mg bid
Tetracycline *plus*	500 mg bid
Clarithromycin or metronidazole	500 mg bid
3. Omeprazole (lansoprazole) *plus*	20 mg bid (30 mg bid)
Clarithromycin *plus*	250 or 500 mg bid
Metronidazole[b] *or*	500 mg bid
Amoxicillin[c]	1 g bid
Quadruple Therapy	
Omeprazole (lansoprazole)	20 mg (30 mg) daily
Bismuth subsalicylate	2 tablets qid
Metronidazole	250 mg qid
Tetracycline	500 mg qid

[a]Alternative: use prepacked Helidac (see text).
[b]Alternative: use prepacked Prevpac (see text).
[c]Use either metronidazole or amoxicillin, not both.

success rates. Addition of acid suppression assists in providing early symptom relief and may enhance bacterial eradication.

Triple therapy, although effective, has several drawbacks, including the potential for poor patient compliance and drug-induced side effects. Compliance is being addressed by simplifying the regimens so that patients can take the medications twice a day. Simpler (dual therapy) and shorter regimens (7 and 10 days) are not as effective as triple therapy for 14 days. Two anti-*H. pylori* regimens are available in prepackaged formulation: Prevpac (lansoprazole, clarithromycin, and amoxicillin) and Helidac (bismuth subsalicylate, tetracycline, and metronidazole). The contents of the Prevpac are to be taken twice per day for 14 days, whereas Helidac constituents are taken four times per day with an antisecretory agent (PPI or H_2 blocker), also for at least 14 days.

Side effects have been reported in up to 20–30% of patients on triple therapy. Bismuth may cause black stools, constipation, or darkening of the tongue. The most feared complication with amoxicillin is pseudomembranous colitis, but this occurs in <1–2% of patients. Amoxicillin can also lead to antibiotic-associated diarrhea, nausea, vomiting, skin rash, and allergic reaction. Tetracycline has been reported to cause rashes and, very rarely, hepatotoxicity and anaphylaxis.

One important concern with treating patients who may not need treatment is the potential for development of antibiotic-resistant strains. The incidence and type of antibiotic-resistant *H. pylori* strains vary worldwide. Strains resistant to metronidazole, clarithromycin, amoxicillin, and tetracycline have been described, with the latter two being uncommon. Antibiotic-resistant strains are the most common cause for treatment failure in compliant patients. Unfortunately, in vitro resistance does not predict outcome in patients. Culture and sensitivity testing of *H. pylori* is not performed routinely. Although resistance to metronidazole has been found in as many as 30% of isolates in North America and 80% in developing countries, triple therapy is effective in eradicating the organism in >50% of patients infected with a resistant strain. Clarithromycin resistance is seen in 13% of individuals in the United States, with resistance to amoxicillin being <1% and resistance to both metronidazole and clarithromycin in the 5% range.

Failure of *H. pylori* eradication with triple therapy in a compliant patient is usually due to infection with a resistant organism. Quadruple therapy (Table 14-4), where clarithromycin is substituted for metronidazole (or vice versa), should be the next step. The combination of pantoprazole, amoxicillin, and rifabutin for 10 days has also been used successfully (86% cure rate) in patients infected with resistant strains. Additional regimens considered for second-line therapy include levofloxin-based triple therapy (levofloxin, amoxicillin, PPI) for 10 days and furazolidone-based triple therapy (furazolidone, amoxicillin, and a PPI) for 14 days. Unfortunately, there is no universally accepted treatment regimen recommended for patients who have failed two courses of antibiotics. If eradication is still not achieved in a compliant patient, then culture and sensitivity of the organism should be considered. Additional factors that may lower eradication rates include the patient's country of origin (higher in Northeast Asia than other parts of Asia or Europe) and cigarette smoking.

In view of the observation that between 15 and 25% of patients treated with first-line therapy may still remain infected with the organism, new approaches to treatment have been explored. One promising approach is sequential therapy. This regimen consists of 5 days of amoxicillin and a PPI, followed by an additional 5 days of PPI plus tinidazole and clarithromycin. Initial studies have demonstrated eradication rates of >90% with good patient tolerance. Confirmation of these findings and applicability of this approach in the United States are needed.

Reinfection after successful eradication of *H. pylori* is rare in the United States (<1%/year). If recurrent infection occurs within the first 6 months after completing therapy, the most likely explanation is recrudescence as opposed to reinfection.

THERAPY OF NSAID-RELATED GASTRIC OR DUODENAL INJURY Medical intervention for NSAID-related mucosal injury includes treatment of an active ulcer and primary prevention of future injury. Recommendations for the treatment and primary prevention of NSAID-related mucosal injury are listed in Table 14-5. Ideally, the injurious agent should be stopped as the first step in the therapy of an active NSAID-induced ulcer. If that is possible, then treatment with one of the

TABLE 14-5

RECOMMENDATIONS FOR TREATMENT OF NSAID-RELATED MUCOSAL INJURY	
CLINICAL SETTING	**RECOMMENDATION**
Active ulcer	
NSAID discontinued	H_2 receptor antagonist or PPI
NSAID continued	PPI
Prophylactic therapy	Misoprostol
	PPI
	Selective COX-2 inhibitor
H. pylori infection	Eradication if active ulcer present or there is a past history of peptic ulcer disease

Note: PPI, proton pump inhibitor; COX-2, isoenzyme of cyclooxygenase.

acid inhibitory agents (H$_2$ blockers, PPIs) is indicated. Cessation of NSAIDs is not always possible because of the patient's severe underlying disease. Only PPIs can heal GUs or DUs, independent of whether NSAIDs are discontinued.

The approach to primary prevention has included avoiding the agent, using NSAIDs that are theoretically less injurious, and/or the use of concomitant medical therapy to prevent NSAID-induced injury. Primary prevention of NSAID-induced ulceration can be accomplished by misoprostol (200 μg qid) or a PPI. High-dose H$_2$ blockers (famotidine, 40 mg bid) have also shown some promise in preventing endoscopically documented ulcers, although PPIs are superior. The highly selective COX-2 inhibitors, celecoxib and rofecoxib, are 100 times more selective inhibitors of COX-2 than standard NSAIDs, leading to gastric or duodenal mucosal injury that is comparable to placebo; their utilization led to an increase in cardiovascular events and withdrawal from the market. Additional caution was engendered when the CLASS study demonstrated that the advantage of celecoxib in preventing gastrointestinal complications was offset when low-dose aspirin was used simultaneously. Therefore, gastric protection therapy is required in individuals taking COX-2 inhibitors and aspirin prophylaxis. Finally, much of the work performed demonstrating the benefit of COX-2 inhibitors and PPIs on gastrointestinal injury has been performed in individuals of average risk; it is unclear if the same level of benefit will be achieved in high-risk patients. For example, concomitant use of warfarin and a COX-2 inhibitor was associated with rates of gastrointestinal bleeding similar to those observed in patients taking nonselective NSAIDs. A combination of factors, including withdrawal of the majority of COX-2 inhibitors from the market, the observation that low-dose aspirin appears to diminish the beneficial effect of COX-2 selective inhibitors, and the growing use of aspirin for prophylaxis of cardiovascular events, have significantly altered the approach to gastric protective therapy during the use of NSAIDs. A guide for the approach to the use of NSAIDs is shown in **Table 14-6**. Individuals who are not at risk for cardiovascular events, do not use aspirin, and are without risk for GI complications can receive nonselective NSAIDs without gastric protection. In those without cardiovascular risk factors but with a high potential risk for NSAID-induced GI toxicity, cautious use of a selective COX-2 inhibitor or a nonselective NSAID with gastric protection with a PPI is in order. Individuals with cardiovascular risk factors who require low-dose aspirin and have low potential for NSAID-induced toxicity should be considered for a non-NSAID agent or use of a traditional NSAID in combination with gastric protection, if warranted. Finally, individuals with cardiovascular and GI risks who require

TABLE 14-6

GUIDE TO NSAID THERAPY

	NO/LOW NSAID GI RISK	NSAID GI RISK
No CV risk (no aspirin)	Traditional NSAID	Coxib or Traditional NSAID + PPI Consider non-NSAID therapy
CV risk (consider aspirin)	Traditional NSAID + PPI if GI risk warrants gastroprotection Consider non-NSAID therapy	A gastroprotective agent must be added if a traditional NSAID is prescribed Consider non-NSAID therapy

Note: NSAID, nonsteroidal anti-inflammatory drug; GI, gastrointestinal; CV, cardiovascular; PPI, proton pump inhibitor.
Source: Adapted from AM Fendrick: Am J Manag Care 10:740, 2004.

aspirin must be considered for non-NSAID therapy, but if that is not an option, then gastric protection with any type of NSAID must be considered.

APPROACH AND THERAPY: SUMMARY Controversy continues regarding the best approach to the patient who presents with dyspepsia (Chap. 5). The discovery of *H. pylori* and its role in pathogenesis of ulcers has added a new variable to the equation. Previously, if a patient <50 years old presented with dyspepsia and without alarming signs or symptoms suggestive of an ulcer complication or malignancy, an empirical therapeutic trial with acid suppression was commonly recommended. Although this approach is practiced by some today, an approach presently gaining approval for the treatment of patients with dyspepsia is outlined in **Fig. 14-12**. The referral to a gastroenterologist is for the potential need of endoscopy and subsequent evaluation and treatment if the endoscopy is negative.

Once an ulcer (GU or DU) is documented, the main issue at stake is whether *H. pylori* or an NSAID is involved. With *H. pylori* present, independent of the NSAID status, triple therapy is recommended for 14 days, followed by continued acid-suppressing drugs (H$_2$ receptor antagonist or PPIs) for a total of 4–6 weeks. Selection of patients for documentation of *H. pylori* eradication (organisms gone at least 4 weeks after completing antibiotics) is an area of some debate. The test of choice for documenting eradication is the urea breath test (UBT). The stool antigen assay may also hold promise for this purpose, but the data have not been as clear-cut as in the case of using the stool antigen test for primary diagnosis, especially if one considers patients who live in areas of low *H. pylori* prevalence. Further studies are warranted, but if the UBT is not available, a stool antigen should be considered to document eradication. The patient must be

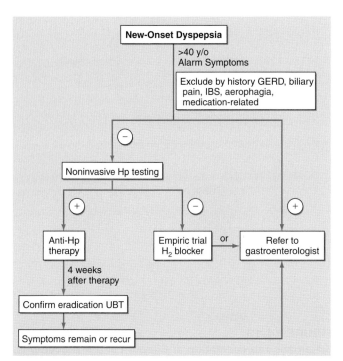

FIGURE 14-12
Overview of new-onset dyspepsia. Hp, *Helicobacter pylori*; UBT, urea breath test; IBS, irritable bowel syndrome. *(Adapted from BS Anand and DY Graham: Endoscopy 31:215, 1999.)*

off antisecretory agents when being tested for eradication of *H. pylori* with UBT or stool antigen. Serologic testing is not useful for the purpose of documenting eradication since antibody titers fall slowly and often do not become undetectable. Two approaches toward documentation of eradication exist: (1) test for eradication only in individuals with a complicated course or in individuals who are frail or with multisystem disease who would do poorly with an ulcer recurrence, and (2) test all patients for successful eradication. Some recommend that patients with complicated ulcer disease or who are frail should be treated with long-term acid suppression, thus making documentation of *H. pylori* eradication a moot point. In view of this discrepancy in practice, it would be best to discuss with the patient the different options available.

Several issues differentiate the approach to a GU versus a DU. GUs, especially of the body and fundus, have the potential of being malignant. Multiple biopsies of a GU should be taken initially; even if these are negative for neoplasm, repeat endoscopy to document healing at 8–12 weeks should be performed, with biopsy if the ulcer is still present. About 70% of GUs eventually found to be malignant undergo significant (usually incomplete) healing.

The majority (>90%) of GUs and DUs heal with the conventional therapy outlined above. A GU that fails to heal after 12 weeks and a DU that does not heal after

8 weeks of therapy should be considered refractory. Once poor compliance and persistent *H. pylori* infection have been excluded, NSAID use, either inadvertent or surreptitious, must be excluded. In addition, cigarette smoking must be eliminated. For a GU, malignancy must be meticulously excluded. Next, consideration should be given to a gastric acid hypersecretory state such as ZES (see "Zollinger-Ellison Syndrome," later in the chapter) or the idiopathic form, which can be excluded with gastric acid analysis. Although a subset of patients have gastric acid hypersecretion of unclear etiology as a contributing factor to refractory ulcers, ZES should be excluded with a fasting gastrin or secretin stimulation test (described later in the chapter under "Diagnosis"). More than 90% of refractory ulcers (either DUs or GUs) heal after 8 weeks of treatment with higher doses of PPI (omeprazole, 40 mg/d; lansoprazole 30–60 mg/d). This higher dose is also effective in maintaining remission. Surgical intervention may be a consideration at this point; however, other rare causes of refractory ulcers must be excluded before recommending surgery. Rare etiologies of refractory ulcers that may be diagnosed by gastric or duodenal biopsies include ischemia, Crohn's disease, amyloidosis, sarcoidosis, lymphoma, eosinophilic gastroenteritis, or infection [cytomegalovirus (CMV), tuberculosis, or syphilis].

SURGICAL THERAPY   Surgical intervention in PUD can be viewed as being either elective, for treatment of medically refractory disease, or as urgent/emergent, for the treatment of an ulcer-related complication. The development of pharmacologic and endoscopic approaches for the treatment of peptic disease and its complications has led to a substantial decrease in the number of operations needed for this disorder. Refractory ulcers are an exceedingly rare occurrence. Surgery is more often required for treatment of an ulcer-related complication. Gastrointestinal bleeding (Chap. 8), perforation, and gastric outlet obstruction are the three complications that may require surgical intervention.

Hemorrhage is the most common ulcer-related complication, occurring in ~15–25% of patients. Bleeding may occur in any age group but is most often seen in older patients (sixth decade or beyond). The majority of patients stop bleeding spontaneously, but endoscopic therapy (Chap. 12) is necessary in some. Parenterally and orally administered PPIs also decrease ulcer rebleeding in patients who have undergone endoscopic therapy. Patients unresponsive or refractory to endoscopic intervention will require surgery (~5% of transfusion-requiring patients).

Free peritoneal perforation occurs in ~2–3% of DU patients. As in the case of bleeding, up to 10% of these patients will not have antecedent ulcer symptoms. Concomitant bleeding may occur in up to 10% of patients with perforation, with mortality being increased substantially. Peptic ulcer can also penetrate into adjacent organs, especially with a posterior DU, which can penetrate into the pancreas, colon, liver, or biliary tree.

Pyloric channel ulcers or DUs can lead to gastric outlet obstruction in ~2–3% of patients. This can result from chronic scarring or from impaired motility due to inflammation and/or edema with pylorospasm. Patients may present with early satiety, nausea, vomiting of undigested food, and weight loss. Conservative management with nasogastric suction, intravenous hydration/nutrition, and antisecretory agents is indicated for 7–10 days with the hope that a functional obstruction will reverse. If a mechanical obstruction persists, endoscopic intervention with balloon dilation may be effective. Surgery should be considered if all else fails.

SPECIFIC OPERATIONS FOR DUODENAL ULCERS Surgical treatment is designed to decrease gastric acid secretion. Operations most commonly performed include (1) vagotomy and drainage (by pyloroplasty, gastroduodenostomy, or gastrojejunostomy), (2) highly selective vagotomy (which does not require a drainage procedure), and (3) vagotomy with antrectomy. The specific procedure performed is dictated by the underlying circumstances: elective vs. emergency, the degree and extent of duodenal ulceration, and the expertise of the surgeon. Moreover, the trend has been toward minimally invasive and anatomy-preserving operations.

Vagotomy is a component of each of these procedures and is aimed at decreasing acid secretion through ablating cholinergic input to the stomach. Unfortunately, both truncal and selective vagotomy (preserves the celiac and hepatic branches) result in gastric atony despite successful reduction of both basal acid output (BAO, decreased by 85%) and maximal acid output (MAO, decreased by 50%). Drainage through pyloroplasty or gastroduodenostomy is required in an effort to compensate for the vagotomy-induced gastric motility disorder. This procedure has an intermediate complication rate and a 10% ulcer recurrence rate. To minimize gastric dysmotility, highly selective vagotomy (also known as parietal cell, super-selective, or proximal vagotomy) was developed. Only the vagal fibers innervating the portion of the stomach that contains parietal cells is transected, thus leaving fibers important for regulating gastric motility intact. Although this procedure leads to an immediate decrease in both BAO and stimulated acid output, acid secretion recovers over time. By the end of the first postoperative year, basal and stimulated acid output are ~30 and 50%, respectively, of preoperative levels. Ulcer recurrence rates are higher with highly selective vagotomy ($\geq$10%), although the overall complication rates are the lowest of the three procedures.

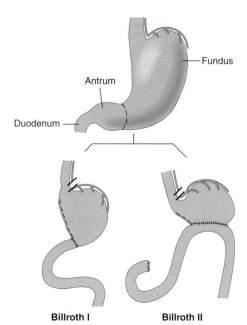

FIGURE 14-13
Schematic representation of Billroth I and II procedures.

The procedure that provides the lowest rates of ulcer recurrence (1%) but has the highest complication rate is vagotomy (truncal or selective) in combination with antrectomy. Antrectomy is aimed at eliminating an additional stimulant of gastric acid secretion, gastrin. Two principal types of reanastomoses are used after antrectomy: gastroduodenostomy (Billroth I) or gastrojejunostomy (Billroth II) (**Fig. 14-13**). Although Billroth I is often preferred over II, severe duodenal inflammation or scarring may preclude its performance.

Of these procedures, highly selective vagotomy may be the one of choice in the elective setting, except in situations where ulcer recurrence rates are high (prepyloric ulcers and those refractory to medical therapy). Selection of vagotomy and antrectomy may be more appropriate in these circumstances.

These procedures have been traditionally performed by standard laparotomy. The advent of laparoscopic surgery has led several surgical teams to successfully perform highly selective vagotomy, truncal vagotomy/pyloroplasty, and truncal vagotomy/antrectomy through this approach. An increase in the number of laparoscopic procedures for treatment of PUD has occurred.

Specific Operations for Gastric Ulcers The location and the presence of a concomitant DU dictate the operative procedure performed for a GU. Antrectomy (including the ulcer) with a Billroth I anastomosis is the treatment of choice for an antral ulcer. Vagotomy is performed only if a DU is present. Although ulcer excision with vagotomy and drainage procedure has been proposed, the higher incidence of ulcer recurrence makes this a less desirable approach. Ulcers located near the esophagogastric junction may require a more radical approach, a subtotal gastrectomy with a Roux-en-Y esophagogastrojejunostomy (Csende's procedure). A less aggressive approach, including antrectomy, intraoperative ulcer biopsy, and vagotomy (Kelling-Madlener procedure), may be indicated in fragile patients with a high GU. Ulcer recurrence approaches 30% with this procedure.

Surgery-Related Complications Complications seen after surgery for PUD are related primarily to the extent of the anatomical modification performed. Minimal alteration (highly selective vagotomy) is associated with higher rates of ulcer recurrence and less gastrointestinal disturbance. More aggressive surgical procedures have a lower rate of ulcer recurrence but a greater incidence of gastrointestinal dysfunction. Overall, morbidity and mortality related to these procedures are quite low. Morbidity associated with vagotomy and antrectomy or pyloroplasty is ≤5%, with mortality ~1%. Highly selective vagotomy has lower morbidity and mortality rates of 1 and 0.3%, respectively.

In addition to the potential early consequences of any intraabdominal procedure (bleeding, infection, thromboembolism), gastroparesis, duodenal stump leak, and efferent loop obstruction can be observed.

Recurrent Ulceration The risk of ulcer recurrence is directly related to the procedure performed. Ulcers that recur after partial gastric resection tend to develop at the anastomosis (stomal or marginal ulcer). Epigastric abdominal pain is the most frequent presenting complaint (>90%). Severity and duration of pain tend to be more progressive than observed with DUs before surgery.

Ulcers may recur for several reasons, including incomplete vagotomy, inadequate drainage, retained antrum, and, less likely, persistent or recurrent *H. pylori* infection. ZES should have been excluded preoperatively. Surreptitious use of NSAIDs is an important reason for recurrent ulcers after surgery, especially if the initial procedure was done for an NSAID-induced ulcer. Once *H. pylori* and NSAIDs have been excluded as etiologic factors, the question of incomplete vagotomy or retained gastric antrum should be explored. For the latter, fasting plasma gastrin levels should be determined. If elevated, retained antrum or ZES (see "Zollinger-Ellison Syndrome" later in the chapter) should be considered. A combination of acid secretory analysis and secretin stimulation (see "Diagnosis" later in the chapter) can assist in this differential diagnosis. Incomplete vagotomy can be ruled out by gastric acid analysis coupled with sham feeding. In this test, gastric acid output is measured while the patient sees, smells, and chews a meal (without swallowing). The cephalic phase of gastric secretion, which is mediated by the vagus, is being assessed with this study. An increase in gastric acid output in response to sham feeding is evidence that the

vagus nerve is intact. A rise in serum pancreatic polypeptide >50% within 30 min of sham feeding is also suggestive of an intact vagus nerve.

Medical therapy with H_2 blockers will heal postoperative ulceration in 70–90% of patients. The efficacy of PPIs has not been fully assessed in this group, but one may anticipate greater rates of ulcer healing compared to those obtained with H_2 blockers. Repeat operation (complete vagotomy, partial gastrectomy) may be required in a small subgroup of patients who have not responded to aggressive medical management.

Afferent Loop Syndromes Two types of afferent loop syndrome can occur in patients who have undergone partial gastric resection with Billroth II anastomosis. The more common of the two is bacterial overgrowth in the afferent limb secondary to stasis. Patients may experience postprandial abdominal pain, bloating, and diarrhea with concomitant malabsorption of fats and vitamin B_{12}. Cases refractory to antibiotics may require surgical revision of the loop. The less-common afferent loop syndrome can present with severe abdominal pain and bloating that occur 20–60 min after meals. Pain is often followed by nausea and vomiting of bile-containing material. The pain and bloating may improve after emesis. The cause of this clinical picture is theorized to be incomplete drainage of bile and pancreatic secretions from an afferent loop that is partially obstructed. Cases refractory to dietary measures may need surgical revision.

Dumping Syndrome Dumping syndrome consists of a series of vasomotor and gastrointestinal signs and symptoms and occurs in patients who have undergone vagotomy and drainage (especially Billroth procedures). Two phases of dumping, early and late, can occur. Early dumping takes place 15–30 min after meals and consists of crampy abdominal discomfort, nausea, diarrhea, belching, tachycardia, palpitations, diaphoresis, light-headedness, and, rarely, syncope. These signs and symptoms arise from the rapid emptying of hyperosmolar gastric contents into the small intestine, resulting in a fluid shift into the gut lumen with plasma volume contraction and acute intestinal distention. Release of vasoactive gastrointestinal hormones (vasoactive intestinal polypeptide, neurotensin, motilin) is also theorized to play a role in early dumping.

The late phase of dumping typically occurs 90 min to 3 h after meals. Vasomotor symptoms (light-headedness, diaphoresis, palpitations, tachycardia, and syncope) predominate during this phase. This component of dumping is thought to be secondary to hypoglycemia from excessive insulin release.

Dumping syndrome is most noticeable after meals rich in simple carbohydrates (especially sucrose) and high osmolarity. Ingestion of large amounts of fluids may also contribute. Up to 50% of postvagotomy and drainage patients will experience dumping syndrome to some degree. Signs and symptoms often improve with time, but a severe protracted picture can occur in up to 1% of patients.

Dietary modification is the cornerstone of therapy for patients with dumping syndrome. Small, multiple (six) meals devoid of simple carbohydrates coupled with elimination of liquids during meals is important. Antidiarrheals and anticholinergic agents are complementary to diet. Guar and pectin, which increase the viscosity of intraluminal contents, may be beneficial in more symptomatic individuals. Acarbose, an α-glucosidase inhibitor that delays digestion of ingested carbohydrates, has also been shown to be beneficial in the treatment of the late phases of dumping. The somatostatin analogue octreotide has been successful in diet-refractory cases. This drug is administered subcutaneously (50 µg tid), titrated according to clinical response. A long-acting depot formulation of octreotide can be administered once every 28 days and provides symptom relief comparable to the short-acting agent. In addition, patient weight gain and quality of life appear to be superior with the long-acting form.

Postvagotomy Diarrhea Up to 10% of patients may seek medical attention for the treatment of postvagotomy diarrhea. This complication is most commonly observed after truncal vagotomy. Patients may complain of intermittent diarrhea that occurs typically 1–2 h after meals. Occasionally the symptoms may be severe and relentless. This is due to a motility disorder from interruption of the vagal fibers supplying the luminal gut. Other contributing factors may include decreased absorption of nutrients (see later), increased excretion of bile acids, and release of luminal factors that promote secretion. Diphenoxylate or loperamide is often useful in symptom control. The bile salt–binding agent cholestyramine may be helpful in severe cases. Surgical reversal of a 10-cm segment of jejunum may yield a substantial improvement in bowel frequency in a subset of patients.

Bile Reflux Gastropathy A subset of post-partial gastrectomy patients who present with abdominal pain, early satiety, nausea, and vomiting will have mucosal erythema of the gastric remnant as the only finding. Histologic examination of the gastric mucosa reveals minimal inflammation but the presence of epithelial cell injury. This clinical picture is categorized as bile or alkaline reflux gastropathy/gastritis. Although reflux of bile is implicated as the reason for this disorder, the mechanism is unknown. Prokinetic agents, cholestyramine, and sucralfate have been somewhat effective treatments. Severe refractory symptoms may require using either nuclear scanning with ^{99m}Tc-HIDA to document reflux or an alkaline challenge test, where 0.1 N NaOH is infused into the stomach in an effort to reproduce the patient's symptoms. Surgical diversion of pancreaticobiliary secretions away from the gastric remnant with a Roux-en-Y gastrojejunostomy consisting of a long (50–60 cm) Roux limb has been used in severe cases. Bilious vomiting improves, but early satiety and bloating may persist in up to 50% of patients.

Maldigestion and Malabsorption Weight loss can be observed in up to 60% of patients after partial gastric resection. A significant component of this weight reduction is due to decreased oral intake. However, mild steatorrhea can also develop. Reasons for maldigestion/malabsorption include decreased gastric acid production, rapid gastric emptying, decreased food dispersion in the stomach, reduced luminal bile concentration, reduced pancreatic secretory response to feeding, and rapid intestinal transit.

Decreased serum vitamin B_{12} levels can be observed after partial gastrectomy. This is usually not due to deficiency of IF, since a minimal amount of parietal cells (source of IF) are removed during antrectomy. Reduced vitamin B_{12} may be due to competition for the vitamin by bacterial overgrowth or inability to split the vitamin from its protein-bound source due to hypochlorhydria.

Iron-deficiency anemia may be a consequence of impaired absorption of dietary iron in patients with a Billroth II gastrojejunostomy. Absorption of iron salts is normal in these individuals; thus, a favorable response to oral iron supplementation can be anticipated. Folate deficiency with concomitant anemia can also develop in these patients. This deficiency may be secondary to decreased absorption or diminished oral intake.

Malabsorption of vitamin D and calcium resulting in osteoporosis and osteomalacia is common after partial gastrectomy and gastrojejunostomy (Billroth II). Osteomalacia can occur as a late complication in up to 25% of post-partial gastrectomy patients. Bone fractures occur twice as commonly in men after gastric surgery as in a control population. It may take years before x-ray findings demonstrate diminished bone density. Elevated alkaline phosphatase, reduced serum calcium, bone pain, and pathologic fractures may be seen in patients with osteomalacia. The high incidence of these abnormalities in this subgroup of patients justifies treating them with vitamin D and calcium supplementation indefinitely. Therapy is especially important in females.

Gastric Adenocarcinoma The incidence of adenocarcinoma in the gastric stump is increased 15 years after resection. Some have reported a four- to fivefold increase in gastric cancer 20–25 years after resection. The pathogenesis is unclear but may involve alkaline reflux, bacterial proliferation, or hypochlorhydria. The role of endoscopic screening is not clear, and most guidelines do not support its use.

RELATED CONDITIONS

ZOLLINGER-ELLISON SYNDROME

Severe peptic ulcer diathesis secondary to gastric acid hypersecretion due to unregulated gastrin release from a non-β cell endocrine tumor (gastrinoma) defines the components of ZES. Initially, ZES was typified by aggressive and refractory ulceration in which total gastrectomy provided the only chance for enhancing survival. Today it can be cured by surgical resection in up to 30% of patients.

Epidemiology

The incidence of ZES varies from 0.1 to 1% of individuals presenting with PUD. Males are more commonly affected than females, and the majority of patients are diagnosed between ages 30 and 50. Gastrinomas are classified into sporadic tumors (more common) and those associated with multiple endocrine neoplasia (MEN) type I (see later).

Pathophysiology

Hypergastrinemia originating from an autonomous neoplasm is the driving force responsible for the clinical manifestations in ZES. Gastrin stimulates acid secretion through gastrin receptors on parietal cells and by inducing histamine release from ECL cells. Gastrin also has a trophic action on gastric epithelial cells. Long-standing hypergastrinemia leads to markedly increased gastric acid secretion through both parietal cell stimulation and increased parietal cell mass. The increased gastric acid output leads to peptic ulcer diathesis, erosive esophagitis, and diarrhea.

Tumor Distribution

Although early studies suggested that the vast majority of gastrinomas occurred within the pancreas, a significant number of these lesions are extrapancreatic. Over 80% of these tumors are found within the hypothetical gastrinoma triangle (confluence of the cystic and common bile ducts superiorly, junction of the second and third portions of the duodenum inferiorly, and junction of the neck and body of the pancreas medially). Duodenal tumors constitute the most common nonpancreatic lesion; between 50% and 75% of gastrinomas are found here. Duodenal tumors are smaller, slower-growing, and less likely to metastasize than pancreatic lesions. Less-common extrapancreatic sites include stomach, bones, ovaries, heart, liver, and lymph nodes. More than 60% of tumors are considered malignant, with up to 30–50% of patients having multiple lesions or metastatic disease at presentation. Histologically, gastrin-producing cells appear well-differentiated, expressing markers typically found in endocrine neoplasms (chromogranin, neuron-specific enolase).

Clinical Manifestations

Gastric acid hypersecretion is responsible for the signs and symptoms observed in patients with ZES. Peptic ulcer is the most common clinical manifestation, occurring in >90% of gastrinoma patients. Initial presentation and ulcer location (duodenal bulb) may be indistinguishable from common PUD. Clinical situations that should create suspicion of gastrinoma are ulcers in unusual locations (second part of the duodenum and beyond), ulcers refractory to standard medical therapy, ulcer recurrence after acid-reducing surgery, ulcers presenting with frank complications (bleeding, obstruction, and perforation), or ulcers in the absence of *H. pylori* or NSAID ingestion. Symptoms of esophageal origin are present in up to two-thirds of patients with ZES, with a spectrum ranging from mild esophagitis to frank ulceration with stricture and Barrett's mucosa.

Diarrhea, the next most common clinical manifestation, is found in up to 50% of patients. Although diarrhea often occurs concomitantly with acid peptic disease, it may also occur independent of an ulcer. Etiology of the diarrhea is multifactorial, resulting from marked volume overload to the small bowel, pancreatic enzyme inactivation by acid, and damage of the intestinal epithelial surface by acid. The epithelial damage can lead to a mild degree of maldigestion and malabsorption of nutrients. The diarrhea may also have a secretory component due to the direct stimulatory effect of gastrin on enterocytes or the cosecretion of additional hormones from the tumor, such as vasoactive intestinal peptide.

Gastrinomas can develop in the presence of MEN I syndrome (Chap. 50) in ~25% of patients. This autosomal dominant disorder involves primarily three organ sites: the parathyroid glands (80–90%), pancreas (40–80%), and pituitary gland (30–60%). The genetic defect in MEN I is in the long arm of chromosome 11 (11q11-q13). In view of the stimulatory effect of calcium on gastric secretion, the hyperparathyroidism and hypercalcemia seen in MEN I patients may have a direct effect on ulcer disease. Resolution of hypercalcemia by parathyroidectomy reduces gastrin and gastric acid output in gastrinoma patients. An additional distinguishing feature in ZES patients with MEN I is the higher incidence of gastric carcinoid tumor development (as compared to patients with sporadic gastrinomas). Gastrinomas tend to be smaller, multiple, and located in the duodenal wall more often than is seen in patients with sporadic ZES. Establishing the diagnosis of MEN I is critical not only from the standpoint of providing genetic counseling to the patient and his or her family but also to the surgical approach recommended.

TABLE 14-7

WHEN TO OBTAIN A FASTING SERUM GASTRIN LEVEL
Multiple ulcers
Ulcers in unusual locations; associated with severe esophagitis; resistant to therapy with frequent recurrences; in the absence of NSAID ingestion or *H. pylori* infection
Ulcer patients awaiting surgery
Extensive family history for peptic ulcer disease
Postoperative ulcer recurrence
Basal hyperchlorhydria
Unexplained diarrhea or steatorrhea
Hypercalcemia
Family history of pancreatic islet, pituitary, or parathyroid tumor
Prominent gastric or duodenal folds

Diagnosis

The first step in the evaluation of a patient suspected of having ZES is to obtain a fasting gastrin level. A list of clinical scenarios that should arouse suspicion regarding this diagnosis is shown in **Table 14-7**. Fasting gastrin levels are usually <150 pg/mL. Virtually all gastrinoma patients will have a gastrin level >150–200 pg/mL. Measurement of fasting gastrin should be repeated to confirm the clinical suspicion.

Multiple processes can lead to an elevated fasting gastrin level: gastric hypochlorhydria or achlorhydria (the most frequent), with or without pernicious anemia; retained gastric antrum; G cell hyperplasia; gastric outlet obstruction; renal insufficiency; massive small-bowel obstruction; and conditions such as rheumatoid arthritis, vitiligo, diabetes mellitus, and pheochromocytoma. Gastric acid induces feedback inhibition of gastrin release. A decrease in acid production will subsequently lead to failure of the feedback inhibitory pathway, resulting in net hypergastrinemia. Gastrin levels will thus be high in patients using antisecretory agents for the treatment of acid peptic disorders and dyspepsia. *H. pylori* infection can also cause hypergastrinemia. Although a fasting gastrin >10 times normal is highly suggestive of ZE, two-thirds of patients will have fasting gastrin levels that overlap with levels found in the more common disorders outlined above.

The next step in establishing a biochemical diagnosis of gastrinoma is to assess acid secretion. Nothing further needs to be done if decreased acid output is observed. In contrast, normal or elevated gastric acid output suggests a need for additional tests. Up to 12% of patients with common PUD may have comparable levels of acid secretion. A BAO/MAO ratio >0.6 is highly suggestive of ZES, but a ratio <0.6 does not exclude the diagnosis. Pentagastrin is no longer available in the United States, making measurement of MAO virtually impossible. An endoscopic method for measuring gastric acid output has been developed but requires further validation. If the technology for measuring gastric acid secretion is not available, a basal gastric pH ≥3 virtually excludes a gastrinoma.

Gastrin provocative tests have been developed in an effort to differentiate between the causes of hypergastrinemia and are especially helpful in patients with indeterminate acid secretory studies. The tests are the secretin stimulation test and the calcium infusion study. The most sensitive and specific gastrin provocative test for the diagnosis of gastrinoma is the secretin study. An increase in gastrin of ≥200 pg within 15 min of secretin injection has a sensitivity and specificity of >90% for ZES. The calcium infusion study is less sensitive and specific than the secretin test, with a rise of >400 pg/mL observed in ~80% of gastrinoma patients. The lower accuracy, coupled with it being a more cumbersome study with greater potential for adverse effects, makes calcium infusion less useful. It is used in the rare cases where the patient's clinical characteristics are highly suggestive of ZES, but the secretin stimulation is inconclusive.

Tumor Localization

Once the biochemical diagnosis of gastrinoma has been confirmed, the tumor must be located. Multiple imaging studies have been utilized in an effort to enhance tumor localization (**Table 14-8**). The broad range of sensitivity is due to the variable success rates achieved by the different investigative groups. Endoscopic ultrasound (EUS) permits imaging of the pancreas with a high degree of resolution (<5 mm). This modality is particularly helpful in excluding small neoplasms within the pancreas and in assessing the presence of surrounding lymph nodes and

TABLE 14-8

SENSITIVITY OF IMAGING STUDIES IN ZOLLINGER-ELLISON SYNDROME		
	SENSITIVITY, %	
STUDY	**PRIMARY GASTRINOMA**	**METASTATIC GASTRINOMA**
Ultrasound	21–28	14
CT scan	35–59	35–72
Selective angiography	35–68	33–86
Portal venous sampling	70–90	N/A
SASI	55–78	41
MRI	30–60	71
Octreoscan	67–86	80–100
EUS	80–100	N/A

Note: CT, computed tomography; SASI, selective arterial secretin injection; MRI, magnetic resonance imaging; octreoscan, imaging with ^{111}In-pentreotide; EUS, endoscopic ultrasonography.

vascular involvement, but it is not very sensitive for finding duodenal lesions. Several types of endocrine tumors express cell-surface receptors for somatostatin. This permits the localization of gastrinomas by measuring the uptake of the stable somatostatin analogue ^{111}In-pentreotide (octreoscan) with sensitivity and specificity rates of >75%.

Up to 50% of patients have metastatic disease at diagnosis. Success in controlling gastric acid hypersecretion has shifted the emphasis of therapy toward providing a surgical cure. Detecting the primary tumor and excluding metastatic disease are critical in view of this paradigm shift. Once a biochemical diagnosis has been confirmed, the patient should first undergo an abdominal CT scan, MRI, or octreoscan (depending on availability) to exclude metastatic disease. Once metastatic disease has been excluded, an experienced endocrine surgeon may opt for exploratory laparotomy with intraoperative ultrasound or transillumination. In other centers, careful examination of the peripancreatic area with EUS, accompanied by endoscopic exploration of the duodenum for primary tumors, will be performed before surgery. Selective arterial secretin injection may be a useful adjuvant for localizing tumors in a subset of patients.

Rx Treatment:
ZOLLINGER-ELLISON SYNDROME

Treatment of functional endocrine tumors is directed at ameliorating the signs and symptoms related to hormone overproduction, curative resection of the neoplasm, and attempts to control tumor growth in metastatic disease.

PPIs are the treatment of choice and have decreased the need for total gastrectomy. Initial PPI doses tend to be higher than those used for treatment of GERD or PUD. The initial dose of omeprazole or lansoprazole should be in the range of 60 mg in divided doses in a 24-h period. Dosing can be adjusted to achieve a BAO <10 meq/h (at the drug trough) in surgery-naive patients and to <5 meq/h in individuals who have previously undergone an acid-reducing operation. Although the somatostatin analogue has inhibitory effects on gastrin release from receptor-bearing tumors and inhibits gastric acid secretion to some extent, PPIs have the advantage of reducing parietal cell activity to a greater degree. Despite this, octreotide may be considered as adjunctive therapy to the PPI in patients with tumors that express somatostatin receptors and have peptic symptoms that are difficult to control with high-dose PPI.

The ultimate goal of surgery would be to provide a definitive cure. Improved understanding of tumor

distribution has led to 10-year disease-free intervals as high as 34% in sporadic gastrinoma patients undergoing surgery. A positive outcome is highly dependent on the experience of the surgical team treating these rare tumors. Surgical therapy of gastrinoma patients with MEN I remains controversial because of the difficulty in rendering these patients disease-free with surgery. In contrast to the encouraging postoperative results observed in patients with sporadic disease, only 6% of MEN I patients are disease-free 5 years after an operation. Some groups suggest surgery only if a clearly identifiable, nonmetastatic lesion is documented by structural studies. Others advocate a more aggressive approach, where all patients free of hepatic metastasis are explored and all detected tumors in the duodenum are resected; this is followed by enucleation of lesions in the pancreatic head, with a distal pancreatectomy to follow. The outcome of the two approaches has not been clearly defined. Laparoscopic surgical interventions may provide attractive approaches in the future.

Therapy of metastatic endocrine tumors in general remains suboptimal; gastrinomas are no exception. Medical approaches including chemotherapy (streptozotocin, 5-fluorouracil, and doxorubicin), IFN-α, and hepatic artery embolization lead to significant toxicity without a substantial improvement in overall survival. ^{111}In-pentreotide has been used in the therapy of metastatic neuroendocrine tumors; further studies are needed. Several novel therapies are being explored, including radiofrequency or cryoablation of liver lesions and use of agents that block the vascular endothelial growth receptor pathway (bevacizumab, sunitinib) (Chap. 50).

Surgical approaches including debulking surgery and liver transplantation for hepatic metastasis have also produced limited benefit. Therefore, early recognition and surgery are the only chances for curing this disease.

The overall 5- and 10-year survival rates for gastrinoma patients are 62–75% and 47–53%, respectively. Individuals with the entire tumor resected or those with a negative laparotomy have 5- and 10-year survival rates >90%. Patients with incompletely resected tumors have 5- and 10-year survival of 43% and 25%, respectively. Patients with hepatic metastasis have <20% survival at 5 years. Favorable prognostic indicators include primary duodenal wall tumors, isolated lymph node tumor, and undetectable tumor upon surgical exploration. Poor outcome is seen in patients with shorter disease duration; higher gastrin levels (>10,000 pg/mL); large pancreatic primary tumors (>3 cm); metastatic disease to lymph nodes, liver, and bone; and Cushing's syndrome. Rapid growth of hepatic metastases is also predictive of poor outcome.

STRESS-RELATED MUCOSAL INJURY

Patients suffering from shock, sepsis, massive burns, severe trauma, or head injury can develop acute erosive gastric mucosal changes or frank ulceration with bleeding. Classified as stress-induced gastritis or ulcers, injury is most commonly observed in the acid-producing (fundus and body) portions of the stomach. The most common presentation is gastrointestinal bleeding, which is usually minimal but can occasionally be life-threatening. Respiratory failure requiring mechanical ventilation and underlying coagulopathy are risk factors for bleeding, which tends to occur 48–72 h after the acute injury or insult.

Histologically, stress injury does not contain inflammation or *H. pylori*; thus, "gastritis" is a misnomer. Although elevated gastric acid secretion may be noted in patients with stress ulceration after head trauma (Cushing's ulcer) and severe burns (Curling's ulcer), mucosal ischemia and breakdown of the normal protective barriers of the stomach also play an important role in the pathogenesis. Acid must contribute to injury in view of the significant drop in bleeding noted when acid inhibitors are used as prophylaxis for stress gastritis.

Improvement in the general management of intensive care unit patients has led to a significant decrease in the incidence of gastrointestinal bleeding due to stress ulceration. The estimated decrease in bleeding is from 20–30% to <5%. This improvement has led to some debate regarding the need for prophylactic therapy. The limited benefit of medical (endoscopic, angiographic) and surgical therapy in a patient with hemodynamically compromising bleeding associated with stress ulcer/gastritis supports the use of preventive measures in high-risk patients (mechanically ventilated, coagulopathy, multiorgan failure, or severe burns). Maintenance of gastric pH >3.5 with continuous infusion of H_2 blockers or liquid antacids administered every 2–3 h are viable options. Tolerance to the H_2 blocker is likely to develop; thus, careful monitoring of the gastric pH and dose adjustment is important if H_2 blockers are used. Moreover, administration of antacids is cumbersome, requiring use of a gastric tube, and the agent may lead to diarrhea and electrolyte abnormalities. Sucralfate slurry (1 g every 4–6 h) has also been somewhat successful but requires a gastric tube and may lead to constipation and aluminum toxicity. Sucralfate use in endotracheal intubated patients has also been associated with aspiration pneumonia. PPIs are the treatment of choice for stress prophylaxis. Oral PPI is the best option if the patient can tolerate enteral administration. Pantoprazole is available as an intravenous formulation for individuals in whom enteral administration is not possible. If bleeding occurs despite these measures, endoscopy, intraarterial vasopressin, or embolization are options. If all else fails, then surgery should be considered. Although vagotomy and antrectomy may be used, the better approach would be a total gastrectomy, which has an exceedingly high mortality rate in this setting.

GASTRITIS

The term *gastritis* should be reserved for histologically documented inflammation of the gastric mucosa. Gastritis is not the mucosal erythema seen during endoscopy and is not interchangeable with "dyspepsia." The etiologic factors leading to gastritis are broad and heterogeneous. Gastritis has been classified based on time course (acute vs chronic), histologic features, and anatomic distribution or proposed pathogenic mechanism (Table 14-9).

The correlation between the histologic findings of gastritis, the clinical picture of abdominal pain or dyspepsia, and endoscopic findings noted on gross inspection of the gastric mucosa is poor. Therefore, there is no typical clinical manifestation of gastritis.

Acute Gastritis

The most common causes of acute gastritis are infectious. Acute infection with *H. pylori* induces gastritis. However, *H. pylori* acute gastritis has not been extensively studied. It is reported as presenting with sudden onset of epigastric pain, nausea, and vomiting, and limited mucosal histologic studies demonstrate a marked infiltrate of neutrophils with edema and hyperemia. If not treated, this picture will evolve into one of chronic gastritis. Hypochlorhydria lasting for up to 1 year may follow acute *H. pylori* infection.

The highly acidic gastric environment may be one reason why infectious processes of the stomach are rare. Bacterial infection of the stomach or phlegmonous gastritis is a rare, potentially life-threatening disorder characterized

TABLE 14-9

CLASSIFICATION OF GASTRITIS	

I. Acute gastritis
  A. Acute *H. pylori* infection
  B. Other acute infectious gastritides
    1. Bacterial (other than *H. pylori*)
    2. *Helicobacter helmanni*
    3. Phlegmonous
    4. Mycobacterial
    5. Syphilitic
    6. Viral
    7. Parasitic
    8. Fungal
	II. Chronic atrophic gastritis
	  A. Type A: Autoimmune, body-predominant
	  B. Type B: *H. pylori*–related, antral-predominant
	  C. Indeterminant
	III. Uncommon forms of gastritis
	  A. Lymphocytic
	  B. Eosinophilic
	  C. Crohn's disease
	  D. Sarcoidosis
	  E. Isolated granulomatous gastritis

by marked and diffuse acute inflammatory infiltrates of the entire gastric wall, at times accompanied by necrosis. Elderly individuals, alcoholics, and AIDS patients may be affected. Potential iatrogenic causes include polypectomy and mucosal injection with India ink. Organisms associated with this entity include streptococci, staphylococci, *Escherichia coli*, *Proteus*, and *Haemophilus* sp. Failure of supportive measures and antibiotics may result in gastrectomy.

Other types of infectious gastritis may occur in immunocompromised individuals such as AIDS patients. Examples include herpetic (herpes simplex) or CMV gastritis. The histologic finding of intranuclear inclusions would be observed in the latter.

Chronic Gastritis

Chronic gastritis is identified histologically by an inflammatory cell infiltrate consisting primarily of lymphocytes and plasma cells, with very scant neutrophil involvement. Distribution of the inflammation may be patchy, initially involving superficial and glandular portions of the gastric mucosa. This picture may progress to more severe glandular destruction, with atrophy and metaplasia. Chronic gastritis has been classified according to histologic characteristics. These include superficial atrophic changes and gastric atrophy.

The early phase of chronic gastritis is *superficial gastritis*. The inflammatory changes are limited to the lamina propria of the surface mucosa, with edema and cellular infiltrates separating intact gastric glands. Additional findings may include decreased mucus in the mucous cells and decreased mitotic figures in the glandular cells. The next stage is *atrophic gastritis*. The inflammatory infiltrate extends deeper into the mucosa, with progressive distortion and destruction of the glands. The final stage of chronic gastritis is *gastric atrophy*. Glandular structures are lost, and there is a paucity of inflammatory infiltrates. Endoscopically, the mucosa may be substantially thin, permitting clear visualization of the underlying blood vessels.

Gastric glands may undergo morphologic transformation in chronic gastritis. Intestinal metaplasia denotes the conversion of gastric glands to a small intestinal phenotype with small-bowel mucosal glands containing goblet cells. The metaplastic changes may vary in distribution from patchy to fairly extensive gastric involvement. Intestinal metaplasia is an important predisposing factor for gastric cancer (Chap. 47).

Chronic gastritis is also classified according to the predominant site of involvement. Type A refers to the body-predominant form (autoimmune) and type B is the antral-predominant form (*H. pylori*–related). This classification is artificial in view of the difficulty in distinguishing these two entities. The term *AB gastritis* has been used to refer to a mixed antral/body picture.

Type A Gastritis

The less common of the two forms involves primarily the fundus and body, with antral sparing. Traditionally, this form of gastritis has been associated with pernicious anemia in the presence of circulating antibodies against parietal cells and IF; thus, it is also called *autoimmune gastritis*. *H. pylori* infection can lead to a similar distribution of gastritis. The characteristics of an autoimmune picture are not always present.

Antibodies to parietal cells have been detected in >90% of patients with pernicious anemia and in up to 50% of patients with type A gastritis. The parietal cell antibody is directed against H^+,K^+-ATPase. T cells are also implicated in the injury pattern of this form of gastritis.

Parietal cell antibodies and atrophic gastritis are observed in family members of patients with pernicious anemia. These antibodies are observed in up to 20% of individuals over age 60 and in ~20% of patients with vitiligo and Addison's disease. About half of patients with pernicious anemia have antibodies to thyroid antigens, and about 30% of patients with thyroid disease have circulating antiparietal cell antibodies. Anti-IF antibodies are more specific than parietal cell antibodies for type A gastritis, being present in ~40% of patients with pernicious anemia. Another parameter consistent with this form of gastritis being autoimmune in origin is the higher incidence of specific familial histocompatibility haplotypes such as HLA-B8 and -DR3.

The parietal cell–containing gastric gland is preferentially targeted in this form of gastritis, and achlorhydria results. Parietal cells are the source of IF, lack of which will lead to vitamin B_{12} deficiency and its sequelae (megaloblastic anemia, neurologic dysfunction).

Gastric acid plays an important role in feedback inhibition of gastrin release from G cells. Achlorhydria, coupled with relative sparing of the antral mucosa (site of G cells), leads to hypergastrinemia. Gastrin levels can be markedly elevated (>500 pg/mL) in patients with pernicious anemia. ECL cell hyperplasia with frank development of gastric carcinoid tumors may result from gastrin trophic effects. The role of gastrin in carcinoid development is confirmed by the observation that antrectomy leads to regression of these lesions. Hypergastrinemia and achlorhydria may also be seen in non-pernicious anemia-associated type A gastritis.

Type B Gastritis

Type B, or antral-predominant, gastritis is the more common form of chronic gastritis. *H. pylori* infection is the cause of this entity. Although described as "antral-predominant," this is likely a misnomer in view of studies documenting the progression of the inflammatory process toward the body and fundus of infected individuals. The conversion to a pan-gastritis is time-dependent—estimated to require 15–20 years. This form of gastritis increases with age, being present in up to

150

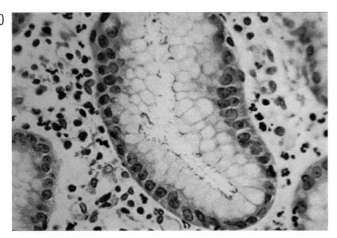

FIGURE 14-14

Chronic gastritis and *H. pylori* organisms. Steiner silver stain of superficial gastric mucosa, showing abundant darkly staining microorganisms layered over the apical portion of the surface epithelium. Note that there is no tissue invasion.

100% of persons over age 70. Histology improves after *H. pylori* eradication. The number of *H. pylori* organisms decreases dramatically with progression to gastric atrophy, and the degree of inflammation correlates with the level of these organisms. Early on, with antral-predominant findings, the quantity of *H. pylori* is highest and a dense chronic inflammatory infiltrate of the lamina propria is noted, accompanied by epithelial cell infiltration with polymorphonuclear leukocytes (**Fig. 14-14**).

Multifocal atrophic gastritis, gastric atrophy with subsequent metaplasia, has been observed in chronic *H. pylori*–induced gastritis. This may ultimately lead to development of gastric adenocarcinoma (Fig. 14-8; Chap. 47). *H. pylori* infection is now considered an independent risk factor for gastric cancer. Worldwide epidemiologic studies have documented a higher incidence of *H. pylori* infection in patients with adenocarcinoma of the stomach as compared to control subjects. Seropositivity for *H. pylori* is associated with a three- to sixfold increased risk of gastric cancer. This risk may be as high as ninefold after adjusting for the inaccuracy of serologic testing in the elderly. The mechanism by which *H. pylori* infection leads to cancer is unknown, but it appears to be related to the chronic inflammation induced by the organism. Eradication of *H. pylori* as a general preventative measure for gastric cancer is being evaluated but is not yet recommended.

Infection with *H. pylori* is also associated with development of a low-grade B cell lymphoma, gastric MALT lymphoma. The chronic T cell stimulation caused by the infection leads to production of cytokines that promote the B cell tumor. The tumor should be initially staged with a CT scan of the abdomen and EUS. Tumor growth remains dependent on the presence of *H. pylori*, and its eradication is often associated with complete regression of the tumor. The tumor may take more than a year to regress after treating the infection. Such patients should be followed by EUS every 2–3 months. If the tumor is stable or decreasing in size, no other therapy is necessary. If the tumor grows, it may have become a high-grade B cell lymphoma. When the tumor becomes a high-grade aggressive lymphoma histologically, it loses responsiveness to *H. pylori* eradication.

**Rx Treatment:
CHRONIC GASTRITIS**

Treatment in chronic gastritis is aimed at the sequelae and not the underlying inflammation. Patients with pernicious anemia will require parenteral vitamin B$_{12}$ supplementation on a long-term basis. Eradication of *H. pylori* is not routinely recommended unless PUD or a low-grade MALT lymphoma is present.

Miscellaneous Forms of Gastritis

Lymphocytic gastritis is characterized histologically by intense infiltration of the surface epithelium with lymphocytes. The infiltrative process is primarily in the body of the stomach and consists of mature T cells and plasmacytes. The etiology of this form of chronic gastritis is unknown. It has been described in patients with celiac sprue, but whether there is a common factor associating these two entities is unknown. No specific symptoms suggest lymphocytic gastritis. A subgroup of patients have thickened folds noted on endoscopy. These folds are often capped by small nodules that contain a central depression or erosion; this form of the disease is called *varioliform gastritis*. *H. pylori* probably plays no significant role in lymphocytic gastritis. Therapy with glucocorticoids or sodium cromoglycate has obtained unclear results.

Marked eosinophilic infiltration involving any layer of the stomach (mucosa, muscularis propria, and serosa) is characteristic of *eosinophilic gastritis*. Affected individuals will often have circulating eosinophilia with clinical manifestation of systemic allergy. Involvement may range from isolated gastric disease to diffuse eosinophilic gastroenteritis. Antral involvement predominates, with prominent edematous folds being observed on endoscopy. These prominent antral folds can lead to outlet obstruction. Patients can present with epigastric discomfort, nausea, and vomiting. Treatment with glucocorticoids has been successful.

Several systemic disorders may be associated with *granulomatous gastritis*. Gastric involvement has been observed in Crohn's disease. Involvement may range from granulomatous infiltrates noted only on gastric biopsies to frank ulceration and stricture formation. Gastric Crohn's disease usually occurs in the presence of small-intestinal disease. Several rare infectious processes can lead to granulomatous gastritis, including histoplasmosis, candidiasis, syphilis, and tuberculosis. Other unusual causes of this form of gastritis include sarcoidosis, idiopathic granulomatous gastritis, and eosinophilic granulomas involving the stomach. Establishing the specific etiologic agent in this form of gastritis can be difficult, at times requiring repeat endoscopy with biopsy and cytology. Occasionally a surgically obtained full-thickness biopsy of the stomach may be required to exclude malignancy.

MÉNÉTRIER'S DISEASE

Ménétrier's disease is a rare entity characterized by large, tortuous gastric mucosal folds. The differential diagnosis of large gastric folds includes ZES, malignancy, infectious etiologies (CMV, histoplasmosis, syphilis), and infiltrative disorders such as sarcoidosis. The mucosal folds in Ménétrier's disease are often most prominent in the body and fundus. Histologically, massive foveolar hyperplasia (hyperplasia of surface and glandular mucous cells) is noted, which replaces most of the chief and parietal cells. This hyperplasia produces the prominent folds observed. The pits of the gastric glands elongate and may become extremely tortuous. Although the lamina propria may contain a mild chronic inflammatory infiltrate, Ménétrier's disease is not considered a form of gastritis. The etiology of this unusual clinical picture is unknown. Overexpression of growth factors such as TGF-α may be involved in the process.

Epigastric pain, at times accompanied by nausea, vomiting, anorexia, and weight loss, are signs and symptoms in patients with Ménétrier's disease. Occult gastrointestinal bleeding may occur, but overt bleeding is unusual and, when present, is due to superficial mucosal erosions. Twenty to 100% of patients (depending on time of presentation) develop a protein-losing gastropathy accompanied by hypoalbuminemia and edema. Gastric acid secretion is usually reduced or absent because of the replacement of parietal cells. Large gastric folds are readily detectable by either radiographic (barium meal) or endoscopic methods. Endoscopy with deep mucosal biopsy (and cytology) is required to establish the diagnosis and exclude other entities that may present similarly. A nondiagnostic biopsy may lead to a surgically obtained full-thickness biopsy to exclude malignancy.

℞ **Treatment:**
MÉNÉTRIER'S DISEASE

Medical therapy with anticholinergic agents, prostaglandins, PPIs, prednisone, and H_2 receptor antagonists yields varying results. Anticholinergics decrease protein loss. A high-protein diet should be recommended to replace protein loss in patients with hypoalbuminemia. Ulcers should be treated with a standard approach. Severe disease with persistent and substantial protein loss may require total gastrectomy. Subtotal gastrectomy is performed by some; it may be associated with higher morbidity and mortality secondary to the difficulty in obtaining a patent and long-lasting anastomosis between normal and hyperplastic tissues.

ACKNOWLEDGMENT

The author acknowledges the contribution of material to this chapter by Dr. Lawrence Friedman and Dr. Walter Peterson from their chapter on this subject in the 14th edition of Harrison's Principles of Internal Medicine.

FURTHER READINGS

BESWICK EJ et al: *H pylori* and host interactions that influence pathogenesis. World J Gastroenterol 12:5599, 2006

CHAN FK et al: Preventing recurrent upper gastrointestinal bleeding in patients with *Helicobacter pylori* infection who are taking low-dose aspirin or naproxen. N Engl J Med 344:967, 2001

CHAN FK, LEUNG WK: Peptic-ulcer disease. Lancet 360:933, 2002

COVER TL, BLASER MJ: *Helicobacter pylori* in health and disease. Gastroenterology 136:1863, 2009

ERNST PB et al: The translation of *Helicobacter pylori* basic research to patient care. Gastroenterology 130:188, 2006

FOX JG, WANG TC: Inflammation, atrophy, and gastric cancer. J Clin Invest 117:60, 2007

LAI KC et al: Lansoprazole for the prevention of recurrences of ulcer complications from long-term low-dose aspirin use. N Engl J Med 346:2033, 2002

LAINE L: Approaches to nonsteroidal anti-inflammatory drug use in the high-risk patient. Gastroenterology 120:594, 2001

———: Gastrointestinal effects of NSAIDs and coxibs. J Pain Symptom Manage 25(Suppl 2):532, 2003

LEONG RW: Differences in peptic ulcer between the East and the West. Gastroenterol Clin North Am 38:363, 2009

MCCOLL KE: Helicobacter pylori-negative nonsteroidal anti-inflammatory drug-negative ulcer. Gastroenterol Clin North Am 38:353, 2009

MOAYYEDI P et al: An update of the Cochrane systematic review of *Helicobacter pylori* eradication therapy in nonulcer dyspepsia: Resolving the discrepancy between systematic reviews. Am J Gastroenterol 98:2621, 2003

NAPOLITANO L: Refractory peptic ulcer disease. Gastroenterol Clin North Am 38:267, 2009

SUERBAUM S, MICHETTI P: *Helicobacter pylori* infection. N Engl J Med 347:1175, 2002

VILAICHONE RK et al: *Helicobacter pylori* diagnosis and management. Gastroenterol Clin North Am 35:229, 2006

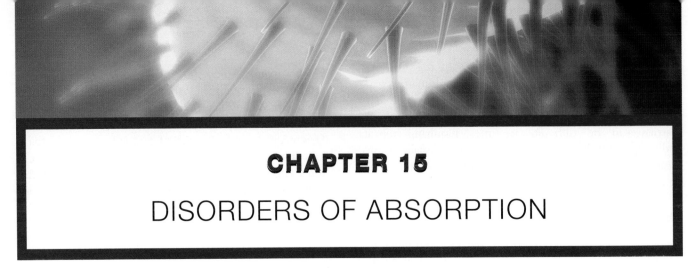

CHAPTER 15

DISORDERS OF ABSORPTION

Henry J. Binder

Disorders of absorption constitute a broad spectrum of conditions with multiple etiologies and varied clinical manifestations. Almost all of these clinical problems are associated with *diminished* intestinal absorption of one or more dietary nutrients and are often referred to as the *malabsorption syndrome*. This term is not ideal as it represents a pathophysiologic state, does *not* provide an etiologic explanation for the underlying problem, and should not be considered an adequate final diagnosis. The only clinical situations in which absorption is *increased* are hemochromatosis and Wilson's disease, in which absorption of iron and copper, respectively, are increased.

Most, but not all, malabsorption syndromes are associated with *steatorrhea*, an increase in stool fat excretion of >6% of dietary fat intake. Some malabsorption disorders are not associated with steatorrhea: primary lactase deficiency, a congenital absence of the small intestinal brush border disaccharidase enzyme lactase, is associated with lactose "malabsorption," and pernicious anemia is associated with a marked decrease in intestinal absorption of cobalamin (vitamin B_{12}) due to an absence of gastric parietal cell intrinsic factor required for cobalamin absorption.

Disorders of absorption must be included in the differential diagnosis of diarrhea (Chap. 6). First, diarrhea is frequently associated with and/or is a consequence of the diminished absorption of one or more dietary nutrients. The diarrhea may be secondary either to the

intestinal process that is responsible for the steatorrhea or to steatorrhea per se. Thus, celiac sprue (see later) is associated with both extensive morphologic changes in the small intestinal mucosa and reduced absorption of several dietary nutrients; in contrast, the diarrhea of steatorrhea is the result of the effect of nonabsorbed dietary fatty acids on intestinal, usually colonic, ion transport. For example, oleic acid and ricinoleic acid (a bacterially hydroxylated fatty acid that is also the active ingredient in castor oil, a widely used laxative) induce active colonic Cl ion secretion, most likely secondary to increasing intracellular Ca. In addition, diarrhea per se may result in mild steatorrhea (<11 g fat excretion while on a 100-g fat diet). Second, most patients will indicate that they have diarrhea, not that they have fat malabsorption. Third, many intestinal disorders that have diarrhea as a prominent symptom (e.g., ulcerative colitis, traveler's diarrhea secondary to an enterotoxin produced by *Escherichia coli*) do not necessarily have diminished absorption of any dietary nutrient.

Diarrhea as a *symptom* (i.e., when used by patients to describe their bowel movement pattern) may be a decrease in stool consistency, an increase in stool volume, an increase in number of bowel movements, or any combination of these three changes. In contrast, diarrhea as a *sign* is a quantitative increase in stool water or weight of >200–225 mL, or gram per 24 h, when a western-type diet is consumed. Individuals consuming a diet with higher fiber content may normally have a stool weight of up to 400 g/24 h. Thus, the clinician must clarify what an individual patient means by diarrhea. Some 10% of patients referred to gastroenterologists for further evaluation of unexplained diarrhea do not have an increase in stool water when it is determined quantitatively. Such patients may have small, frequent, somewhat loose bowel movements with stool urgency that is indicative of proctitis but do not have an increase in stool weight or volume.

It is also critical to establish whether a patient's diarrhea is secondary to diminished absorption of one or more dietary nutrients, in contrast to diarrhea that is due to small- and/or large-intestinal fluid and electrolyte secretion. The former has often been termed *osmotic diarrhea*, while the latter has been referred to as *secretory diarrhea*. Unfortunately, both secretory and osmotic elements can be present simultaneously in the same disorder; thus, this separation is not always precise. Nonetheless, two studies—determination of stool electrolytes and observation of the effect of a fast on stool output—can help make this distinction.

The demonstration of the effect of prolonged (>24 h) fasting on stool output can be very effective in suggesting that a *dietary nutrient* is responsible for the individual's diarrhea. A secretory diarrhea associated with enterotoxin-induced traveler's diarrhea would not be affected by prolonged fasting, as enterotoxin-induced stimulation of intestinal fluid and electrolyte secretion is not altered by eating. In contrast, diarrhea secondary to lactose malabsorption in primary lactase deficiency would undoubtedly cease during a prolonged fast. Thus, a substantial decrease in stool output while fasting during a quantitative stool collection of at least 24 h is presumptive evidence that the diarrhea is related to malabsorption of a dietary nutrient. The persistence of stool output while fasting indicates that the diarrhea is likely secretory and that the cause of diarrhea is *not* a dietary nutrient. Either a luminal (e.g., *E. coli* enterotoxin) or circulating (e.g., vasoactive intestinal peptide) secretagogue could be responsible for the patient's diarrhea persisting unaltered during a prolonged fast. The observed effects of fasting can be compared and correlated with stool electrolyte and osmolality determinations.

Measurement of stool electrolytes and osmolality requires the comparison of stool Na^+ and K^+ concentrations determined in liquid stool to the stool osmolality to determine the presence or absence of a so-called stool osmotic gap. The following formula is used:

$$2 \times (\text{stool } [Na^+] + \text{stool } [K^+]) \leq \text{stool osmolality}$$

The cation concentrations are doubled to estimate stool anion concentrations. The presence of a significant osmotic gap suggests the presence in stool water of a substance (or substances) other than Na/K/anions that is

presumably responsible for the patient's diarrhea. Originally, stool osmolality was measured, but it is almost invariably greater than the required 290–300 mosmol/kg H_2O, reflecting bacterial degradation of nonabsorbed carbohydrate either immediately before defecation or in the stool jar while awaiting chemical analysis, even when the stool is refrigerated. As a result, the stool osmolality should be assumed to be 300 mosmol/kg H_2O. A low stool osmolality (<290 mosmol/kg H_2O) reflects the addition of either dilute urine or water indicating either collection of urine and stool together or so-called factitious diarrhea, a form of Munchausen's syndrome. When the calculated difference is >50, an osmotic gap is present, suggesting that the diarrhea is due to a nonabsorbed dietary nutrient, e.g., a fatty acid and/or carbohydrate. When this difference is <25, it is presumed that a dietary nutrient is not responsible for the diarrhea. Since elements of both osmotic (i.e., malabsorption of a dietary nutrient) and secretory diarrhea may be present, this separation at times is less clear-cut at the bedside than when used as a teaching example. Ideally, the presence of an osmotic gap will be associated with a marked decrease in stool output during a prolonged fast, while the absence of an osmotic gap will likely be present in an individual whose stool output had not been reduced substantially during a period of fasting.

NUTRIENT DIGESTION AND ABSORPTION

The lengths of the small intestine and colon are ~300 cm and ~80 cm, respectively. However, the effective functional surface area is approximately 600-fold greater than that of a hollow tube as a result of the presence of folds, villi (in the small intestine), and microvilli. The functional surface area of the small intestine is somewhat greater than that of a doubles tennis court. In addition to nutrient digestion and absorption, the intestinal epithelia have several other functions:

1. *Barrier and immune defense*. The intestine is exposed to a large number of potential antigens and enteric and invasive microorganisms, and it is extremely effective in preventing the entry of almost all these agents. The intestinal mucosa also synthesizes and secretes secretory IgA.
2. *Fluid and electrolyte absorption and secretion*. The intestine absorbs ~7–8 L of fluid daily, comprising dietary fluid intake (1–2 L/d) and salivary, gastric, pancreatic, biliary, and intestinal fluid (6–7 L/d). Several stimuli, especially bacteria and bacterial enterotoxins, induce fluid and electrolyte secretion that may lead to diarrhea (Chap. 22).
3. *Synthesis and secretion of several proteins*. The intestinal mucosa is a major site for the production of proteins, including apolipoproteins.

4. *Production of several bioactive amines and peptides.* The intestine is one of the largest endocrine organs in the body and produces several amines and peptides that serve as paracrine and hormonal mediators of intestinal function.

The small and large intestines are distinct anatomically (villi are present in the small intestine but are absent in the colon) and functionally (nutrient digestion and absorption take place in the small intestine but not in the colon). No precise anatomic characteristics separate duodenum, jejunum, and ileum, although certain nutrients are absorbed exclusively in specific areas of the small intestine. However, villous cells in the small intestine (and surface epithelial cells in the colon) and crypt cells have distinct anatomic and functional characteristics. Intestinal epithelial cells are continuously renewed, with new proliferating epithelial cells at the base of the crypt migrating over 48–72 h to the tip of the villus (or surface of the colon), where they are well-developed epithelial cells with digestive and absorptive function. This high rate of cell turnover explains the relatively rapid resolution of diarrhea and other digestive tract side effects during chemotherapy as new cells not exposed to these toxic agents are produced. Equally important is the paradigm of separation of villous/surface cell and crypt cell function: digestive hydrolytic enzymes are present primarily in the brush border of villous epithelial cells. Absorptive and secretory functions are also separated, with villous/surface cells primarily, but not exclusively, being the site for absorptive function, while secretory function is present in crypts of both the small and large intestine.

Nutrients, minerals, and vitamins are absorbed by one or more active transport mechanisms. Active transport mechanisms are energy-dependent and mediated by membrane transport proteins. These processes will result in the *net* movement of a substance against or in the absence of an electrochemical concentration gradient. Intestinal absorption of amino acids and monosaccharides, e.g., glucose, is also a specialized form of active transport— *secondary active transport.* The movement of these actively transported nutrients against a concentration gradient is Na^+-dependent and is due to a Na^+ gradient across the apical membrane. The Na^+ gradient is maintained by Na^+,K^+-ATPase, the so-called Na^+ pump located on the basolateral membrane, which extrudes Na^+ and maintains low intracellular [Na] as well as the Na^+ gradient across the apical membrane. As a result, active glucose absorption and glucose-stimulated Na^+ absorption require both the apical membrane transport protein, SGLT1, and the basolateral Na^+,K^+-ATPase. In addition to glucose absorption being Na^+-dependent, glucose also stimulates Na^+ and fluid absorption, which is the physiologic basis of oral rehydration therapy for the treatment of diarrhea (Chap. 6).

The mechanisms of intestinal fluid and electrolyte absorption and secretion are discussed in Chap. 6.

Although the intestinal epithelial cells are crucial mediators of absorption and ion and water flow, the several cell types in the lamina propria (e.g., mast cells, macrophages, myofibroblasts) and the enteric nervous system interact with the epithelium to regulate mucosal cell function. The function of the intestine is the result of the integrated responses of and interactions between both intestinal epithelial cells and intestinal muscle.

ENTEROHEPATIC CIRCULATION OF BILE ACIDS

Bile acids are not present in the diet but are synthesized in the liver by a series of enzymatic steps that also include cholesterol catabolism. Indeed, interruption of the enterohepatic circulation of bile acids can reduce serum cholesterol levels by 10% before a new steady state is established. Bile acids are either primary or secondary: primary bile acids are synthesized in the liver from cholesterol, and secondary bile acids are synthesized from primary bile acids in the intestine by colonic bacterial enzymes. The two primary bile acids in humans are cholic acid and chenodeoxycholic acid; the two most abundant secondary bile acids are deoxycholic acid and lithocholic acid. Approximately 500-mg bile acids are synthesized in the liver daily, conjugated to either taurine or glycine to form tauro-conjugated or glyco-conjugated bile acids, respectively, and are secreted into the duodenum in bile. The primary functions of bile acids are (1) to promote bile flow, (2) to solubilize cholesterol and phospholipid in the gallbladder by mixed micelle formation, and (3) to enhance dietary lipid digestion and absorption by forming mixed micelles in the proximal small intestine.

Bile acids are primarily absorbed by an active, Na^+-dependent process that is located exclusively in the ileum, though bile acids can also be absorbed to a lesser extent by non-carrier-mediated transport processes in the jejunum, ileum, and colon. Conjugated bile acids that enter the colon are deconjugated by colonic bacterial enzymes to unconjugated bile acids and are rapidly absorbed. Colonic bacterial enzymes also dehydroxylate bile acids to secondary bile acids.

Bile acids absorbed from the intestine return to the liver via the portal vein where they are resecreted (**Fig. 15-1**). Bile acid synthesis is largely autoregulated by 7α-hydroxylase, the initial enzyme in cholesterol degradation. A decrease in the amount of bile acids returning to the liver from the intestine is associated with an increase in bile acid synthesis/cholesterol catabolism, which helps keep the bile acid pool size relatively constant. However, the capacity to increase bile acid synthesis is limited to about two to two and a half-fold (see later). The bile acid pool size is approximately 4 g and is circulated via the enterohepatic circulation about twice during each meal, or six to eight times during a 24-h period. A relatively small quantity of bile

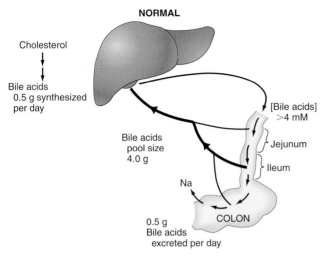

FIGURE 15-1

Schematic representation of the enterohepatic circulation of bile acids. Bile acid synthesis is cholesterol catabolism and occurs in the liver. Bile acids are secreted in bile and are stored in the gallbladder between meals and at night. Food in the duodenum induces the release of cholecystokinin, a potent stimulus for gallbladder contraction resulting in bile acid entry into the duodenum. Bile acids are primarily absorbed via a Na-dependent transport process that is located only in the ileum. A relatively small quantity of bile acids (~500 mg) is not absorbed in a 24-h period and is lost in stool. Fecal bile acid losses are matched by bile acid synthesis. The bile acid pool (the total amount of bile acids in the body) is ~4 g and is circulated twice during each meal or six to eight times in a 24-h period.

acids is not absorbed and is excreted in stool daily; this fecal loss is matched by hepatic bile acid synthesis.

Defects in any of the steps of the enterohepatic circulation of bile acids can result in a decrease in duodenal concentration of conjugated bile acids and, as a result, steatorrhea. Thus, steatorrhea can be caused by abnormalities in bile acid synthesis and excretion, their physical state in the intestinal lumen, and reabsorption (Table 15-1).

TABLE 15-1

DEFECTS IN ENTEROHEPATIC CIRCULATION OF BILE ACIDS

PROCESS	PATHOPHYSIOLOGIC DEFECT	DISEASE EXAMPLE
Synthesis	Decreased hepatic function	Cirrhosis
Biliary secretion	Altered canalicular function	Primary biliary cirrhosis
Maintenance of conjugated bile acids	Bacterial overgrowth	Jejunal diverticulosis
Reabsorption	Abnormal ileal function	Crohn's disease

Synthesis

Decreased bile acid synthesis and steatorrhea have been demonstrated in chronic liver disease, but steatorrhea is often not a major component of the illness of these patients.

Secretion

Although bile acid secretion may be reduced or absent in biliary obstruction, steatorrhea is rarely a significant medical problem in these patients. In contrast, primary biliary cirrhosis represents a defect in canalicular excretion of organic anions, including bile acids, and not infrequently is associated with steatorrhea and its consequences, e.g., chronic bone disease. Thus, the osteomalacia and other chronic bone abnormalities often present in patients with primary biliary cirrhosis and other cholestatic syndromes are secondary to steatorrhea that then leads to calcium and vitamin D malabsorption.

Maintenance of Conjugated Bile Acids

In bacterial overgrowth syndromes associated with diarrhea, steatorrhea, and macrocytic anemia, a colonic type of bacterial flora is increased in the small intestine. The steatorrhea is primarily a result of the decrease in conjugated bile acids secondary to their deconjugation by colonic-type bacteria. Two complementary explanations account for the resulting impairment of micelle formation: (1) unconjugated bile acids are rapidly absorbed in the jejunum by nonionic diffusion, resulting in a reduced concentration of duodenal bile acids; and (2) the critical micellar concentration (CMC) of unconjugated bile acids is higher than that of conjugated bile acids, and therefore unconjugated bile acids are less effective than conjugated bile acids in micelle formation.

Reabsorption

Ileal dysfunction caused by either Crohn's disease or surgical resection results in a decrease in bile acid reabsorption in the ileum and an *increase* in the delivery of bile acids to the large intestine. The resulting clinical consequences—diarrhea with or without steatorrhea—are determined by the *degree* of ileal dysfunction and the *response* of the enterohepatic circulation to bile acid losses (Table 15-2). Patients with limited ileal disease or resection will often have diarrhea but not steatorrhea. The diarrhea, a result of bile acids in the colon stimulating active Cl secretion, has been called *bile acid diarrhea*, or cholorrheic enteropathy, and responds promptly to cholestyramine, an anion-binding resin. Such patients do not develop steatorrhea because hepatic synthesis of bile acids increases to compensate for the rate of fecal bile acid losses, resulting in maintenance of both the bile acid pool size and the intraduodenal concentrations of bile

TABLE 15-2

COMPARISON OF BILE ACID AND FATTY ACID DIARRHEA

	BILE ACID DIARRHEA	FATTY ACID DIARRHEA
Extent of ileal disease	Limited	Extensive
Ileal bile acid absorption	Reduced	Reduced
Fecal bile acid excretion	Increased	Increased
Fecal bile acid loss compensated by hepatic synthesis	Yes	No
Bile acid pool size	Normal	Reduced
Intraduodenal [bile acid]	Normal	Reduced
Steatorrhea	None or mild	>20 g
Response to cholestyramine	Yes	No
Response to low-fat diet	No	Yes

TABLE 15-3

COMPARISON OF DIFFERENT TYPES OF FATTY ACIDS

	LONG-CHAIN	MEDIUM-CHAIN	SHORT-CHAIN
Carbon chain length	>12	8–12	<8
Present in diet	In large amounts	In small amounts	No
Origin	In diet as triglycerides	Only in small amounts in diet as triglycerides	Bacterial degradation in colon of nonabsorbed carbohydrate to fatty acids
Primary site of absorption	Small intestine	Small intestine	Colon
Requires pancreatic lipolysis	Yes	No	No
Requires micelle formation	Yes	No	No
Presence in stool	Minimal	No	Substantial

acids. In contrast, patients with greater degrees of ileal disease and/or resection will often have diarrhea and steatorrhea that do not respond to cholestyramine. In this situation, ileal disease is also associated with increased amounts of bile acids entering the colon; however, hepatic synthesis can no longer increase sufficiently to maintain the bile acid pool size. As a consequence, the intraduodenal concentration of bile acids is also reduced to less than the CMC, resulting in impaired micelle formation and steatorrhea. This second situation is often called *fatty acid diarrhea*. Cholestyramine may not be effective (and may even increase the diarrhea by further depleting the intraduodenal bile acid concentration); however, a low-fat diet to reduce fatty acids entering the colon can be effective. Two clinical features, the length of ileum removed and the degree of steatorrhea, can predict whether an individual patient will respond to cholestyramine. Unfortunately, these predictors are imperfect, and a therapeutic trial of cholestyramine is often necessary to establish whether an individual patient will benefit from cholestyramine. Table 15-2 contrasts the characteristics of bile acid diarrhea (small ileal dysfunction) and fatty acid diarrhea (large ileal dysfunction).

LIPIDS

Steatorrhea is caused by one or more defects in the digestion and absorption of dietary fat. Average intake of dietary fat in the United States is approximately 120–150 g/d, and fat absorption is linear to dietary fat intake. The total load of fat presented to the small intestine is considerably greater, as substantial amounts of lipid are secreted in bile each day. (See earlier in the chapter for discussion of enterohepatic circulation of bile acids.) Three types of fatty acids compose fats: long-chain fatty acids (LCFAs), medium-chain fatty acids (MCFAs), and short-chain fatty acids (SCFAs) (Table 15-3). Dietary fat is exclusively

composed of long-chain triglycerides (LCTs), i.e., glycerol that is bound via ester-linkages to three LCFAs. While the majority of dietary LCFAs have carbon chain lengths of 16 or 18, fatty acids of carbon chain length >12 are metabolized in the same manner; saturated and unsaturated fatty acids are handled identically.

Assimilation of dietary lipid requires three integrated processes: (1) an intraluminal, or digestive, phase; (2) a mucosal, or absorptive, phase; and (3) a delivery, or postabsorptive, phase. An abnormality at any site of this process can cause steatorrhea (Table 15-4). Therefore it is essential that any patient with steatorrhea be evaluated to identify the specific physiologic defect in overall lipid digestion-absorption, as therapy will be determined by the specific cause of the steatorrhea.

The digestive phase has two components, *lipolysis* and *micellar formation*. Although dietary lipid is in the form of LCTs, the intestinal mucosa does not absorb triglycerides; they must first be hydrolyzed (Fig. 15-2). The initial step in lipid digestion is the formation of emulsions of finely dispersed lipid, which is accomplished by mastication and gastric contractions. Lipolysis, the hydrolysis of triglycerides to free fatty acids, monoglycerides, and glycerol by lipase, is initiated in the stomach by a gastric lipase that has a pH optimum of 4.5–6.0. About 20–30% of total lipolysis occurs in the stomach. Lipolysis is completed in the duodenum and jejunum by pancreatic lipase, which is inactivated by a pH <7.0. Pancreatic lipolysis is greatly enhanced by the presence of a second pancreatic enzyme, colipase, which facilitates the movement of lipase to the triglyceride.

TABLE 15-4

DEFECTS IN LIPID DIGESTION AND ABSORPTION IN STEATORRHEA

PHASE: PROCESS	PATHOPHYSIOLOGIC DEFECT	DISEASE EXAMPLE
Digestive		
Lipolysis formation	Decrease lipase secretion	Chronic pancreatitis
Micelle formation	Decreased intraduodenal bile acids	See Table 15-1
Absorptive		
Mucosal uptake and resterification	Mucosal dysfunction	Celiac sprue
Post-Absorptive		
Chylomicron formation	Absent betalipoproteins	Abetalipoproteinemia
Delivery from intestine	Abnormal lymphatics	Intestinal lymphangiectasia

Impaired lipolysis can lead to steatorrhea and can occur in the presence of pancreatic insufficiency due to chronic pancreatitis in adults or cystic fibrosis in children and adolescents. Normal lipolysis can be maintained by approximately 5% of maximal pancreatic lipase secretion; thus, steatorrhea is a late manifestation of these disorders. A reduction in intraduodenal pH can also result in altered lipolysis as pancreatic lipase is inactivated at pH <7. Thus, ~15% of patients with gastrinoma (Chap. 14) with substantial increases in gastric acid secretion from ectopic production of gastrin (usually from an islet cell adenoma) have diarrhea, and some will have steatorrhea believed secondary to acid-inactivation of pancreatic lipase. Similarly, patients with chronic pancreatitis (who have reduced lipase secretion) often have a decrease in pancreatic bicarbonate secretion, which will also result in a decrease in intraduodenal pH and inactivation of endogenous pancreatic lipase or of therapeutically administered lipase.

Overlying the microvillus membrane of the small intestine is the so-called unstirred water layer, a relatively stagnant aqueous phase that must be traversed by the products of lipolysis that are primarily water-insoluble. Water-soluble mixed micelles provide a mechanism for the water-insoluble products of lipolysis to reach the luminal plasma membrane of villous epithelial cells, the site for lipid absorption. Mixed micelles are molecular aggregates composed of fatty acids, monoglycerides, phospholipids, cholesterol, and conjugated bile acids. Mixed micelles are formed when the concentration of conjugated bile acids is greater than its CMC, which differs among the several bile acids present in the small intestinal lumen. Conjugated bile acids, synthesized in the liver and excreted into the duodenum in bile, are regulated by the enterohepatic circulation (see earlier). Steatorrhea can result from impaired movement of fatty acids across the unstirred aqueous fluid layer in two situations: (1) an increase in the relative thickness of the unstirred water layer that occurs in bacterial overgrowth syndromes (see later) secondary to functional stasis (e.g., scleroderma); and (2) a decrease in the *duodenal* concentration of conjugated bile acids below its CMC, resulting in impaired micelle formation. Thus, steatorrhea can be caused by one or more defects in the enterohepatic circulation of bile acids.

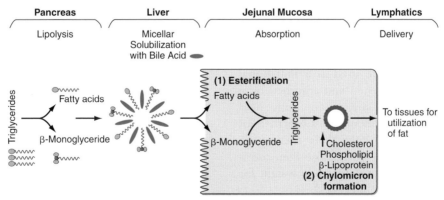

FIGURE 15-2

Schematic representation of lipid digestion and absorption. Dietary lipid is in the form of long-chain triglycerides (LCTs). The overall process can be divided into (1) a digestive phase that includes both lipolysis and micelle formation requiring pancreatic lipase and conjugated bile acids, respectively, in the duodenum; (2) an absorptive phase for mucosal uptake and reesterification; and (3) a postabsorptive phase that includes chylomicron formation and exit from the intestinal epithelial cell via lymphatics. *(Courtesy of John M. Dietschy, MD; with permission.)*

Uptake and reesterification constitute the *absorptive phase* of lipid digestion-absorption. Although passive diffusion has been thought responsible, a carrier-mediated process may mediate fatty acid and monoglyceride uptake. Regardless of the uptake process, fatty acids and monoglycerides are reesterified by a series of enzymatic steps in the endoplasmic reticulum and Golgi to form triglycerides, the form in which lipid exits from the intestinal epithelial cell. Impaired lipid absorption as a result of either mucosal inflammation (e.g., celiac sprue) and/or intestinal resection can also lead to steatorrhea.

The reesterified triglycerides require the formation of *chylomicrons* to permit their exit from the small-intestinal epithelial cell and their delivery to the liver via the *lymphatics*. Chylomicrons are composed of β-lipoprotein and contain triglycerides, cholesterol, cholesterol esters, and phospholipids and enter the lymphatics, not the portal vein. Defects in the *postabsorptive phase* of lipid digestion-absorption can also result in steatorrhea, but these disorders are uncommon. Abetalipoproteinemia, or acanthocytosis, is a rare disorder of impaired synthesis of β-lipoprotein associated with abnormal erythrocytes (acanthocytes), neurologic problems, and steatorrhea. Lipolysis, micelle formation, and lipid uptake are all normal in patients with abetalipoproteinemia, but the reesterified triglyceride cannot exit from the epithelial cell because of the failure to produce chylomicrons. Small-intestinal biopsies of these rare patients in the postprandial state reveal lipid-laden small-intestinal epithelial cells that become perfectly normal in appearance following a 72–96 h fast. Similarly, abnormalities of intestinal lymphatics (e.g., intestinal lymphangiectasia) may also be associated with steatorrhea as well as protein loss (see later). Steatorrhea can result from defects at any of the several steps in lipid digestion-absorption.

The mechanism of lipid digestion-absorption outlined above is limited to *dietary* lipid that is almost exclusively in the form of LCTs (Table 15-3). Medium-chain triglycerides (MCTs), composed of fatty acids with carbon chain lengths of 8–10, are present in large amounts in coconut oil and are used as a nutritional supplement. MCTs can be digested and absorbed by a different pathway from LCTs and at one time held promise as an important treatment of steatorrhea of almost all etiologies. Unfortunately, their therapeutic effects have been less than expected because their use is often not associated with an increase in body weight for reasons that are not completely understood.

MCTs, in contrast to LCTs, do not require pancreatic lipolysis as the triglyceride can be absorbed intact by the intestinal epithelial cell. Further, micelle formation is not necessary for the absorption of MCTs or medium-chain fatty acids, if hydrolyzed by pancreatic lipase. MCTs are absorbed more efficiently than LCTs for the following reasons: (1) the rate of MCT absorption is greater than that of long-chain fatty acids; (2) medium-chain fatty

acids following absorption are not reesterified; (3) following absorption, MCTs are hydrolyzed to medium-chain fatty acids; (4) MCTs do not require chylomicron formation for their exit from the intestinal epithelial cells; and (5) their route of exit is via the portal vein and not via lymphatics. Thus, the absorption of MCTs is greater than that of LCTs in pancreatic insufficiency, conditions with reduced intraduodenal bile acid concentrations, small-intestinal mucosal disease, abetalipoproteinemia, and intestinal lymphangiectasia.

SCFAs are not dietary lipids but are synthesized by colonic bacterial enzymes from nonabsorbed carbohydrate and are the anions in highest concentration in stool (between 80 and 130 mM). The SCFAs present in stool are primarily acetate, propionate, and butyrate, whose carbon chain lengths are 2, 3, and 4, respectively. Butyrate is the primary nutrient for colonic epithelial cells, and its deficiency may be associated with one or more colitides. SCFAs conserve calories and carbohydrate, because carbohydrates not completely absorbed in the small intestine will not be absorbed in the large intestine due to the absence of both disaccharidases and SGLT1, the transport protein that mediates monosaccharide absorption. In contrast, SCFAs are rapidly absorbed and stimulate colonic Na-Cl and fluid absorption. Most non–*Clostridium difficile* antibiotic-associated diarrhea is due to antibiotic suppression of colonic microflora, with a resulting decrease in SCFA production. As *C. difficile* accounts for about 10–15% of all antibiotic-associated diarrhea, a relative decrease in colonic production of SCFAs is likely the cause of most antibiotic-associated diarrhea.

The clinical manifestations of steatorrhea are a consequence of both the underlying disorder responsible for the development of steatorrhea and steatorrhea per se. Depending on the degree of steatorrhea and the level of dietary intake, significant fat malabsorption may lead to weight loss. Steatorrhea per se can be responsible for diarrhea; if the primary cause of the steatorrhea has not been identified, a low-fat diet can often ameliorate the diarrhea by decreasing fecal fat excretion. Steatorrhea is often associated with fat-soluble vitamin deficiency, which will require replacement with water-soluble preparations of these vitamins.

Disorders of absorption may also be associated with malabsorption of other dietary nutrients, most often carbohydrates, with or without a decrease in dietary lipid digestion and absorption. Therefore, knowledge of the mechanism of the digestion and absorption of carbohydrates, proteins, and other minerals and vitamins is useful in the evaluation of patients with altered intestinal nutrient absorption.

CARBOHYDRATES

Carbohydrates in the diet are present in the form of starch, disaccharides (sucrose and lactose), and glucose.

Carbohydrates are absorbed only in the small intestine and only in the form of monosaccharides. Therefore, before their absorption, starch and disaccharides must first be digested by pancreatic amylase and intestinal brush border disaccharidases to monosaccharides. Monosaccharide absorption occurs by a Na-dependent process mediated by the brush border transport protein SGLT1.

Lactose malabsorption is the only clinically important disorder of carbohydrate absorption. Lactose, the disaccharide present in milk, requires digestion by brush border lactase to its two constituent monosaccharides, glucose and galactose. Lactase is present in almost all species in the postnatal period but then disappears throughout the animal kingdom, except in humans. Lactase activity persists in many individuals throughout life. Two different types of lactase deficiency exist—primary and secondary. In *primary lactase deficiency*, a genetically determined decrease or absence of lactase is noted, while all other aspects of both intestinal absorption and brush border enzymes are normal. In a number of non-Caucasian groups, primary lactase deficiency is common in adulthood. Table 15-5 presents the incidence of primary lactase deficiency in several ethnic groups. Northern European and North American Caucasians are the only groups to maintain small-intestinal lactase activity throughout adult life. The persistence of lactase is the abnormality due to a defect in the regulation of its maturation. In contrast, *secondary lactase deficiency* occurs in association with small-intestinal mucosal disease with abnormalities in both structure and function of other brush border enzymes and transport processes. Secondary lactase deficiency is often seen in celiac sprue.

As lactose digestion is rate-limiting compared to glucose/galactose absorption, lactase deficiency is associated with significant lactose malabsorption. Some individuals with lactose malabsorption develop symptoms such as diarrhea, abdominal pain, cramps, and/or flatus. Most individuals with primary lactase deficiency do not have symptoms. Since lactose intolerance may be associated with symptoms suggestive of irritable bowel syndrome, persistence of such symptoms in an individual with lactose intolerance while on a strict lactose-free diet would suggest that the individual's symptoms were related to irritable bowel syndrome.

Development of symptoms of lactose intolerance is related to several factors:

1. *Amount of lactose in the diet.*
2. *Rate of gastric emptying.* Symptoms are more likely when gastric emptying is rapid than when gastric emptying is slower. Therefore it is more likely that skim milk will be associated with symptoms of lactose intolerance than will whole milk, as the rate of gastric emptying following skim milk intake is more rapid. Similarly, the diarrhea observed following subtotal gastrectomy is often a result of lactose intolerance, as gastric emptying is accelerated in patients with a gastrojejunostomy.
3. *Small-intestinal transit time.* Although the small and large intestine contribute to the development of symptoms, many of the symptoms of lactase deficiency are related to the interaction of colonic bacteria and nonabsorbed lactose. More rapid small-intestinal transit makes symptoms more likely.
4. *Colonic compensation by production of SCFAs from nonabsorbed lactose.* Reduced levels of colonic microflora, which can occur following antibiotic use, will also be associated with increased symptoms following lactose ingestion, especially in a lactase-deficient individual.

Glucose-galactose or monosaccharide malabsorption may also be associated with diarrhea and is due to a congenital absence of SGLT1. Diarrhea is present when individuals with this disorder ingest carbohydrates that contain actively transported monosaccharides (e.g., glucose, galactose) but not monosaccharides that are not actively transported (e.g., fructose). Fructose is absorbed by the brush border transport protein GLUT 5, a facilitated diffusion process that is not Na-dependent and is distinct from SGLT1. In contrast, some individuals develop diarrhea as a result of consuming large quantities of sorbitol, a sugar used in diabetic candy; sorbitol is only minimally absorbed due to the absence of an intestinal absorptive transport mechanism for sorbitol.

PROTEINS

Protein is present in food almost exclusively as polypeptides and requires extensive hydrolysis to di- and tripeptides and amino acids before absorption. Proteolysis occurs in both the stomach and small intestine; it is mediated by pepsin secreted as pepsinogen by gastric chief cells and trypsinogen and other peptidases from pancreatic acinar cells. These proenzymes, pepsinogen and trypsinogen, must be activated to pepsin (by pepsin

TABLE 15-5

PRIMARY LACTASE DEFICIENCY IN DIFFERENT ADULT ETHNIC GROUPS	
ETHNIC GROUP	**PREVALENCE OF LACTASE DEFICIENCY, %**
Northern European	5–15
Mediterranean	60–85
African black	85–100
American black	45–80
American Caucasian	10–25
Native American	50–95
Mexican American	40–75
Asian	90–100

Source: From FJ Simons: Am J Dig Dis 23:963, 1978.

in the presence of a pH <5) and trypsin (by the intestinal brush border enzyme enterokinase and subsequently by trypsin). Proteins are absorbed by separate transport systems for di- and tripeptides and for different types of amino acids, e.g., neutral and dibasic. Alterations in either protein or amino acid digestion and absorption are rarely observed clinically, even in the presence of extensive small-intestinal mucosal inflammation. However, three rare genetic disorders involve protein digestion-absorption: (1) *Enterokinase deficiency* is due to an absence of the brush border enzyme that converts the proenzyme trypsinogen to trypsin and is associated with diarrhea, growth retardation, and hypoproteinemia. (2) *Hartnup syndrome*, a defect in neutral amino acid transport, is characterized by a pellagra-like rash and neuropsychiatric symptoms. (3) *Cystinuria*, a defect in dibasic amino acid transport, is associated with renal calculi and chronic pancreatitis.

Approach to the Patient:
MALABSORPTION

The clues provided by the history, symptoms, and initial preliminary observations will serve to limit extensive, ill-focused, and expensive laboratory and imaging studies. For example, a clinician evaluating a patient with symptoms suggestive of malabsorption who recently had extensive small-intestinal resection for mesenteric ischemia should direct the initial assessment almost exclusively to define whether a short bowel syndrome might explain the entire clinical picture. Similarly, the development of a pattern of bowel movements suggestive of steatorrhea in a patient with long-standing alcohol abuse and chronic pancreatitis should lead toward assessing pancreatic exocrine function.

The classic picture of malabsorption is rarely seen today in most parts of the United States. As a consequence, diseases with malabsorption must be suspected in individuals with less severe symptoms and signs and with subtle evidence of the altered absorption of only a *single* nutrient rather than obvious evidence of the malabsorption of multiple nutrients.

Although diarrhea can be caused by changes in fluid and electrolyte movement in either the small or the large intestine, dietary nutrients are absorbed almost exclusively in the small intestine. Therefore the demonstration of diminished absorption of a dietary nutrient provides unequivocal evidence of small-intestinal disease, although colonic dysfunction may also be present (e.g., Crohn's disease may involve both small and large intestine). Dietary nutrient absorption may be segmental or diffuse along the small intestine and is site-specific. Thus, for example, calcium, iron, and folic acid are exclusively absorbed by active transport processes in the proximal small intestine, especially the duodenum;

in contrast, the active transport mechanisms for both cobalamin and bile acids are present only in the ileum. Therefore, in an individual who years previously had had an intestinal resection, the details of which are not presently available, a presentation with evidence of calcium, folic acid, and iron malabsorption but without cobalamin deficiency would make it likely that the duodenum and jejunum, but not ileum, had been resected.

Some nutrients, e.g., glucose, amino acids, and lipids, are absorbed throughout the small intestine, though their rate of absorption is greater in the proximal than in the distal segments. However, following segmental resection of the small intestine, the remaining segments undergo both morphologic and functional "adaptation" to enhance absorption. Such adaptation is secondary to the presence of luminal nutrients and hormonal stimuli and may not be complete in humans for several months following the resection. Adaptation is critical for survival in individuals who have undergone massive resection of the small intestine and/or colon.

Establishing the presence of steatorrhea and identifying its specific cause are often quite difficult. The "gold standard" still remains a timed, quantitative stool fat determination. On a practical basis, stool collections are invariably difficult and often incomplete, as nobody wants to handle stool. A qualitative test—Sudan III stain—has long been available to establish the presence of an increase in stool fat. This test is rapid and inexpensive but, as a qualitative test, does not establish the degree of fat malabsorption and is best used as a preliminary screening study. Many of the blood, breath, and isotopic tests that have been developed (1) do not directly measure fat absorption; (2) have excellent sensitivity when steatorrhea is obvious and severe but have poor sensitivity when steatorrhea is mild (e.g., stool chymotrypsin, elastase, that can potentially distinguish pancreatic from nonpancreatic etiologies of steatorrhea); or (3) have not survived the transition from the research laboratory to commercial application.

Despite this situation, the use of routine laboratory studies (i.e., complete blood count, prothrombin time, serum protein determination, alkaline phosphatase) may suggest the presence of dietary nutrient depletion, especially iron, folate, cobalamin, and vitamins D and K. Additional studies include measurement of serum carotene, cholesterol, albumin, iron, folate, and cobalamin levels. The serum carotene level can also be reduced if the patient has poor dietary intake of leafy vegetables.

If steatorrhea and/or altered absorption of other nutrients are suspected, the history, clinical observations, and laboratory testing can help detect deficiency of a nutrient, especially the fat-soluble vitamins A, D, E, or K.

Thus, evidence of metabolic bone disease with elevated alkaline phosphatase and/or reduced serum calcium levels would suggest vitamin D malabsorption. A deficiency of vitamin K would be suggested by an elevated prothrombin time in an individual without liver disease who was not taking anticoagulants. Macrocytic anemia would lead to evaluation of whether cobalamin or folic acid malabsorption was present. The presence of iron-deficiency anemia in the absence of occult bleeding from the gastrointestinal tract in either a male or a nonmenstruating female would require evaluation of iron malabsorption and the exclusion of celiac sprue, as iron is absorbed exclusively in the proximal small intestine.

At times, however, a timed (72 h) quantitative stool collection, preferably on a defined diet, must be obtained to determine stool fat content and establish the presence of steatorrhea. The presence of steatorrhea then requires further assessment to establish the pathophysiologic process(es) responsible for the defect in dietary lipid digestion-absorption (Table 15-4). Some of the other studies include the Schilling test, D-xylose test, duodenal mucosal biopsy, small-intestinal radiologic examination, and tests of pancreatic exocrine function.

The Schilling Test This test is performed to determine the cause for cobalamin malabsorption. Since cobalamin absorption requires multiple steps, including gastric, pancreatic, and ileal processes, the Schilling test can also be used to assess the integrity of these other organs. Cobalamin is present primarily in meat. Except in strict vegans, *dietary* cobalamin deficiency is exceedingly uncommon. Dietary cobalamin is bound in the stomach to a glycoprotein called *R-binder protein*, which is synthesized in both the stomach and salivary glands. This cobalamin–R binder complex is formed in the acid milieu of the stomach. Cobalamin absorption has an absolute requirement for intrinsic factor, another glycoprotein synthesized and released by gastric parietal cells, to promote its uptake by specific cobalamin receptors on the brush border of ileal enterocytes. Pancreatic protease enzymes split the cobalamin–R binder complex to release cobalamin in the proximal small intestine, where cobalamin is then bound by intrinsic factor.

As a consequence, cobalamin absorption may be abnormal in the following:

1. *Pernicious anemia*, a disease in which immunologically mediated atrophy of gastric parietal cells leads to an absence of both gastric acid and intrinsic factor secretion.
2. *Chronic pancreatitis* as a result of deficiency of pancreatic proteases to split the cobalamin–R binder complex. Although 50% of patients with chronic pancreatitis have been reported to have an abnormal Schilling test that was corrected by pancreatic enzyme replacement, the presence of a cobalamin-responsive macrocytic anemia in chronic pancreatitis is extremely rare. Although this probably reflects a difference in the digestion/absorption of cobalamin in food versus that in a crystalline form, the Schilling test can still be used to assess pancreatic exocrine function.
3. *Achlorhydria*, or absence of another factor secreted with acid that is responsible for splitting cobalamin away from the proteins in food to which it is bound. Up to one-third of individuals >60 years of age have marginal vitamin B_{12} absorption because of the inability to release cobalamin from food; these people have no defects in absorbing crystalline vitamin B_{12}.
4. *Bacterial overgrowth syndromes*, which are most often secondary to stasis in the small intestine, leading to bacterial utilization of cobalamin (often referred to as *stagnant bowel syndrome*; see later).
5. *Ileal dysfunction* (as a result of either inflammation or prior intestinal resection) due to impaired function of the mechanism of cobalamin–intrinsic factor uptake by ileal intestinal epithelial cells.

The Schilling test is performed by administering [58]Co-labeled cobalamin orally and collecting urine for 24 h, and it is dependent on normal renal and bladder function. Urinary excretion of cobalamin will reflect cobalamin absorption provided that intrahepatic binding sites for cobalamin are fully occupied. To ensure saturation of hepatic cobalamin binding sites so that all absorbed radiolabeled cobalamin will be excreted in urine, 1 mg cobalamin is administered intramuscularly 1 h following ingestion of the radiolabeled cobalamin. The Schilling test may be abnormal (usually defined as <10% excretion in 24 h) in pernicious anemia, chronic pancreatitis, blind loop syndrome, and ileal disease (**Table 15-6**). Therefore, whenever an abnormal

TABLE 15-6

DIFFERENTIAL RESULTS OF SCHILLING TEST IN SEVERAL DISEASES ASSOCIATED WITH COBALAMIN (CBL) MALABSORPTION

	[58]CO-CBL	WITH INTRINSIC FACTOR	WITH PANCREATIC ENZYMES	AFTER 5 DAYS OF ANTIBIOTICS
Pernicious anemia	Reduced	Normal	Reduced	Reduced
Chronic pancreatitis	Reduced	Reduced	Normal	Reduced
Bacterial overgrowth	Reduced	Reduced	Reduced	Normal
Ileal disease	Reduced	Reduced	Reduced	Reduced

Schilling test is found, [58]Co-labeled cobalamin should be administered on another occasion either bound to intrinsic factor, with pancreatic enzymes, or following a 5-day course of antibiotics (often tetracycline). A variation of the Schilling test can detect failure to split cobalamin from food proteins. The labeled cobalamin is cooked together with a scrambled egg and administered orally. People with achlorhydria will excrete <10% of the labeled cobalamin in the urine. In addition to establishing the etiology for cobalamin deficiency, the Schilling test can be used to help delineate the pathologic process responsible for steatorrhea by assessing ileal, pancreatic, and small-intestinal luminal function. Unfortunately, the Schilling test is infrequently performed because of the unavailability of human intrinsic factor.

Urinary D-Xylose Test The urinary D-xylose test for carbohydrate absorption provides an assessment of proximal small-intestinal mucosal function. D-Xylose, a pentose, is absorbed almost exclusively in the proximal small intestine. The D-xylose test is usually performed by giving 25 g D-xylose and collecting urine for 5 h. An abnormal test (<4.5 g excretion) primarily reflects the presence of duodenal/jejunal mucosal disease. The D-xylose test can also be abnormal in patients with blind loop syndrome (as a consequence primarily of abnormal intestinal mucosa) and, as a false-positive study, in patients with large collections of fluid in a third space (i.e., ascites, pleural fluid). The ease of obtaining a mucosal biopsy of the small intestine by endoscopy and the false-negative rate of the D-xylose test have led to its diminished use. When small-intestinal mucosal disease is suspected, a small-intestinal mucosal biopsy should be performed.

Radiologic Examination Radiologic examination of the small intestine using barium contrast (small-bowel series or study) can provide important information in the evaluation of the patient with presumed or suspected malabsorption. These studies are most often performed in conjunction with the examination of the esophagus, stomach, and duodenal bulb, and insufficient barium is given to the patient to permit an adequate examination

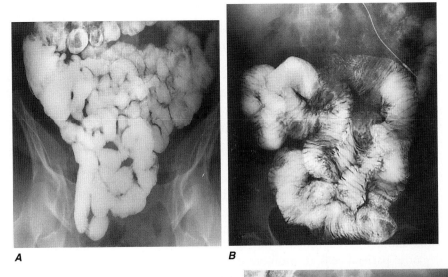

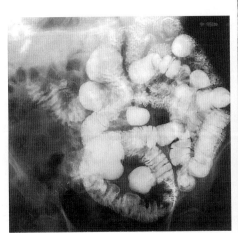

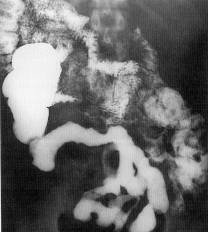

FIGURE 15-3

Barium contrast small-intestinal radiologic examinations. *A.* Normal individual. *B.* Celiac sprue. *C.* Jejunal diverticulosis. *D.* Crohn's disease. *(Courtesy of Morton Burrell, MD, Yale University; with permission.)*

of the small-intestinal mucosa, especially the ileum. As a result, many gastrointestinal radiologists alter the procedure of a barium contrast examination of the small intestine by performing either a small-bowel series in which a large amount of barium is given by mouth without concurrent examination of the esophagus and stomach or an enteroclysis study in which a large amount of barium is introduced into the duodenum via a fluoroscopically placed tube. In addition, many of the diagnostic features initially described by radiologists to denote the presence of small-intestinal disease (e.g., flocculation, segmentation) are rarely seen with current barium suspensions. Nonetheless, in skilled hands barium contrast examination of the small intestine can yield important information. For example, with extensive mucosal disease, dilation of intestine can be seen, as dilution of barium from increased intestinal fluid secretion (**Fig. 15-3**). A normal barium contrast study does *not* exclude the possibility of small-intestinal disease. However, a small-bowel series remains a useful examination to look for anatomic abnormalities, such as strictures and fistulas (as in Crohn's disease) or blind loop syndrome (e.g., multiple jejunal diverticula), and to define the extent of a previous surgical resection. Noninvasive capsule endoscopy and double-barrel enteroscopy are useful aids in the diagnostic assessment of small intestinal pathology.

Biopsy of Small-Intestinal Mucosa A small-intestinal mucosal biopsy is essential in the evaluation of a patient with documented steatorrhea or chronic diarrhea (lasting >3 weeks) (Chap. 6). The ready availability of endoscopic equipment to examine the stomach and duodenum has led to its almost uniform use as the preferred method to obtain histologic material of proximal small-intestinal mucosa. The primary indications for a small-intestinal biopsy are (1) evaluation of a patient either with documented or suspected steatorrhea or with chronic diarrhea, and (2) diffuse or focal abnormalities of the small intestine defined on a small-intestinal series. Lesions seen on small-bowel biopsy can be classified into three different categories (**Table 15-7**):

1. *Diffuse, specific lesions.* Relatively few diseases associated with altered nutrient absorption have specific histopathologic abnormalities on small-intestinal mucosal biopsy, and they are uncommon. Whipple's disease is characterized by the presence of periodic acid-Schiff (PAS)–positive macrophages in the lamina propria, while the bacilli that are also present may require electron-microscopic examination for identification (**Fig. 15-4**). *Abetalipoproteinemia* is characterized by a normal mucosal appearance except for the presence of mucosal absorptive cells that contain lipid postprandial and disappear

TABLE 15-7

DISEASE THAT CAN BE DIAGNOSED BY SMALL-INTESTINAL MUCOSAL BIOPSIES

LESIONS	PATHOLOGIC FINDINGS
Diffuse, Specific	
Whipple's disease	Lamina propria contains macrophages containing PAS+ material
Agammaglobulinemia	No plasma cells; either normal or absent villi ("flat mucosa")
Abetalipoproteinemia	Normal villi; epithelial cells vacuolated with fat postprandially
Patchy, Specific	
Intestinal lymphoma	Malignant cells in lamina propria and submucosa
Intestinal lymphangiectasia	Dilated lymphatics; clubbed villi
Eosinophilic gastroenteritis	Eosinophil infiltration of lamina propria and mucosa
Amyloidosis	Amyloid deposits
Crohn's disease	Noncaseating granulomas
Infection by one or more microorganisms (see text)	Specific organisms
Mastocytosis	Mast cell infiltration of lamina propria
Diffuse, Nonspecific	
Celiac sprue	Short or absent villi; mononuclear infiltrate; epithelial cell damage; hypertrophy of crypts
Tropical sprue	Similar to celiac sprue
Bacterial overgrowth	Patchy damage to villi; lymphocyte infiltration
Folate deficiency	Short villi; decreased mitosis in crypts; megalocytosis
Vitamin B_{12} deficiency	Similar to folate deficiency
Radiation enteritis	Similar to folate deficiency
Zollinger-Ellison syndrome	Mucosal ulceration and erosion from acid
Protein-calorie malnutrition	Villous atrophy; secondary bacterial overgrowth
Drug-induced enteritis	Variable histology

Note: PAS+, periodic acid–Schiff positive.

CHAPTER 15

Disorders of Absorption

following a prolonged period of either fat-free intake or fasting. *Immune globulin deficiency* is associated with a variety of histopathologic findings on small-intestinal mucosal biopsy. The characteristic feature is the absence of or substantial reduction in the number of plasma cells in the lamina propria; the mucosal architecture may be either perfectly normal

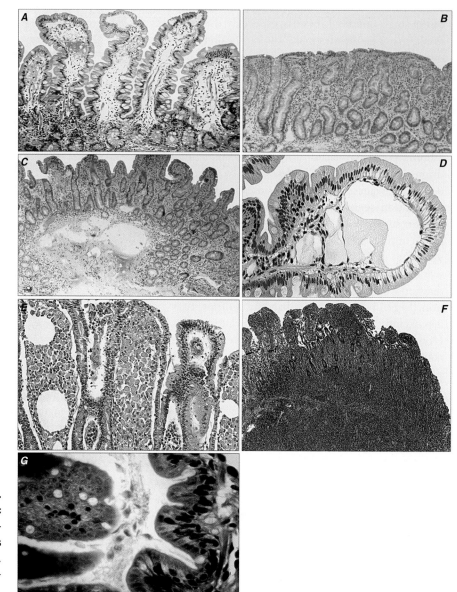

FIGURE 15-4

Small-intestinal mucosal biopsies.
A. Normal individual. ***B.*** Untreated celiac sprue. ***C.*** Treated celiac sprue. ***D.*** Intestinal lymphangiectasia. ***E.*** Whipple's disease. ***F.*** Lymphoma. ***G.*** Giardiasis. *(Courtesy of Marie Robert, MD, Yale University; with permission.)*

or flat (i.e., villous atrophy). As patients with immune globulin deficiency are often infected with *Giardia lamblia*, *Giardia* trophozoites may also be seen in the biopsy.

2. *Patchy, specific lesions.* Several diseases show abnormal small–intestinal mucosa with a patchy distribution. As a result, biopsies obtained randomly or in the absence of abnormalities visualized endoscopically may not reveal the diagnostic features. Intestinal *lymphoma* can at times be diagnosed on mucosal biopsy by the identification of malignant lymphoma cells in the lamina propria and submucosa. The presence of dilated lymphatics in the submucosa and sometimes in the lamina propria indicates the presence of *lymphangiectasia* associated with hypoproteinemia secondary to protein loss into the intestine. *Eosinophilic*

gastroenteritis comprises a heterogeneous group of disorders with a spectrum of presentations and symptoms with an eosinophilic infiltrate of the lamina propria, with or without peripheral eosinophilia. The patchy nature of the infiltrate as well as its presence in the submucosa often leads to an absence of histopathologic findings on mucosal biopsy. As the involvement of the duodenum in *Crohn's disease* is also submucosal and not necessarily continuous, mucosal biopsies are not the most direct approach to the diagnosis of duodenal Crohn's disease (Chap. 16). Amyloid deposition can be identified by Congo Red stain in some patients with *amyloidosis* involving the duodenum.

3. Several microorganisms can be identified on small-intestinal biopsies, establishing a correct diagnosis.

Many of these microorganisms are associated with diarrhea that occurs in immunodeficient individuals, especially those with HIV infection, and include *Cryptosporidium, Isospora belli,* cytomegalovirus, *Mycobacterium avium-intracellulare,* and *G. lamblia.*

4. *Diffuse, nonspecific lesions. Celiac sprue* presents with a characteristic mucosal appearance on duodenal/proximal jejunal mucosal biopsy that is not diagnostic of the disease. The diagnosis of celiac sprue is established by clinical, histologic, and immunologic response to a gluten-free diet. *Tropical sprue* is associated with histologic findings similar to those of celiac sprue after a tropical or subtropical exposure but does not respond to gluten restriction; most often symptoms improve with antibiotics and folate administration.

Patients with steatorrhea require assessment of *pancreatic exocrine function*, which is often abnormal in chronic pancreatitis. The secretin test that collects pancreatic secretions by duodenal intubation following intravenous administration of secretin is the only test that directly measures pancreatic exocrine function and is available at few specialized centers. Endoscopic approaches provide excellent assessment of pancreatic duct anatomy but do *not* assess exocrine function (Chap. 45).

Table 15–8 summarizes the results of the D-xylose test, Schilling test, and small-intestinal mucosal biopsy in patients with five different causes of steatorrhea.

TABLE 15-8

RESULTS OF DIAGNOSTIC STUDIES IN DIFFERENT CAUSES OF STEATORRHEA

	D-XYLOSE TEST	SCHILLING TEST	DUODENAL MUCOSAL BIOPSY
Chronic pancreatitis	Normal	50% abnormal; if abnormal, normal with pancreatic enzymes	Normal
Bacterial overgrowth syndrome	Normal or only modestly abnormal	Often abnormal; if abnormal, normal after antibiotics	Usually normal
Ileal disease	Normal	Abnormal	Normal
Celiac sprue	Decreased	Normal	Abnormal: probably "flat"
Intestinal lymphangiectasia	Normal	Normal	Abnormal: "dilated lymphatics"

CELIAC SPRUE

Celiac sprue is a common cause of malabsorption of one or more nutrients in Caucasians, especially those of European descent. Estimated incidence in the United States may be as high as 1:113 people. Celiac sprue has had several other names, including nontropical sprue, celiac disease (in children), adult celiac disease, and gluten-sensitive enteropathy. The etiology of celiac sprue is not known, but environmental, immunologic, and genetic factors are important. Celiac sprue has protean manifestations, almost all of which are secondary to nutrient malabsorption, and a varied natural history, with the onset of symptoms occurring at ages ranging from the first year of life through the eighth decade.

The hallmark of celiac sprue is the presence of an abnormal small-intestinal biopsy (Fig. 15-4) and the response of the condition—malabsorption and the histologic changes on the small-intestinal biopsy—to the elimination of gluten from the diet. The histologic changes have a proximal-to-distal intestinal distribution of severity, which probably reflects the exposure of the intestinal mucosa to varied amounts of dietary gluten; the symptoms correlate with histologic changes.

The symptoms of celiac sprue may appear with the introduction of cereals in an infant's diet, although spontaneous remissions often occur during the second decade of life that may be either permanent or followed by the reappearance of symptoms over several years. Alternatively, the symptoms of celiac sprue may first become evident at almost any age throughout adulthood. In many patients, frequent spontaneous remissions and exacerbations occur. The symptoms range from significant malabsorption of multiple nutrients, with diarrhea, steatorrhea, weight loss, and the consequences of nutrient depletion (i.e., anemia and metabolic bone disease), to the absence of any gastrointestinal symptoms but with evidence of the depletion of a single nutrient (e.g., iron or folate deficiency, osteomalacia, edema from protein loss). Asymptomatic relatives of patients with celiac sprue have been identified as having this disease either by small-intestinal biopsy or by serologic studies [e.g., antiendomysial antibodies, tissue transglutaminase (tTG)]. The availability of these "celiac serologies" has led to a substantial increase in the diagnosis of celiac sprue and the diagnosis is now being made primarily in patients without "classic" symptoms but with atypical and subclinical presentations.

Etiology

The etiology of celiac sprue is not known, but environmental, immunologic, and genetic factors all appear to contribute to the disease. One *environmental* factor is the clear association of the disease with gliadin, a component of gluten that is present in wheat, barley, and rye. In addition to the role of gluten restriction in treatment, the instillation of gluten into both normal-appearing rectum and distal ileum of patients with celiac sprue results in morphologic changes within hours.

An *immunologic* component to etiology is suspected. Serum antibodies—IgA antigliadin, IgA antiendomysial, and IgA anti-tTG antibodies—are present, but it is not known whether such antibodies are primary or secondary to the tissue damage. The antiendomysial antibody has 90–95% sensitivity and 90–95% specificity; the antigen recognized by the antiendomysial antibody is tTG. Antibody studies are frequently used to identify patients with celiac sprue; patients with these antibodies should undergo duodenal biopsy. This autoantibody has not been linked to a pathogenetic mechanism (or mechanisms) responsible for celiac sprue. Nonetheless, this antibody is useful in establishing the true prevalence of celiac sprue in the general population. A 4-week treatment with prednisolone of a patient with celiac sprue who continues to eat gluten will induce a remission and convert the "flat" abnormal duodenal biopsy to a more normal-appearing one. In addition, gliadin peptides may interact with gliadin-specific T cells that may either mediate tissue injury or induce the release of one or more cytokines that cause tissue injury.

Genetic factor(s) also appear to be involved in celiac sprue. The incidence of celiac sprue varies widely in different population groups (high in Caucasians, low in blacks and Asians) and is 10% in first-degree relatives of celiac sprue patients. Furthermore, almost all patients with celiac sprue express the HLA-DQ2 allele, though only a minority of people expressing DQ2 have celiac sprue. Absence of DQ2 excludes the diagnosis of celiac sprue.

Diagnosis

A small-intestinal biopsy is required to establish a diagnosis of celiac sprue (Fig. 15-4). A biopsy should be performed in patients with symptoms and laboratory findings suggestive of nutrient malabsorption and/or deficiency and with a positive tTG serology. Since the presentation of celiac sprue is often subtle, without overt evidence of malabsorption or nutrient deficiency, it is important to have a relatively low threshold to perform a biopsy. It is more prudent to perform a biopsy than to obtain another test of intestinal absorption, which can never completely exclude or establish this diagnosis.

The diagnosis of celiac sprue requires the presence of characteristic histologic changes on small-intestinal biopsy together with a prompt clinical and histologic response following the institution of a gluten-free diet. If serologic studies have detected the presence of IgA antiendomysial or tTG antibodies, they too should disappear after a gluten-free diet is started. The changes seen on duodenal/jejunal biopsy are restricted to the mucosa

and include (1) absence or reduced height of villi, resulting in a flat appearance; (2) increased loss of villous cells in association with increased crypt cell proliferation, resulting in crypt hyperplasia and loss of villous structure, with consequent villous, but not mucosal, atrophy; (3) cuboidal appearance and nuclei that are no longer oriented basally in surface epithelial cells and increased intraepithelial lymphocytes; and (4) increased lymphocytes and plasma cells in the lamina propria (Fig. 15-4B). Although these features are characteristic of celiac sprue, they are *not* diagnostic because a similar appearance can be seen in tropical sprue, eosinophilic enteritis, and milk-protein intolerance in children and occasionally in lymphoma, bacterial overgrowth, Crohn's disease, and gastrinoma with acid hypersecretion. However, the presence of a characteristic histologic appearance that reverts toward normal following the initiation of a gluten-free diet establishes the diagnosis of celiac sprue (Fig. 15-4C). Readministration of gluten with or without an additional small-intestinal biopsy is not necessary.

Failure to Respond to Gluten Restriction

The most common cause of persistent symptoms in a patient who fulfills all the criteria for diagnosing celiac sprue is continued intake of gluten. Gluten is ubiquitous, and significant effort must be made to exclude all gluten from the diet. Use of rice in place of wheat flour is very helpful, and several support groups provide important aid to patients with celiac sprue and to their families. More than 90% of patients who have the characteristic findings of celiac sprue will respond to complete dietary gluten restriction. The remainder constitute a heterogeneous group (whose condition is often called *refractory sprue*) that includes some patients who (1) respond to restriction of other dietary protein, e.g., soy; (2) respond to glucocorticoids; (3) are "temporary" (i.e., the clinical and morphologic findings disappear after several months or years); or (4) fail to respond to all measures and have a fatal outcome, with or without documented complications of celiac sprue, such as development of intestinal T cell lymphoma.

Mechanism of Diarrhea

The diarrhea in celiac sprue has several pathogenetic mechanisms. Diarrhea may be secondary to (1) steatorrhea, which is primarily a result of the changes in jejunal mucosal function; (2) secondary lactase deficiency, a consequence of changes in jejunal brush border enzymatic function; (3) bile acid malabsorption resulting in bile acid–induced fluid secretion in the colon, in cases with more extensive disease involving the ileum; and (4) endogenous fluid secretion resulting from crypt hyperplasia. Patients with more severe involvement with celiac sprue may obtain temporary improvement with *dietary lactose and fat restriction* while awaiting the full effects of total gluten restriction, which is primary therapy.

Associated Diseases

Celiac sprue is associated with dermatitis herpetiformis (DH), though the association has not been explained. Patients with DH have characteristic papulovesicular lesions that respond to dapsone. Almost all patients with DH have histologic changes in the small intestine consistent with celiac sprue, although usually much milder and less diffuse in distribution. Most patients with DH have mild or no gastrointestinal symptoms. In contrast, relatively few patients with celiac sprue have DH.

Celiac sprue is also associated with diabetes mellitus type 1 and IgA deficiency. The clinical importance of the former association is that although severe watery diarrhea without evidence of malabsorption is most often seen in patients with "diabetic diarrhea," assay of antiendomysial antibodies and/or a small-intestinal biopsy must at times be considered to exclude this association.

Complications

The most important complication of celiac sprue is the development of cancer. An increased incidence of both gastrointestinal and nongastrointestinal neoplasms as well as intestinal lymphoma exists in patients with celiac sprue. For unexplained reasons the occurrence of lymphoma in patients with celiac sprue is higher in Ireland and the United Kingdom than in the United States. The possibility of lymphoma must be considered whenever a patient with celiac sprue previously doing well on a gluten-free diet is no longer responsive to gluten restriction or a patient who presents with clinical and histologic features consistent with celiac sprue does not respond to a gluten-free diet. Other complications of celiac sprue include the development of intestinal ulceration independent of lymphoma and so-called refractory sprue (see earlier) and collagenous sprue. In *collagenous sprue*, a layer of collagen-like material is present beneath the basement membrane; patients with collagenous sprue generally do not respond to a gluten-free diet and often have a poor prognosis.

TROPICAL SPRUE

Tropical sprue is a poorly understood syndrome that affects both expatriates and natives in certain but not all tropical areas and is manifested by chronic diarrhea, steatorrhea, weight loss, and nutritional deficiencies, including those of both folate and cobalamin. This disease affects 5–10% of the population in some tropical areas.

Chronic diarrhea in a tropical environment is most often caused by infectious agents including *G. lamblia*, *Yersinia enterocolitica*, *C. difficile*, *Cryptosporidium parvum*, and *Cyclospora cayetanensis*, among other organisms. Tropical sprue should not be entertained as a possible diagnosis until the presence of cysts and trophozoites has been excluded in three stool samples.

Chronic infections of the gastrointestinal tract and diarrhea are discussed in Chap. 22.

The small-intestinal mucosa in individuals living in tropical areas is not identical to that of individuals who reside in temperate climates. Biopsies reveal a mild alteration of villous architecture with a modest increase in mononuclear cells in the lamina propria, which on occasion can be as severe as that seen in celiac sprue. These changes are observed both in native residents and in expatriates living in tropical regions and are usually associated with mild decreases in absorptive function, but they revert to "normal" when an individual moves or returns to a temperate area. Some have suggested that the changes seen in tropical enteropathy and in tropical sprue represent different ends of the spectrum of a single entity, but convincing evidence to support this concept is lacking.

Etiology

Because tropical sprue responds to antibiotics, the consensus is that it may be caused by one or more infectious agents. Nonetheless, the etiology and pathogenesis of tropical sprue are uncertain. First, its occurrence is not evenly distributed in all tropical areas; rather, it is found in specific locations, including southern India, the Philippines, and several Caribbean islands (e.g., Puerto Rico, Haiti), but is rarely observed in Africa, Jamaica, or Southeast Asia. Second, an occasional individual will not develop symptoms of tropical sprue until long after having left an endemic area. This is the reason why the original term for celiac sprue was *nontropical sprue* to distinguish it from tropical sprue. Third, multiple microorganisms have been identified on jejunal aspirate with relatively little consistency among studies. *Klebsiella pneumoniae*, *Enterobacter cloacae*, or *E. coli* have been implicated in some studies of tropical sprue, while other studies have favored a role for a toxin produced by one or more of these bacteria. Fourth, the incidence of tropical sprue appears to have decreased substantially during the past two decades. One speculation for the reduced occurrence is the wider use of antibiotics in acute diarrhea, especially in travelers to tropical areas from temperate countries. Fifth, the role of folic acid deficiency in the pathogenesis of tropical sprue requires clarification. Folic acid is absorbed exclusively in the duodenum and proximal jejunum, and most patients with tropical sprue have evidence of folate malabsorption and depletion. Although folate deficiency can cause changes in small-intestinal mucosa that are corrected by folate replacement, several earlier studies reporting that tropical sprue could be cured by folic acid did not provide an explanation for the "insult" that was initially responsible for folate malabsorption.

The clinical pattern of tropical sprue varies in different areas of the world (e.g., India vs Puerto Rico). Not infrequently, individuals in South India initially will report the occurrence of an acute enteritis before the development of steatorrhea and malabsorption. In contrast, in Puerto Rico a most insidious onset of symptoms and a more dramatic response to antibiotics is seen when compared to some other locations. Tropical sprue in different areas of the world may not be the same disease, and similar clinical entities may have different etiologies.

Diagnosis

The diagnosis of tropical sprue is best made by the presence of an abnormal small-intestinal mucosal biopsy in an individual with chronic diarrhea and evidence of malabsorption who is either residing or has recently lived in a tropical country. The small-intestinal biopsy in tropical sprue does not have pathognomonic features but resembles, and can often be indistinguishable from, that seen in celiac sprue (Fig. 15-4). The biopsy in tropical sprue will have less villous architectural alteration and more mononuclear cell infiltrate in the lamina propria. In contrast to celiac sprue, the histologic features of tropical sprue are present with a similar degree of severity throughout the small intestine, and a gluten-free diet does not result in either clinical or histologic improvement in tropical sprue.

℞ Treatment:
TROPICAL SPRUE

Broad-spectrum antibiotics and folic acid are most often curative, especially if the patient leaves the tropical area and does not return. Tetracycline should be used for up to 6 months and may be associated with improvement within 1–2 weeks. Folic acid alone will induce a hematologic remission as well as improvement in appetite, weight gain, and some morphologic changes in small intestinal biopsy. Because of the presence of marked folate deficiency, folic acid is most often given together with antibiotics.

SHORT BOWEL SYNDROME

This is a descriptive term for the myriad clinical problems that occur following resection of varying lengths of small intestine. The factors that determine both the type and degree of symptoms include (1) the specific segment (jejunum vs ileum) resected, (2) the length of the resected segment, (3) the integrity of the ileocecal valve, (4) whether any large intestine has also been removed, (5) residual disease in the remaining small and/or large intestine (e.g., Crohn's disease, mesenteric artery disease), and (6) the degree of adaptation in the remaining

intestine. Short bowel syndrome can occur at any age from neonates through the elderly.

Three different situations in adults demand intestinal resections: (1) mesenteric vascular disease, including atherosclerosis, thrombotic phenomena, and vasculitides; (2) primary mucosal and submucosal disease, e.g., Crohn's disease; and (3) operations without preexisting small intestinal disease, such as trauma and jejunoileal bypass for obesity.

Following resection of the small intestine, the residual intestine undergoes adaptation of both structure and function that may last for up to 6–12 months. Continued intake of dietary nutrients and calories is required to stimulate adaptation via direct contact with intestinal mucosa, the release of one or more intestinal hormones, and pancreatic and biliary secretions. Thus, enteral nutrition and calorie administration must be maintained, especially in the early postoperative period, even if an extensive intestinal resection requiring total parenteral nutrition (TPN) had been performed. The subsequent ability of such patients to absorb nutrients will not be known for several months, until adaptation is completed.

Multiple factors besides the absence of intestinal mucosa (required for lipid, fluid, and electrolyte absorption) contribute to the diarrhea and steatorrhea in these patients. Removal of the ileum and especially the ileocecal valve is often associated with more severe diarrhea than jejunal resection. Without part or all of the ileum, diarrhea can be caused by an increase in bile acids entering the colon, leading to their stimulation of colonic fluid and electrolyte secretion. Absence of the ileocecal valve is also associated with a decrease in intestinal transit time and bacterial overgrowth from the colon. Lactose intolerance as a result of the removal of lactase-containing mucosa as well as gastric hypersecretion will also contribute to the diarrhea.

In addition to diarrhea and/or steatorrhea, a range of nonintestinal symptoms is also observed in some patients. A significant increase in renal calcium oxalate calculi is observed in patients with a small-intestinal resection with an intact colon and is due to an increase in oxalate absorption by the large intestine, with subsequent hyperoxaluria (called *enteric hyperoxaluria*). Two possible mechanisms for the increase in oxalate absorption in the colon have been suggested: (1) bile acids and fatty acids that increase colonic mucosal permeability, resulting in increased oxalate absorption; and (2) increased fatty acids that bind calcium, resulting in increased soluble oxalate that is then absorbed. Since oxalate is high in relatively few foods (e.g., spinach, rhubarb, tea), dietary restrictions alone are not adequate treatment. Cholestyramine, an anion-binding resin, and calcium have proved useful in reducing the hyperoxaluria. Similarly, an increase in cholesterol gallstones is related to a decrease in the bile acid pool size, which results in the generation of cholesterol supersaturation in gallbladder bile. Gastric hypersecretion of acid occurs in many patients following large resections of the small intestine. The etiology is unclear but may be related to either reduced hormonal inhibition of acid secretion or increased gastrin levels due to reduced small-intestinal catabolism of circulating gastrin. The resulting gastric acid secretion may be an important factor contributing to the diarrhea and steatorrhea. A reduced pH in the duodenum can inactivate pancreatic lipase and/or precipitate duodenal bile acids, thereby increasing steatorrhea, and an increase in gastric secretion can create a volume overload relative to the reduced small-intestinal absorptive capacity. Inhibition of gastric acid secretion with proton pump inhibitors can help in reducing the diarrhea and steatorrhea.

℞ **Treatment:**
SHORT BOWEL SYNDROME

Treatment of short bowel syndrome depends on the severity of symptoms and whether the individual is able to maintain caloric and electrolyte balance with oral intake alone. Initial treatment includes judicious use of opiates (including codeine) to reduce stool output and to establish an effective diet. An initial diet should be low-fat and high-carbohydrate to minimize the diarrhea from fatty acid stimulation of colonic fluid secretion. MCTs (see earlier), a low-lactose diet, and various fiber-containing diets should also be tried. In the absence of an ileocecal valve, the possibility of bacterial overgrowth must be considered and treated. If gastric acid hypersecretion is contributing to the diarrhea and steatorrhea, a proton pump inhibitor may be helpful. Usually none of these therapeutic approaches will provide an instant solution, but they can reduce disabling diarrhea.

The patient's vitamin and mineral status must also be monitored; replacement therapy should be initiated if indicated. Fat-soluble vitamins, folate, cobalamin, calcium, iron, magnesium, and zinc are the most critical factors to monitor on a regular basis. If these approaches are not successful, home TPN is an established therapy that can be maintained for many years. Intestinal transplantation is becoming established as a possible approach for individuals with extensive intestinal resection who cannot be maintained without TPN, which is often called "intestinal failure." Considerable attention has been directed to the potential effectiveness of trophic hormones, e.g. glucagon-like peptide 2 (GLP-2) to improve absorptive function, and small-intestinal transplantation is also available in selected patients.

BACTERIAL OVERGROWTH SYNDROME

Bacterial overgrowth syndrome comprises a group of disorders with diarrhea, steatorrhea, and macrocytic anemia whose common feature is the proliferation of colonic-type

bacteria within the small intestine. This bacterial proliferation is due to stasis caused by impaired peristalsis (*functional stasis*), changes in intestinal anatomy (*anatomic stasis*), or direct communication between the small and large intestine. These conditions have also been referred to as *stagnant bowel syndrome* or *blind loop syndrome*.

Pathogenesis

The manifestations of bacterial overgrowth syndromes are a direct consequence of the presence of increased amounts of a colonic-type bacterial flora, such as *E. coli* or *Bacteroides*, in the small intestine. *Macrocytic anemia* is due to cobalamin, not folate, deficiency. Most bacteria require cobalamin for growth, and increasing concentrations of bacteria use up the relatively small amounts of dietary cobalamin. *Steatorrhea* is due to impaired micelle formation as a consequence of a reduced intraduodenal concentration of conjugated bile acids and the presence of unconjugated bile acids. Certain bacteria, e.g., *Bacteroides*, deconjugate conjugated bile acids to unconjugated bile acids. Unconjugated bile acids will be absorbed more rapidly than conjugated bile acids, and, as a result, the intraduodenal concentration of bile acids will be reduced. In addition, the CMC of unconjugated bile acids is higher than that of conjugated bile acids, resulting in a decrease in micelle formation. *Diarrhea* is due, at least in part, to the steatorrhea, when it is present. However, some patients manifest diarrhea *without* steatorrhea, and it is assumed that the colonic-type bacteria in these patients are producing one or more bacterial enterotoxins that are responsible for fluid secretion and diarrhea.

Etiology

The etiology of these different disorders is bacterial proliferation in the small intestinal lumen secondary to either anatomic or functional stasis or to a communication between the relatively sterile small intestine and the colon with its high levels of aerobic and anaerobic bacteria. Several examples of *anatomic* stasis have been identified: (1) one or more diverticula (both duodenal and jejunal) (Fig. 15-3C); (2) fistulas and strictures related to Crohn's disease (Fig. 15-3D); (3) a proximal duodenal afferent loop following a subtotal gastrectomy and gastrojejunostomy; (4) a bypass of the intestine, e.g., jejunoileal bypass for obesity; and (5) dilation at the site of a previous intestinal anastomosis. These anatomic derangements are often associated with the presence of a segment (or segments) of intestine out of continuity of propagated peristalsis, resulting in stasis and bacterial proliferation. Bacterial overgrowth syndromes can also occur in the *absence* of an anatomic blind loop when *functional* stasis is present. Impaired peristalsis and bacterial overgrowth in the absence of a blind loop occur in scleroderma, where motility abnormalities exist in both the esophagus and small intestine. Functional stasis and bacterial overgrowth can also occur in association with diabetes mellitus and in the small intestine when a direct connection exists between the small and large intestine, including an ileocolonic resection, or occasionally following an enterocolic anastomosis that permits entry of bacteria into the small intestine as a result of bypassing the ileocecal valve.

Diagnosis

The diagnosis may be suspected from the combination of a low serum cobalamin level and an elevated serum folate level, as enteric bacteria frequently produce folate compounds that will be absorbed in the duodenum. Ideally, the diagnosis of the bacterial overgrowth syndrome is the demonstration of increased levels of aerobic and/or anaerobic colonic-type bacteria in a jejunal aspirate obtained by intubation. This specialized test is rarely available, and bacterial overgrowth is best established by a Schilling test (Table 15-6), which should be abnormal following the administration of ^{58}Co-labeled cobalamin, with or without the administration of intrinsic factor. Following the administration of tetracycline for 5 days, the Schilling test will become normal, confirming the diagnosis of bacterial overgrowth. Breath hydrogen testing or lactulose (nondigestible disaccharide) administration has also been used to detect bacterial overgrowth.

℞ **Treatment:**
BACTERIAL OVERGROWTH SYNDROME

Primary treatment should be directed, if at all possible, to the surgical correction of an anatomic blind loop. In the absence of functional stasis, it is important to define the anatomic relationships responsible for stasis and bacterial overgrowth. For example, bacterial overgrowth secondary to strictures, one or more diverticula, or a proximal afferent loop can potentially be cured by surgical correction of the anatomic state. In contrast, the functional stasis of scleroderma or certain anatomic stasis states (e.g., multiple jejunal diverticula), cannot be corrected surgically, and these conditions should be treated with broad-spectrum antibiotics. Tetracycline used to be the initial treatment of choice; due to increasing resistance, however, other antibiotics such as metronidazole, amoxicillin/clavulanic acid, and cephalosporins have been employed. The antibiotic should be given for approximately 3 weeks or until symptoms remit. Although the natural history of these conditions is chronic, antibiotics should not be given continuously. Symptoms usually remit within 2–3 weeks of initial antibiotic therapy. Therapy need not be repeated until symptoms recur. In the presence of frequent recurrences, several treatment strategies exist, but the use of antibiotics for 1 week per month, whether or not symptoms are present, is often most effective.

Unfortunately, therapy for bacterial overgrowth syndrome is largely empirical, with an absence of clinical trials on which to base decisions regarding the antibiotic choice, the duration of treatment, and/or the best approach for treating recurrences. Bacterial overgrowth may also occur as a component of another chronic disease, e.g., Crohn's disease, radiation enteritis, or short bowel syndrome. Treatment of the bacterial overgrowth in these settings will not cure the underlying problem but may be very important in ameliorating a subset of clinical problems that are related to bacterial overgrowth.

WHIPPLE'S DISEASE

Whipple's disease is a chronic multisystem disease associated with diarrhea, steatorrhea, weight loss, arthralgia, and central nervous system (CNS) and cardiac problems; it is caused by the bacteria *Tropheryma whipplei*. Until the identification of *T. whipplei* by polymerase chain reaction, the hallmark of Whipple's disease had been the presence of PAS-positive macrophages in the small intestine (Fig. 15-4*E*) and other organs with evidence of disease.

Etiology

Whipple's disease is caused by a small gram-positive bacillus, *T. whipplei*. The bacillus, an actinobacterium, has low virulence but high infectivity, and relatively minimal symptoms are observed compared to the extent of the bacilli in multiple tissues.

Clinical Presentation

The onset of Whipple's disease is insidious and is characterized by diarrhea, steatorrhea, abdominal pain, weight loss, migratory large-joint arthropathy, and fever as well as ophthalmologic and CNS symptoms. The development of dementia is a relatively late symptom and an extremely poor prognostic sign, especially in patients who relapse following the induction of a remission with antibiotics. For unexplained reasons, the disease occurs primarily in middle-aged Caucasian men. The steatorrhea in these patients is generally believed secondary to both small-intestinal mucosal injury and lymphatic obstruction secondary to the increased number of PAS-positive macrophages in the lamina propria of the small intestine.

Diagnosis

The diagnosis of Whipple's disease is suggested by a multisystem disease in a patient with diarrhea and steatorrhea. Obtaining tissue biopsies from the small intestine and/or other organs that may be involved (e.g., liver, lymph nodes, heart, eyes, CNS, or synovial membranes), based on the patient's symptoms, is the primary approach to establish the diagnosis of Whipple's disease. The presence of PAS-positive macrophages containing the characteristic small (0.25 × 1–2 mm) bacilli is suggestive of this diagnosis. However, Whipple's disease can be confused with the PAS-positive macrophages containing *M. avium* complex, which may be a cause of diarrhea in AIDS. The presence of the *T. whipplei* bacillus outside of macrophages is a more important indicator of active disease than is their presence within the macrophages. *T. whipplei* has now been successfully grown in culture.

Rx Treatment:
WHIPPLE'S DISEASE

The treatment for Whipple's disease is prolonged use of antibiotics. The current drug of choice is double-strength trimethoprim/sulfamethoxazole for approximately 1 year. PAS-positive macrophages can persist following successful treatment, and the presence of bacilli outside of macrophages is indicative of persistent infection or an early sign of recurrence. Recurrence of disease activity, especially with dementia, is an extremely poor prognostic sign and requires an antibiotic that crosses the blood-brain barrier. If trimethoprim/sulfamethoxazole is not tolerated, chloramphenicol is an appropriate second choice.

PROTEIN-LOSING ENTEROPATHY

Protein-losing enteropathy is not a specific disease but rather a group of gastrointestinal and nongastrointestinal disorders with hypoproteinemia and edema in the absence of either proteinuria or defects in protein synthesis, e.g., chronic liver disease. These diseases are characterized by excess protein loss into the gastrointestinal tract. Normally, about 10% of total protein catabolism occurs via the gastrointestinal tract. Evidence of increased protein loss into the gastrointestinal tract occurs in more than 65 different diseases, which can be classified into three groups: (1) mucosal ulceration, such that the protein loss primarily represents exudation across damaged mucosa, e.g., ulcerative colitis, gastrointestinal carcinomas, and peptic ulcer; (2) nonulcerated mucosa, but with evidence of mucosal damage so that the protein loss represents loss across epithelia with altered permeability, e.g., celiac sprue and Ménétrier's disease in the small intestine and stomach, respectively; and (3) lymphatic dysfunction, representing either primary lymphatic disease or secondary to partial lymphatic obstruction that may occur as a result of enlarged lymph nodes or cardiac disease.

Diagnosis

The diagnosis of protein-losing enteropathy is suggested by the presence of peripheral edema and low serum albumin and globulin levels in the absence of renal and hepatic disease. It is extremely rare for an individual with protein-losing enteropathy to have selective loss of *only* albumin or *only* globulins. Therefore, marked reduction of serum albumin with normal serum globulins should not initiate an evaluation for protein-losing enteropathy but should suggest the presence of renal and/or hepatic disease. Likewise, reduced serum globulins with normal serum albumin levels are more likely a result of reduced globulin synthesis rather than enhanced globulin loss into the intestine. Documentation of an increase in protein loss into the gastrointestinal tract has been established by the administration of one of several radiolabeled proteins and its quantitation in stool during a 24- or 48-h period. Unfortunately, none of these radiolabeled proteins is available for routine clinical use. α_1-Antitrypsin, a protein that accounts for ~4% of total serum proteins and is resistant to proteolysis, can be used to document enhanced rates of serum protein loss into the intestinal tract but cannot be used to assess gastric protein loss due to its degradation in an acid milieu. α_1-Antitrypsin clearance is measured by determining stool volume and both stool and plasma α_1-antitrypsin concentrations. In addition to the loss of protein via abnormal and distended lymphatics, peripheral lymphocytes may also be lost via lymphatics, resulting in a relative lymphopenia. Thus, the presence of lymphopenia in a patient with hypoproteinemia supports the presence of increased loss of protein into the gastrointestinal tract.

Patients with increased protein loss into the gastrointestinal tract from lymphatic obstruction often have steatorrhea and diarrhea. The steatorrhea is a result of altered lymphatic flow as lipid-containing chylomicrons exit from intestinal epithelial cells via intestinal lymphatics (Table 15-4; Fig. 15-4). In the absence of mechanical or anatomic lymphatic obstruction, intrinsic intestinal lymphatic dysfunction, with or without lymphatic dysfunction in the peripheral extremities, has been named *intestinal lymphangiectasia*. Similarly, about 50% of individuals with intrinsic peripheral lymphatic disease (Milroy disease) will also have intestinal lymphangiectasia and hypoproteinemia. Other than steatorrhea and enhanced protein loss into the gastrointestinal tract, all other aspects of intestinal absorptive function are normal in intestinal lymphangiectasia.

Other Causes

Patients who appear to have idiopathic protein-losing enteropathy without any evidence of gastrointestinal disease should be examined for cardiac disease—especially right-sided valvular disease and chronic pericarditis. On occasion, hypoproteinemia can be the only presentation for these two types of heart disease. Ménétrier's disease (also called *hypertrophic gastropathy*) is an uncommon entity that involves the body and fundus of the stomach

TABLE 15-9

CLASSIFICATION OF MALABSORPTION SYNDROMES

Inadequate digestion
  Postgastrectomy[a]
  Deficiency or inactivation of pancreatic lipase
    Exocrine pancreatic insufficiency
      Chronic pancreatitis
      Pancreatic carcinoma
      Cystic fibrosis
      Pancreatic insufficiency—congenital or acquired
    Gastrinoma—acid inactivation of lipase[a]
    Drugs—orlistat
Reduced intraduodenal bile acid concentration/impaired micelle formation
  Liver disease
    Parenchymal liver disease
    Cholestatic liver disease
  Bacterial overgrowth in small intestine:
    Anatomic stasis   Functional stasis
      Afferent loop stasis/blind   Diabetes[a]
      loop/strictures/fistulae   Scleroderma[a]
                                   Intestinal
                                     pseudoobstruction
  Interrupted enterohepatic circulation of bile salts
    Ileal resection
    Crohn's disease[a]
  Drugs (bind or precipitate bile salts)—neomycin, cholestyramine, calcium carbonate
Impaired mucosal absorption/mucosal loss or defect
  Intestinal resection or bypass[a]
  Inflammation, infiltration, or infection:
    Crohn's disease[a]   Celiac sprue
    Amyloidosis   Collagenous sprue
    Scleroderma[a]   Whipple's disease[a]
    Lymphoma[a]   Radiation enteritis[a]
    Eosinophilic enteritis   Folate and vitamin B_{12}
                                  deficiency
    Mastocytosis   Infections—giardiasis
    Tropical sprue   Graft-versus-host
                                 disease
  Genetic disorders
    Disaccharidase deficiency
    Agammaglobulinemia
    Abetalipoproteinemia
    Hartnup disease
    Cystinuria
  Impaired nutrient delivery to and/or from intestine:
    Lymphatic obstruction   Circulatory disorders
    Lymphoma[a]   Congestive heart failure
    Lymphangiectasia   Constrictive pericarditis
                                 Mesenteric artery
                                   atherosclerosis
                                 Vasculitis
  Endocrine and metabolic disorders
    Diabetes[a]
    Hypoparathyroidism
    Adrenal insufficiency
    Hyperthyroidism
    Carcinoid syndrome

[a]Malabsorption caused by more than one mechanism.

and is characterized by large gastric folds, reduced gastric acid secretion, and, at times, enhanced protein loss into the stomach.

℞ Treatment:
PROTEIN-LOSING ENTEROPATHY

As excess protein loss into the gastrointestinal tract is most often secondary to a specific disease, treatment should be directed primarily to the underlying disease process and not to the hypoproteinemia. For example, if significant hypoproteinemia with resulting peripheral edema is secondary to either celiac sprue or ulcerative colitis, a gluten-free diet or mesalamine, respectively, would be the initial therapy. When enhanced protein loss is secondary to lymphatic obstruction, it is critical to establish the nature of this obstruction. Identification of mesenteric

TABLE 15-10

PATHOPHYSIOLOGY OF CLINICAL MANIFESTATIONS OF MALABSORPTION DISORDERS

SYMPTOM OR SIGN	MECHANISM
Weight loss/malnutrition	Anorexia, malabsorption of nutrients
Diarrhea	Impaired absorption or secretion of water and electrolytes; colonic fluid secretion secondary to unabsorbed dihydroxy bile acids and fatty acids
Flatus	Bacterial fermentation of unabsorbed carbohydrate
Glossitis, cheilosis, stomatitis	Deficiency of iron, vitamin B_{12}, folate, and vitamin A
Abdominal pain	Bowel distention or inflammation, pancreatitis
Bone pain	Calcium, vitamin D malabsorption, protein deficiency, osteoporosis
Tetany, paresthesia	Calcium and magnesium malabsorption
Weakness	Anemia, electrolyte depletion (particularly K^+)
Azotemia, hypotension	Fluid and electrolyte depletion
Amenorrhea, decreased libido	Protein depletion, decreased calories, secondary hypopituitarism
Anemia	Impaired absorption of iron, folate, vitamin B_{12}
Bleeding	Vitamin K malabsorption, hypoprothrombinemia
Night blindness/ xerophthalmia	Vitamin A malabsorption
Peripheral neuropathy	Vitamin B_{12} and thiamine deficiency
Dermatitis	Deficiency of vitamin A, zinc, and essential fatty acid

nodes or lymphoma may be possible by imaging studies. Similarly, it is important to exclude cardiac disease as a cause of protein-losing enteropathy either by echosonography or, on occasion, by a right-heart catheterization.

The increased protein loss that occurs in intestinal lymphangiectasia is a result of distended lymphatics associated with lipid malabsorption. Treatment of the hypoproteinemia is accomplished by a low-fat diet and the administration of MCTs (Table 15-3), which do not exit from the intestinal epithelial cells via lymphatics but are delivered to the body via the portal vein.

SUMMARY

A pathophysiologic classification of the many conditions that can produce malabsorption is given in Table 15-9. A summary of the pathophysiology of the various clinical manifestations of malabsorption is given in Table 15-10.

FURTHER READINGS

AMERICAN GASTROENTEROLOGICAL ASSOCIATION: AGA technical review on the evaluation and management of chronic diarrhea. Gastroenterology 116:1464, 1999

BUCHMAN AL: Etiology and initial management of short bowel syndrome. Gastroenterology 130:S5, 2006

COOK SI, SELLIN JH: Short chain fatty acids in health and disease. Aliment Pharmacol Ther 12:499, 1998

FENOLLER F et al: Whipple's disease. N Engl J Med 356:55, 2007

FORD AC et al: Yield of diagnostic tests for celiac disease in individuals with symptoms suggestive of irritable bowel syndrome: systematic review and meta-analysis. Arch Intern Med 169:651, 2009

GASBARRINI G et al: Celiac disease in the 21st century: issues of under- and over-diagnosis. Int J Immunpathol Pharmacol 22:1, 2009

GREENBERGER NJ: Enzymatic therapy in patients with chronic pancreatitis. Gastroenterol Clin North Am 28:687, 1999

Hunt KA van Heel DA. Recent advances in celiac disease genetics. Gut 58:473, 2009

JAMES S: Celiac disease: Proceedings of the NIH Consensus Conference on Celiac Disease. Gastroenterology 128:S1, 2005

HAREWOOD GC, MURRAY JA: Approaching the patient with chronic malabsorption syndrome. Semin Gastrointest Dis 10: 138, 1999

KAGNOFF MF: Celiac disease: pathogenesis of a model immunogenetic disease. J Clin Invest 117:41, 2007

SHAW AD, DAVIES GJ: Lactose intolerance: Problems in diagnosis and treatment. J Clin Gastroenterol 28:208, 1999

VERDU EF: Between celiac disease and irritable bowel syndrome: the "no man's land" of gluten sensitivity. Am J Gastroenterol 104:1587, 2009

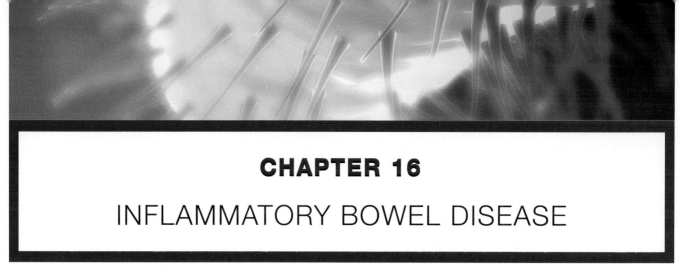

CHAPTER 16

INFLAMMATORY BOWEL DISEASE

Sonia Friedman ■ Richard S. Blumberg

Inflammatory bowel disease (IBD) is an immune-mediated chronic intestinal condition. Ulcerative colitis (UC) and Crohn's disease (CD) are the two major types of IBD.

EPIDEMIOLOGY

The incidence of IBD varies within different geographic areas. CD and UC both occur at the highest incidence in Europe, the United Kingdom, and North America. In North America, incidence rates range from 2.2 to 14.3 cases per 100,000 person-years for UC and from 3.1 to 14.6 cases per 100,000 person-years for CD (Table 16-1). Prevalence ranges from 37 to 246 cases per 100,000 person-years for UC and from 26 to 199 cases per 100,000 person-years for CD. In Europe, incidence ranges from 1.5 to 20.3 cases per 100,000 person-years for UC and from 0.7 to 9.8 cases for CD; prevalence ranges from 21.4 to 243 cases for UC and from 8.3 to 214 cases per 100,000 person-years for CD. IBD has been rare in other areas except Israel,

Australia, and South Africa. The incidence of IBD, especially UC, is rising in Japan, South Korea, Singapore, northern India, and Latin America, areas previously thought to have low incidence. The highest mortality is during the first years of disease and in long-duration disease due to the risk of colon cancer. In a Swedish population study, the standardized mortality ratios for CD and UC were 1.51 and 1.37, respectively.

The peak age of onset of UC and CD is between 15 and 30 years. A second peak occurs between the ages of 60 and 80. The male to female ratio for UC is 1:1 and for CD is 1.1–1.8:1. UC and CD have two- to fourfold increased frequency in Jewish populations in the United States, Europe, and South Africa. Furthermore, disease frequency differs within the Jewish populations. The prevalence of IBD in Ashkenazi Jews is about twice that of Israeli-born, Sephardic, or Oriental Jews. The prevalence decreases progressively in non-Jewish Caucasian, African-American, Hispanic, and Asian populations. Urban areas have a higher prevalence of IBD than rural

TABLE 16-1

EPIDEMIOLOGY OF IBD

	ULCERATIVE COLITIS	CROHN'S DISEASE
Incidence (North America) per person-years	2.2–14.3/100,000	3.1–14.6/100,000
Age of onset	15–30 & 60–80	15–30 & 60–80
Ethnicity	Jewish > Non-Jewish Caucasian > African American > Hispanic > Asian	
Male:female ratio	1:1	1.1–1.8:1
Smoking	May prevent disease	May cause disease
Oral contraceptives	No increased risk	Odds ratio 1.4
Appendectomy	Protective	Not protective
Monozygotic twins	6% concordance	58% concordance
Dizygotic twins	0% concordance	4% concordance

areas, and high socioeconomic classes have a higher prevalence than lower socioeconomic classes.

The effects of cigarette smoking are different in UC and CD. The risk of UC in smokers is 40% that of non-smokers. Additionally, former smokers have a 1.7-fold increased risk for UC than people who have never smoked. In contrast, smoking is associated with a twofold increased risk of CD. Oral contraceptives are also linked to CD; the odds ratio of CD for oral contraceptive users is about 1.4. Appendectomy is protective against UC but increases the risk of CD.

IBD runs in families. If a patient has IBD, the lifetime risk that a first-degree relative will be affected is ~10%. If two parents have IBD, each child has a 36% chance of being affected. In twin studies, 58% of monozygotic twins are concordant for CD and 6% are concordant for UC, whereas 4% of dizygotic twins are concordant for CD and none are concordant for UC. The risks of developing IBD are higher in first-degree relatives of Jewish versus non-Jewish patients: 7.8% versus 5.2% for CD and 4.5% versus 1.6% for UC. Anatomic site and clinical type of CD is also concordant within families.

Additional evidence for genetic predisposition to IBD comes from its association with certain genetic syndromes. UC and CD are both associated with Turner's syndrome, and Hermansky-Pudlak syndrome is associated with granulomatous colitis. Glycogen storage disease type 1b can present with Crohn's-like lesions of the large and small bowel. Other immunodeficiency disorders, such as hypogammaglobulinemia, selective IgA deficiency, and hereditary angioedema, also exhibit an increased association with IBD.

ETIOLOGY AND PATHOGENESIS

A consensus hypothesis is that in genetically predisposed individuals, both exogenous factors (e.g., normal luminal flora) and host factors (e.g., intestinal epithelial cell barrier function, innate and adaptive immune function) cause a chronic state of dysregulated mucosal immune function that is further modified by specific environmental factors (e.g., smoking). Although chronic activation of the mucosal immune system may represent an appropriate response to an unidentified infectious agent, a search for such an agent has thus far been unrewarding. As such, IBD is currently considered an inappropriate response to the endogenous microbial flora within the intestine, with or without some component of autoimmunity. Importantly, the normal intestine contains a large number of immune cells in a chronic state of so-called physiologic inflammation, in which the gut is poised for, but actively restrained from, full immunologic responses. During the course of infections in the normal host, full activation of the gut-associated lymphoid tissue occurs but is rapidly superseded by dampening the immune response and tissue repair. In IBD this process may not be regulated normally.

GENETIC CONSIDERATIONS

IBD is a polygenic disorder that gives rise to multiple clinical subgroups within UC and CD. Genome-wide searches have shown disease-associated loci on many chromosomes (Table 16-2). Some loci are associated with both UC and CD, suggesting some overlap in pathogenesis. Specific gene associations are mostly undefined; however, several predisposing genes have been identified (Table 16-2). *CARD15* (caspase-associated recruitment domain containing protein 15) on chromosome 16 is a cytosolic molecule that senses bacterial muramyl dipeptide and regulates intracellular signaling. CARD15 protein is expressed by intestinal epithelial cells, including Paneth cells, monocytes, macrophages, and dendritic cells. Loss-of-function mutations in CARD15 are highly associated with CD and

176

TABLE 16-2

REPLICATED GENETIC LOCI IN IBD

IBD LOCUS[a]	CHROMOSOME	GENE[b]	PHENOTYPE
IBD1	16q	CARD15	CD
IBD2	12p	—	CD,UC
IBD3	6p	MHC?	CD
IBD4	14q	—	CD
IBD5	5q	OCTN?	CD
IBD6	19p	—	CD,UC
IBD7	1p	—	CD,UC
IBD8	16p	—	CD
IBD9	3p	—	CD
—	10q	DLG5	CD
—	1p	IL-23R	CD,UC
—	2q	ATG16L1	CD
—	5p	PTGER4	CD

[a]Taken from National Center for Biotechnology Information, Online Mendelian Inheritance in Man, *http://www.ncbi.nlm.nih.gov/entrez/query.fcgi?db=OMIM.*

[b]CARD15, caspase-associated recruitment domain containing protein 15; MHC, major histocompatibility complex; DLG5, Drosophila Discs Large Homolog 5; OCTN, novel organic cation transporter protein; IL-23R, Interleukin-23 receptor; ATG16L1, autophagy-related 16-like 1 gene; PTGER4, prostaglandin receptor EP4.

Source: Adapted from S Vermeire, P Rutgeerts: Genes Immun 6:637, 2005.

may account for up to 10% of CD risk. CD-associated CARD15 alleles either allow excess NF-κB activation or decreased intestinal antimicrobial activity by diminishing defensin production by Paneth cells. Homozygosity for these mutant alleles confers up to a fortyfold increased risk for fibrostenosing CD, especially in the ileum.

IBD has also been associated with polymorphisms in DLG5 and the IL-23 receptor. These studies show the importance of both innate and adaptive immunity and the involvement of many different cell types, including the intestinal epithelium and lymphocytes, in IBD. Indeed, patients with IBD and their first-degree relatives may exhibit diminished intestinal epithelial cell barrier function.

DEFECTIVE IMMUNE REGULATION IN IBD

The mucosal immune system is normally unreactive to luminal contents due to oral tolerance. When soluble antigens are administered orally rather than subcutaneously or intramuscularly, antigen-specific nonresponsiveness is induced. Multiple mechanisms are involved in the induction of oral tolerance and include deletion or anergy of antigen-reactive T cells or activation of CD4+ T cells that suppress gut inflammation through secretion of inhibitory cytokines, such as interleukin (IL) 10 and transforming growth factor β (TGF-β). Oral tolerance may be responsible for the lack of immune responsiveness to dietary antigens and the commensal flora in the

intestinal lumen. In IBD this suppression of inflammation is altered, leading to uncontrolled inflammation. The mechanisms of this regulated immune suppression are incompletely known.

Gene knockout (−/−) or transgenic (Tg) mouse models of colitis have revealed that deleting specific cytokines (e.g., IL-2, IL-10, TGF-β) or their receptors, deleting molecules associated with T cell antigen recognition (e.g., T cell antigen receptors) or interfering with intestinal epithelial cell barrier function (e.g., deleting N-cadherin, mucus glycoprotein or NF-κB) leads to colitis or enteritis. Thus, a variety of specific alterations can lead to immune activation and inflammation directed at the colon in mice. How these relate to human IBD remains to be defined.

In both UC and CD, an inflammatory pathway emerges from the genetic predisposition in which activated CD4+ T cells in the lamina propria secrete inflammatory cytokines. Some activate other inflammatory cells (macrophages and B cells) and others act indirectly to recruit other lymphocytes, inflammatory leukocytes, and mononuclear cells from the bloodstream into the gut through interactions between homing receptors on leukocytes (e.g., α4β7 integrin) and addressins on vascular endothelium (e.g., MadCAM1). CD4+ T cells are of three major types, all of which may be associated with colitis in animal models and humans: T_H1 cells [interferon (IFN) γ], T_H2 cells (IL-4, IL-5, IL-13), and T_H17 cells (IL-17). T_H1 cells induce transmural granulomatous inflammation that resembles CD, T_H2 cells and related natural killer T cells that secrete IL-13 induce superficial mucosal inflammation resembling UC, and T_H17 cells may be responsible for neutrophilic recruitment. The T_H1 cytokine pathway is initiated by IL-12, a key cytokine in the pathogenesis of experimental models of mucosal inflammation. IL-4 and IL-23, together with IL-6 and TGF-β, induce T_H2 and T_H17 cells, respectively. Activated macrophages secrete tumor necrosis factor (TNF). Thus, use of antibodies to block proinflammatory cytokines (e.g., anti-TNF, anti-IL-12, anti-IL-23, anti-IL-6, anti-IFN-γ) or molecules associated with leukocyte recruitment (e.g., anti-α4β7) or use of cytokines that inhibit inflammation and promote regulatory T cells (e.g., IL-10) or promote intestinal barrier function (e.g., granulocyte-macrophage colony-stimulating factor) may be beneficial to humans with colitis.

THE INFLAMMATORY CASCADE IN IBD

Once initiated in IBD, the immune inflammatory response is perpetuated by T-cell activation. A sequential cascade of inflammatory mediators extends the response; each step is a potential target for therapy. Inflammatory cytokines, such as IL-1, IL-6, and TNF, have diverse effects on tissues. They promote fibrogenesis, collagen production, activation of tissue metalloproteinases, and

SECTION III Disorders of the Alimentary Tract

the production of other inflammatory mediators; they also activate the coagulation cascade in local blood vessels (e.g., increased production of von Willebrand's factor). These cytokines are normally produced in response to infection but are usually turned off or inhibited at the appropriate time to limit tissue damage. In IBD their activity is not regulated, resulting in an imbalance between the proinflammatory and anti-inflammatory mediators. Therapies such as the 5-ASA (5-aminosalicylic acid) compounds are potent inhibitors of these inflammatory mediators through inhibition of transcription factors such as NF-κB that regulate their expression.

EXOGENOUS FACTORS

IBD may have an as yet undefined infectious etiology. Observational studies suggest that multiple pathogens (e.g., *Salmonella* sp., *Shigella* sp., *Campylobacter* sp., *Clostridium difficile*) may initiate IBD by triggering an inflammatory response that the mucosal immune system may fail to control. However, in an IBD patient, the normal flora is likely perceived as if it were a pathogen. Anaerobic organisms, particularly *Bacteroides* and *Clostridia* species, and some aerobic species such as *Escherichia*, may be responsible for the induction of inflammation. This notion is supported by the immune response in patients with CD to bacterial antigens such as I2, OmpC, and flagellin. In addition, agents that alter the intestinal flora, such as metronidazole, ciprofloxacin, and elemental diets, may improve CD. CD also responds to fecal diversion, demonstrating the ability of luminal contents to exacerbate disease. On the other hand, other organisms, so-called probiotics (e.g., *Lactobacillus* sp., *Bifidobacterium* sp., *Taenia suis*, and *Saccharomyces boulardii*), may inhibit inflammation in animal models and humans.

Psychosocial factors can contribute to worsening of symptoms. Major life events such as illness or death in the family, divorce or separation, interpersonal conflict, or other major loss are associated with an increase in IBD symptoms such as pain, bowel dysfunction, and bleeding. Acute daily stress can worsen bowel symptoms even after controlling for major life events. When the sickness-impact profile, a measurement of overall psychological and physical functioning, is used, IBD patients have functional impairment greater than that of a normal population but less than that of patients with chronic back pain or amyotrophic lateral sclerosis.

PATHOLOGY

ULCERATIVE COLITIS: MACROSCOPIC FEATURES

UC is a mucosal disease that usually involves the rectum and extends proximally to involve all or part of the colon. About 40–50% of patients have disease limited to the rectum and rectosigmoid, 30–40% have disease extending beyond the sigmoid but not involving the whole colon, and 20% have a total colitis. Proximal spread occurs in continuity without areas of uninvolved mucosa. When the whole colon is involved, the inflammation extends 1–2 cm into the terminal ileum in 10–20% of patients. This is called *backwash ileitis* and is of little clinical significance. Although variations in macroscopic activity may suggest skip areas, biopsies from normal-appearing mucosa are usually abnormal. Thus, it is important to obtain multiple biopsies from apparently uninvolved mucosa, whether proximal or distal, during endoscopy.

With mild inflammation, the mucosa is erythematous and has a fine granular surface that looks like sandpaper. In more severe disease, the mucosa is hemorrhagic, edematous, and ulcerated (Fig. 16-1). In long-standing disease, inflammatory polyps (pseudopolyps) may be present as a result of epithelial regeneration. The mucosa may appear normal in remission, but in patients with many years of disease it appears atrophic and featureless and the entire colon becomes narrowed and shortened. Patients with fulminant disease can develop a toxic colitis or megacolon where the bowel wall thins and the mucosa is severely ulcerated; this may lead to perforation.

ULCERATIVE COLITIS: MICROSCOPIC FEATURES

Histologic findings correlate well with the endoscopic appearance and clinical course of UC. The process is limited to the mucosa and superficial submucosa, with deeper layers unaffected except in fulminant disease. In UC, two major histologic features suggest chronicity

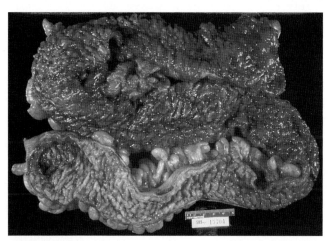

FIGURE 16-1

Pan-ulcerative colitis. Mucosa has a lumpy, bumpy appearance because of areas of inflamed but intact mucosa separated by ulcerated areas. *(Courtesy of Dr. KE Rosado and Dr. CA Parkos, Division of Gastrointestinal Pathology, Department of Pathology, Emory University, Atlanta, Georgia; with permission.)*

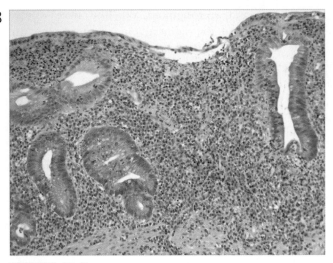

FIGURE 16-2

Medium power view of colonic mucosa in ulcerative colitis showing diffuse mixed inflammation, basal lymphoplasmacytosis, crypt atrophy and irregularity and superficial erosion. These features are typical of chronic active ulcerative colitis. *(Courtesy of Dr. R Odze, Division of Gastrointestinal Pathology, Department of Pathology, Brigham and Women's Hospital, Boston, Massachusetts; with permission.)*

and help distinguish it from infectious or acute self-limited colitis. First, the crypt architecture of the colon is distorted; crypts may be bifid and reduced in number, often with a gap between the crypt bases and the muscularis mucosae. Second, some patients have basal plasma cells and multiple basal lymphoid aggregates. Mucosal vascular congestion, with edema and focal hemorrhage, and an inflammatory cell infiltrate of neutrophils, lymphocytes, plasma cells, and macrophages may be present. The neutrophils invade the epithelium, usually in the crypts, giving rise to cryptitis and, ultimately, to crypt abscesses (**Fig. 16-2**).

CROHN'S DISEASE: MACROSCOPIC FEATURES

CD can affect any part of the gastrointestinal tract from the mouth to the anus. Some 30–40% of patients have small-bowel disease alone, 40–55% have disease involving both the small and large intestines, and 15–25% have colitis alone. In the 75% of patients with small-intestinal disease, the terminal ileum is involved in 90%. Unlike UC, which almost always involves the rectum, the rectum is often spared in CD. CD is segmental with skip areas in the midst of diseased intestine (**Fig. 16-3**). Perirectal fistulas, fissures, abscesses, and anal stenosis are present in one-third of patients with CD, particularly those with colonic involvement. Rarely, CD may also involve the liver and the pancreas.

Unlike UC, CD is a transmural process. Endoscopically, aphthous or small superficial ulcerations characterize mild disease; in more active disease, stellate ulcerations

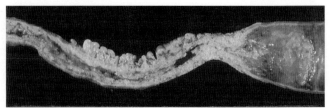

FIGURE 16-3

Portion of colon with stricture in patient with CD. *(Courtesy of Dr. KE Rosado and Dr. CA Parkos, Division of Gastrointestinal Pathology, Department of Pathology, Emory University, Atlanta, Georgia; with permission.)*

fuse longitudinally and transversely to demarcate islands of mucosa that frequently are histologically normal. This "cobblestone" appearance is characteristic of CD, both endoscopically and by barium radiography. As in UC, pseudopolyps can form in CD.

Active CD is characterized by focal inflammation and formation of fistula tracts, which resolve by fibrosis and stricturing of the bowel. The bowel wall thickens and becomes narrowed and fibrotic, leading to chronic, recurrent bowel obstructions. Projections of thickened mesentery encase the bowel ("creeping fat"), and serosal and mesenteric inflammation promotes adhesions and fistula formation.

CROHN'S DISEASE: MICROSCOPIC FEATURES

The earliest lesions are aphthoid ulcerations and focal crypt abscesses with loose aggregations of macrophages, which form noncaseating granulomas in all layers of the bowel wall (**Fig. 16-4**). Granulomas can be seen in

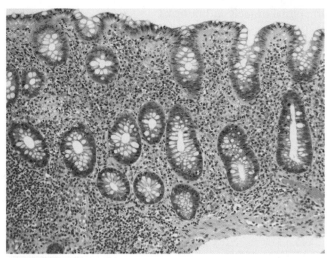

FIGURE 16-4

Medium power view of Crohn's colitis showing mixed acute and chronic inflammation, crypt atrophy, and multiple small epithelioid granulomas in the mucosa. *(Courtesy of Dr. R Odze, Division of Gastrointestinal Pathology, Department of Pathology, Brigham and Women's Hospital, Boston, Massachusetts; with permission.)*

lymph nodes, mesentery, peritoneum, liver, and pancreas. Although granulomas are a pathognomonic feature of CD, they are rarely found on mucosal biopsies. Surgical resection reveals granulomas in about half of cases. Other histologic features of CD include submucosal or subserosal lymphoid aggregates, particularly away from areas of ulceration, gross and microscopic skip areas, and transmural inflammation that is accompanied by fissures that penetrate deeply into the bowel wall and sometimes form fistulous tracts or local abscesses.

CLINICAL PRESENTATION

ULCERATIVE COLITIS

Signs and Symptoms

The major symptoms of UC are diarrhea, rectal bleeding, tenesmus, passage of mucus, and crampy abdominal pain. The severity of symptoms correlates with the extent of disease. Although UC can present acutely, symptoms usually have been present for weeks to months. Occasionally, diarrhea and bleeding are so intermittent and mild that the patient does not seek medical attention.

Patients with proctitis usually pass fresh blood or blood-stained mucus, either mixed with stool or streaked onto the surface of a normal or hard stool. They also have tenesmus, or urgency with a feeling of incomplete evacuation, but rarely have abdominal pain. With proctitis or proctosigmoiditis, proximal transit slows, which may account for the constipation commonly seen in patients with distal disease.

When the disease extends beyond the rectum, blood is usually mixed with stool or grossly bloody diarrhea may be noted. Colonic motility is altered by inflammation with rapid transit through the inflamed intestine. When the disease is severe, patients pass a liquid stool containing blood, pus, and fecal matter. Diarrhea is often nocturnal and/or postprandial. Although severe pain is

not a prominent symptom, some patients with active disease may experience vague lower abdominal discomfort or mild central abdominal cramping. Severe cramping and abdominal pain can occur with severe attacks of the disease. Other symptoms in moderate to severe disease include anorexia, nausea, vomiting, fever, and weight loss.

Physical signs of proctitis include a tender anal canal and blood on rectal examination. With more extensive disease, patients have tenderness to palpation directly over the colon. Patients with a toxic colitis have severe pain and bleeding, and those with megacolon have hepatic tympany. Both may have signs of peritonitis if a perforation has occurred. The classification of disease activity is shown in Table 16-3.

Laboratory, Endoscopic, and Radiographic Features

Active disease can be associated with a rise in acute-phase reactants [C-reactive protein (CRP)], platelet count, and erythrocyte sedimentation rate (ESR), and a decrease in hemoglobin. Fecal calprotectin levels correlate well with histologic inflammation, predict relapses, and detect pouchitis. In severely ill patients, the serum albumin level will fall rather quickly. Leukocytosis may be present but is not a specific indicator of disease activity. Proctitis or proctosigmoiditis rarely causes a rise in CRP. Diagnosis relies upon the patient's history; clinical symptoms; negative stool examination for bacteria, *C. difficile* toxin, and ova and parasites; sigmoidoscopic appearance (see Fig. 12-4*A*); and histology of rectal or colonic biopsy specimens.

Sigmoidoscopy is used to assess disease activity and is often performed before treatment. If the patient is not having an acute flare, colonoscopy is used to assess disease extent and activity. Histologic features change more slowly than clinical features but can also be used to grade disease activity.

TABLE 16-3

ULCERATIVE COLITIS: DISEASE PRESENTATION

	MILD	MODERATE	SEVERE
Bowel movements	<4 per day	4–6 per day	>6 per day
Blood in stool	Small	Moderate	Severe
Fever	None	<37.5°C mean	>37.5°C mean
Tachycardia	None	<90 mean pulse	>90 mean pulse
Anemia	Mild	>75%	≤75%
Sedimentation rate	<30 mm		>30 mm
Endoscopic appearance	Erythema, decreased vascular pattern, fine granularity	Marked erythema, coarse granularity, absent vascular markings, contact bleeding, no ulcerations	Spontaneous bleeding, ulcerations

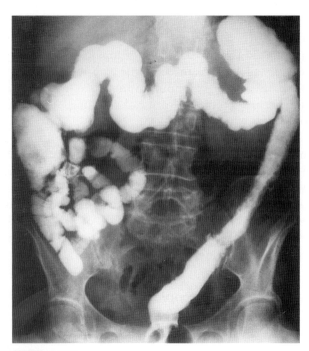

FIGURE 16-5
Barium enema in a patient with acute ulcerative colitis: inflammation of the entire colon. *(Courtesy of Dr. JM Braver, Gastrointestinal Radiology, Department of Radiology, Brigham and Women's Hospital, Boston, Massachusetts; with permission.)*

The earliest radiologic change of UC seen on single-contrast barium enema is a fine mucosal granularity (**Fig. 16-5**). With increasing severity, the mucosa becomes thickened, and superficial ulcers are seen. Deep ulcerations can appear as "collar-button" ulcers, which indicate that the ulceration has penetrated the mucosa. Haustral folds may be normal in mild disease, but as activity progresses they become edematous and thickened. Loss of haustration can occur, especially in patients with long-standing disease. In addition, the colon becomes shortened and narrowed. Polyps in the colon may be postinflammatory polyps or pseudopolyps, adenomatous polyps, or carcinoma.

CT scanning is not as helpful as endoscopy and barium enema in making the diagnosis of UC, but typical findings include mild mural thickening (<1.5 cm), inhomogeneous wall density, absence of small-bowel thickening, increased perirectal and presacral fat, target appearance of the rectum, and adenopathy.

Complications

Only 15% of patients with UC present initially with catastrophic illness. Massive hemorrhage occurs with severe attacks of disease in 1% of patients, and treatment for the disease usually stops the bleeding. However, if a patient requires 6–8 units of blood within 24–48 h, colectomy is indicated. *Toxic megacolon* is defined as a transverse colon with a diameter of >5–6 cm, with loss of haustration in patients with severe attacks of UC. It occurs in about 5% of attacks and can be triggered by electrolyte abnormalities and narcotics. About 50% of acute dilations will resolve with medical therapy alone, but urgent colectomy is required for those that do not improve. Perforation is the most dangerous of the local complications, and the physical signs of peritonitis may not be obvious, especially if the patient is receiving glucocorticoids. Although perforation is rare, the mortality rate for perforation complicating a toxic megacolon is about 15%. In addition, patients can develop a toxic colitis and such severe ulcerations that the bowel may perforate without first dilating.

Strictures occur in 5–10% of patients and are always a concern in UC because of the possibility of underlying neoplasia. Although benign strictures can form from the inflammation and fibrosis of UC, strictures that are impassable with the colonoscope should be presumed malignant until proven otherwise. A stricture that prevents passage of the colonoscope is an indication for surgery. UC patients occasionally develop anal fissures, perianal abscesses, or hemorrhoids, but the occurrence of extensive perianal lesions should suggest CD.

CROHN'S DISEASE

Signs and Symptoms

Although CD usually presents as acute or chronic bowel inflammation, the inflammatory process evolves toward one of two patterns of disease: a fibrostenotic-obstructing pattern or a penetrating-fistulous pattern, each with different treatments and prognoses. The site of disease influences the clinical manifestations.

◼ Ileocolitis

Because the most common site of inflammation is the terminal ileum, the usual presentation of ileocolitis is a chronic history of recurrent episodes of right lower quadrant pain and diarrhea. Sometimes the initial presentation mimics acute appendicitis with pronounced right lower quadrant pain, a palpable mass, fever, and leukocytosis. Pain is usually colicky; it precedes and is relieved by defecation. A low-grade fever is usually noted. High-spiking fever suggests intraabdominal abscess formation. Weight loss is common—typically 10–20% of body weight—and develops as a consequence of diarrhea, anorexia, and fear of eating.

An inflammatory mass may be palpated in the right lower quadrant of the abdomen. The mass is composed of inflamed bowel, adherent and indurated mesentery, and enlarged abdominal lymph nodes. Extension of the mass can cause obstruction of the right ureter or bladder inflammation, manifested by dysuria and fever. Edema, bowel wall thickening, and fibrosis of the bowel wall within the mass account for the radiographic "string sign" of a narrowed intestinal lumen.

Bowel obstruction may take several forms. In the early stages of disease, bowel wall edema and spasm produce intermittent obstructive manifestations and increasing symptoms of postprandial pain. Over several years, persistent inflammation gradually progresses to fibrostenotic narrowing and stricture. Diarrhea will decrease and be replaced by chronic bowel obstruction. Acute episodes of obstruction occur as well, precipitated by bowel inflammation and spasm or sometimes by impaction of undigested food or medication. These episodes usually resolve with intravenous fluids and gastric decompression.

Severe inflammation of the ileocecal region may lead to localized wall thinning, with microperforation and fistula formation to the adjacent bowel, the skin, or the urinary bladder, or to an abscess cavity in the mesentery. Enterovesical fistulas typically present as dysuria or recurrent bladder infections or, less commonly, as pneumaturia or fecaluria. Enterocutaneous fistulas follow tissue planes of least resistance, usually draining through abdominal surgical scars. Enterovaginal fistulas are rare and present as dyspareunia or as a feculent or foul-smelling, often painful vaginal discharge. They are unlikely to develop without a prior hysterectomy.

Jejunoileitis

Extensive inflammatory disease is associated with a loss of digestive and absorptive surface, resulting in malabsorption and steatorrhea. Nutritional deficiencies can also result from poor intake and enteric losses of protein and other nutrients. Intestinal malabsorption can cause hypoalbuminemia, hypocalcemia, hypomagnesemia, coagulopathy, and hyperoxaluria with nephrolithiasis in patients with an intact colon. Vertebral fractures are caused by a combination of vitamin D deficiency, hypocalcemia, and prolonged glucocorticoid use. Pellagra from niacin deficiency can occur in extensive small-bowel disease, and malabsorption of vitamin B_{12} can lead to megaloblastic anemia and neurologic symptoms.

Diarrhea is characteristic of active disease; its causes include (1) bacterial overgrowth in obstructive stasis or fistulization, (2) bile-acid malabsorption due to a diseased or resected terminal ileum, and (3) intestinal inflammation with decreased water absorption and increased secretion of electrolytes.

Colitis and Perianal Disease

Patients with colitis present with low-grade fevers, malaise, diarrhea, crampy abdominal pain, and sometimes hematochezia. Gross bleeding is not as common as in UC and appears in about half of patients with exclusively colonic disease. Only 1–2% bleed massively. Pain is caused by passage of fecal material through narrowed and inflamed segments of large bowel. Decreased rectal compliance is another cause for diarrhea in Crohn's colitis patients. Toxic megacolon is rare but may be seen with severe inflammation and short-duration disease.

Stricturing can occur in the colon in 4–16% of patients and produce symptoms of bowel obstruction. If the endoscopist is unable to traverse a stricture in Crohn's colitis, surgical resection should be considered, especially if the patient has symptoms of chronic obstruction. Colonic disease may fistulize into the stomach or duodenum, causing feculent vomiting, or to the proximal or mid small bowel, causing malabsorption by "short circuiting" and bacterial overgrowth. Ten percent of women with Crohn's colitis will develop a rectovaginal fistula.

Perianal disease affects about one-third of patients with Crohn's colitis and is manifested by incontinence, large hemorrhoidal tags, anal strictures, anorectal fistulae, and perirectal abscesses. Not all patients with perianal fistula will have endoscopic evidence of colonic inflammation.

Gastroduodenal Disease

Symptoms and signs of upper gastrointestinal tract disease include nausea, vomiting, and epigastric pain. Patients usually have a *H. pylori*–negative gastritis. The second portion of the duodenum is more commonly involved than the bulb. Fistulas involving the stomach or duodenum arise from the small or large bowel and do not necessarily signify the presence of upper gastrointestinal tract involvement. Patients with advanced gastroduodenal CD may develop a chronic gastric outlet obstruction.

Laboratory, Endoscopic, and Radiographic Features

Laboratory abnormalities include elevated ESR and CRP. In more severe disease, findings include hypoalbuminemia, anemia, and leukocytosis.

Endoscopic features of CD include rectal sparing, aphthous ulcerations, fistulas, and skip lesions. Endoscopy is useful for biopsy of mass lesions or strictures, or for inspecting filling defects seen on barium enema. Colonoscopy allows examination and biopsy of the terminal ileum, and upper endoscopy is useful in diagnosing gastroduodenal involvement in patients with upper tract symptoms. Ileal or colonic strictures may be dilated with balloons introduced through the colonoscope. Wireless capsule endoscopy (WCE) allows direct visualization of the entire small-bowel mucosa (**Fig. 16-6**). The diagnostic yield of detecting lesions suggestive of active CD is higher with WCE than CT enterography or small-bowel series. WCE cannot be used in the setting of a small-bowel stricture. Capsule retention occurs in <1% of patients with suspected CD, but retention rates of 4–6% are seen in patients with established CD.

In CD, early radiographic findings in the small bowel include thickened folds and aphthous ulcerations. "Cobblestoning" from longitudinal and transverse

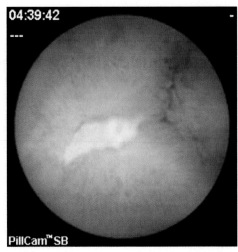

FIGURE 16-6

Wireless capsule endoscopy image in a patient with Crohn's disease of the ileum shows ulcerations and narrowing of the intestinal lumen. *(Courtesy of Dr. S Reddy, Gastroenterology Division, Department of Medicine, Brigham and Women's Hospital, Boston, Massachusetts; with permission.)*

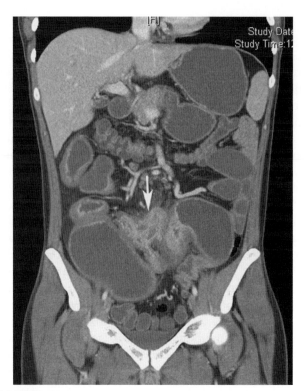

FIGURE 16-7

Coronal contrast-enhanced MDCT image obtained after oral administration of 1350 cc of neutral oral contrast material shows dilation of small-bowel loops, segmental mucosal hyperenhancement, and interloop sinus tracts (*white arrow*) and mesenteric fat stranding. *(Courtesy of Dr. K Mortele, Gastrointestinal Radiology, Department of Radiology, Brigham and Women's Hospital, Boston, Massachusetts; with permission.)*

ulcerations most frequently involves the small bowel. In more advanced disease, strictures, fistulas, inflammatory masses, and abscesses may be detected. The earliest macroscopic findings of colonic CD are aphthous ulcers. These small ulcers are often multiple and separated by normal intervening mucosa. As disease progresses, aphthous ulcers become enlarged, deeper, and occasionally connected to one another, forming longitudinal stellate, serpiginous, and linear ulcers (see Fig. 12-4*B*).

The transmural inflammation of CD leads to decreased luminal diameter and limited distensibility. As ulcers progress deeper, they can lead to fistula formation. The radiographic "string sign" represents long areas of circumferential inflammation and fibrosis, resulting in long segments of luminal narrowing. The segmental nature of CD results in wide gaps of normal or dilated bowel between involved segments.

CT enterography combines the improved spatial and temporal resolution of multidetector-row CT with large volumes of ingested neutral enteric contrast material to permit visualization of the entire small bowel and lumen. Unlike routine CT, which is used to detect the extraenteric complications of CD such as fistula and abscess, CT enterography clearly depicts the small-bowel inflammation associated with CD by displaying mural hyperenhancement, stratification, and thickening; engorged vasa recta; and perienteric inflammatory changes (**Figs. 16-7** and **16-8**). CT enterography is becoming the first-line test for the evaluation of suspected CD and its complications. MRI may prove superior for demonstrating pelvic lesions such as ischiorectal abscesses.

Complications

Because CD is a transmural process, serosal adhesions develop that provide direct pathways for fistula formation and reduce the incidence of free perforation. Perforation occurs in 1–2% of patients, usually in the ileum but occasionally in the jejunum or as a complication of toxic megacolon. The peritonitis of free perforation, especially colonic, may be fatal. Intraabdominal and pelvic abscesses occur in 10–30% of patients with Crohn's disease at some time in the course of their illness. CT-guided percutaneous drainage of the abscess is standard therapy. Despite adequate drainage, most patients need resection of the offending bowel segment. Percutaneous drainage has an especially high failure rate in abdominal wall abscesses. Systemic glucocorticoid therapy increases the risk of intraabdominal and pelvic abscesses in CD patients who have never had an operation. Other complications include intestinal obstruction in 40%, massive hemorrhage, malabsorption, and severe perianal disease.

Serologic Markers

Two antibodies that can be detected in the serum of IBD patients are perinuclear antineutrophil cytoplasmic

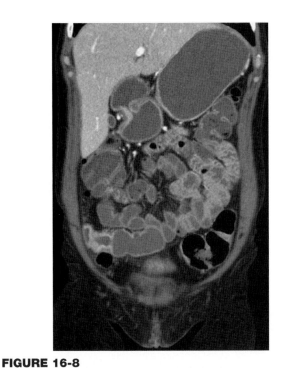

FIGURE 16-8
Coronal contrast-enhanced MDCT image obtained after oral administration of 1350 cc of neutral oral contrast material shows mucosal hyperenhancement of the terminal ileum with narrowing and mild prestenotic dilatation. *(Courtesy of Dr. K Mortele, Gastrointestinal Radiology, Department of Radiology, Brigham and Women's Hospital, Boston, Massachusetts; with permission.)*

based on the prevalence of IBD in a given population. For the patient population with a prevalence of IBD of 62%, the PPV is 94% and the NPV is 63%.

In a referral center population, 55% of CD patients were seroreactive to outer membrane porin C (Omp C) of *E. coli*; 50–54% of CD patients are positive for antibody to I_2, a homologue of the bacterial transcription-factor families from a *Pseudomonas fluorescens*–associated sequence. Combining these diagnostic assays further improves the ability to diagnose CD. In a referral population of CD patients, 85% had an antibody to at least one antigen (pANCA, ASCA, Omp C, and I_2); only 4% responded to all four. Antibody positivity may help predict disease phenotype. ASCA positivity is associated with an increased rate of early CD complications; Omp C–positive patients are more likely to have internal perforating disease; and I_2 positive patients are more likely to have fibrostenosing disease. Patients positive for I_2, Omp C, and ASCA are the most likely to have undergone small-bowel surgery.

Cbir1 flagellin is an immunodominant antigen of the enteric microbial flora to which strong B cell and CD4+ T cell responses occur in colitic mice. Transfer of Cbir1-specific CD4+ T_H1 T cells to C3H/SCID mice generates a severe colitis dependent on exogenous expression of Cbir1 flagellin in the cecum and colon. Around 50% of patients with CD have serum reactivity to Cbir1, whereas UC patients have little or no reactivity to this flagellin. Anti-Cbir1 expression is associated with small-bowel disease, fibrostenosing, and internal penetrating disease. Children with CD positive for all four immune responses (ASCA+, Omp C+, I_2+ and anti-Cbir1+) may have more aggressive disease and a shorter time to progression to internal perforating and/or stricturing disease. In addition, these antibody tests may help decide whether a patient with indeterminate colitis should undergo an IPAA, because patients with predominant features of CD have a more difficult postoperative course.

Other serologic markers in IBD patients include antigoblet cell autoantibodies, pancreatic autoantibodies, and an autoantibody against tropomyosin isoform 5 found in colon epithelial cells. Antibodies to red cell membrane antigens that cross-react with enteropathogens such as *Campylobacter* sp. may be associated with hemolytic anemia in CD. None of these antibodies are useful in the diagnosis and management of patients with IBD.

DIFFERENTIAL DIAGNOSIS OF UC AND CD

UC and CD have similar features to many other diseases. In the absence of a key diagnostic test, a combination of features is used (Table 16-4). Once a diagnosis of IBD is made, distinguishing between UC and CD is impossible in up to 15% of cases. These are termed *indeterminate colitis*.

antibodies (pANCAs) and anti-*Saccharomyces cerevisiae* antibodies (ASCAs). A distinct set of pANCAs is associated with UC. The antigens to which these antibodies are directed have not been identified, but they are distinct from those associated with vasculitis and likely represent cross-reactions with enteric bacterial antigens. pANCA positivity is found in about 60–70% of UC patients and 5–10% of CD patients; 5–15% of first-degree relatives of UC patients are pANCA positive, whereas only 2–3% of the general population is pANCA-positive. pANCA may also identify specific disease phenotypes. pANCA positivity is more often associated with pancolitis, early surgery, pouchitis, or inflammation of the pouch after ileal pouch–anal anastomosis (IPAA) and primary sclerosing cholangitis (PSC). pANCA in CD is associated with colonic disease that resembles UC.

ASCA antibodies recognize mannose sequences in the cell wall of *S. cerevisiae*; 60–70% of CD patients, 10–15% of UC patients, and up to 5% of non-IBD controls are ASCA-positive. The sensitivity and specificity of pANCA/ASCA vary depending upon the prevalence of IBD in a given population. In a patient population with a combined prevalence of UC and CD of 62%, pANCA/ASCA serology showed a sensitivity of 64% and a specificity of 94%. Positive and negative predictive values (PPV and NPV) for pANCA/ASCA also vary

TABLE 16-4

DIFFERENT CLINICAL, ENDOSCOPIC, AND RADIOGRAPHIC FEATURES

	ULCERATIVE COLITIS	CROHN'S DISEASE
Clinical		
Gross blood in stool	Yes	Occasionally
Mucus	Yes	Occasionally
Systemic symptoms	Occasionally	Frequently
Pain	Occasionally	Frequently
Abdominal mass	Rarely	Yes
Significant perineal disease	No	Frequently
Fistulas	No	Yes
Small-intestinal obstruction	No	Frequently
Colonic obstruction	Rarely	Frequently
Response to antibiotics	No	Yes
Recurrence after surgery	No	Yes
ANCA-positive	Frequently	Rarely
ASCA-positive	Rarely	Frequently
Endoscopic		
Rectal sparing	Rarely	Frequently
Continuous disease	Yes	Occasionally
"Cobblestoning"	No	Yes
Granuloma on biopsy	No	Occasionally
Radiographic		
Small bowel significantly abnormal	No	Yes
Abnormal terminal ileum	Occasionally	Yes
Segmental colitis	No	Yes
Asymmetric colitis	No	Yes
Stricture	Occasionally	Frequently

Note: ANCA, antineutrophil cytoplasm antibody; ASCA, anti-*Saccharomyces cerevisiae* antibody.

INFECTIOUS DISEASE

Infections of the small intestines and colon can mimic CD or UC. They may be bacterial, fungal, viral, or protozoal in origin (Table 16-5). *Campylobacter* colitis can mimic the endoscopic appearance of severe UC and can cause a relapse of established UC. *Salmonella* can cause watery or bloody diarrhea, nausea, and vomiting. Shigellosis causes watery diarrhea, abdominal pain, and fever followed by rectal tenesmus and by the passage of blood and mucus per rectum. All three are usually self-limited, but 1% of patients infected with *Salmonella* become asymptomatic carriers. *Yersinia enterocolitica* infection occurs mainly in the terminal ileum and causes mucosal ulceration, neutrophil invasion, and thickening of the ileal wall. Other bacterial infections that may mimic IBD include *C. difficile*, which presents with watery diarrhea, tenesmus, nausea, and vomiting; and *E. coli*, three categories of which can cause colitis. These are enterohemorrhagic, enteroinvasive, and enteroadherent *E. coli*, all of which can cause bloody diarrhea and abdominal tenderness. Diagnosis of bacterial colitis is made by sending stool specimens for bacterial culture and *C. difficile* toxin analysis. Gonorrhea, *Chlamydophila*, and syphilis can also cause proctitis.

Gastrointestinal involvement with mycobacterial infection occurs primarily in the immunosuppressed patient but may occur in patients with normal immunity. Distal ileal and cecal involvement predominates, and patients present with symptoms of small-bowel obstruction and a tender abdominal mass. The diagnosis is made most directly by colonoscopy with biopsy and culture. *Mycobacterium avium-intracellulare* complex infection occurs in advanced stages of HIV infection and in other immunocompromised states; it usually manifests as a systemic infection with diarrhea, abdominal pain, weight loss, fever, and malabsorption. Diagnosis is established by acid-fast smear and culture of mucosal biopsies.

Although most of the patients with viral colitis are immunosuppressed, cytomegalovirus (CMV) and herpes simplex proctitis may occur in immunocompetent

TABLE 16-5

DISEASES THAT MIMIC IBD

INFECTIOUS ETIOLOGIES

Bacterial	**Mycobacterial**	**Viral**
Salmonella	Tuberculosis	Cytomegalovirus
Shigella	*Mycobacterium avium*	Herpes simplex
Toxigenic *Escherichia coli*	**Parasitic**	HIV
Campylobacter	Amebiasis	**Fungal**
Yersinia	*Isospora*	Histoplasmosis
Clostridium difficile	*Trichuris trichura*	*Candida*
Gonorrhea	Hookworm	*Aspergillus*
Chlamydia trachomatis	*Strongyloides*	

NONINFECTIOUS ETIOLOGIES

Inflammatory	**Neoplastic**	**Drugs and chemicals**
Appendicitis	Lymphoma	NSAIDs
Diverticulitis	Metastatic carcinoma	Phosphasoda
Diversion colitis	Carcinoma of the ileum	Cathartic colon
Collagenous/lymphocytic colitis	Carcinoid	Gold
Ischemic colitis	Familial polyposis	Oral contraceptives
Radiation colitis/enteritis		Cocaine
Solitary rectal ulcer syndrome		Chemotherapy
Eosinophilc gastroenteritis		
Neutropenic colitis		
Beçhet's syndrome		
Graft-versus-host disease		

Note: NSAIDs, nonsteroidal anti-inflammatory drugs.

individuals. CMV occurs most commonly in the esophagus, colon, and rectum but may also involve the small intestine. Symptoms include abdominal pain, bloody diarrhea, fever, and weight loss. With severe disease, necrosis and perforation can occur. Diagnosis is made by identification of intranuclear inclusions in mucosal cells on biopsy. Herpes simplex infection of the gastrointestinal tract is limited to the oropharynx, anorectum, and perianal areas. Symptoms include anorectal pain, tenesmus, constipation, inguinal adenopathy, difficulty with urinary voiding, and sacral paresthesias. Diagnosis is made by rectal biopsy. HIV itself can cause diarrhea, nausea, vomiting, and anorexia. Small-intestinal biopsies show partial villus atrophy; small-bowel bacterial overgrowth and fat malabsorption may also be noted.

Protozoan parasites include *Isospora belli*, which can cause a self-limited infection in healthy hosts but causes a chronic profuse, watery diarrhea, and weight loss in AIDS patients. *Entamoeba histolytica* or related species infect about 10% of the world's population; symptoms include abdominal pain, tenesmus, frequent loose stools containing blood and mucus, and abdominal tenderness. Colonoscopy reveals focal punctate ulcers with normal intervening mucosa; diagnosis is made by biopsy or serum amebic antibodies. Fulminant amebic colitis is rare but has a mortality rate of >50%.

Other parasitic infections that may mimic IBD include hookworm (*Necator americanus*), whipworm (*Trichuris trichiura*), and *Strongyloides stercoralis*. In severely immunocompromised patients, *Candida* or *Aspergillus* can be identified in the submucosa. Disseminated histoplasmosis can involve the ileocecal area.

NONINFECTIOUS DISEASE

Diverticulitis can be confused with CD clinically and radiographically. Both diseases cause fever, abdominal pain, tender abdominal mass, leukocytosis, elevated ESR, partial obstruction, and fistulas. Perianal disease or ileitis on small-bowel series favors the diagnosis of CD. Significant endoscopic mucosal abnormalities are more likely in CD than in diverticulitis. Endoscopic or clinical recurrence following segmental resection favors CD. Diverticular-associated colitis is similar to CD, but mucosal abnormalities are limited to the sigmoid and descending colon.

Ischemic colitis is commonly confused with IBD. The ischemic process can be chronic and diffuse, as in UC, or segmental, as in CD. Colonic inflammation due to ischemia may resolve quickly or may persist and result in transmural scarring and stricture formation. Ischemic bowel disease should be considered in the elderly following abdominal aortic aneurysm repair or when a patient has a hypercoagulable state or a severe cardiac or peripheral vascular disorder. Patients usually present with sudden onset of left lower quadrant pain, urgency to defecate, and the passage of bright red blood per rectum. Endoscopic examination often demonstrates a normal-appearing rectum and a sharp transition to an area of inflammation in the descending colon and splenic flexure.

The effects of radiotherapy on the gastrointestinal tract can be difficult to distinguish from IBD. Acute symptoms can occur within 1–2 weeks of starting radiotherapy. When the rectum and sigmoid are irradiated, patients develop bloody, mucoid diarrhea and tenesmus, as in distal UC. With small-bowel involvement, diarrhea is common. Late symptoms include malabsorption and weight loss. Stricturing with obstruction and bacterial overgrowth may occur. Fistulas can penetrate the bladder, vagina, or abdominal wall. Flexible sigmoidoscopy reveals mucosal granularity, friability, numerous telangiectasias, and occasionally discrete ulcerations. Biopsy can be diagnostic.

Solitary rectal ulcer syndrome is uncommon and can be confused with IBD. It occurs in persons of all ages and may be caused by impaired evacuation and failure of relaxation of the puborectalis muscle. Single or multiple ulcerations may arise from anal sphincter overactivity, higher intrarectal pressures during defecation, and digital removal of stool. Patients complain of constipation with straining and pass blood and mucus per rectum. Other symptoms include abdominal pain, diarrhea, tenesmus, and perineal pain. Ulceration as large as 5 cm in diameter is usually seen anteriorly or anteriorlaterally 3–15 cm from the anal verge. Biopsies can be diagnostic.

Several types of colitis are associated with nonsteroidal anti-inflammatory drugs (NSAIDs), including de novo colitis, reactivation of IBD, and proctitis caused by use of suppositories. Most patients with NSAID-related colitis present with diarrhea and abdominal pain, and complications include stricture, bleeding, obstruction, perforation, and fistulization. Withdrawal of these agents is crucial, and in cases of reactivated IBD, standard therapies are indicated.

INDETERMINATE COLITIS

Cases of IBD that cannot be categorized as UC or CD are called *indeterminate colitis*. Long-term follow-up reduces the number of cases labeled indeterminate to about 10%. The disease course of indeterminate colitis is unclear, and surgical recommendations are difficult, especially since up to 20% of pouches fail, requiring

permanent ileostomy. A multistage IPAA (the initial stage consisting of a subtotal colectomy with Hartmann pouch), with careful histologic evaluation of the resected specimen to exclude CD, is advised. Medical therapy is similar to that for UC and CD; most clinicians use 5-ASA drugs, glucocorticoids, and immunomodulators as necessary.

THE ATYPICAL COLITIDES

Two atypical colitides—collagenous colitis and lymphocytic colitis—have completely normal endoscopic appearances. Collagenous colitis has two main histologic components: increased subepithelial collagen deposition and colitis with increased intraepithelial lymphocytes. Female to male ratio is 9:1, and most patients present in the sixth or seventh decades of life. The main symptom is chronic watery diarrhea. Treatments range from sulfasalazine or mesalamine and Lomotil to bismuth to budesonide to prednisone for refractory disease.

Lymphocytic colitis has features similar to collagenous colitis, including age at onset and clinical presentation, but it has almost equal incidence in men and women and no subepithelial collagen deposition on pathologic section. However, intraepithelial lymphocytes are increased. The frequency of celiac disease is increased in lymphocytic colitis and ranges from 9 to 27%. Celiac disease should be excluded in all patients with lymphocytic colitis, particularly if diarrhea does not respond to conventional therapy. Treatment is similar to that of collagenous colitis with the exception of a gluten-free diet for those who have celiac disease.

Diversion colitis is an inflammatory process that arises in segments of the large intestine that are excluded from the fecal stream. It usually occurs in patients with ileostomy or colostomy when a mucus fistula or a Hartmann's pouch has been created. Clinically, patients have mucus or bloody discharge from the rectum. Erythema, granularity, friability, and, in more severe cases, ulceration can be seen on endoscopy. Histopathology shows areas of active inflammation with foci of cryptitis and crypt abscesses. Crypt architecture is normal, which differentiates it from UC. It may be impossible to distinguish from CD. Short-chain fatty acid enemas may help in diversion colitis, but the definitive therapy is surgical reanastomosis.

EXTRAINTESTINAL MANIFESTATIONS

Up to one-third of IBD patients have at least one extraintestinal disease manifestation.

DERMATOLOGIC

Erythema nodosum (EN) occurs in up to 15% of CD patients and 10% of UC patients. Attacks usually correlate with bowel activity; skin lesions develop after the onset of bowel symptoms, and patients frequently have concomitant active peripheral arthritis. The lesions of EN are hot, red, tender nodules measuring 1–5 cm in diameter and are found on the anterior surface of the lower legs, ankles, calves, thighs, and arms. Therapy is directed toward the underlying bowel disease.

Pyoderma gangrenosum (PG) is seen in 1–12% of UC patients and less commonly in Crohn's colitis. Although it usually presents after the diagnosis of IBD, PG may occur years before the onset of bowel symptoms, run a course independent of the bowel disease, respond poorly to colectomy, and even develop years after proctocolectomy. It is usually associated with severe disease. Lesions are commonly found on the dorsal surface of the feet and legs but may occur on the arms, chest, stoma, and even the face. PG usually begins as a pustule and then spreads concentrically to rapidly undermine healthy skin. Lesions then ulcerate, with violaceous edges surrounded by a margin of erythema. Centrally, they contain necrotic tissue with blood and exudates. Lesions may be single or multiple and grow as large as 30 cm. They are sometimes very difficult to treat and often require intravenous antibiotics, intravenous glucocorticoids, dapsone, azathioprine, thalidomide, intravenous cyclosporine, or infliximab.

Other dermatologic manifestations include pyoderma vegetans, which occurs in intertriginous areas; pyostomatitis vegetans, which involves the mucous membranes; Sweet's syndrome, a neutrophilic dermatosis; and metastatic CD, a rare disorder defined by cutaneous granuloma formation. Psoriasis affects 5–10% of patients with IBD and is unrelated to bowel activity. Perianal skin tags are found in 75–80% of patients with CD, especially those with colon involvement. Oral mucosal lesions, seen often in CD and rarely in UC, include aphthous stomatitis and "cobblestone" lesions of the buccal mucosa.

RHEUMATOLOGIC

Peripheral arthritis develops in 15–20% of IBD patients, is more common in CD, and worsens with exacerbations of bowel activity. It is asymmetric, polyarticular, and migratory and most often affects large joints of the upper and lower extremities. Treatment is directed at reducing bowel inflammation. In severe UC, colectomy frequently cures the arthritis.

Ankylosing spondylitis (AS) occurs in about 10% of IBD patients and is more common in CD than UC. About two-thirds of IBD patients with AS express the HLA-B27 antigen. The AS activity is not related to bowel activity and does not remit with glucocorticoids or colectomy. It most often affects the spine and pelvis, producing symptoms of diffuse low-back pain, buttock pain, and morning stiffness. The course is continuous and progressive, leading to permanent skeletal damage and deformity. Infliximab reduces spinal inflammation and improves functional status and quality of life.

Sacroiliitis is symmetric, occurs equally in UC and CD, is often asymptomatic, does not correlate with bowel activity, and does not always progress to AS. Other rheumatic manifestations include hypertrophic osteoarthropathy, pelvic/femoral osteomyelitis, and relapsing polychondritis.

OCULAR

The incidence of ocular complications in IBD patients is 1–10%. The most common are conjunctivitis, anterior uveitis/iritis, and episcleritis. Uveitis is associated with both UC and Crohn's colitis, may be found during periods of remission, and may develop in patients following bowel resection. Symptoms include ocular pain, photophobia, blurred vision, and headache. Prompt intervention, sometimes with systemic glucocorticoids, is required to prevent scarring and visual impairment. Episcleritis is a benign disorder that presents with symptoms of mild ocular burning. It occurs in 3–4% of IBD patients, more commonly in Crohn's colitis, and is treated with topical glucocorticoids.

HEPATOBILIARY

Hepatic steatosis is detectable in about half of the abnormal liver biopsies from patients with CD and UC; patients usually present with hepatomegaly. Fatty liver usually results from a combination of chronic debilitating illness, malnutrition, and glucocorticoid therapy. Cholelithiasis is more common in CD than UC and occurs in 10–35% of patients with ileitis or ileal resection. Gallstone formation is caused by malabsorption of bile acids, resulting in depletion of the bile salt pool and the secretion of lithogenic bile.

PSC shows both intrahepatic and extrahepatic bile duct inflammation and fibrosis, frequently leading to biliary cirrhosis and hepatic failure; 1–5% of patients with IBD have PSC, but 50–75% of patients with PSC have IBD. Although it can be recognized after the diagnosis of IBD, PSC can be detected earlier or even years after proctocolectomy. Most patients have no symptoms at the time of diagnosis; when symptoms are present, they consist of fatigue, jaundice, abdominal pain, fever, anorexia, and malaise. The traditional gold-standard diagnostic test is endoscopic retrograde cholangiopancreatography (ERCP), but magnetic resonance cholangiopancreatography (MRCP) is also sensitive and specific. MRCP is reasonable as an initial diagnostic test in children and can visualize irregularities, multifocal strictures, and dilatations of all levels of the biliary tree. In patients with PSC, both ERCP and MRCP demonstrate multiple bile duct strictures alternating with relatively normal segments.

The bile acid ursodeoxycholic acid (ursodiol) may reduce alkaline phosphatase and serum aminotransferase levels, but histologic improvement has been marginal.

High doses (25–30 mg/kg per day) may decrease the risk of colorectal dysplasia and cancer in patients with UC and PSC. Endoscopic stenting may be palliative for cholestasis secondary to bile duct obstruction. Patients with symptomatic disease develop cirrhosis and liver failure over 5–10 years and eventually require liver transplantation. Ten percent of PSC patients develop cholangiocarcinoma and cannot be transplanted. Patients with IBD and PSC are at increased risk of colon cancer and should be surveyed yearly by colonoscopy and biopsy. Pericholangitis is a subset of PSC found in about 30% of IBD patients; it is confined to small bile ducts and is usually benign.

UROLOGIC

The most frequent genitourinary complications are calculi, ureteral obstruction, and fistulas. The highest frequency of nephrolithiasis (10–20%) occurs in patients with CD following small-bowel resection. Calcium oxalate stones develop secondary to hyperoxaluria, which results from increased absorption of dietary oxalate. Normally, dietary calcium combines with luminal oxalate to form insoluble calcium oxalate, which is eliminated in the stool. In patients with ileal dysfunction, however, nonabsorbed fatty acids bind calcium and leave oxalate unbound. The unbound oxalate is then delivered to the colon, where it is readily absorbed, especially in the presence of inflammation.

METABOLIC BONE DISORDERS

Low bone mass occurs in 3–30% of IBD patients. The risk is increased by glucocorticoids, cyclosporine, methotrexate, and total parenteral nutrition (TPN). Malabsorption and inflammation mediated by IL-1, IL-6, and TNF also contribute to low bone density. An increased incidence of hip, spine, wrist, and rib fractures has been noted: 36% in CD and 45% in UC. The absolute risk of an osteoporotic fracture is about 1% per person per year. Fracture rates, particularly in the spine and hip, were highest among the elderly (age >60). One study noted an odds ratio of vertebral fracture to be 1.72 and hip fracture 1.59. The disease severity predicted the risk of a fracture. Only 13% of IBD patients who had a fracture were on any kind of antifracture treatment. Up to 20% of bone mass can be lost per year with chronic glucocorticoid use. The effect is dosage-dependent. Budesonide may also suppress the pituitary-adrenal axis and thus carries a risk of causing osteoporosis.

Osteonecrosis is characterized by death of osteocytes and adipocytes and eventual bone collapse. The pain is aggravated by motion and swelling of the joints. It affects the hips more often than knees and shoulders, and in one series 4.3% of patients developed osteonecrosis within 6 months of starting glucocorticoids. Diagnosis is made by bone scan or MRI, and treatment consists of pain control, cord decompression, and arthroplasty.

THROMBOEMBOLIC DISORDERS

Patients with IBD have an increased risk of both venous and arterial thrombosis even if the disease is not active. Factors responsible for the hypercoagulable state have included abnormalities of the platelet-endothelial interaction, hyperhomocysteinemia, alterations in the coagulation cascade, impaired fibrinolysis, involvement of tissue factor-bearing microvesicles, disruption of the normal coagulation system by autoantibodies, as well as a genetic predisposition. A spectrum of vasculitides involving small, medium, and large vessels has also been observed.

OTHER DISORDERS

More common cardiopulmonary manifestations include endocarditis, myocarditis, pleuropericarditis, and interstitial lung disease. A secondary or reactive amyloidosis can occur in patients with long-standing IBD, especially in patients with CD. Amyloid material is deposited systemically and can cause diarrhea, constipation, and renal failure. The renal disease can be successfully treated with colchicine. Pancreatitis is a rare extraintestinal manifestation of IBD and results from duodenal fistulas; ampullary CD; gallstones; PSC; drugs such as 6-mercaptopurine, azathioprine, or, very rarely, 5-ASA agents; autoimmune pancreatitis; and primary CD of the pancreas.

℞ **Treatment:**
INFLAMMATORY BOWEL DISEASE

5-ASA AGENTS The mainstay of therapy for mild to moderate UC and Crohn's colitis is sulfasalazine and the other 5-ASA agents. These agents are effective at inducing remission in both UC and CD and in maintaining remission in UC; it remains unclear whether they have a role in remission maintenance in CD.

Sulfasalazine was originally developed to deliver both antibacterial (sulfapyridine) and anti-inflammatory (5-ASA) therapy into the connective tissues of joints and the colonic mucosa. The molecular structure provides a convenient delivery system to the colon by allowing the intact molecule to pass through the small intestine after only partial absorption, and to be broken down in the colon by bacterial azo reductases that cleave the azo bond linking the sulfa and 5-ASA moieties. Sulfasalazine is effective treatment for mild to moderate UC and Crohn's ileocolitis and colitis, but its high rate of side effects limits its use. Although sulfasalazine is more effective at higher doses, at 6 or 8 g/d up to 30% of patients experience allergic reactions or intolerable side effects such as headache, anorexia, nausea, and vomiting that are attributable to the sulfapyridine moiety. Hypersensitivity reactions, independent of sulfapyridine levels, include rash, fever, hepatitis, agranulocytosis, hypersensitivity pneumonitis, pancreatitis, worsening of colitis, and reversible sperm abnormalities. Sulfasalazine can also impair folate absorption, and patients should be given folic acid supplements.

Newer sulfa-free aminosalicylate preparations deliver increased amounts of the pharmacologically active ingredient of sulfasalazine (5-ASA, mesalamine) to the site of active bowel disease while limiting systemic toxicity. Peroxisome proliferator activated receptor γ (PPAR-γ) may mediate 5-ASA therapeutic action by regulating NF-κB. Sulfa-free aminosalicylate formulations include alternative azo-bonded carriers, 5-ASA dimers, pH-dependent tablets, and continuous-release preparations. Each has the same efficacy as sulfasalazine when equimolar concentrations are used. Olsalazine is composed of two 5-ASA radicals linked by an azo bond, which is split in the colon by bacterial reduction and two 5-ASA molecules are released. Olsalazine is similar in effectiveness to sulfasalazine in treating CD and UC, but up to 17% of patients experience nonbloody diarrhea caused by increased secretion of fluid in the small bowel. Balsalazide contains an azo bond binding mesalamine to the carrier molecule 4-aminobenzoyl-β-alanine; it is effective in the colon. Claversal is an enteric-coated form of 5-ASA that consists of mesalamine surrounded by an acrylic-based polymer resin and a cellulose coating that releases mesalamine at pH >6.0, a level that is present from the mid-jejunum continuously to the distal colon.

Asacol is also an enteric-coated form of mesalamine, but it has a slightly different release pattern, with 5-ASA liberated at pH >7.0. The disintegration of Asacol is variable, with complete breakup of the tablet occurring in many different parts of the gut ranging from the small intestine to the splenic flexure; it has increased gastric residence when taken with a meal. Asacol is used to induce and maintain remission in UC and to induce remission in CD ileitis, ileocolitis, and colitis, but meta-analyses have not proven 5-ASA medications superior to placebo for the maintenance of remission in CD. Appropriate doses of Asacol and other 5-ASA compounds are shown in Table 16-6. Some 50–75% of patients with mild to moderate UC and CD improve when treated with 2 g/d of 5-ASA; the dose response continues up to at least 4.8 g/d. Doses of 1.5–4 g/d maintain remission in 50–75% of patients with UC.

Pentasa is another mesalamine formulation that uses an ethylcellulose coating to allow water absorption into small beads containing the mesalamine. Water dissolves the 5-ASA, which then diffuses out of the bead into the lumen. Disintegration of the capsule occurs in the stomach. The microspheres then disperse throughout the entire gastrointestinal tract from the small intestine through the distal colon in both fasted and fed conditions. Controlled trials of Pentasa and Asacol in active

TABLE 16-6

ORAL 5-ASA PREPARATIONS

PREPARATION	FORMULATION	DELIVERY	DOSING PER DAY
Azo-Bond			
Sulfasalazine (500 mg) (Azulfadine)	Sulfapyridine-5-ASA	Colon	3–6 g (acute) 2–4 g (maintenance)
Olsalazine (250 mg) (Dipentum)	5-ASA-5-ASA	Colon	1–3 g
Balsalazide (750 mg) (Colazal)	Aminobenzoyl-alanine-5-ASA	Colon	6.75–9 g
Delayed-Release			
Mesalamine (400, 800 mg) (Asacol)	Eudragit S (pH 7)	Distal ileum-colon	2.4–4.8 g (acute) 1.6–4.8 g (maintenance)
Claversal/Mesasal/Salofalk (250, 500 mg)	Eudragit L (pH 6)	Ileum-colon	1.5–3 g (acute) 1.5–3 g (maintenance)
Sustained-Release			
Mesalamine (250, 500, 1000 mg) (Pentasa)	Ethylcellulose microgranules	Stomach-colon	2–4 g (acute) 1.5–4 g (maintenance)
Extended-Release			
Mesalamine (1.2 gm) (under review by the FDA)	MMX mesalamine (SPD476)	Ileum-colon	2.4–4.8 (acute) 2.4–4.8 (maintenance)

CHAPTER 16 Inflammatory Bowel Disease

CD demonstrate a 40–60% clinical improvement or remission. 5-ASA agents may be effective in postoperative prophylaxis of CD.

Topical mesalamine enemas are effective in mild-to-moderate distal UC and CD. Clinical response occurs in up to 80% of UC patients with colitis distal to the splenic flexure. Combination therapy with mesalamine in both oral and enema form is more effective than either treatment alone for both distal and extensive UC. Mesalamine suppositories are effective in treating proctitis.

GLUCOCORTICOIDS The majority of patients with moderate to severe UC benefit from oral or parenteral glucocorticoids. Prednisone is usually started at doses of 40–60 mg/d for active UC that is unresponsive to 5-ASA therapy. Parenteral glucocorticoids may be administered as intravenous hydrocortisone, 300 mg/d, or methylprednisolone, 40–60 mg/d. Adrenocorticotropic hormone (ACTH) is occasionally preferred for glucocorticoid-naïve patients despite a risk of adrenal hemorrhage. ACTH has equivalent efficacy to intravenous hydrocortisone in both glucocorticoid-naïve and -experienced CD patients.

Topically applied glucocorticoids are also beneficial for distal colitis and may serve as an adjunct in those who have rectal involvement plus more proximal disease. Hydrocortisone enemas or foam may control active disease, although they have no proven role as maintenance therapy. These glucocorticoids are significantly absorbed from the rectum and can lead to adrenal suppression with prolonged administration. Topical 5-ASA therapy is more effective than topical steroid therapy in the treatment of distal UC.

Glucocorticoids are also effective for treatment of moderate-to-severe CD and induce a 60–70% remission rate compared to a 30% placebo response. The systemic effects of standard glucocorticoid formulations have led to the development of more potent formulations that are less well-absorbed and have increased first-pass metabolism. Controlled ileal-release budesonide has been nearly equal to prednisone for ileocolonic CD with fewer glucocorticoid side effects. Budesonide is used for 2–3 months at a dose of 9 mg/d, then tapered. Budesonide 6 mg/d is effective in reducing relapse rates at 3–6 months but not at 12 months in CD patients with a medically induced remission.

Glucocorticoids play no role in maintenance therapy in either UC or CD. Once clinical remission has been induced, they should be tapered according to the clinical activity, normally at a rate of no more than 5 mg/week. They can usually be tapered to 20 mg/d within 4–5 weeks but often take several months to be discontinued altogether. The side effects are numerous, including fluid retention, abdominal striae, fat redistribution, hyperglycemia, subcapsular cataracts, osteonecrosis, myopathy,

emotional disturbances, and withdrawal symptoms. Most of these side effects, aside from osteonecrosis, are related to the dose and duration of therapy.

ANTIBIOTICS Antibiotics have no role in the treatment of active or quiescent UC. However, pouchitis, which occurs in about a third of UC patients after colectomy and IPAA, usually responds to treatment with metronidazole or ciprofloxacin.

Metronidazole is effective in active inflammatory, fistulous, and perianal CD and may prevent recurrence after ileal resection. The most effective dose is 15–20 mg/kg per day in three divided doses; it is usually continued for several months. Common side effects include nausea, metallic taste, and disulfiram-like reaction. Peripheral neuropathy can occur with prolonged administration (several months) and on rare occasions is permanent despite discontinuation. Ciprofloxacin (500 mg bid) is also beneficial for inflammatory, perianal, and fistulous CD. These two antibiotics should be used as second-line drugs in active CD after 5-ASA agents and as first-line drugs in perianal and fistulous CD. Rifaximin has modest activity in CD.

AZATHIOPRINE AND 6-MERCAPTOPURINE Azathioprine and 6-mercaptopurine (6-MP) are purine analogues commonly employed in the management of glucocorticoid-dependent IBD. Azathioprine is rapidly absorbed and converted to 6-MP, which is then metabolized to the active end product, thioinosinic acid, an inhibitor of purine ribonucleotide synthesis and cell proliferation. These agents also inhibit the immune response. Efficacy is seen at 3–4 weeks. Compliance can be monitored by measuring the levels of 6-thioguanine and 6-methyl-mercaptopurine, end products of 6-MP metabolism. Azathioprine (2.0–3.0 mg/kg per day) or 6-MP (1.0–1.5 mg/kg per day) have been employed successfully as glucocorticoid-sparing agents in up to two-thirds of UC and CD patients previously unable to be weaned from glucocorticoids. The role of these immunomodulators as maintenance therapy in UC and CD and for treating active perianal disease and fistulas in CD appears promising. In addition, 6-MP or azathioprine is effective for postoperative prophylaxis of CD.

Although azathioprine and 6-MP are usually well tolerated, pancreatitis occurs in 3–4% of patients, typically presents within the first few weeks of therapy, and is completely reversible when the drug is stopped. Other side effects include nausea, fever, rash, and hepatitis. Bone marrow suppression (particularly leukopenia) is dose-related and often delayed, necessitating regular monitoring of the complete blood cell count (CBC). Additionally, 1 in 300 individuals lacks thiopurine methyltransferase, the enzyme responsible for drug metabolism; an additional 11% of the population are heterozygotes with intermediate enzyme activity. Both are at increased risk of toxicity because of increased accumulation of thioguanine metabolites. Although 6-thioguanine and 6-methylmercaptopurine levels can be followed to determine correct drug dosing and reduce toxicity, weight-based dosing is an acceptable alternative. CBCs and liver function tests should be monitored frequently regardless of dosing strategy. IBD patients treated with azathioprine/6-MP are at a four-fold increased risk of developing a lymphoma. This increased risk could be a result of the medications, the underlying disease, or both.

METHOTREXATE Methotrexate (MTX) inhibits dihydrofolate reductase, resulting in impaired DNA synthesis. Additional anti-inflammatory properties may be related to decreased IL-1 production. Intramuscular or subcutaneous MTX (25 mg/week) is effective in inducing remission and reducing glucocorticoid dosage; 15 mg/week is effective in maintaining remission in active CD. Potential toxicities include leukopenia and hepatic fibrosis, necessitating periodic evaluation of CBCs and liver enzymes. The role of liver biopsy in patients on long-term MTX is uncertain. Hypersensitivity pneumonitis is a rare but serious complication of therapy.

CYCLOSPORINE Cyclosporine (CSA) is a lipophilic peptide with inhibitory effects on both the cellular and humoral immune systems. CSA blocks the production of IL-2 by T-helper lymphocytes. CSA binds to cyclophilin, and this complex inhibits calcineurin, a cytoplasmic phosphatase enzyme involved in the activation of T cells. CSA also indirectly inhibits B cell function by blocking helper T cells. It has a more rapid onset of action than 6-MP and azathioprine.

CSA is most effective given at 2–4 mg/kg per day intravenously in severe UC that is refractory to intravenous glucocorticoids, with 82% of patients responding. CSA can be an alternative to colectomy. The long-term success of oral CSA is not as dramatic, but if patients are started on 6-MP or azathioprine at the time of hospital discharge, remission can be maintained. Intravenous CSA is effective in 80% of patients with refractory fistulas, but 6-MP or azathioprine must be used to maintain remission. Oral CSA alone is effective only at a higher dose (7.5 mg/kg per day) in active disease but is not effective in maintaining remission without 6-MP/azathioprine. For the 2 mg/kg dose, levels as measured by monoclonal radioimmunoassay or by the high performance liquid chromatography assay should be maintained between 150 and 350 ng/mL.

CSA may cause significant toxicity; renal function should be monitored frequently. Hypertension, gingival hyperplasia, hypertrichosis, paresthesias, tremors, headaches, and electrolyte abnormalities are common side effects. Creatinine elevation calls for dose reduction or discontinuation. Seizures may also complicate therapy, especially if the patient is hypomagnesemic or if serum cholesterol levels are <3.1 mmol/L (<120 mg/dL). Opportunistic infections, most notably *Pneumocystis carinii* pneumonia, may occur with combination immunosuppressive treatment; prophylaxis should be given.

TACROLIMUS Tacrolimus is a macrolide antibiotic with immunomodulatory properties similar to CSA. It is 100 times as potent as CSA and is not dependent on bile or mucosal integrity for absorption. These pharmacologic properties enable tacrolimus to have good oral absorption despite proximal small-bowel Crohn's involvement. It has shown efficacy in children with refractory IBD and in adults with extensive involvement of the small bowel. It is also effective in adults with steroid-dependent or refractory UC and CD as well as refractory fistulizing CD.

ANTI-TNF ANTIBODY TNF is a key inflammatory cytokine and mediator of intestinal inflammation. The expression of TNF is increased in IBD. Infliximab is a chimeric mouse-human monoclonal antibody against TNF that is effective in CD. It blocks TNF in the serum and at the cell surface and probably lyses TNF-producing macrophages and T cells through complement fixation and antibody-dependent cytotoxicity. Of active CD patients refractory to glucocorticoids, 6-MP, or 5-ASA, 65% will respond to intravenous infliximab (5 mg/kg); one-third will enter complete remission. Of the patients who experience an initial response, 40% will maintain remission for at least 1 year with repeated infusions of infliximab every 8 weeks.

Infliximab is also effective in CD patients with refractory perianal and enterocutaneous fistulas, with a 68% response rate (50% reduction in fistula drainage) and a 50% complete remission rate. Reinfusion, typically every 8 weeks, is necessary to continue therapeutic benefits in many patients.

The development of antibodies to infliximab (ATI) is associated with an increased risk of infusion reactions and a decreased response to treatment. Patients who receive on-demand or episodic infusions rather than periodic (every 8 weeks) infusions are more likely to develop ATI. If infliximab is used episodically for flares, patients must use concomitant immunosuppression with AZA, 6-MP, or methotrexate in therapeutic doses to decrease the clinical consequences of immunogenicity of the chimeric antibodies. Moreover, prophylaxis with hydrocortisone before each infusion of infliximab will also decrease the formation of antibodies to infliximab. ATI are generally responsible when the quality of response or the response duration to infliximab infusion decreases. Increasing the dosage to 10 mg/kg may restore the efficacy of the drug.

In the CD and rheumatoid arthritis (RA) trials, six lymphomas were diagnosed in 4148 patient-years of follow-up versus none for 691 placebo patient-years. All lymphomas occurred in patients treated with concomitant immunosuppression. Other morbidities of infliximab include acute infusion reactions, severe serum sickness, and increased risk of infections, particularly reactivation of latent tuberculosis. Rarely, infliximab has been associated with optic neuritis, seizures, new-onset or exacerbation of clinical symptoms, and radiographic evidence of central nervous system demyelinating disorders, including multiple sclerosis. It may exacerbate symptoms in patients with New York Heart Association functional class III/IV heart failure.

Infliximab has also shown efficacy in UC. In two large randomized, placebo-controlled trials, 37–49% of patients responded to infliximab and 22 and 20% of patients were able to maintain remission after 30 and 54 weeks, respectively. Patients received infliximab at 0, 2, and 6 weeks and then every 8 weeks until the end of the study.

NUTRITIONAL THERAPIES Dietary antigens may stimulate the mucosal immune response. Patients with active CD respond to bowel rest, along with total parenteral nutrition or TPN. Bowel rest and TPN are as effective as glucocorticoids at inducing remission of active CD but are not effective as maintenance therapy. Enteral nutrition in the form of elemental or peptide-based preparations are also as effective as glucocorticoids or TPN, but these diets are not palatable. Enteral diets may provide the small intestine with nutrients vital to cell growth and do not have the complications of TPN. In contrast to CD, dietary intervention does not reduce inflammation in UC. Standard medical management of UC and CD is shown in **Fig. 16-9.**

NEWER IMMUNOSUPPRESSIVE AGENTS
Thalidomide has been shown to inhibit TNF production by monocytes and other cells. Thalidomide is effective in glucocorticoid-refractory and fistulous CD, but randomized controlled trials are needed.

Adalimumab is a recombinant human monoclonal IgG1 antibody containing only human peptide sequences and is injected subcutaneously. Adalimumab binds TNF-α and neutralizes its function by blocking the interaction between TNF and its cell-surface receptor. Therefore, it seems to have a similar mechanism of action to infliximab but with less immunogenicity. Adalimumab has recently been approved for treatment of

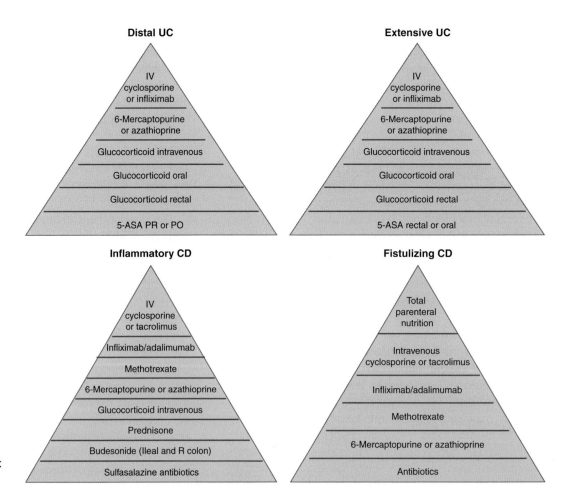

FIGURE 16-9
Medical management of IBD.

CD. It has shown promise in treating CD in several trials and may be useful in infliximab-allergic patients.

Certolizumab Pegol is a PEGylated form of an anti-TNF antibody administered subcutaneously once monthly. Subcutaneous Certolizumab Pegol was effective for induction of clinical response in patients with active inflammatory CD.

SURGICAL THERAPY

Ulcerative Colitis   Nearly half of patients with extensive chronic UC undergo surgery within the first 10 years of their illness. The indications for surgery are listed in Table 16-7. Morbidity is about 20% in elective, 30% for urgent, and 40% for emergency proctocolectomy. The risks are primarily hemorrhage, contamination and sepsis, and neural injury. The operation of choice is an IPAA.

Because UC is a mucosal disease, the rectal mucosa can be dissected and removed down to the dentate line of the anus or about 2 cm proximal to it. The ileum is fashioned into a pouch that serves as a neorectum. This ileal pouch is then sutured circumferentially to the anus in an end-to-end fashion. If performed carefully, this operation preserves the anal sphincter and maintains continence. The overall operative morbidity is 10%, with the major complication being bowel obstruction. Pouch failure necessitating conversion to permanent ileostomy occurs in 5–10% of patients. Some inflamed rectal mucosa is usually left behind, and thus endoscopic surveillance is necessary. Primary dysplasia of the ileal mucosa of the pouch has occurred rarely.

Patients with IPAAs usually have about six to eight bowel movements a day. On validated quality-of-life indices, they report better performance in sports and sexual activities than ileostomy patients. The most

TABLE 16-7

INDICATIONS FOR SURGERY	
ULCERATIVE COLITIS	**CROHN'S DISEASE**
Intractable disease	**Small intestine**
Fulminant disease	Stricture and obstruction
Toxic megacolon	unresponsive to medical
Colonic perforation	therapy
Massive colonic hemorrhage	Massive hemorrhage
Extracolonic disease	Refractory fistula
Colonic obstruction	Abscess
Colon cancer prophylaxis	**Colon and rectum**
Colon dysplasia or cancer	Intractable disease
	Fulminant disease
	Perianal disease
	unresponsive to medical
	therapy
	Refractory fistula
	Colonic obstruction
	Cancer prophylaxis
	Colon dysplasia or cancer

frequent late complication of IPAA is pouchitis in about one-third of patients with UC. This syndrome consists of increased stool frequency, watery stools, cramping, urgency, nocturnal leakage of stool, arthralgias, malaise, and fever. Pouch biopsies may distinguish true pouchitis from underlying CD. Although pouchitis usually responds to antibiotics, 3–5% of patients are refractory and require pouch take-down. A highly concentrated probiotic preparation with four strains of *Lactobacillus*, three strains of *Bifidobacterium*, and one strain of *Streptococcus salivarius* can prevent onset of pouchitis when taken daily.

Crohn's Disease   Most patients with CD require at least one operation in their lifetime. The need for surgery is related to duration of disease and the site of involvement. Patients with small-bowel disease have an 80% chance of requiring surgery. Those with colitis alone have a 50% chance. Surgery is an option only when medical treatment has failed or complications dictate its necessity. The indications for surgery are shown in Table 16-7.

Small Intestinal Disease   Because CD is chronic and recurrent, with no clear surgical cure, as little intestine as possible is resected. Current surgical alternatives for treatment of obstructing CD include resection of the diseased segment and strictureplasty. Surgical resection of the diseased segment is the most frequently performed operation, and in most cases primary anastomosis can be done to restore continuity. If much of the small bowel has already been resected and the strictures are short, with intervening areas of normal mucosa, strictureplasties should be done to avoid a functionally insufficient length of bowel. The strictured area of intestine is incised longitudinally and the incision sutured transversely, thus widening the narrowed area. Complications of strictureplasty include prolonged ileus, hemorrhage, fistula, abscess, leak, and restricture.

Colorectal Disease   A greater percentage of patients with Crohn's colitis require surgery for intractability, fulminant disease, and anorectal disease. Several alternatives are available, ranging from the use of a temporary loop ileostomy to resection of segments of diseased colon or even the entire colon and rectum. For patients with segmental involvement, segmental colon resection with primary anastomosis can be performed. In 20–25% of patients with extensive colitis, the rectum is spared sufficiently to consider rectal preservation. Most surgeons believe that an IPAA is contraindicated in CD due to the high incidence of pouch failure. A diverting colostomy may help heal severe perianal disease or rectovaginal fistulas, but disease almost always recurs with reanastomosis. These patients often require a total proctocolectomy and ileostomy.

INFLAMMATORY BOWEL DISEASE AND PREGNANCY

Patients with quiescent UC and CD have normal fertility rates; the fallopian tubes can be scarred by the inflammatory process of CD, especially on the right side because of the proximity of the terminal ileum. In addition, perirectal, perineal, and rectovaginal abscesses and fistulae can result in dyspareunia. Infertility in men can be caused by sulfasalazine but reverses when treatment is stopped.

In mild or quiescent UC and CD, fetal outcome is nearly normal. Spontaneous abortions, stillbirths, and developmental defects are increased with increased disease activity, not medications. The courses of CD and UC during pregnancy mostly correlate with disease activity at the time of conception. Patients should be in remission for 6 months before conceiving. Most CD patients can deliver vaginally, but cesarean section may be the preferred route of delivery for patients with anorectal and perirectal abscesses and fistulas to reduce the likelihood of fistulas developing or extending into the episiotomy scar.

Sulfasalazine, mesalamine, and balsalazide are safe for use in pregnancy and nursing, but additional folate supplementation must be given with sulfasalazine. Topical 5-ASA agents are also safe during pregnancy and nursing. Glucocorticoids are generally safe for use during pregnancy and are indicated for patients with moderate to severe disease activity. The amount of glucocorticoids received by the nursing infant is minimal. The safest antibiotics to use for CD in pregnancy for short periods of time (weeks, not months) are ampicillin and cephalosporin. Metronidazole can be used in the second or third trimester. Ciprofloxacin causes cartilage lesions in immature animals and should be avoided because of the absence of data on its effects on growth and development in humans.

6-MP and azathioprine pose minimal or no risk during pregnancy, but experience is limited. If the patient cannot be weaned from the drug or has an exacerbation that requires 6-MP/azathioprine during pregnancy, she should continue the drug with informed consent. Their effects during nursing are unknown.

Few data exist on CSA in pregnancy. In a small number of patients with severe IBD treated with intravenous CSA during pregnancy, 80% of pregnancies were successfully completed without development of renal toxicity, congenital malformations, or developmental defects. However, because of the lack of data, CSA should probably be avoided unless the patient would otherwise require surgery. Methotrexate is contraindicated in pregnancy and nursing. No increased risk of stillbirths, miscarriages, or spontaneous abortions has been seen with infliximab.

Surgery in UC should be performed only for emergency indications, including severe hemorrhage, perforation, and megacolon refractory to medical therapy. Total colectomy and ileostomy carry a 50–60% risk of postoperative spontaneous abortion. Fetal mortality is also high in CD requiring surgery. Patients with IPAAs have increased nighttime stool frequency during pregnancy that resolves postpartum. Transient small-bowel obstruction or ileus has been noted in up to 8% of patients with ileostomies.

CANCER IN INFLAMMATORY BOWEL DISEASE

ULCERATIVE COLITIS

Patients with long-standing UC are at increased risk for developing colonic epithelial dysplasia and carcinoma (Fig. 16-9).

The risk of neoplasia in chronic UC increases with duration and extent of disease. The risk of cancer rises 0.5–1% per year after 8–10 years of disease in patients with pancolitis. The only prospective surveillance study reported a lower rate of cancer; 2.5% at 20 years of disease, 7.6% at 30 years of disease, and 10.8% at 40 years. The rates of colon cancer are higher than in the general population, and colonoscopic surveillance is the standard of care.

Annual or biennial colonoscopy with multiple biopsies is recommended for patients with >8–10 years of pancolitis or 12–15 years of left-sided colitis and has been widely employed to screen and survey for subsequent dysplasia and carcinoma. Risk factors for cancer in UC include long-duration disease, extensive disease, family history of colon cancer, PSC, a colon stricture, and the presence of postinflammatory pseudopolyps on colonoscopy.

CROHN'S DISEASE

Risk factors for developing cancer in Crohn's colitis are long-duration and extensive disease, bypassed colon segments, colon strictures, PSC, and family history of colon cancer. The cancer risks in CD and UC are probably equivalent for similar extent and duration of disease. In patients with extensive Crohn's colitis, 22% developed dysplasia or cancer by the fourth surveillance exam after a negative screening colonoscopy. Thus, the same endoscopic surveillance strategy used for UC is recommended for patients with chronic Crohn's colitis. A pediatric colonoscope can be used to pass narrow strictures in CD patients, but surgery should be considered in symptomatic patients with impassable strictures.

MANAGEMENT OF DYSPLASIA AND CANCER

Dysplasia can be flat or polypoid. If flat high-grade dysplasia (HGD) is encountered on colonoscopic surveillance,

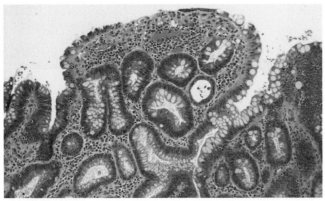

FIGURE 16-10
Medium power view of low-grade dysplasia in a patient with chronic ulcerative colitis. Low-grade dysplastic crypts are interspersed among regenerating crypts. *(Courtesy of Dr. R Odze, Division of Gastrointestinal Pathology, Department of Pathology, Brigham and Women's Hospital, Boston, Massachusetts; with permission.)*

the usual treatment for UC is colectomy and for CD is either colectomy or segmental resection. If flat low-grade dysplasia (LGD) is found (Fig. 16-10), most investigators recommend immediate colectomy. Adenomas may occur coincidently in UC and CD patients with chronic colitis and can be removed endoscopically provided that biopsies of the surrounding mucosa are free of dysplasia.

IBD patients are also at greater risk for other malignancies. Patients with CD may have an increased risk of non-Hodgkin's lymphoma, leukemia, and myelodysplastic syndromes. Severe chronic, complicated perianal disease in CD patients may be associated with an increased risk of cancer in the lower rectum and anal canal (squamous cell cancers). Although the absolute risk of small-bowel adenocarcinoma in CD is low (2.2% at 25 years in one study), patients with long-standing, extensive, small-bowel disease should undergo screening.

QUALITY OF LIFE IN INFLAMMATORY BOWEL DISEASE

The assessment of health-related quality of life plays an important role in the evaluation and treatment of IBD patients. Although clinical trials have generally relied upon traditional disease activity indices such as the Crohn's Disease Activity Index to measure therapeutic

efficacy, these measures do not reflect quality of life. The Inflammatory Bowel Disease Questionnaire is a validated, disease-specific instrument that has been used to measure quality of life. It is a 32-item questionnaire that measures global function, systemic and bowel symptoms, functional and social impairment, and emotional function. When compared to the general population, IBD patients have an impaired quality of life in all six categories. The most frequent concerns of UC patients are having an ostomy bag, developing cancer, effects of medication, the uncertain nature of the disease, and having surgery. The most frequent concerns of CD patients are the uncertain nature of the disease, impaired energy level, effects of medication, the need for surgery, and having an ostomy bag.

FURTHER READINGS

ABREU MT et al: Mutations in NOD2 are associated with fibrostenosing disease in patients with Crohn's disease. Gastroenterology 123:679, 2002

ALLI T et al: Osteoporosis in inflammatory bowel disease. Am J Med 122:599, 2009

AUSTIN G et al: Positive and negative predictive values: Use of inflammatory bowel disease serologic markers. Am J Gastroenterology 101:413, 2006

BAUMGART DC, SANDBORN WJ: Inflammatory bowel disease: Clinical aspects and established and evolving therapies. Lancet 369:1641, 2007

EI-MATARY W et al: Methotrexate for maintenance of remission in ulcerative colitis. Cochrane Database Syst Rev 2009 Jul 8;(3):CD007560

GROSCHWITZ KR, HOGAN SP: Intestinal barrier function: molecular regulation and disease pathogenesis. J Allergy Clin Immunol 124:3, 2009

ITZKOWITZ S et al: Consensus conference: Colorectal cancer screening and surveillance in inflammatory bowel disease. Inflamm Bowel Dis 11:314, 2005

KORNBLUTH A et al: Ulcerative colitis practice guidelines in adults. Am J Gastroenterol 99:1371, 2004

LOFTUS EV: Clinical epidemiology of inflammatory bowel disease: Incidence, prevalence, and environmental influences. Gastroenterology 126:1504, 2004

MULHALL AM et al: Diverticular disease associated with inflammatory bowel disease-like colitis: a systematic review. Dis Colon Rectum 52:1072, 2009

RUTGEERTS P et al: Optimizing anti-TNF treatment in inflammatory bowel disease. Gastroenterology 126:1593, 2004

RUTTER MD et al: Thirty-year analysis of a colonoscopic surveillance program for neoplasia in ulcerative colitis. Gastroenterology 130:1030, 2006

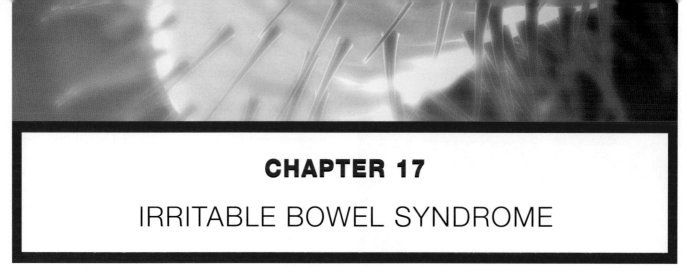

CHAPTER 17

IRRITABLE BOWEL SYNDROME

Chung Owyang

Irritable bowel syndrome (IBS) is a functional bowel disorder characterized by abdominal pain or discomfort and altered bowel habits in the absence of detectable structural abnormalities. No clear diagnostic markers exist for IBS; thus the diagnosis of the disorder is based on clinical presentation. In 2006, the Rome II criteria for the diagnosis of IBS were revised (Table 17-1). IBS is one of the most common conditions encountered in clinical practice but one of the least well understood. Throughout the world, about 10–20% of adults and adolescents have symptoms consistent with IBS, and most studies show a female predominance. IBS symptoms tend to come and go over time and often overlap with other functional disorders such as fibromyalgia, headache, backache, and genitourinary symptoms.

Severity of symptoms varies and can significantly impair quality of life, resulting in high health care costs. Advances in basic, mechanistic, and clinical investigations have improved our understanding of this disorder and its physiologic and psychosocial determinants. Altered gastrointestinal (GI) motility, visceral hyperalgesia, disturbance of brain–gut interaction, abnormal central processing, autonomic and hormonal events, genetic and environmental factors, and psychosocial disturbances are variably involved, depending on the individual. This progress may result in improved methods of treatment.

CLINICAL FEATURES

IBS is a disorder that affects all ages, although most patients have their first symptoms before age 45. Older individuals have a lower reporting frequency. Women are diagnosed with IBS two to three times as often as men and make up 80% of the population with severe IBS. As indicated in Table 17-1, pain or abdominal discomfort is a key symptom for the diagnosis of IBS. These symptoms should be improved with defecation and/or have their onset associated with a change in frequency or form of stool. Painless diarrhea or constipation does not fulfill the diagnostic criteria to be classified as IBS. Supportive symptoms that are not part of the diagnostic criteria include defecation straining, urgency or a feeling of incomplete bowel movement, passing mucus, and bloating.

Abdominal Pain

According to the current IBS diagnostic criteria, abdominal pain or discomfort is a prerequisite clinical

TABLE 17-1

DIAGNOSTIC CRITERIA FOR IRRITABLE BOWEL SYNDROME[a]

Recurrent abdominal pain or discomfort[b] at least 3 days per month in the last 3 months associated with *two or more* of the following:
  1. Improvement with defecation
  2. Onset associated with a change in frequency of stool
  3. Onset associated with a change in form (appearance) of stool

[a]Criteria fulfilled for the last 3 months with symptom onset at least 6 months prior to diagnosis.
[b]Discomfort means an uncomfortable sensation not described as pain. In pathophysiology research and clinical trials, a pain/discomfort frequency of at least 2 days a week during screening evaluation is required for subject eligibility.
Source: Adapted from Longstreth et al.

feature of IBS. Abdominal pain in IBS is highly variable in intensity and location. Pain in IBS is localized to the hypogastrium in 25%, the right side in 20%, to the left side in 20%, and the epigastrium in 10% of patients. It is frequently episodic and crampy, but it may be superimposed on a background of constant ache. Pain may be mild enough to be ignored or it may interfere with daily activities. Despite this, malnutrition due to inadequate caloric intake is exceedingly rare with IBS. Sleep deprivation is also unusual because abdominal pain is almost uniformly present only during waking hours. However, patients with severe IBS frequently wake repeatedly during the night; thus, nocturnal pain is a poor discriminating factor between organic and functional bowel disease. Pain is often exacerbated by eating or emotional stress and improved by passage of flatus or stools. In addition, female patients with IBS commonly report worsening symptoms during the premenstrual and menstrual phases.

Altered Bowel Habits

Alteration in bowel habits is the most consistent clinical feature in IBS. The most common pattern is constipation alternating with diarrhea, usually with one of these symptoms predominating. At first, constipation may be episodic, but eventually it becomes continuous and increasingly intractable to treatment with laxatives. Stools are usually hard with narrowed caliber, possibly reflecting excessive dehydration caused by prolonged colonic retention and spasm. Most patients also experience a sense of incomplete evacuation, thus leading to repeated attempts at defecation in a short time span. Patients whose predominant symptom is constipation may have weeks or months of constipation interrupted with brief periods of diarrhea. In other patients, diarrhea may be the predominant symptom. Diarrhea resulting from IBS usually consists of small volumes of loose stools. Most patients have stool volumes of <200 mL. Nocturnal diarrhea does not occur in IBS. Diarrhea may be aggravated by emotional stress or eating. Stool may be accompanied by passage of large amounts of mucus; hence, the term *mucous colitis* has been used to describe IBS. This is a misnomer, since inflammation is not present. Bleeding is not a feature of IBS unless hemorrhoids are present, and malabsorption or weight loss does not occur.

Bowel pattern subtypes are highly unstable. In a patient population with ~33% prevalence rates of IBS-diarrhea predominant (IBS-D), IBS-constipation predominant (IBS-C), and IBS-mixed (IBS-M) forms, 75% of patients change subtypes and 29% switch between IBS-C and IBS-D over 1 year. The heterogeneity and variable natural history of bowel habits in IBS increase the difficulty of conducting pathophysiology studies and clinical trials.

Gas and Flatulence

Patients with IBS frequently complain of abdominal distention and increased belching or flatulence, all of which they attribute to increased gas. Although some patients with these symptoms actually may have a larger amount of gas, quantitative measurements reveal that most patients who complain of increased gas generate no more than a normal amount of intestinal gas. Most IBS patients have impaired transit and tolerance of intestinal gas loads. In addition, patients with IBS tend to reflux gas from the distal to the more proximal intestine, which may explain the belching.

Upper Gastrointestinal Symptoms

Between 25 and 50% of patients with IBS complain of dyspepsia, heartburn, nausea, and vomiting. This suggests that other areas of the gut apart from the colon may be involved. Prolonged ambulant recordings of small-bowel motility in patients with IBS show a high incidence of abnormalities in the small bowel during the diurnal (waking) period; nocturnal motor patterns are not different from those of healthy controls. The overlap between dyspepsia and IBS is great. The prevalence of IBS is higher among patients with dyspepsia (31.7%) than among those who reported no symptoms of dyspepsia (7.9%). Conversely, among patients with IBS, 55.6% reported symptoms of dyspepsia. In addition the functional abdominal symptoms can change over time. Those with predominant dyspepsia or IBS can flux between the two. Thus it is conceivable that functional dyspepsia and IBS are two manifestations of a single, more extensive digestive system disorder. Furthermore, IBS symptoms are prevalent in noncardiac chest pain patients, suggesting overlap with other functional gut disorders.

PATHOPHYSIOLOGY

The pathogenesis of IBS is poorly understood, although roles of abnormal gut motor and sensory activity, central neural dysfunction, psychological disturbances, stress, and luminal factors have been proposed.

Studies of colonic myoelectrical and motor activity under unstimulated conditions have not shown consistent abnormalities in IBS. In contrast, colonic motor abnormalities are more prominent under stimulated conditions in IBS. IBS patients may exhibit increased rectosigmoid motor activity for up to 3 h after eating. Similarly, inflation of rectal balloons both in IBS-D and IBS-C patients leads to marked distention-evoked contractile activity, which may be prolonged. Recordings from the transverse, descending, and sigmoid colon showed that the motility index and peak amplitude of high-amplitude propagating contractions (HAPCs) in diarrhea-prone IBS patients were greatly increased compared to those in healthy subjects and were associated with rapid colonic transit and accompanied by abdominal pain.

As with studies of motor activity, IBS patients frequently exhibit exaggerated sensory responses to visceral stimulation. Postprandial pain has been temporally related to entry of the food bolus into the cecum in 74% of patients. Rectal balloon inflation produces nonpainful and painful sensations at lower volumes in IBS patients than in healthy controls without altering rectal tension, suggestive of visceral afferent dysfunction in IBS. Similar studies show gastric and esophageal hypersensitivity in patients with nonulcer dyspepsia and noncardiac chest pain, raising the possibility that these conditions have a similar pathophysiologic basis. Lipids lower the thresholds for the first sensation of gas, discomfort, and pain in IBS patients. Furthermore, IBS patients have an increased area of referred pain after lipid ingestion that was not observed in healthy individuals. Hence, postprandial symptoms in IBS patients may be explained in part by a nutrient-dependent exaggerated sensory component of the gastrocolonic response. In contrast to enhanced gut sensitivity, IBS patients do not exhibit heightened sensitivity elsewhere in the body. Thus, the afferent pathway disturbances in IBS appear to be selective for visceral innervation with sparing of somatic pathways. The mechanisms responsible for visceral hypersensitivity are still under investigation. It has been proposed that these exaggerated responses may be due to: (1) increased end-organ sensitivity with recruitment of "silent" nociceptors; (2) spinal hyperexcitability with activation of nitric oxide and possibly other neurotransmitters; (3) endogenous (cortical and brainstem) modulation of caudad nociceptive transmission; and (4) over time, the possible development of long-term hyperalgesia due to development of neuroplasticity, resulting in permanent or semipermanent changes in neural responses to chronic or recurrent visceral stimulation (Table 17–2).

The role of central nervous system (CNS) factors in the pathogenesis of IBS is strongly suggested by the clinical association of emotional disorders and stress with symptom exacerbation and the therapeutic response to therapies that act on cerebral cortical sites. Functional brain imaging studies such as MRI have shown that in response to distal colonic stimulation, the mid-cingulate cortex, a brain region concerned with attention processes and response selection, shows greater activation in IBS patients. Modulation of this region is associated with changes in the subjective unpleasantness of pain. In addition, IBS patients also show preferential activation of the prefrontal lobe, which contains a vigilance network within the brain that increases alertness. These may represent a form of cerebral dysfunction leading to the increased perception of visceral pain.

Abnormal psychiatric features are recorded in up to 80% of IBS patients, especially in referral centers; however, no single psychiatric diagnosis predominates. Most of these patients demonstrated exaggerated symptoms in response to visceral distention, and this abnormality persists even after exclusion of psychological factors. Psychological factors influence pain thresholds in IBS patients, as stress alters sensory thresholds. An association between prior sexual or physical abuse and development of IBS has been reported. The pathophysiologic relationship between IBS and sexual or physical abuse is unknown. Sexual abuse is not associated with lower pain threshold in IBS patients.

Thus, patients with IBS frequently demonstrate increased motor reactivity of the colon and small bowel to a variety of stimuli and altered visceral sensation associated with lowered sensation thresholds. These may result from CNS–enteric nervous system dysregulation (Fig. 17-1).

IBS may be induced by GI infection. In an investigation of 544 patients with confirmed bacterial gastroenteritis,

TABLE 17-2

PROPOSED MECHANISMS FOR VISCERAL HYPERSENSITIVITY	
End-organ sensitivity	Long-term hyperalgesia
"Silent" nociceptors	Tonic cortical regulation
CNS modulation	Neuroplasticity
Cortex	
Brainstem	

Note: CNS, central nervous system.

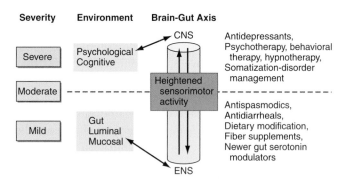

FIGURE 17-1

Therapeutic targets for irritable bowel syndrome. Patients with mild to moderate symptoms usually have intermittent symptoms that correlate with altered gut physiology. Treatments include gut-acting pharmacologic agents such as antispasmodics, antidiarrheals, fiber supplements, and gut serotonin modulators. Patients who have severe symptoms usually have constant pain and psychosocial difficulties. This group of patients is best managed with antidepressants and other psychosocial treatments. CNS, central nervous system; ENS, enteric nervous system.

one-quarter developed IBS subsequently. Conversely, about one-third of IBS patients experienced an acute "gastroenteritis-like" illness at the onset of their chronic IBS symptomatology. This group of "postinfective" IBS occurs more commonly in females and affects younger rather than older patients and those who have a protracted acute diarrheal illness. The microbes involved in the initial infection are *Campylobacter*, *Salmonella*, and *Shigella*. Those patients with *Campylobacter* infection who are toxin-positive are more likely to develop postinfective IBS. Increased rectal mucosal enteroendocrine cells, T lymphocytes, and increased gut permeability are acute changes following *Campylobacter* enteritis that could persist for more than a year and may contribute to postinfective IBS.

The serotonin (5HT)-containing enterochromaffin cells in the colon are increased in a subset of IBS-D patients compared to healthy individuals or patients with ulcerative colitis. Furthermore, postprandial plasma 5HT plasma levels were significantly higher in this group of patients compared to healthy controls. Since serotonin plays an important role in the regulation of GI motility and visceral perception, the increased release of serotonin may contribute to the postprandial symptoms of these patients and provides a rationale for the use of serotonin antagonists in the treatment of this disorder.

Approach to the Patient:
IRRITABLE BOWEL SYNDROME

Because IBS is a disorder for which no pathognomonic abnormalities have been identified, its diagnosis relies on recognition of positive clinical features and elimination of other organic diseases. A careful history and physical examination are frequently helpful in establishing the diagnosis. Clinical features suggestive of IBS include the following: recurrence of lower abdominal pain with altered bowel habits over a period of time without progressive deterioration, onset of symptoms during periods of stress or emotional upset, absence of other systemic symptoms such as fever and weight loss, and small-volume stool without any evidence of blood.

On the other hand, the appearance of the disorder for the first time in old age, progressive course from time of onset, persistent diarrhea after a 48-h fast, and presence of nocturnal diarrhea or steatorrheal stools argue against the diagnosis of IBS.

Because the major symptoms of IBS—abdominal pain, abdominal bloating, and alteration in bowel habits—are common complaints of many GI organic disorders, the list of differential diagnoses is a long one. The quality, location, and timing of pain may be helpful to suggest specific disorders. Pain due to IBS that occurs in the epigastric or periumbilical area must be differentiated from biliary tract disease, peptic ulcer disorders, intestinal ischemia, and carcinoma of the stomach and pancreas. If pain occurs mainly in the lower abdomen, the possibility of diverticular disease of the colon, inflammatory bowel disease (including ulcerative colitis and Crohn's disease), and carcinoma of the colon must be considered. Postprandial pain accompanied by bloating, nausea, and vomiting suggests gastroparesis or partial intestinal obstruction. Intestinal infestation with *Giardia lamblia* or other parasites may cause similar symptoms. When diarrhea is the major complaint, the possibility of lactase deficiency, laxative abuse, malabsorption, celiac sprue, hyperthyroidism, inflammatory bowel disease, and infectious diarrhea must be ruled out. On the other hand, constipation may be a side effect of many different drugs, such as anticholinergic, antihypertensive, and antidepressant medications. Endocrinopathies such as hypothyroidism and hypoparathyroidism must also be considered in the differential diagnosis of constipation, particularly if other systemic signs or symptoms of these endocrinopathies are present. In addition, acute intermittent porphyria and lead poisoning may present in a fashion similar to IBS, with painful constipation as the major complaint. These possibilities are suspected on the basis of their clinical presentations and are confirmed by appropriate serum and urine tests.

Few tests are required for patients who have typical IBS symptoms and no alarm features. Unnecessary investigations may be costly and even harmful. The American Gastroenterological Association has delineated factors to be considered when determining the aggressiveness of the diagnostic evaluation. These include the duration of symptoms, the change in symptoms over time, the age and sex of the patient, the referral status of the patient, prior diagnostic studies, a family history of colorectal malignancy, and the degree of psychosocial dysfunction. Thus, a younger individual with mild symptoms requires a minimal diagnostic evaluation, while an older person or an individual with rapidly progressive symptoms should undergo a more thorough exclusion of organic disease. Most patients should have a complete blood count and sigmoidoscopic examination; in addition, stool specimens should be examined for ova and parasites in those who have diarrhea. In those >40 years, an air-contrast barium enema or colonoscopy should also be performed. If the main symptoms are diarrhea and increased gas, the possibility of lactase deficiency should be ruled out with a hydrogen breath test or with evaluation after a 3-week lactose-free diet. Some patients with IBS-D may have undiagnosed celiac sprue. Because the symptoms of celiac sprue respond to a gluten-free diet, testing for celiac sprue in IBS may prevent years of morbidity and attendant expense. Decision-analysis studies show that serology testing for celiac sprue in patients with IBS-D has an acceptable cost when the prevalence of celiac sprue is >1% and is the dominant strategy when the prevalence is >8%. In patients with concurrent symptoms of dyspepsia, upper GI radiographs or esophagogastroduo-denoscopy may be advisable. In patients with post-prandial right upper quadrant pain, an ultrasonogram of the gallbladder should be obtained. Laboratory features that argue against IBS include evidence of anemia, elevated sedimentation rate, presence of leukocytes or blood in stool, and stool volume >200–300 mL/d. These findings would necessitate other diagnostic considerations.

R︁x Treatment:
IRRITABLE BOWEL SYNDROME

PATIENT COUNSELING AND DIETARY ALTERATIONS Reassurance and careful explanation of the functional nature of the disorder and of how to avoid obvious food precipitants are important first steps in patient counseling and dietary change. Occasionally, a meticulous dietary history may reveal substances (such as coffee, disaccharides, legumes, and cabbage) that aggravate symptoms. Excessive fructose and artificial sweeteners, such as sorbitol or mannitol, may cause diarrhea, bloating, cramping or flatulence. As a therapeutic trial, patients should be encouraged to eliminate any foodstuffs that appear to produce symptoms. However patients should avoid nutritionally depleted diets.

STOOL-BULKING AGENTS High-fiber diets and bulking agents, such as bran or hydrophilic colloid, are frequently used in treating IBS. Studies suggest that dietary fiber has multiple effects on colonic physiology. The water-holding action of fibers may contribute to increased stool bulk because of the ability of fiber to increase fecal output of bacteria. Fiber also speeds up colonic transit in most persons. In diarrhea-prone patients, whole-colonic transit is faster than average; however, dietary fiber can delay transit. Furthermore, because of their hydrophilic properties, stool-bulking agents bind water and thus prevent both excessive hydration or dehydration of stool. The latter observation may explain the clinical experience that a high-fiber diet relieves diarrhea in some IBS patients. More recently, fiber supplementation with psyllium has been shown to reduce perception of rectal distention, indicating that fiber may have positive affect on visceral afferent function.

The beneficial effects of dietary fiber on colonic physiology suggest that dietary fiber should be an effective treatment for IBS patients, but controlled trials of dietary fiber have produced variable results. This is not surprising since IBS is a heterogeneous disorder, with some patients being constipated and other having predominant diarrhea. Most investigations report increases in stool weight, decreases in colonic transit times, and improvement in constipation. Others have noted benefits in patients with alternating diarrhea and constipation, pain, and bloating. However, most studies observe no responses in patients with diarrhea- or pain-predominant IBS. It is possible that different fiber preparations may have dissimilar effects on selected symptoms in IBS. A cross-over comparison of different fiber preparations found that psyllium produced greater improvements in stool pattern and abdominal pain than bran. Furthermore psyllium preparations tend to produce less bloating and distention. Despite the equivocal data regarding efficacy, most gastroenterologists consider stool-bulking agents worth trying in patients with IBS-C.

ANTISPASMODIC Clinicians have observed that anticholinergic drugs may provide temporary relief for symptoms such as painful cramps related to intestinal spasm. Although controlled clinical trials have produced mixed results, evidence generally supports beneficial effects of anticholinergic drugs for pain. A meta-analysis of 26 double-blind clinical trials of antispasmodic agents in IBS reported better global improvement (62%) and abdominal pain reductions (64%) compared to placebo (35% and 45%, respectively), suggesting efficacy in some patients. The drugs are most effective when prescribed in anticipation of predictable pain. Physiologic studies demonstrate that anticholinergic drugs inhibit the gastrocolic reflex; hence, postprandial pain is best managed by giving antispasmodics 30 min before meals so that effective blood levels are achieved shortly before the anticipated onset of pain. Most anticholinergics contain natural belladonna alkaloids, which may cause xerostomia, urinary hesitancy and retention, blurred vision, and drowsiness. They should be used in the elderly with caution. Some physicians prefer to use synthetic anticholinergics such as dicyclomine that have less effect on mucous membrane secretions and produce fewer undesirable side effects.

ANTIDIARRHEAL AGENTS Peripherally acting opiate-based agents are the initial therapy of choice for IBS-D. Physiologic studies demonstrate increases in segmenting colonic contractions, delays in fecal transit, increases in anal pressures, and reductions in rectal perception with these drugs. When diarrhea is severe, especially in the painless diarrhea variant of IBS, small doses of loperamide, 2–4 mg every 4–6 h up to a maximum of 12 g/d, can be prescribed. These agents are less addictive than paregoric, codeine, or tincture of opium. In general, the intestines do not become tolerant of the antidiarrheal effect of opiates, and increasing doses are not required to maintain antidiarrheal potency. These agents are most useful if taken before anticipated stressful events that are known to cause diarrhea. Another anti-diarrhea agent that may be used in IBS patients is the bile acid binder cholestyramine resin.

ANTIDEPRESSANT DRUG In addition to their mood-elevating effects, antidepressant medications have several physiologic effects that suggest they may be beneficial in IBS. In IBS-D patients, the tricyclic antidepressant imipramine slows jejunal migrating motor complex transit propagation and delays orocecal and whole-gut transit, indicative of a motor inhibitory effect. Some studies also suggest that tricyclic agents may alter visceral afferent neural function.

A number of studies indicate that tricyclic antidepressants may be effective in some IBS patients. In a 2-month study of desipramine, abdominal pain improved in 86% of patients compared to 59% given placebo. Another study of desipramine in 28 IBS patients showed improvement in stool frequency, diarrhea, pain, and depression. When stratified according to the predominant symptoms, improvements were observed in IBS-D patients with no improvement being noted in IBS-C patients. The beneficial effects of the tricyclic compounds in the treatment of IBS appear to be independent of their effects on depression. The therapeutic benefits for the bowel symptoms occur faster and at a lower dosage. The efficacy of antidepressant agents in other chemical classes in the management of IBS is less well-evaluated. In contrast to tricyclic agents, the selective serotonin reuptake inhibitor (SSRI) paroxetine accelerates orocecal transit, raising the possibility that this drug class may be useful in IBS-C patients. The SSRI citalopram blunts perception of rectal distention and reduces the magnitude of the gastrocolonic response in healthy volunteers. A small placebo-controlled study of citalopram in IBS patients reported reductions in pain. Mianserin, with serotonin 5-HT2 and 5-HT3 receptor antagonist and α_2-adrenoceptor antagonist effects, reduced pain, distress, and functional disability compared to placebo. Despite these preliminary results, the efficacy of SSRIs in the treatment of IBS needs further confirmation.

ANTIFLATULENCE THERAPY The management of excessive gas is seldom satisfactory, except when there is obvious aerophagia or disaccharidase deficiency. Patients should be advised to eat slowly and not chew gum or drink carbonated beverages. Bloating may decrease if an associated gut syndrome such as IBS or constipation is improved. If bloating is accompanied by diarrhea and worsens after ingesting dairy products, fresh fruits, vegetables, or juices, further investigation or a dietary exclusion trial may be worthwhile. Avoiding

flatogenic foods, exercising, losing excess weight, and taking activated charcoal are safe but unproven remedies. Data regarding the use of surfactants such as simethicone are conflicting. Antibiotics are unlikely to help, but trials of probiotics are encouraging. Beano, an over-the-counter oral β-glycosidase solution, may reduce rectal passage of gas without decreasing bloating and pain. Pancreatic enzymes reduce bloating, gas, and fullness during and after high-calorie, high-fat meal ingestion. Tegaserod improves bloating in some constipated female IBS patients.

SEROTONIN RECEPTOR AGONIST AND ANTAGONISTS Serotonin receptor antagonists have been evaluated as therapies for IBS-D. Serotonin acting on 5-HT3 receptors enhances the sensitivity of afferent neurons projecting from the gut. In humans, a 5-HT3 receptor antagonist such as alosetron reduces perception of painful visceral stimulation in IBS. It also induces rectal relaxation, increases rectal compliance, and delays colonic transit. Large, 12-week placebo-controlled trials of alosetron reported reductions in discomfort and improvements in stool frequency, consistency, and urgency in nonconstipated IBS patients. A follow-up 48-week study confirmed the long-term efficacy of alosetron. For unclear reasons, women with IBS derived greater benefit than men. However, in postrelease surveillance, 84 cases of ischemic colitis were observed, including 44 cases that required surgery and 4 deaths. As a consequence, the medication was voluntarily withdrawn by the manufacturer in 2000. Alosetron has been reintroduced under a new risk-management program where patients have to sign a patient-physician agreement. This has significantly limited its usage.

Novel 5-HT4 receptor agonists such as tegaserod exhibit prokinetic activity by stimulating peristalsis. In IBS patients with constipation, tegaserod accelerated intestinal and ascending colon transit. Clinical trials involving >4000 IBS-C patients reported reductions in discomfort and improvements in constipation and bloating, compared to placebo. Diarrhea is the major side effect. However, tegaserod has been withdrawn from the market; a meta-analysis revealed an increase in serious cardiovascular events.

CHLORIDE CHANNEL ACTIVATORS Lubiprostone is a bicyclic fatty acid that stimulates chloride channels in the apical membrane of intestinal epithelial cells. Chloride secretion induces passive movement of sodium and water into the bowel lumen and improves bowel function. The major side effects are nausea and diarrhea. Lubiprostone is a new class of compounds for treatment of chronic constipation with or without IBS.

SUMMARY The treatment strategy of IBS depends on the severity of the disorder (Table 17-3). Most of the IBS patients have mild symptoms. They are usually cared for in

TABLE 17-3

SPECTRUM OF SEVERITY IN IBS

	MILD	MODERATE	SEVERE
Clinical features			
Prevalence	70%	25%	5%
Correlations with gut physiology	+++	++	+
Symptoms constant	0	+	+++
Psychosocial difficulties	0	+	+++
Health care issues	+	++	+++
Practice type	Primary	Specialty	Referral

primary care practices, have little or no psychosocial difficulties, and do not seek health care often. Treatment usually involves education, reassurance, and dietary/lifestyle changes. A smaller portion have moderate symptoms that are usually intermittent and correlate with altered gut physiology, e.g., worsened with eating or stress and relieved by defecation. Treatments include gut-acting pharmacologic agents such as antispasmodics, antidiarrheals, fiber supplements, and the newer gut serotonin modulators (Table 17-4). A small proportion of IBS patients have severe and refractory symptoms, are usually seen in referral centers, and frequently have constant pain and psychosocial difficulties (Fig. 17-1). This group of patients is best managed with antidepressants and other psychological treatments (Table 17-4).

FURTHER READINGS

AMERICAN COLLEGE OF GASTROENTEROLOGY TASK FORCE ON IRRITABLE BOWEL SYNDROME: An evidence-based position statement on the management of irritable bowel syndrome. Am J Gastroenterol 104(suppl 1):S1, 2009

DROSSMAN DA et al: AGA technical review on irritable bowel syndrome. Gastroenterology 123:2108, 2002

FORD AC et al: Efficacy of 5-HT3 antagonists and 5-HT4 agonists in irritable bowel syndrome: systematic review and meta-analysis. Am J Gastroenterol 104:1831, 2009

GERSHON MD, JACK J: The serotonin signaling system: From basic understanding to drug development for functional GI disorders. Gastroenterology 132:397, 2007

LONGSTRETH GF et al: Functional bowel disorders. Gastroenterology 130:1480, 2006

MAYER EA et al: Neuroimaging of the brain-gut axis: From basic understanding to treatment of functional GI disorders. Gastroenterology 131:1925, 2006

MERTZ H: Irritable bowel syndrome. N Engl J Med 349:2136, 2003

OWYANG C: Irritable bowel syndrome, in *Textbook of Gastroenterology*, 4th ed, T Yamada (ed). Philadelphia, Lippincott Williams and Wilkins, 2003, pp 1817–42

PREIDIS GA, Versalovic J: Targeting the human microbiome with antibiotics, probiotics, and prebiotics: gastroenterology enters the metagenomics era. Gastroenterology 136:2015, 2009

SPIEGEL BM et al: Testing for celiac sprue in irritable bowel syndrome with predominant diarrhea: A cost effectiveness analysis. Gastroenterology 126:1721, 2004

SPILLER R, GARSED K: Postinfectious irritable bowel syndrome. Gastroenterology 136:1979, 2009

TALLEY NJ: Evaluation of drug treatment for irritable bowel syndrome. Br J Clin Pharmacol 56:362, 2003

TABLE 17-4

POSSIBLE DRUGS FOR A DOMINANT SYMPTOM IN IBS

SYMPTOM	DRUG	DOSE
Diarrhea	Loperamide	2–4 mg when necessary/maximum 12 g/d
	Cholestyramine resin	4 g with meals
	Alosetron[a]	0.5–1 mg bid (for severe IBS, women)
Constipation	Psyllium husk	3–4 g bid with meals, then adjust
	Methylcellulose	2 g bid with meals, then adjust
	Calcium polycarbophil	1 g qd to qid
	Lactulose syrup	10–20 g bid
	70% sorbitol	15 mL bid
	Polyethylene glycol 3350	17 g in 250 mL water qd
	Lubiprostone (Amitiza)	24 mg bid
	Magnesium hydroxide	30–60 mL qd
Abdominal pain	Smooth-muscle relaxant	qd to qid ac
	Tricyclic antidepressants	Start 25–50 mg hs, then adjust
	Selective serotonin reuptake inhibitors	Begin small dose, increase as needed

[a]Available only in the United States.
Source: Adapted from Longstreth GF et al.

CHAPTER 18

DIVERTICULAR DISEASE AND COMMON ANORECTAL DISORDERS

Susan L. Gearhart

DIVERTICULAR DISEASE

Incidence and Epidemiology

Among western populations, diverticulosis of the colon affects nearly one-half of individuals over age 60. Fortunately, only 20% of patients with diverticulosis develop symptomatic disease. However, in the United States, diverticular disease results in >200,000 hospitalizations annually, making it the fifth most costly gastrointestinal disorder. The mean hospital stay is 9.7 days, with an average cost of $42,000 per patient. The mean age at presentation of the disease is 59 years. Although the prevalence among females and males is similar, males tend to present at a younger age. Diverticulosis is rare in underdeveloped countries, where diets include more fiber and roughage. However, shortly following migration to the United States, immigrants will develop diverticular disease at the same rate as U.S. natives.

Anatomy and Pathophysiology

Two types of diverticula occur in the intestine: true and false, or pseudodiverticula. A true diverticulum is a saclike herniation of the entire bowel wall, whereas a pseudodiverticulum involves only a protrusion of the mucosa through the muscularis propria of the colon (**Fig. 18-1**). The most common type of diverticulum affecting the colon is the pseudodiverticulum. The protrusion occurs at the point where the nutrient artery, or *vasa recti*, penetrates through the muscularis propria, resulting in a break in the integrity of the colonic wall. Diverticula commonly affect the sigmoid colon; only 5% of persons exhibit pancolonic diverticula. This anatomic restriction may be a result of the relative high-pressure zone within the muscular sigmoid colon. Thus, higher amplitude contractions combined with constipated, high-fat content stool within the sigmoid lumen results in the creation of these diverticula. *Diverticulitis*, or inflammation of a diverticulum, is related to the retention of particulate material within the diverticular sac and the formation of a fecalith. Consequently, the vasa recti is either compressed or eroded, leading to either perforation or bleeding.

Presentation, Evaluation, and Management of Diverticular Bleeding

Hemorrhage from a colonic diverticulum is the most common cause of hematochezia in patients >60 years, yet only 20% of patients with diverticulosis will have gastrointestinal bleeding. Patients at increased risk for bleeding tend to be hypertensive, have atherosclerosis,

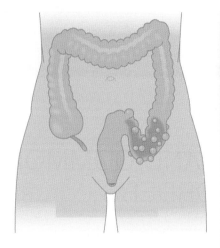
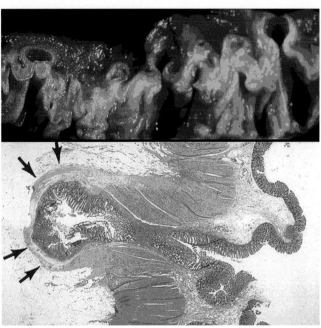

FIGURE 18-1

Gross and microscopic view of sigmoid diverticular disease. Arrows mark an inflamed diverticula with the diverticular wall made up only of mucosa.

and regularly use nonsteroidal anti-inflammatory agents. Most bleeds are self-limited and stop spontaneously with bowel rest. The lifetime risk of rebleeding is 25%.

Localization of diverticular bleeding should include colonoscopy, which may be both diagnostic and therapeutic in the management of mild to moderate diverticular bleeding. If the patient is stable, massive bleeding is best managed by angiography. Mesenteric angiography can localize the bleeding site and occlude the bleeding vessel successfully with a coil in 80% of cases. The patient can then be followed closely with repetitive colonoscopy, if necessary, looking for evidence of colonic ischemia. Alternatively, a segmental resection of the colon can be undertaken to eliminate the risk of further bleeding. This may be advantageous in patients on chronic blood thinners. However, with newer techniques of highly selective coil embolization, the rate of colonic ischemia is <10% and the risk of acute rebleeding is <25%. As another alternative, a selective infusion of vasopressin can be given to stop the hemorrhage, although this has been associated with significant complications, including myocardial infarction and intestinal ischemia. Furthermore, bleeding recurs in 50% of patients once the infusion is stopped. Localization studies indicate that bleeding as a result of colonic diverticulosis is more often seen from the right colon. For this reason, patients with presumed bleeding from diverticular disease requiring emergent surgery without localization should undergo a total abdominal colectomy. If the patient is unstable or has had a 6-unit bleed within 24 h, current recommendations are that surgery should be performed. In patients without severe comorbidities,

surgical resection can be performed with a primary anastomosis. A higher anastomotic leak rate has been reported in patients who received >10 units of blood.

Presentation, Evaluation, and Staging of Diverticulitis

Acute uncomplicated diverticulitis characteristically presents with fever, anorexia, left lower quadrant abdominal pain, and obstipation (Table 18-1). In <25% of cases, patients may present with generalized peritonitis indicating the presence of a diverticular perforation. On examination, the patient may have abdominal distention and signs of localized or generalized peritonitis. Laboratory investigations will demonstrate a leukocytosis. Rarely, a patient may present with an air-fluid level in the left lower quadrant on plain abdominal film. This is a

TABLE 18-1

PRESENTATION OF DIVERTICULAR DISEASE
Uncomplicated Diverticular Disease—75%
Abdominal pain
Fever
Leukocytosis
Anorexia/obstipation
Complicated Diverticular Disease—25%
Abscess 16%
Perforation 10%
Stricture 5%
Fistula 2%

giant diverticulum of the sigmoid colon and is managed with resection to avoid impending perforation.

The diagnosis of diverticulitis is best made on CT with the following findings: sigmoid diverticula, thickened colonic wall >4 mm, and inflammation within the pericolic fat ± the collection of contrast material or fluid. In 16% of patients, an abdominal abscess may be present. Symptoms of irritable bowel syndrome (IBS) may mimic those of diverticulitis. Therefore, suspected diverticulitis that does not meet CT criteria or is not associated with a leukocytosis or fever is not diverticular disease. Other conditions that can mimic diverticular disease include an ovarian cyst, endometriosis, acute appendicitis, and pelvic inflammatory disease.

Barium enema or colonoscopy should not be performed in the acute setting because of the higher risk of colonic perforation associated with insufflation or insertion of barium-based contrast material under pressure. A sigmoid malignancy can masquerade as diverticular disease. Therefore, a barium enema or colonoscopy should be performed ~6 weeks after an attack of diverticular disease.

Complicated diverticular disease is defined as diverticular disease associated with an abscess or perforation and less commonly with a fistula (Table 18-1). Perforated diverticular disease is staged using the Hinchey classification system (**Fig. 18-2**). This staging system was developed to predict outcomes following the surgical management of complicated diverticular disease. In complicated diverticular disease with fistula formation, common locations include cutaneous, vaginal, or vesicle fistulae. These conditions present with either passage of stool through the skin or vagina or the presence of air in the urinary stream (pneumaturia). Colovaginal fistulae are more common in women who have undergone a hysterectomy.

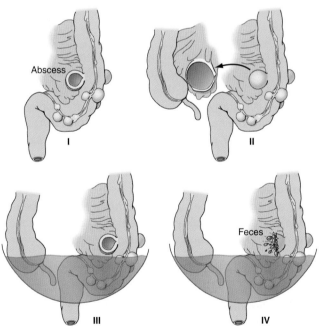

FIGURE 18-2

Hinchey classification of diverticulitis. Stage I: perforated diverticulitis with a confined paracolic abscess. Stage II: perforated diverticulitis that has closed spontaneously with distant abscess formation. Stage III: noncommunicating perforated diverticulitis with fecal peritonitis (the diverticular neck is closed off and therefore contrast will not freely expel on radiographic images). Stage IV: perforation and free communication with the peritoneum, resulting in fecal peritonitis.

℞ Treatment: DIVERTICULAR DISEASE

MEDICAL MANAGEMENT Asymptomatic diverticular disease discovered on imaging studies or at the time of colonoscopy is best managed by diet alterations. Patients should be instructed to eat a fiber-enriched diet that includes 30 g of fiber each day. Supplementary fiber products such as Metamucil, Fibercon, or Citrucel are useful. The patient should also be instructed to avoid nuts and popcorn, which may obstruct the lumen of a diverticulum.

Symptomatic diverticular disease, defined as radiographic and hematologic confirmation of inflammation and infection within the colon, should be treated initially with antibiotics and bowel rest. Nearly 75% of patients hospitalized for acute diverticulitis will respond to nonoperative treatment with a suitable antimicrobial regimen. The current recommended antimicrobial coverage is trimethoprim/sulfamethoxazole or ciprofloxacin and metronidazole targeting aerobic gram-negative rods and anaerobic bacteria. Unfortunately, these agents do not cover enterococci, and the addition of ampicillin to this regimen for nonresponders is recommended. Alternatively, single-agent therapy with a third-generation penicillin such as IV piperacillin or oral penicillin/clavulanic acid may be effective. The usual course of antibiotics is 7–10 d. Rifixamin (a poorly absorbed broad-spectrum antibiotic) in combination with fiber, is associated with less frequent recurrent symptoms from uncomplicated diverticular disease. Patients should remain on a limited diet until their pain resolves. A role for parenteral nutrition has not been established.

SURGICAL MANAGEMENT Preoperative risk factors influencing postoperative mortality rates include higher American Society of Anesthesia (ASA) class and preexisting organ failure. In patients who are low risk (ASA I and II), surgical therapy can be offered to patients who have had at least two documented attacks of diverticulitis requiring hospitalization or those who do not rapidly improve on medical therapy. Studies indicate that medical therapy can be continued beyond two attacks without an increased risk of perforation requiring a colostomy, especially in those >50 years. In contrast, younger patients may experience a more aggressive form of the disease; therefore, waiting beyond two attacks is not recommended. Surgical therapy is indicated in all low surgical risk patients with complicated diverticular disease.

The goals of surgical management of diverticular disease include controlling sepsis, eliminating complications such as fistula or obstruction, removing the diseased colonic segment, and restoring intestinal continuity. These goals must be obtained while minimizing morbidity, length of hospitalization, and cost in addition to maximizing survival and quality of life. Table 18-2 lists the operation most commonly indicated based upon Hinchey classification and the predicted morbidity and mortality. Surgical objectives include removal of the diseased sigmoid down to the rectosigmoid junction. Failure to do this may result in recurrent disease. The current options for uncomplicated diverticular disease include an open sigmoid resection or a laparoscopic sigmoid resection. The benefits of laparoscopic resection over open surgical techniques include early discharge (by at least 1 day), less narcotic use, and an earlier return to work. However, laparoscopic resection is associated with a longer operative procedure and is more costly. The complication rates between open and laparoscopic surgery are similar.

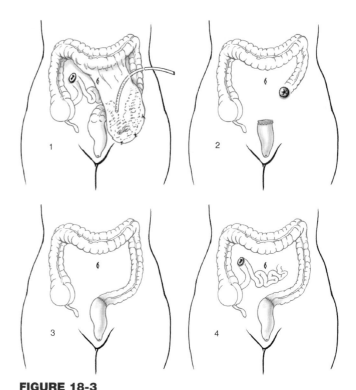

FIGURE 18-3

Methods of surgical management of complicated diverticular disease. *(1)* Drainage, omental pedicle graft, and proximal diversion. *(2)* Hartman's procedure. *(3)* Sigmoid resection with coloproctostomy. *(4)* Sigmoid resection with coloproctostomy and proximal diversion.

TABLE 18-2

	OUTCOME FOLLOWING SURGICAL THERAPY FOR COMPLICATED DIVERTICULAR DISEASE		
HINCHEY STAGE	**OPERATIVE PROCEDURE**	**ANASTOMOTIC LEAK RATE, %**	**OVERALL MORBIDITY, %**
I	Resection with primary anastomosis without diverting stoma	3.8	22
II	Resection with primary anastomosis +/– diversion	3.8	30
III	Hartmann's procedure vs diverting colostomy and omental pedal graft	–	0 vs 6 mortality
IV	Hartmann's procedure vs diverting colostomy and omental pedicle graft	–	6 vs 2 mortality

The options for the surgical management of complicated diverticular disease (Fig. 18-3) include the following: (1) proximal diversion of the fecal stream with an ileostomy or colostomy and sutured omental patch with drainage, (2) resection with colostomy and mucus fistula or closure of distal bowel with formation of a Hartmann's pouch, (3) resection with anastomosis (coloproctostomy), or (4) resection with anastomosis and diversion (coloproctostomy with loop ileostomy or colostomy). Laparoscopic techniques have been employed for complicated diverticular disease; however, higher conversion rates to open techniques have been reported.

Patients with Hinchey stages I and II disease are managed with percutaneous drainage followed by resection with anastomosis about 6 weeks later. Percutaneous drainage is recommended for abscesses ≥5 cm with a well-defined wall that is accessible. Paracolic abscesses <5 cm in size may resolve with antibiotics alone. Contraindications to percutaneous drainage are no percutaneous access route, pneumoperitoneum, and fecal peritonitis. Urgent operative intervention is undertaken if patients develop generalized peritonitis, and most will need to be managed with a Hartmann's procedure. In selected cases, nonoperative therapy may be considered. In one nonrandomized study, nonoperative management of isolated paracolic abscesses (Hinchey stage I) was associated with only a 20% recurrence rate at 2 years. Over 80% of patients with distant abscesses (Hinchey stage II) required surgical resection for recurrent symptoms.

Hinchey stage III disease is managed with a Hartman's procedure or with primary anastomosis and proximal diversion. If the patient has significant comorbidities, making operative intervention risky, a limited procedure including intraoperative peritoneal lavage (irrigation), omental patch to the oversewn perforation, and proximal diversion of the fecal stream with either an ileostomy or transverse colostomy can be performed. No anastomosis of any type should be attempted in Hinchey stage IV disease. A limited approach to these patients is associated with a decreased mortality.

Recurrent Symptoms

Recurrent abdominal symptoms following surgical resection for diverticular disease occurs in 10% of patients. Recurrent diverticular disease develops in patients following inadequate surgical resection. A retained segment of diseased rectosigmoid colon is associated with twice the incidence of recurrence. IBS may also cause recurrence of initial symptoms. Patients undergoing surgical resection for presumed diverticulitis and symptoms of abdominal cramping and irregular loose bowel movements consistent with IBS have functionally poorer outcomes.

COMMON DISEASES OF THE ANORECTUM

RECTAL PROLAPSE (PROCIDENTIA)
Incidence and Epidemiology

Rectal prolapse is six times more common in women than in men. The incidence of rectal prolapse peaks in women >60 years. Women with rectal prolapse have a higher incidence of associated pelvic floor disorders including urinary incontinence, rectocele, cystocele, and enterocele. About 20% of children with rectal prolapse will have cystic fibrosis. All children presenting with prolapse should undergo a sweat chloride test. Less common associations include Ehlers-Danlos syndrome, solitary rectal ulcer syndrome, congenital hypothyroidism, and Hirschsprung's disease.

Anatomy and Pathophysiology

Rectal prolapse (procidentia) is a circumferential, full-thickness protrusion of the rectal wall through the anal orifice. It is often associated with a redundant sigmoid colon, pelvic laxity, and a deep rectovaginal septum (pouch of Douglas). Initially, rectal prolapse was felt to

be the result of early internal rectal intussusception, which occurs in the upper to mid rectum. This was considered to be the first step in an inevitable progression to full-thickness external prolapse. However, only 1 of 38 patients with internal prolapse followed for >5 years developed full-thickness prolapse. Others have suggested that full-thickness prolapse is the result of damage to the nerve supply to the pelvic floor muscles or pudendal nerves from repeated stretching with straining to defecate. Damage to the pudendal nerves would weaken the pelvic floor muscles, including the external anal sphincter muscles. Bilateral pudendal nerve injury is more significantly associated with prolapse and incontinence than unilateral injury.

Presentation and Evaluation

The majority of patient complaints include anal mass, bleeding per rectum, and poor perianal hygiene. Prolapse of the rectum usually occurs following defecation and will spontaneously reduce or require the patient to manually reduce the prolapse. Constipation occurs in ~30–67% of patients with rectal prolapse. Differing degrees of fecal incontinence occur in 50–70% of patients. Other associated findings include outlet obstruction (anismus) in 30%, colonic inertia in 10%, and solitary rectal ulcer syndrome in 12%.

Office evaluation is best performed after the patient has been given an enema, which enables the prolapse to protrude. An important distinction should be made between full-thickness rectal prolapse and isolated mucosal prolapse associated with hemorrhoidal disease (Fig. 18-4). Mucosal prolapse is known for radial grooves rather than circumferential folds around the anus and is due to increased laxity of the connective tissue between the submucosa and underlying muscle of the anal canal. The evaluation of prolapse should also include cystoproctography and colonoscopy. These examinations evaluate for associated pelvic floor disorders and rule out a malignancy or a polyp as the lead point for prolapse. If rectal prolapse is associated with chronic constipation, the patient should undergo a defecating proctogram and a sitzmark study. This will evaluate for the presence of anismus or colonic inertia. Anismus is the result of attempting to defecate against a closed pelvic floor and is also known as *nonrelaxing puborectalis*. This can be seen when straightening of the rectum fails to occur on fluoroscopy while the patient is attempting to defecate. In colonic inertia, a sitzmark study will demonstrate retention of >20% of markers on abdominal x-ray 5 days after swallowing. For patients with fecal incontinence, endoanal ultrasound and manometric evaluation, including pudendal nerve testing of their anal sphincter muscles, may be performed before surgery for prolapse (see "Fecal Incontinence" later in the chapter).

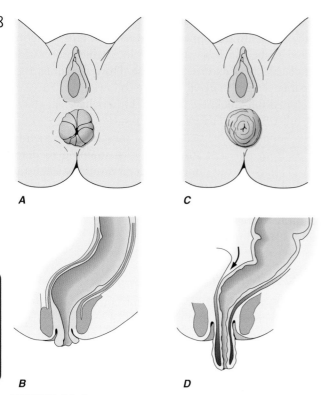

FIGURE 18-4
Degree of rectal prolapse. Mucosal prolapse only (*A, B,* sagittal view). Full-thickness prolapse associated with redundant rectosigmoid and deep pouch of Douglas (*C, D,* sagittal view).

℞ Treatment: RECTAL PROLAPSE

The medical approach to the management of rectal prolapse is limited and includes stool-bulking agents or fiber supplementation to ease the process of evacuation. Surgical correction of rectal prolapse is the mainstay of therapy. Two approaches are commonly considered, transabdominal and transperineal. Transabdominal approaches have been associated with lower recurrence rates, but some patients with significant comorbidities are better served by a transperineal approach.

Common transperineal approaches include a transanal proctectomy (Altemeier procedure), mucosal proctectomy (Delorme procedure), or placement of a Tirsch wire encircling the anus. The goal of the transperineal approach is to remove the redundant rectosigmoid colon. Common transabdominal approaches include presacral suture or mesh rectopexy (Ripstein) with (Frykman-Goldberg) or without resection of the redundant sigmoid. Transabdominal procedures can be performed effectively with laparoscopic techniques without increased incidence of recurrence. The goal of the transabdominal approach is to restore normal anatomy by removing redundant bowel and reattaching the supportive tissue of the rectum to the presacral fascia. The final alternative is abdominal proctectomy with end-sigmoid colostomy. Colon resection, in general,

is reserved for patients with constipation and outlet obstruction. If total colonic inertia is present, as defined by a history of constipation and a positive sitzmark study, a subtotal colectomy with an ileosigmoid or rectal anastomosis may be required at the time of rectopexy.

FECAL INCONTINENCE

Incidence and Epidemiology

The prevalence of fecal incontinence in the United States is 0.5–11%. The majority of patients are women. A higher incidence of incontinence is seen among parous women. One-half of patients with fecal incontinence also suffer from urinary incontinence. The majority of incontinence is a result of obstetric injury to the pelvic floor, either while carrying a fetus or during the delivery. Risk factors at the time of delivery include the use of forceps and the need for an episiotomy. Other causes include congenital abnormalities such as imperforate anus, trauma, or rectal prolapse.

Anatomy and Pathophysiology

The anal sphincter complex is made up of the internal and external anal sphincter. The internal sphincter is smooth muscle and a continuation of the circular fibers of the rectal wall. It is innervated by the intestinal myenteric plexus and is therefore not under voluntary control. The external anal sphincter is formed in continuation with the levator ani muscles and is under voluntary control. The pudendal nerve supplies motor innervation to the external anal sphincter. Obstetric injury may result in tearing of the muscle fibers anteriorly at the time of the delivery. This results in an obvious anterior defect on endoanal ultrasound. Injury may also be the result of stretching of the pudendal nerves. The majority of patients who suffer from fecal incontinence following obstetric injury do so several years following the birth of their last child.

Presentation and Evaluation

Patients may suffer with varying degrees of fecal incontinence. Minor incontinence includes incontinence to flatus and occasional seepage of liquid stool. Major incontinence is frequent inability to control solid waste. As a result of fecal incontinence, patients suffer from poor perianal hygiene. Beyond the immediate problems associated with fecal incontinence, these patients are often withdrawn and suffer from depression. For this reason, quality-of-life measures have become an important component in the evaluation of patients with fecal incontinence.

The evaluation of fecal incontinence should include a thorough history and physical examination, anal manometry, pudendal nerve terminal motor latency (PNTML), and endoanal ultrasound. Unfortunately, all of these investigations are user-dependent. Centers that care for patients with fecal incontinence will have an anorectal physiology laboratory that uses standardized methods of evaluating anorectal physiology. Anal manometry measures resting and squeeze pressures within the anal canal using an intraluminal water-perfused catheter. Pudendal nerve studies evaluate the function of the nerves innervating the anal canal using a finger electrode placed in the anal canal. Stretch injuries to these nerves will result in a delayed response of the sphincter muscle to a stimulus, indicating a prolonged latency. Finally, ultrasound will evaluate the extent of the injury to the sphincter muscles before surgical repair. Only PNTML has been shown to consistently predict outcome following surgical intervention.

Rarely does a pelvic floor disorder exist alone. The majority of patients with fecal incontinence will have a degree of urinary incontinence. Similarly, fecal incontinence is a part of the spectrum of pelvic organ prolapse. For this reason, patients may present with symptoms of obstructed defecation as well as fecal incontinence. Careful evaluation including cinedefecography should be performed to search for other associated defects. Surgical repair of incontinence without attention to other associated defects may decrease the success of the repair.

℞ **Treatment:**
FECAL INCONTINENCE

The "gold standard" for the treatment of fecal incontinence with an isolated sphincter defect is overlapping sphincteroplasty. The external anal sphincter muscle and scar tissue as well as any identifiable internal sphincter muscle are dissected free from the surrounding adipose and connective tissue and then an overlapping repair is performed in an attempt to rebuild the muscular ring and restore its function. Other newer approaches include radiofrequency therapy to the anal canal to aid in the development of collagen fibers and provide tensile strength to the sphincter muscles. Sacral nerve stimulation and the artificial bowel sphincter are both adaptations of procedures developed for the management of urinary incontinence. Sacral nerve stimulation is ideally suited for patients with intact but weak anal sphincters. A temporary nerve stimulator is placed on the third sacral nerve. If there is at least a 50% improvement in symptoms, a permanent nerve stimulator is placed under the skin. The artificial bowel sphincter is a cuff and reservoir apparatus that allows for manual inflation of a cuff placed around the anus, increasing anal tone. This allows the patient to manually close off the anal canal until defecation is necessary.

Long-term results following overlapping sphincteroplasty show about a 50% failure rate over 5 years. Poorer outcome has been seen in patients with prolonged

PNTML. Long-term results for sacral stimulation and the artificial bowel sphincter are limited. However, the artificial bowel sphincter has been associated with a 30% infection rate.

HEMORRHOIDAL DISEASE
Incidence and Epidemiology

Symptomatic hemorrhoids affect >1 million individuals in western civilization per year. The prevalence of hemorrhoidal disease is not selective for age or sex. However, age is known to have a deleterious effect on the anal canal. The prevalence of hemorrhoidal disease is less in underdeveloped countries. The typical low-fiber, high-fat western diet is associated with constipation and straining and the development of symptomatic hemorrhoids.

Anatomy and Pathophysiology

Hemorrhoidal cushions are a normal part of the anal canal. The vascular structures contained within this tissue aid in continence by preventing damage to the sphincter muscle. Three main hemorrhoidal complexes traverse the anal canal—the left lateral, the right anterior, and the right posterior. Engorgement and straining results in prolapse of this tissue into the anal canal. Over time, the anatomic support system of the hemorrhoidal complex weakens, exposing this tissue to the outside of the anal canal where it is susceptible to injury. Hemorrhoids are commonly classified as internal or external. Although small external cushions do exist, the standard classification of hemorrhoidal disease is based on the progression of the disease from their normal internal location to the prolapsing external position (**Table 18-3**).

TABLE 18-3

THE STAGING AND TREATMENT OF HEMORRHOIDS

STAGE	DESCRIPTION OF CLASSIFICATION	TREATMENT
I	Enlargement with bleeding	Fiber supplementation Cortisone suppository Sclerotherapy
II	Protrusion with spontaneous reduction	Fiber supplementation Cortisone suppository
III	Protrusion requiring manual reduction	Fiber supplementation Cortisone suppository Banding Operative hemorrhoidectomy (stapled or traditional)
IV	Irreducible protrusion	Fiber supplementation Cortisone suppository Operative hemorrhoidectomy

Patients commonly present to a physician for two reasons: bleeding and protrusion. Pain is less common than with fissures and, if present, is described as a dull ache from engorgement of the hemorrhoidal tissue. Severe pain may indicate a thrombosed hemorrhoid. Hemorrhoidal bleeding is described as bright red blood seen either in the toilet or upon wiping. Occasional patients can present with significant bleeding, which may be a cause of anemia; however, the presence of a colonic neoplasm must be ruled out. Patients who present with a protruding mass complain about inability to maintain perianal hygiene and are often concerned about the presence of a malignancy.

The diagnosis of hemorrhoidal disease is made on physical examination. Inspection of the perianal region for evidence of thrombosis or excoriation is performed, followed by a careful digital examination. Anoscopy is performed paying particular attention to the known position of hemorrhoidal disease. The patient is asked to strain. If this is difficult for the patient, the maneuver can be performed while sitting on a toilet. The physician is notified when the tissue prolapses. It is important to differentiate the circumferential appearance of a full-thickness rectal prolapse from the radial nature of prolapsing hemorrhoids; see "Rectal Prolapse (Procidentia)" earlier in the chapter. The stage and location of the hemorrhoidal complexes are defined.

℞ **Treatment:**
HEMORRHOIDAL DISEASE

The treatment for bleeding hemorrhoids is based upon the stage of the disease (Table 18-3). In all patients with bleeding, the possibility of other causes must be considered. In young patients without a family history of colorectal cancer, the hemorrhoidal disease may be treated first and a colonoscopic examination performed if the bleeding continues. Older patients who have not had colorectal cancer screening should undergo colonoscopy or flexible sigmoidoscopy.

With rare exceptions, the acutely thrombosed hemorrhoid can be excised within the first 72 h by performing an elliptical excision. Sitz baths, fiber, and stool softeners are prescribed. Additional therapy for bleeding hemorrhoids includes banding, sclerotherapy, excisional hemorrhoidectomy, and stapled hemorrhoidectomy. Sensation begins at the dentate line; therefore, banding or sclerotherapy can be performed without discomfort in the office. Bands are placed around the engorged tissue, causing ischemia and fibrosis. This aids in fixing the tissue proximally in the anal canal. Patients may complain of a dull ache for 24 h following band application. During sclerotherapy, 1–2 mL of a sclerosant (usually sodium tetradechol sulfate)

is injected using a 25-gauge needle into the submucosa of the hemorrhoidal complex. Care must be taken not to inject the anal canal circumferentially or stenosis may occur. The sutured and stapled hemorrhoidectomy are equally effective in the treatment of symptomatic third- and fourth-degree hemorrhoids. However, because the sutured hemorrhoidectomy involves the removal of redundant tissue down to the anal verge, unpleasant anal skin tags are removed as well. The stapled hemorrhoidectomy is associated with less discomfort; however, this procedure does not remove anal skin tags. No procedures on hemorrhoids should be done in patients who are immunocompromised or who have active proctitis. Furthermore, emergent hemorrhoidectomy for bleeding hemorrhoids is associated with a higher complication rate.

Acute complications associated with the treatment of hemorrhoids include pain, infection, recurrent bleeding, and urinary retention. Care should be taken to place bands properly and to avoid overhydration in patients undergoing operative hemorrhoidectomy. Late complications include fecal incontinence as a result of injury to the sphincter during the dissection. Anal stenosis may develop from overzealous excision, with loss of mucosal skin bridges for reepithelialization. Finally, an *ectropion* (prolapse of rectal mucosa from the anal canal) may develop. Patients with an ectropion complain of a "wet" anus as a result of inability to prevent soiling once the rectal mucosa is exposed below the dentate line.

ANORECTAL ABSCESS

Incidence and Epidemiology

The development of a perianal abscess is more common in men than women by a ratio of 3:1. The peak incidence is in the third to fifth decade of life. Perianal pain associated with the presence of an abscess accounts for 15% of office visits to a colorectal surgeon. The disease is more prevalent in immunocompromised patients such as diabetics, those with hematologic disorders or inflammatory bowel disease (IBD), and persons who are HIV positive. These disorders should be considered in patients with recurrent perianal infections.

Anatomy and Pathophysiology

An anorectal abscess is an abnormal fluid–containing cavity in the anorectal region. Anorectal abscess results from an infection involving the glands surrounding the anal canal. Normally, these glands release mucus into the anal canal, which aids in defecation. When stool accidentally enters the anal glands, the glands become infected and an abscess develops. Anorectal abscesses are perianal in 40–50% of patients, ischiorectal in 20–25%, intersphincteric in 2–5%, and supralevator in 2.5% (**Fig. 18–5**).

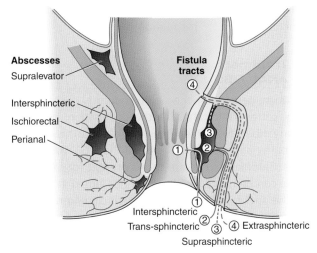

FIGURE 18-5
Common locations of anorectal abscess *(left)* and fistula in ano *(right)*.

Presentation and Evaluation

Perianal pain and fever are the hallmarks of an abscess. Patients may have difficulty voiding and have blood in the stool. A prostatic abscess may present with similar complaints including dysuria. Patients with a prostatic abscess will often have a history of recurrent sexually transmitted diseases. On physical examination, a large fluctuant area is usually readily visible. Routine laboratory evaluation shows an elevated white blood cell count. Diagnostic procedures are rarely necessary unless evaluating a recurrent abscess. A CT scan or MRI has an accuracy of 80% in determining incomplete drainage. If there is a concern about the presence of IBD, a rigid or flexible sigmoidoscopic examination may be done at the time of drainage to evaluate for inflammation within the rectosigmoid region. A more complete evaluation for Crohn's disease would include a full colonoscopy and small-bowel series.

℞ **Treatment:**
ANORECTAL ABSCESS

Office drainage of an uncomplicated anorectal abscess may suffice. A small incision close to the anal verge is made and a Mallenkot drain is advanced into the abscess cavity. For patients who have a complicated abscess or who are diabetic or immunocompromised, drainage should be performed in an operating room under anesthesia. These patients are at greater risk for developing necrotizing fasciitis. The course of antibiotics is controversial but should be at least 2 weeks in patients who are immunocompromised or have prosthetic heart valves, artificial joints, diabetes, or IBD.

Incidence and Epidemiology

The incidence and prevalence of fistulating perianal disease parallels the incidence of anorectal abscess. Some 30–40% of abscesses will give rise to fistula in ano. While the majority of the fistulas are cryptoglandular in origin, 10% are associated with IBD, tuberculosis, malignancy, and radiation.

Anatomy and Pathophysiology

A fistula in ano is defined as a communication of an abscess cavity with an identifiable internal opening within the anal canal. This identifiable opening is most commonly located at the dentate line where the anal glands enter the anal canal. Patients experiencing continuous drainage following the treatment of a perianal abscess likely have a fistula in ano. These fistulas are classified by their relationship to the anal sphincter muscles, with 70% being intersphincteric, 23% transsphincteric, 5% suprasphincteric, and 2% extrasphincteric (Fig. 18-5).

Presentation and Evaluation

A patient with a fistula in ano will complain of constant drainage from the perianal region. The drainage may increase with defecation. Perianal hygiene is difficult to maintain. Examination under anesthesia is the best way to evaluate a fistula. At the time of the examination, anoscopy is performed to look for an internal opening. Diluted hydrogen peroxide will aid in identifying such an opening. In lieu of anesthesia, MRI with an endoanal coil will also identify tracts in 80% of the cases. After drainage of an abscess with insertion of a Mallenkot catheter, a fistulagram through the catheter can be obtained in search of an occult fistula tract. Goodsall's rule states that a posterior external fistula will enter the anal canal in the posterior midline, whereas an anterior fistula will enter at the nearest crypt. A fistula exiting >3 cm from the anal verge may have a complicated upward extension and may not obey Goodsall's rule.

℞ **Treatment:**
FISTULA IN ANO

A newly diagnosed draining fistula is best managed with placement of a seton, a vessel loop or silk tie placed through the fistula tract, which maintains the tract open and quiets down the surrounding inflammation that occurs from repeated blockage of the tract. Once the inflammation is less, the exact relationship of the fistula tract to the anal sphincters can be ascertained. A simple fistulotomy can be performed for intersphincteric and low (less than one-third of the muscle) transsphincteric fistulas without compromising continence. For a higher transsphincteric fistula, an anorectal advancement flap in combination with a drainage catheter or fibrin glue may be used. Very long (>2 cm) and narrow tracts respond better to fibrin glue than shorter tracts. Patients should be maintained on stool-bulking agents, nonnarcotic pain medication, and sitz baths. Early complications from these procedures include urinary retention and bleeding. Later complications include temporary and permanent incontinence. Recurrence following fistulotomy is 0–18% and following anorectal advancement flap is 20–30% and is related to failure to excise and close the internal opening.

ANAL FISSURE

Incidence and Epidemiology

Anal fissures occur at all ages but are more common in the third through the fifth decades. A fissure is the most common cause of rectal bleeding in infancy. The prevalence is equal in males and females. It is associated with constipation, diarrhea, infectious etiologies, perianal trauma, and Crohn's disease.

Anatomy and Pathophysiology

Trauma to the anal canal occurs following defecation. This injury occurs in the anterior or, more commonly, the posterior anal canal. Irritation caused by the trauma to the anal canal results in an increased resting pressure of the internal sphincter. The blood supply to the sphincter and anal mucosa enters laterally. Therefore, increased anal sphincter tone results in a relative ischemia in the region of the fissure and leads to poor healing of the anal injury. A fissure that is not in the posterior or anterior position should raise suspicion for other causes, including tuberculosis, syphilis, Crohn's disease, and malignancy.

Presentation and Evaluation

A fissure can be easily diagnosed on history alone. The classic complaint is pain, which is strongly associated with defecation and is relentless. The bright red bleeding that can be associated with a fissure is less extensive than that associated with hemorrhoids. On examination, most fissures are located in either the posterior or anterior position. A lateral fissure is worrisome as it may have a less benign nature, and systemic disorders should be ruled out. A chronic fissure is indicated by the presence of a hypertrophied anal papilla at the proximal end of the fissure and a sentinel pile or skin tag at the distal end. Often the circular fibers of the hypertrophied internal sphincter are visible within the base of the fissure. If anal manometry is performed, elevation in anal resting pressure and a sawtooth deformity with paradoxical contractions of the sphincter muscles are pathognomonic.

℞ Treatment:
ANAL FISSURE

The management of the acute fissure is conservative. Stool softeners for those with constipation, increased dietary fiber, topical anesthetics, glucocorticoids, and sitz baths are prescribed and will heal 60–90% of fissures. Chronic fissures are those present for >6 weeks. These can be treated with modalities aimed at decreasing the anal canal resting pressure including nifedipine or nitroglycerin ointment applied three times a day, and botulinum toxin type A, up to 20 units, injected into the internal sphincter on each side of the fissure. Surgical management includes anal dilation and lateral internal sphincterotomy. Usually, one-third of the internal sphincter muscle is divided; it is easily identified because it is hypertrophied. Recurrence rates from medical therapy are higher, but this is offset by a risk of incontinence following sphincterotomy. Lateral internal sphincterotomy more commonly leads to incontinence in women.

ACKNOWLEDGMENT

I would like to thank Cory Sandore for providing some illustrations for this chapter. Gregory Bulkley, MD, contributed to this chapter in the 16th edition of Harrison's Principles of Internal Medicine.

FURTHER READINGS

COLECCHIA A et al: Diverticular disease of the colon: New perspectives in symptom development and treatment. World J Gastroenterol 9:1385, 2003

COMMANE DM et al: Diet, ageing and genetic factors in the pathogenesis of diverticular disease. World J Gastroenterol 15:2479, 2009

GATTA L et al: Efficacy of 5-ASA in the treatment of colonic diverticular disease. J Clin Gastroenterol Jul 6, 2009 [epub ahead of print]

JANES S et al: Elective surgery after acute diverticulitis. Br J Surgery 92:133, 2005

———: The place of elective surgery following acute diverticulitis in young patients: when is surgery indicated? An analysis of the literature. Dis Colon Rectum 52:1008, 2009

KARULF R et al: Rectal prolapse. Curr Probl Surg 38:757, 2001

LINDSEY I et al: A randomized, controlled trial of fibrin glue vs. conventional treatment for anal fistula. Dis Colon Rectum 45:1608, 2002

OHNING GV et al: Definitive therapy for internal hemorrhoids—new opportunities and options. Rev Gastroenterol Disord 9:16, 2009

STEIN E: Botulinum toxin and anal fissure. Curr Probl Dermatol 30:218, 2002

SUTHERLAND LM et al: A systematic review of stapled hemorrhoidectomy. Arch Surg 137:1395, 2002

WONG WD et al: Practice parameters for the treatment of sigmoid diverticulitis—supporting documentation. Dis Colon Rectum 43:290, 2000

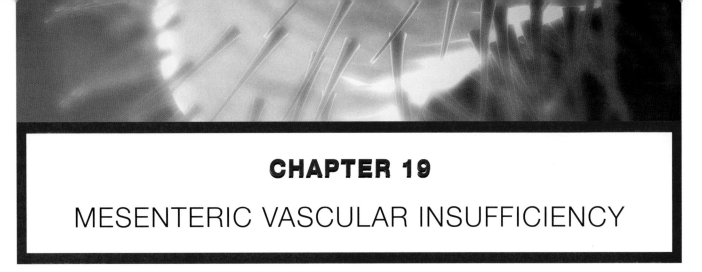

CHAPTER 19

MESENTERIC VASCULAR INSUFFICIENCY

Susan L. Gearhart

INTESTINAL ISCHEMIA

Incidence and Epidemiology

Intestinal ischemia is an uncommon vascular disease associated with a high mortality. It is categorized according to etiology: (1) arteriooclusive mesenteric ischemia (AOMI), (2) nonocclusive mesenteric ischemia (NOMI), and (3) mesenteric venous thrombosis (MVT). Acute intestinal ischemia is more common than its counterpart, chronic arterial ischemia. Risk factors for acute arterial ischemia include atrial fibrillation, recent myocardial infarction, valvular heart disease, and recent cardiac or vascular catheterization. The increased incidence of intestinal ischemia seen in western countries parallels the incidence of atherosclerosis and the aging population. With the exception of strangulated small-bowel obstruction, ischemic colitis is the most common form of acute ischemia and the most prevalent gastrointestinal disease complicating cardiovascular surgery. The incidence of ischemic colitis following elective aortic repair is 5–9%, and the incidence triples in patients following emergent repair. Other less common forms of intestinal ischemia include chronic mesenteric angina associated with atherosclerotic disease and MVT. The latter is associated with the presence of a hypercoagulable state including protein C or S deficiency, antithrombin III deficiency, polycythemia vera, and carcinoma.

Anatomy and Pathophysiology

Intestinal ischemia occurs when insufficient perfusion to intestinal tissue produces ischemic tissue injury. The blood supply to the intestines is depicted in **Fig. 19-1**.

To prevent ischemic injury, extensive collateralization occurs between major mesenteric trunks and branches of the mesenteric arcades (**Table 19-1**). Collateral vessels within the small bowel are numerous and meet within the duodenum and the bed of the pancreas. Collateral vessels within the colon meet at the splenic flexure and descending/sigmoid colon. These areas, which are inherently at risk for decreased blood flow, are known as *Griffiths' point* and *Sudeck's point*, respectively, and are the most common locations for colonic ischemia (Fig. 19-1, shaded area). The splanchnic circulation can receive up to 30% of the cardiac output. Protective responses to prevent intestinal ischemia include abundant collateralization, autoregulation of blood flow, and the ability to increase oxygen extraction from the blood.

Occlusive ischemia is a result of disruption of blood flow by an embolus or progressive thrombosis in a major artery supplying the intestine. Emboli originate from the heart in >75% of cases and lodge preferentially just distal to the origin of the middle colic artery from the superior mesenteric artery. Progressive thrombosis of at least two of the major vessels supplying the intestine is required for the development of chronic intestinal angina. Nonocclusive ischemia is disproportionate mesenteric vasoconstriction (arteriolar vasospasm) in response to a severe physiologic stress such as dehydration or shock. If left untreated, early mucosal stress ulceration will progress to full-thickness injury.

Presentation, Evaluation, and Management

Intestinal ischemia remains one of the most challenging diagnoses. The mortality rate is >50%. The most significant

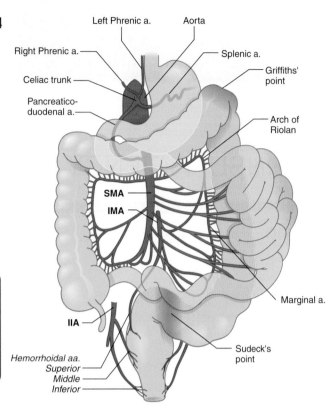

FIGURE 19-1

Blood supply to the intestines includes the celiac artery, superior mesenteric artery (SMA), inferior mesenteric artery (IMA), and branches of the internal iliac artery (IIA). Sudeck's and Griffiths' points, indicated by shaded area, are watershed areas within the colonic blood supply and common locations for ischemia.

indicator of survival is the timeliness of diagnosis and treatment. An overview of diagnosis and management of each form of intestinal ischemia is given in Table 19-2.

Acute mesenteric ischemia resulting from arterial embolus or thrombosis presents with severe acute, nonremitting abdominal pain strikingly out of proportion to the physical findings. Associated symptoms may include nausea and vomiting, transient diarrhea, and bloody stools. With the exception of minimal abdominal distention and hypoactive bowel sounds, early abdominal examination is unimpressive. Later findings will demonstrate peritonitis and cardiovascular collapse. In the evaluation of acute intestinal ischemia, routine laboratory tests should be obtained, including complete blood count, serum chemistry, coagulation profile, arterial blood gas, amylase, lipase, lactic acid, blood type and cross-match, and cardiac enzymes. Regardless of the need for urgent surgery, emergent admission to a monitored bed or intensive care unit is recommended for resuscitation and further evaluation. If the diagnosis of intestinal ischemia is being considered, consultation with a surgical service is necessary.

Other diagnostic modalities that may be useful in diagnosis but should not delay surgical therapy include electrocardiogram (ECG), abdominal radiographs, CT, and mesenteric angiography. More recently, mesentery duplex scanning and visible light spectroscopy during colonoscopy have been demonstrated to be beneficial. The ECG may demonstrate an arrhythmia, indicating the possible source of the emboli. A plain abdominal film may show evidence of free intraperitoneal air, indicating a perforated viscus and the need for emergent exploration. Earlier features of intestinal ischemia seen on abdominal radiographs include bowel-wall edema, known as "thumbprinting." If the ischemia progresses, air can be seen within the bowel wall (*pneumatosis intestinalis*) and within the portal venous system. Other features include calcifications of the aorta and its tributaries, indicating atherosclerotic disease. With the administration of oral and IV contrast, dynamic CT with three-dimensional reconstruction is a highly sensitive test for intestinal ischemia. In acute embolic disease, mesenteric angiography is best performed intraoperatively. A mesenteric duplex scan demonstrating a high peak velocity of flow in the superior mesenteric artery (SMA) is associated with an ~80% positive predictive value of mesenteric ischemia. More significantly, a negative duplex scan virtually precludes the diagnosis of mesenteric ischemia.

TABLE 19-1

COLLATERAL ARTERIAL INTESTINAL BLOOD FLOW			
INVOLVED CIRCULATION	MESENTERIC ARTERY	ADJOINING ARTERY	COLLATERAL ARTERY
Systemic	Celiac	Descending aorta	Phrenic
Systemic	IMA	Hypogastric	Middle hemorrhoidal
Mesenteric	Celiac	SMA	Superior/inferior pancreaticoduodenal
Mesenteric	SMA	IMA	Arch of Riolan
Mesenteric	SMA	Celiac/IMA	Intramesenteric
Mesenteric	SMA	IMA	Marginal

Note: IMA, inferior mesenteric artery; SMA, superior mesenteric artery.

TABLE 19-2

215

OVERVIEW OF THE MANAGEMENT OF ACUTE INTESTINAL ISCHEMIA

CONDITION	KEY TO EARLY DIAGNOSIS	TREATMENT OF UNDERLYING CAUSE	TREATMENT OF SPECIFIC LESION	TREATMENT OF SYSTEMIC CONSEQUENCES

Arterial embolus	Early laparotomy	Anticoagulation
		Cardioversion
		Proximal
		  thrombectomy
		Aneurysmectomy
			Laparotomy
			Embolectomy
			Vascular bypass
			Assess viability and
			  resect dead bowel
				Ensure hydration
				Give antibiotics
				Reverse acidosis
				Optimize oxygen delivery
				Support cardiac output
				Treat other embolic sites
				Avoid vasoconstrictors

Arterial thrombosis	Duplex ultrasound
	Angiography
		Anticoagulation
		Hydration
			Endovascular stent
			Endarterectomy/
			  thrombectomy
			  or vascular
			  bypass
			Assess viability and
			  resect dead bowel
				Give antibiotics
				Reverse acidosis
				Optimize oxygen delivery
				Support cardiac output
				Avoid vasoconstrictors

Venous thrombosis	Spiral CT	Anticoagulation
		Massive hydration
			Anticoagulation +/−
			  laparotomy/thrombectomy/
			  portasystemic shunt
			Assess viability and
			  resect dead bowel
				Give antibiotics
				Reverse acidosis
				Optimize oxygen delivery
				Support cardiac output
				Avoid vasoconstrictors

Nonocclusive mesenteric ischemia	Vasospasm:
	  Angiography
	Hypoperfusion:
	  Spiral CT or
	  colonoscopy
		Ensure hydration
		Support cardiac
		  output
		Avoid
		  vasoconstrictors
		Ablate renin-
		  angiotensin axis
			Vasospasm:
			  Intraarterial vasodilators
			Hypoperfusion:
			  Delayed laparotomy
			Assess viability and
			  resect dead bowel
				Ensure hydration
				Give antibiotics
				Reverse acidosis
				Optimize oxygen delivery
				Support cardiac output
				Avoid vasoconstrictors

Source: Modified from GB Bulkley, in JL Cameron (ed): *Current Surgical Therapy,* 2d ed. Toronto, BC Decker, 1986.

CHAPTER 19 Mesenteric Vascular Insufficiency

Duplex imaging serves as a screening test; further investigations with angiography are needed. Endoscopic techniques using visible light spectroscopy can be used in the diagnosis of chronic ischemia.

The "gold standard" for the diagnosis and management of acute arterial occlusive disease is laparotomy. Surgical exploration should not be delayed if suspicion of acute occlusive mesenteric ischemia is high or evidence of clinical deterioration or frank peritonitis is present. The goal of operative exploration is to resect compromised bowel and restore blood supply. Intraoperative or preoperative arteriography and systemic heparinization may assist the vascular surgeon in restoring blood supply to compromised bowel. The entire length of the small and large bowel beginning at the ligament of Treitz should be evaluated. The pattern of intestinal ischemia may indicate the level of arterial occlusion. In the case of SMA occlusion where the embolus usually lies just proximal to the origin of the middle colic artery, the proximal jejunum is often spared while the remainder of the small bowel to the transverse colon will be ischemic. The surgical management of acute mesenteric ischemia of the small bowel is attempted

embolectomy via intraoperative angiography or arteriotomy. Although more commonly applied to chronic disease, acute thrombosis may be managed with angioplasty, with or without endovascular stent placement. If this is unsuccessful, a bypass from the aorta to the superior mesenteric artery is performed.

Nonocclusive or vasospastic mesenteric ischemia presents with generalized abdominal pain, anorexia, bloody stools, and abdominal distention. Often these patients are obtunded, and physical findings may not assist in the diagnosis. The presence of a leukocytosis, metabolic acidosis, elevated amylase or creatinine phosphokinase levels, and/or lactic acidosis are useful in support of the diagnosis of advanced intestinal ischemia; however, these markers may not be indicative of either reversible ischemia or frank necrosis. Investigational markers for intestinal ischemia include D-dimer, glutathione S-transferase, platelet-activating factor (PAF), and mucosal pH monitoring. Regardless of the need for urgent surgery, emergent admission to a monitored bed or intensive care unit is recommended for resuscitation and further evaluation. Early manifestations of intestinal ischemia include fluid sequestration within the bowel wall leading to a loss of interstitial volume. Aggressive fluid resuscitation may be necessary. To optimize oxygen delivery, nasal O_2 and blood transfusions may be given. Broad-spectrum antibiotics should be given to provide sufficient coverage for enteric pathogens, including gram-negative and anaerobic organisms. Frequent monitoring of the patient's vital signs, urine output, blood gases, and lactate levels is paramount, as is frequent abdominal examination. All vasoconstricting agents should be avoided; fluid resuscitation is the intervention of choice to maintain hemodynamics.

If ischemic colitis is a concern, colonoscopy should be performed to assess the integrity of the colon mucosa. Visualization of the rectosigmoid region may demonstrate decreased mucosal integrity, associated more commonly with nonocclusive mesenteric ischemia, or, on occasion, occlusive disease as a result of acute loss of inferior mesenteric arterial flow following aortic surgery. Ischemia of the colonic mucosa is graded as *mild* with minimal mucosal erythema or as *moderate* with pale mucosal ulcerations and evidence of extension to the muscular layer of the bowel wall. *Severe* ischemic colitis presents with severe ulcerations resulting in black or green discoloration of the mucosa, consistent with full-thickness bowel-wall necrosis. The degree of reversibility can be predicted from the mucosal findings: mild erythema is nearly 100% reversible, moderate ~50%, and frank necrosis is simply dead bowel. Follow-up colonoscopy can be performed to rule out progression of ischemic colitis.

Laparotomy for nonocclusive mesenteric ischemia is warranted for signs of peritonitis or worsening endoscopic findings and if the patient's condition does not improve with aggressive resuscitation. Ischemic colitis is optimally treated with resection of the ischemic bowel and formation of a proximal stoma. Primary anastomosis should not be performed in patients with acute intestinal ischemia.

Patients with MVT may present with a gradual or sudden onset. Symptoms include vague abdominal pain, nausea, and vomiting. Examination findings include abdominal distention with mild to moderate tenderness and signs of dehydration. The diagnosis of mesenteric thrombosis is frequently made on abdominal spiral CT with oral and IV contrast. Findings on CT include bowel-wall thickening and ascites. Intravenous contrast will demonstrate a delayed arterial phase and clot within the superior mesenteric vein. The goal of management is to optimize hemodynamics and correct electrolyte abnormalities with massive fluid resuscitation. Intravenous antibiotics as well as anticoagulation should be initiated. If laparotomy is performed and MVT is suspected, heparin anticoagulation is immediately initiated and compromised bowel is resected. Of all acute intestinal disorders, mesenteric venous insufficiency is associated with the best prognosis.

Chronic intestinal ischemia presents with intestinal angina or abdominal pain associated with need for increased blood flow to the intestine. Patients report abdominal cramping and pain following ingestion of a meal. Weight loss and chronic diarrhea may also be noted. Abdominal pain without weight loss is not chronic mesenteric angina. Physical examination will often reveal the presence of an abdominal bruit as well as other manifestations of atherosclerosis. Duplex ultrasound evaluation of the mesenteric vessels has gained in popularity. In the absence of obesity and an increased bowel gas pattern, the radiologist may be able to identify flow disturbances within the vessels or the lack of a vasodilation response to feeding. This tool is frequently used as a screening test for patients with symptoms suggestive of chronic mesenteric ischemia. The gold standard for confirmation of mesenteric arterial occlusion is mesenteric angiography. Evaluation with mesenteric angiography allows for identification and possible intervention for the treatment of thrombus within the vessel lumen and will also evaluate the patency of remaining mesenteric vessels. The use of mesenteric angiography may be limited in the presence of renal failure or contrast allergy. Magnetic resonance angiography is an alternative if the administration of contrast dye is contraindicated.

The management of chronic intestinal ischemia includes medical management of atherosclerotic disease by lipid-lowering medications, exercise, and cessation of smoking. A full cardiac evaluation should be performed before intervention. Newer endovascular procedures may avoid an operative intervention in selected patient populations. Angioplasty with endovascular stenting in the treatment of chronic mesenteric ischemia is associated with an 80% long-term success rate. In patients requiring surgical exploration, the approach used is determined by the mesenteric angiogram. The entire length of the small and large bowel should be evaluated, beginning at the ligament of Treitz. Restoration of blood flow at the time of laparotomy is accomplished with mesenteric bypass.

Determination of intestinal viability intraoperatively in patients with suspected intestinal ischemia can be challenging. After revascularization, the bowel wall should be observed for return of a pink color and peristalsis. Palpation of major arterial vessels can be performed as well as applying a doppler flowmeter to the antimesenteric border of the bowel wall, but neither is a definitive indicator of viability. In equivocal cases, 1 g of IV sodium fluorescein is administered and the pattern of bowel reperfusion is observed under ultraviolet illumination with a standard (3600 Å) Wood's lamp. An area of nonfluorescence >5 mm in diameter suggests nonviability. If doubt persists, reexploration performed 24–48 h following surgery will allow demarcation of nonviable bowel. Primary intestinal anastomosis in patients with ischemic bowel is always worrisome, and reanastomosis should be deferred to the time of second-look laparotomy.

ACKNOWLEDGMENT

I thank Cory Sandore for providing some illustrations for this chapter. Gregory Bulkley contributed to this chapter in the 16th edition of Harrison's Principles of Internal Medicine.

FURTHER READINGS

CRUZ RJ Jr et al: Regional blood flow distribution and oxygen metabolism during mesenteric ischemia and congestion. J Surg Res Jan 3 2009 [epub ahead of print]

HSU H et al: Impact of etiological factors and APACHE II and POSSUM scores in management and clinical outcomes of acute intestinal ischemic disease after surgical treatment. World J Surg 30:2152, 2006

MATSUMOTO AH et al: Percutaneous transluminal angioplasty and stenting in the treatment of chronic mesenteric ischemia: Results and long-term follow-up. J Am Coll Surg 194(Suppl): S22, 2002

MITCHELL EL, MONETA GL: Mesenteric duplex scanning. Perspect Vasc Surg Endovasc Ther 18:175, 2006

NELSON AL et al: Hepatic portal venous gas: the ABCs of management. Arch Surg 144:575, 2009

SHIH MC et al: CTA and MRA in mesenteric ischemia: Part 2, normal findings and complications after surgical and endovascular treatment. AJR Am J Roentgenol 188:462, 2007

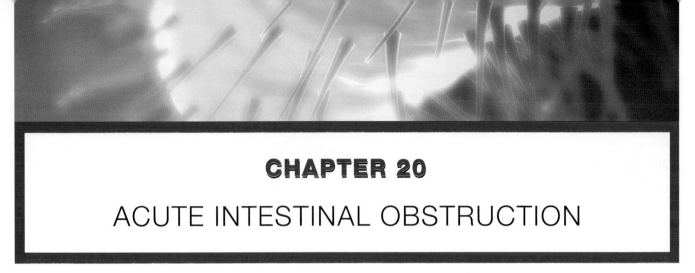

CHAPTER 20

ACUTE INTESTINAL OBSTRUCTION

Susan L. Gearhart ■ William Silen

ETIOLOGY AND CLASSIFICATION

In 75% of patients, acute intestinal obstruction results from previous abdominal surgery secondary to adhesive bands or internal or external hernias. The incidence of acute intestinal obstruction requiring hospital admission within the first few postoperative weeks is 5–25%, and 10–50% of these patients will require surgical intervention. The incidence of postoperative intestinal obstruction may be lower following laparoscopic surgery than open procedures. However, the laparoscopic gastric bypass procedure may be associated with an unexpected high rate of intestinal obstruction, with a higher reoperative rate. The reason for this is unknown. Other causes of intestinal obstruction not related to previous abdominal surgery include lesions *intrinsic* to the wall of the intestine, e.g., diverticulitis, carcinoma, regional enteritis; and luminal obstruction, e.g., gallstone obstruction, intussusception.

Two other conditions that must be differentiated from acute intestinal obstruction include *adynamic ileus* and *primary intestinal pseudoobstruction*. Adynamic ileus is mediated via the hormonal component of the sympathoadrenal system and may occur after any peritoneal insult; its severity and duration will be dependent to some degree on the type of peritoneal injury. Hydrochloric acid, colonic contents, and pancreatic enzymes are among the most irritating substances, whereas blood and urine are less so. Adynamic ileus occurs to some degree after any abdominal operation. Retroperitoneal hematoma, particularly associated with vertebral fracture, may cause severe adynamic ileus, and the latter may occur with other retroperitoneal conditions, such as ureteral calculus or severe pyelonephritis. Thoracic diseases, including lower-lobe pneumonia, fractured ribs, and myocardial infarction, frequently produce adynamic ileus, as do electrolyte disturbances, particularly potassium depletion. Finally, intestinal ischemia, whether from vascular occlusion or intestinal distention itself, may perpetuate an adynamic ileus. Intestinal pseudoobstruction is a chronic motility disorder that frequently mimics mechanical obstruction. This condition is often exacerbated by narcotic use. Unnecessary operations in such patients should be avoided.

PATHOPHYSIOLOGY

Distention of the intestine is caused by the accumulation of gas and fluid proximal to and within the obstructed segment. Between 70 and 80% of intestinal gas consists of swallowed air, and because this is composed mainly of nitrogen, which is poorly absorbed from the intestinal lumen, removal of air by continuous gastric suction is a useful adjunct in the treatment of intestinal distention. The accumulation of fluid proximal to the obstructing mechanism results not only from ingested fluid, swallowed saliva, gastric juice, and biliary and pancreatic secretions but also from interference with normal sodium and water transport. During the first 12–24 h of obstruction, a marked depression of flux from lumen to blood occurs of sodium and consequently water in the distended proximal intestine. After

24 h, sodium and water move into the lumen, contributing further to the distention and fluid losses. Intraluminal pressure rises from a normal of 2–4 cmH$_2$O to 8–10 cmH$_2$O. The loss of fluids and electrolytes may be extreme, and unless replacement is prompt, hypovolemia, renal insufficiency, and shock may result. Vomiting, accumulation of fluids within the lumen, and the sequestration of fluid into the edematous intestinal wall and peritoneal cavity as a result of impairment of venous return from the intestine all contribute to massive loss of fluid and electrolytes.

The most feared complication of acute intestinal obstruction is the presence of a "closed loop." Closed-loop obstruction of the small intestine results when the lumen is occluded at two points by a single mechanism such as a fascial hernia or adhesive band, thus producing a closed loop whose blood supply is often occluded by the hernia or band as well. During peristalsis, when a "closed loop" is present, pressures reach 30–60 cmH$_2$O. Strangulation of the closed loop is common in association with marked distention proximal to the involved loop. A form of closed-loop obstruction is encountered when complete obstruction of the colon exists in the presence of a competent ileocecal valve (85% of individuals). Although the blood supply of the colon is not entrapped within the obstructing mechanism, distention of the cecum is extreme because of its greater diameter (Laplace's law), and impairment of the intramural blood supply is considerable, with consequent gangrene of the cecal wall. Once impairment of blood supply to the gastrointestinal tract occurs, bacterial invasion supervenes, and peritonitis develops. The systemic effects of extreme distention include elevation of the diaphragm with restricted ventilation and subsequent atelectasis. Venous return via the inferior vena cava may also be impaired.

SYMPTOMS

Mechanical intestinal obstruction is characterized by cramping midabdominal pain, which tends to be more severe the higher the obstruction. The pain occurs in paroxysms, and the patient is relatively comfortable in the intervals between the pains. Audible borborygmi are often noted by the patient simultaneously with the paroxysms of pain. The pain may become less severe as distention progresses, probably because motility is impaired in the edematous intestine. When strangulation is present, the pain is usually more localized and may be steady and severe without a colicky component, a fact that often causes delay in diagnosis of obstruction. Vomiting is almost invariable, and it is earlier and more profuse the higher the obstruction. The vomitus initially contains bile and mucus and remains as such if the obstruction is high in the intestine. With low ileal obstruction, the vomitus becomes feculent, i.e., orange-brown in color with a foul odor, which results from the overgrowth of

bacteria proximal to the obstruction. Hiccups (singultus) are common. Obstipation and failure to pass gas by rectum are invariably present when the obstruction is complete, although some stool and gas may be passed spontaneously or after an enema shortly after onset of the complete obstruction. Diarrhea is occasionally observed in partial obstruction. Blood in the stool is rare but does occur in cases of intussusception.

In *adynamic ileus* as well as *colonic pseudoobstruction*, colicky pain is absent and only discomfort from distention is evident. Vomiting may be frequent but is rarely profuse. Complete obstipation may or may not occur. Singultus (hiccups) is common.

PHYSICAL FINDINGS

Abdominal distention is the hallmark of all forms of intestinal obstruction. It is least marked in cases of obstruction high in the small intestine and most marked in colonic obstruction. In early obstruction of the small and large intestine, tenderness and rigidity are usually minimal; the temperature is rarely >37.8°C (100°F). The appearance of shock, tenderness, rigidity, and fever indicates that contamination of the peritoneum with infected intestinal content has occurred. Hernial orifices should always be carefully examined for the presence of a mass. Auscultation may reveal loud, high-pitched borborygmi coincident with colicky pain, but this finding is often absent late in strangulating or nonstrangulating obstruction. A quiet abdomen does not eliminate the possibility of obstruction, nor does it necessarily establish the diagnosis of adynamic ileus. The presence of a palpable abdominal mass usually signifies a closed-loop strangulating small-bowel obstruction; the tense fluid-filled loop is the palpable lesion.

LABORATORY AND X-RAY FINDINGS

Laboratory and radiographic studies are used to help differentiate the two important clinical aspects of this disorder: strangulation versus nonstrangulation and partial versus complete obstruction. Leukocytosis, with shift to the left, usually occurs when strangulation is present, but a normal white blood cell count does not exclude strangulation. Elevation of the serum amylase level is encountered occasionally in all forms of intestinal obstruction. Roentgenographic images demonstrating distention of fluid- and gas-filled loops of small intestine usually arranged in a "stepladder" pattern with air-fluid levels and an absence or paucity of colonic gas are pathognomonic for small-bowel obstruction. Complete obstruction is suggested when passage of gas or stool per rectum has ceased and when gas is absent in the distal intestine by x-ray. A general haze due to peritoneal fluid and sometimes a "coffee bean"–shaped mass are seen in strangulating closed loop obstruction. A thin barium upper gastrointestinal series may help to differentiate partial from complete obstruction. However, thick barium given by mouth should be avoided when the obstruction is considered to be high grade or complete since retained barium sulfate may become inspissated. CT is the most commonly used modality to evaluate postoperative patients for intestinal obstruction because of its ability in differentiating adynamic ileus, partial obstruction, and complete obstruction (**Fig. 20-1**). However, the sensitivity and specificity of CT for strangulating obstruction are low (50 and 80%, respectively).

Common causes of colonic obstruction can be seen on abdominal roentgenographic series. These films may demonstrate a "bird's beak" sign when a sigmoid volvulus has occurred or an enlarged cecum when a cecal torsion or bascule is present. Colonic obstruction with a competent ileocecal valve is easily recognized because distention with gas is mainly confined to the colon. Gastrografin enema may help in demonstrating a complete colonic obstruction. Furthermore, *barium should never be given by mouth to a patient with a possible colonic obstruction* until that possibility has been excluded.

℞ **Treatment:**
ACUTE INTESTINAL OBSTRUCTION

SMALL-INTESTINAL OBSTRUCTION The overall mortality rate for obstruction of the small intestine is about 10%. While the mortality rate for nonstrangulating obstruction is 5–8%, the mortality rate for a strangulating obstruction ranges from 20 to 75%. Since strangulating small-bowel obstruction is always complete, surgical interventions should always be undertaken in such patients after suitable preparation. Before operating, fluid and electrolyte balance should be restored and decompression instituted by means of a nasogastric tube. Replacement of potassium is especially important because intake is nil and losses in vomitus are large. There are few, if any, indications for the use of a long intestinal tube. Operative intervention may be undertaken successfully by laparoscopic techniques with a decreased incidence of wound complications. However, laparoscopic lysis of adhesions is associated with a longer operative time and higher conversion to open rate when compared to other laparoscopic procedures.

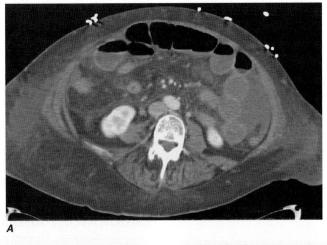

A

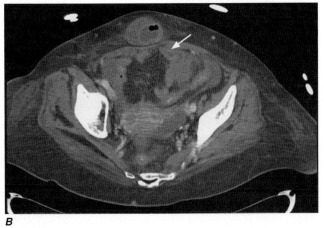

B

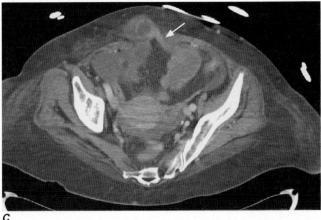

C

FIGURE 20-1

CT with oral and intravenous contrast demonstrating **(A)** evidence of small-bowel dilatation with air-fluid levels consistent with a small-bowel obstruction; **(B)** a partial small-bowel obstruction from an incarcerated ventral hernia (*arrow*); and **(C)** decompressed bowel seen distal to the hernia (*arrow*).

Alternatively, lysis of adhesions can occur through an open abdominal incision. In general, >50% of adhesions that occur are found at the previous incision site. Purely nonoperative therapy is safe only in the presence of incomplete obstruction and is best utilized in patients without increasing abdominal pain or leukocytosis. The overall recurrence of small-bowel obstruction is 16%. Population-based studies show that although the surgical management of small-bowel obstruction is associated with longer hospital stays, the rate of readmission for obstruction is lower. However, regardless of treatment type, following the index admission, only 20% of patients required readmission within a 5-year follow-up period.

COLONIC OBSTRUCTION The mortality rate for colonic obstruction is about 20%. As in small-bowel obstruction, nonoperative treatment is contraindicated unless the obstruction is incomplete. Incomplete obstruction can be treated with colonoscopic decompression and placement of a metallic stent if a malignant lesion is present. The success rate approaches 90% depending on the location of the obstruction, with left-sided lesions being more successfully stented than right-sided lesions. In general, the colonic stent is considered to be a temporary solution or a "bridge to surgery," which allows for colonic preparation before surgical intervention. When obstruction is complete, early operation is mandatory, especially when the ileocecal valve is competent, because of the concern for cecal perforation. Cecal perforation is more likely if the cecal diameter is >10 cm on plain abdominal film.

Decisions regarding the operative management of colonic obstruction are based on the cause of the obstruction and the patient's overall well-being. For obstruction on the left side of the colon, operative management strategies include either decompression by cecostomy or transverse colostomy or resection with end-colostomy formation (Hartmann's procedure).

Primary resection of obstructing left-sided lesions with on-table washout of the colon has also been accomplished safely. For a lesion of the right or transverse colon, primary resection and anastomosis can be performed safely because distention of the ileum with consequent discrepancy in size and hazard in suture are usually not present. Furthermore, the bacterial and stool content is less on the right side of the colon, decreasing the chance of infection.

ADYNAMIC ILEUS This type of ileus usually responds to nonoperative decompression and treatment of the primary disease. The prognosis is usually good. Correction of electrolyte abnormalities should be performed (i.e., potassium, magnesium). Successful decompression of a colonic ileus has been accomplished by repetitive colonoscopy. Neostigmine is also effective in cases of colonic ileus that have not responded to other conservative treatment. Rarely, adynamic colonic distention may become so great that cecostomy is required if cecal gangrene is feared.

FURTHER READINGS

DUBOIS A et al: Postoperative ileus: Physiopathology, etiology and treatment. Ann Surg 178:781, 1973

ESKELINEN M et al: Contributions of history-taking, physical examination, and computer assistance to diagnosis of acute small-bowel obstruction. A prospective study of 1333 patients with acute abdominal pain. Scand J Gastroenterol 29:715, 1994

FEVANG BT et al: Complications and death after surgical treatment of small bowel obstruction: A 35-year institutional experience. Ann Surg 231:529, 2000

JACKSON BR: The diagnosis of colonic obstruction. Dis Colon Rectum 25:603, 1982

LEE IK et al: Selective laparoscopic management of adhesive small bowel obstruction using CT guidance. Am Surg 75:227, 2009

SILEN W: Cope's Early Diagnosis of the Acute Abdomen, 21st ed. London, Oxford, 2005

WANG N et al: Adult intussusception: a retrospective review of 41 cases. World J Gastroenterol 15:3303, 2009

CHAPTER 21

ACUTE APPENDICITIS AND PERITONITIS

Susan L. Gearhart ■ William Silen

ACUTE APPENDICITIS

INCIDENCE AND EPIDEMIOLOGY

With more than 250,000 appendectomies performed annually, appendicitis is the most common abdominal surgical emergency in the United States. The peak incidence of acute appendicitis is in the second and third decades of life; it is relatively rare at the extremes of age. However, perforation is more common in infancy and in the elderly, during which periods mortality rates are highest. Males and females are equally affected, except between puberty and age 25, when males predominate in a 3:2 ratio. The incidence of appendicitis has remained stable in the United States over the last 40 years, while the incidence of appendicitis is much lower in underdeveloped countries, especially parts of Africa, and in lower socioeconomic groups. The mortality rate in the United States decreased eightfold between 1941 and 1970 but has remained at <1 per 100,000 since then.

PATHOGENESIS

Appendicitis is believed to occur as a result of appendiceal luminal obstruction. Obstruction is most commonly caused by a fecalith, which results from accumulation and inspissation of fecal matter around vegetable fibers. Enlarged lymphoid follicles associated with viral infections (e.g., measles), inspissated barium, worms (e.g., pinworms, *Ascaris*, and *Taenia*), and tumors (e.g., carcinoid or carcinoma) may also obstruct the lumen. Other common pathologic findings include appendiceal ulceration. The cause of the ulceration is unknown, although a viral etiology has been postulated. Infection with *Yersinia* organisms may cause the disease, since high complement fixation antibody titers have been found in up to 30% of cases of proven appendicitis. Luminal bacteria multiply and invade the appendiceal wall as venous engorgement and subsequent arterial compromise result from the high intraluminal pressures. Finally, gangrene and perforation occur. If the process evolves slowly, adjacent organs such as the terminal ileum, cecum, and omentum may wall off the appendiceal area so that a localized abscess will develop, whereas rapid progression of vascular impairment may cause perforation with free access to the peritoneal cavity. Subsequent rupture of primary appendiceal abscesses may produce fistulas between the appendix and bladder, small intestine, sigmoid, or cecum. Occasionally, acute appendicitis may be the first manifestation of Crohn's disease.

While chronic infection of the appendix with tuberculosis, amebiasis, and actinomycosis may occur, a useful clinical aphorism states that *chronic appendiceal inflammation is not usually the cause of prolonged abdominal pain of weeks' or months' duration.* In contrast, recurrent acute appendicitis does occur, often with complete resolution of inflammation and symptoms between attacks. Recurrent acute appendicitis may also occur if a long appendiceal stump is left after initial appendectomy.

CLINICAL MANIFESTATIONS

The sequence of abdominal discomfort and anorexia associated with acute appendicitis is pathognomonic. The pain is described as being located in the periumbilical region initially and then migrating to the right lower quadrant. This classic sequence of symptoms occurs in only 66% of patients. However, in a male patient these symptoms are sufficient to advise surgical exploration. The differential diagnoses for periumbilical and right lower quadrant pain is listed in Table 21-1. The periumbilical abdominal pain is of the visceral type, resulting from distention of the appendiceal lumen. This pain is carried on slow-conducting C fibers and is usually poorly localized in the periumbilical or epigastric region. In general, this visceral pain is mild, often cramping, and usually lasting 4–6 h, but it may not be noted by stoic individuals. As inflammation spreads to the parietal peritoneal surfaces, the pain becomes somatic, steady, and more severe and aggravated by motion or cough. Parietal afferent nerves are A delta fibers, which are fast-conducting and unilateral. These fibers localize the pain to the *right lower quadrant. Anorexia is very common; a hungry patient does not have acute appendicitis. Nausea* and *vomiting* occur in 50–60% of cases, but vomiting is usually self-limited. Change in bowel habit is of little diagnostic value, since any or no alteration may be observed, although the

TABLE 21-1

THE ANATOMIC ORIGIN OF PERIUMBILICAL AND RIGHT LOWER QUADRANT PAIN IN THE DIFFERENTIAL DIAGNOSIS OF APPENDICITIS

Periumbilical

Appendicitis
Small-bowel obstruction
Gastroenteritis
Mesenteric ischemia

Right Lower Quadrant

Gastrointestinal causes	Gynecologic causes
Appendicitis	Ovarian tumor/torsion
Inflammatory bowel disease	Pelvic inflammatory disease
Right-sided diverticulitis	Renal causes
Gastroenteritis	Pyelonephritis
Inguinal hernia	Perinephritic abscess
	Nephrolithiasis

presence of diarrhea caused by an inflamed appendix in juxtaposition to the sigmoid may cause diagnostic difficulties. Urinary frequency and dysuria occur if the appendix lies adjacent to the bladder.

Physical findings vary with time after onset of the illness and according to the location of the appendix, which may be situated deep in the pelvic cul-de-sac; in the right lower quadrant in any relation to the peritoneum, cecum, and small intestine; in the right upper quadrant (especially during pregnancy); or even in the left lower quadrant. *The diagnosis cannot be established unless tenderness can be elicited.* While tenderness is sometimes absent in the early visceral stage of the disease, it ultimately always develops and is found in any location corresponding to the position of the appendix. Typically, tenderness to palpation will often occur at McBurney's point, anatomically located on a line one-third of the way between the anterior iliac spine and the umbilicus. Abdominal tenderness may be completely absent if a retrocecal or pelvic appendix is present, in which case the sole physical finding may be tenderness in the flank or on rectal or pelvic examination. Referred rebound tenderness is often present and is most likely to be absent early in the illness. Flexion of the right hip and guarded movement by the patient are due to parietal peritoneal involvement. Hyperesthesia of the skin of the right lower quadrant and a positive psoas or obturator sign are often late findings and are rarely of diagnostic value.

The temperature is usually normal or slightly elevated [37.2°–38°C (99°–100.5°F)], but a temperature >38.3°C (101°F) should suggest perforation. Tachycardia is commensurate with the elevation of the temperature. Rigidity and tenderness become more marked as the disease progresses to perforation and localized or diffuse peritonitis. Distention is rare unless severe diffuse peritonitis has developed. A mass may develop if localized perforation has occurred but will not usually be detectable before 3 days after onset. Earlier presence of a mass suggests carcinoma of the cecum or Crohn's disease. Perforation is rare before 24 h after onset of symptoms, but the rate may be as high as 80% after 48 h.

Although moderate leukocytosis of 10,000–18,000 cells/μL is frequent (with a concomitant left shift), the absence of leukocytosis does not rule out acute appendicitis. Leukocytosis of >20,000 cells/μL suggests probable perforation. Anemia and blood in the stool suggest a primary diagnosis of carcinoma of the cecum, especially in elderly individuals. The urine may contain a few white or red blood cells without bacteria if the appendix lies close to the right ureter or bladder. Urinalysis is most useful in excluding genitourinary conditions that may mimic acute appendicitis.

Radiographs are rarely of value except when an opaque fecalith (5% of patients) is observed in the right lower quadrant (especially in children). Consequently, abdominal films are not routinely obtained unless other conditions

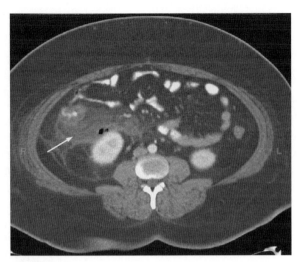

FIGURE 21-1

CT with oral and intravenous contrast of acute appendicitis. There is thickening of the wall of the appendix and periappendiceal stranding (*arrow*).

such as intestinal obstruction or ureteral calculus may be present. The diagnosis may also be established by the ultrasonic demonstration of an enlarged and thick-walled appendix. Ultrasound is most useful to exclude ovarian cysts, ectopic pregnancy, or tuboovarian abscess. Several studies have recently demonstrated the benefit of contrast-enhanced or nonenhanced CT over ultrasound and plain radiographs in the diagnosis of acute appendicitis. The findings on CT will include a thickened appendix with periappendiceal stranding and often the presence of a fecalith (**Figs. 21-1** and **21-2**). The reported positive predictive value of CT is 95–97% and the overall accuracy is 90–98%. Furthermore, nonvisualization of the appendix on CT is associated with the findings of a normal appendix 98% of the time. Free peritoneal air is uncommon, even in perforated appendicitis.

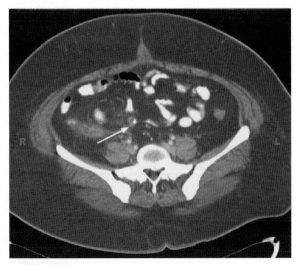

FIGURE 21-2

Appendiceal fecolith (*arrow*).

While the typical historic sequence and physical findings are present in 50–60% of cases, a wide variety of atypical patterns of disease are encountered, especially at the age extremes and during pregnancy. Infants under 2 years of age have a 70–80% incidence of perforation and generalized peritonitis. This is thought to be the result of a delay in diagnosis. Any infant or child with diarrhea, vomiting, and abdominal pain is highly suspect. Fever is much more common in this age group, and abdominal distention is often the only physical finding. In the elderly, pain and tenderness are often blunted, and thus the diagnosis is also frequently delayed and leads to a 30% incidence of perforation in patients over 70. Elderly patients often present initially with a slightly painful mass (a primary appendiceal abscess) or with adhesive intestinal obstruction 5 or 6 days after a previously undetected perforated appendix.

Appendicitis occurs about once in every 500–2000 pregnancies and is the most common extrauterine condition requiring abdominal operation. The diagnosis may be missed or delayed because of the frequent occurrence of mild abdominal discomfort and nausea and vomiting during pregnancy and because of the gradual shift of the appendix from the right lower quadrant to the right upper quadrant during the second and third trimester of pregnancy. Appendicitis tends to be most common during the second trimester. The diagnosis is best made with ultrasound, which has an 80% accuracy; however, if perforation has already occurred, the accuracy of ultrasound decreases to 30%. Early intervention is warranted because the incidence of fetal loss with a normal appendix is 1.5%. With perforation, the incidence of fetal loss is 20–35%.

DIFFERENTIAL DIAGNOSIS

Acute appendicitis has been labeled the *masquerader*, and the diagnosis is often more difficult to make in young females. Obtaining a good history, including sexual activity and the presence of a vaginal discharge, will help differentiate acute appendicitis from pelvic inflammatory disease (PID). The presence of a malodorous vaginal discharge and gram-negative intracellular diplococci are pathognomonic for PID. Pain on movement of the cervix is also more specific for PID but may occur in appendicitis if perforation has occurred or if the appendix lies adjacent to the uterus or adnexa. *Rupture of a graafian follicle* (mittelschmerz) occurs at midcycle and will produce pain and tenderness more diffuse and usually of a less severe degree than in appendicitis. *Rupture of a corpus luteum cyst* is identical clinically to rupture of a graafian follicle but develops about the time of menstruation. The presence of an adnexal mass, evidence of blood loss, and a positive pregnancy test help differentiate *ruptured tubal pregnancy*. *Twisted ovarian cyst* and *endometriosis* are occasionally difficult to distinguish from appendicitis. In all these female conditions, ultrasonography and laparoscopy may be of great value.

Acute mesenteric lymphadenitis and *acute gastroenteritis* are the diagnoses usually given when enlarged, slightly reddened lymph nodes at the root of the mesentery and a normal appendix are encountered at operation in a patient who usually has right lower quadrant tenderness. Retrospectively, these patients may have had a higher temperature, diarrhea, more diffuse pain and abdominal tenderness, and a lymphocytosis. Between cramps, the abdomen is completely relaxed. Children seem to be affected more frequently than adults. Some of these patients have infection with *Y. pseudotuberculosis* or *Y. enterocolitica*, in which case the diagnosis can be established by culture of the mesenteric nodes or by serologic titers. In *Salmonella* gastroenteritis, the abdominal findings are similar, although the pain may be more severe and more localized, and fever and chills are common. The occurrence of similar symptoms among other members of the family may be helpful. *Regional enteritis* (Crohn's disease) is usually associated with a more prolonged history, often with previous exacerbations regarded as episodes of gastroenteritis unless the diagnosis has been established previously. Often an inflammatory mass is palpable. In addition, acute cholecystitis, perforated ulcer, acute pancreatitis, acute diverticulitis, strangulating intestinal obstruction, ureteral calculus, and pyelonephritis may present diagnostic difficulties.

℞ Treatment:
ACUTE APPENDICITIS

If the diagnosis is in question, 4–6 h of observation with serial abdominal exams is always more beneficial than harmful. Antibiotics should not be administered when the diagnosis is in question, since they will only mask the perforation. The treatment of presumed acute appendicitis is early operation and appendectomy as soon as the patient can be prepared. Appendectomy is frequently accomplished laparoscopically and is associated with less postoperative narcotic use and earlier discharge. It is acceptable to have a 15–20% incidence of a normal appendix at the time of appendectomy to avoid perforation. The use of early laparoscopy instead of close clinical observation has not shown a clinical benefit in the management of patients with nonspecific abdominal pain.

A different approach is indicated if a palpable mass is found 3–5 days after the onset of symptoms. This finding usually represents the presence of a phlegmon or abscess, and complications from attempted surgical excision are frequent. Such patients treated with broad-spectrum antibiotics, drainage of abscesses >3 cm, parenteral fluids, and bowel rest usually show resolution of symptoms within 1 week. *Interval appendectomy* can be performed safely 6–12 weeks later. A randomized clinical trial has demonstrated that antibiotics alone can effectively treat acute, nonperforated appendicitis in 86% of male patients. However, antibiotics alone were associated with a higher recurrence rate than surgical intervention. If the mass enlarges or the patient becomes more toxic, the abscess should be drained. Perforation is associated with generalized peritonitis and its complications, including subphrenic, pelvic, or other abscesses, and can be avoided by early diagnosis. The mortality rate for nonperforated appendicitis is 0.1%, little more than the risk of general anesthesia; for perforated appendicitis, mortality is 3% (and can reach 15% in the elderly).

ACUTE PERITONITIS

Peritonitis is an inflammation of the peritoneum; it may be localized or diffuse in location, acute or chronic in natural history, infectious or aseptic in pathogenesis. Acute peritonitis is most often infectious and is usually related to a perforated viscus (and called *secondary peritonitis*). When no intraabdominal source is identified, infectious peritonitis is called *primary* or *spontaneous*. Acute peritonitis is associated with decreased intestinal motor activity, resulting in distention of the intestinal lumen with gas and fluid. The accumulation of fluid in the bowel together with the lack of oral intake leads to rapid intravascular volume depletion with effects on cardiac, renal, and other systems.

ETIOLOGY

Infectious agents gain access to the peritoneal cavity through a perforated viscus, a penetrating wound of the abdominal wall, or external introduction of a foreign object that is or becomes infected (for example, a chronic peritoneal dialysis catheter). In the absence of immune compromise, host defenses are capable of eradicating small contaminations. The conditions that most commonly result in the introduction of bacteria into the peritoneum are ruptured appendix, ruptured diverticulum, perforated peptic ulcer, incarcerated hernia, gangrenous gall bladder, volvulus, bowel infarction, cancer, inflammatory bowel disease, or intestinal obstruction. However, a wide range of mechanisms may play a role (**Table 21-2**). Bacterial peritonitis can also occur in the apparent absence of an intraperitoneal source of bacteria (primary or spontaneous bacterial peritonitis). This condition occurs in the setting of ascites and liver cirrhosis in 90% of the cases, usually in patients with ascites with low protein concentration (<1 g/L) (Chap. 41). Bacterial peritonitis is discussed in detail in Chap. 24.

Aseptic peritonitis may be due to peritoneal irritation by abnormal presence of physiologic fluids (e.g., gastric

TABLE 21-2

CONDITIONS LEADING TO SECONDARY BACTERIAL PERITONITIS

Perforations of bowel	Perforations or leaking of other organs
Trauma, blunt or penetrating	Pancreas—pancreatitis
Inflammation	Gall bladder—cholecystitis
Appendicitis	Urinary bladder—trauma, rupture
Diverticulitis	Liver—bile leak after biopsy
Peptic ulcer disease	Fallopian tubes— salpingitis
Inflammatory bowel disease	Bleeding into the peritoneal cavity
Iatrogenic	**Disruption of integrity of peritoneal cavity**
Endoscopic perforation	
Anastomotic leaks	Trauma
Catheter perforation	Continuous ambulatory peritoneal dialysis (indwelling catheter)
Vascular	
Embolus	Intraperitoneal chemotherapy
Ischemia	
Obstructions	Perinephric abscess
Adhesions	Iatrogenic—postoperative, foreign body
Strangulated hernias	
Volvulus	
Intussusception	
Neoplasms	
Ingested foreign body, toothpick, fish bone	

juice, bile, pancreatic enzymes, blood, or urine) or sterile foreign bodies (e.g., surgical sponges or instruments, starch from surgical gloves) in the peritoneal cavity or as a complication of rare systemic diseases such as lupus erythematosus, porphyria, or familial Mediterranean fever. Chemical irritation of the peritoneum is greatest for acidic gastric juice and pancreatic enzymes. In chemical peritonitis, a major risk of secondary bacterial infection exists.

CLINICAL FEATURES

The cardinal manifestations of peritonitis are acute abdominal pain and tenderness, usually with fever. The location of the pain depends on the underlying cause and whether the inflammation is localized or generalized. Localized peritonitis is most common in uncomplicated appendicitis and diverticulitis, and physical findings are limited to the area of inflammation. Generalized peritonitis is associated with widespread inflammation and diffuse abdominal tenderness and rebound. Rigidity of the abdominal wall is common in both localized and generalized peritonitis. Bowel sounds are usually absent. Tachycardia, hypotension, and signs of dehydration are common. Leukocytosis and marked acidosis are common laboratory findings. Plain abdominal films may show dilation of large and small bowel with edema of the bowel wall. Free air under the diaphragm is associated with a perforated viscus. CT and/or ultrasonography can identify the presence of free fluid or an abscess. When ascites is present, diagnostic paracentesis with cell count (>250 neutrophils/μL is usual in peritonitis), protein and lactate dehydrogenase levels, and culture is essential. In elderly and immunosuppressed patients, signs of peritoneal irritation may be more difficult to detect.

THERAPY AND PROGNOSIS

Treatment relies on rehydration, correction of electrolyte abnormalities, antibiotics, and surgical correction of the underlying defect. Mortality rates are <10% for uncomplicated peritonitis associated with a perforated ulcer or ruptured appendix or diverticulum in an otherwise healthy person. Mortality rates of ≥40% have been reported for elderly people, those with underlying illnesses, and when peritonitis has been present for >48 h.

FURTHER READINGS

ANDERSON RE: The natural history and traditional management of appendicitis revisited: Spontaneous resolution and predominance of prehospital perforations imply that a correct diagnosis is more important than an early diagnosis. World J Surg 31:86, 2007

CHEADLE WG, SPAIN DA: The continuing challenge of intraabdominal infection. Am J Surg 186(Suppl 1):15, 2003

FLUM DR et al: Has misdiagnosis of appendicitis decreased over time? A population-based analysis. JAMA 286:1748, 2001

GANGULI S et al: Right lower quadrant pain: Value of the nonvisualized appendix in patients at multidetector CT. Radiology 214:175, 2006

GRONROOS JM, GRONROOS P: Leucocyte count and C-reactive protein in the diagnosis of acute appendicitis. Br J Surg 86:501, 1999

KILPATRICK CC, OREJUELA FJ: Management of the acute abdomen in pregnancy: a review. Curr Opin Obstet Gynecol 20:534, 2008

MORINO M et al: Acute non-specific abdominal pain: A randomized controlled study comparing early laparoscopy vs. clinical observation. Ann Surg 241:881, 2006

SMITH JE, HALL EJ: The use of plain abdominal x-rays in the emergency department. Emerg Med J 26:160, 2009

STYRUD J et al: Appendectomy vs. antibiotic treatment in acute appendectomy: A prospective multicenter randomized controlled trial. World J Surg 30:1033, 2006

WHITLEY S et al: The appendix on CT. Clin Radiol 64:190, 2009

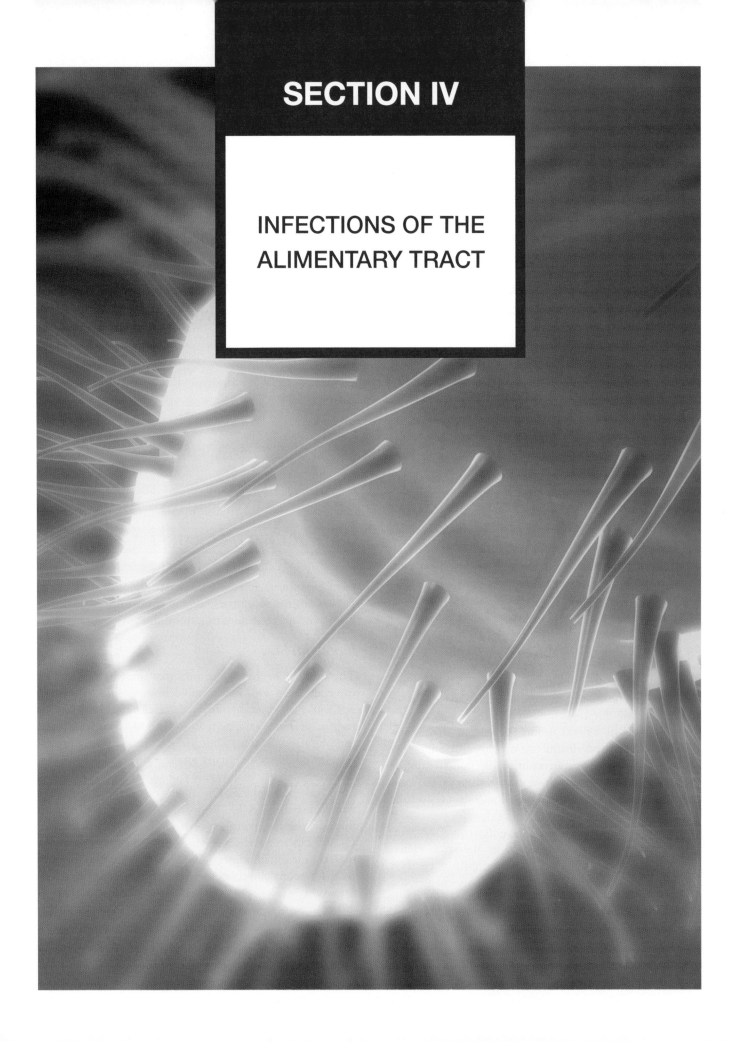

SECTION IV

INFECTIONS OF THE ALIMENTARY TRACT

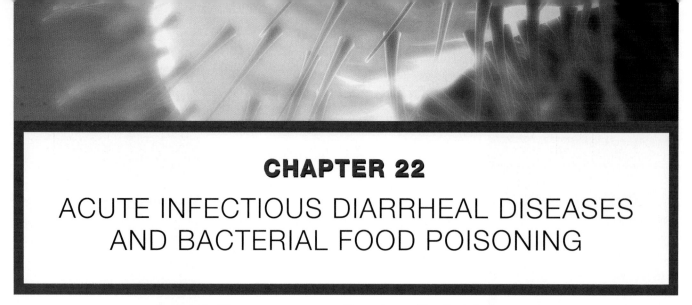

CHAPTER 22

ACUTE INFECTIOUS DIARRHEAL DISEASES AND BACTERIAL FOOD POISONING

Joan R. Butterton ■ Stephen B. Calderwood

Ranging from mild annoyances during vacations to devastating dehydrating illnesses that can kill within hours, acute gastrointestinal illnesses rank second only to acute upper respiratory illnesses as the most common diseases worldwide. In children <5 years old, attack rates range from 2–3 illnesses per child per year in developed countries to as high as 10–18 illnesses per child per year in developing countries. In Asia, Africa, and Latin America, acute diarrheal illnesses are not only a leading cause of morbidity in children—with an estimated 1 billion cases per year—but also a major cause of death. These illnesses are responsible for 4–6 million deaths per year, or a sobering total of 12,600 deaths per day. In some areas, >50% of childhood deaths are directly attributable to acute diarrheal illnesses. In addition, by contributing to malnutrition and thereby reducing resistance to other infectious agents, gastrointestinal illnesses may be indirect factors in a far greater burden of disease.

The wide range of clinical manifestations of acute gastrointestinal illnesses is matched by the wide variety of infectious agents involved, including viruses, bacteria, and parasitic pathogens (Table 22-1). This chapter discusses factors that enable gastrointestinal pathogens to cause disease, reviews host defense mechanisms, and delineates an approach to the evaluation and treatment of patients presenting with acute diarrhea. Individual organisms causing acute gastrointestinal illnesses are discussed in detail in subsequent chapters.

PATHOGENIC MECHANISMS

Enteric pathogens have developed a variety of tactics to overcome host defenses. Understanding the virulence factors employed by these organisms is important in the diagnosis and treatment of clinical disease.

Inoculum Size

The number of microorganisms that must be ingested to cause disease varies considerably from species to species. For *Shigella*, enterohemorrhagic *Escherichia coli*, *Giardia lamblia*, or *Entamoeba*, as few as 10–100 bacteria or cysts can produce infection, while 10^5–10^8 *Vibrio cholerae* organisms must be ingested orally to cause disease. The infective dose of *Salmonella* varies widely, depending on the species, host, and food vehicle. The ability of organisms to overcome host defenses has important implications for transmission; *Shigella*, enterohemorrhagic *E. coli*, *Entamoeba*, and *Giardia* can spread by person-to-person contact, whereas under some circumstances *Salmonella* may have to grow in food for several hours before reaching an effective infectious dose.

Adherence

Many organisms must adhere to the gastrointestinal mucosa as an initial step in the pathogenic process; thus, organisms that can compete with the normal bowel flora

TABLE 22-1

GASTROINTESTINAL PATHOGENS CAUSING ACUTE DIARRHEA

MECHANISM	LOCATION	ILLNESS	STOOL FINDINGS	EXAMPLES OF PATHOGENS INVOLVED
Noninflammatory (enterotoxin)	Proximal small bowel	Watery diarrhea	No fecal leukocytes; mild or no increase in fecal lactoferrin	*Vibrio cholerae*, enterotoxigenic *Escherichia coli* (LT and/or ST), enteroaggregative *E. coli*, *Clostridium perfringens*, *Bacillus cereus*, *Staphylococcus aureus*, *Aeromonas hydrophila*, *Plesiomonas shigelloides*, rotavirus, norovirus, enteric adenoviruses, *Giardia lamblia*, *Cryptosporidium* spp., *Cyclospora* spp., microsporidia
Inflammatory (invasion or cytotoxin)	Colon or distal small bowel	Dysentery or inflammatory diarrhea	Fecal polymorphonuclear leukocytes; substantial increase in fecal lactoferrin	*Shigella* spp., *Salmonella* spp., *Campylobacter jejuni*, enterohemorrhagic *E. coli*, enteroinvasive *E. coli*, *Yersinia enterocolitica*, *Vibrio parahaemolyticus*, *Clostridium difficile*, ?*A. hydrophila*, ?*P. shigelloides*, *Entamoeba histolytica*
Penetrating	Distal small bowel	Enteric fever	Fecal mononuclear leukocytes	*Salmonella typhi*, *Y. enterocolitica*, ?*Campylobacter fetus*

Note: LT, heat-labile enterotoxin; ST, heat-stable enterotoxin.
Source: After Guerrant and Steiner.

and colonize the mucosa have an important advantage in causing disease. Specific cell-surface proteins involved in attachment of bacteria to intestinal cells are important virulence determinants. *V. cholerae*, for example, adheres to the brush border of small-intestinal enterocytes via specific surface adhesins, including the toxin-coregulated pilus and other accessory colonization factors. Enterotoxigenic *E. coli*, which causes watery diarrhea, produces an adherence protein called *colonization factor antigen* that is necessary for colonization of the upper small intestine by the organism prior to the production of enterotoxin. Enteropathogenic *E. coli*, an agent of diarrhea in young children, and enterohemorrhagic *E. coli*, which causes hemorrhagic colitis and the hemolytic-uremic syndrome, produce virulence determinants that allow these organisms to attach to and efface the brush border of the intestinal epithelium.

Toxin Production

The production of one or more exotoxins is important in the pathogenesis of numerous enteric organisms. Such toxins include *enterotoxins*, which cause watery diarrhea by acting directly on secretory mechanisms in the intestinal mucosa; *cytotoxins*, which cause destruction of mucosal cells and associated inflammatory diarrhea;

and *neurotoxins*, which act directly on the central or peripheral nervous system.

The prototypical enterotoxin is cholera toxin, a heterodimeric protein composed of one A and five B subunits. The A subunit contains the enzymatic activity of the toxin, while the B subunit pentamer binds holotoxin to the enterocyte surface receptor, the ganglioside G_{M1}. After the binding of holotoxin, a fragment of the A subunit is translocated across the eukaryotic cell membrane into the cytoplasm, where it catalyzes the ADP-ribosylation of a GTP-binding protein and causes persistent activation of adenylate cyclase. The end result is an increase of cyclic AMP in the intestinal mucosa, which increases Cl^- secretion and decreases Na^+ absorption, leading to loss of fluid and the production of diarrhea.

Enterotoxigenic strains of *E. coli* may produce a protein called *heat-labile enterotoxin* (LT) that is similar to cholera toxin and causes secretory diarrhea by the same mechanism. Alternatively, enterotoxigenic strains of *E. coli* may produce *heat-stable enterotoxin* (ST), one form of which causes diarrhea by activation of guanylate cyclase and elevation of intracellular cyclic GMP. Some enterotoxigenic strains of *E. coli* produce both LT and ST.

Bacterial cytotoxins, in contrast, destroy intestinal mucosal cells and produce the syndrome of dysentery, with bloody stools containing inflammatory cells. Enteric pathogens that produce such cytotoxins include *Shigella dysenteriae* type 1, *Vibrio parahaemolyticus*, and *Clostridium difficile*. *S. dysenteriae* type 1 and Shiga toxin–producing strains of *E. coli* produce potent cytotoxins and have been associated with outbreaks of hemorrhagic colitis and hemolytic-uremic syndrome.

Neurotoxins are usually produced by bacteria outside the host and therefore cause symptoms soon after ingestion. Included are the staphylococcal and *Bacillus cereus* toxins, which act on the central nervous system to produce vomiting.

Invasion

Dysentery may result not only from the production of cytotoxins but also from bacterial invasion and destruction of intestinal mucosal cells. Infections due to *Shigella* and enteroinvasive *E. coli* are characterized by the organisms' invasion of mucosal epithelial cells, intraepithelial multiplication, and subsequent spread to adjacent cells. *Salmonella* causes inflammatory diarrhea by invasion of the bowel mucosa but generally is not associated with the destruction of enterocytes or the full clinical syndrome of dysentery. *Salmonella typhi* and *Yersinia enterocolitica* can penetrate intact intestinal mucosa, multiply intracellularly in Peyer's patches and intestinal lymph nodes, and then disseminate through the bloodstream to cause enteric fever, a syndrome characterized by fever, headache, relative bradycardia, abdominal pain, splenomegaly, and leukopenia.

HOST DEFENSES

Given the enormous number of microorganisms ingested with every meal, the normal host must combat a constant influx of potential enteric pathogens. Studies of infections in patients with alterations in defense mechanisms have led to a greater understanding of the variety of ways in which the normal host can protect itself against disease.

Normal Flora

The large numbers of bacteria that normally inhabit the intestine act as an important host defense by preventing colonization by potential enteric pathogens. Persons with fewer intestinal bacteria, such as infants who have not yet developed normal enteric colonization or patients receiving antibiotics, are at significantly greater risk of developing infections with enteric pathogens. The composition of the intestinal flora is as important as the number of organisms present. More than 99% of the normal colonic flora is made up of anaerobic bacteria, and the acidic pH and volatile fatty acids produced by these organisms appear to be critical elements in resistance to colonization.

Gastric Acid

The acidic pH of the stomach is an important barrier to enteric pathogens, and an increased frequency of infections due to *Salmonella*, *G. lamblia*, and a variety of helminths has been reported among patients who have undergone gastric surgery or are achlorhydric for some other reason. Neutralization of gastric acid with antacids or H_2 blockers—a common practice in the management of hospitalized patients—similarly increases the risk of enteric colonization. In addition, some microorganisms can survive the extreme acidity of the gastric environment; rotavirus, for example, is highly stable to acidity.

Intestinal Motility

Normal peristalsis is the major mechanism for clearance of bacteria from the proximal small intestine. When intestinal motility is impaired (e.g., by treatment with opiates or other antimotility drugs, anatomic abnormalities, or hypomotility states), the frequency of bacterial overgrowth and infection of the small bowel with enteric pathogens is increased. Some patients whose treatment for *Shigella* infection consists of diphenoxylate hydrochloride with atropine (Lomotil) experience prolonged fever and shedding of organisms, while patients treated with opiates for mild *Salmonella* gastroenteritis have a higher frequency of bacteremia than those not treated with opiates.

Immunity

Both cellular immune responses and antibody production play important roles in protection from enteric infections. The wide spectrum of viral, bacterial, parasitic, and fungal gastrointestinal infections in patients with AIDS highlights the significance of cell-mediated immunity in protection from these pathogens. Humoral immunity is also important and consists of systemic IgG and IgM as well as secretory IgA. The mucosal immune system may be the first line of defense against many gastrointestinal pathogens. The binding of bacterial antigens to the luminal surface of M cells in the distal small bowel and the subsequent presentation of antigens to subepithelial lymphoid tissue lead to the proliferation of sensitized lymphocytes. These lymphocytes circulate and populate all of the mucosal tissues of the body as IgA-secreting plasma cells.

Genetic Determinants

The mechanisms underlying genetic variation in host susceptibility remain poorly understood. People with blood group O show increased susceptibility to cholera, shigellosis, and norovirus infection. A polymorphism in the interleukin 8 gene is associated with increased risk of diarrhea from enteroaggregative *E. coli*.

Approach to the Patient:
INFECTIOUS DIARRHEA OR BACTERIAL FOOD POISONING

The approach to the patient with possible infectious diarrhea or bacterial food poisoning is shown in Fig. 22-1.

HISTORY The answers to questions with high discriminating value can quickly narrow the range of potential causes of diarrhea and help determine whether treatment is needed. Important elements of the narrative history are detailed in Fig. 22-1.

PHYSICAL EXAMINATION The examination of patients for signs of dehydration provides essential information about the severity of the diarrheal illness and the need for rapid therapy. Mild dehydration is indicated by thirst, dry mouth, decreased axillary sweat, decreased urine output, and slight weight loss. Signs of moderate dehydration include an orthostatic fall in blood pressure, skin tenting, and sunken eyes (or, in infants, a sunken fontanelle). Signs of severe dehydration range from hypotension and tachycardia to confusion and frank shock.

DIAGNOSTIC APPROACH After the severity of illness is assessed, the clinician must distinguish between *inflammatory* and *noninflammatory* disease. Using the history and epidemiologic features of the case as guides, the clinician can then rapidly evaluate the need for further efforts to define a specific etiology and for therapeutic intervention. Examination of a stool sample may supplement the narrative history. Grossly bloody or mucoid stool suggests an inflammatory process. A test for fecal leukocytes (preparation of a thin smear of stool on a glass slide, addition of a drop of methylene blue, and examination of the

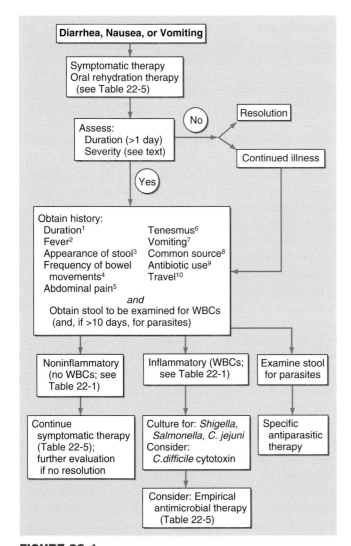

FIGURE 22-1
Clinical algorithm for the approach to patients with community-acquired infectious diarrhea or bacterial food poisoning. Key to superscripts: **1.** Diarrhea lasting >2 weeks

is generally defined as chronic; in such cases, many of the causes of acute diarrhea are much less likely, and a new spectrum of causes needs to be considered. **2.** Fever often implies invasive disease, although fever and diarrhea may also result from infection outside the gastrointestinal tract, as in malaria. **3.** Stools that contain blood or mucus indicate ulceration of the large bowel. Bloody stools without fecal leukocytes should alert the laboratory to the possibility of infection with Shiga toxin–producing enterohemorrhagic *Escherichia coli*. Bulky white stools suggest a small-intestinal process that is causing malabsorption. Profuse "rice-water" stools suggest cholera or a similar toxigenic process. **4.** Frequent stools over a given period can provide the first warning of impending dehydration. **5.** Abdominal pain may be most severe in inflammatory processes like those due to *Shigella*, *Campylobacter*, and necrotizing toxins. Painful abdominal muscle cramps, caused by electrolyte loss, can develop in severe cases of cholera. Bloating is common in giardiasis. An appendicitis-like syndrome should prompt a culture for *Yersinia enterocolitica* with cold enrichment. **6.** Tenesmus (painful rectal spasms with a strong urge to defecate but little passage of stool) may be a feature of cases with proctitis, as in shigellosis or amebiasis. **7.** Vomiting implies an acute infection (e.g., a toxin-mediated illness or food poisoning) but can also be prominent in a variety of systemic illnesses (e.g., malaria) and in intestinal obstruction. **8.** Asking patients whether anyone else they know is sick is a more efficient means of identifying a common source than is constructing a list of recently eaten foods. If a common source seems likely, specific foods can be investigated. See text for a discussion of bacterial food poisoning. **9.** Current antibiotic therapy or a recent history of treatment suggests *Clostridium difficile* diarrhea (Chap. 23). Stop antibiotic treatment if possible and consider tests for *C. difficile* toxins. Antibiotic use may increase the risk of other infections, such as salmonellosis. **10.** See text and Table 22-5 for a discussion of traveler's diarrhea. (*After Guerrant and Steiner; RL Guerrant, DA Bobak: N Engl J Med 325:327, 1991; with permission.*)

TABLE 22-2

POST-DIARRHEA COMPLICATIONS OF ACUTE INFECTIOUS DIARRHEAL ILLNESS	
COMPLICATION	**COMMENTS**
Chronic diarrhea • Lactase deficiency • Small-bowel bacterial overgrowth • Malabsorption syndromes (tropical and celiac sprue)	Occurs in ~1% of travelers with acute diarrhea • Protozoa account for ~1/3 of cases
Initial presentation or exacerbation of inflammatory bowel disease	May be precipitated by traveler's diarrhea
Irritable bowel syndrome	Occurs in ~10% of travelers with traveler's diarrhea
Reiter's syndrome (reactive arthritis)	Particularly likely after infection with invasive organisms (*Shigella*, *Salmonella*, *Campylobacter*)
Hemolytic-uremic syndrome (hemolytic anemia, thrombocytopenia, and renal failure)	Follows infection with Shiga toxin–producing bacteria (*Shigella dysenteriae* type 1 and enterohemorrhagic *Escherichia coli*)

wet mount) can suggest inflammatory disease in patients with diarrhea, although the predictive value of this test is still debated. A test for fecal lactoferrin, which is a marker of fecal leukocytes, is more sensitive and is available in latex agglutination and enzyme-linked immunosorbent assay formats. Causes of acute infectious diarrhea, categorized as inflammatory and noninflammatory, are listed in Table 22-1.

POST-DIARRHEA COMPLICATIONS Chronic complications may follow the resolution of an acute diarrheal episode. The clinician should inquire about prior diarrheal illness if the conditions listed in Table 22-2 are observed.

EPIDEMIOLOGY

Travel History

Of the several million people who travel from temperate industrialized countries to tropical regions of Asia, Africa, and Central and South America each year, 20–50% experience a sudden onset of abdominal cramps, anorexia, and watery diarrhea; thus *traveler's diarrhea* is the most common travel-related illness. The time of onset is usually 3 days to 2 weeks after the traveler's arrival in a tropical area; most cases begin within the first 3–5 days. The illness is generally self-limited, lasting 1–5 days. The high rate of diarrhea among travelers to underdeveloped areas is related to the ingestion of contaminated food or water.

The organisms that cause traveler's diarrhea vary considerably with location (Table 22-3). In all areas, enterotoxigenic and enteroaggregative *E. coli* are the most common isolates from persons with the classic secretory traveler's diarrhea syndrome.

Location

Day-care centers have particularly high attack rates of enteric infections. Rotavirus is most common among children <2 years old, with attack rates of 75–100% among those exposed. *G. lamblia* is more common among older children, with somewhat lower attack rates. Other common organisms, often spread by fecal-oral contact, are *Shigella*, *Campylobacter jejuni*, and *Cryptosporidium*. A characteristic feature of infection among children attending day-care centers is the high rate of secondary cases among family members.

Similarly, hospitals are sites in which enteric infections are concentrated. In medical intensive care units and pediatric wards, diarrhea is one of the most common manifestations of nosocomial infections. *C. difficile* is the predominant cause of nosocomial diarrhea among adults in the United States. Viral pathogens, especially rotavirus, can spread rapidly in pediatric wards. Enteropathogenic *E. coli* has been associated with outbreaks of diarrhea in nurseries for newborns. One-third of elderly patients in chronic-care institutions develop a significant diarrheal illness each year; more than half of these cases are caused by cytotoxin-producing *C. difficile*. Antimicrobial therapy can predispose to pseudomembranous colitis by altering the normal colonic flora and allowing the multiplication of *C. difficile* (Chap. 23).

Age

Most of the morbidity and mortality from enteric pathogens involves children <5 years of age. Breast-fed

TABLE 22-3

233

EPIDEMIOLOGY OF TRAVELER'S DIARRHEA

ETIOLOGIC AGENT	APPROXIMATE PERCENTAGE OF CASES	COMMENTS
Enterotoxigenic *Escherichia coli*	15–50	Single most important agent, particularly in summertime in semitropical areas; percentage of cases ranges from 15% in Asia to 50% in Latin America
Enteroaggregative *E. coli*	20–35	Emerging enteric pathogen of worldwide distribution
Shigella and enteroinvasive *E. coli*	10–25	Major causes of fever and dysentery
Salmonella	5–10	Causes fever and dysentery
Campylobacter jejuni	3–15	More common in winter in semitropical areas; more common in Asia
Aeromonas	5	Important in Thailand
Plesiomonas	5	Related to tropical travel and seafood consumption
Vibrio cholerae	0–10	Most common in India and Asia; also common in Central and South America
Rotavirus and norovirus	10–40	Latin America, Asia, and Africa; norovirus associated with seafood ingestion on cruise ships
Entamoeba histolytica	5	Particularly important in Mexico and Thailand
Giardia lamblia	<2	Zoonotic reservoirs in northern United States; affects hikers and campers who drink from freshwater streams; contaminates water supplies in Russia
Cryptosporidium	2	Affects travelers to Russia, Mexico, and Africa; causes large-scale urban outbreaks in United States
Cyclospora	<1	Affects travelers to Nepal, Haiti, and Peru; contaminates water or food
Unknown	20	Illness improves with antibacterial therapy, implicating bacterial diarrhea

Source: After Dupont.

infants are protected from contaminated food and water and derive some protection from maternal antibodies, but their risk of infection rises dramatically when they begin to eat solid foods. Infants and younger children are more likely than adults to develop rotavirus disease, while older children and adults are more commonly infected with norovirus. Other organisms with higher attack rates among children than among adults include enterotoxigenic, enteropathogenic, and enterohemorrhagic *E. coli*; *C. jejuni*; and *G. lamblia*. In children, the incidence of *Salmonella* infections is highest among those <1 year of age, while the attack rate for *Shigella* infections is greatest among those 6 months to 4 years of age.

Bacterial Food Poisoning

If the history and the stool examination indicate a non-inflammatory etiology of diarrhea and there is evidence of a common-source outbreak, questions concerning the ingestion of specific foods and the time of onset of the diarrhea after a meal can provide clues to the bacterial cause of the illness. Potential causes of bacterial food poisoning are shown in Table 22-4.

Bacterial disease caused by an enterotoxin elaborated outside the host, such as that due to *Staphylococcus aureus* or *B. cereus*, has the shortest incubation period (1–6 h) and generally lasts <12 h. Most cases of staphylococcal food poisoning are caused by contamination from infected human carriers. Staphylococci can multiply at a wide range of temperatures; thus, if food is left to cool slowly and remains at room temperature after cooking, the organisms will have the opportunity to form enterotoxin. Outbreaks following picnics where potato salad, mayonnaise, and cream pastries have been served offer classic examples of staphylococcal food poisoning. Diarrhea, nausea, vomiting,

TABLE 22-4

BACTERIAL FOOD POISONING		
INCUBATION PERIOD, ORGANISM	**SYMPTOMS**	**COMMON FOOD SOURCES**
1–6 h		
Staphylococcus aureus	Nausea, vomiting, diarrhea	Ham, poultry, potato or egg salad, mayonnaise, cream pastries
Bacillus cereus	Nausea, vomiting, diarrhea	Fried rice
8–16 h		
Clostridium perfringens	Abdominal cramps, diarrhea (vomiting rare)	Beef, poultry, legumes, gravies
B. cereus	Abdominal cramps, diarrhea (vomiting rare)	Meats, vegetables, dried beans, cereals
>16 h		
Vibrio cholerae	Watery diarrhea	Shellfish
Enterotoxigenic *Escherichia coli*	Watery diarrhea	Salads, cheese, meats, water
Enterohemorrhagic *E. coli*	Bloody diarrhea	Ground beef, roast beef, salami, raw milk, raw vegetables, apple juice
Salmonella spp.	Inflammatory diarrhea	Beef, poultry, eggs, dairy products
Campylobacter jejuni	Inflammatory diarrhea	Poultry, raw milk
Shigella spp.	Dysentery	Potato or egg salad, lettuce, raw vegetables
Vibrio parahaemolyticus	Dysentery	Mollusks, crustaceans

and abdominal cramping are common, while fever is less so.

B. cereus can produce either a syndrome with a short incubation period—the *emetic* form, mediated by a staphylococcal type of enterotoxin—or one with a longer incubation period (8–16 h)—the *diarrheal* form, caused by an enterotoxin resembling *E. coli* LT, in which diarrhea and abdominal cramps are characteristic but vomiting is uncommon. The emetic form of *B. cereus* food poisoning is associated with contaminated fried rice; the organism is common in uncooked rice, and its heat-resistant spores survive boiling. If cooked rice is not refrigerated, the spores can germinate and produce toxin. Frying before serving may not destroy the preformed, heat-stable toxin.

Food poisoning due to *Clostridium perfringens* also has a slightly longer incubation period (8–14 h) and results from the survival of heat-resistant spores in inadequately cooked meat, poultry, or legumes. After ingestion, toxin is produced in the intestinal tract, causing moderately severe abdominal cramps and diarrhea; vomiting is rare, as is fever. The illness is self-limited, rarely lasting >24 h.

Not all food poisoning has a bacterial cause. Nonbacterial agents of short-incubation food poisoning include capsaicin, which is found in hot peppers, and a variety of toxins found in fish and shellfish.

LABORATORY EVALUATION

Many cases of noninflammatory diarrhea are self-limited or can be treated empirically, and in these instances the clinician may not need to determine a specific etiology. Potentially pathogenic *E. coli* cannot be distinguished from normal fecal flora by routine culture, and tests to detect enterotoxins are not available in most clinical laboratories. In situations in which cholera is a concern, stool should be cultured on thiosulfate–citrate–bile salts–sucrose (TCBS) agar. A latex agglutination test has made the rapid detection of rotavirus in stool practical for many laboratories, while reverse-transcriptase polymerase chain reaction and specific antigen enzyme immunoassays have been developed for the identification of norovirus. At least three stool specimens should be examined for *Giardia* cysts or stained for *Cryptosporidium* if the level of clinical suspicion regarding the involvement of these organisms is high.

All patients with fever and evidence of inflammatory disease acquired outside the hospital should have stool cultured for *Salmonella*, *Shigella*, and *Campylobacter*. *Salmonella* and *Shigella* can be selected on MacConkey's agar as non-lactose-fermenting (colorless) colonies or can be grown on *Salmonella-Shigella* agar or in selenite enrichment broth, both of which inhibit most organisms except these pathogens. Evaluation of nosocomial diarrhea should initially focus on *C. difficile*; stool culture for other pathogens in this setting has an extremely low yield and is not cost-effective. Toxins A and B produced by pathogenic strains of *C. difficile* can be detected by rapid enzyme immunoassays and latex agglutination tests (Chap. 23). Isolation of *C. jejuni* requires inoculation of fresh stool onto selective growth medium and incubation at 42°C in a microaerophilic atmosphere. In many laboratories in the United States, *E. coli* O157:H7 is among the most common pathogens isolated from visibly bloody stools. Strains of this enterohemorrhagic serotype can be identified in specialized laboratories by serotyping but also can be identified presumptively in hospital laboratories as lactose-fermenting, indole-positive colonies of sorbitol nonfermenters (white colonies) on sorbitol MacConkey plates. Fresh stools should be examined for amebic cysts and trophozoites.

Treatment:
℞ INFECTIOUS DIARRHEA OR BACTERIAL FOOD POISONING

In many cases, a specific diagnosis is not necessary or not available to guide treatment. The clinician can proceed with the information obtained from the history, stool examination, and evaluation of dehydration severity. Empirical regimens for the treatment of traveler's diarrhea are listed in Table 22-5.

The mainstay of treatment is adequate rehydration. The treatment of cholera and other dehydrating diarrheal diseases was revolutionized by the promotion of oral rehydration solutions, the efficacy of which depends on the fact that glucose-facilitated absorption of sodium and water in the small intestine remains intact in the presence of cholera toxin. The use of oral rehydration solutions has reduced mortality due to cholera from >50% (in untreated cases) to <1%. The World Health Organization recommends a solution containing 3.5 g sodium chloride, 2.5 g sodium bicarbonate, 1.5 g potassium chloride, and 20 g glucose (or 40 g sucrose) per liter of water. Oral rehydration solutions containing rice or cereal as the carbohydrate source may be even more effective than glucose-based solutions, and the addition of L-histidine may reduce the frequency and volume of stool output. Patients who are severely dehydrated or in whom vomiting precludes the use of oral therapy should receive IV solutions such as Ringer's lactate.

Although most secretory forms of traveler's diarrhea—usually due to enterotoxigenic and enteroaggregative *E. coli*—can be treated effectively with rehydration, bismuth subsalicylate, or antiperistaltic agents, antimicrobial agents can shorten the duration of illness from 3–4 days to 24–36 h. Changes in diet have not been shown to have an impact on the duration of illness, while the efficacy of probiotics continues to be debated.

Antibiotic treatment for children who present with bloody diarrhea raises special concerns. Laboratory studies of enterohemorrhagic *E. coli* strains have demonstrated that a number of antibiotics induce replication of Shiga toxin–producing lambdoid bacteriophages, significantly increasing toxin production by these strains. Clinical studies have supported these laboratory results, and antibiotics are not recommended for the treatment of enterohemorrhagic *E. coli* infections in children.

PROPHYLAXIS

Improvements in hygiene to limit fecal-oral spread of enteric pathogens will be necessary if the prevalence of diarrheal diseases is to be significantly reduced in developing countries. Travelers can reduce their risk of diarrhea by eating only hot, freshly cooked food; by avoiding raw vegetables, salads, and unpeeled fruit; and by drinking only boiled or treated water and avoiding ice. Historically, few travelers to tourist destinations adhere to these dietary restrictions. However, an intensive hygienic effort in Jamaica involving government, hotel, and tourism agencies led to a decrease in the incidence of traveler's diarrhea by 72% from 1996 to 2002.

Bismuth subsalicylate is an inexpensive agent for the prophylaxis of traveler's diarrhea; it is taken at a dosage of 2 tablets (525 mg) four times a day. Treatment appears to be effective and safe for up to 3 weeks. Prophylactic antimicrobial agents, although effective, are not generally recommended for the prevention of traveler's diarrhea, except when travelers are immunosuppressed or have other underlying illnesses that place them at high risk for morbidity from gastrointestinal infection. The risk of side effects and the possibility of developing an infection with a drug-resistant organism or with more harmful, invasive bacteria make it more reasonable to institute an empirical short course of treatment if symptoms develop. The recent availability of effective nonabsorbed antibiotics such as rifaximin may lead to new prophylactic options.

The possibility of exerting a major impact on the worldwide morbidity and mortality associated with diarrheal diseases has led to intense efforts to develop effective

TABLE 22-5

TREATMENT OF TRAVELER'S DIARRHEA ON THE BASIS OF CLINICAL FEATURES

CLINICAL SYNDROME	SUGGESTED THERAPY
Watery diarrhea (no blood in stool, no fever), 1 or 2 unformed stools per day without distressing enteric symptoms	Oral fluids (Pedialyte, Lytren, or flavored mineral water) and saltine crackers
Watery diarrhea (no blood in stool, no fever), 1 or 2 unformed stools per day with distressing enteric symptoms	Bismuth subsalicylate (for adults): 30 mL or 2 tablets (262 mg/tablet) every 30 min for 8 doses; or loperamide[a]: 4 mg initially followed by 2 mg after passage of each unformed stool, not to exceed 8 tablets (16 mg) per day (prescription dose) or 4 caplets (8 mg) per day (over-the-counter dose); drugs can be taken for 2 days
Watery diarrhea (no blood in stool, no distressing abdominal pain, no fever), >2 unformed stools per day	Antibacterial drug[b] plus (for adults) loperamide[a] (see dose above)
Dysentery (passage of bloody stools) or fever (>37.8°C)	Antibacterial drug[b]
Vomiting, minimal diarrhea	Bismuth subsalicylate (for adults; see dose above)
Diarrhea in infants (<2 years old)	Fluids and electrolytes (Pedialyte, Lytren); continue feeding, especially with breast milk; seek medical attention for moderate dehydration, fever lasting >24 h, bloody stools, or diarrhea lasting more than several days
Diarrhea in pregnant women	Fluids and electrolytes; can consider attapulgite, 3 g initially, with dose repeated after passage of each unformed stool or every 2 h (whichever is earlier), for a total dosage of 9 g/d; seek medical attention for persistent or severe symptoms
Diarrhea despite trimethoprim-sulfamethoxazole prophylaxis	Fluoroquinolone—with loperamide[a] (see dose above) if no fever and no blood in stool, alone in cases of fever/dysentery
Diarrhea despite fluoroquinolone prophylaxis	Bismuth subsalicylate (see dose above) for mild to moderate disease; consult physician for moderate to severe disease or if disease persists

[a]Loperamide should not be used by patients with fever or dysentery; its use may prolong diarrhea in patients with infection due to *Shigella* or other invasive organisms.

[b]The recommended antibacterial drugs are as follows:

Travel to high-risk country other than Thailand:

Adults: (1) A fluoroquinolone such as ciprofloxacin, 750 mg as a single dose or 500 mg bid for 3 days; levofloxacin, 500 mg as a single dose or 500 mg qd for 3 days; or norfloxacin, 800 mg as a single dose or 400 mg bid for 3 days. (2) Azithromycin, 1000 mg as a single dose or 500 mg qd for 3 days. (3) Rifaximin, 200 mg tid or 400 mg bid for 3 days (not recommended for use in dysentery).
Children: Azithromycin, 10 mg/kg on day 1, 5 mg/kg on days 2 and 3 if diarrhea persists.
Alternative agent: furazolidone, 7.5 mg/kg per day in four divided doses for 5 days.

Travel to Thailand (with risk of fluoroquinolone-resistant *Campylobacter*):

Adults: Azithromycin (at above dose for adults). Alternative agent: a fluoroquinolone (at above doses for adults).
Children: Same as for children traveling to other areas (see above).
All patients should take oral fluids (Pedialyte, Lytren, or flavored mineral water) plus saltine crackers. If diarrhea becomes moderate or severe, if fever persists, or if bloody stools or dehydration develops, the patient should seek medical attention.
Source: After Dupont.

vaccines against the common bacterial and viral enteric pathogens. Recent research has yielded promising advances in the development of vaccines against rotavirus, *Shigella*, *V. cholerae*, *S. typhi*, and enterotoxigenic *E. coli*.

FURTHER READINGS

AL-ABRI SS et al: Traveller's diarrhoea. Lancet Infect Dis 5:349, 2005

BARTLETT JG: Clinical practice. Antibiotic-associated diarrhea. N Engl J Med 346:334, 2002

DUPONT HL: Travelers' diarrhea, in *Infections of the Gastrointestinal Tract*, 2d ed, MJ Blaser et al (eds). Philadelphia, Lippincott Williams & Wilkins, 2002, Chap 19

FLORES J, OKHUYSEN PC: Genetics of susceptibility to infection with enteric pathogens. Curr Opin Infect Dis Jul 23, 2009 [epub ahead of print]

GREIG JD, LEE MB: Enteric outbreaks in long-term care facilities and recommendations for prevention: a review. Epidemiol Infect 137:145, 2009

GUERRANT RL, STEINER TS: Principles and syndromes of enteric infection, in *Mandell, Douglas and Bennett's Principles and Practice of Infectious Diseases*, 5th ed, GL Mandell et al (eds). Philadelphia, Churchill Livingstone, 2000, Chap 81

KOO HL, DUPONT HL: Current and future developments in travelers' diarrhea therapy. Expert Rev Anti Infect Ther 4:417, 2006

LYNCH MF et al: The growing burden of foodborne outbreaks due to contaminated fresh produce: risks and opportunities. Epidemiol Infect 137:307, 2009

MUSHER DM, MUSHER BL: Contagious acute gastrointestinal infections. N Engl J Med 351:2417, 2004

OKHUYSEN PC: Current concepts in travelers' diarrhea: Epidemiology, antimicrobial resistance and treatment. Curr Opin Infect Dis 18:522, 2005

SAZAWAL S et al: Efficacy of probiotics in prevention of acute diarrhoea: A meta-analysis of masked, randomised, placebo-controlled trials. Lancet Infect Dis 6:374, 2006

TAUXE RV et al: Foodborne disease, in *Mandell, Douglas and Bennett's Principles and Practice of Infectious Diseases*, 5th ed, GL Mandell et al (eds). Philadelphia, Churchill Livingstone, 2000, Chap 87

WONG CS et al: The risk of the hemolytic-uremic syndrome after antibiotic treatment of *Escherichia coli* O157:H7 infections. N Engl J Med 342:1930, 2000

Acute Infectious Diarrheal Diseases and Bacterial Food Poisoning

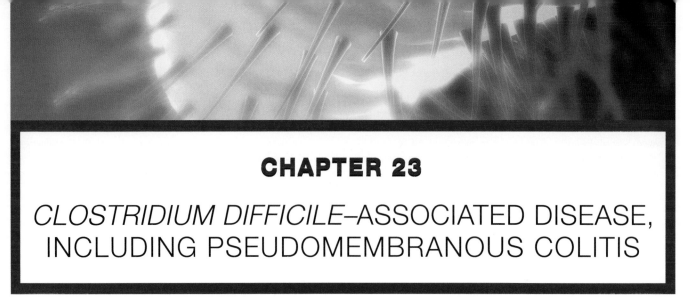

CHAPTER 23

CLOSTRIDIUM DIFFICILE–ASSOCIATED DISEASE, INCLUDING PSEUDOMEMBRANOUS COLITIS

Dale N. Gerding ■ Stuart Johnson

DEFINITION

Clostridium difficile–associated disease (CDAD) is a unique colon infection that is acquired almost exclusively in association with antimicrobial use and the consequent disruption of the normal colonic flora. The most commonly diagnosed diarrheal illness acquired in the hospital, CDAD results from the ingestion of spores of *C. difficile* that vegetate, multiply, and secrete toxins, causing diarrhea and pseudomembranous colitis (PMC).

ETIOLOGY AND EPIDEMIOLOGY

C. difficile is an obligately anaerobic, gram-positive, spore-forming bacillus whose spores are found widely in nature, particularly in the environment of hospitals and chronic-care facilities. CDAD occurs most frequently in hospitals and nursing homes where the level of antimicrobial use is high and the environment is contaminated by *C. difficile* spores.

Clindamycin, ampicillin, and cephalosporins were the first antibiotics associated with CDAD. The second- and third-generation cephalosporins, particularly cefotaxime, ceftriaxone, cefuroxime, and ceftazidime, are agents frequently responsible for this condition, and the fluoroquinolones (ciprofloxacin, levofloxacin, gatifloxacin,

and moxifloxacin) are the most recent drug class to be implicated in hospital outbreaks. Penicillin/β-lactamase-inhibitor combinations such as ticarcillin/clavulanate and piperacillin/tazobactam pose significantly less risk. However, all antibiotics, including vancomycin and metronidazole (the agents most commonly used to treat CDAD), have been found to carry a risk of subsequent CDAD. Rare cases are reported in patients without prior antibiotic exposure.

C. difficile is acquired exogenously, most frequently in the hospital, and is carried in the stool of symptomatic and asymptomatic patients. The rate of fecal colonization is often ≥20% among adult patients hospitalized for >1 week; in contrast, the rate is 1–3% among community residents. The risk of *C. difficile* acquisition increases in proportion to length of hospital stay. Asymptomatic fecal carriage of *C. difficile* in healthy neonates is very common, with rates often exceeding 50% during the first 6 months of life, but associated disease in this population is rare. Spores of *C. difficile* are found on environmental surfaces (where the organism can persist for months) and on the hands of hospital personnel who fail to practice good hand hygiene. Hospital epidemics of CDAD have been attributed to a single *C. difficile* strain and to multiple strains present simultaneously. Other identified risk factors for CDAD include older

238

age, greater severity of underlying illness, gastrointestinal surgery, use of electronic rectal thermometers, enteral tube feeding, and antacid treatment. Use of proton pump inhibitors may be a risk factor.

PATHOLOGY AND PATHOGENESIS

Spores of toxigenic *C. difficile* are ingested, survive gastric acidity, germinate in the small bowel, and colonize the lower intestinal tract, where they elaborate two large toxins: toxin A, an enterotoxin, and toxin B, a cytotoxin. These toxins initiate processes resulting in the disruption of epithelial-cell barrier function, diarrhea, and pseudomembrane formation. Toxin A is a potent neutrophil chemoattractant, and both toxins glucosylate the GTP-binding proteins of the Rho subfamily that regulate the actin cell cytoskeleton. Disruption of the cytoskeleton results in loss of cell shape, adherence, and tight junctions, with consequent fluid leakage. A third toxin, binary toxin CDT, was previously found in only ~6% of strains but is present in all isolates of the newly recognized epidemic strain (see "Global Considerations" later in the chapter); this toxin is related to *C. perfringens* iota toxin. Its role in the pathogenesis of CDAD has not yet been defined.

The pseudomembranes of PMC are confined to the colonic mucosa and initially appear as 1- to 2-mm whitish-yellow plaques. The intervening mucosa appears unremarkable, but, as the disease progresses, the pseudomembranes coalesce to form larger plaques and become confluent over the entire colon wall (**Fig. 23-1**).

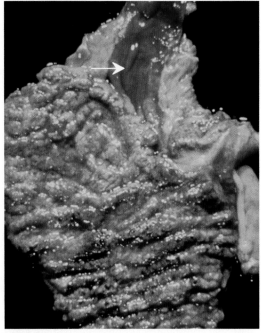

FIGURE 23-1
Autopsy specimen showing confluent pseudomembranes covering the cecum of a patient with pseudomembranous colitis. Note the sparing of the terminal ileum (*arrow*).

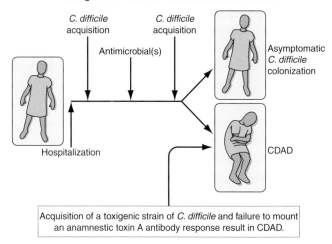

Pathogenesis model for *C. difficile* enteric disease

FIGURE 23-2
Pathogenesis model for hospital-acquired Clostridium difficile–associated diarrhea (CDAD). At least three events are integral to *C. difficile* pathogenesis. Exposure to antibiotics establishes susceptibility to infection. Once susceptible, the patient may acquire nontoxigenic (nonpathogenic) or toxigenic strains of *C. difficile* as a second event. Acquisition of toxigenic *C. difficile* may be followed by asymptomatic colonization or CDAD, depending on one or more additional events, including an inadequate host anamnestic IgG response to *C. difficile* toxin A.

The whole colon is usually involved, but 10% of patients have rectal sparing. Viewed microscopically, the pseudomembranes have a mucosal attachment point and contain necrotic leukocytes, fibrin, mucus, and cellular debris. The epithelium is eroded and necrotic in focal areas, with neutrophil infiltration of the mucosa.

Patients colonized with *C. difficile* were initially thought to be at high risk for CDAD. However, four prospective studies have shown that colonized patients actually have a decreased risk of subsequent CDAD. At least three events are proposed as essential for the development of CDAD (**Fig. 23-2**). Exposure to antimicrobial agents is the first event and establishes susceptibility to *C. difficile* infection. The second event is exposure to toxigenic *C. difficile*. Given that the majority of patients do not develop CDAD after the first two events, a third event is clearly essential for its occurrence. Candidate third events include exposure to a *C. difficile* strain of particular virulence, exposure to antimicrobial agents especially likely to cause CDAD, and an inadequate host immune response. The host anamnestic serum IgG antibody response to toxin A of *C. difficile* is the most likely third event that determines which patients develop diarrhea and which patients remain asymptomatic. The majority of humans first develop antibody to *C. difficile* toxins when colonized asymptomatically during the first year of life. Infants are thought not to develop symptomatic CDAD because they lack suitable mucosal toxin

CHAPTER 23

Clostridium Difficile-Associated Disease

receptors that develop later in life. In adulthood, serum levels of IgG antibody to toxin A increase more in response to infection in individuals who become asymptomatic carriers than in those who develop CDAD. For persons who develop CDAD, increasing levels of antitoxin A during treatment correlate with a lower risk of recurrence of CDAD.

GLOBAL CONSIDERATIONS

Rates and severity of CDAD in the United States, Canada, and Europe have increased markedly since the year 2000. Rates in U.S. hospitals tripled between 2000 and 2005. Hospitals in Montreal, Quebec, have reported rates four times higher than the 1997 baseline, with directly attributable mortality of 6.9% (increased from 1.5% previously). An epidemic strain, variously known as toxinotype III, REA type BI, PCR ribotype 027, and pulsed-field type NAP1, is thought to account for much of the increase in incidence and has been found in the United States, Canada, and Europe. The epidemic organism is characterized by (1) an ability to produce 16–23 times as much toxin A and toxin B as control strains in vitro; (2) the presence of a third toxin (binary toxin CDT); and (3) high-level resistance to all fluoroquinolones.

CLINICAL MANIFESTATIONS

Diarrhea is the most common manifestation caused by *C. difficile*. Stools are almost never grossly bloody and range from soft and unformed to watery or mucoid in consistency, with a characteristic odor. Patients may have as many as 20 bowel movements per day. Clinical and laboratory findings include fever in 28% of cases, abdominal pain in 22%, and leukocytosis in 50%. When adynamic ileus (which is seen on x-ray in ~20% of cases) results in cessation of stool passage, the diagnosis of CDAD is frequently overlooked. A clue to the presence of unsuspected CDAD in these patients is unexplained leukocytosis, with ≥15,000 cells/μL. Such patients are at high risk for complications of *C. difficile* infection, particularly toxic megacolon and sepsis.

C. difficile diarrhea recurs after treatment in ~15–30% of cases, and this figure may be increasing. Recurrences may represent either relapses due to the same strain or reinfections with a new strain. Recurrence of clinical CDAD is likely to be a result of continued disruption of the normal fecal flora by the antibiotic used to treat CDAD.

DIAGNOSIS

The diagnosis of CDAD is based on a combination of clinical criteria: (1) diarrhea (≥3 unformed stools per 24 h for ≥2 days), with no other recognized cause; plus (2) toxin A or B detected in the stool, toxin-producing *C. difficile* detected by stool culture, or pseudomembranes seen in the colon. PMC is a more advanced form of CDAD and is visualized at endoscopy in only ~50% of patients with diarrhea who have a positive stool culture and toxin assay for *C. difficile* (Table 23-1). Endoscopy is a rapid diagnostic tool in seriously ill patients with suspected PMC and an acute abdomen, but a negative result in this examination does not rule out CDAD.

Despite the array of tests available for *C. difficile* and its toxins (Table 23-1), no single test has high sensitivity, high specificity, and rapid turnaround. The turnaround

TABLE 23-1

RELATIVE SENSITIVITY AND SPECIFICITY OF DIAGNOSTIC TESTS FOR *CLOSTRIDIUM DIFFICILE*–ASSOCIATED DISEASE (CDAD)

TYPE OF TEST	RELATIVE SENSITIVITY[a]	RELATIVE SPECIFICITY[a]	COMMENT
Stool culture for *C. difficile*	++++	+++	Most sensitive test; specificity is ++++ if the *C. difficile* isolate tests positive for toxin; with clinical data, is diagnostic of CDAD
Cell culture cytotoxin test on stool	+++	++++	With clinical data, is diagnostic of CDAD; highly specific but not as sensitive as stool culture
Enzyme immunoassay for toxin A or toxins A and B in stool	++ to +++	+++	With clinical data, is diagnostic of CDAD; rapid results, but not as sensitive as stool culture or cell culture cytotoxin test
Latex test for *C. difficile* antigen in stool	++	+++	Detects glutamate dehydrogenase found in toxigenic and nontoxigenic strains of *C. difficile* and other stool organisms; less sensitive and specific than other tests; rapid results
Colonoscopy or sigmoidoscopy	+	++++	Highly specific if pseudomembranes are seen; insensitive compared with other tests

[a] According to both clinical and test-based criteria.

Note: ++++, >90%; +++, 71–90%; ++, 51–70%; +, ~50%.

time for reporting of a positive result in the cell cytotoxicity test can be shortened to <24 h if cell cultures are examined at intervals as short as 4 h. However, this approach is labor intensive, and observation for 48 h is required for a conclusive test result. Most laboratory tests for toxins lack sensitivity. However, testing of multiple additional stool specimens is not recommended. Empirical treatment is appropriate if CDAD is strongly suspected on clinical grounds. Testing of asymptomatic patients is not recommended except for epidemiologic study purposes. In particular, so-called tests of cure following treatment are not recommended because many patients continue to harbor the organism and toxin after diarrhea has ceased and test results do not always predict recurrence of CDAD. Thus these results should not be used to restrict placement of patients in long-term-care or nursing home facilities.

Treatment:
℞ *CLOSTRIDIUM DIFFICILE*-ASSOCIATED DISEASE

PRIMARY CDAD When possible, discontinuation of any ongoing antimicrobial administration is recommended as the first step in treatment of CDAD. Earlier studies indicated that 15-23% of patients respond to this simple measure. However, with the advent of the current epidemic strain and the associated rapid clinical deterioration of some patients, prompt initiation of specific CDAD treatment has become the standard. General treatment guidelines include hydration and the avoidance of antiperistaltic agents and opiates, which may mask symptoms and possibly worsen disease. Nevertheless, antiperistaltic agents have been used safely with vancomycin or metronidazole for mild to moderate CDAD.

Although limited prospective randomized clinical trials showed no statistical differences among treatment agents for cessation of diarrhea (the primary outcome endpoint; Table 23-2), later observational studies suggest that response rates to metronidazole may have decreased. The clinical response rate for bacitracin is 10–20% lower than that for vancomycin; therefore, bacitracin use for first-line therapy is discouraged. All drugs, particularly vancomycin, should be given orally if possible. When IV metronidazole is administered, fecal bactericidal drug concentrations are achieved during acute diarrhea, and CDAD treatment has been successful; however, in the presence of adynamic ileus, IV metronidazole treatment of PMC has failed. In previous randomized trials, diarrhea response rates to oral therapy with vancomycin or metronidazole were ≥94%, but two recent observational studies found that metronidazole response rates had declined to 74% and 78%. Although the mean time to resolution of diarrhea is 2–4 days, the response to metronidazole may be much slower. Treatment should not be deemed a failure until a drug has been given for at least 6 days. On the basis of data for shorter courses of vancomycin (Table 23-2), it is recommended that metronidazole and vancomycin be given for at least 10 days, although no controlled comparisons

TABLE 23-2

EXPECTED TREATMENT OUTCOMES BASED ON RANDOMIZED COMPARATIVE TRIALS OF ORAL THERAPY FOR *CLOSTRIDIUM DIFFICILE*-ASSOCIATED DISEASE

TREATMENT	DOSE AND DURATION	RESOLUTION OF DIARRHEA, %	RECURRENCE, %
Placebo or discontinuation of offending antibiotics	None	21	Unknown
Metronidazole	250 mg qid × 10 d	95	5
	250 mg qid × 10 d[a]	82	30
	500 mg tid × 10 d	94	17
Vancomycin	500 mg tid × 10 d	94	17
	500 mg qid × 10 d	100	15
	125 mg qid × 10 d[a]	91	19
	125 mg qid × 7 d	86	33
	125 mg qid × 5 d	75	Unknown
Teicoplanin	400 mg bid × 10 d	96	7
	100 mg bid × 10 d	96	8
Nitazoxanide	500 mg bid × 10 d[a]	89	22
Fusidic acid	500 mg tid × 10 d	93	28
Bacitracin	25,000 U qid × 10 d	80	42

[a]Data from randomized trials reported in 2006.

are available. Although metronidazole is not approved for this indication by the U.S. Food and Drug Administration (FDA), most patients with mild to moderate illness respond to 500 mg given by mouth three times a day for 10 days; extension of the treatment period may be needed for slow responders. Because of the recent increase in metronidazole failures, patients treated with this drug should be monitored carefully for progressive defervescence (if fever is present), alleviation of abdominal pain and tenderness, decreases in the number of daily bowel movements, and decreases in the white blood cell (WBC) count. Clinical deterioration, with worsening signs and symptoms, or an unexplained increase in the WBC count during treatment are indications for a switch to vancomycin (usual dose, 125 mg orally four times a day). Although the use of vancomycin is discouraged for treatment of mildly to moderately ill patients, it is appropriate to use this agent for the initial treatment of patients who appear seriously ill, particularly if they have a high WBC count (>15,000/μL); controlled clinical outcome data on vancomycin use against the epidemic strain are not available. A randomized prospective trial of the antiparasitic drug nitazoxanide showed that (although not approved by the FDA for this indication) it was at least as effective as metronidazole for the treatment of CDAD, providing a potential alternative to vancomycin and metronidazole.

RECURRENT CDAD Overall, ~15–30% of patients experience recurrences of CDAD, either as relapses caused by the original organism or as reinfections following treatment (Table 23-2). Recurrence rates are higher among patients ≥65 years old and among patients who remain in the hospital after the initial episode of CDAD. Patients who have a first recurrence of CDAD have a high rate of second recurrence (33–65%). In the first recurrence, retreatment with metronidazole is comparable to treatment with vancomycin. Recurrent disease, once thought to be relatively mild, has been documented to pose a significant (11%) risk of serious complications (shock, megacolon, perforation, colectomy, or death within 30 days). There is no standard treatment for multiple recurrences, but long or repeated metronidazole courses should be avoided because of potential neurotoxicity. Approaches include the administration of vancomycin followed by the yeast *Saccharomyces boulardii*; the administration of vancomycin followed by synthetic fecal bacterial enema; and the intentional colonization of the patient with a nontoxigenic strain of *C. difficile*. None of these biotherapeutic approaches has been approved by the FDA for use in the United States. Other strategies include (1) the use of vancomycin in tapering doses or with pulse dosing every other day for 4–6 weeks and (2) sequential treatment with vancomycin (125 mg four times daily) followed by rifaximin (400 mg twice daily) for 14 days. IV immunoglobulin, which has also been used with some success, presumably provides antibodies to *C. difficile* toxins.

FULMINANT CDAD Fulminant (rapidly progressive and severe) CDAD presents the most difficult treatment challenge. Patients with fulminant disease often do not have diarrhea, and their illness mimics an acute surgical abdomen. Sepsis (hypotension, fever, tachycardia, leukocytosis) may result from severe CDAD. An acute abdomen (with or without toxic megacolon) may include signs of obstruction, ileus, colon-wall thickening, and ascites on abdominal CT, often with peripheral-blood leukocytosis (≥20,000 cells/μL). Whether or not the patient has diarrhea, the differential diagnosis of an acute abdomen, sepsis, or toxic megacolon should include CDAD if the patient has received antibiotics in the past 2 months. Cautious sigmoidoscopy or colonoscopy to visualize PMC and an abdominal CT examination are the best diagnostic tests in patients without diarrhea.

Medical management of fulminant CDAD is suboptimal because of the difficulty of delivering metronidazole or vancomycin to the colon by the oral route in the presence of ileus. Vancomycin (given via nasogastric tube and by retention enema) plus IV metronidazole have been used in uncontrolled studies with some success, but surgical colectomy may be life-saving if there is no response to medical management. The incidence of fulminant CDAD requiring colectomy appears to be increasing in the evolving epidemic.

PROGNOSIS

The mortality rate attributed to CDAD, previously found to be 0.6–3.5%, has reached 6.9% in recent outbreaks and is progressively higher with increasing age. Most patients recover, but recurrences are common.

PREVENTION AND CONTROL

Strategies for the prevention of CDAD are of two types: those aimed at preventing transmission of the organism to the patient and those aimed at reducing the risk of CDAD if the organism is transmitted. Transmission of *C. difficile* in clinical practice has been prevented by gloving of personnel, elimination of the use of contaminated electronic thermometers, and use of hypochlorite (bleach) solution for environmental decontamination of patients' rooms. Hand hygiene is critical; hand washing is recommended in CDAD outbreaks because alcohol hand gels are not sporicidal. CDAD outbreaks have been best controlled by restricting the use of specific antibiotics, such as clindamycin and second- and third-generation cephalosporins. Outbreaks of CDAD due to clindamycin-resistant strains have resolved promptly when clindamycin use was restricted.

FURTHER READINGS

HOOKMAN P, BARKIN JS: Clostridium difficile associated infection, diarrhea and colitis. World J Gastroenterol 15:1554, 2009

HUBERT B et al: A portrait of the geographic dissemination of the *Clostridium difficile* North American pulsed-field type 1 strain and the epidemiology of *C. difficile*–associated disease in Quebec. Clin Infect Dis 44:238, 2007

JOHNSON S: Recurrent *Clostridium difficile* infection: a review of risk factors, treatments and outcomes. J Infect 58:403, 2009

——— et al: Interruption of recurrent *Clostridium difficile*–associated diarrhea episodes by serial therapy with vancomycin and rifaximin. Clin Infect Dis 44:846, 2007

KYNE L et al: Association between antibody response to toxin A and protection against recurrent *Clostridium difficile* diarrhea. Lancet 357:189, 2001

——— et al: Asymptomatic carriage of *Clostridium difficile* and serum levels of IgG antibody against toxin A. N Engl J Med 342:390, 2000

LEFFLET DA, LAMONT JT. Treatment of *Clostridium difficile*-associated disease. Gastroenterology 136:1899, 2009

LOO VG et al: A predominantly clonal multi-institutional outbreak of *Clostridium difficile*–associated diarrhea with high morbidity and mortality. N Engl J Med 353:2442, 2005

MCDONALD LC et al: *Clostridium difficile* infection in patients discharged from US short-stay hospitals, 1996–2003. Emerg Infect Dis 12:409, 2006

——— et al: An epidemic, toxin gene–variant strain of *Clostridium difficile*. N Engl J Med 353:2433, 2005

MCFARLAND LV: Alternative treatments for *Clostridium difficile* disease: What really works? J Med Microbiol 54:101, 2005

PARKES GC et al: The mechanisms and efficacy of probiotics in the prevention of *Clostridium difficile*-associated diarrhoea. Lancet Infect Dis 9:237, 2009

PEPIN J et al: The management and outcomes of a first recurrence of *Clostridium difficile* associated disease in Quebec. Clin Infect Dis 42:758, 2006

ZAR FA et al: A comparison of vancomycin and metronidazole for the treatment of *Clostridium difficile*–associated diarrhea, stratified by disease severity. Clin Infect Dis 45:302, 2007

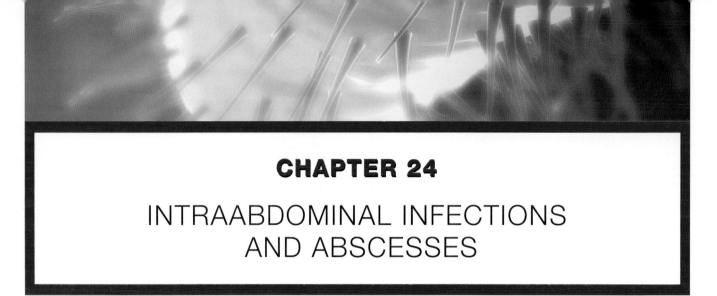

CHAPTER 24

INTRAABDOMINAL INFECTIONS AND ABSCESSES

Miriam J. Baron ■ Dennis L. Kasper

Intraperitoneal infections generally arise because a normal anatomic barrier is disrupted. This disruption may occur when the appendix, a diverticulum, or an ulcer ruptures; when the bowel wall is weakened by ischemia, tumor, or inflammation (e.g., in inflammatory bowel disease); or with adjacent inflammatory processes, such as pancreatitis or pelvic inflammatory disease, in which enzymes (in the former case) or organisms (in the latter) may leak into the peritoneal cavity. Whatever the inciting event, once inflammation develops and organisms usually contained within the bowel or another organ enter the normally sterile peritoneal space, a predictable series of events takes place. Intraabdominal infections occur in two stages: peritonitis and—if the patient survives this stage and goes untreated—abscess formation. The types of microorganisms predominating in each stage of infection are responsible for the pathogenesis of disease.

PERITONITIS

Peritonitis is a life-threatening event that is often accompanied by bacteremia and sepsis syndrome. The peritoneal cavity is large but is divided into compartments. The upper and lower peritoneal cavities are divided by the transverse mesocolon; the greater omentum extends from the transverse mesocolon and from the lower pole of the stomach to line the lower peritoneal cavity. The

pancreas, duodenum, and ascending and descending colon are located in the anterior retroperitoneal space; the kidneys, ureters, and adrenals are found in the posterior retroperitoneal space. The other organs, including liver, stomach, gallbladder, spleen, jejunum, ileum, transverse and sigmoid colon, cecum, and appendix, are within the peritoneal cavity. The cavity is lined with a serous membrane that can serve as a conduit for fluids—a property exploited in peritoneal dialysis (Fig. 24-1). A small amount of serous fluid is normally present in the peritoneal space, with a protein content (consisting mainly of albumin) of <30 g/L and <300 white blood cells (WBCs, generally mononuclear cells) per microliter. In bacterial infections, leukocyte recruitment into the infected peritoneal cavity consists of an early influx of polymorphonuclear leukocytes (PMNs) and a prolonged subsequent phase of mononuclear cell migration. The phenotype of the infiltrating leukocytes during the course of inflammation is regulated primarily by resident-cell chemokine synthesis.

PRIMARY (SPONTANEOUS) BACTERIAL PERITONITIS

Peritonitis is either primary (without an apparent source of contamination) or secondary. The types of organisms found and the clinical presentations of these two processes are different. In adults, primary bacterial

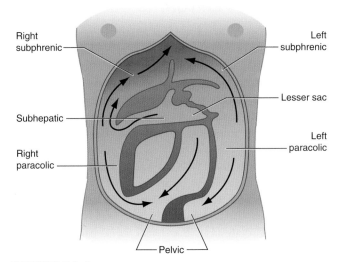

FIGURE 24-1
Diagram of the intraperitoneal spaces, showing the circulation of fluid and potential areas for abscess formation. Some compartments collect fluid or pus more often than others. These compartments include the pelvis (the lowest portion), the subphrenic spaces on the right and left sides, and Morrison's pouch, which is a posterosuperior extension of the subhepatic spaces and is the lowest part of the paravertebral groove when a patient is recumbent. The falciform ligament separating the right and left subphrenic spaces appears to act as a barrier to the spread of infection; consequently, it is unusual to find bilateral subphrenic collections. *[Reprinted with permission from B Lorber (ed): Atlas of Infectious Diseases, vol VII: Intra-abdominal Infections, Hepatitis, and Gastroenteritis. Philadelphia, Current Medicine, 1996, p 1.13.]*

peritonitis (PBP) occurs most commonly in conjunction with cirrhosis of the liver (frequently the result of alcoholism). However, the disease has been reported in adults with metastatic malignant disease, postnecrotic cirrhosis, chronic active hepatitis, acute viral hepatitis, congestive heart failure, systemic lupus erythematosus, and lymphedema as well as in patients with no underlying disease. Although PBP virtually always develops in patients with preexisting ascites, it is, in general, an uncommon event, occurring in ≤10% of cirrhotic patients. The cause of PBP has not been established definitively but is believed to involve hematogenous spread of organisms in a patient in whom a diseased liver and altered portal circulation result in a defect in the usual filtration function. Organisms multiply in ascites, a good medium for growth. The proteins of the complement cascade have been found in peritoneal fluid, with lower levels in cirrhotic patients than in patients with ascites of other etiologies. The opsonic and phagocytic properties of PMNs are diminished in patients with advanced liver disease.

The presentation of PBP differs from that of secondary peritonitis. The most common manifestation is fever, which is reported in up to 80% of patients. Ascites is found but virtually always predates infection. Abdominal pain, an acute onset of symptoms, and peritoneal irritation during physical examination can be helpful diagnostically, but the absence of any of these findings does not exclude this often-subtle diagnosis. Nonlocalizing symptoms (such as malaise, fatigue, or encephalopathy) without another clear etiology should also prompt consideration of PBP in a susceptible patient. It is vital to sample the peritoneal fluid of any cirrhotic patient with ascites and fever. The finding of >250 PMNs/μL is diagnostic for PBP, according to Conn (*http://jac.oxford-journals.org/cgi/content/full/47/3/369*). This criterion does not apply to secondary peritonitis (see "Secondary Peritonitis" later in the chapter). The microbiology of PBP is also distinctive. While enteric gram-negative bacilli such as *Escherichia coli* are most commonly encountered, gram-positive organisms such as streptococci, enterococci, or even pneumococci are sometimes found. In PBP, a single organism is typically isolated; anaerobes are found less frequently in PBP than in secondary peritonitis, in which a mixed flora including anaerobes is the rule. In fact, if PBP is suspected and multiple organisms including anaerobes are recovered from the peritoneal fluid, the diagnosis must be reconsidered and a source of secondary peritonitis sought.

The diagnosis of PBP is not easy. It depends on the exclusion of a primary intraabdominal source of infection. Contrast-enhanced CT is useful in identifying an intraabdominal source for infection. It may be difficult to recover organisms from cultures of peritoneal fluid, presumably because the burden of organisms is low. However, the yield can be improved if 10 mL of peritoneal fluid is placed directly into a blood culture bottle. Since bacteremia frequently accompanies PBP, blood should be cultured simultaneously. No specific radiographic studies are helpful in the diagnosis of PBP. A plain film of the abdomen would be expected to show ascites. Chest and abdominal radiography should be performed in patients with abdominal pain to exclude free air, which signals a perforation (**Fig. 24-2**).

℞ **Treatment:**
PRIMARY BACTERIAL PERITONITIS

Treatment for PBP is directed at the isolate from blood or peritoneal fluid. Gram's staining of peritoneal fluid often gives negative results in PBP. Therefore, until culture results become available, therapy should cover gram-negative aerobic bacilli and gram-positive cocci. Third-generation cephalosporins such as cefotaxime (2 g q8h, administered IV) provide reasonable initial

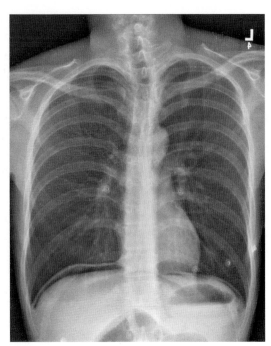

FIGURE 24-2

Pneumoperitoneum. Free air under the diaphragm on an upright chest film suggests the presence of a bowel perforation and associated peritonitis. *(Image courtesy of Dr. John Braver; with permission.)*

coverage in moderately ill patients. Broad-spectrum antibiotics, such as penicillin/β-lactamase inhibitor combinations (e.g., piperacillin/tazobactam, 3.375 g q6h IV for adults with normal renal function) or ceftriaxone (2 g q24h IV), are also options. Empirical coverage for anaerobes is not necessary. After the infecting organism is identified, therapy should be narrowed to target the specific pathogen. Patients with PBP usually respond within 72 h to appropriate antibiotic therapy. Antimicrobial therapy can be administered for as little as 5 days if rapid improvement occurs and blood cultures are negative, but a course of up to 2 weeks may be required for patients with bacteremia and for those whose improvement is slow. Persistence of WBCs in the ascitic fluid after therapy should prompt a search for additional diagnoses.

Prevention

PBP has a high rate of recurrence. Up to 70% of patients experience a recurrence within 1 year. Antibiotic prophylaxis reduces this rate to to <20%. Prophylactic regimens for adults with normal renal function include fluoroquinolones (ciprofloxacin, 750 mg weekly; norfloxacin, 400 mg/d) or trimethoprim-sulfamethoxazole (one double-strength tablet daily). However, long-term administration of broad-spectrum antibiotics in this setting has been shown to increase the risk of severe staphylococcal infections.

SECONDARY PERITONITIS

Secondary peritonitis develops when bacteria contaminate the peritoneum as a result of spillage from an intraabdominal viscus. The organisms found almost always constitute a mixed flora in which facultative gram-negative bacilli and anaerobes predominate, especially when the contaminating source is colonic. Early in the course of infection, when the host response is directed toward containment of the infection, exudate containing fibrin and PMNs is found. Early death in this setting is attributable to gram-negative bacillary sepsis and to potent endotoxins circulating in the bloodstream. Gram-negative bacilli, particularly *E. coli*, are common bloodstream isolates, but *Bacteroides fragilis* bacteremia also occurs. The severity of abdominal pain and the clinical course depend on the inciting process. The organisms isolated from the peritoneum also vary with the source of the initial process and the normal flora at that site. Secondary peritonitis can result primarily from chemical irritation and/or bacterial contamination. For example, as long as the patient is not achlorhydric, a ruptured gastric ulcer will release low-pH gastric contents that will serve as a chemical irritant. The normal flora of the stomach comprises the same organisms found in the oropharynx but in lower numbers. Thus, the bacterial burden in a ruptured ulcer is negligible compared with that in a ruptured appendix. The normal flora of the colon below the ligament of Treitz contains ~10^{11} anaerobic organisms/g of feces but only 10^8 aerobes/g; therefore, anaerobic species account for 99.9% of the bacteria. Leakage of colonic contents (pH 7–8) does not cause significant chemical peritonitis, but infection is intense because of the heavy bacterial load.

Depending on the inciting event, local symptoms may occur in secondary peritonitis—for example, epigastric pain from a ruptured gastric ulcer. In appendicitis (Chap. 21), the initial presenting symptoms are often vague, with periumbilical discomfort and nausea followed in a number of hours by pain more localized to the right lower quadrant. Unusual locations of the appendix (including a retrocecal position) can complicate this presentation further. Once infection has spread to the peritoneal cavity, pain increases, particularly with infection involving the parietal peritoneum, which is innervated extensively. Patients usually lie motionless, often with knees drawn up to avoid stretching the nerve fibers of the peritoneal cavity. Coughing and sneezing, which increase pressure within the peritoneal cavity, are associated with sharp pain. There may or may not be pain localized to the infected or diseased organ from which secondary peritonitis has arisen. Patients with secondary peritonitis generally have abnormal findings on abdominal examination, with marked voluntary and involuntary guarding of the anterior abdominal musculature. Later findings include tenderness, especially rebound tenderness. In addition, there may be localized findings in the area of the inciting event. In general, patients are febrile, with marked leukocytosis and a left shift of the WBCs to band forms.

While recovery of organisms from peritoneal fluid is easier in secondary than in primary peritonitis, a tap of the abdomen is rarely the procedure of choice in secondary peritonitis. An exception is in cases involving trauma, where the possibility of a hemoperitoneum may need to be excluded early. Emergent studies (such as abdominal CT) to find the source of peritoneal contamination should be undertaken if the patient is hemodynamically stable; unstable patients may require surgical intervention without prior imaging.

℞ **Treatment:**
SECONDARY PERITONITIS

Treatment for secondary peritonitis includes early administration of antibiotics aimed particularly at aerobic gram-negative bacilli and anaerobes (see below). Mild to moderate disease can be treated with many drugs covering these organisms, including broad-spectrum penicillin/β-lactamase inhibitor combinations (e.g., ticarcillin/clavulanate, 3.1 g q4–6h IV) or cefoxitin (2 g q4–6h IV). Patients in intensive care units should receive imipenem (500 mg q6h IV), meropenem (1 g q8h IV), or combinations of drugs, such as ampicillin plus metronidazole plus ciprofloxacin. The role of enterococci and *Candida* spp. in mixed infections is controversial. Secondary peritonitis usually requires both surgical intervention to address the inciting process and antibiotics to treat early bacteremia, to decrease the incidence of abscess formation and wound infection, and to prevent distant spread of infection. While surgery is rarely indicated in PBP in adults, it may be life-saving in secondary peritonitis.

Peritonitis may develop as a complication of abdominal surgeries. These infections may be accompanied by localizing pain and/or nonlocalizing symptoms such as fever, malaise, anorexia, and toxicity. As a nosocomial infection, postoperative peritonitis may be associated with organisms such as staphylococci, components of the gram-negative hospital microflora, and the microbes that cause PBP and secondary peritonitis, as described above.

PERITONITIS IN PATIENTS UNDERGOING CAPD

A third type of peritonitis arises in patients who are undergoing continuous ambulatory peritoneal dialysis (CAPD). Unlike PBP and secondary peritonitis, which are caused by endogenous bacteria, CAPD-associated peritonitis usually involves skin organisms. The pathogenesis of infection is similar to that of intravascular device–related infection, in which skin organisms migrate along the catheter, which both serves as an entry point and exerts the effects of a foreign body. Exit-site or tunnel infection may or may not accompany CAPD-associated peritonitis. Like PBP, CAPD-associated peritonitis is usually caused by a single organism. Peritonitis is, in fact, the most common reason for discontinuation of CAPD. Improvements in equipment design, especially the Y-set connector, have resulted in a decrease from one case of peritonitis per 9 months of CAPD to one case per 15 months.

The clinical presentation of CAPD peritonitis resembles that of secondary peritonitis in that diffuse pain and peritoneal signs are common. The dialysate is usually cloudy and contains >100 WBCs/μL, >50% of which are neutrophils. The most common organisms are *Staphylococcus* spp., which accounted for ~45% of cases in one recent series. Historically, coagulase-negative staphylococcal species were identified most commonly in these infections, but more recently these isolates have been decreasing in frequency. *Staphylococcus aureus* is more often involved among patients who are nasal carriers of the organism than among those who are not, and this organism is the most common pathogen in overt exit-site infections. Gram-negative bacilli and fungi such as *Candida* spp. are also found. Vancomycin-resistant enterococci and vancomycin-intermediate *S. aureus* have been reported to produce peritonitis in CAPD patients. The finding of more than one organism in dialysate culture should prompt evaluation for secondary peritonitis. As with PBP, culture of dialysate fluid in blood culture bottles improves the yield. To facilitate diagnosis, several hundred milliliters of removed dialysis fluid should be concentrated by centrifugation before culture.

℞ **Treatment:**
CAPD PERITONITIS

Empirical therapy for CAPD peritonitis should be directed at *S. aureus*, coagulase-negative *Staphylococcus*, and gram-negative bacilli until the results of cultures are available. Guidelines issued in 2005 suggest that agents should be chosen on the basis of local experience with resistant organisms. In some centers, a first-generation cephalosporin such as cefazolin (for gram-positive bacteria) and a fluoroquinolone or a third-generation cephalosporin such as ceftazidime (for gram-negative bacteria) may be reasonable; in areas with high rates of infection with methicillin-resistant *S. aureus*, vancomycin should be used instead of cefazolin, and gram-negative coverage may need to be broadened. Broad coverage including vancomycin should be particularly considered for toxic patients and for those with exit-site infections. Loading doses are administered intraperitoneally; doses depend on the dialysis method and the patient's renal function. Antibiotics are given either continuously (i.e., with each exchange) or intermittently (i.e., once daily, with the dose allowed to remain in the peritoneal cavity for at least 6 h). If the patient is severely ill, IV antibiotics should be added at doses appropriate for the patient's degree of renal failure. The clinical response to an empirical treatment regimen should be rapid; if the patient has not responded after 48 h of treatment, catheter removal should be considered.

INTRAABDOMINAL ABSCESSES

INTRAPERITONEAL ABSCESSES

Abscess formation is common in untreated peritonitis if overt gram-negative sepsis either does not develop or develops but is not fatal. In experimental models of abscess formation, mixed aerobic and anaerobic organisms have been implanted intraperitoneally. Without therapy directed at anaerobes, animals develop intraabdominal abscesses. As in humans, these experimental abscesses may stud the peritoneal cavity, lie within the omentum or mesentery, or even develop on the surface of or within viscera such as the liver.

Pathogenesis and Immunity

There is often disagreement about whether an abscess represents a disease state or a host response. In a sense, it represents both: while an abscess is an infection in which viable infecting organisms and PMNs are contained in a fibrous capsule, it is also a process by which the host confines microbes to a limited space, thereby preventing further spread of infection. In any event, abscesses do cause significant symptoms, and patients with abscesses can be quite ill. Experimental work has helped to define both the host cells and the bacterial virulence factors responsible—most notably, in the case of *B. fragilis*. This organism, although accounting for only 0.5% of the normal colonic flora, is the anaerobe most frequently isolated from intraabdominal infections, is especially prominent in abscesses, and is the most common anaerobic bloodstream isolate. On clinical grounds, therefore, *B. fragilis* appears to be uniquely virulent. Moreover, *B. fragilis* acts alone to cause abscesses in animal models of intraabdominal infection, whereas most other *Bacteroides* species must act synergistically with a facultative organism to induce abscess formation.

Of the several virulence factors identified in *B. fragilis*, one is critical: the capsular polysaccharide complex (CPC) found on the bacterial surface. The CPC comprises at least eight distinct surface polysaccharides. Structural analysis of these polysaccharides has shown an unusual motif of oppositely charged sugars. Polysaccharides having these *zwitterionic* characteristics, such as

polysaccharide A (PSA), evoke a host response in the peritoneal cavity that localizes bacteria into abscesses. *B. fragilis* and PSA have been found to adhere to primary mesothelial cells in vitro; this adherence, in turn, stimulates the production of tumor necrosis factor α (TNF-α) and intercellular adhesion molecule 1 (ICAM-1) by peritoneal macrophages. Although abscesses characteristically contain PMNs, the process of abscess induction depends on the stimulation of T lymphocytes by these unique zwitterionic polysaccharides. The stimulated CD4+ T lymphocytes secrete leukoattractant cytokines and chemokines. The alternative pathway of complement and fibrinogen also participate in abscess formation.

While antibodies to the CPC enhance bloodstream clearance of *B. fragilis*, CD4+ T cells are critical in immunity to abscesses. When administered subcutaneously, *B. fragilis* PSA has immunomodulatory characteristics and stimulates CD4+ T regulatory cells via an interleukin (IL) 2–dependent mechanism to produce IL-10. IL-10 downregulates the inflammatory response, thereby preventing abscess formation.

Clinical Presentation

Of all intraabdominal abscesses, 74% are intraperitoneal or retroperitoneal and are not visceral. Most intraperitoneal abscesses result from fecal spillage from a colonic source, such as an inflamed appendix. Abscesses can also arise from other processes. They usually form within weeks of the development of peritonitis and may be found in a variety of locations—from omentum to mesentery, pelvis to psoas muscles, and subphrenic space to a visceral organ such as the liver, where they may develop either on the surface of the organ or within it. Periappendiceal and diverticular abscesses occur commonly. Diverticular abscesses are least likely to rupture. Infections of the female genital tract and pancreatitis are also among the more common causative events. When abscesses occur in the female genital tract—either as a primary infection (e.g., tuboovarian abscess) or as an infection extending into the pelvic cavity or peritoneum—*B. fragilis* figures prominently among the organisms isolated. *B. fragilis* is not found in large numbers in the normal vaginal flora. For example, it is encountered less commonly in pelvic inflammatory disease and endometritis without an associated abscess. In pancreatitis with leakage of damaging pancreatic enzymes, inflammation is prominent. Therefore, clinical findings such as fever, leukocytosis, and even abdominal pain do not distinguish pancreatitis itself from complications such as pancreatic pseudocyst, pancreatic abscess (Chap. 46), or intraabdominal collections of pus. Especially in cases of necrotizing pancreatitis, in which the incidence of local pancreatic infection may be as high as 30%, needle aspiration under CT guidance is performed to sample fluid for culture. Many centers prescribe preemptive antibiotics for patients with necrotizing pancreatitis. Imipenem is frequently used for this purpose since it reaches high tissue levels in the pancreas (although it is not unique in this regard). If needle aspiration yields infected fluid, most experts agree that surgery is superior to percutaneous drainage.

Diagnosis

Scanning procedures have considerably facilitated the diagnosis of intraabdominal abscesses. Abdominal CT probably has the highest yield, although ultrasonography is particularly useful for the right upper quadrant, kidneys, and pelvis. Both indium-labeled WBCs and gallium tend to localize in abscesses and may be useful in finding a collection. Since gallium is taken up in the bowel, indium-labeled WBCs may have a slightly greater yield for abscesses near the bowel. Neither indium-labeled WBC nor gallium scans serve as a basis for a definitive diagnosis, however; both need to be followed by other, more specific studies, such as CT, if an area of possible abnormality is identified. Abscesses contiguous with or contained within diverticula are particularly difficult to diagnose with scanning procedures. Occasionally, a barium enema may detect a diverticular abscess not diagnosed by other procedures, although barium should not be injected if a perforation is suspected. If one study is negative, a second study sometimes reveals a collection. Although exploratory laparotomy has been less commonly used since the advent of CT, this procedure still must be undertaken on occasion if an abscess is strongly suspected on clinical grounds.

℞ Treatment:
INTRAPERITONEAL ABSCESSES

An algorithm for the management of patients with intraabdominal (including intraperitoneal) abscesses is presented in **Fig. 24-3**. The treatment of intraabdominal infections involves the determination of the initial focus of infection, the administration of broad-spectrum antibiotics targeting the organisms involved, and the performance of a drainage procedure if one or more definitive abscesses have formed. Antimicrobial therapy, in general, is adjunctive to drainage and/or surgical correction of an underlying lesion or process in intraabdominal abscesses. Unlike the intraabdominal abscesses resulting from most causes, for which drainage of some kind is generally required, abscesses associated with diverticulitis usually wall off locally after rupture of a diverticulum, so that surgical intervention is not routinely required.

A number of agents exhibit excellent activity against aerobic gram-negative bacilli. Since mortality in

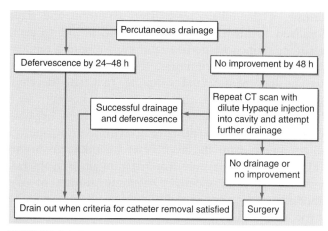

FIGURE 24-3

Algorithm for the management of patients with intraabdominal abscesses using percutaneous drainage. Antimicrobial therapy should be administered concomitantly. *[Reprinted with permission from B Lorber (ed): Atlas of Infectious Diseases, vol VII: Intra-abdominal Infections, Hepatitis, and Gastroenteritis. Philadelphia, Current Medicine, 1996, p 1.30, as adapted from OD Rotstein, RL Simmons, in SL Gorbach et al (eds): Infectious Diseases. Philadelphia, Saunders, 1992, p 668.]*

intraabdominal sepsis is linked to gram-negative bacteremia, empirical therapy for intraabdominal infection always needs to include adequate coverage of gram-negative aerobic, facultative, and anaerobic organisms. Even if anaerobes are not cultured from clinical specimens, they still must be covered by the therapeutic regimen. Empirical antibiotic therapy should be the same as that discussed earlier in the chapter for secondary peritonitis.

VISCERAL ABSCESSES

Liver Abscesses

The liver is the organ most subject to the development of abscesses. In one study of 540 intraabdominal abscesses, 26% were visceral. Liver abscesses made up 13% of the total number, or 48% of all visceral abscesses. Liver abscesses may be solitary or multiple; they may arise from hematogenous spread of bacteria or from local spread from contiguous sites of infection within the peritoneal cavity. In the past, appendicitis with rupture and subsequent spread of infection was the most common source for a liver abscess. Currently, associated disease of the biliary tract is most common. Pylephlebitis (suppurative thrombosis of the portal vein), usually arising from infection in the pelvis but sometimes from infection elsewhere in the peritoneal cavity, is another common source for bacterial seeding of the liver.

Fever is the most common presenting sign of liver abscess. Some patients, particularly those with associated disease of the biliary tract, have symptoms and signs localized to the right upper quadrant, including pain, guarding, punch tenderness, and even rebound tenderness. Nonspecific symptoms, such as chills, anorexia, weight loss, nausea, and vomiting, may also develop. Only 50% of patients with liver abscesses, however, have hepatomegaly, right-upper-quadrant tenderness, or jaundice; thus, half of patients have no symptoms or signs to direct attention to the liver. Fever of unknown origin (FUO) may be the only manifestation of liver abscess, especially in the elderly. Diagnostic studies of the abdomen, especially the right upper quadrant, should be a part of any FUO workup. The single most reliable laboratory finding is an elevated serum concentration of alkaline phosphatase, which is documented in 70% of patients with liver abscesses. Other tests of liver function may yield normal results, but 50% of patients have elevated serum levels of bilirubin, and 48% have elevated concentrations of aspartate aminotransferase. Other laboratory findings include leukocytosis in 77% of patients, anemia (usually normochromic, normocytic) in 50%, and hypoalbuminemia in 33%. Concomitant bacteremia is found in one-third of patients. A liver abscess is sometimes suggested by chest radiography, especially if a new elevation of the right hemidiaphragm is seen; other suggestive findings include a right basilar infiltrate and a right pleural effusion.

Imaging studies are the most reliable methods for diagnosing liver abscesses. These studies include ultrasonography, CT (**Fig. 24-4**), indium-labeled WBC or gallium scan, and MRI. More than one such study may be required. Organisms recovered from liver abscesses vary with the source. In liver infection arising from the

biliary tree, enteric gram–negative aerobic bacilli and enterococci are common isolates. Unless previous surgery has been performed, anaerobes are not generally involved in liver abscesses arising from biliary infections. In contrast, in liver abscesses arising from pelvic and other intraperitoneal sources, a mixed flora including both aerobic and anaerobic species is common; *B. fragilis* is the species most frequently isolated. With hematogenous spread of infection, usually only a single organism is encountered; this species may be *S. aureus* or a streptococcal species such as *S. milleri*. Results of cultures obtained from drain sites are not reliable for defining the etiology of infections. Liver abscesses may also be caused by *Candida* spp.; such abscesses usually follow fungemia in patients receiving chemotherapy for cancer and often present when PMNs return after a period of neutropenia. Amebic liver abscesses are not an uncommon problem (Chap. 31). Amebic serologic testing gives positive results in >95% of cases; thus, a negative result helps to exclude this diagnosis.

℞ Treatment:
LIVER ABSCESSES

(Fig. 24-3) While drainage—either percutaneous (with a pigtail catheter kept in place) or surgical—is the mainstay of therapy for intraabdominal abscesses (including liver abscesses), there is growing interest in medical management alone for pyogenic liver abscesses. The drugs used for empirical therapy include the same ones used in intraabdominal sepsis and secondary bacterial peritonitis. Usually, a diagnostic aspirate of abscess contents should be obtained before the initiation of empirical therapy, with antibiotic choices adjusted when the results of Gram's staining and culture become available. Cases treated without definitive drainage generally require longer courses of antibiotic therapy. When percutaneous drainage was compared with open surgical drainage, the average length of hospital stay for the former was almost twice that for the latter, although both the time required for fever to resolve and the mortality rate were the same for the two procedures. Mortality was appreciable despite treatment, averaging 15%. Several factors predict the failure of percutaneous drainage and therefore may favor primary surgical intervention. These factors include the presence of multiple, sizable abscesses; viscous abscess contents that tend to plug the catheter; associated disease (e.g., disease of the biliary tract) requiring surgery; or the lack of a clinical response to percutaneous drainage in 4–7 days.

Treatment of candidal liver abscesses often entails initial administration of amphotericin B or liposomal amphotericin, with subsequent fluconazole therapy.

In some cases, therapy with fluconazole alone (6 mg/kg daily) may be used—e.g., in clinically stable patients whose infecting isolate is susceptible to this drug.

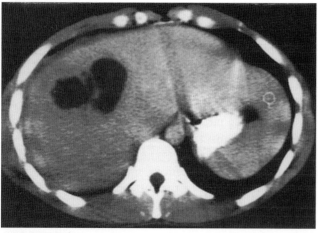

FIGURE 24-4

Multilocular liver abscess on CT scan. Multiple or multilocular abscesses are more common than solitary abscesses. *[Reprinted with permission from B Lorber (ed): Atlas of Infectious Diseases, Vol VII: Intra-abdominal Infections, Hepatitis, and Gastroenteritis. Philadelphia, Current Medicine, 1996, Fig. 1.22.]*

Splenic Abscesses

Splenic abscesses are much less common than liver abscesses. The incidence of splenic abscesses has ranged from 0.14% to 0.7% in various autopsy series. The clinical setting and the organisms isolated usually differ from those for liver abscesses. The degree of clinical suspicion for splenic abscess needs to be high, as this condition is frequently fatal if left untreated. Even in the most recently published series, diagnosis was made only at autopsy in 37% of cases. While splenic abscesses may arise occasionally from contiguous spread of infection or from direct trauma to the spleen, hematogenous spread of infection is more common. Bacterial endocarditis is the most common associated infection. Splenic abscesses can develop in patients who have received extensive immunosuppressive therapy (particularly those with malignancy involving the spleen) and in patients with hemoglobinopathies or other hematologic disorders (especially sickle cell anemia).

While ~50% of patients with splenic abscesses have abdominal pain, the pain is localized to the left upper quadrant in only half of these cases. Splenomegaly is found in ~50% of cases. Fever and leukocytosis are generally present; the development of fever preceded diagnosis by an average of 20 days in one series. Left-sided chest findings may include abnormalities to auscultation, and chest radiographic findings may include an infiltrate or a left-sided pleural effusion. CT scan of the abdomen has been the most sensitive diagnostic tool. Ultrasonography can yield the diagnosis but is less sensitive. Liver-spleen scan or gallium scan may also be useful. Streptococcal species are the most common bacterial isolates from splenic abscesses, followed by *S. aureus*—presumably reflecting the associated endocarditis. An increase in the prevalence of gram-negative aerobic isolates from splenic abscesses has been reported; these organisms often derive from a urinary tract focus, with associated bacteremia, or from another intraabdominal source. *Salmonella* species are seen fairly commonly, especially in patients with sickle cell hemoglobinopathy. Anaerobic species accounted for only 5% of isolates in the largest collected series, but the reporting of a number of "sterile abscesses" may indicate that optimal techniques for the isolation of anaerobes were not employed.

Rx Treatment:
SPLENIC ABSCESSES

Because of he high mortality figures reported for splenic abscesses, splenectomy with adjunctive antibiotics has traditionally been considered standard treatment and remains the best approach for complex, multilocular abscesses or multiple abscesses. However, percutaneous drainage has worked well for single, small (<3 cm)

abscesses in some studies and may also be useful for patients with high surgical risk. Patients undergoing splenectomy should be vaccinated against encapsulated organisms (*Streptococcus pneumoniae*, *Haemophilus influenzae*, *Neisseria meningitidis*). The most important factor in successful treatment of splenic abscesses is early diagnosis.

Perinephric and Renal Abscesses

Perinephric and renal abscesses are not common: The former accounted for only ~0.02% of hospital admissions and the latter for ~0.2% in Altemeier's series of 540 intraabdominal abscesses. Before antibiotics became available, most renal and perinephric abscesses were hematogenous in origin, usually complicating prolonged bacteremia, with *S. aureus* most commonly recovered. Now, in contrast, >75% of perinephric and renal abscesses arise from a urinary tract infection. Infection ascends from the bladder to the kidney, with pyelonephritis occurring prior to abscess development. Bacteria may directly invade the renal parenchyma from medulla to cortex. Local vascular channels within the kidney may also facilitate the transport of organisms. Areas of abscess developing within the parenchyma may rupture into the perinephric space. The kidneys and adrenal glands are surrounded by a layer of perirenal fat that, in turn, is surrounded by Gerota's fascia, which extends superiorly to the diaphragm and inferiorly to the pelvic fat. Abscesses extending into the perinephric space may track through Gerota's fascia into the psoas or transversalis muscles, into the anterior peritoneal cavity, superiorly to the subdiaphragmatic space, or inferiorly to the pelvis. Of the risk factors that have been associated with the development of perinephric abscesses, the most important is concomitant nephrolithiasis obstructing urinary flow. Of patients with perinephric abscess, 20–60% have renal stones. Other structural abnormalities of the urinary tract, prior urologic surgery, trauma, and diabetes mellitus have also been identified as risk factors.

The organisms most frequently encountered in perinephric and renal abscesses are *E. coli*, *Proteus* spp., and *Klebsiella* spp. *E. coli*, the aerobic species most commonly found in the colonic flora, seems to have unique virulence properties in the urinary tract, including factors promoting adherence to uroepithelial cells. The urease of *Proteus* spp. splits urea, thereby creating a more alkaline and more hospitable environment for bacterial proliferation. *Proteus* spp. are frequently found in association with large struvite stones caused by the precipitation of magnesium ammonium sulfate in an alkaline environment. These stones serve as a nidus for recurrent urinary tract infection. While a single bacterial species is usually recovered from a perinephric or renal abscess, multiple species may also be found. If a urine culture is not contaminated with periurethral flora and is found to contain more than one organism, a perinephric abscess or renal abscess should be considered in the differential diagnosis. Urine cultures may also be polymicrobial in cases of bladder diverticulum.

Candida spp. can cause renal abscesses. This fungus may spread to the kidney hematogenously or by ascension from the bladder. The hallmark of the latter route of infection is ureteral obstruction with large fungal balls.

The presentation of perinephric and renal abscesses is quite nonspecific. Flank pain and abdominal pain are common. At least 50% of patients are febrile. Pain may be referred to the groin or leg, particularly with extension of infection. The diagnosis of perinephric abscess, like that of splenic abscess, is frequently delayed, and the mortality rate in some series is appreciable, although lower than in the past. Perinephric or renal abscess should be most seriously considered when a patient presents with symptoms and signs of pyelonephritis and remains febrile after 4 or 5 days of treatment. Moreover, when a urine culture yields a polymicrobial flora, when a patient is known to have renal stones, or when fever and pyuria coexist with a sterile urine culture, these diagnoses should be entertained.

Renal ultrasonography and abdominal CT are the most useful diagnostic modalities. If a renal or perinephric abscess is diagnosed, nephrolithiasis should be excluded, especially when a high urinary pH suggests the presence of a urea-splitting organism.

Rx Treatment: PERINEPHRIC AND RENAL ABSCESSES

Treatment for perinephric and renal abscesses, like that for other intraabdominal abscesses, includes drainage of pus and antibiotic therapy directed at the organism(s) recovered. For perinephric abscesses, percutaneous drainage is usually successful.

Psoas Abscesses

The psoas muscle is another location in which abscesses are encountered. Psoas abscesses may arise from a hematogenous source, by contiguous spread from an intraabdominal or pelvic process, or by contiguous spread from nearby bony structures (e.g., vertebral bodies). Associated osteomyelitis due to spread from bone to muscle or from muscle to bone is common in psoas abscesses. When Pott's disease was common, *Mycobacterium tuberculosis* was a frequent cause of psoas abscess. Currently, either *S. aureus* or a mixture of enteric organisms including aerobic and anaerobic gram-negative bacilli is usually isolated from psoas abscesses in the United States. *S. aureus* is most likely to be isolated

when a psoas abscess arises from hematogenous spread or a contiguous focus of osteomyelitis; a mixed enteric flora is the most likely etiology when the abscess has an intraabdominal or pelvic source. Patients with psoas abscesses frequently present with fever, lower abdominal or back pain, or pain referred to the hip or knee. CT is the most useful diagnostic technique.

Rx Treatment: PSOAS ABSCESSES

Treatment includes surgical drainage and the administration of an antibiotic regimen directed at the inciting organism(s).

Pancreatic Abscesses

See Chap. 46.

ACKNOWLEDGMENT

The substantial contributions of Dori F. Zaleznik, MD, to this chapter in previous editions are gratefully acknowledged.

FURTHER READINGS

CAMPILLO B et al: Epidemiology of severe hospital-acquired infections in patients with liver cirrhosis: Effect of long-term administration of norfloxacin. Clin Infect Dis 26:1066, 1998

GIBSON FC III et al: Cellular mechanism of intraabdominal abscess formation by *Bacteroides fragilis*. J Immunol 160:5000, 1998

JOHANSSEN EC, MADOFF LC: Infections of the liver and biliary system, in *Principles and Practice of Infectious Diseases,* 6th ed, GL Mandell et al (eds). Philadelphia, Elsevier Churchill Livingstone, 2005, pp 951–959

LEVISON ME, BUSH LM: Peritonitis and intraperitoneal abscesses, in *Principles and Practice of Infectious Diseases,* 6th ed, GL Mandell et al (eds). Philadelphia, Elsevier Churchill Livingstone, 2005, pp 927–945

MAZUSKI JE, SOLOMKIN JS: Intra-abdominal infections. Surg Clin North Am 89:421, 2009 PMID:19281892

PAPPAS PG et al: Guidelines for treatment of candidiasis. Clin Infect Dis 38:161, 2004

PIRAINO B et al: Peritoneal dialysis–related infections recommendations: 2005 update. Perit Dial Int 25:107, 2005

RAHIMIAN J et al: Pyogenic liver abscess: Recent trends in etiology and mortality. Clin Infect Dis 39:1654, 2004

SOLOMKIN JS et al: Guidelines for the selection of anti-infective agents for complicated intra-abdominal infections. Clin Infect Dis 37:997, 2003

TZIANABOS AO, KASPER DL: Anaerobic infections: General concepts, in *Principles and Practice of Infectious Diseases,* 6th ed, GL Mandell et al (eds). Philadelphia, Elsevier Churchill Livingstone, 2005, pp 2810–2816

TZIANABOS AO et al: T cells activated by zwitterionic molecules prevent abscesses induced by pathogenic bacteria. J Biol Chem 275:6733, 2000

VAN RULER O et al: Comparison of on-demand vs planned relaparotomy strategy in patients with severe peritonitis: A randomized trial. JAMA 298:865, 2007

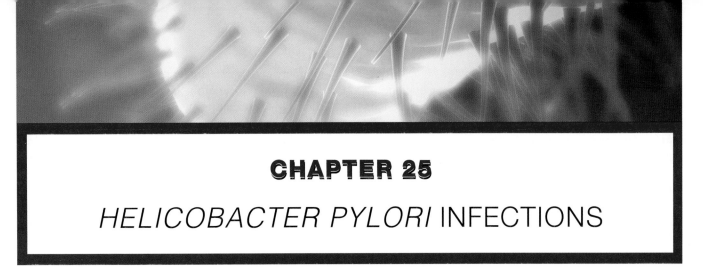

CHAPTER 25

HELICOBACTER PYLORI INFECTIONS

John C. Atherton   ■   Martin J. Blaser

DEFINITION

Helicobacter pylori, which persistently colonizes the stomachs of ~50% of the world's human population, is the main risk factor for peptic ulceration (Chap. 14) as well as for gastric adenocarcinoma and gastric MALT (mucosa-associated lymphoid tissue) lymphoma (Chap. 47). Treatment for *H. pylori* has revolutionized the management of peptic ulcer disease, providing a permanent cure in many cases. The prevention of *H. pylori* colonization could potentially represent primary prevention of gastric malignancy and peptic ulceration. However, controversial but increasing evidence indicates that *H. pylori* may in fact offer some protection against recently emergent diseases—most notably gastroesophageal reflux disease (GERD) and its complications (e.g., esophageal adenocarcinoma). Thus, clearance of *H. pylori* from human populations may not be without negative repercussions.

ETIOLOGIC AGENT

H. pylori is a gram-negative bacillus that has naturally colonized humans for at least tens of thousands of years. It is noninvasive and lives in gastric mucus, with a small proportion of the bacteria adherent to the mucosa. Its spiral shape and flagella render *H. pylori* motile in the mucus environment. This organism has several acid-resistance mechanisms, most notably a highly expressed urease that catalyzes urea hydrolysis to produce buffering ammonia. *H. pylori* is microaerophilic (requiring low levels of oxygen), is slow-growing, and requires complex growth media in vitro. Publication of several complete genomic sequences of *H. pylori* since 1997 has led to significant advances in the understanding of the organism's biology.

A very small proportion of gastric *Helicobacter* infections are due to species other than *H. pylori*, which probably are acquired most often as zoonoses. Whether these non-*pylori* gastric helicobacters cause disease remains controversial. In immunocompromised hosts, several nongastric (intestinal) *Helicobacter* species can cause disease with clinical features resembling those of *Campylobacter* infections; these species are covered in Chap. 28.

EPIDEMIOLOGY

The prevalence of *H. pylori* among adults is ~30% in the United States and other developed countries as opposed to >80% in most developing countries. In the United States, prevalence varies with age: ~50% of 60-year-old persons and ~20% of 30-year-old persons are colonized. *H. pylori* is usually acquired in childhood. The age association is due mostly to a birth-cohort effect whereby current 60-year-olds were more commonly colonized as children than current 30-year-olds. Spontaneous acquisition or loss of *H. pylori* in adulthood is uncommon. Other strong risk factors for *H. pylori* colonization are markers of crowding and poor hygiene in childhood. The very low incidence among children in developed countries at present is probably due, at least in part, to improved living standards and increased use of antibiotics.

Humans are the only important reservoir of *H. pylori*. Children may acquire the organism from their parents (more often from the mother) or from other children. Whether transmission usually takes place by the fecal-oral or the oral-oral route is unknown, but *H. pylori* is easily cultured from vomitus and gastroesophageal refluxate and is less easily cultured from stool.

PATHOLOGY AND PATHOGENESIS

H. pylori colonization induces a tissue response in the stomach; termed *chronic superficial gastritis*, this response includes infiltration of the mucosa by both mononuclear and polymorphonuclear cells. (The term *gastritis* should be used specifically to describe histologic features; it has also been used to describe endoscopic appearances and even symptoms, which do not correlate with microscopic findings or even with the presence of *H. pylori*.) Although *H. pylori* is capable of numerous adaptations that prevent excessive stimulation of the immune system, colonization is accompanied by a considerable persistent immune response, including the production of both local and systemic antibodies as well as cell-mediated responses. However, these responses are ineffective in clearing the bacterium. This inefficient clearing appears to be due in part to *H. pylori*'s down-regulation of the immune system, which fosters its own persistence.

Most *H. pylori*–colonized persons do not develop clinical sequelae. That some persons develop overt disease whereas others do not is related to a combination of factors: bacterial strain differences, host susceptibility to disease, and environmental factors. Several *H. pylori* virulence factors are more common among strains that are associated with disease than among those that are not. The *cag* pathogenicity island (PaI) is a group of genes that encodes a secretion system through which a specific protein, CagA, is translocated into epithelial cells. CagA affects host cell signal transduction, inducing proliferative and cytoskeletal changes. The secretion system also induces a proinflammatory cytokine response, which results in enhanced inflammation. Patients with peptic ulcer disease or gastric adenocarcinoma are more likely than persons without these conditions to be colonized by *cag* PaI-positive strains. The secreted *H. pylori* protein VacA occurs in several forms. Strains with the more active forms are more commonly isolated from patients with peptic ulcer disease or gastric carcinoma than from persons without these conditions. BabA and SabA, adhesins expressed by only some strains, are associated with increased gastric inflammation and with increased risk of peptic ulceration and gastric adenocarcinoma. Other *H. pylori* factors that may affect disease risk are still being described.

The best-characterized host determinants of disease are genetic polymorphisms leading to enhanced *H. pylori*–stimulated secretion of proinflammatory cytokines such as interleukin 1β. *H. pylori*–positive individuals with these polymorphisms are at increased risk of hypochlorhydria and gastric adenocarcinoma. In addition, environmental cofactors are important in pathogenesis. Smoking increases the risks of ulcers and cancer in *H. pylori*–positive individuals. Diets high in salt and preserved foods increase cancer risk, whereas diets high in antioxidants and vitamin C are protective.

The pattern of gastric inflammation is associated with disease risk: antral-predominant gastritis is most closely linked with duodenal ulceration, whereas pangastritis is linked with gastric ulceration and adenocarcinoma. This difference probably explains why patients with duodenal ulceration rarely develop gastric adenocarcinoma later in life, despite being colonized by *H. pylori*.

How gastric colonization causes duodenal ulceration is now becoming clearer. *H. pylori*–induced gastritis diminishes the number of somatostatin-producing D cells. Since somatostatin inhibits gastrin release, gastrin levels are higher than in *H. pylori*–negative persons. These increased gastrin levels lead to increased meal-stimulated acid secretion in the gastric corpus, which is only mildly inflamed in antral-predominant gastritis. In turn, increased acid secretion eventually induces protective gastric metaplasia in the duodenum; the duodenum can then become colonized by *H. pylori*, inflamed, and ulcerated.

The pathogenesis of gastric ulceration and that of gastric adenocarcinoma are less well understood, although both conditions arise in association with pan- or corpus-predominant gastritis. The hormonal changes described above still occur, but the inflamed acid-producing gastric corpus produces less acid, with consequent relative hypochlorhydria, despite the hypergastrinemia. Gastric ulcers usually occur at the junction of antral and corpus-type mucosa, and this region is particularly inflamed. Gastric cancer probably stems from progressive DNA damage and the survival of abnormal epithelial cell clones. The DNA damage is thought to be due principally to reactive oxygen and nitrogen species arising from inflammatory cells and perhaps from other bacteria that survive in hypochlorhydric stomachs. Longitudinal analyses of gastric biopsy specimens taken years apart from the same patient show that the common *intestinal* type of gastric adenocarcinoma follows the stepwise changes from simple gastritis to gastric atrophy, intestinal metaplasia, and dysplasia. A second, *diffuse* type of gastric adenocarcinoma may arise directly from simple chronic gastritis.

CLINICAL MANIFESTATIONS

Essentially all *H. pylori*–colonized persons have gastric tissue responses, but fewer than 15% develop associated illnesses such as peptic ulceration, gastric adenocarcinoma, or gastric lymphoma (**Fig. 25-1**). Worldwide, >80% of duodenal ulcers and >60% of gastric ulcers are related to *H. pylori* colonization (Chap. 14), although the proportion of ulcers due to aspirin and nonsteroidal anti-inflammatory drugs (NSAIDs) is increasing, especially in developed countries. The main lines of evidence for an ulcer-promoting role for *H. pylori* are (1) that the presence of the organism is a risk factor for the development of ulcers, (2) that non-NSAID-induced ulcers rarely develop in the absence of *H. pylori*, (3) that eradication of *H. pylori* markedly reduces rates of ulcer relapse, and (4) that experimental *H. pylori* infection of gerbils causes gastric ulceration.

Prospective nested case-control studies have shown that *H. pylori* colonization is a risk factor for adenocarcinomas of the distal (noncardia) stomach (Chap. 47). Long-term experimental infection of gerbils also may result in gastric adenocarcinoma. Moreover, the presence of *H. pylori* is strongly associated with primary gastric lymphoma, although this condition is less common. Many low-grade gastric B cell lymphomas arising from MALT are driven by T cell stimulation, which in turn is driven by *H. pylori* antigen stimulation; *H. pylori* antigen–driven tumors may regress either fully or partially after *H. pylori* eradication.

Many patients have upper gastrointestinal symptoms but have normal results in upper gastrointestinal endoscopy (so-called functional or nonulcer dyspepsia; Chap. 14). Because *H. pylori* is common, some of these patients will be positive for the organism. *H. pylori* eradication leads to symptom resolution only a little (<10%) more commonly than does placebo treatment. Whether such patients have peptic ulcers in remission at the time of endoscopy or whether a small subgroup of patients with true functional dyspepsia respond to *H. pylori* treatment is unclear.

Much interest has focused on a possible protective role for *H. pylori* against GERD (Chap. 13) and adenocarcinoma of the esophagus and gastric cardia (Chap. 47). The main lines of evidence for this role are (1) that there is a temporal relationship between a falling prevalence of

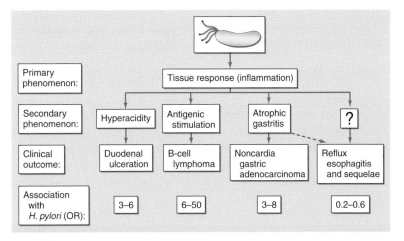

FIGURE 25-1

Schematic of the relationships between colonization with *Helicobacter pylori* and diseases of the upper gastrointestinal tract among persons in developed countries. Essentially all persons colonized with *H. pylori* develop a host response, which is generally termed *chronic gastritis*. The nature of the interaction of the host with the particular bacterial population determines the clinical outcome. *H. pylori* colonization increases the lifetime risk of peptic ulcer disease, noncardia gastric cancer, and B cell non-Hodgkin's gastric lymphoma [odds ratios (ORs) for all, >3]. In contrast, a growing body of evidence indicates that *H. pylori* colonization (especially with *cagA*⁺ strains) protects against adenocarcinoma of the esophagus (and the sometimes related gastric cardia) and premalignant lesions such as Barrett's esophagus (OR, <1). While the incidences of peptic ulcer disease (cases not due to nonsteroidal anti-inflammatory drugs) and noncardia gastric cancer are declining in developed countries, the incidence of adenocarcinoma of the esophagus is rapidly increasing. (*Adapted from Blaser MJ: Hypothesis: The changing relationships of Helicobacter pylori and humans: Implications for health and disease. J Infect Dis 179:1523, 1999; with permission.*)

H. pylori colonization and a rising incidence of these conditions, and (2) that, in most studies, the prevalence of *H. pylori* colonization (especially with proinflammatory *cagA*$^+$ strains) is significantly lower among patients with these esophageal diseases than among control subjects. The mechanism underlying this protective effect appears to include *H. pylori*–induced hypochlorhydria. Since, at the individual level, GERD symptoms may decrease, worsen, or remain unchanged after treatment targeting *H. pylori*, concerns about GERD should not affect decisions about *H. pylori* treatment when a definite indication exists.

H. pylori has an increasingly recognized role in other gastric pathologies. It may be one initial precipitant of autoimmune gastritis and pernicious anemia and also may predispose some patients to iron deficiency through hypochlorhydria and reduced iron absorption. In addition, several extragastrointestinal pathologies have been linked with *H. pylori* colonization, although evidence of causality is less strong. Several small studies have documented improvement or resolution of idiopathic thrombocytopenic purpura after treatment for *H. pylori* colonization. A potentially important but even more controversial association is with ischemic heart disease and cerebrovascular disease. However, the strength of these associations is reduced if confounding factors are taken into account, and most authorities consider the associations to be noncausal.

DIAGNOSIS

Tests for *H. pylori* can be divided into two groups: invasive tests, which require upper gastrointestinal endoscopy and are based on the analysis of gastric biopsy specimens, and noninvasive tests (Table 25-1). Endoscopy often is not performed in the initial management of young dyspeptic patients without "alarm" symptoms but is commonly used to exclude malignancy in older patients. If endoscopy is performed, the most convenient biopsy-based test is the biopsy urease test, in which one large or two small antral biopsy specimens are placed into a gel containing urea and an indicator. The presence of *H. pylori* urease elicits a color change, which often occurs within minutes but can require up to 24 h. Histologic examination of biopsy specimens for *H. pylori* is also accurate, provided that a special stain (e.g., a modified Giemsa or silver stain) permitting optimal visualization of the organism is used. If biopsy specimens are obtained from both antrum and corpus, histologic study yields additional information, including the degree and pattern of inflammation, atrophy, metaplasia, and dysplasia. Microbiologic culture is most specific but may be insensitive because of difficulty with *H. pylori* isolation. Once the organism is cultured, its identity as *H. pylori* can be confirmed by its typical appearance on Gram's stain and its positive reactions in oxidase, catalase, and urease tests. Moreover, the organism's susceptibility to antibiotics can be determined; this information can be clinically useful in difficult cases. The occasional biopsy specimens containing the less common non-*pylori* gastric helicobacters give only weakly positive results in the biopsy urease test. Positive identification of these bacteria requires visualization of the characteristic long, tight spirals in histologic sections.

Noninvasive *H. pylori* testing is the norm if gastric cancer does not need to be excluded by endoscopy. The most consistently accurate test is the urea breath test. In this simple test, the patient drinks a labeled urea solution and then blows into a tube. The urea is labeled with either the nonradioactive isotope ^{13}C or a minute dose of the radioactive isotope ^{14}C. If *H. pylori* urease is present,

TABLE 25-1

TESTS COMMONLY USED TO DETECT *HELICOBACTER PYLORI*		
TEST	ADVANTAGES	DISADVANTAGES
Invasive (Based on Endoscopic Biopsy)		
Biopsy urease test	Quick, simple	Some commercial tests not fully sensitive before 24 h
Histology	May give additional histologic information	Sensitivity dependent on experience and use of special stains
Culture	Permits determination of antibiotic susceptibility	Sensitivity dependent on experience
Noninvasive		
Serology	Inexpensive and convenient	Cannot be used for early follow-up; some commercial kits inaccurate
^{13}C or ^{14}C urea breath test	Inexpensive and simpler than endoscopy; useful for follow-up after treatment	Low-dose irradiation in ^{14}C test (although ^{14}C is rarely used)
Stool antigen test	Inexpensive and convenient; useful for follow-up after treatment; may be useful in children	New test; role not fully established; appears less accurate than urea breath test, particularly when used to assess treatment success

the urea is hydrolyzed and labeled carbon dioxide is detected in breath samples. The stool antigen test, another simple assay, is more convenient and potentially less expensive than the urea breath test but has been slightly less accurate in some comparative studies. The simplest tests for ascertaining *H. pylori* status are serologic assays measuring specific IgG levels in serum by enzyme-linked immunosorbent assay or immunoblot. The best of these tests are as accurate as other diagnostic methods, but many commercial tests—especially rapid office tests—do not perform well.

The urea breath test, the stool antigen test, and biopsy-based tests can all be used to assess the success of treatment (**Fig. 25-2**). However, because these tests are dependent on *H. pylori* load, their use <4 weeks after treatment may lead to false-negative results. Furthermore, these tests are unreliable if performed within 4 weeks of intercurrent treatment with antibiotics or bismuth compounds or within 2 weeks of the discontinuation of proton pump inhibitor (PPI) treatment. In the assessment of treatment success, noninvasive tests are normally preferred; however, after gastric ulceration, endoscopy should be repeated to ensure healing and to exclude gastric carcinoma by further histologic sampling.

Serologic tests are not used to monitor treatment success, as the gradual drop in titer of *H. pylori*–specific antibodies is too slow to be of practical use.

R͟x Treatment: *H. PYLORI* INFECTIONS

The most clear-cut indications for treatment are *H. pylori*–related duodenal or gastric ulceration or low-grade gastric B cell lymphoma. *H. pylori* should be eradicated in patients with documented ulcer disease, whether or not the ulcers are currently active, to reduce the likelihood of relapse (Fig. 25-2). Many guidelines now recommend *H. pylori* treatment in uninvestigated simple dyspepsia following noninvasive diagnosis; others also recommend treatment in functional dyspepsia, in case the patient is one of the perhaps 5–10% to benefit (beyond placebo effects) from such treatment. People with a strong family history of gastric cancer should be treated to eradicate *H. pylori* in the hope that their risk will be reduced. For several reasons, widespread community screening for and treatment of *H. pylori* as primary prophylaxis for gastric cancer and peptic ulcers are not currently recommended. To begin with, it is unclear whether treatment for *H. pylori* reduces the risk of cancer from that in persons who have never acquired the organism. The largest study to date (performed in China) showed no such risk reduction during the 7 years of follow-up. Moreover, treatment has side effects that can be severe in rare cases. Antibiotic resistance may arise in *H. pylori* or other incidentally carried bacteria. Otherwise

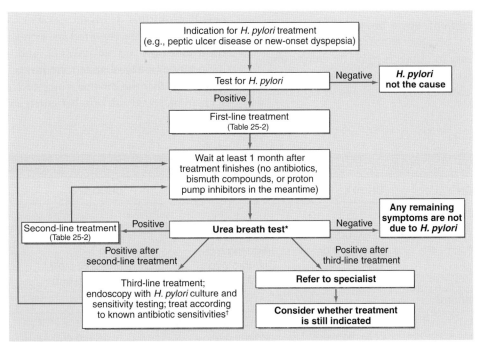

FIGURE 25-2

Algorithm for the management of *Helicobacter pylori* infection. *Occasionally, an endoscopy and a biopsy-based test are used instead of a urea breath test in follow-up after treatment. The main indication for these invasive tests is gastric ulceration; in this condition, as opposed to duodenal ulceration, it is important to check healing and to exclude underlying gastric adenocarcinoma. †Some authorities now use empirical third-line regimens, several of which have been described.

healthy people may become anxious, especially if treatment is unsuccessful. Finally, it is possible that treatment for *H. pylori* will provoke or exacerbate GERD.

Although *H. pylori* is susceptible to a wide range of antibiotics in vitro, monotherapy has been disappointing in vivo, probably because of inadequate antibiotic delivery to the colonization niche. Failure of monotherapy has prompted the development of multidrug regimens, the most successful of which are triple and quadruple combinations that produce *H. pylori* eradication rates of >90% in many trials and >75% in clinical practice. Current regimens consist of a PPI or ranitidine bismuth citrate and two or three antimicrobial agents given for 7–14 days (Table 25-2).

The two most important factors in successful *H. pylori* treatment are the patient's close compliance with the regimen and the use of drugs to which *H. pylori* has not acquired resistance. Treatment failure following minor lapses in compliance is common and often leads to acquired resistance to metronidazole or clarithromycin. To stress the importance of compliance, written instructions should be given to the patient, and minor side effects of the regimen should be explained. Resistance to metronidazole and clarithromycin is of growing concern. Clarithromycin resistance is less prevalent but, if present, usually results in treatment failure. Metronidazole-resistant strains of *H. pylori* are more common, but these strains still may be cleared by metronidazole-containing regimens. Assessment of antibiotic susceptibilities before treatment would be optimal but is not usually undertaken because endoscopy and mucosal biopsy are necessary to obtain *H. pylori* for culture and because most microbiology laboratories are inexperienced in *H. pylori* culture. In the absence of susceptibility

information, a history of the patient's antibiotic use should be obtained, and, even if only distant exposure is identified (e.g., previous metronidazole consumption for giardiasis or trichomoniasis), use of the agent should be avoided if possible. If initial *H. pylori* treatment fails, two strategies are commonly used (Fig. 25-2). One is re-treatment with a quadruple-drug regimen (Table 25-2). The second is endoscopy, biopsy, and culture plus treatment based on documented antibiotic sensitivities. If re-treatment fails, susceptibility testing should usually be performed, although empirical third-line therapies have been described.

Clearance of non-*pylori* gastric helicobacters can follow the use of bismuth compounds alone or of triple-drug regimens. However, in the absence of trials, it is unclear whether this outcome represents successful treatment or natural clearance of the bacterium.

PREVENTION

Carriage of *H. pylori* has considerable public health significance in developed countries, where it is associated with peptic ulcer disease and gastric adenocarcinoma, and in developing countries, where gastric adenocarcinoma is an even more common cause of cancer death late in life. However, given that *H. pylori* has co-evolved with its human host over millennia, preventing or eliminating colonization on a population basis may have distinct disadvantages. For example, absence of *H. pylori* has been reported to increase the risk of diarrheal diseases and of GERD and its complications, including esophageal adenocarcinoma. Recently, we have speculated that the disappearance of *H. pylori* is associated with an increased risk of other emerging diseases reflecting

TABLE 25-2

RECOMMENDED TREATMENT REGIMENS FOR *HELICOBACTER PYLORI*

REGIMEN, DURATION	DRUG 1	DRUG 2	DRUG 3	DRUG 4
First-Line Treatment				
Regimen 1: OCA (7–14 days)[a]	Omeprazole[b] (20 mg bid)	Clarithromycin (500 mg bid)	Amoxicillin (1 g bid)	—
Regimen 2: OCM (7–14 days)	Omeprazole[b] (20 mg bid)	Clarithromycin (500 mg bid)	Metronidazole (500 mg bid)	—
Second-Line Treatment[c]				
Regimen 3: OBTM (14 days)[d]	Omeprazole[b] (20 mg bid)	Bismuth subsalicylate (2 tabs qid)	Tetracycline HCl (500 mg qid)	Metronidazole (500 mg tid)

[a]Meta-analyses show that a 14-day course of therapy is slightly superior to a 7-day course. However, the success rate for 7-day therapy is so high in northern Europe (>80%) that 7-day treatment is recommended in most guidelines.
[b]Omeprazole may be replaced with any proton pump inhibitor at an equivalent dosage or, in Regimens 1 and 2, with ranitidine bismuth citrate (400 mg).
[c]An alternative to this second-line therapy is to culture *H. pylori* and to be guided by antibiotic susceptibility data. Patients in whom second-line therapy fails should undergo endoscopy for *H. pylori* culture and antibiotic susceptibility testing.
[d]Data supporting this regimen come mainly from Europe and are based on the use of bismuth subcitrate and metronidazole (400 mg tid).

aspects of the current Western lifestyle, such as asthma, obesity, and type 2 diabetes mellitus. If mass prevention were contemplated, vaccination would be the most obvious method, and experimental immunization of animals has given promising results. However, in the United States and other developed countries, rates of *H. pylori* carriage, peptic ulceration, and gastric adenocarcinoma are falling, while rates of esophageal reflux disease and its sequelae are increasing. Thus, prevention of colonization in these countries may be unnecessary or even unwise.

FURTHER READINGS

BLASER MJ: Who are we? Indigenous microbes and the ecology of human diseases. EMBO Rep 7:956, 2006

BLASER MJ, ATHERTON JC: *Helicobacter pylori* persistence: Biology and disease. J Clin Invest 113:321, 2004

CHEN Y, BLASER MJ: Inverse associations of *Helicobacter pylori* with asthma and allergies. Arch Intern Med 167:821, 2007

COVER TL, BLASER MJ: *Helicobacter pylori* in health and disease. Gastroenterology 136:1863, 2009

DUBE C: *Helicobacter pylori* in water sources: a global environmental health concern. Rev Environ Health 24:1, 2009

FRANCO AT et al: Activation of beta-catenin by carcinogenic *Helicobacter pylori*. Proc Natl Acad Sci USA 102:10646, 2005

HANSSON LE et al: The risk of stomach cancer in patients with gastric or duodenal ulcer disease. N Engl J Med 335:242, 1996

KAMANGAR F et al: Opposing risks of gastric cardia and noncardia gastric adenocarcinomas associated with *Helicobacter pylori* seropositivity. J Natl Cancer Inst 98:1445, 2006

MARSHALL BJ, Warren JR: Unidentified curved bacilli in the stomach of patients with gastritis and peptic ulceration. Lancet 1:1311, 1984

ODENBREIT S et al: Translocation of *Helicobacter pylori* CagA into gastric epithelial cells by type IV secretion. Science 287:1497, 2000

PARSONNET J et al: *Helicobacter pylori* infection and gastric lymphoma. N Engl J Med 330:1267, 1994

RIEDER G et al: *Helicobacter pylori* cag-type IV secretion system facilitates corpus colonization to induce precancerous conditions in Mongolian gerbils. Gastroenterology 128:1229, 2005

SOUZA RC, LIMA JH: *Helicobacter pylori* and gastroesophageal reflux disease: a review of this intriguing relationship. Dis Esophagus 22:256, 2009

TOMB JF et al: The complete genome sequence of the gastric pathogen *Helicobacter pylori*. Nature 388:539, 1997

WONG BC et al: *Helicobacter pylori* eradication to prevent gastric cancer in a high-risk region of China: A randomized controlled trial. JAMA 291:187, 2004

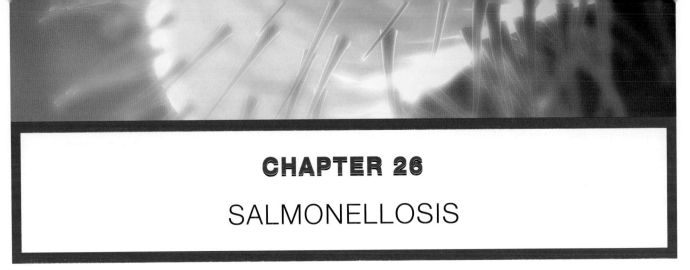

CHAPTER 26

SALMONELLOSIS

David A. Pegues ■ Samuel I. Miller

Bacteria of the genus *Salmonella* are highly adapted for growth in both humans and animals and cause a wide spectrum of disease. The growth of serotypes *S.* Typhi and *S.* Paratyphi is restricted to human hosts, in whom these organisms cause enteric (typhoid) fever. The remaining serotypes (nontyphoidal *Salmonella*, or NTS) can colonize the gastrointestinal tracts of a broad range of animals, including mammals, reptiles, birds, and insects. More than 200 serotypes are pathogenic to humans, in whom they often cause gastroenteritis and can be associated with localized infections and/or bacteremia.

ETIOLOGY

This large genus of gram-negative bacilli within the family Enterobacteriaceae consists of two species: *S. choleraesuis*, which contains six subspecies, and *S. bongori*. *S. choleraesuis* subspecies I contains almost all the serotypes pathogenic for humans. Because the designation *S. choleraesuis* refers to both a species and a serotype, the species designation *S. enterica* has been recommended and widely adopted. According to the current *Salmonella* nomenclature system, the full taxonomic designation *Salmonella enterica* subspecies *enterica* serotype Typhimurium can be shortened to *Salmonella* serotype Typhimurium or simply *Salmonella* Typhimurium.

Members of the seven *Salmonella* subspecies are classified into >2400 serotypes (serovars) according to the somatic O antigen [lipopolysaccharide (LPS) cell-wall components], the surface Vi antigen (restricted to *S.* Typhi and *S.* Paratyphi C), and the flagellar H antigen. For simplicity, most *Salmonella* serotypes are named for the city where they were identified, and the serotype is often used as the species designation.

Salmonellae are gram-negative, non-spore-forming, facultatively anaerobic bacilli that measure 2–3 by 0.4–0.6 μm. The initial identification of salmonellae in the clinical microbiology laboratory is based on growth characteristics. Salmonellae, like other Enterobacteriaceae, produce acid on glucose fermentation, reduce nitrates, and do not produce cytochrome oxidase. In addition, all salmonellae except *S.* Gallinarum-Pullorum are motile by means of peritrichous flagella, and all but *S.* Typhi produce gas (H_2S) on sugar fermentation. Notably, only 1% of clinical isolates ferment lactose; a high level of suspicion must be maintained to detect these rare clinical lactose-fermenting isolates.

Although serotyping of all surface antigens can be used for formal identification, most laboratories perform a few simple agglutination reactions that define specific O-antigen serogroups, designated A, B, C_1, C_2, D, and E. Strains in these six serogroups cause ~99% of *Salmonella* infections in humans and warm-blooded animals. Molecular typing methods, including pulsed-field gel electrophoresis, are used in epidemiologic investigations to differentiate *Salmonella* strains of a common serotype.

PATHOGENESIS

All *Salmonella* infections begin with ingestion of organisms in contaminated food or water. The infectious dose is 10^3–10^6 colony-forming units. Conditions that decrease either stomach acidity (an age of <1 year, antacid ingestion, or achlorhydric disease) or intestinal integrity (inflammatory bowel disease, prior gastrointestinal surgery, or alteration of the intestinal flora by antibiotic administration) increase susceptibility to *Salmonella* infection.

Once salmonellae reach the small intestine, they penetrate the mucous layer of the gut and traverse the intestinal layer through phagocytic microfold (M) cells that reside within Peyer's patches. Salmonellae can trigger the formation of membrane ruffles in normally nonphagocytic epithelial cells. These ruffles reach out and enclose adherent bacteria within large vesicles by a process referred to as *bacteria-mediated endocytosis* (BME). BME is dependent on the direct delivery of *Salmonella* proteins into the cytoplasm of epithelial cells by a specialized bacterial secretion system (*type III secretion*). These bacterial proteins mediate alterations in the actin cytoskeleton that are required for *Salmonella* uptake.

After crossing the epithelial layer of the small intestine, *S.* Typhi and *S.* Paratyphi, which cause enteric (typhoid) fever, are phagocytosed by macrophages. These salmonellae survive the antimicrobial environment of the macrophage by sensing environmental signals that trigger alterations in regulatory systems of the phagocytosed bacteria. For example, PhoP/PhoQ (the best-characterized regulatory system) triggers the expression of outer-membrane proteins and mediates modifications in LPS so that the altered bacterial surface can resist microbicidal activities and potentially alter host cell signaling. In addition, salmonellae encode a second type III secretion system that directly delivers bacterial proteins across the phagosome membrane into the macrophage cytoplasm. This secretion system functions to remodel the *Salmonella*-containing vacuole, promoting bacterial survival and replication.

Once phagocytosed, salmonellae disseminate throughout the body in macrophages via the lymphatics and colonize reticuloendothelial tissues (liver, spleen, lymph nodes, and bone marrow). Patients have relatively few or no signs and symptoms during this initial incubation stage. Signs and symptoms, including fever and abdominal pain, probably result from secretion of cytokines by macrophages and epithelial cells in response to bacterial products that are recognized by innate immune receptors when a critical number of organisms have replicated. Over time, the development of hepatosplenomegaly is likely to be related to the recruitment of mononuclear cells and the development of a specific acquired cell-mediated immune response to *S. typhi* colonization. The recruitment of additional mononuclear cells and lymphocytes to Peyer's patches during the several weeks after initial colonization/infection can result in marked enlargement and necrosis of the Peyer's patches, which may be mediated by bacterial products that promote cell death as well as the inflammatory response.

In contrast to enteric fever, which is characterized by an infiltration of mononuclear cells into the small-bowel mucosa, NTS gastroenteritis is characterized by massive polymorphonuclear leukocyte (PMN) infiltration into both the large- and small-bowel mucosa. This response appears to depend on the induction of interleukin (IL) 8, a strong neutrophil chemotactic factor, which is secreted by intestinal cells as a result of *Salmonella* colonization and translocation of bacterial proteins into host cell cytoplasm. The degranulation and release of toxic substances by neutrophils may result in damage to the intestinal mucosa, causing the inflammatory diarrhea observed with nontyphoidal gastroenteritis.

ENTERIC (TYPHOID) FEVER

Typhoid fever is a systemic disease characterized by fever and abdominal pain and caused by dissemination of *S.* Typhi or *S.* Paratyphi. The disease was initially called *typhoid fever* because of its clinical similarity to typhus. However, in the early 1800s, typhoid fever was clearly defined pathologically as a unique illness on the basis of its association with enlarged Peyer's patches and mesenteric lymph nodes. In 1869, given the anatomic site of infection, the term *enteric fever* was proposed as an alternative designation to distinguish typhoid fever from typhus. However, to this day, the two designations are used interchangeably.

EPIDEMIOLOGY

In contrast to other *Salmonella* serotypes, the etiologic agents of enteric fever—*S.* Typhi and *S.* Paratyphi serotypes A, B, and C—have no known hosts other than humans. Most commonly, foodborne or waterborne transmission results from fecal contamination by ill or asymptomatic chronic carriers. Sexual transmission between male partners has been described. Health care workers occasionally acquire enteric fever after exposure to infected patients or during processing of clinical specimens and cultures.

 With improvements in food handling and water/sewage treatment, enteric fever has become rare in developed nations. Worldwide, however, there were an estimated 22 million cases of enteric fever, with 200,000 deaths, in 2002. The incidence is highest (>100 cases per 100,000 population per year) in south-central and Southeast Asia; medium

(10–100 cases per 100,000) in the rest of Asia, Africa, Latin America, and Oceania (excluding Australia and New Zealand); and low in other parts of the world. A high incidence of enteric fever correlates with poor sanitation and lack of access to clean drinking water. In endemic regions, enteric fever is more common in urban than rural areas and among young children and adolescents. Risk factors include contaminated water or ice, flooding, food and drinks purchased from street vendors, raw fruits and vegetables grown in fields fertilized with sewage, ill household contacts, lack of hand washing and toilet access, and evidence of prior *Helicobacter pylori* infection (an association probably related to chronically reduced gastric acidity). It is estimated that there is one case of paratyphoid fever for every four cases of typhoid fever, but the incidence of infection associated with *S.* Paratyphi A appears to be increasing, especially in India.

Multidrug-resistant (MDR) strains of *S.* Typhi emerged in 1989 in China and Southeast Asia and have since disseminated widely (**Fig. 26-1**). These strains contain plasmids encoding resistance to chloramphenicol, ampicillin, and trimethoprim—antibiotics long used to treat enteric fever. With the increased use of fluoroquinolones to treat MDR enteric fever, strains of *S.* Typhi and *S.* Paratyphi with reduced susceptibility to ciprofloxacin [minimal inhibitory concentration (MIC), 0.125–1.0 μg/mL] have emerged in India and Vietnam and have been associated with clinical treatment failure. Testing of isolates for resistance to the first-generation quinolone nalidixic acid detects most but not all strains with reduced susceptibility to ciprofloxacin.

The incidence of enteric fever among U.S. travelers is estimated at 3–30 cases per 100,000. Of 1393 cases reported to the Centers for Disease Control and Prevention (CDC) in 1994–1999, 74% were associated with recent international travel, most commonly to India (30%), Pakistan (13%), Mexico (12%), Bangladesh (8%), the Philippines (8%), and Haiti (5%). Likewise, of 356 cases reported in the United States in 2003, ~74% occurred in persons who reported international travel during the preceding 6 weeks. Only 4% of travelers diagnosed with enteric fever gave a history of *S.* Typhi vaccination within the previous 5 years. Increased rates of MDR *S.* Typhi and *S.* Paratyphi have been reported among travelers. In 1996– 1997, 80% of U.S. travelers with enteric fever acquired in Vietnam were infected with MDR *S.* Typhi strains. Of the 25–30% of reported cases of enteric fever in the United States that are domestically acquired, the majority are sporadic, but 7% have occurred in recognized outbreaks linked to contaminated food products and previously unrecognized chronic carriers. An increasing proportion of cases (currently ~80%) are associated with foreign-born U.S. residents visiting friends and relatives in their native countries.

CLINICAL COURSE

Enteric fever is a misnomer, in that the hallmark features of this disease—fever and abdominal pain—are variable. While fever is documented at presentation in >75% of cases, abdominal pain is reported in only 30–40%. Thus, a high index of suspicion for this potentially fatal systemic illness is necessary when a person presents with fever and a history of recent travel to a developing country.

The incubation period for *S.* Typhi averages 10–14 days but ranges from 3 to 21 days, with the duration likely reflecting the inoculum size and the host's health and immune status. The most prominent symptom is

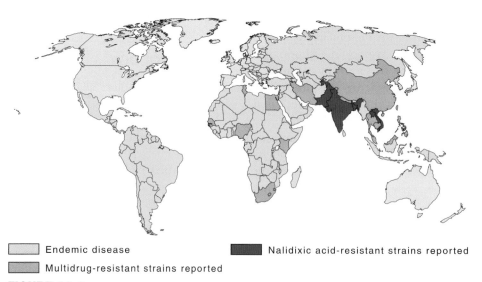

Endemic disease   Nalidixic acid-resistant strains reported

Multidrug-resistant strains reported

FIGURE 26-1

Global distribution of resistance to S. Typhi, 1990–2002. *(Reprinted with permission from Parry CM et al: Typhoid fever. N Engl J Med 347: 1770, 2002. © 2002 Massachusetts Medical Society. All rights reserved.)*

prolonged fever (38.8°–40.5°C; 101.8°–104.9°F), which can continue for up to 4 weeks if untreated. *S.* Paratyphi A is thought to cause milder disease than *S.* Typhi, with predominantly gastrointestinal symptoms. However, a prospective study of 669 consecutive cases of enteric fever in Kathmandu, Nepal, found that the infections were clinically indistinguishable. In this series, symptoms reported on initial medical evaluation included headache (80%), chills (35–45%), cough (30%), sweating (20–25%), myalgias (20%), malaise (10%), and arthralgia (2–4%). Gastrointestinal symptoms included anorexia (55%), abdominal pain (30–40%), nausea (18–24%), vomiting (18%), and diarrhea (22–28%) more commonly than constipation (13–16%). Physical findings included coated tongue (51–56%), splenomegaly (5–6%), and abdominal tenderness (4–5%).

Early physical findings of enteric fever include rash ("rose spots"), hepatosplenomegaly (3–6%), epistaxis, and relative bradycardia at the peak of high fever. Rose spots (Fig. 26-2) make up a faint, salmon-colored, blanching, maculopapular rash located primarily on the trunk and chest. The rash is evident in ~30% of patients at the end of the first week and resolves without a trace after 2–5 days. Patients can have two or three crops of lesions, and *Salmonella* can be cultured from punch biopsies of these lesions. The faintness of the rash makes it difficult to detect in highly pigmented patients.

The development of severe disease (which occurs in ~10–15% of patients) depends on host factors (immunosuppression, antacid therapy, previous exposure, and vaccination), strain virulence and inoculum, and choice of antibiotic therapy. Gastrointestinal bleeding (10–20%) and intestinal perforation (1–3%) most commonly occur in the third and fourth weeks of illness and result from hyperplasia, ulceration, and necrosis of the ileocecal Peyer's patches at the initial site of *Salmonella* infiltration. Both complications are life-threatening and require immediate fluid resuscitation and surgical intervention, with broadened antibiotic coverage for polymicrobial peritonitis (Chap. 24) and treatment of gastrointestinal hemorrhages, including bowel resection. Neurologic manifestations occur in 2–40% of patients and include meningitis, Guillain-Barré syndrome, neuritis, and neuropsychiatric symptoms (described as "muttering delirium" or "coma vigil"), with picking at bedclothes or imaginary objects.

Rare complications whose incidences are reduced by prompt antibiotic treatment include disseminated intravascular coagulation, hematophagocytic syndrome, pancreatitis, hepatic and splenic abscesses and granulomas, endocarditis, pericarditis, myocarditis, orchitis, hepatitis, glomerulonephritis, pyelonephritis and hemolytic uremic syndrome, severe pneumonia, arthritis, osteomyelitis, and parotitis. Up to 10% of patients develop mild relapse, usually within 2–3 weeks of fever resolution and in association with the same strain type and susceptibility profile.

Up to 10% of untreated patients with typhoid fever excrete *S.* Typhi in the feces for up to 3 months, and 1–4% develop chronic asymptomatic carriage, shedding *S.* Typhi in either urine or stool for >1 year. Chronic carriage is more common among women, infants, and persons with biliary abnormalities or concurrent bladder infection with *Schistosoma haematobium*. The anatomic abnormalities associated with the latter conditions presumably allow prolonged colonization.

DIAGNOSIS

Since the clinical presentation of enteric fever is relatively nonspecific, the diagnosis needs to be considered in any febrile traveler returning from a developing country, especially the Indian subcontinent, the Philippines, or Latin America. Other diagnoses that should be considered in these travelers include malaria, hepatitis, bacterial enteritis, dengue fever, rickettsial infections, leptospirosis, amebic liver abscesses, and acute HIV infection. Other than a positive culture, no specific laboratory test is diagnostic for enteric fever. In 15–25% of cases, leukopenia and neutropenia are detectable. Leukocytosis is more common among children, during the first 10 days of illness, and in cases complicated by intestinal perforation or secondary infection. Other nonspecific laboratory findings include moderately elevated liver function tests and muscle enzyme levels.

The definitive diagnosis of enteric fever requires the isolation of *S.* Typhi or *S.* Paratyphi from blood, bone marrow, other sterile sites, rose spots, stool, or intestinal secretions. The yield of blood cultures is quite variable; sensitivity is as high as 90% during the first week of infection and decreases to 50% by the third week. A low yield in infected patients is related to low numbers of salmonellae (<15 organisms/mL) and/or to recent antibiotic treatment. Since almost all *S.* Typhi organisms in blood are associated with the mononuclear-cell/platelet

FIGURE 26-2
"Rose spots," the rash of enteric fever due to *S.* Typhi or *S.* Paratyphi.

fraction, centrifugation of blood and culture of the buffy coat can substantially reduce the time to isolation of the organism but does not increase sensitivity.

Unlike blood culture, bone marrow culture remains highly (90%) sensitive despite ≤5 days of antibiotic therapy. Culture of intestinal secretions (best obtained by a noninvasive duodenal string test) can be positive despite a negative bone marrow culture. If blood, bone marrow, and intestinal secretions are all cultured, the yield is >90%. Stool cultures, while negative in 60–70% of cases during the first week, can become positive during the third week of infection in untreated patients.

Several serologic tests, including the classic Widal test for "febrile agglutinins," are available. None of these tests is sufficiently sensitive or specific to replace culture-based methods for the diagnosis of enteric fever in developed countries. Polymerase chain reaction and DNA probe assays to detect S. Typhi in blood are being developed.

℞ Treatment:
ENTERIC (TYPHOID) FEVER

Prompt administration of appropriate antibiotic therapy prevents severe complications of enteric fever and results in a case-fatality rate of <1%. The initial choice of antibiotics depends on the susceptibility of the S. Typhi and S. Paratyphi strains in the area of residence or travel (Table 26-1). For treatment of drug-susceptible typhoid fever, fluoroquinolones are the most effective class of agents, with cure rates of ~98% and relapse and fecal carriage rates of <2%. Experience is most extensive with ciprofloxacin. Short-course ofloxacin therapy is similarly successful against infection caused by nalidixic acid–susceptible strains. However, the increased incidence of nalidixic acid–resistant (NAR) S. Typhi in Asia, which is probably related to the widespread availability of fluoroquinolones over the counter, is now limiting the use of this drug class for empirical therapy. Patients infected with NAR S. Typhi strains should be treated with ceftriaxone, azithromycin, or high-dose ciprofloxacin. However, high-dose fluoroquinolone therapy for NAR enteric fever has been associated with delayed resolution of fever and high rates of fecal carriage during convalescence.

Ceftriaxone, cefotaxime, and (oral) cefixime are effective for treatment of MDR enteric fever, including NAR and fluoroquinolone-resistant strains. These agents clear fever in ~1 week, with failure rates of ~5–10%, fecal carriage rates of <3%, and relapse rates of 3–6%. Oral azithromycin results in defervescence in 4–6 days, with rates of relapse and convalescent stool carriage of <3%. Despite efficient in vitro killing of *Salmonella*, first- and second-generation cephalosporins as well as aminoglycosides are ineffective in treating clinical infections.

TABLE 26-1

ANTIBIOTIC THERAPY FOR ENTERIC FEVER IN ADULTS

INDICATION	AGENT	DOSAGE (ROUTE)	DURATION, DAYS
Empirical Treatment			
	Ceftriaxone[a]	1–2 g/d (IV)	7–14
	Azithromycin	1 g/d (PO)	5
Fully Susceptible			
	Ciprofloxacin[b] (first line)	500 mg bid (PO) or 400 mg q12h (IV)	5–7
	Amoxicillin (second line)	1 g tid (PO) or 2 g q6h (IV)	14
	Chloramphenicol	25 mg/kg tid (PO or IV)	14–21
	Trimethoprim-sulfamethoxazole	160/800 mg bid (PO)	14
Multidrug-Resistant			
	Ciprofloxacin	500 mg bid (PO) or 400 mg q12h (IV)	5–7
	Ceftriaxone	2–3 g/d (IV)	7–14
	Azithromycin	1 g/d (PO)[c]	5
Nalidixic Acid-Resistant			
	Ceftriaxone	1–2 g/d (IV)	7–14
	Azithromycin	1 g/d (PO)	5
	High-dose ciprofloxacin	750 mg bid (PO) or 400 mg q8h (IV)	10–14

[a]Or another third-generation cephalosporin [e.g., cefotaxime, 2 g q8h (IV), or cefixime, 400 mg bid (PO)].
[b]Or ofloxacin, 400 mg bid (PO) for 2–5 days.
[c]Or 1 g on day 1 followed by 500 mg/d PO for 6 days.

Patients with persistent vomiting, diarrhea, and/or abdominal distension should be hospitalized and given supportive therapy as well as a parenteral third-generation cephalosporin or fluoroquinolone, depending on the susceptibility profile. Therapy should be administered for at least 10 days or for 5 days after fever resolution.

In a randomized, prospective, double-blind study of critically ill patients with enteric fever (i.e., those with shock and obtundation) in Indonesia in the early 1980s, the administration of dexamethasone (3-mg initial dose followed by eight doses of 1 mg/kg every 6 h) with chloramphenicol was associated with a substantially lower mortality rate than treatment with chloramphenicol alone (10% vs 55%). Although this study has not been repeated in the "post-chloramphenicol era," severe enteric fever remains one of the few indications for glucocorticoid treatment of an acute bacterial infection.

The 1–5% of patients who develop chronic carriage of *Salmonella* can be treated for 4–6 weeks with an appropriate oral antibiotic. Treatment with oral amoxicillin, trimethoprim-sulfamethoxazole (TMP-SMX), ciprofloxacin, or norfloxacin is ~80% effective in eradicating chronic carriage of susceptible organisms. However, in cases of anatomic abnormality (e.g., biliary or kidney stones), eradication often requires both antibiotic therapy and surgical correction.

PREVENTION AND CONTROL

Theoretically, it is possible to eliminate the salmonellae that cause enteric fever since they survive only in human hosts and are spread by contaminated food and water. However, given the high prevalence of the disease in developing countries that lack adequate sewage disposal and water treatment, this goal is currently unrealistic. Thus, travelers to developing countries should be advised to monitor their food and water intake carefully and to consider vaccination.

Two typhoid vaccines are commercially available: (1) Ty21a, an oral live attenuated *S.* Typhi vaccine (given on days 1, 3, 5, and 7, with a booster every 5 years); and (2) Vi CPS, a parenteral vaccine consisting of purified Vi polysaccharide from the bacterial capsule (given in 1 dose, with a booster every 2 years). The old parenteral whole-cell typhoid/paratyphoid A and B vaccine is no longer licensed, largely because of significant side effects (see later). An acetone-killed whole-cell vaccine is available only for use by the U.S. military. The minimal age for vaccination is 6 years for Ty21a and 2 years for Vi CPS. Currently, there is no licensed vaccine for paratyphoid fever.

A large-scale meta-analysis of vaccine trials comparing whole-cell vaccine, Ty21a, and Vi CPS in populations in endemic areas indicates that, while all three vaccines are similarly effective for the first year, the 3-year cumulative efficacy of the whole-cell vaccine (73%) exceeds that of both Ty21a (51%) and Vi CPS (55%). In addition, the heat-killed whole-cell vaccine maintains its efficacy for 5 years, whereas Ty21a and Vi CPS maintain their efficacy for 4 and 2 years, respectively. However, the whole-cell vaccine is associated with a much higher incidence of side effects (especially fever: 16% vs 1–2%) than the other two vaccines.

Vi CPS typhoid vaccine is poorly immunogenic in children <5 years of age because of T cell–independent properties. In the recently developed Vi-rEPA vaccine, Vi is bound to a nontoxic recombinant protein that is identical to *Pseudomonas aeruginosa* exotoxin A. In 2- to 4-year-olds, two injections of Vi-rEPA induced higher T-cell responses and higher levels of serum IgG antibody to Vi than did Vi CPS in 5- to 14-year-olds. In a two-dose trial in 2- to 5-year-old children in Vietnam, Vi-rEPA provided 91% efficacy at 27 months and 88% efficacy at 43 months and was very well tolerated. Similar results were obtained in a trial in Cambodia. This vaccine is not yet commercially available in the United States. At least three new live vaccines are in clinical development and may prove more efficacious and longer-lasting than previous live vaccines.

Although data on typhoid vaccines in travelers are limited, some evidence suggests that efficacy rates may be substantially lower than those for local populations in endemic areas. Both the CDC and the World Health Organization recommend typhoid vaccination for travelers to typhoid-endemic countries. Recent analyses from the CDC found that 16% of travel-associated cases occurred among persons who stayed at their travel destination for ≤2 weeks. Thus, vaccination should be strongly considered even for persons planning short-term travel to high-risk areas such as the Indian subcontinent. In the United States, persons who have intimate or household contact with a chronic carrier or laboratory workers who frequently deal with *S.* Typhi also should receive typhoid vaccine.

Enteric fever is a notifiable disease in the United States. Individual health departments have their own guidelines for allowing ill or colonized food handlers or health care workers to return to their jobs. The reporting system enables public health departments to identify potential source patients and to treat chronic carriers in order to prevent further outbreaks. In addition, since 1–4% of patients with *S.* Typhi infection become chronic carriers, it is important to monitor patients (especially child-care providers and food handlers) for chronic carriage and to treat this condition if indicated.

NONTYPHOIDAL SALMONELLOSIS

EPIDEMIOLOGY

During 1996-1999, there were an estimated 1.4 million cases of nontyphoidal salmonellosis in the United States, resulting in 168,000 physician office visits, 15,000 hospitalizations, and 400 deaths annually. In 2004, the incidence of NTS infection in this country was 14.7 per 100,000 persons—the highest rate among the nine food-borne enteric pathogens under active surveillance. Five serotypes accounted for 57% of U.S. infections in 2004: Typhimurium (20%), Enteritidis (15%), Newport (10%), Javiana (7%), and Heidelberg (5%).

The incidence of nontyphoidal salmonellosis is highest during the rainy season in tropical climates and during the warmer months in temperate climates, coinciding with the peak in food-borne outbreaks. Rates of morbidity and mortality associated with NTS are highest among the elderly, infants, and immunocompromised individuals, including those with hemoglobinopathies, HIV infection, or infections that cause blockade of the reticuloendothelial system (e.g., bartonellosis, malaria, schistosomiasis, and histoplasmosis).

Unlike S. Typhi and S. Paratyphi, whose only reservoir is humans, NTS can be acquired from multiple animal reservoirs. Transmission is most commonly associated with animal food products, especially eggs, poultry, undercooked ground meat, and dairy products and fresh produce contaminated with animal waste.

S. Enteritidis infection associated with chicken eggs emerged as a major cause of foodborne disease during the 1980s and 1990s. S. Enteritidis infection of the ovaries and upper oviduct tissue of hens results in contamination of egg contents before shell deposition. Infection is spread to egg-laying hens from breeding flocks and through contact with rodents and manure. Of the 360 outbreaks of S. Enteritidis with a confirmed source that were reported to the CDC in 1985-1998, 279 (78%) were associated with raw or undercooked eggs. After peaking at 3.9 cases per 100,000 U.S. population in 1995, the incidence of S. Enteritidis infection declined dramatically to 1.98 per 100,000 in 1999; this decrease probably reflected improved on-farm control measures, refrigeration, and education of consumers and food-service workers. Transmission via contaminated eggs can be prevented by cooking eggs until the yolk is solidified and through pasteurization of egg products.

Centralization of food processing and widespread food distribution have contributed to the increased incidence of NTS in developing countries. Manufactured foods to which recent Salmonella outbreaks have been traced include pasteurized milk, infant formula, powdered milk products, and various processed foods. Large outbreaks have also been linked to fresh produce, including alfalfa sprouts, cantaloupe, fresh-squeezed orange juice, and tomatoes; these items become contaminated by manure or water at a single site and then are widely distributed.

An estimated 6% of sporadic Salmonella infections in the United States are attributed to contact with reptiles and amphibians, especially iguanas, snakes, turtles, and lizards. Reptile-associated Salmonella infection more commonly leads to hospitalization and more frequently involves infants than do other Salmonella infections. Other pets, including African hedgehogs, snakes, birds, rodents, baby chicks, ducklings, dogs, and cats, are also potential sources of NTS.

Increasing antibiotic resistance in NTS species is a global problem and has been linked to the widespread use of antimicrobial agents in food animals and especially in animal feed. In the early 1990s, S. Typhimurium definitive phage type 104 (DT104), characterized by resistance to ≥5 antibiotics (ampicillin, chloramphenicol, streptomycin, sulfonamides, and tetracyclines; R-type ACSSuT), emerged worldwide. From 1979–1980 to 2001, the prevalence of S. Typhimurium ACSSuT increased in the United States from 0.6% to 7% of all NTS isolates, and most (65%) of these ACSSuT isolates were phage type DT104. Acquisition is associated with exposure to ill farm animals and to various meat products, including uncooked or undercooked ground beef. In an analysis of U.S. surveillance data for 1996–2001, antibiotic-resistant NTS strains, especially S. Typhimurium DT104, were associated with an increased risk of bloodstream infection and hospitalization. NAR and trimethoprim-resistant DT104 strains are emerging, especially in the United Kingdom.

Because of increased resistance to conventional antibiotics such as ampicillin and TMP-SMX, extended-spectrum cephalosporins and fluoroquinolones have emerged as the agents of choice for the treatment of MDR NTS infections. With the increased use of these agents, the CDC reported that the prevalence of ceftriaxone-resistant NTS strains rose from 0 in 1995 to 0.5% in 1998. Of the ceftriaxone-resistant isolates, 77% were from children <18 years of age, in whom ceftriaxone is the antibiotic of choice for treatment of invasive infection. These strains contained plasmid-encoded AmpC β-lactamases that were probably acquired by horizontal genetic transfer from Escherichia coli strains in food-producing animals—an event linked to the widespread use of the veterinary cephalosporin ceftiofur.

Resistance to nalidixic acid and fluoroquinolones also has begun to emerge and is most commonly associated with point mutations in the DNA gyrase genes gyrA and gyrB. Nalidixic acid resistance is a good predictor of reduced susceptibility to clinically useful fluoroquinolones. From 1994–1995 to 2000, the rate of NAR NTS isolates in the United States increased fivefold (from 0.5% to 2.5%). In Denmark, infection with NAR S. Typhimurium DT104 has been linked to swine and associated with a threefold higher risk of invasive disease or death within 90 days. In Taiwan in 2000, a strain of ciprofloxacin-resistant (MIC, ≥4 μg/mL) S. Choleraesuis caused a large outbreak of invasive infections that was linked to the use of enrofloxacin in swine feed.

CLINICAL MANIFESTATIONS

Gastroenteritis

Infection with NTS most often results in gastroenteritis indistinguishable from that caused by other enteric pathogens. Nausea, vomiting, and diarrhea occur 6–48 h after the ingestion of contaminated food or water. Patients often experience abdominal cramping and fever (38–39°C; 100.5–102.2°F). Diarrheal stools are usually loose, nonbloody, and of moderate volume. However, large-volume watery stools, bloody stools, or symptoms of dysentery may occur. Rarely, NTS causes pseudoappendicitis or an illness that mimics inflammatory bowel disease.

Gastroenteritis caused by NTS is usually self-limited. Diarrhea resolves within 3–7 days and fever within 72 h. Stool cultures remain positive for 4–5 weeks after infection and—in rare cases of chronic carriage (<1%)—for >1 year. Antibiotic treatment usually is not recommended and in some studies has prolonged fecal carriage. Neonates, the elderly, and immunosuppressed patients (e.g., transplant recipients, HIV-infected persons) with NTS gastroenteritis are especially susceptible to dehydration and dissemination and may require hospitalization and antibiotic therapy. Acute NTS gastroenteritis was associated with a threefold increased risk of dyspepsia and irritable bowel syndrome at 1 year in a recent study from Spain.

Bacteremia and Endovascular Infections

Up to 5% of patients with NTS gastroenteritis develop bacteremia; of these, 5–10% develop localized infections. Bacteremia and metastatic infection are most common with *S. Choleraesuis* and *S. Dublin* and among infants, the elderly, and immunocompromised patients. NTS endovascular infection should be suspected in high-grade bacteremia, especially with preexisting valvular heart disease, atherosclerotic vascular disease, prosthetic vascular graft, or aortic aneurysm. Arteritis should be suspected in elderly patients with prolonged fever and back, chest, or abdominal pain developing after an episode of gastroenteritis. Endocarditis and arteritis are rare (<1% of cases) but are associated with potentially fatal complications, including valve perforation, endomyocardial abscess, infected mural thrombus, pericarditis, mycotic aneurysms, aneurysm rupture, aortoenteric fistula, and vertebral osteomyelitis.

Localized Infections

Intraabdominal Infections

Intraabdominal infections due to NTS are rare and usually manifest as hepatic or splenic abscesses or as cholecystitis. Risk factors include hepatobiliary anatomic abnormalities (e.g., gallstones), abdominal malignancy, and sickle cell disease (especially with splenic abscesses). Eradication of the infection often requires surgical correction of abnormalities and percutaneous drainage of abscesses.

Central Nervous System Infections

Meningitis most commonly develops in infants 1–4 months of age. It often results in severe sequelae (including seizures, hydrocephalus, brain infarction, and mental retardation) with death in up to 60% of cases. Other rare central nervous system infections include ventriculitis, subdural empyema, and brain abscesses.

Pulmonary Infections

NTS pulmonary infections usually present as lobar pneumonia, and complications include lung abscess, empyema, and bronchopleural fistula formation. The majority of cases occur in patients with lung cancer, structural lung disease, sickle cell disease, or glucocorticoid use.

Urinary and Genital Tract Infections

Urinary tract infections caused by NTS present as either cystitis or pyelonephritis. Risk factors include malignancy, urolithiasis, structural abnormalities, HIV infection, and renal transplantation. NTS genital infections are rare and include ovarian and testicular abscesses, prostatitis, and epididymitis. Like other focal infections, both genital and urinary tract infections can be complicated by abscess formation.

Bone, Joint, and Soft Tissue Infections

Salmonella osteomyelitis most commonly affects the femur, tibia, humerus, or lumbar vertebrae and is most often seen in association with sickle cell disease, hemoglobinopathies, or preexisting bone disease (e.g., fractures). Prolonged antibiotic treatment is recommended to decrease the risk of relapse and chronic osteomyelitis. Septic arthritis occurs in the same patient population as osteomyelitis and usually involves the knee, hip, or shoulder joints. Reactive arthritis (Reiter's syndrome) can follow NTS gastroenteritis and is seen most frequently in persons with the HLA-B27 histocompatibility antigen. NTS rarely can cause soft tissue infections, usually at sites of local trauma in immunosuppressed patients.

DIAGNOSIS

The diagnosis of NTS infection is based on the isolation of the organism from freshly passed stool or from blood or another ordinarily sterile body fluid. All salmonellae isolated in clinical laboratories should be sent to local public health departments for serotyping. Blood cultures should be done whenever a patient has prolonged or recurrent fever. Endovascular infection should be suspected if there is high-grade bacteremia (>50% of three or more blood cultures positive). Echocardiography, computed tomography, and indium-labeled white cell scanning are used to identify localized infection. When another localized infection is suspected, joint fluid, abscess drainage, or cerebrospinal fluid should be cultured, as clinically indicated.

℞ **Treatment:**
NONTYPHOIDAL SALMONELLOSIS

Antibiotics should not be used routinely to treat uncomplicated NTS gastroenteritis. The symptoms are usually self-limited, and the duration of fever and diarrhea is not significantly decreased by antibiotic therapy. In addition, antibiotic treatment has been associated with increased rates of relapse and prolonged gastrointestinal carriage. Dehydration secondary to diarrhea should be treated with fluid and electrolyte replacement.

Preemptive antibiotic treatment (**Table 26-2**) should be considered for patients at increased risk for invasive NTS infection, including neonates (probably up to 3 months of age); persons >50 years of age with suspected atherosclerosis; and patients with immunosuppression, cardiac valvular or endovascular abnormalities, or significant joint disease. Treatment should consist of an oral or IV antibiotic administered for 48–72 h or until the patient becomes afebrile. Immunocompromised persons may require up to 7–14 days of therapy. The <1% of persons who develop chronic carriage of NTS should receive a prolonged antibiotic course, as described above for chronic carriage of *S.* Typhi.

Because of the increasing prevalence of antibiotic resistance, empirical therapy for life-threatening NTS bacteremia or focal NTS infection should include a third-generation cephalosporin or a fluoroquinolone (Table 26-2). If the bacteremia is low-grade (<50% of blood cultures positive), the patient should be treated for 7–14 days. Patients with AIDS and NTS bacteremia should receive 1–2 weeks of IV antibiotic therapy followed by 4 weeks of oral therapy with a fluoroquinolone. Patients whose infections relapse after this

TABLE 26-2

ANTIBIOTIC THERAPY FOR NONTYPHOIDAL *SALMONELLA* INFECTION IN ADULTS

INDICATION	AGENT	DOSAGE (ROUTE)	DURATION, DAYS
Preemptive Treatment[a]			
	Ciprofloxacin[b]	500 mg bid (PO)	2–3
Severe Gastroenteritis[c]			
	Ciprofloxacin	500 mg bid (PO) or 400 mg q12h (IV)	3–7
	Trimethoprim-sulfamethoxazole	160/800 mg bid (PO)	
	Amoxicillin	1 g tid (PO)	
	Ceftriaxone	1–2 g/d (IV)	
Bacteremia			
	Ceftriaxone[d]	2 g/d (IV)	7–14
	Ciprofloxacin	400 mg q12h (IV), then 500 mg bid (PO)	
Endocarditis or Arteritis			
	Ceftriaxone	2 g/d (IV)	42
	Ciprofloxacin	400 mg q8h (IV), then 750 mg bid (PO)	
	Ampicillin	2 g q4h (IV)	
Meningitis			
	Ceftriaxone	2 g q12 h (IV)	14–21
	Ampicillin	2 g q4h (IV)	
Other Localized Infection			
	Ceftriaxone	2 g/d (IV)	14–28
	Ciprofloxacin	500 mg bid (PO) or 400 mg q12h (IV)	
	Ampicillin	2 g q6h (IV)	

[a]Consider for neonates; persons >50 years of age with possible atherosclerotic vascular disease; and patients with immunosuppression, endovascular graft, or joint prosthesis.
[b]Or ofloxacin, 400 mg bid (PO).
[c]Consider on an individualized basis for patients with severe diarrhea and high fever who require hospitalization.
[d]Or cefotaxime, 2 g q8h (IV).

regimen should receive long-term suppressive therapy with a fluoroquinolone or TMP-SMX, as indicated by bacterial sensitivities.

If the patient has endocarditis or arteritis, treatment for 6 weeks with an IV β-lactam antibiotic (such as ceftriaxone or ampicillin) is indicated. IV ciprofloxacin followed by prolonged oral therapy is an option, but published experience is limited. Early surgical resection of infected aneurysms or other infected endovascular sites is recommended. Patients with infected prosthetic vascular grafts that cannot be resected have been maintained successfully on chronic suppressive oral therapy. For extraintestinal nonvascular infections, a 2- to 4-week course of antibiotic therapy (depending on the infection site) is usually recommended. In chronic osteomyelitis, abscess, or urinary or hepatobiliary infection associated with anatomic abnormalities, surgical resection or drainage may be required in addition to prolonged antibiotic therapy for eradication of infection.

PREVENTION AND CONTROL

Despite widespread efforts to prevent or reduce bacterial contamination of animal-derived food products and to improve food-safety education and training, recent declines in the incidence of NTS in the United States have been modest compared with those of other foodborne pathogens. This observation probably reflects the complex epidemiology of NTS. Identifying effective risk-reduction strategies requires monitoring of every step of food production, from handling of raw animal or plant products to preparation of finished foods. Contaminated food can be made safe for consumption by pasteurization, irradiation, or proper cooking. All cases of NTS infection should be reported to local public health departments, since tracking and monitoring of these cases can identify the source(s) of infection and help authorities anticipate large outbreaks. Lastly, the prudent use of antimicrobial agents in both humans and animals is needed to limit the emergence of MDR *Salmonella*.

FURTHER READINGS

COHEN JI et al: Extra-intestinal manifestations of *Salmonella* infections. Medicine 66:349, 1987

GLYNN MK et al: Emergence of multidrug-resistant *Salmonella enterica* serotype *typhimurium* DT104 infections in the United States. N Engl J Med 338:1333, 1998

HOFFMAN SL et al: Reduction in mortality in chloramphenicol-treated severe typhoid fever by high-dose dexamethasone. N Engl J Med 310:82, 1984

LIN FY et al: The efficacy of a *Salmonella typhi* Vi conjugate vaccine in two-to-five-year-old children. N Engl J Med 344:1263, 2001

MASKEY AP et al: *Salmonella* enteric serovar Paratyphi A and *S. enterica* serovar Typhi cause indistinguishable clinical syndromes in Kathmandu, Nepal. Clin Infect Dis 42:1247, 2006

OHL ME, MILLER SI: *Salmonella*: A model for bacterial pathogenesis. Annu Rev Med 52:259, 2001

STEINBERG EB et al: Typhoid fever in travelers: Who should be targeted for prevention. Clin Infect Dis 39:186, 2004

SU LH et al: Antimicrobial resistance in nontyphoid *Salmonella* serotypes: A global challenge. Clin Infect Dis 39:546, 2004

TSOLIS RM et al: From bench to bedside: stealth of enteroinvasive pathogens. Nat Rev Microbiol 6:883, 2008

VARMA JK et al: Antimicrobial-resistant nontyphoidal *Salmonella* is associated with excess bloodstream infections and hospitalizations. J Infect Dis 191:554, 2005

WHITAKER JA et al: Rethinking typhoid fever vaccines: implications for travelers and people living in highly endemic areas. J Travel Med 16:46, 2009

CHAPTER 26

Salmonellosis

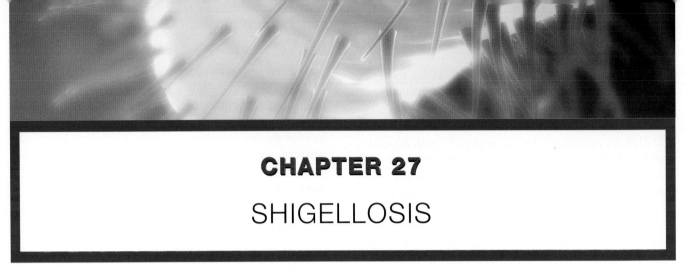

CHAPTER 27

SHIGELLOSIS

Philippe Sansonetti ■ Jean Bergounioux

The discovery of *Shigella* as the etiologic agent of dysentery—a clinical syndrome of fever, intestinal cramps, and frequent passage of small, bloody, mucopurulent stools—is attributed to the Japanese microbiologist Kiyoshi Shiga, who isolated the Shiga bacillus (now known as *Shigella dysenteriae* type 1) from patients' stools in 1897 during a large and devastating dysentery epidemic. *Shigella* cannot be distinguished from *Escherichia coli* by DNA hybridization and remains a separate species only on historical and clinical grounds.

DEFINITION

Shigella is a non-spore-forming, gram-negative bacterium that, unlike *E. coli,* is nonmotile and does not produce gas from sugars, decarboxylate lysine, or hydrolyze arginine. Some serovars produce indole, and occasional strains utilize sodium acetate. *S. dysenteriae, S. flexneri, S. boydii,* and *S. sonnei* (serogroups A, B, C, and D, respectively) can be differentiated on the basis of biochemical and serologic characteristics. Genome sequencing of *E. coli* K12, *S. flexneri* 2a, *S. sonnei, S. dysenteriae* type 1, and S. boydii has revealed that these species have ~93% of genes in common. The three major genomic "signatures" of *Shigella* are (1) a 215-kb virulence plasmid that carries most of the genes required for pathogenicity (particularly invasive capacity); (2) the lack or alteration of genetic sequences encoding products (e.g., lysine decarboxylase) that, if expressed, would attenu-

ate pathogenicity; and (3) in *S. dysenteriae* type 1, the presence of genes encoding Shiga toxin, a potent cytotoxin.

EPIDEMIOLOGY

The human intestinal tract represents the major reservoir of *Shigella*, which is also found (albeit rarely) in the higher primates. Because excretion of shigellae is greatest in the acute phase of disease, the bacteria are transmitted most efficiently by the fecal-oral route. Most cases of shigellosis are caused by person-to-person transmission, although some outbreaks reflect contamination of water or food. *Shigella* can also be transmitted by flies and, given its capacity to survive in foodstuffs, can be a significant cause of food-borne infection. The high-level infectivity of *Shigella* is reflected by the very small inoculum required for experimental infection of volunteers [100 colony-forming units (CFU)], by the very high attack rates during outbreaks in day care centers (33–73%), and by the high rates of secondary cases among family members of sick children (26–33%). Shigellosis can also be transmitted sexually.

In a review published under the auspices of the World Health Organization (WHO), the total annual number of cases in 1966–1997 was estimated at 165 million, and 69% of these cases occurred in children <5 years of age. In this review, the annual number of deaths was calculated to range between 500,000 and 1.1 million. More recent data (2000–2004) from six Asian countries (Bangladesh, China, Pakistan, Indonesia, Vietnam, and Thailand) indicate that even though the incidence of shigellosis remains stable, mortality rates associated with this disease may have decreased significantly, possibly as a result of improved nutritional standards. However, extensive and essentially uncontrolled use of antibiotics has increased the risk of emergence of multidrug-resistant *Shigella* strains.

Throughout history, *Shigella* epidemics have often occurred in settings of human crowding under poor hygienic conditions—e.g., among soldiers in campaigning armies, inhabitants of besieged cities, groups on pilgrimages, and refugees in camps. Epidemics follow a cyclic pattern in areas such as the Indian subcontinent and sub-Saharan Africa. These devastating epidemics, which are most often caused by *S. dysenteriae* type 1, are characterized by high attack rates and high mortality rates. In Bangladesh, for instance, an epidemic caused by *S. dysenteriae* type 1 was associated with a 42% increase in mortality rates among children 1–4 years of age. Apart from these epidemics, shigellosis is essentially an endemic disease, with 99% of cases occurring in the developing world and particularly high prevalences in the most impoverished areas, where personal and general hygiene is substandard. *S. flexneri* isolates predominate in less well-developed areas, whereas *S. sonnei* is more prevalent in economically emerging regions and in the industrialized world.

An often-overlooked complication of shigellosis is the short- and long-term impairment of the nutritional status of infected children in endemic areas. Combined with anorexia, the exudative enteropathy resulting from mucosal abrasions contributes to rapid exacerbation of the patient's nutritional status. Shigellosis is thus a major contributor to stunted growth among children in developing countries.

PATHOGENESIS AND PATHOLOGY

271

Shigella infection occurs through oral contamination. Direct fecal-oral transmission predominates since the organism is not well adapted to survive in the environment. Resistance to low-pH conditions allows shigellae to survive passage through the gastric barrier, an ability that may explain in part why a small inoculum (as few as 100 CFU) is sufficient to cause infection.

The watery diarrhea that usually precedes the dysenteric syndrome is attributable to active secretion and abnormal water reabsorption, a secretory effect at the jejunal level described in experimentally infected rhesus monkeys. This initial purge is probably due to the combined action of an enterotoxin (ShET-1) and mucosal inflammation. The dysenteric syndrome, manifested by bloody and mucopurulent stools, reflects invasion of the mucosa.

The pathogenesis of *Shigella* is essentially determined by a large virulence plasmid of 214 kb comprising ~100 genes, of which 25 encode a type III secretion system that inserts into the membrane of the host cell to allow effectors to transit from the bacterial cytoplasm to the cell cytoplasm (Fig. 27-1). Bacteria are thereby able to invade intestinal epithelial cells by inducing their own uptake after the initial crossing of the epithelial barrier through M cells (the specialized translocating epithelial cells in the follicle-associated epithelium that covers mucosal lymphoid nodules). The organisms induce apoptosis of subepithelial resident macrophages. Once inside the cytoplasm of intestinal epithelial cells, *Shigella* effectors trigger the cytoskeletal rearrangements necessary to direct uptake of the organism into the epithelial cell. The *Shigella*-containing vacuole is then quickly lysed, releasing bacteria into the cytosol.

Intracellular shigellae next use cytoskeletal components to propel themselves inside the infected cell; when

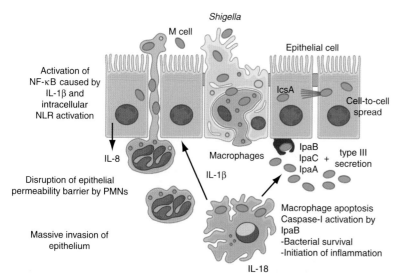

FIGURE 27-1

Invasive strategy of *Shigella flexneri*. IL, interleukin; NLR, nod-like receptor; PMN, polymorphonuclear leukocyte.

the moving organism and the host cell membrane come into contact, cellular protrusions form and are engulfed by neighboring cells. This series of events permits bacterial cell-to-cell spread that is protected from immune effector mechanisms.

Cytokines released by a growing number of infected intestinal epithelial cells attract increased numbers of immune cells [particularly polymorphonuclear leukocytes (PMNs)] to the infected site, thus further destabilizing the epithelial barrier, exacerbating inflammation, and leading to the acute colitis that characterizes shigellosis. Recent evidence indicates that some of the type III secretion system–injected effectors can control the extent of inflammation, thus facilitating bacterial survival.

Shiga toxin produced by *S. dysenteriae* type 1 increases disease severity. Shiga toxin and Shiga-like toxins belong to a group of A1-B5 protein toxins whose B subunit binds to the cell surface and whose catalytic A subunit expresses an RNA N-glycosidase on 28S ribosomal RNA. These events lead to inhibition of binding of the amino-acyl-tRNA to the 60S ribosomal subunit and thus to a general shutoff of cell protein biosynthesis. Shiga toxins are translocated from the bowel into the circulation. After binding to the receptor globotriaosylceramide on target cells in the kidney, toxin is internalized by receptor-mediated endocytosis and interacts with the subcellular machinery to inhibit protein synthesis. The consequent pathophysiologic changes may result in hemolytic-uremic syndrome (HUS; see later).

CLINICAL MANIFESTATIONS

The presentation and severity of shigellosis depend to some extent on the infecting species but even more on the age and the immunologic and nutritional status of the host. Poverty and a poor hygienic environment are strongly related to the number and severity of diarrheal episodes, especially in children <5 years old.

Shigellosis typically evolves through four phases: incubation, watery diarrhea, dysentery, and the postinfectious phase. The incubation period usually lasts 1–4 days but may be as long as 8 days. Typical initial manifestations are transient fever, limited watery diarrhea, malaise, and anorexia. Signs and symptoms may range from mild abdominal discomfort to severe cramps, diarrhea, fever, vomiting, and tenesmus. The manifestations are usually exacerbated in children, with temperatures up to 40°–41°C and more severe anorexia and watery diarrhea. Unlike most diarrheal syndromes, dysenteric syndromes do not have dehydration as a major feature. This initial phase may represent the only clinical manifestation of shigellosis, especially in developed countries. Otherwise, dysentery follows within hours or days and is characterized by small volumes of bloody mucopurulent

stools with increased tenesmus and abdominal cramps. At this stage, *Shigella* produces acute colitis involving mainly the distal colon and the rectum. Endoscopy demonstrates an edematous and hemorrhagic mucosa, with ulcerations and possibly overlying exudates resembling pseudomembranes. The extent of the lesions correlates with the number and frequency of stools and with the degree of protein loss by exudative mechanisms. Most episodes are self-limited and resolve without treatment in 1 week. With appropriate treatment, recovery takes place within a few days to a week, with no sequelae.

Acute life-threatening complications are seen most often in children <5 years of age, particularly affecting malnourished children in developing countries. Risk factors for death include nonbloody diarrhea, moderate to severe dehydration, bacteremia, absence of fever, abdominal tenderness, and rectal prolapse. Major complications are predominantly intestinal (e.g., toxic megacolon, intestinal perforations, rectal prolapse) or metabolic (e.g., hypoglycemia, hyponatremia, dehydration). Bacteremia is rare and is reported most frequently in severely malnourished children, HIV-infected patients, and patients with defects in innate immunity. Alterations of consciousness, including seizures, delirium, and coma, may occur, especially in children <5 years old, and are associated with a poor prognosis; fever and severe metabolic alterations are more often the major causes of altered consciousness than is meningitis or the Ekiri syndrome (toxic encephalopathy associated with bizarre posturing, cerebral edema, and fatty degeneration of viscera), which has been reported in Japanese children. Pneumonia, vaginitis, and keratoconjunctivitis due to *Shigella* are rarely reported. In the absence of serious malnutrition, severe and very unusual clinical manifestations, such as meningitis, may be linked to disorders of immune function and require relevant investigations.

Two complications of particular importance are toxic megacolon and HUS. Toxic megacolon is a consequence of severe inflammation extending to the colonic smooth-muscle layer and causing paralysis and dilatation. The patient presents with abdominal distention and tenderness, with or without signs of localized or generalized peritonitis. The abdominal x-ray characteristically shows marked dilatation of the transverse colon (with the greatest distention in the ascending and descending colons); thumbprinting caused by mucosal inflammatory edema; and loss of the normal haustral pattern associated with pseudopolyps, often extending into the lumen. Pneumatosis coli is an occasional finding. If perforation occurs, radiographic signs of pneumoperitoneum may be apparent. Predisposing factors (e.g., hypokalemia and use of opioids, anticholinergics, loperamide, psyllium seeds, and antidepressants) should be sought.

Shiga toxin produced by *S. dysenteriae* type 1 has been linked to HUS in developing countries but rarely in industrialized countries. HUS is an early complication that most often develops after several days of diarrhea. Clinical examination shows pallor, asthenia, and irritability and, in some cases, bleeding of the nose and gums, oliguria, and increasing edema. HUS is a nonimmune (Coombs test–negative) hemolytic anemia defined by a diagnostic triad: microangiopathic hemolytic anemia [hemoglobin level typically <80 g/L (<8 g/dL)], thrombocytopenia (mild to moderate in severity; typically <60,000 platelets/μL), and acute renal failure due to thrombosis of the glomerular capillaries (with markedly elevated creatinine levels). Anemia is severe, with fragmented red blood cells (schizocytes) in the peripheral smear, high serum concentrations of lactate dehydrogenase and free circulating hemoglobin, and elevated reticulocyte counts. Acute renal failure occurs in 55–70% of cases; however, renal function recovers in most of these cases (up to 70% in various series). Leukemoid reactions, with leukocyte counts of 50,000/μL, are sometimes noted in association with HUS.

The postinfectious immunologic complication known as reactive arthritis (Reiter's syndrome) can develop weeks or months after shigellosis, especially in patients expressing the histocompatibility antigen HLA-B27. About 3% of patients infected with *S. flexneri* later develop Reiter's syndrome, with arthritis, ocular inflammation, and urethritis—a condition that can last for months or years and progress to difficult-to-treat chronic arthritis. Postinfectious arthropathy occurs only after infection with *S. flexneri* and not after infection with the other *Shigella* serotypes.

LABORATORY DIAGNOSIS

The differential diagnosis in patients with a dysenteric syndrome depends on the clinical and environmental context. In developing areas, infectious diarrhea caused by other invasive pathogenic bacteria (*Salmonella enteritidis, Campylobacter jejuni, Clostridium difficile, Yersinia enterocolitica*) or parasites (*Entamoeba histolytica*) should be considered. Only bacteriologic and parasitologic examinations of stool can truly differentiate among these pathogens. A first flare of inflammatory bowel disease, such as Crohn's disease or ulcerative colitis (Chap. 16), should be considered in patients in industrialized countries. Despite similar symptoms, anamnesis discriminates between shigellosis, which usually follows recent travel in an endemic zone, and these other conditions.

Microscopic examination of stool smears shows the presence of erythrophagocytic trophozoites with very few PMNs in *E. histolytica* infection, whereas bacterial enteroinvasive infections (particularly shigellosis) are characterized by high PMN counts in each microscopic field. However, because shigellosis often manifests only as watery diarrhea, systematic attempts to isolate *Shigella* are necessary.

The "gold standard" for the diagnosis of *Shigella* infection remains the isolation and identification of the pathogen from fecal material. One major difficulty, particularly in endemic areas where laboratory facilities are not immediately available, is the fragility of *Shigella* and its common disappearance during transport, especially with rapid changes in temperature and pH. In the absence of a reliable enrichment medium, buffered glycerol saline or Cary-Blair medium can be used as a holding medium, but prompt inoculation onto isolation medium is essential. The probability of isolation is higher if the portion of stools that contains bloody and/or mucopurulent material is directly sampled. Rectal swabs can be used as they offer the highest rate of successful isolation during the acute phase of disease. Blood cultures are positive in <5% of cases and should be done only when a patient presents with a clinical picture of severe sepsis.

In addition to quick processing, the use of several media increases the likelihood of successful isolation: a nonselective medium such as bromocresol-purple agar lactose; a low-selectivity medium such as MacConkey or eosin-methylene blue; and a high-selectivity medium such as Hektoen, *Salmonella-Shigella*, or xylose-lysine-deoxycholate agar. After incubation on these media for 12–18 h at 37°C, shigellae appear as non-lactose-fermenting colonies that measure 0.5–1 mm in diameter and have a convex, translucent, smooth surface. Suspected colonies on nonselective or low-selectivity medium can be subcultured on a high-selectivity medium before being specifically identified or can be identified directly by standard commercial systems on the basis of four major characteristics: glucose positivity (usually without production of gas), lactose negativity, H_2S negativity, and lack of motility. The four *Shigella* serogroups (A–D) can then be differentiated by additional characteristics. This approach adds time and difficulty to the identification process, however; thus, after presumptive diagnosis, the use of serologic methods—e.g., slide agglutination, with group- and then type-specific antisera—should be considered. Group-specific antisera are widely available; in contrast, because of the large number of serotypes and sub-serotypes that must be considered, type-specific antisera are rare and more expensive and are often restricted to reference laboratories.

℞ **Treatment:**
SHIGELLOSIS

ANTIBIOTIC SUSCEPTIBILITY OF *SHIGELLA*
As an enteroinvasive disease, shigellosis requires antibiotic treatment. Since the mid-1960s, however, increasing

resistance to multiple drugs has been a dominant factor in treatment decisions. Resistance rates are highly dependent on the geographic area. Clonal spread of particular strains and horizontal transfer of resistance determinants, particularly via plasmids and transposons, contribute to multidrug resistance. Quinolone resistance is essentially due to chromosomal mutations affecting DNA gyrase and topoisomerase IV. A review of the antibiotic resistance history of Shigella in India found that, after their introduction in the late 1980s, the second-generation quinolones norfloxacin, ciprofloxacin, and ofloxacin were highly effective in the treatment of shigellosis, including cases caused by multidrug-resistant strains of *S. dysenteriae* type 1. In contrast, investigations of recent outbreaks in India and Bangladesh have shown high levels of resistance (generally 5%) to norfloxacin, ciprofloxacin, and ofloxacin among certain isolates. The incidence of multidrug resistance parallels widespread uncontrolled use of antibiotics (particularly in developing areas), calls for the rational use of effective drugs, and underscores the need for alternative drugs to treat infections caused by resistant strains.

ANTIBIOTIC TREATMENT OF SHIGELLOSIS

(Table 27-1) Because of the ready transmissibility of *Shigella*, current public health recommendations in the United States are that every case be treated with antibiotics. Ciprofloxacin is recommended as first-line treatment. A number of other drugs have been tested and shown to be effective, including ceftriaxone, azithromycin, pivmecillinam, and some fifth-generation

quinolones. While infections caused by non-*dysenteriae* *Shigella* in immunocompetent individuals are routinely treated with a 3-day course of antibiotics, it is recommended that *S. dysenteriae* infections be treated for 5 days and that *Shigella* infections in immunocompromised patients be treated for 7–10 days.

Treatment for shigellosis must be adapted to the clinical context, with the recognition that the most fragile patients are children <5 years old, who represent two-thirds of all cases worldwide. There are few data on the use of quinolones in children. The half-life of ciprofloxacin is longer in infants than in older individuals. The ciprofloxacin dose generally recommended for children is 30 mg/kg per day in two divided doses. Adults living in areas with high hygienic standards are likely to develop milder, shorter-duration disease, whereas infants in endemic areas can develop severe, sometimes fatal dysentery. In the former setting, treatment will remain minimal and bacteriologic proof of infection will often come after symptoms have resolved; in the latter setting, more aggressive measures, possibly including resuscitation, may be required.

REHYDRATION AND NUTRITION *Shigella* infection rarely causes significant dehydration. Cases requiring aggressive rehydration (particularly in industrialized countries) are uncommon. In developing countries, malnutrition remains the primary indicator for diarrhea-related death, highlighting the importance of nutrition in early management. Rehydration should be oral unless the patient is comatose or presents in shock. Because of

TABLE 27-1

RECOMMENDED ANTIMICROBIAL THERAPY FOR SHIGELLOSIS

| ANTIMICROBIAL AGENT | TREATMENT SCHEDULE | | LIMITATIONS |
	IN CHILDREN	IN ADULTS	
First Line			
Ciprofloxacin	15 mg/kg 2 times per day for 3 days, PO	500 mg	
Second Line			
Pivmecillinam	20 mg/kg 4 times per day for 5 days, PO	100 mg No pediatric formulation	Cost
			Frequent administration Resistance emerging
Ceftriaxone	50–100 mg/kg Once a day IM for 2–5 days	— Must be injected	Efficacy not validated
Azithromycin	6–20 mg/kg Once a day for 1–5 days, PO	1–1.5 g Efficacy not validated	Cost
			MIC near serum concentration Resistance emerges rapidly and spreads to other bacteria

Source: WHO Library Cataloguing-in-Publication Data: Guidelines for the control of shigellosis, including epidemics due to *Shigella dysenteriae* type 1 (*www.searo.who.int/LinkFiles/CAH_Publications_shigella.pdf*).

the improved effectiveness of reduced-osmolarity oral rehydration solution (especially for children with acute noncholera diarrhea), the WHO and UNICEF now recommend a standard solution of 245 mOsm/L [sodium, 75 mmol/L; chloride, 65 mmol/L; glucose (anhydrous), 75 mmol/L; potassium, 20 mmol/L; citrate, 10 mmol/L]. In shigellosis, as in acute infectious diarrhea of most etiologies (including cholera), the coupled transport of sodium to glucose or other solutes is largely unaffected, and oral rehydration therapy represents the easiest and most efficient form of rehydration, especially in severe cases.

Nutrition should be started as soon as possible after completion of initial rehydration. Early refeeding is safe, well tolerated, and clinically beneficial. Because breast-feeding reduces diarrheal losses and the need for oral rehydration in infants, it should be maintained in the absence of contraindications (e.g., maternal HIV infection).

NONSPECIFIC, SYMPTOM-BASED THERAPY
Antimotility agents have been implicated in prolonged fever in volunteers with shigellosis. These agents are suspected of increasing the risk of toxic megacolon and are thought to have been responsible for HUS in children infected by Shiga toxin–producing strains of *E. coli*. For safety reasons, it is better to avoid antimotility agents in bloody diarrhea.

TREATMENT OF COMPLICATIONS There is no consensus regarding the best treatment for toxic megacolon. The patient should be assessed frequently by both medical and surgical teams. Anemia, dehydration, and electrolyte deficits (particularly hypokalemia) may aggravate colonic atony and should be actively treated. Nasogastric aspiration helps to deflate the colon. Parenteral nutrition has not been proved to be beneficial. Fever persisting beyond 48–72 h raises the possibility of local perforation or abscess. Most studies recommend colectomy if, after 48–72 h, colonic distention persists. However, some physicians recommend continuation of medical therapy for up to 7 days if the patient seems to be improving clinically despite persistent megacolon without free perforation. Intestinal perforation, either isolated or complicating toxic megacolon, requires surgical treatment and intensive medical support.

Rectal prolapse must be treated as soon as possible. With the health care provider using surgical gloves or a soft warm wet cloth and the patient in the knee-chest position, the prolapsed rectum is gently pushed back into place. If edema of the rectal mucosa is evident (rendering reintegration difficult), it can be osmotically reduced by applying gauze impregnated with a warm solution of saturated magnesium sulfate.

Rectal prolapse often relapses but usually resolves along with the resolution of dysentery.

HUS must be treated by water restriction, including discontinuation of oral rehydration solution and potassium-rich alimentation. Hemofiltration is usually required.

PREVENTION
Hand washing after defecation or handling of children's feces and before handling of food is recommended. However, this protocol entails an average of 32 hand washes per day, with consumption of 20 L of water. If soap is too costly, ash or mud can be used, but access to water remains essential. Stool precautions, together with a cleaning protocol for medical staff as well as for patients, have proven useful in limiting the spread of infection during *Shigella* outbreaks. Ideally, patients should have a negative stool culture before their infection is considered cured. Recurrences are rare if treatment and prevention are correctly implemented.

Although several live attenuated oral and subunit parenteral vaccine candidates have been produced and are undergoing clinical trials, no vaccine against shigellosis is currently available. Especially given the rapid progression of antibiotic resistance in *Shigella*, a vaccine is urgently needed.

FURTHER READINGS
BENNISH ML, WOJTYNIAK BJ: Mortality due to shigellosis: Community and hospital data. Rev Infect Dis 13(Suppl 4):S245, 1991

COSSART P, SANSONETTI PJ: Bacterial invasion: The paradigms of enteroinvasive pathogens. Science 304:242, 2004

KOTLOFF KL et al: Overview of live vaccine strategies against *Shigella*, in *New Generation Vaccines*, 3d ed, MM Levine et al (eds). London, Informa Healthcare, 2004, pp 723–735

——— et al: Global burden of Shigella infections: Implications for vaccine development and implementation of control strategies. Bull World Health Organ 77:651, 1999

NIYOGI SK: Shigellosis. J Microbiol 43:133, 2005

PHALIPON A: Vaccination against shigellosis: is it the path that is difficult or is it the difficult that is the path? Microbes Infect 10:1057, 2008

PHALIPON A, SANSONETTI PJ: Shigella's ways of manipulating the host intestinal innate and adaptive immune system: A tool box for survival? Immunol Cell Biol 85:119, 2007

VON SEIDLEIN L et al: A multicentre study of Shigella diarrhoea in six Asian countries: Disease burden, clinical manifestations, and microbiology. PLoS Med 3(9):e353, 2006

WORLD HEALTH ORGANIZATION: Guidelines for the control of shigellosis, including epidemics due to *Shigella dysenteriae* type 1. WHO Library Cataloguing-in-Publication Data (*www.searo.who.int/LinkFiles/CAH_Publications_shigella.pdf*)

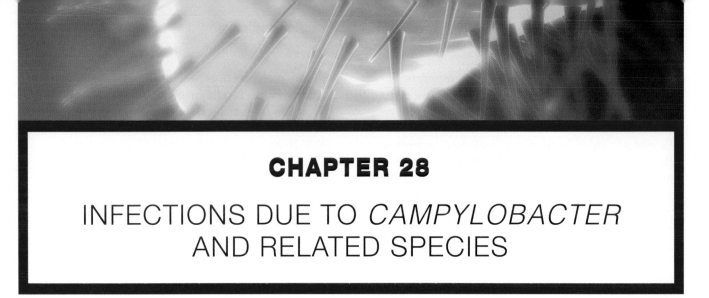

CHAPTER 28

INFECTIONS DUE TO *CAMPYLOBACTER* AND RELATED SPECIES

Martin J. Blaser

DEFINITION

Bacteria of the genus *Campylobacter* and of the related genera *Arcobacter* and *Helicobacter* (Chap. 25) cause a variety of inflammatory conditions. Although acute diarrheal illnesses are most common, these organisms may cause infections in virtually all parts of the body, especially in compromised hosts, and these infections may have late nonsuppurative sequelae. The designation *Campylobacter* comes from the Greek for "curved rod" and refers to the organism's vibrio-like morphology.

ETIOLOGY

Campylobacters are motile, non-spore-forming, curved, gram-negative rods. Originally known as *Vibrio fetus*, these bacilli were reclassified as a new genus in 1973, after their dissimilarity to other vibrios was recognized. More than 15 species have since been identified. These species are currently divided into three genera: *Campylobacter*, *Arcobacter*, and *Helicobacter*. Not all of the species are pathogens of humans. The human pathogens fall into two major groups: those that primarily cause diarrheal disease and those that cause extraintestinal infection. The principal diarrheal pathogen is *C. jejuni*, which accounts for 80–90% of all cases of recognized illness due to campylobacters and related genera. Other organisms that cause diarrheal disease include *C. coli*, *C. upsaliensis*, *C. lari*, *C. hyointestinalis*, *C. fetus*, *A. butzleri*, *A. cryaerophilus*, *H. cinaedi*, and *H. fennelliae*. The two *Helicobacter* species causing diarrheal disease, *H. cinaedi* and *H. fennelliae*, are intestinal rather than gastric organisms; in terms of the clinical features of the illnesses they cause, these species most closely resemble *Campylobacter* rather than *H. pylori* (Chap. 25) and thus are considered in this chapter.

The major species causing extraintestinal illnesses is *C. fetus*. However, any of the diarrheal agents listed above may cause systemic or localized infection as well. Neither aerobes nor strict anaerobes, these microaerophilic organisms are adapted for survival in the gastrointestinal mucous layer. This chapter focuses on *C. jejuni* and *C. fetus* as the major pathogens in and prototypes for their groups. The key features of infection are listed by species (excluding *C. jejuni*, described in detail in the text below) in **Table 28-1**.

EPIDEMIOLOGY

Campylobacters are found in the gastrointestinal tract of many animals used for food (including poultry, cattle, sheep, and swine) and many household pets (including birds, dogs, and cats). These microorganisms usually do not cause illness in their animal hosts. In most cases,

TABLE 28-1   277

CLINICAL FEATURES ASSOCIATED WITH INFECTION DUE TO "ATYPICAL" *CAMPYLOBACTER* AND RELATED SPECIES IMPLICATED AS CAUSES OF HUMAN ILLNESS

SPECIES	COMMON CLINICAL FEATURES	LESS COMMON CLINICAL FEATURES	ADDITIONAL INFORMATION
Campylobacter coli	Fever, diarrhea, abdominal pain	Bacteremia[a]	Clinically indistinguishable from *C. jejuni*
Campylobacter fetus	Bacteremia,[a] sepsis, meningitis, vascular infections	Diarrhea, relapsing fevers	Not usually isolated from media containing cephalothin or incubated at 42°C
Campylobacter upsaliensis	Watery diarrhea, low-grade fever, abdominal pain	Bacteremia, abscesses	Difficult to isolate because of cephalothin susceptibility
Campylobacter lari	Abdominal pain, diarrhea	Colitis, appendicitis	Seagulls frequently colonized; organism often transmitted to humans via contaminated water
Campylobacter hyointestinalis	Watery or bloody diarrhea, vomiting, abdominal pain	Bacteremia	Causes proliferative enteritis in swine
Helicobacter fennelliae	Chronic mild diarrhea, abdominal cramps, proctitis	Bacteremia[a]	Best treated with fluoroquinolones
Helicobacter cinaedi	Chronic mild diarrhea, abdominal cramps, proctitis	Bacteremia[a]	Best treated with fluoroquinolones; identified in healthy hamsters
Campylobacter jejuni subspecies *doylei*	Diarrhea	Chronic gastritis, bacteremia[b]	Uncertain role as human pathogen
Arcobacter cryaerophilus	Diarrhea	Bacteremia	Cultured under aerobic conditions
Arcobacter butzleri	Fever, diarrhea, abdominal pain, nausea	Bacteremia, appendicitis	Cultured under aerobic conditions; enzootic in nonhuman primates
Campylobacter sputorum	Pulmonary, perianal, groin, and axillary abscesses	Bacteremia	Three clinically relevant biovars: *C. sputorum* subspecies *sputorum*, *C. sputorum* subspecies *bubulus*, and *Campylobacter mucosalis*

[a]In immunocompromised hosts, especially HIV-infected persons.
[b]In children.
Source: Adapted from BM Allos, MJ Blaser: *Campylobacter jejuni* and the expanding spectrum of related infections. Clin Infect Dis 20:1092, 1995.

campylobacters are transmitted to humans in raw or undercooked food products or through direct contact with infected animals. In the United States and other developed countries, ingestion of contaminated poultry that has not been sufficiently cooked is the most common mode of acquisition (30–70% of cases). Other modes include ingestion of raw (unpasteurized) milk or untreated water, contact with infected household pets, travel to developing countries (campylobacters being among the leading causes of traveler's diarrhea; Chap. 22), oral-anal sexual contact, and (occasionally) contact with an index case who is incontinent of stool.

Campylobacter infections are common. Several studies indicate that, in the United States, diarrheal disease due to campylobacters is more common than that due to *Salmonella* and *Shigella* combined. Infections occur throughout the year, but their incidence peaks during summer and early autumn. Persons of all ages are affected; however, attack rates for *C. jejuni* are highest among young children and young adults, while those for *C. fetus* are highest at the extremes of age. Systemic infections due to *C. fetus* (and to other *Campylobacter* and related species) are most common among compromised hosts. Persons at increased risk include those with AIDS, hypogammaglobulinemia,

neoplasia, liver disease, diabetes mellitus, and generalized atherosclerosis as well as neonates and pregnant women. However, apparently healthy nonpregnant persons occasionally develop transient *Campylobacter* bacteremia as part of a gastrointestinal illness.

 In developing countries, *C. jejuni* infections are hyperendemic, with the highest rates among children <2 years old. Infection rates fall with age, as does the illness-to-infection ratio. These observations suggest that frequent exposure to *C. jejuni* leads to the acquisition of immunity.

PATHOLOGY AND PATHOGENESIS

Many *C. jejuni* infections are subclinical, especially in hosts in developing countries who have had multiple prior infections and thus are partially immune. Most illnesses occur within 2–4 days (range, 1–7 days) of exposure to the organism in food or water. The sites of tissue injury include the jejunum, ileum, and colon. Biopsies show an acute nonspecific inflammatory reaction, with neutrophils, monocytes, and eosinophils in the lamina propria, as well as damage to the epithelium, including loss of mucus, glandular degeneration, and crypt abscesses. Biopsy findings may be consistent with Crohn's disease or ulcerative colitis, but these "idiopathic" chronic inflammatory diseases should not be diagnosed unless infectious colitis, *specifically including* that due to infection with *Campylobacter* species and related organisms, has been ruled out.

The high frequency of *C. jejuni* infections and their severity and recurrence among hypogammaglobulinemic patients suggest that antibodies are important in protective immunity. The pathogenesis of infection is uncertain. Both the motility of the strain and its capacity to adhere to host tissues appear to favor disease, but classic enterotoxins and cytotoxins (although described and including cytolethal distending toxin, or CDT) appear not to play substantial roles in tissue injury or disease production. The organisms have been visualized in the epithelium, albeit in low numbers. The documentation of a significant tissue response and occasionally of *C. jejuni* bacteremia further suggests that tissue invasion is clinically significant, and in vitro studies are consistent with this pathogenetic feature.

The pathogenesis of *C. fetus* infections is better defined. Virtually all clinical isolates of *C. fetus* possess a proteinaceous capsule-like structure (an S-layer) that renders the organisms resistant to complement-mediated killing and opsonization. As a result, *C. fetus* can cause bacteremia and can seed sites beyond the intestinal tract. The ability of the organism to switch the S-layer proteins expressed—a phenomenon that results in antigenic variability—may contribute to the chronicity and high rate of recurrence of *C. fetus* infections in compromised hosts.

CLINICAL MANIFESTATIONS

The clinical features of infections due to *Campylobacter* and the related *Arcobacter* and intestinal *Helicobacter* species causing enteric disease appear to be highly similar. *C. jejuni* can be considered the prototype, in part because it is by far the most common enteric pathogen. A prodrome of fever, headache, myalgia, and/or malaise often occurs 12–48 h before the onset of diarrheal symptoms. The most common signs and symptoms of the intestinal phase are diarrhea, abdominal pain, and fever. The degree of diarrhea varies from several loose stools to grossly bloody stools; most patients presenting for medical attention have ≥10 bowel movements on the worst day of illness. Abdominal pain usually consists of cramping and may be the most prominent symptom. Pain is usually generalized but may become localized; *C. jejuni* infection may cause pseudoappendicitis. Fever may be the only initial manifestation of *C. jejuni* infection, a situation mimicking the early stages of typhoid fever. Febrile young children may develop convulsions. *Campylobacter* enteritis is generally self-limited; however, symptoms persist for >1 week in 10–20% of patients seeking medical attention, and clinical relapses occur in 5–10% of untreated patients.

C. fetus may cause a diarrheal illness similar to that due to *C. jejuni*, especially in normal hosts. This organism may also cause either intermittent diarrhea or nonspecific abdominal pain without localizing signs. Sequelae are uncommon, and the outcome is benign. *C. fetus* may also cause a prolonged relapsing systemic illness (with fever, chills, and myalgias) that has no obvious primary source; this manifestation is especially common among compromised hosts. Secondary seeding of an organ (e.g., meninges, brain, bone, urinary tract, or soft tissue) complicates the course, which may be fulminant. *C. fetus* infections have a tropism for vascular sites: endocarditis, mycotic aneurysm, and septic thrombophlebitis may all occur. Infection during pregnancy often leads to fetal death. A variety of *Campylobacter* species and *H. cinaedi* can cause recurrent cellulitis with fever and bacteremia in immunocompromised hosts.

COMPLICATIONS

Except in infection with *C. fetus*, bacteremia is uncommon, developing most often in immunocompromised hosts and at the extremes of age. Three patterns of extraintestinal infection have been noted: (1) transient bacteremia in a normal host with enteritis (benign course, no specific treatment needed); (2) sustained bacteremia or focal infection in a normal host (bacteremia originating from enteritis, with patients responding well to antimicrobial therapy); and (3) sustained bacteremia or focal infection in a compromised host. Enteritis may not be clinically apparent. Antimicrobial therapy, possibly prolonged, is necessary for suppression or cure of the infection.

Campylobacter, Arcobacter, and intestinal *Helicobacter* infections in patients with AIDS or hypogammaglobulinemia may be severe, persistent, and extraintestinal; relapse after cessation of therapy is common. Hypogammaglobulinemic patients may also develop osteomyelitis and an erysipelas-like rash or cellulitis.

Local suppurative complications of infection include cholecystitis, pancreatitis, and cystitis; distant complications include meningitis, endocarditis, arthritis, peritonitis, cellulitis, and septic abortion. All these complications are rare, except in immunocompromised hosts. Hepatitis, interstitial nephritis, and the hemolytic-uremic syndrome occasionally complicate acute infection. Reactive arthritis and other rheumatologic complaints may develop several weeks after infection, especially in persons with the HLA-B27 phenotype. Guillain-Barré syndrome (or its Miller Fisher or cranial polyneuropathy variant) follows *Campylobacter* infections uncommonly—i.e., in 1 of every 1000–2000 cases or, for certain *C. jejuni* serotypes (such as O19), in 1 of every 100–200 cases. Despite the low frequency of this complication, it is now estimated that *Campylobacter* infections, because of their high incidence, may trigger 20–40% of all cases of Guillain-Barré syndrome. Immunoproliferative small-intestinal disease (*alpha chain disease*), a form of lymphoma that originates in small-intestinal mucosa-associated lymphoid tissue, has been associated with *C. jejuni*; antimicrobial therapy has led to marked clinical improvement.

DIAGNOSIS

In patients with *Campylobacter* enteritis, peripheral leukocyte counts reflect the severity of the inflammatory process. However, stools from nearly all *Campylobacter*-infected patients presenting for medical attention in the United States contain leukocytes or erythrocytes. Fecal smears should be treated with Gram's or Wright's stain and examined in all suspected cases. When the diagnosis of *Campylobacter* enteritis is suspected on the basis of findings indicating inflammatory diarrhea (fever, fecal leukocytes), clinicians can ask the laboratory to attempt the visualization of organisms with characteristic vibrioid morphology by direct microscopic examination of stools with Gram's staining or to use phase-contrast or dark-field microscopy to identify the organisms' characteristic "darting" motility. Confirmation of the diagnosis of *Campylobacter* infection is based on identification of an isolate from cultures of stool, blood, or another site. *Campylobacter*-specific media should be used to culture stools from all patients with inflammatory or bloody diarrhea. Since all *Campylobacter* species are fastidious, they will not be isolated unless selective media or other selective techniques are used. Not all media are equally useful for isolation of the broad array of campylobacters; therefore, failure to isolate campylobacters from stool does not entirely rule out their presence. The detection of the organisms in stool almost always implies infection; there is a brief period of postconvalescent fecal carriage and no commensalism in humans. In contrast, *C. sputorum* and related organisms found in the oral cavity are commensals with rare pathogenic significance. Because of low levels of metabolic activity in standard blood culture media, *Campylobacter* bacteremia may be difficult to detect unless laboratorians are looking for low-positive results in quantitative assays.

DIFFERENTIAL DIAGNOSIS

The symptoms of *Campylobacter* enteritis are not sufficiently unusual to distinguish this illness from that due to *Salmonella*, *Shigella*, *Yersinia*, and other pathogens. The combination of fever and fecal leukocytes or erythrocytes is indicative of inflammatory diarrhea, and definitive diagnosis is based on culture or demonstration of the characteristic organisms on stained fecal smears. Similarly, extraintestinal *Campylobacter* illness is diagnosed by culture. Infection due to *Campylobacter* should be suspected in the setting of septic abortion, and that due to *C. fetus* should be suspected specifically in the setting of septic thrombophlebitis. It is important to reiterate that (1) the

presentation of *Campylobacter* enteritis may mimic that of ulcerative colitis or Crohn's disease, (2) *Campylobacter* enteritis is much more common than either of the latter (especially among young adults), and (3) biopsy may not distinguish among these entities. Thus a diagnosis of inflammatory bowel disease should not be made until *Campylobacter* infection has been ruled out, especially in persons with a history of foreign travel, significant animal contact, immunodeficiency, or exposure incurring a high risk of transmission.

℞ Treatment: INFECTIONS DUE TO *CAMPYLOBACTER* AND RELATED SPECIES

Fluid and electrolyte replacement is central to the treatment of diarrheal illnesses (Chap. 22). Even among patients presenting for medical attention with *Campylobacter* enteritis, not all clearly benefit from specific antimicrobial therapy. Indications for therapy include high fever, bloody diarrhea, severe diarrhea, persistence for >1 week, and worsening of symptoms. A 5- to 7-day course of erythromycin (250 mg orally four times daily or—for children—30–50 mg/kg per day, in divided doses) is the regimen of choice. Both clinical trials and in vitro susceptibility testing indicate that other macrolides, including clarithromycin and azithromycin, also are useful therapeutic agents. An alternative regimen for adults is ciprofloxacin (500 mg orally twice daily) or another fluoroquinolone for 5–7 days, but resistance to this class of agents as well as to tetracyclines has been increasing. Patients infected with antibiotic-resistant strains are at increased risk of adverse outcomes. Use of antimotility agents, which may prolong the duration of symptoms and have been associated with toxic megacolon and with death, is not recommended.

For systemic infections, treatment with gentamicin (1.7 mg/kg IV every 8 h after a loading dose of 2 mg/kg), imipenem (500 mg IV every 6 h), or chloramphenicol (50 mg/kg IV each day in three or four divided doses) should be started empirically, but susceptibility testing should then be performed. Ciprofloxacin and amoxicillin/clavulanate are alternative agents for susceptible strains. In the absence of immunocompromise or endovascular infections, therapy should be administered for 14 days. For immunocompromised patients with systemic infections due to *C. fetus* and for patients with endovascular infections, prolonged therapy (for up to 4 weeks) is usually necessary. For recurrent infections in immunocompromised hosts, lifelong therapy/prophylaxis is sometimes necessary.

PROGNOSIS

Nearly all patients recover fully from *Campylobacter* enteritis, either spontaneously or after antimicrobial therapy. Volume depletion probably contributes to the few deaths that are reported. As stated earlier, occasional patients develop reactive arthritis or Guillain-Barré syndrome or its variants. Systemic infection with *C. fetus* is much more often fatal than that due to related species; this higher mortality rate reflects in part the population affected. Prognosis depends on the rapidity with which appropriate therapy is begun. Otherwise-healthy hosts usually survive *C. fetus* infections without sequelae. Compromised hosts often have recurrent and/or life-threatening infections due to a variety of *Campylobacter* species.

FURTHER READINGS

HAVELAAR AH et al: Immunity to *Campylobacter*: its role in risk assessment and epidemiology. Crit Rev Microbiol 35:1, 2009

HELMS M et al: Adverse health events associated with antimicrobial drug resistance in *Campylobacter* species: A registry-based cohort study. J Infect Dis 191:1050, 2005

JAGUSZTYN-KRYNICKA EK et al: Update on *Campylobacter jejuni* vaccine development for preventing human campylobacteriosis. Expert Rev Vaccines 8:625, 2009

LANG DR et al (eds): Development of Guillain-Barré syndrome following *Campylobacter* infection. J Infect Dis 176(Suppl 2):S91, 1997

LECUIT M et al: Immunoproliferative small intestinal disease associated with *Campylobacter jejuni*. N Engl J Med 350:239, 2004

LUANGTONGKUM T et al: Antibiotic resistance in *Campylobacter*: emergence, transmission and persistence. Future Microbiol 4:189, 2009

MEAD PS et al: Food-related illness and death in the United States. Emerg Infect Dis 5:607, 1999

NACHAMKIN I, BLASER MJ (eds): *Campylobacter jejuni*, 2d ed. Washington, American Society for Microbiology, 2000

SMITH KE et al: Quinolone-resistant *Campylobacter jejuni* infections in Minnesota, 1992–1998. Investigation Team. N Engl J Med 340:1525, 1999

CHAPTER 29

CHOLERA AND OTHER VIBRIOSES

Matthew K. Waldor ■ Gerald T. Keusch

Members of the genus *Vibrio* cause a number of important infectious syndromes. Classic among them is cholera, a devastating diarrheal disease caused by *V. cholerae* that has been responsible for seven global pandemics and much suffering over the past two centuries. Epidemic cholera remains a significant public health concern in the developing world today. Other vibrioses caused by other *Vibrio* species include syndromes of diarrhea, soft tissue infection, or primary sepsis. All *Vibrio* species are highly motile, facultatively anaerobic, curved gram-negative rods with one or more flagella. In nature, vibrios most commonly reside in tidal rivers and bays under conditions of moderate salinity. They proliferate in the summer months when water temperatures exceed 20°C. As might be expected, the illnesses they cause also increase in frequency during the warm months.

CHOLERA

DEFINITION

Cholera is an acute diarrheal disease that can, in a matter of hours, result in profound, rapidly progressive dehydration and death. Accordingly, cholera gravis (the severe form of cholera) is a much-feared disease, particularly in its epidemic presentation. Fortunately, prompt aggressive fluid repletion and supportive care can obviate the high mortality that cholera has historically wrought. While the term *cholera* has occasionally been applied to any severely dehydrating secretory diarrheal illness, whether infectious in etiology or not, it has generally referred to disease caused by *V. cholerae* serogroup O1. In 1992, however, a new serogroup (O139) that causes epidemic cholera emerged on the Indian subcontinent and has since killed thousands of people.

MICROBIOLOGY AND EPIDEMIOLOGY

The species *V. cholerae* comprises a host of organisms classified on the basis of the carbohydrate determinants of their lipopolysaccharide (LPS) O antigens. Some 200 serogroups have now been recognized. They are divided into those that agglutinate in antisera to the O1 group antigen (*V. cholerae* O1) and those that do not (non-O1 *V. cholerae*). Although some non-O1 *V. cholerae* serogroups have occasionally caused sporadic outbreaks of diarrhea, serogroup O1 was, until the emergence of serogroup O139, the exclusive cause of epidemic cholera. Two biotypes of *V. cholerae* O1, classical and El Tor, are distinguished. Each biotype is further subdivided into two serotypes, termed *Inaba* and *Ogawa*.

The natural habitat of *V. cholerae* is coastal salt water and brackish estuaries, where the organism lives in close relation to plankton. Humans become infected incidentally but, once infected, can act as vehicles for spread. Ingestion of water contaminated by human feces is the most common means of acquisition of *V. cholerae*. Consumption of contaminated food can also contribute to spread. There is no known animal reservoir. While the infectious dose is relatively high, it is markedly reduced in hypochlorhydric persons, in those using antacids, and when gastric acidity is buffered by a meal. Cholera is predominantly a pediatric disease in endemic areas, but it affects adults and children equally when newly introduced into a population. Children <2 years of age are less likely to develop severe cholera than are older children, perhaps because of passive immunity acquired from breast milk. In endemic areas, the disease is more common in the summer and fall months. For unexplained reasons, susceptibility to cholera is significantly influenced by ABO blood group status; persons with type O blood are at greatest risk, while those with type AB are at least risk.

Cholera is native to the Ganges delta in the Indian subcontinent. Since 1817, seven global pandemics have occurred. The current (seventh) pandemic—the first due to the El Tor biotype—began in Indonesia in 1961 and spread throughout Asia as *V. cholerae* El Tor displaced the endemic classical strain. In the early 1970s, El Tor cholera erupted in Africa, causing major epidemics before becoming a persistent endemic problem. Currently, >90% of cholera cases reported annually to the World Health Organization (WHO) are from Africa (**Fig. 29-1**). In the period 2000–2004, the annual worldwide number of cholera cases reported to the WHO remained stable at ~100,000. This number is certainly a significant underestimate, as several nations with endemic cholera do not report cholera cases to the WHO.

The recent history of cholera has been punctuated by severe outbreaks. Such outbreaks are often precipitated by war or other circumstances that lead to the breakdown of public health measures. Such was the case in the camps for Rwandan refugees set up in 1994 around Goma, Zaire. Since 1973, sporadic endemic infections due to *V. cholerae* O1 strains related to the seventh-pandemic strain have been recognized along the U.S. Gulf Coast of Louisiana and Texas. These infections are typically associated with the consumption of contaminated, locally harvested shellfish. Occasionally, cases in U.S. locations remote from the Gulf Coast have been linked to shipped-in Gulf Coast seafood.

It was not until 1991 that the current cholera pandemic reached Latin America. Beginning along the Peruvian coast in January 1991, the disease spread in an explosive epidemic to virtually all of South and Central America and to Mexico (**Fig. 29-2**). About 400,000 cases were reported in the first year of the outbreak, and >1 million had been reported by the end of 1994. While the cumulative mortality rate has been <1%, the mortality rate approached 30% in the communities first affected, where a lack of familiarity with the disease led initially to the deployment of ineffective treatment. Intensive education of health care providers and of the community at large has enhanced awareness of the disease and its appropriate management and has greatly diminished mortality. As it did in Africa two decades earlier, the epidemic El Tor strain proved capable of establishing itself in inland waters rather than in its classic niche of coastal salt waters; the organism has already become endemic in many of the Latin American countries into which it was recently introduced. Cases linked to the Latin American epidemic have occurred (via importation of contaminated seafood) in the United States. Although secondary spread of this strain has not taken place in the United States, these events underscore the need for vigilance among health care professionals, even in locations remote from an epidemic.

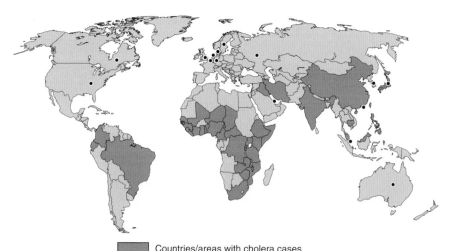

FIGURE 29-1

World distribution of cholera in 2004.

(Adapted from WHO: Cholera, 2004.)

☐ Countries/areas with cholera cases

● Imported cholera cases

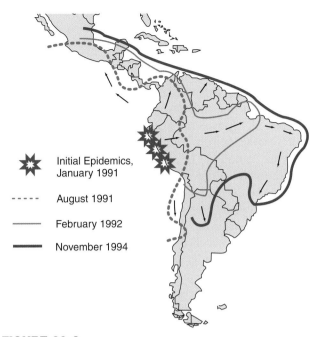

FIGURE 29-2
Spread of *Vibrio cholerae* O1 in the Americas, 1991–1994. *(Courtesy of Dr. Robert V. Tauxe, Centers for Disease Control and Prevention, Atlanta; with permission.)*

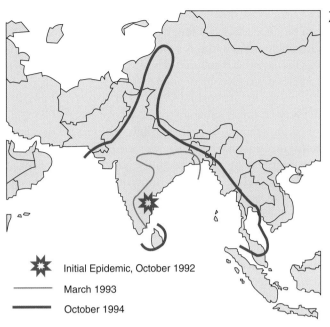

FIGURE 29-3
Spread of *Vibrio cholerae* O139 in the Indian subcontinent and elsewhere in Asia, 1992–1994. *(Courtesy of Dr. Robert V. Tauxe, CDC, Atlanta; with permission.)*

In October 1992, a large-scale outbreak of clinical cholera occurred in southeastern India. The etiologic agent proved to be of a novel *V. cholerae* serogroup. This strain spread rapidly up and down the coast of the Bay of Bengal, reaching Bangladesh in December 1992. There alone, it caused more than 100,000 cases of cholera in the first 3 months of 1993. It subsequently spread across the Indian subcontinent and to neighboring countries, affecting Pakistan, Nepal, western China, Thailand, and Malaysia by the end of 1994 (Fig. 29–3). The organism has since been designated *V. cholerae* O139 Bengal in recognition of its novel O antigen and its geographic origin. The clinical manifestations and epidemiologic features of the disease caused by *V. cholerae* O139 Bengal are indistinguishable from those of O1 cholera. Immunity to the latter, however, is not protective against the former. Because naturally acquired immunity to *V. cholerae* O1 does not cross-protect against *V. cholerae* O139 Bengal, vaccines being developed against the former are unlikely to be effective against the latter.

Some authorities believed that the emergence of *V. cholerae* O139 signaled the beginning of the eighth global cholera pandemic. Indeed, just as O1 El Tor replaced the classical biotype that preceded it, O139 Bengal in 1993 rapidly replaced O1 El Tor as the most common environmental isolate and the predominant cause of clinical cholera in the areas in which it had appeared. However, by the beginning of 1994, O1 El Tor had resumed its dominance in Bangladesh. *V. cholerae* O139 has not spread outside of Asia, and currently, in

most regions of Southeast Asia, *V. cholerae* O1 remains dominant.

PATHOGENESIS

In the final analysis, cholera is a toxin-mediated disease. Its characteristic watery diarrhea is due to the action of cholera toxin, a potent protein enterotoxin elaborated by the organism after it colonizes the small intestine. For *V. cholerae* to colonize the small intestine and produce cholera toxin, it must first recognize, contend with, and traverse several hostile environments. The first of these is the acidic milieu of the stomach. To elude the bactericidal effects of gastric acidity, *V. cholerae* relies, at least in part, on a relatively large inoculum size (compared to that needed for colonization by *Shigella*, for instance). The organism must next traverse the mucous layer lining the small bowel. *V. cholerae* chemotaxis and motility and the action of a variety of proteases may allow the organism to traverse this gel covering the intestinal epithelium. The toxin-coregulated pilus (TCP), so named because its synthesis is regulated in parallel with that of cholera toxin, is essential for *V. cholerae* intestinal colonization. Cholera toxin, TCP, and several other virulence factors are coordinately regulated by ToxR. This protein modulates the expression of virulence genes in response to environmental signals via a cascade of regulatory proteins. Additional regulatory processes, including bacterial responses to the density of the bacterial population (in a phenomenon known as *quorum sensing*), control the virulence of *V. cholerae*.

Once established in the human small bowel, the organism produces cholera toxin, which consists of a monomeric enzymatic moiety (the A subunit) and a pentameric binding moiety (the B subunit). The B pentamer binds to G_{M1} ganglioside, a glycolipid on the surface of epithelial cells that serves as the toxin receptor and makes possible the delivery of the A subunit to its cytosolic target. The activated A subunit (A_1) irreversibly transfers ADP-ribose from nicotinamide adenine dinucleotide to its specific target protein, the GTP-binding regulatory component of adenylate cyclase. The ADP-ribosylated G protein upregulates the activity of adenylate cyclase; the result is the intracellular accumulation of high levels of cyclic AMP. In intestinal epithelial cells, cyclic AMP inhibits the absorptive sodium transport system in villus cells and activates the secretory chloride transport system in crypt cells, and these events lead to the accumulation of sodium chloride in the intestinal lumen. Since water moves passively to maintain osmolality, isotonic fluid accumulates in the lumen. When the volume of that fluid exceeds the capacity of the rest of the gut to resorb it, watery diarrhea results. Unless the wasted fluid and electrolytes are adequately replaced, shock (due to profound dehydration) and acidosis (due to loss of bicarbonate) follow. Although perturbation of the adenylate cyclase pathway is the primary mechanism by which cholera toxin causes excess fluid secretion, increasing evidence indicates that cholera toxin also enhances intestinal secretion via prostaglandins and/or neural histamine receptors.

The genes encoding cholera toxin (*ctxAB*) are part of the genome of a bacteriophage designated CTXΦ. The receptor for this phage on the *V. cholerae* surface is the intestinal colonization factor TCP. Since *ctxAB* is part of a mobile genetic element (CTXΦ), horizontal transfer of this bacteriophage may account for the emergence of new toxigenic *V. cholerae* serogroups. Many of the other genes important for *V. cholerae* pathogenicity, including the genes encoding the biosynthesis of TCP, those encoding accessory colonization factors, and those regulating virulence gene expression, are clustered together in the *V. cholerae* pathogenicity island. Similar clustering of virulence genes is found in other bacterial pathogens. It is believed that pathogenicity islands are acquired by horizontal gene transfer.

V. cholerae O139 Bengal is closely related to the O1 El Tor strains of the seventh pandemic and seems to have arisen from them by horizontal gene transfer. It shares the virulence attributes and general pathogenic mechanisms of O1 vibrios. *V. cholerae* O139 Bengal is in fact virtually identical to the seventh-pandemic strains of *V. cholerae* O1 El Tor except for two important differences: production of the novel O139 LPS and of an immunologically related O-antigen polysaccharide capsule. Encapsulation is not a feature of O1 strains and may explain the resistance of O139 strains to human serum in vitro as well as the occasional development of O139 bacteremia.

CLINICAL MANIFESTATIONS

After a 24- to 48-h incubation period, cholera begins with the sudden onset of painless watery diarrhea that may quickly become voluminous and is often followed shortly by vomiting. In severe cases, stool volume can exceed 250 mL/kg in the first 24 h. If fluids and electrolytes are not replaced, hypovolemic shock and death ensue. Fever is usually absent. Muscle cramps due to electrolyte disturbances are common. The stool has a characteristic appearance: a nonbilious, gray, slightly cloudy fluid with flecks of mucus, no blood, and a somewhat sweet, inoffensive odor. It has been called "rice-water" stool because of its resemblance to the water in which rice has been washed. Clinical symptoms parallel volume contraction: At losses of 3–5% of normal body weight, thirst develops; at 5–8%, postural hypotension, weakness, tachycardia, and decreased skin turgor are documented; and at >10%, oliguria, weak or absent pulses, sunken eyes (and, in infants, sunken fontanelles), wrinkled ("washerwoman") skin, somnolence, and coma are characteristic. Complications derive exclusively from the effects of volume and electrolyte depletion and include renal failure due to acute tubular necrosis. Thus, if the patient is adequately treated with fluid and electrolytes, complications are averted and the process is self-limited, resolving in a few days.

Laboratory data usually reveal an elevated hematocrit (due to hemoconcentration) in nonanemic patients; mild neutrophilic leukocytosis; elevated levels of blood urea nitrogen and creatinine consistent with prerenal azotemia; normal sodium, potassium, and chloride levels; a markedly reduced bicarbonate level (<15 mmol/L); and an elevated anion gap (due to increases in serum lactate, protein, and phosphate). Arterial pH is usually low (~7.2).

DIAGNOSIS

The clinical suspicion of cholera can be confirmed by the identification of *V. cholerae* in stool; however, the organism must be specifically sought. With experience, it can be detected directly by dark-field microscopy on a wet mount of fresh stool, and its serotype can be discerned by immobilization with specific antiserum. Laboratory isolation of the organism requires the use of a selective medium. The best of these is thiosulfate–citrate–bile salts–sucrose (TCBS) agar, on which the organism grows as a flat yellow colony. If a delay in sample processing is expected, Carey-Blair transport medium and/or alkaline-peptone water-enrichment medium should be inoculated as well. In endemic areas, there is little need for biochemical confirmation and characterization, although these tasks may be worthwhile in places where *V. cholerae* is an uncommon isolate. Standard microbiologic biochemical testing for Enterobacteriaceae will suffice for identification of *V. cholerae*. All vibrios are oxidase-positive.

The yield of stool cultures for the diagnosis of *V. cholerae* infection declines late in the course of the illness or when effective antibacterial therapy is initiated. Monoclonal antibody–based diagnostic kits and methods based on the polymerase chain reaction and on DNA probes have been developed for detection of *V. cholerae* O1 and O139.

℞ Treatment: CHOLERA

Cholera is simple to treat; only the rapid and adequate replacement of fluids, electrolytes, and base is required. The mortality rate for appropriately treated disease is usually <1%. However, analysis of a large outbreak of cholera among airline travelers from an endemic country to the United States revealed frequent misdiagnoses by U.S. health professionals and poor appreciation on their part of the principles of management. Fluid replacement may be given orally, but oral rehydration is not always feasible in the presence of significant vomiting. Oral rehydration takes advantage of the hexose-Na^+ cotransport mechanism to move Na^+ across the gut mucosa together with an actively transported molecule such as glucose. For the sake of simplicity, the WHO advises routine use of a single solution of oral rehydration salts (ORS) for diarrheal disease rather than encouraging attempts to choose among multiple formulations according to etiology (Table 29-1). If available, rice-based ORS is considered superior to standard ORS in the treatment of cholera.

For initial management of severely dehydrated patients, IV fluid replacement is preferable. Because profound acidosis (pH <7.2) is common in this group, Ringer's lactate is the best choice among commercial products (Table 29-2). It must be used with additional potassium supplements, preferably given by mouth. The total fluid deficit in severely dehydrated patients (≥10% of body weight) can be replaced safely within the first

TABLE 29-1

COMPOSITION OF WORLD HEALTH ORGANIZATION ORAL REHYDRATION SOLUTION (ORS)[a,b]

CONSTITUENT	CONCENTRATION, mmol/L
Na^+	75
K^+	20
Cl-	65
Citrate[c]	10
Glucose	75

[a]Contains (per package, to be added to 1 L of drinking water): NaCl, 2.6 g; $Na_3C_6H_5O_7 \cdot 2H_2O$, 2.9 g; KCl, 1.5 g; and glucose, 15 g.
[b]If prepackaged ORS is unavailable, a simple homemade alternative can be prepared by combining 5 g NaCl (about 1 level teaspoon) with either 50 g precooked rice cereal or 40 g sucrose in 1 L of drinking water. In that case, potassium must be supplied separately (e.g., in orange juice or coconut water).
[c]10 mmol citrate per liter, which supplies 30 mmol HCO_3/L.

TABLE 29-2

ELECTROLYTE COMPOSITION OF CHOLERA STOOL AND OF INTRAVENOUS REHYDRATION SOLUTION

	CONCENTRATION, mmol/L			
SUBSTANCE	Na^+	K^+	Cl-	BASE
Stool				
Adult	135	15	90	30
Child	100	25	90	30
Ringer's lactate	130	4[a]	109	28

[a]Potassium supplements, preferably administered by mouth, are required to replace the usual potassium losses from stool.

4 h of therapy, half within the first hour. Thereafter, oral therapy can usually be initiated, with the goal of maintaining fluid intake equal to fluid output. However, patients with continued large-volume diarrhea may require prolonged IV treatment to keep up with gastrointestinal fluid losses. Severe hypokalemia can develop but will respond to potassium given either IV or orally. In the absence of adequate staff to monitor the patient's progress, the oral route of rehydration and potassium replacement is safer than the IV route.

Although not necessary for cure, the use of an antibiotic to which the organism is susceptible diminishes the duration and volume of fluid loss and hastens clearance of the organism from the stool. Single-dose tetracycline (2 g) or doxycycline (300 mg) is effective in adults but is not recommended for children <8 years of age because of possible deposition in bone and developing teeth. Emerging drug resistance is an ever-present concern. For adults with cholera in areas where tetracycline resistance is prevalent, ciprofloxacin [either in a single dose (30 mg/kg, not to exceed a total dose of 1 g) or in a short course (15 mg/kg bid for 3 days, not to exceed a total daily dose of 1 g)], erythromycin (a total of 40 mg/kg daily in three divided doses for 3 days), or a single 1-g dose of azithromycin is a clinically effective substitute. These drugs are highly effective in reducing total stool output and are significantly better than trimethoprim-sulfamethoxazole. For children, furazolidone has been the recommended agent and trimethoprim-sulfamethoxazole the second choice. Because of cost and/or toxicity issues related to the other drugs, erythromycin is a good choice for pediatric cholera.

PREVENTION

Provision of safe water and facilities for sanitary disposal of feces, improved nutrition, and attention to food preparation and storage in the household can significantly reduce the incidence of cholera.

Much effort has been devoted to the development of an effective cholera vaccine over the past two decades, with a particular focus on oral vaccine strains. Traditional killed cholera vaccine given intramuscularly provides little protection to nonimmune subjects and predictably causes adverse effects, including pain at the injection site, malaise, and fever. The vaccine's limited efficacy is due, at least in part, to its failure to induce a local immune response at the intestinal mucosal surface.

Two types of oral cholera vaccines have been developed. The first is a killed whole-cell (WC) vaccine. Two formulations of the killed WC vaccine have been prepared: one that also contains the nontoxic B subunit of cholera toxin (WC/BS) and one composed solely of killed bacteria. In field trials in Bangladesh, both of the killed vaccines offered significant protection from cholera compared with placebo for the first 6 months after vaccination, with protection rates of ~58% for WC and 85% for WC/BS. Protective efficacy rates for both vaccines declined to ~50% by 3 years after vaccine administration. Immunity was relatively sustained in persons vaccinated at an age of >5 years but was not well sustained in younger vaccinees. The WC/BS vaccine proved effective in a trial conducted in a sub-Saharan African population with a high prevalence of HIV infection. Killed oral vaccines also confer herd protection to unvaccinated individuals living in proximity to vaccinated individuals. Serious consideration should be given to the administration of the WC/BS vaccine in high-risk environments such as refugee camps. The WC/BS vaccine is available in Europe but not in the United States.

The second approach is a live attenuated vaccine strain developed, for example, by the isolation or creation of mutants lacking the genes encoding cholera toxin. Strain CVD 103-HgR, an oral live cholera vaccine licensed for immunization of travelers in Europe, is derived from a classical biotype strain of *V. cholerae* and contains a deletion of the cholera toxin A subunit gene. This strain has been extensively tested in volunteers; a single dose yielded a high degree of protection against experimental challenge with classical *V. cholerae* strains,

with almost no side effects. Protective efficacy was not as great against challenge with El Tor *V. cholerae*. Unfortunately, in a large field trial in Indonesian children, this vaccine failed to induce protection against clinical cholera. Other live attenuated vaccine candidate strains have been prepared from El Tor and O139 *V. cholerae* and are now undergoing clinical trials. Because of the minimal efficacy of existing parenteral vaccines, cholera immunization is recommended for U.S. travelers only if it is mandated by the countries they plan to visit.

OTHER *VIBRIO* SPECIES

 The genus *Vibrio* includes several human pathogens that do not cause cholera. Abundant in coastal waters throughout the world, noncholera vibrios can reach high concentrations in the tissues of filter-feeding mollusks. As a result, human infection commonly follows the ingestion of seawater or of raw or undercooked shellfish (Table 29-3). Most noncholera vibrios can be cultured on blood or MacConkey agar, which contains enough salt to support the growth of these halophilic species. In the microbiology laboratory, the species of noncholera vibrios are distinguished by standard biochemical tests. The most important of these organisms are *V. parahaemolyticus* and *V. vulnificus*.

The two major types of syndromes for which these species are responsible are gastrointestinal illness (due to *V. parahaemolyticus*, non-O1 *V. cholerae*, *V. mimicus*, *V. fluvialis*, *V. hollisae*, and *V. furnissii*) and soft tissue infections (due to *V. vulnificus*, *V. alginolyticus*, and *V. damselae*). *V. vulnificus* is also a cause of primary sepsis in some compromised individuals. *V. parahaemolyticus* causes rare cases of wound infection and otitis and very rare cases of sepsis.

SPECIES ASSOCIATED PRIMARILY WITH GASTROINTESTINAL ILLNESS

V. Parahaemolyticus

Widespread in marine environments, *V. parahaemolyticus* grows in saline concentrations up to 8–10%. This species

TABLE 29-3

FEATURES OF SELECTED NONCHOLERA VIBRIOSES			
ORGANISM	**VEHICLE OR ACTIVITY**	**HOST AT RISK**	**SYNDROME**
V. parahaemolyticus	Shellfish, seawater	Normal	Gastroenteritis
	Seawater	Normal	Wound infection
Non-O1 *V. cholerae*	Shellfish, travel	Normal	Gastroenteritis
	Seawater	Normal	Wound infection, otitis media
V. vulnificus	Shellfish	Immunosuppressed[a]	Sepsis, secondary cellulitis
	Seawater	Normal	Wound infection, cellulitis
V. alginolyticus	Seawater	Normal	Wound infection, cellulitis, otitis
	Seawater	Burned, other immunosuppressed	Sepsis

[a]Especially with liver disease or hemochromatosis.

Source: Table 161-3 in *Harrison's Principles of Internal Medicine,* 14th edition.

was originally implicated in enteritis in Japan in 1953, accounting for 24% of reported cases in one study—a rate that presumably was due to the common practice of eating raw seafood in that country. *V. parahaemolyticus* has since been identified as a significant intestinal pathogen in many regions of the world. In the United States, common-source outbreaks of diarrhea caused by this organism have been linked to the consumption of undercooked or improperly handled seafood or of other foods contaminated by seawater. Since the mid-1990s, the incidence of *V. parahaemolyticus* infections has increased in several countries, including the United States. Serotypes O3:K6, O4:K68, and O1:K-untypable, which are genetically related to one another, account for this increase. The enteropathogenicity of *V. parahaemolyticus* is closely linked to its ability to cause hemolysis on Wagatsuma agar (i.e., the *Kanagawa phenomenon*). Although the mechanism by which the organism causes diarrhea remains unclear, the genome sequence of *V. parahaemolyticus* contains a pathogenicity island—a cluster of likely virulence-associated genes. *V. parahaemolyticus* should be considered a possible etiologic agent in all cases of diarrhea that can be linked epidemiologically to seafood consumption or to the sea itself.

Infections with *V. parahaemolyticus* can result in two distinct gastrointestinal presentations. The more common of the two presentations (including nearly all cases in North America) is characterized by watery diarrhea, usually occurring in conjunction with abdominal cramps, nausea, and vomiting and accompanied in ~25% of cases by fever and chills. After an incubation period of 4 h to 4 days, symptoms develop and persist for a median of 3 days. Dysentery, the less common presentation, is characterized by severe abdominal cramps, nausea, vomiting, and bloody or mucoid stools.

Most cases of *V. parahaemolyticus*–associated gastrointestinal illness, regardless of the presentation, are self-limited and require neither antimicrobial treatment nor hospitalization. Deaths are extremely rare. Severe infections are associated with underlying diseases, including diabetes, preexisting liver disease, iron-overload states, or immunosuppression. The occasional severe case should be treated with fluid replacement and antibiotics, as described above for cholera.

Non-O1 V. Cholerae

The heterogeneous non-O1 *V. cholerae* organisms cannot be distinguished from *V. cholerae* O1 by routine biochemical tests but do not agglutinate in O1 antiserum. Non-O1 strains have caused several well-studied food-borne outbreaks of gastroenteritis and have also been responsible for sporadic cases of otitis media, wound infection, and bacteremia. Like other vibrios, non-O1 *V. cholerae* organisms are widely distributed in marine environments. In most instances, recognized cases in the United States have been associated with the consumption of raw oysters or with recent travel, typically to Mexico. The broad clinical spectrum of diarrheal illness caused by these organisms is probably due to the group's heterogeneous virulence attributes. *V. cholerae* O139 Bengal, although technically a non-O1 vibrio, is not grouped with these pathogens because it can cause epidemic cholera.

In the United States, about half of all non-O1 *V. cholerae* isolates are from stool samples. The typical incubation period for gastroenteritis due to these organisms is <2 days, and the illness lasts for ~2–7 days. Patients' stools may be copious and watery or may be partly formed, less voluminous, and bloody or mucoid. Diarrhea can result in severe dehydration. Many cases include abdominal cramps, nausea, vomiting, and fever. Like those with cholera, patients who are seriously dehydrated should receive oral or IV fluids; the value of antibiotics is not clear.

Extraintestinal infections due to non-O1 *V. cholerae* commonly follow occupational or recreational exposure to seawater. Around 10% of non-O1 *V. cholerae* isolates come from cases of wound infection, 10% from cases of otitis media, and 20% from cases of bacteremia (which is particularly likely to develop in patients with liver disease). Extraintestinal infections should be treated with antibiotics. Information to guide antibiotic selection and dosing is limited, but most strains are sensitive in vitro to tetracycline, ciprofloxacin, and third-generation cephalosporins.

V. Vulnificus

V. vulnificus is the most common cause of severe vibrio infections in the United States. Like most vibrios, this organism proliferates in the warm summer months and requires a saline environment for growth. In this country, infections in humans typically occur in coastal states between May and October and most commonly affect men >40 years of age. *V. vulnificus* has been linked to two distinct syndromes: primary sepsis, which usually occurs in patients with underlying liver disease, and primary wound infection, which generally affects people without underlying disease. Some authors have suggested that *V. vulnificus* also causes gastroenteritis independent of other clinical manifestations. *V. vulnificus* is endowed with a number of virulence attributes, including a capsule that confers resistance to phagocytosis and to the bactericidal activity of human serum as well as a cytolysin. Measured as the 50% lethal dose in mice, the organism's virulence is considerably increased under conditions of iron overload; this observation is consistent with the propensity of *V. vulnificus* to infect patients who have hemochromatosis.

Primary sepsis most often develops in patients who have cirrhosis or hemochromatosis. However, *V. vulnificus* bacteremia can also affect individuals who have hematopoietic disorders or chronic renal insufficiency, those who are using immunosuppressive medications or alcohol, or (in rare instances) those who have no known underlying disease. After a median incubation period of 16 h, the patient develops malaise, chills, fever, and prostration. One-third of patients develop hypotension, which is often apparent at admission. Cutaneous manifestations develop in most cases (usually within 36 h of onset) and characteristically involve the extremities (the lower more often than the upper). In a common sequence, erythematous patches are followed by ecchymoses, vesicles, and bullae. In fact, sepsis and bullous skin lesions suggest the diagnosis in appropriate settings. Necrosis and sloughing may also be evident. Laboratory studies reveal leukopenia more often than leukocytosis, thrombocytopenia, or elevated levels of fibrin split products. *V. vulnificus* can be cultured from blood or cutaneous lesions. The mortality rate approaches 50%, with most deaths due to uncontrolled sepsis. Accordingly, prompt treatment is critical and should include empirical antibiotic administration, aggressive debridement, and general supportive care. *V. vulnificus* is sensitive in vitro to a number of antibiotics, including tetracycline, fluoroquinolones, and third-generation cephalosporins. Data from animal models suggest that either a fluoroquinolone or the combination of minocycline and cefotaxime should be used in the treatment of *V. vulnificus* septicemia.

V. vulnificus can infect either a fresh or an old wound that comes into contact with seawater; the patient may or may not have underlying disease. After a short incubation period (4 h to 4 days; mean, 12 h), the disease begins with swelling, erythema, and (in many cases) intense pain around the wound. These signs and symptoms are followed by cellulitis, which spreads rapidly and is sometimes accompanied by vesicular, bullous, or necrotic lesions. Metastatic events are uncommon. Most patients have a fever and leukocytosis. *V. vulnificus* can be cultured from skin lesions and occasionally from the blood. Prompt antibiotic therapy and debridement are usually curative.

V. Alginolyticus

First identified as a pathogen of humans in 1973, *V. alginolyticus* occasionally causes eye, ear, and wound infections. This species is the most salt-tolerant of the vibrios and can grow in salt concentrations of >10%. Most clinical isolates come from superinfected wounds that presumably become contaminated at the beach. Although severity varies, *V. alginolyticus* infection tends not to be serious and generally responds well to antibiotic therapy and drainage. A few cases of otitis externa, otitis media, and conjunctivitis due to this pathogen have been described. Tetracycline treatment usually results in cure. *V. alginolyticus* is a rare cause of bacteremia in immunocompromised hosts.

ACKNOWLEDGMENT

The authors gratefully acknowledge the valuable contributions of Dr. Robert Deresiewicz, a coauthor of this chapter for the 14th edition of Harrison's Principles of Internal Medicine.

FURTHER READINGS

BASAK S et al: Influence of domain architecture and codon usage pattern on the evolution of virulence factors of *Vibrio cholerae*. Biochem Biophys Res Commun 379:803, 2009

GREGORIO GV et al: Polymer-based oral rehydration solution for treating acute watery diarrhea. Cochrane Database Syst Rev Apr 15;(2):CD006519, 2009

KOELLE K: The impact of climate on the disease dynamics of cholera. Clin Microbiol Infect 15 (Suppl 1):29, 2009

LUCAS MES et al: Effectiveness of mass oral cholera vaccination in Beira, Mozambique. N Engl J Med 352:757, 2005

SACK DA et al: Cholera. Lancet 363:223, 2004

SAHA D et al: Single-dose azithromycin for the treatment of cholera in adults. N Engl J Med 354:2452, 2006

TANG HJ et al: In vitro and in vivo activities of newer fluoroquinolones against *Vibrio vulnificus*. Antimicrob Agents Chemother 46:3580, 2002

WORLD HEALTH ORGANIZATION: *The Treatment of Diarrhoea: A Manual for Physicians and Other Senior Health Workers.* Geneva, World Health Organization, 2005 (*www.who.int/child-adolescent-health/New_Publications/CHILD_HEALTH/ISBN_92_4_159318_0.pdf*)

———: Cholera, 2004. Wkly Epidemiol Rec 80:261, 2005 (*www.who.int/wer*)

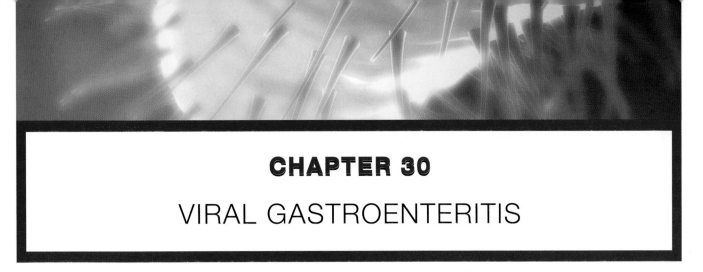

CHAPTER 30

VIRAL GASTROENTERITIS

Umesh D. Parashar ■ Roger I. Glass

Acute infectious gastroenteritis is a common illness that affects persons of all ages worldwide. It is a leading cause of mortality among children in developing countries, accounting for an estimated 2 million deaths each year, and is responsible for up to 10–12% of all hospitalizations among children in industrialized countries, including the United States. Elderly persons, especially those with debilitating health conditions, are also at risk of severe complications and death from acute gastroenteritis. Among healthy young adults, acute gastroenteritis is rarely fatal but incurs substantial medical and social costs, including those of time lost from work.

Several enteric viruses have been recognized as important etiologic agents of acute infectious gastroenteritis (Table 30-1, Fig. 30-1). Illness caused by these viruses is characterized by the acute onset of vomiting and/or diarrhea, which may be accompanied by fever, nausea, abdominal cramps, anorexia, and malaise. As shown in Table 30-2, several features can help distinguish gastroenteritis caused by viruses from that caused by bacterial agents. However, the distinction based on clinical and epidemiologic parameters alone is often difficult, and laboratory tests may be required to confirm the diagnosis.

HUMAN CALICIVIRUSES

Etiologic Agent

The Norwalk virus is the prototype strain of a group of nonenveloped, small (27–40 nm), round, icosahedral viruses with relatively amorphous surface features on visualization

TABLE 30-1

VIRAL CAUSES OF GASTROENTERITIS AMONG HUMANS					
VIRUS	**FAMILY**	**GENOME**	**PRIMARY AGE GROUP AT RISK**	**CLINICAL SEVERITY**	**DETECTION ASSAYS**[a]
Group A rotavirus	Reoviridae	Double-strand segmented RNA	Children <5 years	+++	EM, EIA (commercial), PAGE, RT-PCR
Norovirus	Caliciviridae	Positive-sense single-strand RNA	All ages	++	EM, EIA, RT-PCR
Sapovirus	Caliciviridae	Positive-sense single-strand RNA	Children <5 years	+	EM, EIA, RT-PCR
Astrovirus	Astroviridae	Positive-sense single-strand RNA	Children <5 years	+	EM, EIA, RT-PCR
Adenovirus (types 40 and 41)	Adenoviridae	Double-strand DNA	Children <5 years	+/++	EM, EIA (commercial), PCR

[a]EIA, enzyme immunoassay; EM, electron microscopy; PAGE, polyacrylamide gel electrophoresis; PCR, polymerase chain reaction; RT-PCR, reverse-transcriptase PCR.

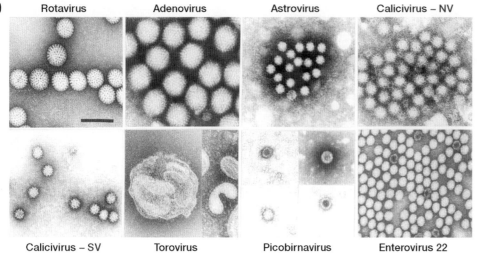

Rotavirus | Adenovirus | Astrovirus | Calicivirus – NV

Calicivirus – SV | Torovirus | Picobirnavirus | Enterovirus 22

FIGURE 30-1
Viral agents of gastroenteritis. NV, Norwalk-like virus; SV, Sapporo-like virus.

by electron microscopy. These viruses have been difficult to classify because they have not been adapted to cell culture, they often are shed in low titers for only a few days, and no animal models are available. Molecular cloning and characterization have demonstrated that these viruses have a single, positive-strand RNA genome ~7.5 kb in length and that they possess a single virion-associated protein—similar to that of typical caliciviruses—with a molecular

TABLE 30-2

CHARACTERISTICS OF GASTROENTERITIS CAUSED BY VIRAL AND BACTERIAL AGENTS

FEATURE	VIRAL GASTROENTERITIS	BACTERIAL GASTROENTERITIS
Setting	Incidence similar in developing and developed countries	More common in settings with poor hygiene and sanitation
Infectious dose	Low (10–100 viral particles) for most agents	High (>10^5 bacteria) for *Escherichia coli*, *Salmonella*, *Vibrio*; medium (10^2–10^5 bacteria) for *Campylobacter jejuni*; low (10–100 bacteria) for *Shigella*
Seasonality	In temperate climates, winter seasonality for most agents; year-round occurrence in tropical areas	More common in summer or rainy months, particularly in developing countries with a high disease burden
Incubation period	1–3 days for most agents; can be shorter for norovirus	1–7 days for common agents (e.g., *Campylobacter*, *E. coli*, *Shigella*, *Salmonella*); a few hours for bacteria producing preformed toxins (e.g., *Staphylococcus aureus*, *Bacillus cereus*)
Reservoir	Primarily humans	Depending on species, human (e.g., *Shigella*, *Salmonella*), animal (e.g., *Campylobacter*, *Salmonella*, *E. coli*), and water (e.g., *Vibrio*) reservoirs exist.
Fever	Common with rotavirus and norovirus; uncommon with other agents	Common with agents causing inflammatory diarrhea (e.g., *Salmonella*, *Shigella*)
Vomiting	Prominent and can be the only presenting feature, especially in children	Common with bacteria producing preformed toxins; less prominent in diarrhea due to other agents
Diarrhea	Common; nonbloody in almost all cases	Prominent and frequently bloody with agents causing inflammatory diarrhea
Duration	1–3 days for norovirus and sapovirus; 2–8 days for other viruses	1–2 days for bacteria producing preformed toxins; 2–8 days for most other bacteria
Diagnosis	This is often a diagnosis of exclusion in clinical practice. Commercial enzyme immunoassays are available for detection of rotavirus and adenovirus, but identification of other agents is limited to research and public health laboratories.	Fecal examination for leukocytes and blood is helpful in differential diagnosis. Culture of stool specimens, sometimes on special media, can identify several pathogens. Molecular techniques are useful epidemiologic tools but are not routinely used in most laboratories.
Treatment	Supportive therapy to maintain adequate hydration and nutrition should be given. Antibiotics and antimotility agents are contraindicated.	Supportive hydration therapy is adequate for most patients. Antibiotics are recommended for patients with dysentery caused by *Shigella* or *Vibrio cholerae* and for some patients with *Clostridium difficile* colitis.

mass of 60 kDa. On the basis of these molecular characteristics, these viruses are presently classified in two genera belonging to the family Caliciviridae: the *noroviruses* and the *sapoviruses* (previously called Norwalk-like viruses and Sapporo-like viruses, respectively).

Epidemiology

Infections with the Norwalk and related human caliciviruses are common worldwide, and most adults have antibodies to these viruses. Antibody is acquired at an earlier age in developing countries—a pattern consistent with the presumed fecal-oral mode of transmission. Infections occur year-round, although, in temperate climates, a distinct increase has been noted in cold-weather months. Noroviruses may be the most common infectious agents of mild gastroenteritis in the community and affect all age groups, whereas sapoviruses primarily cause gastroenteritis in children. Noroviruses also cause traveler's diarrhea, and outbreaks have occurred among military personnel deployed to various parts of the world. The etiologic role of noroviruses in moderate and severe gastroenteritis requiring a visit to a physician or hospitalization is still being studied. However, the limited data available indicate that norovirus may be the second most common viral agent (after rotavirus) among young children and the most common agent among older children and adults. Noroviruses are also recognized as the major cause of epidemics of gastroenteritis worldwide. In the United States, >90% of outbreaks of nonbacterial gastroenteritis are caused by noroviruses. Epidemics occur throughout the year, in all age groups, and in a variety of settings.

Virus is transmitted predominantly by the fecal-oral route but is also present in vomitus. Because an inoculum with very few viruses can be infectious, transmission can occur by aerosolization, by contact with contaminated fomites, and by person-to-person contact. Viral shedding and infectivity are greatest during the acute illness, but challenge studies with Norwalk virus in volunteers indicate that viral antigen may be shed by asymptomatically infected persons and also by symptomatic persons before the onset of symptoms and for up to 2 weeks after the resolution of illness. In one study, 11 of 15 norovirus-infected children <2 years of age shed the virus for >2 weeks after onset; this group included 3 infants <6 months of age who shed virus for 42–47 days or even longer.

Pathogenesis

The exact sites and cellular receptors for attachment of viral particles have not been determined. Data suggest that carbohydrates that are similar to human histo-blood group antigens and are present on the gastroduodenal epithelium of individuals with the secretor phenotype may serve as ligands for the attachment of Norwalk virus. Additional studies must more fully elucidate norovirus-carbohydrate interactions, including potential strain-specific variations. After the infection of volunteers, reversible lesions are noted in the upper jejunum, with broadening and blunting of the villi, shortening of the microvilli, vacuolization of the lining epithelium, crypt hyperplasia, and infiltration of the lamina propria by polymorphonuclear neutrophils and lymphocytes. The lesions persist for at least 4 days after the resolution of symptoms and are associated with malabsorption of carbohydrates and fats and a decreased level of brush-border enzymes. Adenylate cyclase activity is not altered. No histopathologic changes are seen in the stomach or colon, but gastric motor function is delayed, and this alteration is believed to contribute to the nausea and vomiting that are typical of this illness.

Clinical Manifestations

Gastroenteritis caused by Norwalk and related human caliciviruses has a sudden onset, following an average incubation period of 24 h (range, 12–72 h). The illness generally lasts 12–60 h and is characterized by one or more of the following symptoms: nausea, vomiting, abdominal cramps, and diarrhea. Vomiting is more prevalent among children, whereas a greater proportion of adults develop diarrhea. Constitutional symptoms are common, including headache, fever, chills, and myalgias. Noroviruses appear to cause more severe illness than sapoviruses, although both illnesses are less severe than that due to rotavirus. The stools are characteristically loose and watery, without blood, mucus, or leukocytes. White cell counts are generally normal; rarely, leukocytosis with relative lymphopenia may be observed. Death is a rare outcome and usually results from severe dehydration in vulnerable persons (e.g., elderly patients with debilitating health conditions).

Immunity

Approximately 50% of persons challenged with Norwalk virus become ill and acquire short-term immunity against the infecting strain. Immunity to Norwalk virus appears to correlate inversely with level of antibody; i.e., persons with higher levels of preexisting antibody to Norwalk virus are more susceptible to illness. This observation suggests that some individuals have a genetic predisposition to illness. Recent data indicate that specific ABO, Lewis, and secretor blood group phenotypes may influence susceptibility to norovirus infection.

Diagnosis

Cloning and sequencing of the genomes of Norwalk and several other human caliciviruses have allowed the development of assays based on polymerase chain reaction (PCR) for detection of virus in stool and vomitus.

Virus-like particles produced by expression of capsid proteins in a recombinant baculovirus vector have been used to develop enzyme immunoassays (EIAs) for detection of virus in stool or a serologic response to a specific viral antigen. These newer diagnostic techniques are considerably more sensitive than previous detection methods, such as electron microscopy, immune electron microscopy, and EIAs based on reagents derived from humans. However, no currently available single assay can detect all human caliciviruses because of their great genetic and antigenic diversity. In addition, the assays are still cumbersome and are available primarily in research laboratories, although they are increasingly being adopted by public health laboratories for routine screening of fecal specimens from patients affected by outbreaks of gastroenteritis. Commercial EIA kits have been developed but are still being evaluated to determine their optimal use for both outbreak-related and sporadic acute gastroenteritis cases.

℞ **Treatment:**
INFECTIONS WITH NORWALK AND RELATED HUMAN CALICIVIRUSES

The disease is self-limited, and oral rehydration therapy is generally adequate. If severe dehydration develops, IV fluid therapy is indicated. No specific antiviral therapy is available.

Prevention

Epidemic prevention relies on situation-specific measures, such as control of contamination of food and water, exclusion of ill food handlers, and reduction of person-to-person spread through good personal hygiene and disinfection of contaminated fomites. The role of immunoprophylaxis is not clear, given the lack of long-term immunity from natural disease and the paradoxical inverse association between the level of immune response and protection from disease.

ROTAVIRUS

Etiologic Agent

Rotaviruses are members of the family Reoviridae. The viral genome consists of 11 segments of double-strand RNA that are enclosed in a triple-layered, nonenveloped, icosahedral capsid 75 nm in diameter. Viral protein 6 (VP6), the major structural protein, is the target of commercial immunoassays and determines the group specificity of rotaviruses. There are seven major groups of rotavirus (A through G); human illness is caused primarily by group A and, to a much lesser extent, by groups B and C. Two outer-capsid proteins, VP7 (G-protein) and VP4 (P-protein), determine serotype specificity, induce neutralizing antibodies, and form the basis for binary

classification of rotaviruses (G and P types). The segmented genome of rotavirus allows genetic reassortment (i.e., exchange of genome segments between viruses) during co-infection—a property that may play a role in viral evolution and has been utilized in the development of reassortant animal-human rotavirus–based vaccines.

Epidemiology

Worldwide, nearly all children are infected with rotavirus by 3–5 years of age. Neonatal infections are common but are often asymptomatic or mild, presumably because of protection from maternal antibody or breast-feeding. First infections after 3 months of age are likely to be symptomatic, and the incidence of disease peaks among children 4–23 months of age. Reinfections are common, but the severity of disease decreases with each repeat infection. Therefore, severe rotavirus infections are relatively uncommon among older children and adults. Nevertheless, rotavirus can cause illness in parents and caretakers of children with rotavirus diarrhea, immunocompromised persons, travelers, and elderly individuals and should be considered in the differential diagnosis of gastroenteritis among adults. In temperate climates, rotavirus disease occurs predominantly during the cooler fall and winter months. In the United States, the rotavirus season each year begins in the Southwest during the autumn (October through December) and migrates across the continent, peaking in the Northeast during the spring (March through May) (**Fig. 30-2**); the reasons for this characteristic pattern are not clear. In tropical settings, rotavirus disease occurs year-round, with less pronounced seasonal peaks.

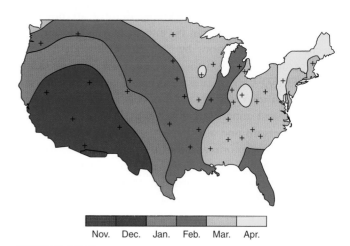

Nov. Dec. Jan. Feb. Mar. Apr.

FIGURE 30-2

Time of peak rotavirus activity in the contiguous 48 states: United States, July 1991 to June 1997. Data are from ~90 U.S. laboratories. *(Adapted from TJ Torok et al: Visualizing geographic and temporal trends in rotavirus activity in the United States, 1991 to 1996. National Respiratory and Enteric Virus Surveillance System Collaborating Laboratories. Pediatr Infect Dis J 16:941, 1997.)*

Rotavirus gastroenteritis is more frequently associated with dehydration than is gastroenteritis caused by other pathogens. Therefore, the proportion of gastroenteritis cases that are attributable to rotavirus increases with increasing severity of illness, ranging from a median of 8% in the community to 18% among outpatients and 40% among hospitalized patients. Each year, rotavirus is estimated to cause ~500,000 childhood deaths worldwide.

During episodes of rotavirus-associated diarrhea, virus is shed in large quantities in stool (10^7–10^{12}/g). Viral shedding detectable by EIA usually subsides within 1 week but may persist for >30 days in immunocompromised individuals. Viral shedding may be detected for longer periods by sensitive molecular assays, such as PCR. The virus is transmitted predominantly through the fecal-oral route. Spread through respiratory secretions, person-to-person contact, or contaminated environmental surfaces has also been postulated to explain the rapid acquisition of antibody in the first 3 years of life, regardless of sanitary conditions.

At least 10 different G serotypes of group A rotavirus have been identified in humans, but only five types (G1 through G4 and G9) are common. While human rotavirus strains that possess a high degree of genetic homology with animal strains have been identified, animal-to-human transmission appears to be uncommon.

 Group B rotaviruses have been associated with several large epidemics of severe gastroenteritis among adults in China since 1982 and have recently been identified in India but not in other parts of the world. Group C rotaviruses have been associated with a small proportion of pediatric gastroenteritis cases in several countries worldwide.

Pathogenesis

Rotaviruses infect and ultimately destroy mature enterocytes in the villous epithelium of the proximal small intestine. The loss of absorptive villous epithelium, coupled with the proliferation of secretory crypt cells, results in secretory diarrhea. Brush-border enzymes characteristic of differentiated cells are reduced, and this change leads to the accumulation of unmetabolized disaccharides and consequent osmotic diarrhea. Studies in mice indicate that a nonstructural rotavirus protein, NSP4, functions as an enterotoxin and contributes to secretory diarrhea by altering epithelial cell function and permeability. In addition, rotavirus may evoke fluid secretion through activation of the enteric nervous system in the intestinal wall. Recent data indicate that rotavirus antigenemia and viremia are common among children with acute rotavirus infection, although the antigen and RNA levels in serum are substantially lower than those in stool.

Clinical Manifestations

The clinical spectrum of rotavirus infection ranges from subclinical infection to severe gastroenteritis leading to life-threatening dehydration. After an incubation period of 1–3 days, the illness has an abrupt onset, with vomiting frequently preceding the onset of diarrhea. Up to one-third of patients may have a temperature of >39°C. The stools are characteristically loose and watery and only infrequently contain red or white cells. Gastrointestinal symptoms generally resolve in 3–7 days.

Respiratory and neurologic features in children with rotavirus infection have been reported, but causal associations have not been proven. Moreover, rotavirus infection has been associated with a variety of other clinical conditions (e.g., sudden infant death syndrome, necrotizing enterocolitis, intussusception, Kawasaki disease, and type 1 diabetes), but no causal relationship has been confirmed with any of these syndromes.

Rotavirus does not appear to be a major opportunistic pathogen in children with HIV infection. In severely immunodeficient children, rotavirus can cause protracted diarrhea with prolonged viral excretion and, in rare instances, can disseminate systemically. Persons who are immunosuppressed for bone marrow transplantation are also at risk for severe or even fatal rotavirus disease.

Immunity

Protection against rotavirus disease is correlated with the presence of virus-specific secretory IgA antibodies in the intestine and, to some extent, the serum. Because virus-specific IgA production at the intestinal surface is short-lived, complete protection against disease is only temporary. However, each infection and subsequent reinfection confers progressively greater immunity; thus severe disease is most common among young children with first or second infections. Immunologic memory is believed to be important in the attenuation of disease severity upon reinfection.

Diagnosis

Illness caused by rotavirus is difficult to distinguish clinically from that caused by other enteric viruses. Because large quantities of virus are shed in feces, the diagnosis can usually be confirmed by a wide variety of commercially available EIAs or by techniques for detecting viral RNA, such as gel electrophoresis, probe hybridization, or PCR.

℞ **Treatment:**
ROTAVIRUS INFECTIONS

Rotavirus gastroenteritis can lead to severe dehydration. Thus appropriate treatment should be instituted early. Standard oral rehydration therapy is successful in most children who can take oral fluids, but IV fluid replacement may be required for patients who are severely dehydrated or are unable to tolerate oral therapy because of frequent vomiting. The therapeutic role of probiotics, bismuth subsalicylate, enkephalinase inhibitors, and nitazoxanide has been evaluated in clinical studies but is not clearly defined. Antibiotics and antimotility agents should be avoided. In immunocompromised children with chronic symptomatic rotavirus disease, orally administered immunoglobulins or colostrum may resolve symptoms, but the choice of agents and their doses have not been well studied and are often empirical.

Prevention

Efforts to develop rotavirus vaccines were pursued because it was apparent—given the similar rates in less developed and industrialized nations—that improvements in hygiene and sanitation were unlikely to reduce disease incidence. The first rotavirus vaccine licensed in the United States in 1998 was withdrawn from the market within 1 year because it was linked with intussusception, a severe bowel obstruction.

In 2006, promising safety and efficacy results for two new rotavirus vaccines were reported from large clinical trials conducted in North America, Europe, and Latin America. One of these vaccines, a multivalent bovine-human reassortant rotavirus-based preparation, was recommended for routine immunization of all U.S. infants in early 2006. The second vaccine, based on a single attenuated human rotavirus strain, is not licensed in the United States but has been introduced in immunization programs in several countries in Latin America and Europe.

Global Considerations

Rotavirus is ubiquitous and infects nearly all children worldwide by 5 years of age. However, compared with rotavirus disease in industrialized countries, that in developing countries occurs at a younger age, is less seasonal, is more often associated with severe outcomes (including death), and is more frequently caused by uncommon rotavirus strains. The different epidemiology of rotavirus disease and the greater prevalence of co-infection with other enteric pathogens, of comorbidities, and of malnutrition in developing countries may adversely affect the performance of rotavirus vaccines. Therefore, before global recommendations for vaccine use can be issued, it is vital to evaluate the efficacy of rotavirus vaccines in resource-poor settings of Africa and Asia. Trials in these areas are under way.

OTHER VIRAL AGENTS OF GASTROENTERITIS

Enteric *adenoviruses* of serotypes 40 and 41 belonging to subgroup F are 70- to 80-nm viruses with double-strand DNA that cause ~2–12% of all diarrhea episodes in young children. Unlike adenoviruses that cause respiratory illness, enteric adenoviruses are difficult to cultivate in cell lines, but they can be detected with commercially available EIAs.

Astroviruses, 28- to 30-nm viruses with a characteristic icosahedral structure, contain a positive-sense, single-strand RNA. At least seven serotypes have been identified, of which serotype 1 is most common. Astroviruses are primarily pediatric pathogens, causing ~2–10% of cases of mild to moderate gastroenteritis in children. The availability of simple immunoassays to detect virus in fecal specimens and of molecular methods to confirm and characterize strains will permit more comprehensive assessment of the etiologic role of these agents.

Toroviruses are 100- to 140-nm, enveloped, positive-strand RNA viruses that are recognized as causes of gastroenteritis in horses (Berne virus) and cattle (Breda virus). Their role as a cause of diarrhea in humans is still unclear, but studies from Canada have demonstrated associations between torovirus excretion and both nosocomial gastroenteritis and necrotizing enterocolitis in neonates. These associations require further evaluation.

Picobirnaviruses are small, bisegmented, double-strand RNA viruses that cause gastroenteritis in a variety of animals. Their role as primary causes of gastroenteritis in humans remains unclear, but several studies have found an association between picobirnaviruses and gastroenteritis in HIV-infected adults.

Several other viruses (e.g., enteroviruses, reoviruses, pestiviruses, and parvovirus B) have been identified in the feces of patients with diarrhea, but their etiologic role in gastroenteritis has not been proven. Diarrhea has also been noted as a manifestation of infection with two recently recognized viruses that primarily cause severe respiratory illness: the severe acute respiratory syndrome–associated coronavirus (SARS-CoV) and influenza A/H5N1 virus.

FURTHER READINGS

GREENBERG HB, ESTES MK: Rotaviruses: from pathogenesis to vaccination. Gastroenterology 136:1939, 2009

HUANG P et al: Norovirus and histo-blood group antigens: Demonstration of a wide spectrum of strain specificities and classification of two major binding groups among multiple binding patterns. J Virol 79:6714, 2005

KO G et al: Noroviruses as a cause of traveler's diarrhea among students from the United States visiting Mexico. J Clin Microbiol 43:6126, 2005

LEUNG WK et al: Enteric involvement of severe acute respiratory syndrome–associated coronavirus infection. Gastroenterology 125:1011, 2003

LODHA A et al: Human torovirus: A new virus associated with neonatal necrotizing enterocolitis. Acta Paediatr 94:1085, 2005

MURATA T et al: Prolonged norovirus shedding in infants <or = 6 months of age with gastroenteritis. Pediatr Infect Dis J 26:46, 2007

PATEL MM et al: Noroviruses: A comprehensive review. J Clin Virol 44:1, 2009

RAY P et al: Quantitative evaluation of rotaviral antigenemia in children with acute rotaviral diarrhea. J Infect Dis 194:588, 2006

ROSSIGNOL JF et al: Effect of nitazoxanide for treatment of severe rotavirus diarrhoea: Randomised double-blind placebo-controlled trial. Lancet 368:124, 2006

RUIZ-PALACIOS G et al: Safety and efficacy of an attenuated vaccine against severe rotavirus gastroenteritis. N Engl J Med 354:11, 2006

SCHLENKER C, SURAWICZ CM: Emerging infections of the gastrointestinal tract. Best Pract Res Clin Gastroenterol 23:89, 2009

TRAN TH et al: Avian influenza A (H5N1) in 10 patients in Vietnam. N Engl J Med 350:1179, 2004

VESIKARI T et al: Safety and efficacy of a pentavalent human-bovine (WC3) reassortant rotavirus vaccine. N Engl J Med 354:23, 2006

CHAPTER 30

Viral Gastroenteritis

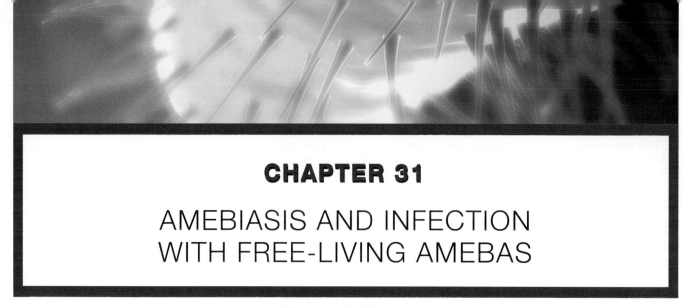

CHAPTER 31

AMEBIASIS AND INFECTION WITH FREE-LIVING AMEBAS

Sharon L. Reed

AMEBIASIS

DEFINITION

Amebiasis is an infection with the intestinal protozoan *Entamoeba histolytica*. About 90% of infections are asymptomatic, and the remaining 10% produce a spectrum of clinical syndromes ranging from dysentery to abscesses of the liver or other organs.

LIFE CYCLE AND TRANSMISSION

E. histolytica is acquired by ingestion of viable cysts from fecally contaminated water, food, or hands. Food-borne exposure is most prevalent and is particularly likely when food handlers are shedding cysts or food is being grown with feces-contaminated soil, fertilizer, or water. Besides the drinking of contaminated water, less common means of transmission include oral and anal sexual practices and—in rare instances—direct rectal inoculation through colonic irrigation devices. Motile trophozoites are released from cysts in the small intestine and, in most patients, remain as harmless commensals in the large bowel. After encystation, infectious cysts are shed in the stool and can survive for several weeks in a moist environment. In some patients, the trophozoites invade either the bowel mucosa,

causing symptomatic colitis, or the bloodstream, causing distant abscesses of the liver, lungs, or brain. The trophozoites may not encyst in patients with active dysentery, and motile hematophagous trophozoites are frequently present in fresh stools. Trophozoites are rapidly killed by exposure to air or stomach acid, however, and therefore cannot transmit infection.

EPIDEMIOLOGY

About 10% of the world's population is infected with *Entamoeba*, the majority with noninvasive *Entamoeba dispar*. Amebiasis results from infection with *E. histolytica* and is the third most common cause of death from parasitic disease (after schistosomiasis and malaria). The wide spectrum of clinical disease caused by *Entamoeba* is due in part to the differences between these two infecting species. Cysts of *E. histolytica* and *E. dispar* are morphologically identical, but *E. histolytica* has unique isoenzymes, surface antigens, DNA markers, and virulence properties (**Table 31-1**). Most asymptomatic carriers, including homosexual men and patients with AIDS, harbor *E. dispar* and have self-limited infections. These observations indicate that *E. dispar* is incapable of causing invasive disease, since *Cryptosporidium* and *Isospora belli*, which also cause only self-limited illnesses

296

TABLE 31-1

E. HISTOLYTICA AND E. DISPAR, COMPARED AND CONTRASTED

Similarities

1. Both species are spread through ingestion of infectious cysts.
2. Cysts of the two species are morphologically identical.
3. Both species colonize the large intestine.

Differences

1. Only *E. histolytica* causes invasive disease.
2. Only *E. histolytica* infections elicit a positive amebic serology.
3. The two species have distinct rRNA sequences.
4. The two species have distinct surface antigens and isoenzyme markers.
5. Gal/GalNAc lectin can be used to differentiate the two species in stool ELISA.

Note: ELISA, enzyme-linked immunosorbent assay; Gal/GalNAc, galactose *N*-acetylgalactosamine. See text.

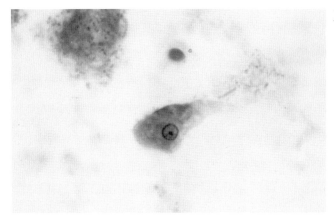

FIGURE 31-1
Trophozoite of *E. histolytica* demonstrating a single nucleus with a central, dot-like nucleolus (trichrome stain).

in immunocompetent people, cause devastating diarrhea in patients with AIDS. However, host factors play a role as well. In one study, 10% of asymptomatic patients who were colonized with *E. histolytica* went on to develop amebic colitis, while the rest remained asymptomatic and cleared the infection within 1 year.

Areas of highest incidence (due to inadequate sanitation and crowding) include most developing countries in the tropics, particularly Mexico, India, and nations of Central and South America, tropical Asia, and Africa. In a 4-year follow-up study of preschool children in a highly endemic area of Bangladesh, 80% of children had at least one episode of infection with *E. histolytica* and 53% had more than one episode. Naturally acquired immunity did develop but was usually short-lived and correlated with the presence in the stool of secretory IgA antibody to the major adherence lectin galactose *N*-acetylgalactosamine (Gal/GalNAc). The main groups at risk for amebiasis in developed countries are returned travelers, recent immigrants, homosexual men, and inmates of institutions.

PATHOGENESIS AND PATHOLOGY

Both trophozoites (Fig. 31-1) and cysts (Fig. 31-2) are found in the intestinal lumen, but only trophozoites of *E. histolytica* invade tissue. The trophozoite is 20–60 μm in diameter and contains vacuoles and a nucleus with a characteristic central nucleolus. In animals, depletion of intestinal mucus, diffuse inflammation, and disruption of the epithelial barrier occur before trophozoites actually come into contact with the colonic mucosa. Trophozoites attach to colonic mucus and epithelial cells by Gal/GalNAc. The earliest intestinal lesions are microulcerations of the mucosa of the cecum, sigmoid colon, or

rectum that release erythrocytes, inflammatory cells, and epithelial cells. Proctoscopy reveals small ulcers with heaped-up margins and normal intervening mucosa. Submucosal extension of ulcerations under viable-appearing surface mucosa causes the classic "flask-shaped" ulcer containing trophozoites at the margins of dead and viable tissues. Although neutrophilic infiltrates may accompany the early lesions in animals, human intestinal infection is marked by a paucity of inflammatory cells, probably in part because of the killing of neutrophils by trophozoites (Fig. 31-3). Treated ulcers characteristically heal with little or no scarring. Occasionally, however, full-thickness necrosis and perforation occur.

Rarely, intestinal infection results in the formation of a mass lesion, or *ameboma*, in the bowel lumen. The overlying mucosa is usually thin and ulcerated, while other layers of the wall are thickened, edematous, and hemorrhagic; this condition results in exuberant formation of granulation tissue with little fibrous-tissue response.

A number of virulence factors have been linked to the ability of *E. histolytica* to invade through the interglandular

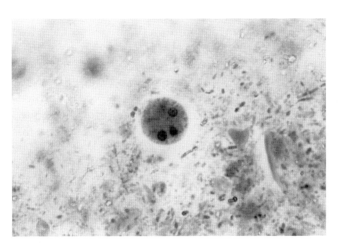

FIGURE 31-2
Cyst of *E. histolytica* showing three of the four nuclei (trichrome stain).

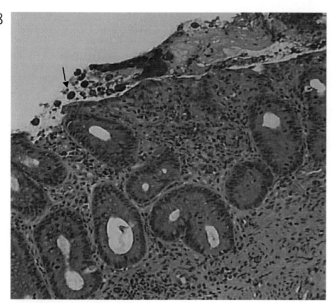

FIGURE 31-3
Pathology of amebic ulcer with colonic invasion. Arrow points to trophozoites (hematoxylin and eosin, 400X).

epithelium. One consists of the extracellular cysteine proteinases that degrade collagen, elastin, IgA, IgG, and the anaphylatoxins C3a and C5a. Other enzymes may disrupt glycoprotein bonds between mucosal epithelial cells in the gut. Amebas can lyse neutrophils, monocytes, lymphocytes, and cells of colonic and hepatic lines. The cytolytic effect of amebas appears to require direct contact with target cells and may be linked to the release of phospholipase A and pore-forming peptides. *E. histolytica* trophozoites also cause apoptosis of human cells.

Liver abscesses are always preceded by intestinal colonization, which may be asymptomatic. Blood vessels may be compromised early by wall lysis and thrombus formation. Trophozoites invade veins to reach the liver through the portal venous system. *E. histolytica* is resistant to complement-mediated lysis—a property critical to survival in the bloodstream. In contrast, *E. dispar* is rapidly lysed by complement and is thus restricted to the bowel lumen. Inoculation of amebas into the portal system of hamsters results in an acute cellular infiltrate consisting predominantly of neutrophils. Later, the neutrophils are lysed by contact with amebas, and the release of neutrophil toxins may contribute to necrosis of hepatocytes. The liver parenchyma is replaced by necrotic material that is surrounded by a thin rim of congested liver tissue. The necrotic contents of a liver abscess are classically described as "anchovy paste," although the fluid is variable in color and is composed of bacteriologically sterile granular debris with few or no cells. Amebas, if seen, tend to be found near the capsule of the abscess.

A study in Bangladeshi schoolchildren revealed that an intestinal IgA response to Gal/GalNAc reduced the risk of new *E. histolytica* infection by 64%. Serum IgG

antibody is not protective; titers correlate with the duration of illness rather than with the severity of disease. Indeed, Bangladeshi children with a serum IgG response were more likely than those without such a response to develop new *E. histolytica* infection. Studies of animals suggest that cell-mediated immunity may be important for protection, although patients with AIDS appear not to be predisposed to more severe disease.

CLINICAL SYNDROMES
Intestinal Amebiasis

The most common type of amebic infection is asymptomatic cyst passage. Even in highly endemic areas, most patients harbor *E. dispar.*

Symptomatic amebic colitis develops 2–6 weeks after the ingestion of infectious cysts. A gradual onset of lower abdominal pain and mild diarrhea is followed by malaise, weight loss, and diffuse lower abdominal or back pain. Cecal involvement may mimic acute appendicitis. Patients with full-blown dysentery may pass 10–12 stools per day. The stools contain little fecal material and consist mainly of blood and mucus. In contrast to those with bacterial diarrhea, fewer than 40% of patients with amebic dysentery are febrile. Virtually all patients have heme-positive stools.

More fulminant intestinal infection, with severe abdominal pain, high fever, and profuse diarrhea, is rare and occurs predominantly in children. Patients may develop toxic megacolon, in which there is severe bowel dilation with intramural air. Patients receiving glucocorticoids are at risk for severe amebiasis. Uncommonly, patients develop a chronic form of amebic colitis, which can be confused with inflammatory bowel disease. The association between severe amebiasis complications and glucocorticoid therapy emphasizes the importance of excluding amebiasis when inflammatory bowel disease is suspected. An occasional patient presents with only an asymptomatic or tender abdominal mass caused by an ameboma, which is easily confused with cancer on barium studies. A positive serologic test or biopsy can prevent unnecessary surgery in this setting. The syndrome of postamebic colitis—persistent diarrhea following documented cure of amebic colitis—is controversial; no evidence of recurrent amebic infection can be found, and re-treatment usually has no effect.

Amebic Liver Abscess

Extraintestinal infection by *E. histolytica* most often involves the liver. Of travelers who develop an amebic liver abscess after leaving an endemic area, 95% do so within 5 months. Young patients with an amebic liver abscess are more likely than older patients to present in the acute phase with prominent symptoms of <10 days' duration. Most patients are febrile and have right-upper-quadrant pain, which may be dull or pleuritic in nature and may radiate to the shoulder. Point tenderness over the liver and right-sided pleural effusion are common. Jaundice is rare. Although the initial site of infection is the colon, fewer than one-third of patients with an amebic abscess have active diarrhea. Older patients from endemic areas are more likely to have a subacute course lasting 6 months, with weight loss and hepatomegaly. About one-third of patients with chronic presentations are febrile. Thus, the clinical diagnosis of an amebic liver abscess may be difficult to establish because the symptoms and signs are often nonspecific. Since 10–15% of patients present only with fever, amebic liver abscess must be considered in the differential diagnosis of fever of unknown origin.

Complications of Amebic Liver Abscess

Pleuropulmonary involvement, which is reported in 20–30% of patients, is the most frequent complication of amebic liver abscess. Manifestations include sterile effusions, contiguous spread from the liver, and rupture into the pleural space. Sterile effusions and contiguous spread usually resolve with medical therapy, but frank rupture into the pleural space requires drainage. A hepatobronchial fistula may cause cough productive of large amounts of necrotic material that may contain amebas. This dramatic complication carries a good prognosis. Abscesses that rupture into the peritoneum may present as an indolent leak or an acute abdomen and require both percutaneous catheter drainage and medical therapy. Rupture into the pericardium, usually from abscesses of the left lobe of the liver, carries the gravest prognosis; it can occur during medical therapy and requires surgical drainage.

Other Extraintestinal Sites

The genitourinary tract may become involved by direct extension of amebiasis from the colon or by hematogenous spread of the infection. Painful genital ulcers, characterized by a punched-out appearance and profuse discharge, may develop secondary to extension from either the intestine or the liver. Both these conditions respond well to medical therapy. Cerebral involvement has been reported in fewer than 0.1% of patients in large clinical series. Symptoms and prognosis depend on the size and location of the lesion.

DIAGNOSTIC TESTS

Laboratory Diagnosis

Stool examinations, serologic tests, and noninvasive imaging of the liver are the most important procedures in the diagnosis of amebiasis. Fecal findings suggestive of amebic colitis include a positive test for heme, a paucity of neutrophils, and amebic cysts or trophozoites. The definitive diagnosis of amebic colitis is made by the demonstration

of hematophagous trophozoites of *E. histolytica* (Fig. 31-1). Because trophozoites are killed rapidly by water, drying, or barium, it is important to examine at least three fresh stool specimens. Examination of a combination of wet mounts, iodine-stained concentrates, and trichrome-stained preparations of fresh stool and concentrates for cysts (Fig. 31-2) or trophozoites (Fig. 31-1) confirms the diagnosis in 75–95% of cases. Cultures of amebas are more sensitive but are not routinely available. If stool examinations are negative, sigmoidoscopy with biopsy of the edge of ulcers may increase the yield, but this procedure is dangerous during fulminant colitis because of the risk of perforation. Trophozoites in a biopsy specimen from a colonic mass confirm the diagnosis of ameboma, but trophozoites are rare in liver aspirates because they are found in the abscess capsule and not in the readily aspirated necrotic center. Accurate diagnosis requires experience, since the trophozoites may be confused with neutrophils and the cysts must be differentiated morphologically from *Entamoeba hartmanni*, *Entamoeba coli*, and *Endolimax nana*, which do not cause clinical disease and do not warrant therapy. Unfortunately, the cysts of *E. histolytica* cannot be distinguished microscopically from those of *E. dispar*. Therefore, the microscopic diagnosis of *E. histolytica* can be made only by the detection of *Entamoeba* trophozoites that have ingested erythrocytes. In terms of sensitivity, stool diagnostic tests based on the detection of the Gal/GalNAc lectin of *E. histolytica* compare favorably with the polymerase chain reaction and with isolation in culture followed by isoenzyme analysis.

Serology is an important addition to the methods used for parasitologic diagnosis of invasive amebiasis. Enzyme-linked immunosorbent assays (ELISAs) and agar gel diffusion assays are positive in more than 90% of patients with colitis, amebomas, or liver abscess. Positive results in conjunction with the appropriate clinical syndrome suggest active disease because serologic findings usually revert to negative within 6–12 months. Even in highly endemic areas such as South Africa, fewer than 10% of asymptomatic individuals have a positive amebic serology. The interpretation of the indirect hemagglutination test is more difficult because titers may remain positive for as long as 10 years.

Up to 10% of patients with acute amebic liver abscess may have negative serologic findings; in suspected cases with an initially negative result, testing should be repeated in a week. In contrast to carriers of *E. dispar*, most asymptomatic carriers of *E. histolytica* develop antibodies. Thus, serologic tests are helpful in assessing the risk of invasive amebiasis in asymptomatic, cyst-passing individuals in nonendemic areas. Serologic tests also should be performed in patients with ulcerative colitis before the institution of glucocorticoid therapy to prevent the development of severe colitis or toxic megacolon owing to unsuspected amebiasis.

Routine hematology and chemistry tests usually are not very helpful in the diagnosis of invasive amebiasis. About three-fourths of patients with an amebic liver abscess have leukocytosis (>10,000 cells/μL); this condition is particularly likely if symptoms are acute or complications have developed. Invasive amebiasis does not elicit eosinophilia. Anemia, if present, is usually multifactorial. Even with large liver abscesses, liver enzyme levels are normal or minimally elevated. The alkaline phosphatase level is most often elevated and may remain so for months. Aminotransferase elevations suggest acute disease or a complication.

Radiographic Studies

Radiographic barium studies are potentially dangerous in acute amebic colitis. Amebomas are usually identified first by a barium enema, but biopsy is necessary for differentiation from carcinoma.

Radiographic techniques such as ultrasonography, CT, and MRI are all useful for detection of the round or oval hypoechoic cyst. More than 80% of patients who have had symptoms for >10 days have a single abscess of the right lobe of the liver (Fig. 31-4). Approximately 50% of patients who have had symptoms for <10 days have multiple abscesses. Findings associated with complications include large abscesses (>10 cm) in the superior part of the right lobe, which may rupture into the pleural space; multiple lesions, which must be differentiated from pyogenic abscesses; and lesions of the left lobe, which may rupture into the pericardium. Because abscesses resolve slowly and may increase in size in patients who are responding clinically to therapy, frequent follow-up ultrasonography may prove confusing. Complete resolution of a liver abscess within 6 months

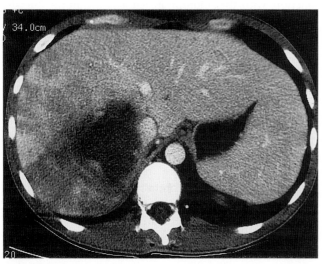

FIGURE 31-4
Abdominal CT scan of a large amebic abscess of the right lobe of the liver. *(Courtesy of the Department of Radiology, UCSD Medical Center, San Diego; with permission.)*

can be anticipated in two-thirds of patients, but 10% may have persistent abnormalities for a year.

DIFFERENTIAL DIAGNOSIS

The differential diagnosis of intestinal amebiasis includes bacterial diarrheas (Chap. 22) caused by *Campylobacter* (Chap. 28); enteroinvasive *Escherichia coli*; and species of *Shigella* (Chap. 27), *Salmonella* (Chap. 26), and *Vibrio* (Chap. 29). Although the typical patient with amebic colitis has less prominent fever than in these other conditions as well as heme-positive stools with few neutrophils, correct diagnosis requires bacterial cultures, microscopic examination of stools, and amebic serologic testing. As has already been mentioned, amebiasis must be ruled out in any patient thought to have inflammatory bowel disease.

Because of the variety of presenting signs and symptoms, amebic liver abscess can easily be confused with pulmonary or gallbladder disease or with any febrile illness with few localizing signs, such as malaria or typhoid fever (Chap. 26). The diagnosis should be considered in members of high-risk groups who have recently traveled outside the United States and in inmates of institutions. Once radiographic studies have identified an abscess in the liver, the most important differential diagnosis is between amebic and pyogenic abscess. Patients with pyogenic abscess typically are older and have a history of underlying bowel disease or recent surgery. Amebic serology is helpful, but aspiration of the abscess, with Gram's staining and culture of the material, may be required for differentiation of the two diseases.

℞ **Treatment:**
AMEBIASIS

INTESTINAL DISEASE (Table 31-2) The drugs used to treat amebiasis can be classified according to their primary site of action. Luminal amebicides are poorly absorbed and reach high concentrations in the bowel, but their activity is limited to cysts and trophozoites close to the mucosa. Only two luminal drugs are available in the United States: iodoquinol and paromomycin. Indications for the use of luminal agents include eradication of cysts in patients with colitis or a liver abscess and treatment of asymptomatic carriers. The majority of asymptomatic individuals who pass cysts are colonized with *E. dispar*, which does not warrant specific therapy. However, it is prudent to treat asymptomatic individuals who pass cysts unless *E. dispar* colonization can be definitively demonstrated by specific antigen-detection tests.

Tissue amebicides reach high concentrations in the blood and tissue after oral or parenteral administration. The development of nitroimidazole compounds, especially metronidazole, was a major advance in the

TABLE 31-2

DRUG THERAPY FOR AMEBIASIS

INDICATION	THERAPY
Asymptomatic carriage	Luminal agent: iodoquinol (650-mg tablets), 650 mg tid for 20 days; *or* paromomycin (250-mg tablets), 500 mg tid for 10 days
Acute colitis	Metronidazole (250- or 500-mg tablets), 750 mg PO or IV tid for 5–10 days, *plus* Luminal agent as above
Amebic liver abscess	Metronidazole, 750 mg PO or IV for 5–10 days, *or* Tinidazole, 2 g PO once, *or* Ornidazole,[a] 2 g PO once, *plus* Luminal agent as above

[a]Not available in the United States.

treatment of invasive amebiasis. Patients with amebic colitis should be treated with intravenous or oral metronidazole. Side effects include nausea, vomiting, abdominal discomfort, and a disulfiram-like reaction. Another longer-acting imidazole compound, tinidazole, is also effective and was recently approved in the United States. All patients should also receive a full course of therapy with a luminal agent, since metronidazole does not eradicate cysts. Resistance to metronidazole has been selected in the laboratory but has not been found in clinical isolates. Relapses are not uncommon and probably represent reinfection or failure to eradicate amebas from the bowel because of an inadequate dosage or duration of therapy.

AMEBIC LIVER ABSCESS Metronidazole is the drug of choice for amebic liver abscess. Longer-acting nitroimidazoles (tinidazole and ornidazole) have been effective as single-dose therapy in developing countries. With early diagnosis and therapy, mortality rates from uncomplicated amebic liver abscess are <1%. The second-line therapeutic agents emetine and chloroquine should be avoided if possible because of the potential cardiovascular and gastrointestinal side effects of the former and the higher relapse rates with the latter. There is no evidence that combined therapy with two drugs is more effective than the single-drug regimen. Studies of South Africans with liver abscesses demonstrated that 72% of patients without intestinal symptoms had bowel infection with *E. histolytica*; thus, all treatment regimens should include a luminal agent to eradicate cysts and prevent further transmission. Amebic liver abscess recurs rarely.

ASPIRATION OF LIVER ABSCESSES More than 90% of patients respond dramatically to metronidazole therapy with decreases in both pain and fever within 72 h. Indications for aspiration of liver abscesses are (1) the need to rule out a pyogenic abscess, particularly in patients with multiple lesions; (2) the lack of a clinical response in 3–5 days; (3) the threat of imminent rupture; and (4) the need to prevent rupture of left-lobe abscesses into the pericardium. There is no evidence that aspiration, even of large abscesses (up to 10 cm), accelerates healing. Percutaneous drainage may be successful even if the liver abscess has already ruptured. Surgery should be reserved for instances of bowel perforation and rupture into the pericardium.

PREVENTION

Amebic infection is spread by ingestion of food or water contaminated with cysts. Since an asymptomatic carrier may excrete up to 15 million cysts per day, prevention of infection requires adequate sanitation and eradication of cyst carriage. In high-risk areas, infection can be minimized by the avoidance of unpeeled fruits and vegetables and the use of bottled water. Because cysts are resistant to readily attainable levels of chlorine, disinfection by iodination (tetraglycine hydroperiodide) is recommended. There is no effective prophylaxis.

INFECTION WITH FREE-LIVING AMEBAS
EPIDEMIOLOGY

Free-living amebas of the genera *Acanthamoeba* and *Naegleria* are distributed throughout the world and have been isolated from a wide variety of fresh and brackish water, including that from lakes, taps, hot springs, swimming pools, and heating and air-conditioning units, and even from the nasal passages of healthy children. Encystation may protect the protozoa from desiccation and food deprivation. The persistence of *Legionella pneumophila* in water supplies may be attributable in part to chronic infection of free-living amebas, particularly *Naegleria*. Free-living amebas of the genus *Balamuthia* have only recently been isolated from soil samples, including a sample from a flowerpot linked to a fatal infection in a child.

NAEGLERIA INFECTIONS

Primary amebic meningoencephalitis caused by *Naegleria fowleri* follows the aspiration of water contaminated with trophozoites or cysts or the inhalation of contaminated dust, leading to invasion of the olfactory neuroepithelium. After an incubation period of 2–15 days, severe headache, high fever, nausea, vomiting, and meningismus develop. Photophobia and palsies of the third, fourth, and sixth cranial nerves are common. Rapid progression to seizures and coma may follow. The prognosis is uniformly poor: most patients die within a week. Only a few survivors, treated with high-dose amphotericin B and rifampin, have been reported. Infection is most common in otherwise-healthy children or young adults, who often report recent swimming in lakes or heated swimming pools.

The diagnosis of *Naegleria* infection should be considered in any patient who has purulent meningitis without evidence of bacteria on Gram's staining, antigen detection assay, and culture. Other laboratory findings resemble those for fulminant bacterial meningitis, with elevated intracranial pressure, high white blood cell counts (up to 20,000/μL), and elevated protein concentrations and low glucose levels in cerebrospinal fluid (CSF). Diagnosis depends on the detection of motile trophozoites in wet mounts of fresh spinal fluid. Antibodies to *Naegleria* spp. have been detected in normal adults; serologic testing is not useful in the diagnosis of acute infection.

ACANTHAMOEBA INFECTIONS
Granulomatous Amebic Encephalitis

Infection with *Acanthamoeba* species follows a more indolent course and typically occurs in chronically ill or debilitated patients. Risk factors include lymphoproliferative disorders, chemotherapy, glucocorticoid therapy, lupus erythematosus, and AIDS. Infection usually reaches the central nervous system (CNS) hematogenously from a primary focus in the sinuses, skin, or lungs. In the CNS, the onset is insidious, and the syndrome often mimics a space-occupying lesion. Altered mental status, headache, and stiff neck may be accompanied by focal findings such as cranial nerve palsies, ataxia, and hemiparesis. Cutaneous ulcers or hard nodules containing amebas are frequently detected in AIDS patients with disseminated *Acanthamoeba* infection.

Examination of the CSF for trophozoites may be diagnostically helpful, but lumbar puncture may be contraindicated because of increased intracerebral pressure. CT frequently reveals cortical and subcortical lesions of decreased density consistent with embolic infarcts. In other patients, multiple enhancing lesions with edema may mimic the computed tomographic appearance of toxoplasmosis. Demonstration of the trophozoites and cysts of *Acanthamoeba* on wet mounts or in biopsy specimens establishes the diagnosis. Culture on nonnutrient agar plates seeded with *E. coli* may also be helpful. Fluorescein-labeled antiserum is available from the Centers for Disease Control and Prevention (CDC) for the detection of protozoa in biopsy specimens. Granulomatous amebic encephalitis in patients with AIDS may have an accelerated course (with survival for only 3–40 days) because of the difficulty these individuals have in forming granulomas. Various antimicrobial agents have

been used to treat *Acanthamoeba* infection, including pentamidine, trimethoprim-sulfamethoxazole, and fluconazole, but the infection is almost uniformly fatal.

Keratitis

The incidence of keratitis caused by *Acanthamoeba* has increased in the past 20 years, in part as a result of improved diagnosis. Earlier infections were associated with trauma to the eye and exposure to contaminated water. At present, most infections are linked to extended-wear contact lenses, and rare cases are associated with laser-assisted in situ keratomileusis (LASIK). Risk factors include the use of homemade saline, the wearing of lenses while swimming, and inadequate disinfection. Since contact lenses presumably cause microscopic trauma, the early corneal findings may be nonspecific. The first symptoms usually include tearing and the painful sensation of a foreign body. Once infection is established, progression is rapid; the characteristic clinical sign is an annular, paracentral corneal ring representing a corneal abscess. Deeper corneal invasion and loss of vision may follow.

The differential diagnosis includes bacterial, mycobacterial, and herpetic infection. The irregular polygonal cysts of *Acanthamoeba* (**Fig. 31-5**) may be identified in corneal scrapings or biopsy material, and trophozoites can be grown on special media. Cysts are resistant to available drugs, and the results of medical therapy have been disappointing. Some reports have suggested partial responses to propamidine isethionate eyedrops. Severe infections usually require keratoplasty.

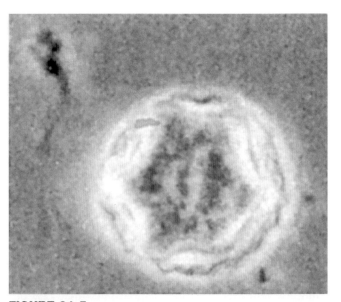

FIGURE 31-5
Double-walled cyst of *Acanthamoeba castellani*, as seen by phase-contrast microscopy. *[From DJ Krogstad et al, in A Balows et al (eds): Manual of Clinical Microbiology, 5th ed. Washington, DC, American Society for Microbiology, 1991.]*

BALAMUTHIA INFECTIONS

Balamuthia mandrillaris, a free-living ameba previously referred to as a leptomyxid ameba, is an important etiologic agent of amebic meningoencephalitis in immunocompetent hosts. The course is typically subacute, with focal neurologic signs, fever, seizures, and headaches leading to death within 1 week to several months after onset. Examination of CSF reveals mononuclear or neutrophilic pleocytosis, elevated protein levels, and normal to low glucose concentrations. Multiple hypodense lesions are usually detected with imaging studies. This mixed picture of space-occupying lesions with CSF pleocytosis is suggestive of *Balamuthia*. Detection of an indirect fluorescent antibody response may be helpful in noninvasive diagnosis, but usually a definitive diagnosis is made postmortem. Fluorescent antibody is available from the CDC. The variety of drugs used to treat the few surviving patients (numbering fewer than five in the United States) include pentamidine, flucytosine, sulfadiazine, and macrolides. The differential diagnosis includes tuberculomas and neurocysticercosis.

FURTHER READINGS

DEETZ TR et al: Successful treatment of *Balamuthia* amoebic encephalitis: Presentation of two cases. Clin Infect Dis 37:1304, 2003

GONZALES ML et al: Antiamoebic drugs for treating amoebic colitis. Cochrane Database Syst Rev Apr 15;(2):CD006085, 2009

HAQUE R et al: *Entamoeba histolytica* infection in children and protection from subsequent amebiasis. Infect Immun 37:1304, 2003

HUSTON CD et al: Caspase-3-dependent killing of host cells by the parasite *Entamoeba histolytica*. Cell Microbiol 2:617, 2000

KUMAR R, LLOYD D: Recent advances in the treatment of *Acanthamoeba* keratitis. Clin Infect Dis 35:434, 2002

LEJEUNE M et al: Recent discoveries in the pathogenesis and immune response toward *Entamoeba histolytica*. Future Microbiol 4:105, 2009

PETRI WA et al: The bittersweet interface of parasite and host lectin-carbohydrate interactions during human invasion by the parasite *Entamoeba histolytica*. Annu Rev Microbiol 56:39, 2002

QUE X, REED SL: Cysteine proteinases and the pathogenesis of amebiasis. Clin Microbiol Rev 13:196, 2002

SHUSTER FL, VISVESVARA GS: Free-living amoebae as opportunistic and non-opportunistic pathogens of humans and animals. Int J Parasitol 345:1001, 2004

SOLAYMANI-MOHAMMADI S et al: Comparison of a stool antigen detection kit and PCR for diagnosis of *Entamoeba histolytica* and *Entamoeba dispar* infections in asymptomatic cyst passers in Iran. J Clin Microbiol 44:2258, 2006

STANLEY SL: Amebiasis. Lancet 361:1025, 2006

———, REED SL: Microbes and microbial toxins: Paradigms for microbial-mucosal interactions. VI. *Entamoeba histolytica*: Parasite-host interactions. Am J Physiol Gastrointest Liver Physiol 280: G1049, 2001

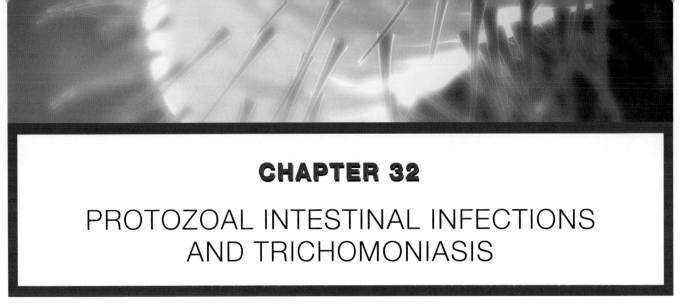

CHAPTER 32

PROTOZOAL INTESTINAL INFECTIONS AND TRICHOMONIASIS

Peter F. Weller

PROTOZOAL INFECTIONS

GIARDIASIS

Giardia lamblia (also known as *G. intestinalis*) is a cosmopolitan protozoal parasite that inhabits the small intestines of humans and other mammals.

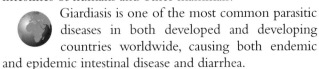 Giardiasis is one of the most common parasitic diseases in both developed and developing countries worldwide, causing both endemic and epidemic intestinal disease and diarrhea.

Life Cycle and Epidemiology

(**Fig. 32-1**) Infection follows the ingestion of environmentally hardy cysts, which excyst in the small intestine, releasing flagellated trophozoites (**Fig. 32-2**) that multiply by binary fission. *Giardia* remains a pathogen of the proximal small bowel and does not disseminate hematogenously. Trophozoites remain free in the lumen or attach to the mucosal epithelium by means of a ventral sucking disk. As a trophozoite encounters altered conditions, it forms a morphologically distinct cyst, which is the stage of the parasite usually found in the feces. Trophozoites may be present and even predominate in loose or watery stools, but it is the resistant cyst that survives outside the body and is responsible for transmission. Cysts do not tolerate heating, desiccation, or continued exposure to feces but do remain viable for months in cold fresh water. The number of cysts excreted varies widely but can approach 10^7 per gram of stool.

Ingestion of as few as 10 cysts is sufficient to cause infection in humans. Because cysts are infectious when excreted, person-to-person transmission occurs where fecal hygiene is poor. Giardiasis, as symptomatic or asymptomatic infections, is especially prevalent in day-care centers; person-to-person spread also takes place in other institutional settings with poor fecal hygiene and during anal-oral contact. If food is contaminated with *Giardia* cysts after cooking or preparation, food-borne transmission can occur. Waterborne transmission accounts for episodic infections (e.g., in campers and travelers) and for major epidemics in metropolitan areas. Surface water, ranging from mountain streams to large municipal reservoirs, can become contaminated with fecally derived *Giardia* cysts; outmoded water systems are subject to cross-contamination from leaking sewer lines. The efficacy of water as a means of transmission is enhanced by the small infectious inoculum of *Giardia*, the prolonged survival of cysts in cold water, and the resistance of cysts to killing by routine chlorination methods that are adequate for controlling bacteria. Viable cysts can be eradicated from water by either boiling or filtration. In the United States, *Giardia* (like *Cryptosporidium*; see later) is a common cause of waterborne epidemics of gastroenteritis. *Giardia* is

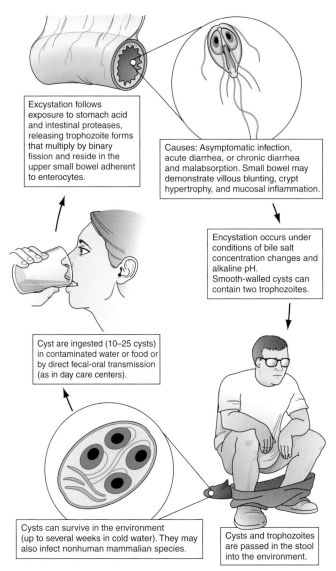

FIGURE 32-1
Life cycle of *Giardia*. (*Reprinted from RL Guerrant et al: Tropical Infectious Disease: Principles, Pathogens and Practice, 2d ed, 2006, p 987; with permission from Elsevier Science.*)

The following text boxes appear in Figure 32-1:

Excystation follows exposure to stomach acid and intestinal proteases, releasing trophozoite forms that multiply by binary fission and reside in the upper small bowel adherent to enterocytes.

Causes: Asymptomatic infection, acute diarrhea, or chronic diarrhea and malabsorption. Small bowel may demonstrate villous blunting, crypt hypertrophy, and mucosal inflammation.

Encystation occurs under conditions of bile salt concentration changes and alkaline pH. Smooth-walled cysts can contain two trophozoites.

Cyst are ingested (10–25 cysts) in contaminated water or food or by direct fecal-oral transmission (as in day care centers).

Cysts can survive in the environment (up to several weeks in cold water). They may also infect nonhuman mammalian species.

Cysts and trophozoites are passed in the stool into the environment.

common in developing countries, and infections may be acquired by travelers.

The importance of animal reservoirs as sources of infection for humans is unclear. *Giardia* parasites morphologically similar to those in humans are found in many mammals, including beavers from reservoirs implicated in epidemics, dogs, and cats.

Giardiasis, like cryptosporidiosis, creates a significant economic burden because of the costs incurred in the installation of water filtration systems required to prevent waterborne epidemics, in the management of epidemics that involve large communities, and in the evaluation and treatment of endemic infections.

Pathophysiology

The reasons that some, but not all, infected patients develop clinical manifestations and the mechanisms by

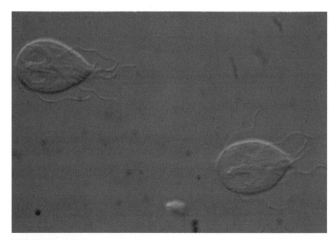

FIGURE 32-2
Flagellated, binucleate *Giardia* trophozoite.

which *Giardia* causes alterations in small-bowel function are largely unknown. Although trophozoites adhere to the epithelium, they do not cause invasive or locally destructive alterations. The lactose intolerance and, in a minority of infected adults and children, significant malabsorption that develop are clinical signs of the loss of brush-border enzyme activities. In most infections, the morphology of the bowel is unaltered; however, in a few cases (usually in chronically infected, symptomatic patients), the histopathologic findings (including flattened villi) and the clinical manifestations resemble those of tropical sprue and gluten-sensitive enteropathy. The pathogenesis of diarrhea in giardiasis is not known.

The natural history of *Giardia* infection varies markedly. Infections may be aborted, transient, recurrent, or chronic. Parasite as well as host factors may be important in determining the course of infection and disease. Both cellular and humoral responses develop in human infections, but their precise roles in the control of infection and/or disease are unknown. Because patients with hypogammaglobulinemia suffer from prolonged, severe infections that are poorly responsive to treatment, humoral immune responses appear to be important. The greater susceptibility of the young than of the old and of newly exposed persons than of chronically exposed populations suggests that at least partial protective immunity may develop. *Giardia* isolates vary genotypically, biochemically, and biologically, and variations among isolates may contribute to different courses of infection.

Clinical Manifestations

Disease manifestations of giardiasis range from asymptomatic carriage to fulminant diarrhea and malabsorption. Most infected persons are asymptomatic, but in epidemics the proportion of symptomatic cases may be higher. Symptoms may develop suddenly or gradually. In persons with acute giardiasis, symptoms develop after an incubation period that lasts at least 5–6 days and usually 1–3 weeks. Prominent early symptoms include diarrhea, abdominal pain, bloating, belching, flatus, nausea, and vomiting. Although diarrhea is common, upper intestinal manifestations such as nausea, vomiting, bloating, and abdominal pain may predominate. The duration of acute giardiasis is usually >1 week, although diarrhea often subsides. Individuals with chronic giardiasis may present with or without having experienced an antecedent acute symptomatic episode. Diarrhea is not necessarily prominent, but increased flatus, loose stools, sulfurous belching, and (in some instances) weight loss occur. Symptoms may be continual or episodic and can persist for years. Some persons who have relatively mild symptoms for long periods recognize the extent of their discomfort only in retrospect. Fever, the presence of blood and/or mucus in the stools, and other signs and symptoms of colitis are uncommon and suggest a different diagnosis or a concomitant illness. Symptoms tend to be intermittent yet recurring and gradually debilitating, in contrast with the acute disabling symptoms associated with many enteric bacterial infections. Because of the less severe illness and the propensity for chronic infections, patients may seek medical advice late in the course of the illness; however, disease can be severe, resulting in malabsorption, weight loss, growth retardation, and dehydration. A number of extraintestinal manifestations have been described, such as urticaria, anterior uveitis, and arthritis; whether these are caused by giardiasis or concomitant processes is unclear.

Giardiasis can be severe in patients with hypogammaglobulinemia and can complicate other preexisting intestinal diseases, such as that occurring in cystic fibrosis. In patients with AIDS, *Giardia* can cause enteric illness that is refractory to treatment.

Diagnosis

(**Table 32–1**) Giardiasis is diagnosed by detection of parasite antigens in the feces or by identification of cysts in the feces or of trophozoites in the feces or small intestines. Cysts are oval, measure 8–12 μm × 7–10 μm, and characteristically contain four nuclei. Trophozoites are pear-shaped, dorsally convex, flattened parasites with two nuclei and four pairs of flagella (Fig. 32-2). The diagnosis is sometimes difficult to establish. Direct examination of fresh or properly preserved stools as well as concentration methods should be used. Because cyst excretion is variable and may be undetectable at times, repeated examination of stool, sampling of duodenal fluid, and biopsy of the small intestine may be required to detect the parasite. Tests for parasitic antigens in stool are at least as sensitive and specific as good microscopic examinations and are easier to perform. All of these methods occasionally yield false-negative results.

Rx Treatment: GIARDIASIS

Cure rates with metronidazole (250 mg thrice daily for 5 days) are usually >90%. Tinidazole (2 g once by mouth) is reportedly more effective than metronidazole. Nitazoxanide (500 mg twice daily for 3 days) is an alternative agent for treatment of giardiasis. Paromomycin, an oral aminoglycoside that is not well absorbed, can be given to symptomatic pregnant patients, although information is limited on how effectively this agent eradicates infection.

Almost all patients respond to therapy and are cured, although some with chronic giardiasis experience delayed resolution of symptoms after eradication of *Giardia*. For many of the latter patients, residual symptoms probably reflect delayed regeneration of intestinal brush-border enzymes. Continued infection should be documented by stool examinations before treatment is repeated. Patients who remain infected after repeated treatments should be evaluated for reinfection through family members, close personal contacts, and environmental sources as well as for hypogammaglobulinemia. In cases refractory to multiple treatment courses, prolonged therapy with metronidazole (750 mg thrice daily for 21 days) has been successful.

Prevention

Although *Giardia* is extremely infectious, disease can be prevented by consumption of noncontaminated food and water and by personal hygiene when caring for infected children. Boiling or filtering potentially contaminated water prevents infection.

TABLE 32-1

DIAGNOSIS OF INTESTINAL PROTOZOAL INFECTIONS

PARASITE	STOOL O+P[a]	FECAL ACID-FAST STAIN	STOOL ANTIGEN IMMUNOASSAYS	OTHER
Giardia	+		+	
Cryptosporidium	−	+	+	
Isospora	−	+		
Cyclospora	−	+		
Microsporidia	−			Special fecal stains, tissue biopsies

[a]O+P, ova and parasites.

CRYPTOSPORIDIOSIS

The coccidian parasite *Cryptosporidium* causes diarrheal disease that is self-limited in immunocompetent human hosts but can be severe in persons with AIDS or other forms of immunodeficiency. Two species of *Cryptosporidium, C. hominis* and *C. parvum,* cause most human infections.

Life Cycle and Epidemiology

Cryptosporidium species are widely distributed in the world. Cryptosporidiosis is acquired by the consumption of oocysts (50% infectious dose: ~132 oocysts in nonimmune individuals), which excyst to liberate sporozoites that in turn enter and infect intestinal epithelial cells. The parasite's further development involves both asexual and sexual cycles, which produce forms capable of infecting other epithelial cells and of generating oocysts that are passed in the feces. *Cryptosporidium* species infect a number of animals, and *C. parvum* can spread from infected animals to humans. Since oocysts are immediately infectious when passed in feces, person-to-person transmission takes place in day-care centers and among household contacts and medical providers. Waterborne transmission (especially that of *C. hominis*) accounts for infections in travelers and for common-source epidemics. Oocysts are quite hardy and resist killing by routine chlorination. Both drinking water and recreational water (e.g., pools, waterslides) have been increasingly recognized as sources of infection.

Pathophysiology

Although intestinal epithelial cells harbor cryptosporidia in an intracellular vacuole, the means by which secretory diarrhea is elicited remain uncertain. No characteristic pathologic changes are found by biopsy. The distribution of infection can be spotty within the principal site of infection, the small bowel. Cryptosporidia are found in the pharynx, stomach, and large bowel of some patients and at times in the respiratory tract. Especially in patients with AIDS, involvement of the biliary tract can cause papillary stenosis, sclerosing cholangitis, or cholecystitis.

Clinical Manifestations

Asymptomatic infections can occur in both immunocompetent and immunocompromised hosts. In immunocompetent persons, symptoms develop after an incubation period of ~1 week and consist principally of watery nonbloody diarrhea, sometimes in conjunction with abdominal pain, nausea, anorexia, fever, and/or weight loss. In these hosts, the illness usually subsides after 1–2 weeks. In contrast, in immunocompromised hosts (especially those with AIDS and CD4+ T cell counts <100/μL), diarrhea can be chronic, persistent, and remarkably profuse, causing clinically significant fluid and electrolyte depletion. Stool

volumes may range from 1 to 25 L/d. Weight loss, wasting, and abdominal pain may be severe. Biliary tract involvement can manifest as midepigastric or right upper quadrant pain.

Diagnosis

(Table 32-1) Evaluation starts with fecal examination for small oocysts, which are smaller (4–5 μm in diameter) than the fecal stages of most other parasites. Because conventional stool examination for ova and parasites does not detect *Cryptosporidium*, specific testing must be requested. Detection is enhanced by evaluation of stools (obtained on multiple days) by several techniques, including modified acid-fast and direct immunofluorescent stains and enzyme immunoassays. Cryptosporidia can also be identified by light and electron microscopy at the apical surfaces of intestinal epithelium from biopsy specimens of the small bowel and, less frequently, the large bowel.

℞ Treatment:
CRYPTOSPORIDIOSIS

Nitazoxanide is approved by the U.S. Food and Drug Administration for the treatment of cryptosporidiosis and is available in tablet form for adults (500 mg twice daily for 3 days) and as an elixir for children. To date, however, this agent has not been effective for the treatment of HIV-infected patients, in whom improved immune status due to antiretroviral therapy can lead to amelioration of cryptosporidiosis. Otherwise, treatment includes supportive care with replacement of fluids and electrolytes and administration of antidiarrheal agents. Biliary tract obstruction may require papillotomy or T-tube placement. Prevention requires minimizing exposure to infectious oocysts in human or animal feces. Use of submicron water filters may minimize acquisition of infection from drinking water.

ISOSPORIASIS

The coccidian parasite *Isospora belli* causes human intestinal disease. Infection is acquired by the consumption of oocysts, after which the parasite invades intestinal epithelial cells and undergoes both sexual and asexual cycles of development. Oocysts excreted in stool are not immediately infectious but must undergo further maturation.

Although *I. belli* infects many animals, little is known about the epidemiology or prevalence of this parasite in humans. It appears to be most common in tropical and subtropical countries. Acute infections can begin abruptly with fever, abdominal pain, and watery nonbloody diarrhea and can last for weeks or months. In patients who have AIDS or are immunocompromised for other reasons, infections often are not self-limited but rather resemble cryptosporidiosis, with chronic, profuse watery diarrhea. Eosinophilia, which is not found in other enteric protozoan infections, may be detectable. The diagnosis (Table 32-1) is usually made by detection of the large (~25 μm) oocysts in stool by modified acid-fast staining. Oocyst excretion may be low-level and intermittent; if repeated stool examinations are unrevealing, sampling of duodenal contents by aspiration or small-bowel biopsy (often with electron-microscopic examination) may be necessary.

Rx Treatment:
ISOSPORIASIS

Trimethoprim-sulfamethoxazole (TMP-SMX; 160/800 mg four times daily for 10 days, and for HIV-infected patients, then three times daily for 3 weeks) is effective. For patients intolerant of sulfonamides, pyrimethamine (50–75 mg/d) can be used. Relapses can occur in persons with AIDS and necessitate maintenance therapy with TMP-SMX (160/800 mg three times per week).

CYCLOSPORIASIS

Cyclospora cayetanensis, a cause of diarrheal illness, is globally distributed: illness due to *C. cayetanensis* has been reported in the United States, Asia, Africa, Latin America, and Europe. The epidemiology of this parasite has not yet been fully defined, but waterborne transmission and food-borne transmission by basil and imported raspberries have been recognized. The full spectrum of illness attributable to *Cyclospora* has not been delineated. Some patients may harbor the infection without symptoms, but many have diarrhea, flulike symptoms, and flatulence and belching. The illness can be self-limited, can wax and wane, or in many cases can involve prolonged diarrhea, anorexia, and upper gastrointestinal symptoms, with sustained fatigue and weight loss in some instances. Diarrheal illness may persist for >1 month. *Cyclospora* can cause enteric illness in patients infected with HIV.

The parasite is detectable in epithelial cells of small-bowel biopsy samples and elicits secretory diarrhea by unknown means. The absence of fecal blood and leukocytes indicates that disease due to *Cyclospora* is not caused by destruction of the small-bowel mucosa. The diagnosis (Table 32-1) can be made by detection of spherical 8- to 10-μm oocysts in the stool, although routine stool O and P examinations are not sufficient. Specific fecal examinations must be requested to detect the oocysts, which are variably acid-fast and are fluorescent when viewed with ultraviolet light microscopy. Cyclosporiasis should be considered in the differential diagnosis of prolonged diarrhea, with or without a history of travel by the patient to other countries.

Rx Treatment:
CYCLOSPORIASIS

Cyclosporiasis is treated with TMP-SMX (160/800 mg twice daily for 7 days). HIV-infected patients may experience relapses after such treatment and thus may require longer-term suppressive maintenance therapy.

MICROSPORIDIOSIS

Microsporidia are obligate intracellular spore-forming protozoa that infect many animals and cause disease in humans, especially as opportunistic pathogens in AIDS. Microsporidia are members of a distinct phylum, Microspora, which contains dozens of genera and hundreds of species. The various microsporidia are differentiated by their developmental life cycles, ultrastructural features, and molecular taxonomy based on ribosomal RNA. The complex life cycles of the organisms result in the production of infectious spores (Fig. 32-3). Currently, eight genera of microsporidia—*Encephalitozoon*, *Pleistophora*, *Nosema*, *Vittaforma*, *Trachipleistophora*, *Brachiola*, *Microsporidium*, and *Enterocytozoon*—are recognized as causes of human disease. Although some microsporidia are probably prevalent causes of self-limited or asymptomatic infections in immunocompetent patients, little is known about how microsporidiosis is acquired.

Microsporidiosis is most common among patients with AIDS, less common among patients with other types of immunocompromise, and rare among immunocompetent hosts. In patients with AIDS, intestinal infections with *Enterocytozoon bieneusi* and *Encephalitozoon* (formerly *Septata*) *intestinalis* are recognized to contribute to chronic diarrhea and wasting; these infections are found in 10–40% of patients with chronic diarrhea. Both organisms have been found in the biliary tracts of patients with cholecystitis. *E. intestinalis* may also disseminate to cause fever, diarrhea, sinusitis, cholangitis, and bronchiolitis. In patients with AIDS, *Encephalitozoon hellem* has caused superficial keratoconjunctivitis as well as sinusitis, respiratory tract disease, and disseminated infection. Myositis due to *Pleistophora* has been documented. *Nosema*, *Vittaforma*, and *Microsporidium* have caused stromal keratitis associated with trauma in immunocompetent patients.

Microsporidia are small gram-positive organisms with mature spores measuring 0.5–2 μm × 1–4 μm. Diagnosis of microsporidial infections in tissue often requires electron microscopy, although intracellular spores can be visualized by light microscopy with hematoxylin and eosin, Giemsa, or tissue Gram's stain. For the diagnosis of intestinal microsporidiosis, modified trichrome or chromotrope 2R-based staining and Uvitex 2B or calcofluor fluorescent staining reveal spores in smears of feces or duodenal aspirates. Definitive therapies for microsporidial

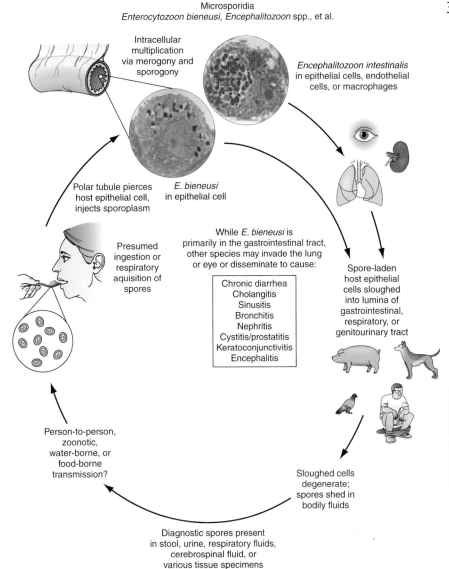

Microsporidia
Enterocytozoon bieneusi, Encephalitozoon spp., et al.

Intracellular
multiplication
via merogony and
sporogony

Encephalitozoon intestinalis
in epithelial cells, endothelial
cells, or macrophages

Polar tubule pierces
host epithelial cell,
injects sporoplasm

E. bieneusi
in epithelial cell

Presumed
ingestion or
respiratory
aquisition of
spores

While *E. bieneusi* is
primarily in the gastrointestinal tract,
other species may invade the lung
or eye or disseminate to cause:

Chronic diarrhea
Cholangitis
Sinusitis
Bronchitis
Nephritis
Cystitis/prostatitis
Keratoconjunctivitis
Encephalitis

Spore-laden
host epithelial
cells sloughed
into lumina of
gastrointestinal,
respiratory, or
genitourinary tract

Person-to-person,
zoonotic,
water-borne, or
food-borne
transmission?

Sloughed cells
degenerate;
spores shed in
bodily fluids

Diagnostic spores present
in stool, urine, respiratory fluids,
cerebrospinal fluid, or
various tissue specimens

FIGURE 32-3
Life cycle of microsporidia. (*Reprinted from RL Guerrant et al: Tropical Infectious Disease: Principles, Pathogens and Practice, 2d ed, 2006, p 1128; with permission from Elsevier Science.*)

infections remain to be established. For superficial keratoconjunctivitis due to *E. hellem*, topical therapy with fumagillin suspension has shown promise. For enteric infections with *E. bieneusi* and *E. intestinalis* in HIV-infected patients, therapy with albendazole may be efficacious.

OTHER INTESTINAL PROTOZOA

Balantidiasis

Balantidium coli is a large ciliated protozoal parasite that can produce a spectrum of large-intestinal disease analogous to amebiasis.

The parasite is widely distributed in the world. Since it infects pigs, cases in humans are more common where pigs are raised. Infective cysts can be transmitted from person to person and through water, but many cases are due to the ingestion of cysts derived from porcine feces in association with slaughtering, with use of pig feces for fertilizer, or with contamination of water supplies by pig feces.

Ingested cysts liberate trophozoites, which reside and replicate in the large bowel. Many patients remain asymptomatic, but some have persisting intermittent diarrhea, and a few develop more fulminant dysentery. In symptomatic individuals, the pathology in the bowel—both gross and microscopic—is similar to that seen in amebiasis, with varying degrees of mucosal invasion, focal necrosis, and ulceration. Balantidiasis, unlike amebiasis, does not spread hematogenously to other organs. The diagnosis is made by detection of the trophozoite stage in stool or sampled colonic tissue. Tetracycline (500 mg four times daily for 10 days) is an effective therapeutic agent.

Blastocystis Hominis Infection

B. hominis, while believed by some to be a protozoan capable of causing intestinal disease, remains an organism of uncertain pathogenicity. Some patients who pass *B. hominis* in their stools are asymptomatic, whereas others have diarrhea and associated intestinal symptoms. Diligent

310 evaluation reveals other potential bacterial, viral, or protozoal causes of diarrhea in some but not all patients with symptoms. Because the pathogenicity of *B. hominis* is uncertain and because therapy for *Blastocystis* infection is neither specific nor uniformly effective, patients with prominent intestinal symptoms should be fully evaluated for other infectious causes of diarrhea. If diarrheal symptoms associated with *Blastocystis* are prominent, either metronidazole (750 mg thrice daily for 10 days) or TMP-SMX (160 mg/800 mg twice daily for 7 days) can be used.

Dientamoeba Fragilis Infection

D. fragilis is unique among intestinal protozoa in that it has a trophozoite stage but not a cyst stage. How trophozoites survive to transmit infection is not known. When symptoms develop in patients with *D. fragilis* infection, they are generally mild and include intermittent diarrhea, abdominal pain, and anorexia. The diagnosis is made by the detection of trophozoites in stool; the lability of these forms accounts for the greater yield when fecal samples are preserved immediately after collection. Since fecal excretion rates vary, examination of several samples obtained on alternate days increases the rate of detection. Iodoquinol (650 mg three times daily for 20 days), paromomycin (25–35 mg/kg per day in three doses for 7 days), metronidazole (500–750 mg three times daily for 10 days), or tetracycline (500 mg four times daily for 10 days) is appropriate for treatment.

TRICHOMONIASIS

Various species of trichomonads can be found in the mouth (in association with periodontitis) and occasionally in the gastrointestinal tract. *Trichomonas vaginalis*—one of the most prevalent protozoal parasites in the United States—is a pathogen of the genitourinary tract and a major cause of symptomatic vaginitis.

LIFE CYCLE AND EPIDEMIOLOGY

T. vaginalis is a pear-shaped, actively motile organism that measures about 10 × 7 μm, replicates by binary fission, and inhabits the lower genital tract of females and the urethra and prostate of males. In the United States, it accounts for ~3 million infections per year in women. While the organism can survive for a few hours in moist environments and could be acquired by direct contact, person-to-person venereal transmission accounts for virtually all cases of trichomoniasis. Its prevalence is greatest among persons with multiple sexual partners and among those with other sexually transmitted diseases.

CLINICAL MANIFESTATIONS

Many men infected with *T. vaginalis* are asymptomatic, although some develop urethritis and a few have epididymitis or prostatitis. In contrast, infection in women, which has an incubation period of 5–28 days, is usually symptomatic and manifests with malodorous vaginal discharge (often yellow), vulvar erythema and itching, dysuria or urinary frequency (in 30–50% of patients), and dyspareunia. These manifestations, however, do not clearly distinguish trichomoniasis from other types of infectious vaginitis.

DIAGNOSIS

Detection of motile trichomonads by microscopic examination of wet mounts of vaginal or prostatic secretions has been the conventional means of diagnosis. Although this approach provides an immediate diagnosis, its sensitivity for the detection of *T. vaginalis* is only ~50–60% in routine evaluations of vaginal secretions. Direct immunofluorescent antibody staining is more sensitive (70–90%) than wet-mount examinations. *T. vaginalis* can be recovered from the urethra of both males and females and is detectable in males after prostatic massage. Culture of the parasite is the most sensitive means of detection; however, the facilities for culture are not generally available, and detection of the organism takes 3–7 days.

℞ Treatment: TRICHOMONIASIS

Metronidazole, given either as a single 2-g dose or in 500-mg doses twice daily for 7 days, is usually effective. Tinidazole (a single 2-g dose) is also effective. All sexual partners must be treated concurrently to prevent reinfection, especially from asymptomatic males. In males with persistent symptomatic urethritis after therapy for nongonococcal urethritis, metronidazole therapy should be considered for possible trichomoniasis. Alternatives to metronidazole for treatment during pregnancy are not readily available, although use of 100-mg clotrimazole vaginal suppositories nightly for 2 weeks may cure some infections in pregnant women. Reinfection often accounts for apparent treatment failures, but strains of *T. vaginalis* exhibiting high-level resistance to metronidazole have been encountered. Treatment of these resistant infections with higher oral doses, parenteral doses, or concurrent oral and vaginal doses of metronidazole or with tinidazole has been successful.

FURTHER READINGS

CDC Division of Parasitic Diseases: http://www.cdc.gov/ncidod/dpd/default.htm

Chex XM et al: Cryptosporidiosis. N Engl J Med 346:1723, 2002

Didier ES: Microsporidiosis: An emerging and opportunistic infection in humans and animals. Acta Trop 94:61, 2005

Leder K et al: No correlation between clinical symptoms and *Blastocystis hominis* in immunocompetent individuals. J Gastroenterol Hepatol 20:1390, 2005

Roxstrom-Lindquist K et al: Giardia immunity—an update. Trends Parasitol 22:26, 2006

Vandenberg O et al: Clinical and microbiological features of dientamoebiasis in patients suspected of suffering from a parasitic gastrointestinal illness: A comparison of *Dientamoeba fragilis* and *Giardia lamblia* infections. Int J Infect Dis 10:255, 2006

Van Der Pol B et al: Prevalence, incidence, natural history, and response to treatment of *Trichomonas vaginalis* infection among adolescent women. J Infect Dis 192:2039, 2005

Ward HD: Intestinal protozoal parasites and diarrheal disease in Bangladesh. Clin Infect Dis 48:1190, 2009

Weiss LM, Schwartz DA: Microsporidiosis, in *Tropical Infectious Diseases: Principles, Pathogens and Practice*, 2d ed, RL Guerrant et al (eds). Elsevier, Philadelphia, 2006, pp 1126–1140

Weitzel T et al: Epidemiological and clinical features of travel-associated cryptosporidiosis. Clin Microbiol Infect 12:921, 2006

Yoder JS, Beach MJ: Cryptosporidiosis surveillance—United States, 2003–2005. MMWR Surveil Sum 56:1, 2007

———— et al: Giardiasis surveillance—United States, 2003–2005. MMWR Surveil Sum 56:11, 2007

Protozoal Intestinal Infections and Trichomoniasis

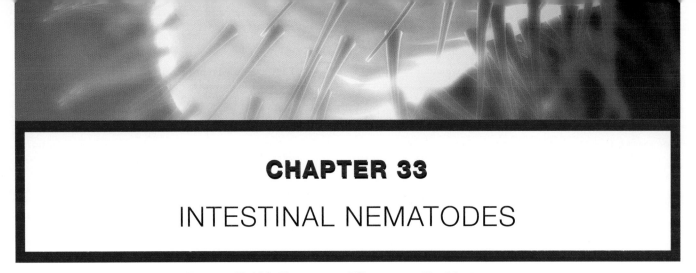

CHAPTER 33

INTESTINAL NEMATODES

Peter F. Weller ■ Thomas B. Nutman

More than a billion persons worldwide are infected with one or more species of intestinal nematodes. **Table 33-1** summarizes biologic and clinical features of infections due to the major intestinal parasitic nematodes. These parasites are most common in regions with poor fecal sanitation, particularly in resource-poor countries in the tropics and subtropics, but they have also been seen with increasing frequency among immigrants and refugees to resource-rich countries. Although nematode infections are not usually fatal, they contribute to malnutrition and diminished work capacity. It is interesting that these helminth infections may protect some individuals from allergic disease. Humans may on occasion be infected with nematode parasites that ordinarily infect animals; these zoonotic infections produce diseases such as trichostrongyliasis, anisakiasis, capillariasis, and abdominal angiostrongyliasis.

Intestinal nematodes are roundworms; they range in length from 1 mm to many centimeters when mature (Table 33-1). Their life cycles are complex and highly varied; some species, including *Strongyloides stercoralis* and *Enterobius vermicularis*, can be transmitted directly from person to person, while others, such as *Ascaris lumbricoides*, *Necator americanus*, and *Ancylostoma duodenale*, require a soil phase for development. Because most helminth parasites do not self-replicate, the acquisition of a heavy burden of adult worms requires repeated exposure to the parasite in its infectious stage, whether larva or egg. Hence, clinical disease, as opposed to asymptomatic infection, generally develops only with prolonged residence in an endemic area. In persons with marginal nutrition, intestinal helminth infections may impair growth and development. Eosinophilia and elevated serum IgE levels are features of many helminthic infections and, when unexplained, should always prompt a search for occult helminthiasis. Significant protective immunity to intestinal nematodes appears not to develop in humans, although mechanisms of parasite immune evasion and host immune responses to these infections have not been elucidated in detail.

ASCARIASIS

A. lumbricoides is the largest intestinal nematode parasite of humans, reaching up to 40 cm in length. Most infected individuals have low worm burdens and are asymptomatic. Clinical disease arises from larval migration in the lungs or effects of the adult worms in the intestines.

Life Cycle

Adult worms live in the lumen of the small intestine. Mature female *Ascaris* worms are extraordinarily

TABLE 33-1

MAJOR HUMAN INTESTINAL PARASITIC NEMATODES

		PARASITIC NEMATODE			
FEATURE	*ASCARIS LUMBRICOIDES* (ROUNDWORM)	*NECATOR AMERICANUS, ANCYLOSTOMA DUODENALE* (HOOKWORM)	*STRONGYLOIDES STERCORALIS*	*TRICHURIS TRICHIURA* (WHIPWORM)	*ENTEROBIUS VERMICULARIS* (PINWORM)
Global prevalence in humans (millions)	1221	740	50	795	300
Endemic areas	Worldwide	Hot, humid regions	Hot, humid regions	Worldwide	Worldwide
Infective stage	Egg	Filariform larva	Filariform larva	Egg	Egg
Route of infection	Oral	Percutaneous	Percutaneous or autoinfection	Oral	Oral
Gastrointestinal location of worms	Jejunal lumen	Jejunal mucosa	Small-bowel mucosa	Cecum, colonic mucosa	Cecum, appendix
Adult worm size	15–40 cm	7–12 mm	2 mm	30–50 mm	8–13 mm (female)
Pulmonary passage of larvae	Yes	Yes	Yes	No	No
Incubation period[a] (days)	60–75	40–100	17–28	70–90	35–45
Longevity	1 year	*N. americanus:* 2–5 years *A. duodenale:* 6–8 years	Decades (owing to autoinfection)	5 years	2 months
Fecundity (eggs/day/ worm)	240,000	*N. americanus:* 4000–10,000 *A. duodenale:* 10,000–25,000	5000–10,000	3000–7000	2000
Principal symptoms	Rarely gastrointestinal or biliary obstruction	Iron-deficiency anemia in heavy infection	Gastrointestinal symptoms; malabsorption or sepsis in hyperinfection	Gastrointestinal symptoms, anemia	Perianal pruritus
Diagnostic stage	Eggs in stool	Eggs in fresh stool, larvae in old stool	Larvae in stool or duodenal aspirate; sputum in hyperinfection	Eggs in stool	Eggs from perianal skin on cellulose acetate tape
Treatment	Mebendazole Albendazole Pyrantel pamoate Ivermectin	Mebendazole Pyrantel pamoate Albendazole	1. Ivermectin 2. Albendazole	Mebendazole Albendazole Ivermectin	Mebendazole Pyrantel pamoate Albendazole

[a]Time from infection to egg production by mature female worm.

CHAPTER 33

Intestinal Nematodes

fecund, each producing up to 240,000 eggs a day, which pass with the feces. Ascarid eggs, which are remarkably resistant to environmental stresses, become infective after several weeks of maturation in the soil and can remain infective for years. After infective eggs are swallowed, larvae hatched in the intestine invade the mucosa, migrate through the circulation to the lungs, break into the alveoli, ascend the bronchial tree, and return via swallowing to the small intestine, where they develop into adult worms. Between 2 and 3 months

elapse between initial infection and egg production. Adult worms live for 1–2 years.

Epidemiology

Ascaris is widely distributed in tropical and subtropical regions as well as in other humid areas, including the rural southeastern United States. Transmission typically occurs through fecally contaminated soil and is due either to a lack of sanitary facilities or to the use of human feces as fertilizer. With their propensity for hand-to-mouth fecal carriage, younger children are most affected. Infection outside endemic areas, though uncommon, can occur when eggs on transported vegetables are ingested.

Clinical Features

During the lung phase of larval migration, ~9–12 days after egg ingestion, patients may develop an irritating nonproductive cough and burning substernal discomfort that is aggravated by coughing or deep inspiration. Dyspnea and blood-tinged sputum are less common. Fever is usually reported. Eosinophilia develops during this symptomatic phase and subsides slowly over weeks. Chest x-rays may reveal evidence of eosinophilic pneumonitis (Löffler's syndrome), with rounded infiltrates a few millimeters to several centimeters in size. These infiltrates may be transient and intermittent, clearing after several weeks. Where there is seasonal transmission of the parasite, seasonal pneumonitis with eosinophilia may develop in previously infected and sensitized hosts.

In established infections, adult worms in the small intestine usually cause no symptoms. In heavy infections, particularly in children, a large bolus of entangled worms can cause pain and small-bowel obstruction, sometimes complicated by perforation, intussusception, or volvulus. Single worms may cause disease when they migrate into aberrant sites. A large worm can enter and occlude the biliary tree, causing biliary colic, cholecystitis, cholangitis, pancreatitis, or (rarely) intrahepatic abscesses. Migration of an adult worm up the esophagus can provoke coughing and oral expulsion of the worm. In highly endemic areas, intestinal and biliary ascariasis can rival acute appendicitis and gallstones as causes of surgical acute abdomen.

Laboratory Findings

Most cases of ascariasis can be diagnosed by microscopic detection of characteristic *Ascaris* eggs (65 by 45 μm) in fecal samples. Occasionally, patients present after passing an adult worm—identifiable by its large size and smooth cream-colored surface—in the stool or through the mouth or nose. During the early transpulmonary migratory phase, when eosinophilic pneumonitis occurs, larvae can be found in sputum or gastric aspirates before diagnostic eggs appear in the stool. The eosinophilia that is prominent during this early stage usually decreases to minimal levels in established infection. Adult worms may be visualized, occasionally serendipitously, on contrast studies of the gastrointestinal tract. A plain abdominal film may reveal masses of worms in gas-filled loops of bowel in patients with intestinal obstruction. Pancreaticobiliary worms can be detected by ultrasound and endoscopic retrograde cholangiopancreatography; the latter method also has been used to extract biliary *Ascaris* worms.

℞ Treatment:
ASCARIASIS

Ascariasis should always be treated to prevent potentially serious complications. Albendazole (400 mg once), mebendazole (500 mg once), or ivermectin (150–200 μg/kg once) is effective. These medications are contraindicated in pregnancy, however. Pyrantel pamoate (11 mg/kg once; maximum, 1 g) is safe in pregnancy. Mild diarrhea and abdominal pain are uncommon side effects of these agents. Partial intestinal obstruction should be managed with nasogastric suction, IV fluid administration, and instillation of piperazine through the nasogastric tube, but complete obstruction and its severe complications require immediate surgical intervention.

HOOKWORM

Two hookworm species (*A. duodenale* and *N. americanus*) are responsible for human infections. Most infected individuals are asymptomatic. Hookworm disease develops from a combination of factors—a heavy worm burden, a prolonged duration of infection, and an inadequate iron intake—and results in iron-deficiency anemia and, on occasion, hypoproteinemia.

Life Cycle

Adult hookworms, which are ~1 cm long, use buccal teeth (*Ancylostoma*) or cutting plates (*Necator*) to attach to the small-bowel mucosa and suck blood (0.2 mL/d per *Ancylostoma* adult) and interstitial fluid. The adult hookworms produce thousands of eggs daily. The eggs are deposited with feces in soil, where rhabditiform larvae hatch and develop over a 1-week period into infectious filariform larvae. Infective larvae penetrate the skin and reach the lungs by way of the bloodstream. There they invade alveoli and ascend the airways before being swallowed and reaching the small intestine. The prepatent period from skin invasion to appearance of eggs in the feces is ~6–8 weeks, but it may be longer with *A. duodenale*. Larvae of *A. duodenale*, if swallowed, can survive and develop directly in the intestinal mucosa. Adult hookworms may survive over a decade but usually live ~6–8 years for *A. duodenale* and 2–5 years for *N. americanus*.

Epidemiology

A. duodenale is prevalent in southern Europe, North Africa, and northern Asia, and *N. americanus* is the predominant species in the western hemisphere and equatorial Africa. The two species overlap in many tropical regions, particularly Southeast Asia. In most areas, older children have the highest incidence and greatest intensity of hookworm infection. In rural areas where fields are fertilized with human feces, older working adults also may be heavily affected.

Clinical Features

Most hookworm infections are asymptomatic. Infective larvae may provoke pruritic maculopapular dermatitis ("ground itch") at the site of skin penetration as well as serpiginous tracks of subcutaneous migration (similar to those of cutaneous larva migrans) in previously sensitized hosts. Larvae migrating through the lungs occasionally cause mild transient pneumonitis, but this condition develops less frequently in hookworm infection than in ascariasis. In the early intestinal phase, infected persons may develop epigastric pain (often with postprandial accentuation), inflammatory diarrhea, or other abdominal symptoms accompanied by eosinophilia. The major consequence of chronic hookworm infection is iron deficiency. Symptoms are minimal if iron intake is adequate, but marginally nourished individuals develop symptoms of progressive iron-deficiency anemia and hypoproteinemia, including weakness and shortness of breath.

Laboratory Findings

The diagnosis is established by the finding of characteristic 40- by 60-μm oval hookworm eggs in the feces. Stool-concentration procedures may be required to detect light infections. Eggs of the two species are indistinguishable by light microscopy. In a stool sample that is not fresh, the eggs may have hatched to release rhabditiform larvae, which need to be differentiated from those of *S. stercoralis*. Hypochromic microcytic anemia, occasionally with eosinophilia or hypoalbuminemia, is characteristic of hookworm disease.

℞ Treatment:
HOOKWORM INFECTION

Hookworm infection can be eradicated with several safe and highly effective anthelmintic drugs, including albendazole (400 mg once), mebendazole (500 mg once), and pyrantel pamoate (11 mg/kg for 3 days). Mild iron-deficiency anemia can often be treated with oral iron alone. Severe hookworm disease with protein loss and malabsorption necessitates nutritional support and oral iron replacement along with deworming.

Ancylostoma caninum *and* Ancylostoma braziliense

A. caninum, the canine hookworm, has been identified as a cause of human eosinophilic enteritis, especially in northeastern Australia. In this zoonotic infection, adult hookworms attach to the small intestine (where they may be visualized by endoscopy) and elicit abdominal pain and intense local eosinophilia. Treatment with mebendazole (100 mg twice daily for 3 days) or albendazole (400 mg once) or endoscopic removal is effective. Both of these animal hookworm species can cause cutaneous larva migrans ("creeping eruption").

STRONGYLOIDIASIS

S. stercoralis is distinguished by its ability—unusual among helminths—to replicate in the human host. This capacity permits ongoing cycles of autoinfection as infective larvae are internally produced. Strongyloidiasis can thus persist for decades without further exposure of the host to exogenous infective larvae. In immunocompromised hosts, large numbers of invasive *Strongyloides* larvae can disseminate widely and can be fatal.

Life Cycle

In addition to a parasitic cycle of development, *Strongyloides* can undergo a free-living cycle of development in the soil (Fig. 33-1). This adaptability facilitates the parasite's survival in the absence of mammalian hosts. Rhabditiform larvae passed in feces can transform into infectious filariform larvae either directly or after a free-living phase of development. Humans acquire strongyloidiasis when filariform larvae in fecally contaminated soil penetrate the skin or mucous membranes. The larvae then travel through the bloodstream to the lungs, where they break into the alveolar spaces, ascend the bronchial tree, are swallowed, and thereby reach the small intestine. There the larvae mature into adult worms that penetrate the mucosa of the proximal small bowel. The minute (2-mm-long) parasitic adult female worms reproduce by parthenogenesis; adult males do not exist. Eggs hatch in the intestinal mucosa, releasing rhabditiform larvae that migrate to the lumen and pass with the feces into soil. Alternatively, rhabditiform larvae in the bowel can develop directly into filariform larvae that penetrate the colonic wall or perianal skin and enter the circulation to repeat the migration that establishes ongoing internal reinfection. This autoinfection cycle allows strongyloidiasis to persist for decades.

🌐 Epidemiology

S. stercoralis is spottily distributed in tropical areas and other hot, humid regions and is particularly common in Southeast Asia, sub-Saharan Africa, and Brazil. In the United States, the parasite is endemic in parts of the South and is found in immigrants and military veterans who have lived in endemic areas abroad.

Clinical Features

In uncomplicated strongyloidiasis, many patients are asymptomatic or have mild cutaneous and/or abdominal

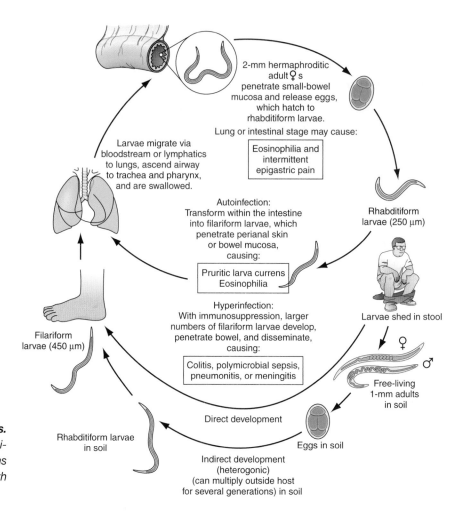

FIGURE 33-1
Life cycle of *Strongyloides stercoralis.*
[Adapted from Guerrant RL et al (eds): Tropical Infectious Diseases: Principles, Pathogens and Practice, 2d ed, p 1276. © 2006, with permission from Elsevier Science.]

symptoms. Recurrent urticaria, often involving the buttocks and wrists, is the most common cutaneous manifestation. Migrating larvae can elicit a pathognomonic serpiginous eruption, *larva currens* ("running larva"). This pruritic, raised, erythematous lesion advances as rapidly as 10 cm/h along the course of larval migration. Adult parasites burrow into the duodenojejunal mucosa and can cause abdominal (usually midepigastric) pain, which resembles peptic ulcer pain except that it is aggravated by food ingestion. Nausea, diarrhea, gastrointestinal bleeding, mild chronic colitis, and weight loss can occur. Small-bowel obstruction may develop with early, heavy infection. Pulmonary symptoms are rare in uncomplicated strongyloidiasis. Eosinophilia is common, with levels fluctuating over time.

The ongoing autoinfection cycle of strongyloidiasis is normally contained by unknown factors of the host's immune system. Abrogation of host immunity, especially with glucocorticoid therapy and much less commonly with other immunosuppressive medications, leads to hyperinfection, with the generation of large numbers of filariform larvae. Colitis, enteritis, or malabsorption may develop. In disseminated strongyloidiasis, larvae may invade not only gastrointestinal tissues and the lungs but also the central nervous system, peritoneum, liver, and

kidneys. Moreover, bacteremia may develop because of the passage of enteric flora through disrupted mucosal barriers. Gram-negative sepsis, pneumonia, or meningitis may complicate or dominate the clinical course. Eosinophilia is often absent in severely infected patients. Disseminated strongyloidiasis, particularly in patients with unsuspected infection who are given glucocorticoids, can be fatal. Strongyloidiasis is a frequent complication of infection with human T cell lymphotropic virus type I, but disseminated strongyloidiasis is not common among patients infected with HIV.

Diagnosis

In uncomplicated strongyloidiasis, the finding of rhabditiform larvae in feces is diagnostic. Rhabditiform larvae are ~250 μm long, with a short buccal cavity that distinguishes them from hookworm larvae. In uncomplicated infections, few larvae are passed and single stool examinations detect only about one-third of cases. Serial examinations and the use of the agar plate detection method improve the sensitivity of stool diagnosis. In uncomplicated strongyloidiasis (but not in hyperinfection), stool examinations may be repeatedly negative. *Strongyloides* larvae may also be found by sampling of the duodenojejunal contents by aspiration or biopsy. An enzyme-linked immunosorbent assay for serum antibodies to antigens of *Strongyloides* is a sensitive method of diagnosing uncomplicated infections. Such serologic testing should be performed for patients whose geographic histories indicate potential exposure, especially those who exhibit eosinophilia and/or are candidates for glucocorticoid treatment of other conditions. In disseminated strongyloidiasis, filariform larvae should be sought in stool as well as in samples obtained from sites of potential larval migration, including sputum, bronchoalveolar lavage fluid, or surgical drainage fluid.

Rx Treatment: STRONGYLOIDIASIS

Even in the asymptomatic state, strongyloidiasis must be treated because of the potential for subsequent fatal hyperinfection. Ivermectin (200 μg/kg daily for 2 days) is more effective than albendazole (400 mg daily for 3 days). For disseminated strongyloidiasis, treatment with ivermectin should be extended for at least 5–7 days or until the parasites are eradicated.

TRICHURIASIS

Most infections with the *Trichuris trichiura* are asymptomatic, but heavy infections may cause gastrointestinal symptoms. Like the other soil-transmitted helminths, whipworm is distributed globally in the tropics and subtropics and is most common among poor children from resource-poor regions of the world.

Life Cycle

Adult *Trichuris* worms reside in the colon and cecum, the anterior portions threaded into the superficial mucosa. Thousands of eggs laid daily by adult female worms pass with the feces and mature in the soil. After ingestion, infective eggs hatch in the duodenum, releasing larvae that mature before migrating to the large bowel. The entire cycle takes ~3 months, and adult worms may live for several years.

Clinical Features

Tissue reactions to *Trichuris* are mild. Most infected individuals have no symptoms or eosinophilia. Heavy infections may result in abdominal pain, anorexia, and bloody or mucoid diarrhea resembling inflammatory bowel disease. Rectal prolapse can result from massive infections in children, who often suffer from malnourishment and other diarrheal illnesses. Moderately heavy *Trichuris* burdens also contribute to growth retardation.

Diagnosis and Treatment

The characteristic 50- by 20-μm lemon-shaped *Trichuris* eggs are readily detected on stool examination. Adult worms, which are 3–5 cm long, are occasionally seen on proctoscopy. Mebendazole (500 mg once) or albendazole (400 mg daily for 3 doses) is safe and effective for treatment. Ivermectin (200 μg/kg daily for 3 doses) is also safe but is not quite as efficacious as the benzimidazoles.

ENTEROBIASIS (PINWORM)

E. vermicularis is more common in temperate countries than in the tropics. In the United States, ~40 million persons are infected with pinworms, with a disproportionate number of cases among children.

Life Cycle and Epidemiology

Enterobius adult worms are ~1 cm long and dwell in the cecum. Gravid female worms migrate nocturnally into the perianal region and release up to 10,000 immature eggs each. The eggs become infective within hours and are transmitted by hand-to-mouth passage. From ingested eggs, larvae hatch and mature into adults. This life cycle takes ~1 month, and adult worms survive for ~2 months. Self-infection results from perianal scratching and transport of infective eggs on the hands or under the nails to the mouth. Because of the ease of person-to-person spread, pinworm infections are common among family members.

Clinical Features

Most pinworm infections are asymptomatic. Perianal pruritus is the cardinal symptom. The itching, which is often worse at night as a result of the nocturnal migration of the female worms, may lead to excoriation and bacterial superinfection. Heavy infections have been claimed to cause abdominal pain and weight loss. On rare occasions, pinworms invade the female genital tract, causing vulvovaginitis and pelvic or peritoneal granulomas. Eosinophilia is uncommon.

Diagnosis

Since pinworm eggs are not released in feces, the diagnosis cannot be made by conventional fecal ova and parasites tests. Instead, eggs are detected by the application of clear cellulose acetate tape to the perianal region in the morning. After the tape is transferred to a slide, microscopic examination will detect pinworm eggs, which are oval, measure 55 by 25 μm, and are flattened along one side.

Rx **Treatment:**
ENTEROBIASIS

Infected children and adults should be treated with mebendazole (100 mg once), albendazole (400 mg once), or pyrantel pamoate (11 mg/kg once; maximum, 1 g), with the same treatment repeated after 2 weeks. Treatment of household members is advocated to eliminate asymptomatic reservoirs of potential reinfection.

TRICHOSTRONGYLIASIS

Trichostrongylus species, which are normally parasites of herbivorous animals, occasionally infect humans, particularly in Asia and Africa. Humans acquire the infection by accidentally ingesting *Trichostrongylus* larvae on contaminated leafy vegetables. The larvae do not migrate in humans but mature directly into adult worms in the small bowel. These worms ingest far less blood than hookworms; most infected persons are asymptomatic, but heavy infections may give rise to mild anemia and eosinophilia. *Trichostrongylus* eggs in stool examinations resemble those of hookworms but are larger (85 by 115 μm). Treatment consists of mebendazole or albendazole.

ANISAKIASIS

Anisakiasis is a gastrointestinal infection caused by the accidental ingestion in uncooked saltwater fish of nematode larvae belonging to the family Anisakidae. The incidence of anisakiasis in the United States has increased as a result of the growing popularity of raw fish dishes. Most cases occur in Japan, the Netherlands, and Chile, where raw fish—sashimi, pickled green herring, and ceviche, respectively—are national culinary staples. Anisakid nematodes parasitize large sea mammals such as whales, dolphins, and seals. As part of a complex parasitic life cycle involving marine food chains, infectious larvae migrate to the musculature of a variety of fish. Both *Anisakis simplex* and *Pseudoterranova decipiens* have been implicated in human anisakiasis, but an identical gastric syndrome may be caused by the red larvae of eustrongylid parasites of fish-eating birds.

When humans consume infected raw fish, live larvae may be coughed up within 48 h. Alternatively, larvae may immediately penetrate the mucosa of the stomach. Within hours, violent upper abdominal pain accompanied by nausea and occasionally vomiting ensues, mimicking an acute abdomen. The diagnosis can be established by direct visualization on upper endoscopy, outlining of the worm by contrast radiographic studies, or histopathologic examination of extracted tissue. Extraction of the burrowing larvae during endoscopy is curative. In addition, larvae may pass to the small bowel, where they penetrate the mucosa and provoke a vigorous eosinophilic granulomatous response.

Symptoms may appear 1–2 weeks after the infective meal, with intermittent abdominal pain, diarrhea, nausea, and fever resembling the manifestations of Crohn's disease. The diagnosis may be suggested by barium studies and confirmed by curative surgical resection of a granuloma in which the worm is embedded. Anisakid eggs are not found in the stool, since the larvae do not mature in humans. Anisakid larvae in saltwater fish are killed by cooking to 60°C, freezing at −20°C for 3 days, or commercial blast freezing, but not usually by salting, marinating, or cold smoking. No medical treatment is available; surgical or endoscopic removal should be undertaken.

CAPILLARIASIS

Intestinal capillariasis is caused by ingestion of raw fish infected with *Capillaria philippinensis*. Subsequent autoinfection can lead to a severe wasting syndrome. The disease occurs in the Philippines and Thailand and, on occasion, elsewhere in Asia. The natural cycle of *C. philippinensis* involves fish from fresh and brackish water. When humans eat infected raw fish, the larvae mature in the intestine into adult worms, which produce invasive larvae that cause intestinal inflammation and villus loss. Capillariasis has an insidious onset with nonspecific abdominal pain and watery diarrhea. If untreated, progressive autoinfection can lead to protein-losing enteropathy and severe malabsorption and ultimately to death from cachexia, cardiac failure, or superinfection. The diagnosis is established by identification of the characteristic peanut-shaped (20- by 40-μm) eggs on stool examination. Severely ill patients require hospitalization and supportive therapy in addition to prolonged anthelmintic treatment with mebendazole or albendazole.

ABDOMINAL ANGIOSTRONGYLIASIS

Abdominal angiostrongyliasis is found in Latin America and Africa. The zoonotic parasite *Angiostrongylus costaricensis* causes eosinophilic ileocolitis after the ingestion of contaminated vegetation. *A. costaricensis* normally parasitizes the cotton rat and other rodents, with slugs and snails serving as intermediate hosts. Humans become infected by accidentally ingesting infective larvae in mollusk slime deposited on fruits and vegetables; children are at highest risk. The larvae penetrate the gut wall and migrate to the mesenteric artery, where they develop into adult worms. Eggs deposited in the gut wall provoke an intense eosinophilic granulomatous reaction, and adult worms may cause mesenteric arteritis, thrombosis, or frank bowel infarction. Symptoms may mimic those of appendicitis, including abdominal pain and tenderness, fever, vomiting, and a palpable mass in the right iliac fossa. Leukocytosis and eosinophilia are prominent. A barium enema may reveal ileocecal-filling defects, but a definitive diagnosis is usually made surgically with partial bowel resection. Pathologic study reveals a thickened bowel wall with eosinophilic granulomas surrounding the *Angiostrongylus* eggs. In nonsurgical cases, the diagnosis rests solely on clinical grounds because larvae and eggs cannot be detected in the stool. Medical therapy for abdominal angiostrongyliasis (mebendazole, thiabendazole) is of uncertain efficacy. Careful observation and surgical resection for severe symptoms are the mainstays of treatment.

FURTHER READINGS

ARTIS D, GRENCIS RK: The intestinal epithelium: sensors to effectors in nematode infection. Mucosal Immunol 1:252, 2008

BETHONY J et al: Soil-transmitted helminth infections: Ascariasis, trichuriasis, and hookworm. Lancet 367:1521, 2006

HOTEZ PJ et al: Hookworm infection. N Engl J Med 351:799, 2004

JOHNSTONG MH: Parasitic helminthes: a pharmacopeia of anti-inflammatory molecules. Parasitology 136:125, 2009

KEISER PB et al: *Strongyloides stercoralis* in the immunocompromised population. Clin Microbiol Rev 17:208, 2004

LAM CS et al: Disseminated strongyloidiasis: A retrospective study of clinical course and outcome. Eur J Clin Microbiol Infect Dis 25:14, 2006

LIM S et al: Complicated and fatal *Strongyloides* infection in Canadians: Risk factors, diagnosis and management. CMAJ 171:479, 2004

LU LH et al: Human intestinal capillariasis (*Capillaria philippinensis*) in Taiwan. Am J Trop Med Hyg 74:810, 2006

SHAH OJ et al: Biliary ascariasis: A review. World J Surg 30:1500, 2006

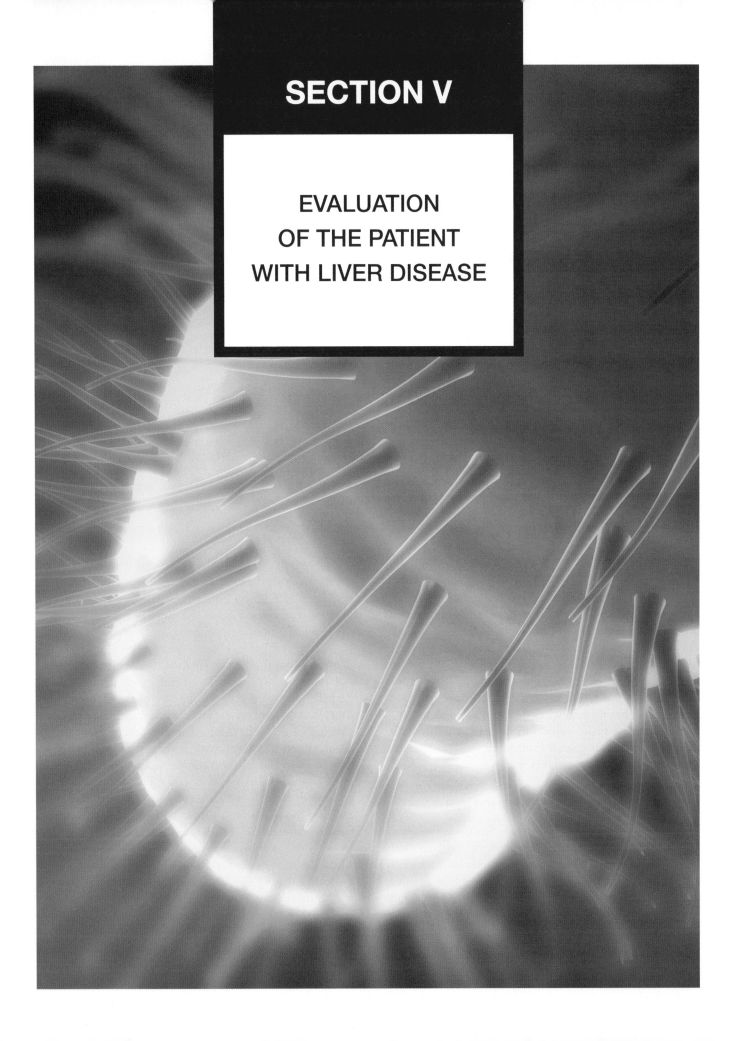

SECTION V

EVALUATION OF THE PATIENT WITH LIVER DISEASE

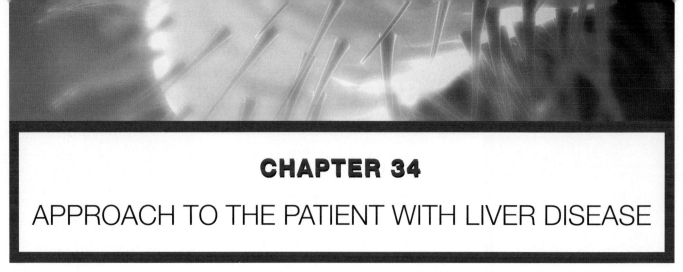

CHAPTER 34

APPROACH TO THE PATIENT WITH LIVER DISEASE

Marc Ghany ■ Jay H. Hoofnagle

In most instances, a diagnosis of liver disease can be made accurately by a careful history, physical examination, and application of a few laboratory tests. In some circumstances, radiologic examinations are helpful or, indeed, diagnostic. Liver biopsy is considered the "gold standard" in evaluation of liver disease but is now needed less for diagnosis than for grading and staging disease. This chapter provides an introduction to diagnosis and management of liver disease, briefly reviewing the structure and function of the liver; the major clinical manifestations of liver disease; and the use of clinical history, physical examination, laboratory tests, imaging studies, and liver biopsy.

LIVER STRUCTURE AND FUNCTION

The liver is the largest organ of the body, weighing 1–1.5 kg and representing 1.5–2.5% of the lean body mass. The size and shape of the liver vary and generally match the general body shape—long and lean or squat and square. The liver is located in the right upper quadrant of the abdomen under the right lower rib cage against the diaphragm and projects for a variable extent into the left upper quadrant. The liver is held in place by ligamentous attachments to the diaphragm, peritoneum, great vessels, and upper gastrointestinal organs.

It receives a dual blood supply; ~20% of the blood flow is oxygen-rich blood from the hepatic artery, and 80% is nutrient-rich blood from the portal vein arising from the stomach, intestines, pancreas, and spleen.

The majority of cells in the liver are hepatocytes, which constitute two-thirds of the mass of the liver. The remaining cell types are Kupffer cells (members of the reticuloendothelial system), stellate (Ito or fat-storing) cells, endothelial cells and blood vessels, bile ductular cells, and supporting structures. Viewed by light microscopy, the liver appears to be organized in lobules, with portal areas at the periphery and central veins in the center of each lobule. However, from a functional point of view, the liver is organized into acini, with both hepatic arterial and portal venous blood entering the acinus from the portal areas (zone 1) and then flowing through the sinusoids to the terminal hepatic veins (zone 3); the intervening hepatocytes constitute zone 2. The advantage of viewing the acinus as the physiologic unit of the liver is that it helps to explain the morphologic patterns and zonality of many vascular and biliary diseases not explained by the lobular arrangement.

Portal areas of the liver consist of small veins, arteries, bile ducts, and lymphatics organized in a loose stroma of supporting matrix and small amounts of collagen. Blood flowing into the portal areas is distributed through the sinusoids, passing from zone 1 to zone 3 of the acinus and draining into the terminal hepatic veins ("central veins"). Secreted bile flows in the opposite direction, in a counter-current pattern from zone 3 to zone 1. The sinusoids are lined by unique endothelial cells that have prominent fen-estrae of variable size, allowing the free flow of plasma but not cellular elements. The plasma is thus in direct contact with hepatocytes in the subendothelial space of Disse.

Hepatocytes have distinct polarity. The basolateral side of the hepatocyte lines the space of Disse and is richly lined with microvilli; it demonstrates endocytotic and pinocytotic activity, with passive and active uptake of nutrients, proteins, and other molecules. The apical pole of the hepatocyte forms the cannicular membranes through which bile components are secreted. The canniculi of hepatocytes form a fine network, which fuses into the bile ductular elements near the portal areas. Kupffer cells usu-ally lie within the sinusoidal vascular space and represent the largest group of fixed macrophages in the body. The stellate cells are located in the space of Disse but are not usually prominent unless activated, when they produce collagen and matrix. Red blood cells stay in the sinusoidal space as blood flows through the lobules, but white blood cells can migrate through or around endothelial cells into the space of Disse and from there to portal areas, where they can return to the circulation through lymphatics.

Hepatocytes perform numerous and vital roles in main-taining homeostasis and health. These functions include the synthesis of most essential serum proteins (albumin, carrier proteins, coagulation factors, many hormonal and growth factors), the production of bile and its carriers (bile acids, cholesterol, lecithin, phospholipids), the regulation of nutrients (glucose, glycogen, lipids, cholesterol, amino acids), and metabolism and conjugation of lipophilic com-pounds (bilirubin, anions, cations, drugs) for excretion in the bile or urine. Measurement of these activities to assess liver function is complicated by the multiplicity and vari-ability of these functions. The most commonly used liver "function" tests are measurements of serum bilirubin, albumin, and prothrombin time. The serum bilirubin level is a measure of hepatic conjugation and excretion, and the serum albumin level and prothrombin time are measures of protein synthesis. Abnormalities of bilirubin, albumin, and prothrombin time are typical of hepatic dysfunction. Frank liver failure is incompatible with life, and the func-tions of the liver are too complex and diverse to be sub-served by a mechanical pump; dialysis membrane; or con-coction of infused hormones, proteins, and growth factors.

LIVER DISEASES

While there are many causes of liver disease (Table 34-1), they generally present clinically in a few distinct patterns, usually classified as hepatocellular, cholestatic (obstructive),

or mixed. In *hepatocellular diseases* (such as viral hepatitis or alcoholic liver disease), features of liver injury, inflammation, and necrosis predominate. In *cholestatic diseases* (such as gall stone or malignant obstruction, primary biliary cirrhosis, some drug-induced liver diseases), features of inhibition of bile flow predominate. In a mixed pattern, features of both hepatocellular and cholestatic injury are present (such as in cholestatic forms of viral hepatitis and many drug-induced liver diseases). The pattern of onset and prominence of symptoms can rapidly suggest a diagnosis, particularly if major risk factors are considered, such as the age and sex of the patient and a history of exposure or risk behaviors.

Typical presenting symptoms of liver disease include jaundice, fatigue, itching, right upper quadrant pain, abdominal distention, and intestinal bleeding. At present, however, many patients are diagnosed with liver disease who have no symptoms and who have been found to have abnormalities in biochemical liver tests as a part of a routine physical examination or screening for blood donation or for insurance or employment. The wide availability of batteries of liver tests makes it relatively simple to demonstrate the presence of liver injury as well as to rule it out in someone suspected of liver disease.

Evaluation of patients with liver disease should be directed at (1) establishing the etiologic diagnosis, (2) esti-mating the disease severity (grading), and (3) establishing the disease stage (staging). *Diagnosis* should focus on the category of disease, such as hepatocellular, cholestatic, or mixed injury, as well as on the specific etiologic diagnosis. *Grading* refers to assessing the severity or activity of disease—active or inactive, and mild, moderate, or severe. *Staging* refers to estimating the place in the course of the natural history of the disease, whether acute or chronic; early or late; precirrhotic, cirrhotic, or end-stage.

The goal of this chapter is to introduce general, salient concepts in the evaluation of patients with liver disease that help lead to the diagnoses discussed in sub-sequent chapters.

CLINICAL HISTORY

The clinical history should focus on the symptoms of liver disease—their nature, pattern of onset, and progression—and on potential risk factors for liver disease. The symp-toms of liver disease include constitutional symptoms such as fatigue, weakness, nausea, poor appetite, and malaise and the more liver-specific symptoms of jaun-dice, dark urine, light stools, itching, abdominal pain, and bloating. Symptoms can also suggest the presence of cirrhosis, end-stage liver disease, or complications of cirrhosis such as portal hypertension. Generally, the constellation of symptoms and their pattern of onset rather than a specific symptom points to an etiology.

Fatigue is the most common and most characteristic symptom of liver disease. It is variously described as lethargy, weakness, listlessness, malaise, increased need for

TABLE 34-1

LIVER DISEASES

Inherited hyperbilirubinemia
  Gilbert syndrome
  Crigler-Najjar syndrome, types I and II
  Dubin-Johnson syndrome
  Rotor syndrome
Viral hepatitis
  Hepatitis A
  Hepatitis B
  Hepatitis C
  Hepatitis D
  Hepatitis E
  Others (mononucleosis, herpes, adenovirus
    hepatitis)
  Cryptogenic hepatitis
Immune and autoimmune liver diseases
  Primary biliary cirrhosis
  Autoimmune hepatitis
  Sclerosing cholangitis
  Overlap syndromes
  Graft-versus-host disease
  Allograft rejection
Genetic liver diseases
  α_1 Antitrypsin deficiency
  Hemochromatosis
  Wilson disease
  Benign recurrent intrahepatic cholestasis (BRIC)
  Progressive familial intrahepatic cholestasis
    (PFIC), types I–III
  Others (galactosemia, tyrosinemia, cystic
    fibrosis, Newman-Pick disease, Gaucher
    disease)
Alcoholic liver disease
  Acute fatty liver
  Acute alcoholic hepatitis
  Laennec cirrhosis
Nonalcoholic fatty liver
  Steatosis
  Steatohepatitis
Acute fatty liver of pregnancy

Liver involvement in systemic diseases
  Sarcoidosis
  Amyloidosis
  Glycogen storage diseases
  Celiac disease
  Tuberculosis
  Mycobacterium avium intracellulare
Cholestatic syndromes
  Benign postoperative cholestasis
  Jaundice of sepsis
  Total parenteral nutrition (TPN)–induced jaundice
  Cholestasis of pregnancy
  Cholangitis and cholecystitis
  Extrahepatic biliary obstruction (stone, stricture, cancer)
  Biliary atresia
  Caroli disease
  Cryptosporidiosis
Drug-induced liver disease
  Hepatocellular patterns (isoniazid, acetaminophen)
  Cholestatic patterns (methyltestosterone)
  Mixed patterns (sulfonamides, phenytoin)
  Micro- and macrovesicular steatosis
    (methotrexate, fialuridine)
Vascular injury
  Venoocclusive disease
  Budd-Chiari syndrome
  Ischemic hepatitis
  Passive congestion
  Portal vein thrombosis
  Nodular regenerative hyperplasia
Mass lesions
  Hepatocellular carcinoma
  Cholangiocarcinoma
  Adenoma
  Focal nodular hyperplasia
  Metastatic tumors
  Abscess
  Cysts
  Hemangioma

sleep, lack of stamina, and poor energy. The fatigue of liver disease typically arises after activity or exercise and is rarely present or severe in the morning after adequate rest (afternoon vs. morning fatigue). Fatigue in liver disease is often intermittent and variable in severity from hour to hour and day to day. In some patients, it may not be clear whether fatigue is due to the liver disease or to other problems such as stress, anxiety, sleep disturbance, or a concurrent illness.

Nausea occurs with more severe liver disease and may accompany fatigue or be provoked by odors of food or eating fatty foods. Vomiting can occur but is rarely persistent or prominent. Poor appetite with weight loss occurs commonly in acute liver diseases but is rare in chronic disease, except when cirrhosis is present and

advanced. Diarrhea is uncommon in liver disease, except with severe jaundice, where lack of bile acids reaching the intestine can lead to steatorrhea.

Right upper quadrant discomfort or ache ("liver pain") occurs in many liver diseases and is usually marked by tenderness over the liver area. The pain arises from stretching or irritation of Glisson's capsule, which surrounds the liver and is rich in nerve endings. Severe pain is most typical of gall bladder disease, liver abscess, and severe venoocclusive disease but is an occasional accompaniment of acute hepatitis.

Itching occurs with acute liver disease, appearing early in obstructive jaundice (from biliary obstruction or drug-induced cholestasis) and somewhat later in hepatocellular disease (acute hepatitis). Itching also occurs in chronic liver diseases, typically the cholestatic forms such as primary biliary cirrhosis and sclerosing cholangitis where it is often the presenting symptom, occurring before the onset of jaundice. However, itching can occur in any liver disease, particularly once cirrhosis is present.

Jaundice is the hallmark symptom of liver disease and perhaps the most reliable marker of severity. Patients usually report darkening of the urine before they notice scleral icterus. Jaundice is rarely detectable with a bilirubin level <43 μmol/L (2.5 mg/dL). With severe cholestasis there will also be lightening of the color of the stools and steatorrhea. Jaundice without dark urine usually indicates indirect (unconjugated) hyperbilirubinemia and is typical of hemolytic anemia and the genetic disorders of bilirubin conjugation, the common and benign form being Gilbert syndrome and the rare and severe form being Crigler-Najjar syndrome. Gilbert syndrome affects up to 5% of the population; the jaundice is more noticeable after fasting and with stress.

Major risk factors for liver disease that should be sought in the clinical history include details of alcohol use, medications (including herbal compounds, birth control pills, and over-the-counter medications), personal habits, sexual activity, travel, exposure to jaundiced or other high-risk persons, injection drug use, recent surgery, remote or recent transfusion with blood and blood products, occupation, accidental exposure to blood or needlestick, and familial history of liver disease.

For assessing the risk of viral hepatitis, a careful history of sexual activity is of particular importance and should include number of lifetime sexual partners and, for men, a history of having sex with men. Sexual exposure is a common mode of spread of hepatitis B but is rare for hepatitis C. A family history of hepatitis, liver disease, and liver cancer is also important. Maternal-infant transmission occurs with both hepatitis B and C. Vertical spread of hepatitis B can now be prevented by passive and active immunization of the infant at birth. Vertical spread of hepatitis C is uncommon, but there are no reliable means of prevention. Transmission is more common in HIV-co-infected mothers and is also linked to prolonged and difficult labor and delivery, early rupture of membranes, and internal fetal monitoring. A history of injection drug use, even in the remote past, is of great importance in assessing the risk for hepatitis B and C. Injection drug use is now the single most common risk factor for hepatitis C. Transfusion with blood or blood products is no longer an important risk factor for acute viral hepatitis. However, blood transfusions received before the introduction of sensitive enzyme immunoassays for antibody to hepatitis C virus (anti-HCV) in 1992 is an important risk factor for chronic hepatitis C. Blood transfusion before 1986, when screening for antibody to hepatitis B core antigen (anti-HBc) was introduced, is also a risk factor for hepatitis B. Travel to an underdeveloped area of the world, exposure to persons with jaundice, and exposure to young children in day-care centers are risk factors for hepatitis A. Hepatitis E is uncommon in the United States; however, it is one of the more common causes of jaundice in Asia and Africa. Tattooing and body piercing (for hepatitis B and C) and eating shellfish (for hepatitis A) are frequently mentioned but are actually quite rare types of exposure for acquiring hepatitis.

A history of alcohol intake is important in assessing the cause of liver disease and also in planning management and recommendations. In the United States, for example, at least 70% of adults drink alcohol to some degree, but significant alcohol intake is less common; in population-based surveys, only 5% have more than two drinks per day, the average drink representing 11–15 g alcohol. Alcohol consumption associated with an increased rate of alcoholic liver disease is probably more than two drinks (22–30 g) per day in women and three drinks (33–45 g) in men. Most patients with alcoholic cirrhosis have a much higher daily intake and have drunk excessively for ≥10 years before onset of liver disease. In assessing alcohol intake, the history should also focus upon whether alcohol abuse or dependence is present. Alcoholism is usually defined on the behavioral patterns and consequences of alcohol intake, not on the basis of the amount of alcohol intake. *Abuse* is defined by a repetitive pattern of drinking alcohol that has adverse effects on social, family, occupational, or health status. *Dependence* is defined by alcohol-seeking behavior, despite its adverse effects. Many alcoholics demonstrate both dependence and abuse, and dependence is considered the more serious and advanced form of alcoholism. A clinically helpful approach to diagnosis of alcohol dependence and abuse is the use of the CAGE questionnaire (Table 34-2), which is recommended in all medical history taking.

Family history can be helpful in assessing liver disease. Familial causes of liver disease include Wilson disease; hemochromatosis and α₁ antitrypsin (α₁AT) deficiency; and the more uncommon inherited pediatric liver

TABLE 34-2

CAGE QUESTIONS[a]	
ACRONYM	**QUESTION**
C	Have you ever felt you ought to *C*ut down on your drinking?
A	Have people *A*nnoyed you by criticizing your drinking?
G	Have you ever felt *G*uilty or bad about your drinking?
E	Have you ever had a drink first thing in the morning to steady your nerves or get rid of a hangover (*E*yeopener)?

[a]One "yes" response should raise suspicion of an alcohol use problem, and more than one is a strong indication that abuse or dependence exists.

diseases of familial intrahepatic cholestasis, benign recurrent intrahepatic cholestasis, and Alagille syndrome. Onset of severe liver disease in childhood or adolescence with a family history of liver disease or neuropsychiatric disturbance should lead to investigation for Wilson disease. A family history of cirrhosis, diabetes, or endocrine failure and the appearance of liver disease in adulthood should suggest hemochromatosis and lead to investigation of iron status. Patients with abnormal iron studies warrant genotyping of the *HFE* gene for the C282Y and H63D mutations typical of genetic hemochromatosis. A family history of emphysema should provoke investigation of α_1AT levels and, if low, for Pi genotype.

PHYSICAL EXAMINATION

The physical examination rarely demonstrates evidence of liver dysfunction in a patient without symptoms or laboratory findings, nor are most signs of liver disease specific to one diagnosis. Thus, the physical examination usually complements rather than replaces the need for other diagnostic approaches. In many patients, the physical examination is normal unless the disease is acute or severe and advanced. Nevertheless, the physical examination is important in that it can be the first evidence for the presence of hepatic failure, portal hypertension, and liver decompensation. In addition, the physical examination can reveal signs that point to a specific diagnosis, either in risk factors or in associated diseases or findings.

Typical physical findings in liver disease are icterus, hepatomegaly, hepatic tenderness, splenomegaly, spider angiomata, palmar erythema, and excoriations. Signs of advanced disease include muscle-wasting, ascites, edema, dilated abdominal veins, hepatic fetor, asterixis, mental confusion, stupor, and coma. In males with cirrhosis, particularly when related to alcohol, signs of hyperestrogenemia such as gynecomastia, testicular atrophy, and loss of male-pattern hair distribution may be found.

Icterus is best appreciated by inspecting the sclera under natural light. In fair-skinned individuals, a yellow color of the skin may be obvious. In dark-skinned individuals, the mucous membranes below the tongue can demonstrate jaundice. Jaundice is rarely detectable if the serum bilirubin level is <43 μmol/L (2.5 mg/dL) but may remain detectable below this level during recovery from jaundice (because of protein and tissue binding of conjugated bilirubin).

Spider angiomata and palmar erythema occur in both acute and chronic liver disease and may be especially prominent in persons with cirrhosis, but they can occur in normal individuals and are frequently present during pregnancy. Spider angiomata are superficial, tortuous arterioles and, unlike simple telangiectases, typically fill from the center outwards. Spider angiomata occur only on the arms, face, and upper torso; they can be pulsatile and may be difficult to detect in dark-skinned individuals.

Hepatomegaly is not a very reliable sign of liver disease, because of the variability of the size and shape of the liver and the physical impediments to assessing liver size by percussion and palpation. Marked hepatomegaly is typical of cirrhosis, venoocclusive disease, infiltrative disorders such as amyloidosis, metastatic or primary cancers of the liver, and alcoholic hepatitis. Careful assessment of the liver edge may also demonstrate unusual firmness, irregularity of the surface, or frank nodules. Perhaps the most reliable physical finding in examining the liver is hepatic tenderness. Discomfort on touching or pressing on the liver should be carefully sought with percussive comparison of the right and left upper quadrants.

Splenomegaly occurs in many medical conditions but can be a subtle but significant physical finding in liver disease. The availability of ultrasound (US) assessment of the spleen allows for confirmation of the physical finding.

Signs of advanced liver disease include muscle-wasting and weight loss as well as hepatomegaly, bruising, ascites, and edema. Ascites is best appreciated by attempts to detect shifting dullness by careful percussion. US examination will confirm the finding of ascites in equivocal cases. Peripheral edema can occur with or without ascites. In patients with advanced liver disease, other factors frequently contribute to edema formation, including hypoalbuminemia, venous insufficiency, heart failure, and medications.

Hepatic failure is defined as the occurrence of signs or symptoms of hepatic encephalopathy in a person with severe acute or chronic liver disease. The first signs of hepatic encephalopathy can be subtle and nonspecific—change in sleep patterns, change in personality, irritability, and mental dullness. Thereafter, confusion, disorientation, stupor, and eventually coma supervene. In acute liver failure, excitability and mania may be present. Physical findings include asterixis and flapping tremors of the body and tongue. *Fetor hepaticus* refers to the slightly sweet, ammoniacal odor that can occur in patients with liver failure, particularly if there is portal-venous shunting of blood around the liver. Other causes of coma and confusion should be excluded, mainly electrolyte imbalances, sedative use, and renal or respiratory failure. The appearance of hepatic encephalopathy during acute hepatitis is the major criterion for diagnosis of fulminant hepatitis and indicates a poor prognosis. In chronic liver disease, encephalopathy is usually triggered by a medical complication, such as gastrointestinal bleeding, over-diuresis, uremia, dehydration, electrolyte imbalance, infection, constipation, or use of narcotic analgesics.

A helpful measure of hepatic encephalopathy is a careful mental status examination and use of the trail-making test, which consists of a series of 25 numbered circles that the patient is asked to connect as rapidly as possible using a pencil. The normal range for the connect-the-dot test is 15–30 s; it is considerably delayed in patients with early hepatic encephalopathy. Other tests include drawing abstract objects or comparison of a signature to previous examples. More sophisticated testing such as with electroencephalography and visual evoked potentials can detect mild forms of encephalopathy, but are rarely clinically useful.

Other signs of advanced liver disease include umbilical hernia from ascites, hydrothorax, prominent veins over the abdomen, and *caput medusa*, which consists of collateral veins seen radiating from the umbilicus and resulting from the recanulation of the umbilical vein. Widened pulse pressure and signs of a hyperdynamic circulation can occur in patients with cirrhosis as a result of fluid and sodium retention, increased cardiac output, and reduced peripheral resistance. Patients with longstanding cirrhosis and portal hypertension are prone to develop the hepatopulmonary syndrome, defined by the triad of liver disease, hypoxemia, and pulmonary arteriovenous shunting. The hepatopulmonary syndrome is characterized by platypnea and orthodeoxia, representing shortness of breath and oxygen desaturation that occur paradoxically upon assuming an upright position.

Several skin disorders and changes occur commonly in liver disease. Hyperpigmentation is typical of advanced chronic cholestatic diseases such as primary biliary cirrhosis and sclerosing cholangitis. In these same conditions, xanthelasma and tendon xanthomata occur as a result of retention and high serum levels of lipids and cholesterol. A slate-gray pigmentation to the skin also occurs with hemochromatosis if iron levels are high for a prolonged period. Mucocutaneous vasculitis with palpable purpura, especially on the lower extremities, is typical of cryoglobulinemia of chronic hepatitis C but can also occur in chronic hepatitis B.

Some physical signs point to specific liver diseases. Kayser-Fleischer rings occur in Wilson's disease and consist of a golden-brown copper pigment deposited in Descemet's membrane at the periphery of the cornea; they are best seen by slit-lamp examination. Dupuytren contracture and parotid enlargement are suggestive of chronic alcoholism and alcoholic liver disease. In metastatic liver disease or primary hepatocellular carcinoma, signs of cachexia and wasting may be prominent, as well as firm hepatomegaly and a hepatic bruit.

LABORATORY TESTING

Diagnosis in liver disease is greatly aided by the availability of reliable and sensitive tests of liver injury and function. A typical battery of blood tests used for initial assessment of liver disease includes measuring levels of serum alanine and aspartate aminotransferases (ALT and AST), alkaline phosphatase, direct and total serum bilirubin, and albumin and assessing prothrombin time. The pattern of abnormalities generally points to hepatocellular versus cholestatic liver disease and will help to decide whether the disease is acute or chronic and

whether cirrhosis and hepatic failure are present. Based on these results, further testing over time may be necessary. Other laboratory tests may be helpful, such as γ-glutamyl transpeptidase (GGT) to define whether alkaline phosphatase elevations are due to liver disease; hepatitis serology to define the type of viral hepatitis; and autoimmune markers to diagnose primary biliary cirrhosis (antimitochondrial antibody; AMA), sclerosing cholangitis (peripheral antineutrophil cytoplasmic antibody; pANCA), and autoimmune hepatitis (antinuclear, smooth-muscle, and liver-kidney microsomal antibody). A simple delineation of laboratory abnormalities and common liver diseases is given in Table 34-3. The use and interpretation of liver function tests is summarized in Chap. 35.

TABLE 34-3

IMPORTANT DIAGNOSTIC TESTS IN COMMON LIVER DISEASES

DISEASE	DIAGNOSTIC TEST
Hepatitis A	Anti-HAV IgM
Hepatitis B	
Acute	HBsAg and anti-HBc IgM
Chronic	HBsAg and HBeAg and/or HBV DNA
Hepatitis C	Anti-HCV and HCV RNA
Hepatitis D (delta)	HBsAg and anti-HDV
Hepatitis E	Anti-HEV
Autoimmune hepatitis	ANA or SMA, elevated IgG levels, and compatible histology
Primary biliary cirrhosis	Mitochondrial antibody, elevated IgM levels, and compatible histology
Primary sclerosing cholangitis	pANCA, cholangiography
Drug-induced liver disease	History of drug ingestion
Alcoholic liver disease	History of excessive alcohol intake and compatible histology
Nonalcoholic steatohepatitis	Ultrasound or CT evidence of fatty liver and compatible histology
α_1 Antitrypsin disease	Reduced α_1 antitrypsin levels, phenotypes PiZZ or PiSZ
Wilson disease	Decreased serum ceruloplasmin and increased urinary copper; increased hepatic copper level
Hemochromatosis	Elevated iron saturation and serum ferritin; genetic testing for *HFE* gene mutations
Hepatocellular cancer	Elevated α-fetoprotein level >500; ultrasound or CT image of mass

Note: HAV, HBV, HCV, HDV, HEV: hepatitis A, B, C, D, or E virus; HBsAg, hepatitis B surface antigen; anti-HBc, antibody to hepatitis B core (antigen); HBeAg, hepatitis e antigen; ANA, antinuclear antibodies; SMA, smooth-muscle antibody; pANCA, peripheral antineutrophil cytoplasmic antibody.

DIAGNOSTIC IMAGING

There have been great advances made in hepatic imaging, although no method is suitably accurate in demonstrating underlying cirrhosis. There are many modalities available for imaging the liver. US, CT, and MRI are the most commonly employed and are complementary to each other. In general, US and CT have a high sensitivity for detecting biliary duct dilatation and are the first-line options for investigating the patient with suspected obstructive jaundice. Both US and CT can detect a fatty liver, which appears bright on both studies. Magnetic resonance cholangiopancreatography (MRCP) and endoscopic retrograde cholangiopancreatography (ERCP) are the procedures of choice for visualization of the biliary tree. MRCP offers several advantages over ERCP; there is no need for contrast media or ionizing radiation, images can be acquired faster, it is less operator dependent, and it carries no risk of pancreatitis. MRCP is superior to US and CT for detecting choledocholithiasis but less specific. It is useful in the diagnosis of bile duct obstruction and congenital biliary abnormalities, but ERCP is more valuable in evaluating ampullary lesions and primary sclerosing cholangitis. ERCP allows for biopsy, direct visualization of the ampulla and common bile duct, and intraductal ultrasonography. It also provides several therapeutic options in patients with obstructive jaundice, such as sphincterotomy, stone extraction, and placement of nasobiliary catheters and biliary stents. Doppler US and MRI are used to assess hepatic vasculature and hemodynamics and to monitor surgically or radiologically placed vascular shunts such as transjugular intrahepatic portosystemic shunts. CT and MRI are indicated for the identification and evaluation of hepatic masses, staging of liver tumors, and preoperative assessment. With regard to mass lesions, sensitivity of hepatic imaging continues to increase; unfortunately, specificity remains a problem, and often two and sometimes three studies are needed before a diagnosis can be reached. Recently, methods using elastrography have been developed to measure hepatic stiffness as a means of assessing hepatic fibrosis. US elastrography is now undergoing evaluation for its ability to detect different degrees of hepatic fibrosis and to obviate the need for liver biopsy in assessing disease stage. If found to be reliable, hepatic elastrography may be an appropriate means of monitoring fibrosis and disease progression. Finally, interventional radiologic techniques allow the biopsy of solitary lesions, insertion of drains into hepatic abscesses, measurement of portal pressure, and creation of vascular shunts in patients with portal hypertension. Which modality to use depends on factors such as availability, cost, and experience of the radiologist with each technique.

LIVER BIOPSY

Liver biopsy remains the gold standard in the evaluation of patients with liver disease, particularly in patients with chronic liver diseases. In selected instances, liver biopsy is necessary for diagnosis but is more often useful in assessing the severity (grade) and stage of liver damage, in predicting prognosis, and in monitoring response to treatment. The size of the liver biopsy is an important determinant of its reliability; a length of 1.5–2 cm being necessary for accurate assessment of fibrosis. In the future, noninvasive means of assessing disease activity (batteries of blood tests) and fibrosis (elastrography and fibrosis markers) may replace liver biopsy in assessing stage and grade of disease.

DIAGNOSIS OF LIVER DISEASE

The major causes of liver disease and key diagnostic features are outlined in Table 34-3, and an algorithm for evaluation of the patient with suspected liver disease is given in **Fig. 34-1**. Specifics of diagnosis are discussed in later chapters. The most common causes of acute liver disease are viral hepatitis (particularly hepatitis A, B, and C), drug-induced liver injury, cholangitis, and alcoholic liver disease. Liver biopsy is usually not needed in the diagnosis and management of acute liver disease, exceptions being situations where the diagnosis remains unclear despite thorough clinical and laboratory investigation. Liver biopsy can be helpful in the diagnosis of drug-induced liver disease and in establishing the diagnosis of acute alcoholic hepatitis.

The most common causes of chronic liver disease in general order of frequency are chronic hepatitis C, alcoholic liver disease, nonalcoholic steatohepatitis, chronic hepatitis B, autoimmune hepatitis, sclerosing cholangitis, primary biliary cirrhosis, hemochromatosis, and Wilson disease. Strict diagnostic criteria have not been developed for most liver diseases, but liver biopsy plays an important role in the diagnosis of autoimmune hepatitis, primary biliary cirrhosis, nonalcoholic and alcoholic steatohepatitis, and Wilson disease (with a quantitative hepatic copper level).

GRADING AND STAGING OF LIVER DISEASE

Grading refers to an assessment of the severity or activity of liver disease, whether acute or chronic; active or inactive; and mild, moderate, or severe. Liver biopsy is the most accurate means of assessing severity, particularly in chronic liver disease. Serum aminotransferase levels are used as a convenient and noninvasive means to follow disease activity, but aminotransferase levels are not always reliable in reflecting disease severity. Thus, normal serum aminotransferase levels in patients with hepatitis B surface antigen (HBsAg) in serum may indicate the inactive HBsAg carrier state or may reflect mild chronic hepatitis B or hepatitis B with fluctuating disease activity. Serum testing for hepatitis B e antigen and hepatitis B virus DNA can help resolve these different patterns, but these markers can also fluctuate and change over time. Similarly, in chronic hepatitis C, serum aminotransferase levels

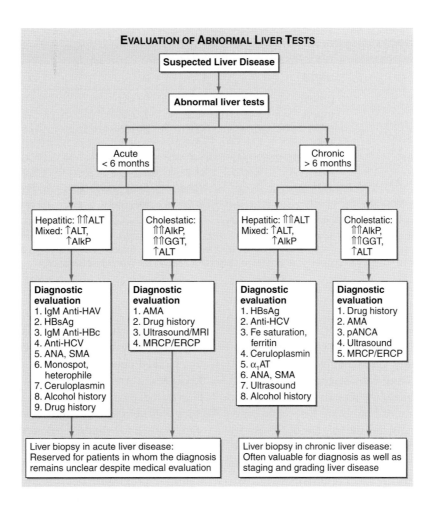

FIGURE 34-1

Algorithm for evaluation of abnormal liver tests. For patients with suspected liver disease, an appropriate approach to evaluation is initial testing for routine liver tests such as bilirubin, albumin, alanine aminotransferase (ALT), aspartate aminotransferase (AST), and alkaline phosphatase (AlkP). These results (sometimes complemented by testing of γ-glutamyl transpeptidase; GGT) will establish whether the pattern of abnormalities is hepatic, cholestatic, or mixed. In addition, the duration of symptoms or abnormalities will show whether the disease is acute or chronic. If the disease is acute and if history, laboratory tests, and imaging studies do not reveal a diagnosis, liver biopsy is appropriate to help to establish the diagnosis. If the disease is chronic, liver biopsy can be helpful not only for diagnosis but also to grade the activity and stage the progression of disease. This approach is largely applicable to patients without immune deficiency. In patients with HIV infection or after bone marrow or solid organ transplantation, diagnostic evaluation should also include evaluation of opportunistic infections (adenovirus, cytomegalovirus, coccidioidomycosis, etc.) as well as vascular and immunologic conditions (venoocclusive disease, graft-vs-host disease). HAV, HCV: hepatitis A or C virus; HBsAg, hepatitis B surface antigen; anti-HBc, antibody to hepatitis B core (antigen); ANA, antinuclear antibodies; SMA, smooth-muscle antibody; MRCP, magnetic resonance cholangiopancreatography; ERCP, endoscopic retrograde cholangiopancreatography; α_1AT, α_1 antitrypsin; AMA, antimitochondrial antibody; pANCA, perinuclear antineutrophil cytoplasmic antibody.

can be normal despite moderate activity of disease. Finally, in both alcoholic and nonalcoholic steatohepatitis, aminotransferase levels are quite unreliable in reflecting severity. In these conditions, liver biopsy is helpful in guiding management and recommending therapy, particularly if therapy is difficult, prolonged, and expensive as is often the case in chronic viral hepatitis. There are several well-verified numerical scales for grading activity in chronic liver disease, the most common being the histology activity index and the Ishak histology scale.

Liver biopsy is also the most accurate means of assessing stage of disease as early or advanced, precirrhotic, and cirrhotic. Staging of disease pertains largely to chronic liver diseases in which progression to cirrhosis and end-stage liver disease can occur, but which may require years or decades to develop. Clinical features, biochemical tests, and hepatic imaging studies are helpful in assessing stage but generally become abnormal only in the middle to late stages of cirrhosis. Noninvasive tests that suggest advanced fibrosis include mild elevations of bilirubin, prolongation of prothrombin time, slight decreases in serum albumin, and mild thrombocytopenia (which is often the first indication of worsening fibrosis). Combinations of blood test results have been used to create models for predicting

TABLE 34-4

CHILD-PUGH CLASSIFICATION OF CIRRHOSIS

FACTOR	UNITS	1	2	3
Serum bilirubin	μmol/L	<34	34–51	>51
	mg/dL	<2.0	2.0–3.0	>3.0
Serum albumin	g/L	>35	30–35	<30
	g/dL	>3.5	3.0–3.5	<3.0
Prothrombin time	Seconds prolonged	0–4	4–6	>6
	INR	<1.7	1.7–2.3	>2.3
Ascites		None	Easily controlled	Poorly controlled
Hepatic encephalopathy		None	Minimal	Advanced

Note: The Child-Pugh score is calculated by adding the scores of the five factors and can range from 5–15. Child-Pugh class is either A (a score of 5–6), B (7–9), or C (10 or above). Decompensation indicates cirrhosis with a Child-Pugh score of 7 or more (class B). This level has been the accepted criterion for listing for liver transplantation.

advanced liver disease, but these are not reliable enough to use on a regular basis and they only separate advanced from early disease. Recently, elastography has been proposed as a means of detecting early stages of fibrosis, but its reliability and reproducibility remain to be proven. Thus, at present early stages of fibrosis are detectable only by liver biopsy. In assessing stage, the degree of fibrosis is usually used as its quantitative measure. The amount of fibrosis is generally staged on a 0 to 4+ (histology activity index) or 0 to 6+ scale (Ishak scale). The importance of staging relates primarily to prognosis and to guiding management of complications. Patients with cirrhosis are candidates for screening and surveillance for esophageal varices and hepatocellular carcinoma. Patients without advanced fibrosis need not undergo screening.

Cirrhosis can also be staged clinically. A reliable staging system is the modified Child-Pugh classification with a scoring system of 5–15: scores of 5 and 6 being Child-Pugh class A (consistent with "compensated cirrhosis"), scores of 7–9 indicating class B, and 10–15 class C (Table 34-4). This scoring system was initially devised to stratify patients into risk groups prior to undergoing portal decompressive surgery. The Child-Pugh score is a reasonably reliable predictor of survival in many liver diseases and predicts the likelihood of major complications of cirrhosis such as bleeding from varices and spontaneous bacterial peritonitis. It was used to assess prognosis in cirrhosis and to provide the standard criteria for listing for liver transplantation (Child-Pugh class B). Recently the Child-Pugh system has been replaced by the model for end-stage liver disease (MELD) score for assessing the need for liver transplantation. The MELD score is a prospectively derived scoring system designed to predict prognosis of patients with liver disease and portal hypertension. It is calculated using three noninvasive variables—the prothrombin time expressed as international normalized ratio (INR), serum bilirubin, and serum creatinine (http://www.unos.org/resources/meldPeldCalculator.asp).

MELD provides a more objective means of assessing disease severity and has less center-to-center variation than the Child-Pugh score and has a wider range of values. MELD is currently used to establish priority listing for liver transplantation in the United States. A similar system using bilirubin, INR, serum albumin, age, and nutritional status is used for children below the age of 12 (PELD).

Thus, liver biopsy is helpful not only in diagnosis but also in management of chronic liver disease and assessment of prognosis. Because liver biopsy is an invasive procedure and not without complications, it should be used only when it will contribute materially to management and therapeutic decisions.

NONSPECIFIC ISSUES IN MANAGEMENT OF PATIENTS WITH LIVER DISEASE

Specifics on management of different forms of acute or chronic liver disease are given in subsequent chapters, but certain issues are applicable to any patient with liver disease. These include advice regarding alcohol use, medications, vaccination, and surveillance for complications of liver disease. Alcohol should be used sparingly, if at all, by patients with liver disease. Abstinence from alcohol should be encouraged for all patients with alcohol-related liver disease and in patients with cirrhosis and those receiving interferon-based therapy for hepatitis B or C. Regarding vaccinations, all patients with liver disease should receive hepatitis A vaccine and those with risk factors should receive hepatitis B vaccination as well. Influenza and pneumococcal vaccination should also be encouraged. Patients with liver disease should be careful in use of any medications, other than the most necessary. Drug-induced hepatotoxicity can mimic many forms of liver disease and can cause exacerbations of chronic hepatitis and cirrhosis; drugs should be suspected in any situation where the cause of exacerbation is unknown. Finally, consideration should be given to surveillance for complications of chronic liver disease such as variceal hemorrhage and hepatocellular carcinoma. Patients with cirrhosis warrant upper endoscopy to assess the presence of varices and should be given chronic therapy with beta blockers or offered endoscopic obliteration if large varices are found. Patients with cirrhosis also warrant screening and long-term surveillance for development of hepatocellular carcinoma. While the optimal regimen for such surveillance has not been established, an appropriate approach is US of the liver at 6- to 12-month intervals.

FURTHER READINGS

BOYER TD et al (eds): *Zakim and Boyer's Hepatology: A Textbook of Liver Disease*, 5th ed. Philadelphia, Saunders, 2006

CASTERA L et al: Prospective comparison of transient elastography, Fibrotest, APRI, and liver biopsy for the assessment of fibrosis in chronic hepatitis C. Gastroenterology 128:343, 2005

KAPLOWITZ N, DELEVE LD (eds): *Drug-Induced Liver Disease*. New York, Marcel Dekker, 2003

KLEINER DE: The liver biopsy in chronic hepatitis C: A view from the other side of the microscope. Semin Liver Dis 25:52, 2005

MANI H, KLEINER DE: Liver biopsy findings in chronic hepatitis B. Hepatology 49:S61, 2009

MARIN D at al: Imaging approach for evaluation of focal liver lesions. Clin Gastroenterol Hepatol 7:624, 2009

SAINI S: Imaging of the hepatobiliary tract. N Engl J Med 336:1880, 1997

TAOULI B et al: Advanced MRI methods for assessment of chronic liver disease. AJR Am J Roentgenol 193:14, 2009

WIESNER R et al: United Network for Organ Sharing Liver Disease Severity Score Committee. Model for end-stage liver disease (MELD) and allocation of donor livers. Gastroenterology 124:91:2003

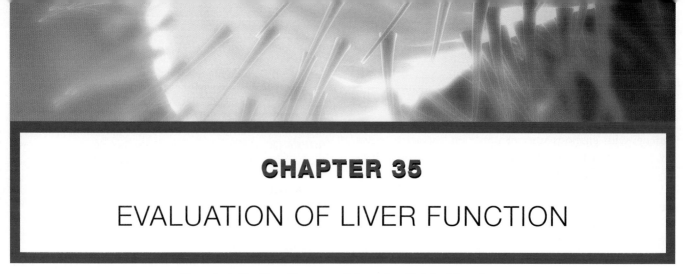

CHAPTER 35

EVALUATION OF LIVER FUNCTION

Daniel S. Pratt ■ Marshall M. Kaplan

Several biochemical tests are useful in the evaluation and management of patients with hepatic dysfunction. These tests can be used to (1) detect the presence of liver disease, (2) distinguish among different types of liver disorders, (3) gauge the extent of known liver damage, and (4) follow the response to treatment.

Liver tests have shortcomings. They can be normal in patients with serious liver disease and abnormal in patients with diseases that do not affect the liver. Liver tests rarely suggest a specific diagnosis; rather, they suggest a general category of liver disease, such as hepatocellular or cholestatic, which then further directs the evaluation.

The liver carries out thousands of biochemical functions, most of which cannot be easily measured by blood tests. Laboratory tests measure only a limited number of these functions. In fact, many tests, such as the aminotransferases or alkaline phosphatase, do not measure liver function at all. Rather, they detect liver cell damage or interference with bile flow. Thus, no one test enables the clinician to accurately assess the liver's total functional capacity.

To increase both the sensitivity and the specificity of laboratory tests in the detection of liver disease, it is best to use them as a battery. Those tests usually employed in clinical practice include the bilirubin, aminotransferases, alkaline phosphatase, albumin, and prothrombin time tests. When more than one of these tests provide abnormal findings, or the findings are persistently abnormal on serial determinations, the probability of liver disease is high. When all test results are normal, the probability of missing occult liver disease is low.

When evaluating patients with liver disorders, it is helpful to group these tests into general categories. The classification we have found most useful is followed in the next sections.

TESTS BASED ON DETOXIFICATION AND EXCRETORY FUNCTIONS

Serum Bilirubin

Bilirubin, a breakdown product of the porphyrin ring of heme-containing proteins, is found in the blood in two fractions—conjugated and unconjugated. The unconjugated fraction, also termed the *indirect fraction,* is insoluble in water and is bound to albumin in the blood. The conjugated (direct) bilirubin fraction is water soluble and can therefore be excreted by the kidney. When measured by the original van den Bergh method, the normal total serum bilirubin concentration is <17 μmol/L (1 mg/dL). Up to 30%, or 5.1 μmol/L (0.3 mg/dL), of the total is direct-reacting (or conjugated) bilirubin.

Elevation of the unconjugated fraction of bilirubin is rarely due to liver disease. An isolated elevation of unconjugated bilirubin is seen primarily in hemolytic disorders and in a number of genetic conditions such as Crigler-Najjar and Gilbert's syndromes. Isolated unconjugated hyperbilirubinemia (bilirubin elevated but <15% direct) should prompt a workup for hemolysis (Fig. 35-1). In the absence of hemolysis, an isolated unconjugated

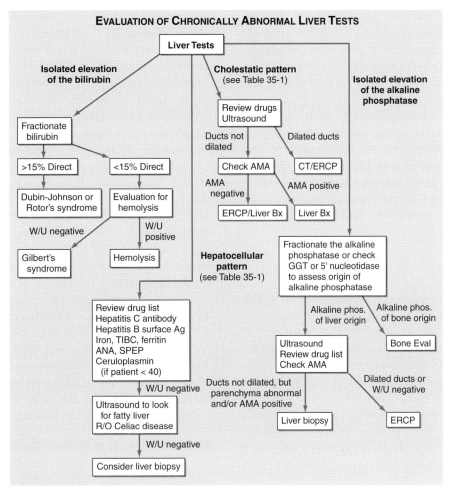

FIGURE 35-1

Algorithm for the evaluation of chronically abnormal liver tests. ERCP, endoscopic retrograde cholangiopancreatography; CT, computed tomography; AMA, antimito-chondrial antibody; ANA, antinuclear antibody; SPEP, serum protein electrophoresis; TIBC, total iron-binding capacity; GGT, γ glutamyl transpeptidase; W/U, workup.

hyperbilirubinemia in an otherwise healthy patient can be attributed to Gilbert's syndrome and no further evaluation is required.

In contrast, conjugated hyperbilirubinemia almost always implies liver or biliary tract disease. The rate-limiting step in bilirubin metabolism is not conjugation of bilirubin, but rather the transport of conjugated bilirubin into the bile canaliculi. Thus, elevation of the conjugated fraction may be seen in any type of liver disease. In most liver diseases, both conjugated and unconjugated fractions of the bilirubin tend to be elevated. Except in the presence of a purely unconjugated hyperbilirubinemia, fractionation of the bilirubin is rarely helpful in determining the cause of jaundice.

Urine Bilirubin

Unconjugated bilirubin always binds to albumin in the serum and is not filtered by the kidney. Therefore, any bilirubin found in the urine is conjugated bilirubin; the presence of bilirubinuria implies the presence of liver disease. A urine dipstick test can theoretically give the same information as fractionation of the serum bilirubin. This test is almost 100% accurate. Phenothiazines may give a false-positive reading with the Ictotest tablet. In patients recovering from jaundice, the urine bilirubin clears prior to the serum bilirubin.

Blood Ammonia

Ammonia is produced in the body during normal protein metabolism and by intestinal bacteria, primarily those in the colon. The liver plays a role in the detoxification of ammonia by converting it to urea, which is excreted by the kidneys. Striated muscle also plays a role in detoxification of ammonia, which is combined with glutamic acid to form glutamine. Patients with advanced liver disease typically have significant muscle wasting, which likely contributes to hyperammonemia in these patients. Some physicians use the blood ammonia for detecting encephalopathy or for monitoring hepatic synthetic function, although its use for either of these indications has problems. There is very poor correlation between either the presence or the severity of acute encephalopathy and elevation of blood ammonia; it can be occasionally useful for identifying occult liver disease in patients with mental status changes. There is also a poor correlation of the blood serum ammonia and hepatic function. The ammonia can be elevated in patients with severe portal hypertension and portal blood shunting around the liver even in the presence of normal or near-normal hepatic function. Elevated arterial ammonia levels have been shown to correlate with outcome in fulminant hepatic failure.

Serum Enzymes

The liver contains thousands of enzymes, some of which are also present in the serum in very low concentrations. These enzymes have no known function in the serum and behave like other serum proteins. They are distributed in the plasma and in interstitial fluid and have characteristic half-lives, usually measured in days. Very little is known about the catabolism of serum enzymes, although they are probably cleared by cells in the reticuloendothelial system. The elevation of a given enzyme activity in the serum is thought to primarily reflect its increased rate of entrance into serum from damaged liver cells.

Serum enzyme tests can be grouped into three categories: (1) enzymes whose elevation in serum reflects damage to hepatocytes, (2) enzymes whose elevation in serum reflects cholestasis, and (3) enzyme tests that do not fit precisely into either pattern.

Enzymes That Reflect Damage to Hepatocytes

The aminotransferases (transaminases) are sensitive indicators of liver cell injury and are most helpful in recognizing acute hepatocellular diseases such as hepatitis. They include the aspartate aminotransferase (AST) and the alanine aminotransferase (ALT). AST is found in the liver, cardiac muscle, skeletal muscle, kidneys, brain, pancreas, lungs, leukocytes, and erythrocytes in decreasing order of concentration. ALT is found primarily in the liver. The aminotransferases are normally present in the serum in low concentrations. These enzymes are released into the blood in greater amounts when there is damage to the liver cell membrane resulting in increased permeability. Liver cell necrosis is not required for the release of the aminotransferases, and there is a poor correlation between the degree of liver cell damage and the level of the aminotransferases. Thus, the absolute elevation of the aminotransferases is of no prognostic significance in acute hepatocellular disorders.

Any type of liver cell injury can cause modest elevations in the serum aminotransferases. Levels of up to 300 U/L are nonspecific and may be found in any type of liver disorder. Minimal ALT elevations in asymptomatic blood donors rarely indicate severe liver disease; studies have shown that fatty liver disease is the most likely explanation. Striking elevations—i.e., aminotransferases >1000 U/L—occur almost exclusively in disorders associated with extensive hepatocellular injury such as (1) viral hepatitis, (2) ischemic liver injury (prolonged hypotension or acute heart failure), or (3) toxin- or drug-induced liver injury.

The pattern of the aminotransferase elevation can be helpful diagnostically. In most acute hepatocellular disorders, the ALT is higher than or equal to the AST. An AST:ALT ratio >2:1 is suggestive while a ratio >3:1 is highly suggestive of alcoholic liver disease. The AST in alcoholic liver disease is rarely >300 U/L and the ALT is often normal. A low level of ALT in the serum is due to an alcohol-induced deficiency of pyridoxal phosphate.

The aminotransferases are usually not greatly elevated in obstructive jaundice. One notable exception occurs during the acute phase of biliary obstruction caused by the passage of a gallstone into the common bile duct. In this setting, the aminotransferases can briefly be in the 1000–2000 U/L range. However, aminotransferase levels decrease quickly, and the liver function tests rapidly evolve into one typical of cholestasis.

Enzymes That Reflect Cholestasis

The activities of three enzymes—alkaline phosphatase, 5′-nucleotidase, and γ-glutamyl transpeptidase (GGT)—are usually elevated in cholestasis. Alkaline phosphatase and 5′-nucleotidase are found in or near the bile canalicular membrane of hepatocytes, while GGT is located in the endoplasmic reticulum and in bile duct epithelial cells. Reflecting its more diffuse localization in the liver, GGT elevation in serum is less specific for cholestasis than are elevations of alkaline phosphatase or 5′-nucleotidase. Some have advocated the use of GGT to identify patients with occult alcohol use. Its lack of specificity makes its use in this setting questionable.

The normal serum alkaline phosphatase consists of many distinct isoenzymes found in the liver, bone, placenta, and, less commonly, small intestine. Patients over age 60 can have a mildly elevated alkaline phosphatase (1–1½ times normal), while individuals with blood types O and B can have an elevation of the serum alkaline phosphatase after eating a fatty meal due to the influx of intestinal alkaline phosphatase into the blood. It is also nonpathologically elevated in children and adolescents undergoing rapid bone growth, because of bone alkaline phosphatase, and late in normal pregnancies due to the influx of placental alkaline phosphatase.

Elevation of liver-derived alkaline phosphatase is not totally specific for cholestasis, and a less than threefold elevation can be seen in almost any type of liver disease. Alkaline phosphatase elevations greater than four times normal occur primarily in patients with cholestatic liver disorders, infiltrative liver diseases such as cancer and amyloidosis, and bone conditions characterized by rapid bone turnover (e.g., Paget's disease). In bone diseases, the elevation is due to increased amounts of the bone isoenzymes. In liver diseases, the elevation is almost always due to increased amounts of the liver isoenzyme.

If an elevated serum alkaline phosphatase is the only abnormal finding in an apparently healthy person, or if the degree of elevation is higher than expected in the clinical setting, identification of the source of elevated isoenzymes is helpful (Fig. 35-1). This problem can be approached in several ways. First, and most precise, is the fractionation of the alkaline phosphatase by electrophoresis. The second approach is based on the observation that alkaline phosphatases from individual tissues differ in susceptibility to inactivation by heat. The finding of an elevated serum alkaline phosphatase level in a patient with a heat-stable fraction strongly suggests that the placenta or a tumor is the source of the elevated enzyme in serum. Susceptibility to inactivation by heat increases, respectively, for the intestinal, liver, and bone alkaline phosphatases, bone being by far the most sensitive. The third, best substantiated, and most available approach involves the measurement of serum 5′-nucleotidase or GGT. These enzymes are rarely elevated in conditions other than liver disease.

In the absence of jaundice or elevated aminotransferases, an elevated alkaline phosphatase of liver origin often, but not always, suggests early cholestasis and, less often, hepatic infiltration by tumor or granulomata. Other conditions that cause isolated elevations of the alkaline phosphatase include Hodgkin's disease, diabetes, hyperthyroidism, congestive heart failure, amyloidosis, and inflammatory bowel disease.

The level of serum alkaline phosphatase elevation is not helpful in distinguishing between intrahepatic and extrahepatic cholestasis. There is essentially no difference among the values found in obstructive jaundice due to cancer, common duct stone, sclerosing cholangitis, or bile duct stricture. Values are similarly increased in patients with intrahepatic cholestasis due to drug-induced hepatitis, primary biliary cirrhosis, rejection of transplanted livers, and, rarely, alcohol-induced steatonecrosis. Values are also greatly elevated in hepatobiliary disorders seen in patients with AIDS (e.g., AIDS cholangiopathy due to cytomegalovirus or cryptosporidial infection and tuberculosis with hepatic involvement).

TESTS THAT MEASURE BIOSYNTHETIC FUNCTION OF THE LIVER

Serum Albumin

Serum albumin is synthesized exclusively by hepatocytes. Serum albumin has a long half-life: 18–20 days, with ~4% degraded per day. Because of this slow turnover, the serum albumin is not a good indicator of acute or mild hepatic dysfunction; only minimal changes in the serum albumin are seen in acute liver conditions such as viral hepatitis, drug-related hepatoxicity, and obstructive jaundice. In hepatitis, albumin levels <3 g/dL should raise the possibility of chronic liver disease. Hypoalbuminemia is more common in chronic liver disorders such as cirrhosis and usually reflects severe liver damage and decreased albumin synthesis. One exception is the patient with ascites in whom synthesis may be normal or even increased, but levels are low because of the increased volume of distribution. However, hypoalbuminemia is not specific for liver disease and may occur in protein malnutrition of any cause, as well as protein-losing enteropathies, nephrotic syndrome, and chronic infections that are associated with prolonged increases in levels of serum interleukin 1 and/or tumor necrosis factor, cytokines that inhibit albumin synthesis. Serum albumin should not be measured for screening in patients in whom there is no suspicion of liver disease. A general medical clinic study of consecutive patients in whom no indications were present for albumin measurement showed that while 12% of patients had abnormal test results, the finding was of clinical importance in only 0.4%.

Serum Globulins

Serum globulins are a group of proteins made up of γ globulins (immunoglobulins) produced by B lymphocytes and α and β globulins produced primarily in hepatocytes. γ Globulins are increased in chronic liver disease, such as chronic hepatitis and cirrhosis. In cirrhosis, the increased serum gamma globulin concentration is due to the increased synthesis of antibodies, some of which are directed against intestinal bacteria. This occurs because the cirrhotic liver fails to clear bacterial antigens that normally reach the liver through the hepatic circulation.

Increases in the concentration of specific isotypes of γ globulins are often helpful in the recognition of certain chronic liver diseases. Diffuse polyclonal increases in IgG levels are common in autoimmune hepatitis; increases >100% should alert the clinician to this possibility. Increases in the IgM levels are common in primary biliary cirrhosis, while increases in the IgA levels occur in alcoholic liver disease.

COAGULATION FACTORS

With the exception of factor VIII, the blood clotting factors are made exclusively in hepatocytes. Their serum half-lives are much shorter than albumin, ranging from 6 h for factor VII to 5 days for fibrinogen. Because of their rapid turnover, measurement of the clotting factors is the single best acute measure of hepatic synthetic function and helpful in both the diagnosis and assessing the prognosis of acute parenchymal liver disease. Useful for this purpose is the *serum prothrombin time,* which

TABLE 35-1

LIVER TEST PATTERNS IN HEPATOBILIARY DISORDERS

TYPE OF DISORDER	BILIRUBIN	AMINOTRANSFERASES	ALKALINE PHOSPHATASE	ALBUMIN	PROTHROMBIN TIME
Hemolysis/Gilbert's syndrome	Normal to 86 µmol/L (5 mg/dL) 85% due to indirect fractions No bilirubinuria	Normal	Normal	Normal	Normal
Acute hepatocellular necrosis (viral and drug hepatitis, hepatotoxins, acute heart failure)	Both fractions may be elevated Peak usually follows aminotransferases Bilirubinuria	Elevated, often >500 IU ALT >AST	Normal to <3 times normal elevation	Normal	Usually normal. If >5X above control and not corrected by parenteral vitamin K, suggests poor prognosis
Chronic hepato-cellular disorders	Both fractions may be elevated Bilirubinuria	Elevated, but usually <300 IU	Normal to <3 times normal elevation	Often decreased	Often prolonged Fails to correct with parenteral vitamin K
Alcoholic hepatitis Cirrhosis	Both fractions may be elevated Bilirubinuria	AST:ALT >2 suggests alcoholic hepatitis or cirrhosis	Normal to <3 times normal elevation	Often decreased	Often prolonged Fails to correct with parenteral vitamin K
Intra- and extra-hepatic cholestasis (Obstructive jaundice)	Both fractions may be elevated Bilirubinuria	Normal to moderate elevation Rarely >500 IU	Elevated, often >4 times normal elevation	Normal, unless chronic	Normal If prolonged, will correct with parenteral vitamin K
Infiltrative diseases (tumor, granulomata); partial bile duct obstruction	Usually normal	Normal to slight elevation	Elevated, often >4 times normal elevation Fractionate, or confirm liver origin with 5' nucleotidase or γ glutamyl transpeptidase	Normal	Normal

collectively measures factors II, V, VII, and X. Biosynthesis of factors II, VII, IX, and X depends on vitamin K. The prothrombin time may be elevated in hepatitis and cirrhosis as well as in disorders that lead to vitamin K deficiency such as obstructive jaundice or fat malabsorption of any kind. Marked prolongation of the prothrombin time, >5 s above control and not corrected by parenteral vitamin K administration, is a poor prognostic sign in acute viral hepatitis and other acute and chronic liver diseases.

OTHER DIAGNOSTIC TESTS

While tests may direct the physician to a category of liver disease, additional radiologic testing and procedures are often necessary to make the proper diagnosis, as shown in Fig. 35-1. The two most commonly used ancillary tests are reviewed here.

Percutaneous Liver Biopsy

Percutaneous biopsy of the liver is a safe procedure that can be easily performed at the bedside with local anesthesia. Liver biopsy is of proven value in the following situations: (1) hepatocellular disease of uncertain cause, (2) prolonged hepatitis with the possibility of chronic active hepatitis, (3) unexplained hepatomegaly, (4) unexplained splenomegaly, (5) hepatic filling defects by radiologic imaging, (6) fever of unknown origin, and (7) staging of malignant lymphoma. Liver biopsy is most accurate in disorders causing diffuse changes throughout the liver and is subject to sampling error in focal infiltrative disorders such as hepatic metastases. Liver biopsy should not be the initial procedure in the diagnosis of cholestasis. The biliary tree should first be assessed for signs of obstruction. Contraindications to performing a percutaneous liver biopsy include significant ascites and prolonged INR. Under these circumstances the biopsy can be performed via the transjugular approach.

Ultrasonography

Ultrasonography is the first diagnostic test to use in patients whose liver tests suggest cholestasis, to look for the presence of a dilated intrahepatic or extrahepatic biliary tree or to identify gallstones. In addition, it shows space-occupying lesions within the liver, enables the clinician to distinguish between cystic and solid masses, and helps direct percutaneous biopsies. Ultrasound with Doppler imaging can detect the patency of the portal vein, hepatic artery, and hepatic veins and determine the direction of blood flow. This is the first test ordered in patients suspected of having Budd-Chiari syndrome.

USE OF LIVER TESTS

As previously noted, the best way to increase the sensitivity and specificity of laboratory tests in the detection of liver disease is to employ a battery of tests that include the aminotransferases, alkaline phosphatase, bilirubin, albumin, and prothrombin time along with the judicious use of the other tests described in this chapter. Table 35-1 shows how patterns of liver tests can lead the clinician to a category of disease that will direct further evaluation. However, it is important to remember that no single set of liver tests will necessarily provide a diagnosis. It is often necessary to repeat these tests on several occasions over days to weeks for a diagnostic pattern to emerge. Figure 35-1 is an algorithm for the evaluation of chronically abnormal liver tests.

FURTHER READINGS

BHATIA V et al: Predictive value of arterial ammonia for complications and outcome in acute liver failure. Gut 55:98, 2006

BOSMA PJ et al: The genetic basis of the reduced expression of bilirubin UDP-glucuronosyltransferase 1 in Gilbert's syndrome. N Engl J Med 333:1171, 1995

BRENSILVER HL, KAPLAN MM: Significance of elevated liver alkaline phosphatase in serum. Gastroenterology 68:1556, 1975

BURKE MD: Liver function: test selection and interpretation of results. Clin Lab Med 22:377, 2002

COHEN JA, KAPLAN MM: The SGOT/SGPT ratio: An indicator of alcoholic liver disease. Dig Dis Sci 24:835, 1979

NG VL: Liver disease, coagulation testing, and hemostasis. Clin Lab Med 29:265, 2009

PRATT DS, KAPLAN MM: Evaluation of abnormal liver-enzyme tests in the asymptomatic patient. N Engl J Med 342:1266, 2000

———: Laboratory tests, in *Schiff's Diseases of the Liver,* 9th ed, ER Schiff et al (eds). Philadelphia, Lippincott Williams & Wilkins, 2003

TOREZAN-FILHO MA et al: Clinical significance of elevated alanine aminotransferase in blood donors: A follow-up study. Liver Int 24:575, 2004

WEISS JS et al: The clinical importance of a protein bound fraction of serum bilirubin in patients with hyperbilirubinemia. N Engl J Med 309:147, 1983

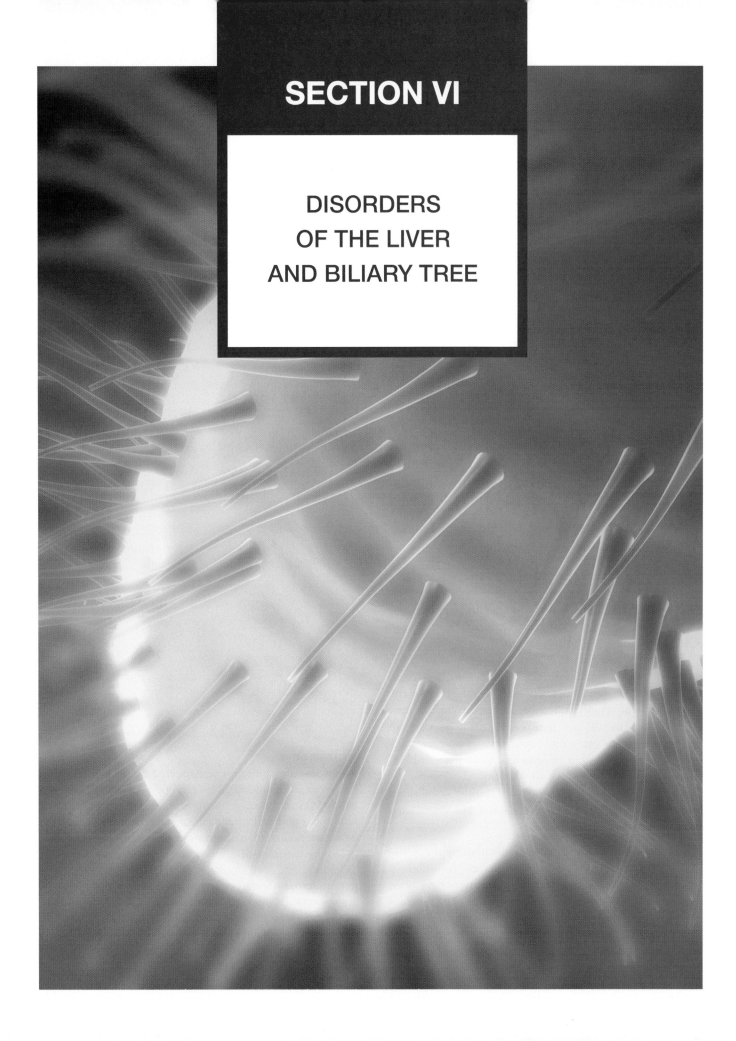

SECTION VI

DISORDERS
OF THE LIVER
AND BILIARY TREE

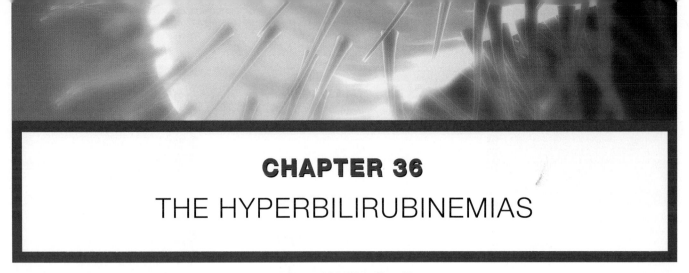

CHAPTER 36
THE HYPERBILIRUBINEMIAS

Allan W. Wolkoff

BILIRUBIN METABOLISM

The hyperbilirubinemias are best understood in terms of perturbations of specific aspects of bilirubin metabolism (Chap. 9) and transport, and these will be briefly reviewed here as depicted in **Fig. 36-1**.

Bilirubin is the end product of heme degradation. From 70–90% of bilirubin is derived from degradation of the hemoglobin of senescent red blood cells. Bilirubin produced in the periphery is transported to the liver within the plasma, where, due to its insolubility in aqueous solutions, it is tightly bound to albumin. Under normal circumstances, bilirubin is removed from the circulation rapidly and efficiently by hepatocytes. Transfer of bilirubin from blood to bile involves four distinct but interrelated steps (Fig. 36-1):

1. *Hepatocellular uptake:* Uptake of bilirubin by the hepatocyte has carrier-mediated kinetics. Although a number of candidate bilirubin transporters have been proposed, the actual transporter remains elusive.
2. *Intracellular binding:* Within the hepatocyte, bilirubin is kept in solution by binding as a nonsubstrate ligand to several of the glutathione–S-transferases, formerly called ligandins.

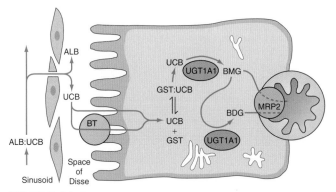

FIGURE 36-1

Hepatocellular bilirubin transport. Albumin-bound bilirubin in sinusoidal blood passes through endothelial cell fenestrae to reach the hepatocyte surface, entering the cell by both facilitated and simple diffusional processes. Within the cell it is bound to glutathione-S-transferases and conjugated by bilirubin-UDP-glucuronosyltransferase (UGT1A1) to mono- and diglucuronides, which are actively transported across the canalicular membrane into the bile. ALB, albumin; UCB, unconjugated bilirubin, UGT1A1, bilirubin-UDP-glucuronosyltransferase; BMG, bilirubin monoglucuronide; GST, glutathione-S-transferase; MRP2, multidrug resistance–associated protein 2; BDG, bilirubin diglucuronide; BT, proposed bilirubin transporter.

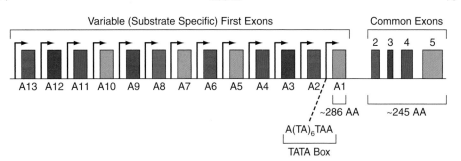

FIGURE 36-2

Structural organization of the human *UGT1* gene complex. This large complex on chromosome 2 contains at least 13 substrate-specific first exons (A1, A2, etc.). Since four of these are pseudogenes, nine UGT1 isoforms with differing substrate specificities are expressed. Each exon 1 has its own promoter and encodes the amino-terminal substrate-specific ~286 amino acids of the various *UGT1*-encoded isoforms, and common exons 2–5 that encode the 245 carboxyl-terminal amino acids common to all of the isoforms. mRNAs for specific isoforms are assembled by splicing a particular first exon such as the bilirubin-specific exon A1 to exons 2 to 5. The resulting message encodes a complete enzyme, in this particular case bilirubin-UDP-glucuronosyltransferase (UGT1A1). Mutations in a first exon affect only a single isoform. Those in exons 2–5 affect all enzymes encoded by the UGT1 complex.

3. *Conjugation:* Bilirubin is conjugated with one or two glucuronic acid moieties by a specific UDP-glucuronosyltransferase to form bilirubin mono- and diglucuronide, respectively. Conjugation disrupts the internal hydrogen bonding that limits aqueous solubility of bilirubin, and the resulting glucuronide conjugates are highly soluble in water. Conjugation is obligatory for excretion of bilirubin across the bile canalicular membrane into bile. The UDP-glucuronosyltransferases have been classified into gene families based on the degree of homology among the mRNAs for the various isoforms. Those that conjugate bilirubin and certain other substrates have been designated the *UGT1* family. These are expressed from a single gene complex by alternative promoter usage. This gene complex contains multiple substrate-specific first exons, designated A1, A2, etc. (Fig. 36-2), each with its own promoter and each encoding the amino-terminal half of a specific isoform. In addition, there are four common exons (exons 2–5) that encode the shared carboxyl-terminal half of all of the *UGT1* isoforms. The various first exons encode the specific aglycone substrate–binding sites for each isoform, while the shared exons encode the binding site for the sugar donor, UDP-glucuronic acid, and the transmembrane domain. Exon A1 and the four common exons, collectively designated the *UGT1A1* gene (Fig. 36-2), encode the physiologically critical enzyme bilirubin-UDP-glucuronosyltransferase (UGT1A1). A functional corollary of the organization of the *UGT1* gene is that a mutation in one of the first exons will affect only a single enzyme isoform. By contrast, a mutation in exons 2–5 will alter all isoforms encoded by the *UGT1* gene complex.

4. *Biliary excretion:* Bilirubin mono- and diglucuronides are excreted across the canalicular plasma membrane into the bile canaliculus by an ATP-dependent transport process mediated by a canalicular membrane protein called *multidrug resistance–associated protein 2* (MRP2). Mutations of MRP2 result in the Dubin-Johnson syndrome (described later in the chapter).

EXTRAHEPATIC ASPECTS OF BILIRUBIN DISPOSITION

Bilirubin in the Gut

Following secretion into bile, conjugated bilirubin reaches the duodenum and passes down the gastrointestinal tract without reabsorption by the intestinal mucosa. An appreciable fraction is converted by bacterial metabolism in the gut to the water-soluble colorless compound, urobilinogen. Urobilinogen undergoes enterohepatic cycling. Urobilinogen not taken up by the liver reaches the systemic circulation, from which some is cleared by the kidneys. Unconjugated bilirubin ordinarily does not reach the gut except in neonates or, by ill-defined alternative pathways, in the presence of severe unconjugated hyperbilirubinemia [e.g., Crigler-Najjar syndrome, type I (CN-I)]. Unconjugated bilirubin that reaches the gut is partly reabsorbed, amplifying any underlying hyperbilirubinemia. Recent reports suggest that oral administration of calcium phosphate with or without the lipase inhibitor orlistat may be an efficient means to interrupt bilirubin enterohepatic cycling to reduce serum bilirubin levels in this situation; however, this remains to be validated in larger clinical trials.

Renal Excretion of Bilirubin Conjugates

Unconjugated bilirubin is not excreted in urine as it is too tightly bound to albumin for effective glomerular filtration and there is no tubular mechanism for its renal secretion. In contrast, the bilirubin conjugates are readily filtered at the glomerulus and can appear in urine in disorders characterized by increased bilirubin conjugates in the circulation.

DISORDERS OF BILIRUBIN METABOLISM LEADING TO UNCONJUGATED HYPERBILIRUBINEMIA

INCREASED BILIRUBIN PRODUCTION

Hemolysis

Increased destruction of erythrocytes leads to increased bilirubin turnover and unconjugated hyperbilirubinemia; the hyperbilirubinemia is usually modest in the presence of normal liver function. In particular, the bone marrow is only capable of a sustained eightfold increase in erythrocyte production in response to a hemolytic stress. Therefore, hemolysis alone cannot result in a sustained hyperbilirubinemia of more than ~68 μmol/L (4 mg/dL). Higher values imply concomitant hepatic dysfunction. When hemolysis is the only abnormality in an otherwise healthy individual, the result is a purely unconjugated hyperbilirubinemia, with the direct-reacting fraction as measured in a typical clinical laboratory being ≤15% of the total serum bilirubin. In the presence of systemic disease, which may include a degree of hepatic dysfunction, hemolysis may produce a component of conjugated hyperbilirubinemia in addition to an elevated unconjugated bilirubin concentration. Prolonged hemolysis may lead to the precipitation of bilirubin salts within the gall bladder or biliary tree, resulting in the formation of gallstones in which bilirubin, rather than cholesterol, is the major component. Such pigment stones may lead to acute or chronic cholecystitis, biliary obstruction, or any other biliary tract consequence of calculous disease.

Ineffective Erythropoiesis

During erythroid maturation, small amounts of hemoglobin may be lost at the time of nuclear extrusion, and a fraction of developing erythroid cells is destroyed within the marrow. These processes normally account for a small proportion of bilirubin that is produced. In various disorders, including thalassemia major, megaloblastic anemias due to folate or vitamin B_{12} deficiency, congenital erythropoietic porphyria, lead poisoning, and various congenital and acquired dyserythropoietic anemias, the fraction of total bilirubin production derived from ineffective erythropoiesis is increased, reaching as

much as 70% of the total. This may be sufficient to produce modest degrees of unconjugated hyperbilirubinemia.

Miscellaneous

Degradation of the hemoglobin of extravascular collections of erythrocytes, such as those seen in massive tissue infarctions or large hematomas, may lead transiently to unconjugated hyperbilirubinemia.

DECREASED HEPATIC BILIRUBIN CLEARANCE

Decreased Hepatic Uptake

Decreased hepatic bilirubin uptake is believed to contribute to the unconjugated hyperbilirubinemia of Gilbert's syndrome (GS), although the molecular basis for this finding remains unclear (see later). Several drugs, including flavaspidic acid, novobiocin, rifampin, and various cholecystographic contrast agents, have been reported to inhibit bilirubin uptake. The resulting unconjugated hyperbilirubinemia resolves with cessation of the medication.

Impaired Conjugation

■ Physiologic Neonatal Jaundice

Bilirubin produced by the fetus is cleared by the placenta and eliminated by the maternal liver. Immediately after birth, the neonatal liver must assume responsibility for bilirubin clearance and excretion. However, many hepatic physiologic processes are incompletely developed at birth. Levels of UGT1A1 are low, and alternative excretory pathways allow passage of unconjugated bilirubin into the gut. Since the intestinal flora that convert bilirubin to urobilinogen are also undeveloped, an enterohepatic circulation of unconjugated bilirubin ensues. As a consequence, most neonates develop mild unconjugated hyperbilirubinemia between days 2 and 5 after birth. Peak levels are typically <85–170 μmol/L (5–10 mg/dL) and decline to normal adult concentrations within 2 weeks, as mechanisms required for bilirubin disposition mature. Prematurity, with more profound immaturity of hepatic function, or hemolysis, result in higher levels of unconjugated hyperbilirubinemia. A rapidly rising unconjugated bilirubin concentration, or absolute levels >340 μmol/L (20 mg/dL), puts the infant at risk for bilirubin encephalopathy, or kernicterus. Under these circumstances, bilirubin crosses an immature blood-brain barrier and precipitates in the basal ganglia and other areas of the brain. The consequences range from appreciable neurologic deficits to death. Treatment options include phototherapy, which converts bilirubin into water-soluble photoisomers that are excreted directly into bile, and exchange transfusion. The canalicular mechanisms responsible for bilirubin excretion are also immature at birth, and their maturation may lag behind that of UGT1A1; this can lead to transient conjugated neonatal hyperbilirubinemia, especially in infants with hemolysis.

Acquired Conjugation Defects

A modest reduction in bilirubin-conjugating capacity may be observed in advanced hepatitis or cirrhosis. However, in this setting, conjugation is better preserved than other aspects of bilirubin disposition, such as canalicular excretion. Various drugs, including pregnanediol, novobiocin, chloramphenicol, and gentamicin, may produce unconjugated hyperbilirubinemia by inhibiting UGT1A1 activity. Finally, bilirubin conjugation may be inhibited by certain fatty acids that are present in breast milk but not serum of mothers whose infants have excessive neonatal hyperbilirubinemia (*breast milk jaundice*). The pathogenesis of breast milk jaundice appears to differ from that of transient familial neonatal hyperbilirubinemia (Lucey-Driscoll syndrome), in which there is a UGT1A1 inhibitor in maternal serum.

HEREDITARY DEFECTS IN BILIRUBIN CONJUGATION

Three familial disorders characterized by differing degrees of unconjugated hyperbilirubinemia have long been recognized. The defining clinical features of each are described in the next sections (Table 36-1). While these disorders have been recognized for decades to reflect differing degrees of deficiency in the ability to conjugate bilirubin, recent advances in the molecular biology of the *UGT1* gene complex have elucidated their interrelationships and clarified previously puzzling features.

Crigler-Najjar Syndrome, Type I (CN-I)

CN-I is characterized by striking unconjugated hyperbilirubinemia of about 340–765 μmol/L (20–45 mg/dL) that appears in the neonatal period and persists for life. Other conventional hepatic biochemical tests such as serum aminotransferases and alkaline phosphatase are normal, and there is no evidence of hemolysis. Hepatic histology is also essentially normal except for the occasional presence of bile plugs within canaliculi. Bilirubin glucuronides are virtually absent from the bile, and there is no detectable constitutive expression of UGT1A1 activity in hepatic tissue. Neither UGT1A1 activity nor the serum bilirubin concentration responds to administration of phenobarbital or other enzyme inducers. In the absence of conjugation, unconjugated bilirubin accumulates in plasma, from which it is eliminated very slowly by alternative pathways that include direct passage into the bile and small intestine. These account for the small amounts of urobilinogen found in feces. No bilirubin is found in the urine. First described in 1952, the disorder is rare (estimated prevalence of 0.6–1.0 per million). Many patients are from geographically or socially isolated communities in which consanguinity is common, and pedigree analyses show an autosomal recessive pattern of inheritance. The majority of patients (type IA) exhibit defects in the glucuronide conjugation of a spectrum of substrates in addition to bilirubin,

TABLE 36-1

PRINCIPAL DIFFERENTIAL CHARACTERISTICS OF GILBERT'S AND CRIGLER-NAJJAR SYNDROMES			
	CRIGLER-NAJJAR SYNDROME		
FEATURE	**TYPE I**	**TYPE II**	**GILBERT'S SYNDROME**
Total serum bilirubin, μmol/L [mg/dL]	310–755 (usually >345) [18–45 (usually >20)]	100–430 (usually ≤345) [6–25 (usually ≤20)]	Typically ≤70 μmol/L (≤4 mg/dL) in absence of fasting or hemolysis
Routine liver tests	Normal	Normal	Normal
Response to phenobarbital	None	Decreases bilirubin by >25%	Decreases bilirubin to normal
Kernicterus	Usual	Rare	No
Hepatic histology	Normal	Normal	Usually normal; increased lipofuscin pigment in some
Bile characteristics			
Color	Pale or colorless	Pigmented	Normal dark color
Bilirubin fractions	>90% unconjugated	Largest fraction (mean: 57%) monoconjugates	Mainly diconjugates but monoconjugates increased (mean: 23%)
Bilirubin UDP-glucuronosyl-transferase activity	Typically absent; traces in some patients	Markedly reduced: 0–10% of normal	Reduced: typically 10–33% of normal
Inheritance (all autosomal)	Recessive	Predominantly recessive	Promoter mutation: recessive Missense mutations: 7 of 8 dominant; 1 reportedly recessive

including various drugs and other xenobiotics. These individuals have mutations in one of the common exons (2–5) of the *UGT1* gene (Fig. 36-2). In a smaller subset (type IB), the defect is limited largely to bilirubin conjugation, and the causative mutation is in the bilirubin-specific exon A1. Estrogen glucuronidation is mediated by UGT1A1 and is defective in all CN-I patients. More than 30 different genetic lesions of *UGT1A1* responsible for CN-I have been identified, including deletions, insertions, alterations in intronic splice donor and acceptor sites, exon skipping, and point mutations that introduce premature stop codons or alter critical amino acids. Their common feature is that they all encode proteins with absent or, at most, traces of bilirubin-UDP-glucuronosyltransferase enzymatic activity.

Prior to the availability of phototherapy, most patients with CN-I died of bilirubin encephalopathy (*kernicterus*) in infancy or early childhood. A few lived as long as early adult life without overt neurologic damage, although more subtle testing usually indicated mild but progressive brain damage. In the absence of liver transplantation, death eventually supervened from late-onset bilirubin encephalopathy, which often followed a nonspecific febrile illness. Although isolated hepatocyte transplantation has been used in a small number of cases of CN-I, early liver transplantation (Chap. 44) remains the best hope to prevent brain injury and death.

Crigler-Najjar Syndrome, Type II (CN-II)

This condition was recognized as a distinct entity in 1962 and is characterized by marked unconjugated hyperbilirubinemia in the absence of abnormalities of other conventional hepatic biochemical tests, hepatic histology, or hemolysis. It differs from CN-I in several specific ways (Table 36-1): (1) Although there is considerable overlap, average bilirubin concentrations are lower in CN-II; (2) accordingly, CN-II is only infrequently associated with kernicterus; (3) bile is deeply colored, and bilirubin glucuronides are present, with a striking, characteristic increase in the proportion of monoglucuronides; (4) UGT1A1 in liver is usually present at reduced levels (typically ≤10% of normal) but may be undetectable by older, less sensitive assays; (5) while typically detected in infancy, hyperbilirubinemia was not recognized in some cases until later in life and, in one instance, at age 34. As with CN-I, most CN-II cases exhibit abnormalities in the conjugation of other compounds, such as salicylamide and menthol, but in some instances the defect appears limited to bilirubin. Reduction of serum bilirubin concentrations by >25% in response to enzyme inducers such as phenobarbital distinguishes CN-II from CN-I, although this response may not be elicited in early infancy and often is not accompanied by measurable UGT1A1 induction. Bilirubin concentrations during phenobarbital administration do not return to normal but are typically in the range of 51–86 μmol/L (3–5 mg/dL). Although the incidence of kernicterus in CN-II is low, instances have occurred, not only in infants but also in adolescents and adults, often in the setting of an intercurrent illness, fasting, or another factor that temporarily raises the serum bilirubin concentration above baseline and reduces serum albumin levels. For this reason, phenobarbital therapy is widely recommended, a single bedtime dose often sufficing to maintain clinically safe plasma bilirubin concentrations.

Over 77 different mutations in the *UGT1* gene have been identified as causing CN-I or CN-II. It was found that missense mutations are more common in CN-II patients as would be expected in this less severe phenotype. Their common feature is that they encode for a bilirubin-UDP-glucuronosyltransferase with markedly reduced, but detectable, enzymatic activity. The spectrum of residual enzyme activity explains the spectrum of phenotypic severity of the resulting hyperbilirubinemia. Molecular analysis has established that a large majority of CN-II patients are either homozygotes or compound heterozygotes for CN-II mutations and that individuals carrying one mutated and one entirely normal allele have normal bilirubin concentrations.

Gilbert's Syndrome

This syndrome is characterized by mild unconjugated hyperbilirubinemia, normal values for standard hepatic biochemical tests, and normal hepatic histology other than a modest increase of lipofuscin pigment in some patients. Serum bilirubin concentrations are most often <51 μmol/L (<3 mg/dL), although both higher and lower values are frequent. The clinical spectrum of hyperbilirubinemia fades into that of CN-II at serum bilirubin concentrations of 86–136 μmol/L (5–8 mg/dL). At the other end of the scale, the distinction between mild cases of GS and a normal state is often blurred. Bilirubin concentrations may fluctuate substantially in any given individual, and at least 25% of patients will exhibit temporarily normal values during prolonged follow-up. More elevated values are associated with stress, fatigue, alcohol use, reduced caloric intake, and intercurrent illness, while increased caloric intake or administration of enzyme-inducing agents produce lower bilirubin levels. GS is most often diagnosed at or shortly after puberty or in adult life during routine examinations that include multichannel biochemical analyses. UGT1A1 activity is typically reduced to 10–35% of normal, and bile pigments exhibit a characteristic increase in bilirubin monoglucuronides. Studies of radiobilirubin kinetics indicate that hepatic bilirubin clearance is reduced to an average of one-third of normal. Administration of phenobarbital normalizes both the serum bilirubin concentration and hepatic bilirubin clearance; however, failure of UGT1A1 activity to improve in many such instances suggests the possible coexistence of an additional defect. Compartmental analysis of bilirubin kinetic data suggests that GS patients have a defect in bilirubin uptake as well as in conjugation. Defect(s) in the hepatic uptake of other organic anions that at least partially share an uptake mechanism with bilirubin, such as sulfobromophthalein and indocyanine green (ICG), are observed in a minority of patients. The metabolism and transport of bile acids, which do not utilize the bilirubin uptake mechanism, are normal. The magnitude of changes in the plasma bilirubin concentration induced by provocation tests such as 48 h of fasting or the IV administration of nicotinic acid have been reported to be of help in separating GS patients from normal individuals. Other studies dispute this assertion. Moreover, on theoretical grounds, the results of such studies should provide no more information than simple measurements of the baseline plasma bilirubin concentration. Family studies indicate that GS and hereditary hemolytic anemias such as hereditary spherocytosis, glucose-6-phosphate dehydrogenase deficiency, and β-thalassemia trait sort independently. Reports of hemolysis in up to 50% of GS patients are believed to reflect better case finding, since patients with both GS and hemolysis have higher bilirubin concentrations, and are more likely to be jaundiced, than patients with either defect alone.

GS is common, with many series placing its prevalence at ≥8%. Males predominate over females by reported ratios ranging from 1.5:1 to >7:1. However, these ratios may have a large artifactual component since normal males have higher mean bilirubin levels than normal females, but the diagnosis of GS is often based on comparison to normal ranges established in men. The high prevalence of GS in the general population may explain the reported frequency of mild unconjugated hyperbilirubinemia in liver transplant recipients. The disposition of most xenobiotics metabolized by glucuronidation appears to be normal in GS, as is oxidative drug metabolism in the majority of reported studies. The principal exception is the metabolism of the antitumor agent irinotecan (CPT-11), whose active metabolite (SN-38) is glucuronidated specifically by bilirubin-UDP-glucuronosyltransferase. Administration of CPT-11 to patients with GS has resulted in several toxicities, including intractable diarrhea and myelosuppression. Some reports also suggest abnormal disposition of menthol, estradiol benzoate, acetaminophen, tolbutamide, and rifamycin SV. Although some of these studies have been disputed, and there have been no reports of clinical complications from use of these agents in GS, prudence should be exercised in prescribing them, or any agents metabolized primarily by glucuronidation, in this condition. It should also be noted that the HIV protease inhibitors indinavir and atazanavir can inhibit UGT1A1, resulting in hyperbilirubinemia that is most pronounced in patients with preexisting GS.

Most older pedigree studies of GS were consistent with autosomal dominant inheritance with variable expressivity. However, studies of the *UGT1* gene in GS have indicated a variety of molecular genetic bases for the phenotypic picture and several different patterns of inheritance. Studies in Europe and the United States found that nearly all patients had normal coding regions for UGT1A1 but were homozygous for the insertion of an extra TA (i.e., A[TA]$_7$TAA rather than A[TA]$_6$TAA) in the promoter region of the first exon. This appeared to be necessary, but not sufficient, for clinically expressed GS, since 15% of normal controls were also homozygous for this variant. While normal by standard criteria, these individuals had somewhat higher bilirubin concentrations than the rest of the controls studied. Heterozygotes for this abnormality had bilirubin concentrations identical to those homozygous for the normal A[TA]$_6$TAA allele. The prevalence of the A[TA]$_7$TAA allele in a general western population is 30%, in which case 9% would be homozygotes. This is slightly higher than the prevalence of GS based on purely phenotypic parameters. It was suggested that additional variables, such as mild hemolysis or a defect in bilirubin uptake, might be among the factors enhancing phenotypic expression of the defect.

Phenotypic expression of GS due solely to the A[TA]$_7$TAA promoter abnormality is inherited as an autosomal recessive trait. A number of CN-II kindreds have been identified in which there is also an allele containing a normal coding region but the A[TA]$_7$TAA promoter abnormality. CN-II heterozygotes who have the A[TA]$_6$TAA promoter are phenotypically normal, whereas those with the A[TA]$_7$TAA promoter express the phenotypic picture of GS. GS in such kindreds may also result from homozygosity for the A[TA]$_7$TAA promoter abnormality. Seven different missense mutations in the *UGT1* gene that reportedly cause GS with dominant inheritance have been found in Japanese individuals. Another Japanese patient with mild unconjugated hyperbilirubinemia was homozygous for a missense mutation in exon 5. GS in her family appeared to be recessive. Missense mutations causing GS have not been reported outside of certain Asian populations.

DISORDERS OF BILIRUBIN METABOLISM LEADING TO MIXED OR PREDOMINANTLY CONJUGATED HYPERBILIRUBINEMIA

In hyperbilirubinemia due to acquired liver disease (e.g., acute hepatitis, common bile duct stone), there are usually elevations in the serum concentrations of both conjugated and unconjugated bilirubin. Although biliary tract obstruction or hepatocellular cholestatic injury may present on occasion with a predominantly conjugated hyperbilirubinemia, it is generally not possible to differentiate intrahepatic from extrahepatic causes of jaundice based upon the serum levels or relative proportions of unconjugated and conjugated bilirubin. The major reason for determining the amounts of conjugated and unconjugated bilirubin in the serum is for the initial differentiation of hepatic parenchymal and obstructive disorders (mixed conjugated and unconjugated hyperbilirubinemia) from the inheritable and hemolytic disorders discussed above that are associated with unconjugated hyperbilirubinemia.

FAMILIAL DEFECTS IN HEPATIC EXCRETORY FUNCTION

Dubin-Johnson Syndrome (DJS)

This benign, relatively rare disorder is characterized by low-grade, predominantly conjugated hyperbilirubinemia (**Table 36-2**). Total bilirubin concentrations are typically between 34 and 85 µmol/L (2 and 5 mg/dL) but on occasion can be in the normal range or as high as 340–430 µmol/L (20–25 mg/dL) and can fluctuate widely in any given patient. The degree of hyperbilirubinemia may be increased by intercurrent illness, oral contraceptive use, and pregnancy. As the hyperbilirubinemia is due to a predominant rise in conjugated bilirubin, bilirubinuria is characteristically present. Aside from elevated serum bilirubin levels, other routine laboratory tests are normal. Physical examination is usually normal except for jaundice, although an occasional patient may have hepatosplenomegaly.

Patients with DJS are usually asymptomatic, although some may have vague constitutional symptoms. These latter patients have usually undergone extensive and often unnecessary diagnostic examinations for unexplained jaundice and have high levels of anxiety. In women, the condition may be subclinical until the patient becomes pregnant or receives oral contraceptives, at which time chemical hyperbilirubinemia becomes frank jaundice. Even in these situations, other routine liver function tests, including serum alkaline phosphatase and transaminase activities, are normal.

A cardinal feature of DJS is the accumulation in the lysosomes of centrilobular hepatocytes of dark, coarsely granular pigment. As a result, the liver may be grossly black in appearance. This pigment is thought to be derived from epinephrine metabolites that are not excreted normally. The pigment may disappear during bouts of viral hepatitis, only to reaccumulate slowly after recovery.

Biliary excretion of a number of anionic compounds is compromised in DJS. These include various cholecystographic agents, as well as sulfobromophthalein (Bromsulphalein, BSP), a synthetic dye formerly used in a test of liver function. In this test, the rate of disappearance of BSP from plasma was determined following bolus intravenous administration. BSP is conjugated with glutathione in the hepatocyte; the resulting conjugate is normally excreted rapidly into the bile canaliculus. Patients with DJS exhibit a characteristic rise in its plasma concentration at 90 min after injection, due to reflux of conjugated BSP into the circulation from the hepatocyte. Dyes such as ICG that are taken up by hepatocytes but are not further metabolized prior to biliary

TABLE 36-2

PRINCIPAL DIFFERENTIAL CHARACTERISTICS OF INHERITABLE DISORDERS OF BILE CANALICULAR FUNCTION							
	DJS	**ROTOR**	**PFIC1**	**BRIC1**	**PFIC2**	**BRIC2**	**PFIC3**
Gene	ABCCA	?	ATP8B1	ATP8B1	ABCB11	ABCB11	ABCB4
Protein	MRP2	?	FIC1	FIC1	BSEP	BSEP	MDR3
Cholestasis	No	No	Yes	Episodic	Yes	Episodic	Yes
Serum γ-GT	Normal	Normal	Normal	Normal	Normal	Normal	↑↑
Serum bile acids	Normal	Normal	↑↑	↑↑ during episodes	↑↑	↑↑ during episodes	↑↑
Clinical features	Mild conjugated hyperbilirubinemia; otherwise normal liver function; dark pigment in liver; characteristic pattern of urinary coproporphyrins	Mild conjugated hyperbilirubinemia; otherwise normal liver function; liver without abnormal pigmentation	Severe cholestasis beginning in childhood	Recurrent episodes of cholestasis beginning at any age	Severe cholestasis beginning in childhood	Recurrent episodes of cholestasis beginning at any age	Severe cholestasis beginning in childhood; decreased phospholipids in bile

excretion do not show this reflux phenomenon. Continuous BSP infusion studies suggest a reduction in the t_{max} for biliary excretion. Bile acid disposition, including hepatocellular uptake and biliary excretion, is normal in DJS. These patients have normal serum and biliary bile acid concentrations and do not have pruritus.

By analogy with findings in several mutant rat strains, the selective defect in biliary excretion of bilirubin conjugates and certain other classes of organic compounds, but not of bile acids that characterizes DJS in humans was found to reflect defective expression of MRP2, an ATP-dependent canalicular membrane transporter. Several different mutations in the MRP2 gene produce the Dubin-Johnson phenotype, which has an autosomal recessive pattern of inheritance. Although MRP2 is undoubtedly important in the biliary excretion of conjugated bilirubin, the fact that this pigment is still excreted in the absence of MRP2 suggests that other, as yet uncharacterized, transport proteins may serve in a secondary role in this process.

Patients with DJS also have a diagnostic abnormality in urinary coproporphyrin excretion. There are two naturally occurring coproporphyrin isomers, I and III. Normally, ~75% of the coproporphyrin in urine is isomer III. In urine from DJS patients, total coproporphyrin content is normal, but >80% is isomer I. Heterozygotes for the syndrome show an intermediate pattern. The molecular basis for this phenomenon remains unclear.

Rotor Syndrome

This benign, autosomal recessive disorder is clinically similar to DJS (Table 36-2), although it is seen even less frequently. A major phenotypic difference is that the liver in patients with Rotor syndrome has no increased pigmentation and appears totally normal. The only abnormality in routine laboratory tests is an elevation of total serum bilirubin, due to a predominant rise in conjugated bilirubin. This is accompanied by bilirubinuria. Several additional features differentiate Rotor syndrome and DJS. In Rotor syndrome, the gallbladder is usually visualized on oral cholecystography, in contrast to the nonvisualization that is typical of DJS. The pattern of urinary coproporphyrin excretion also differs. The pattern in Rotor syndrome resembles that of many acquired disorders of hepatobiliary function, in which coproporphyrin I, the major coproporphyrin isomer in bile, refluxes from the hepatocyte back into the circulation and is excreted in urine. Thus, total urinary coproporphyrin excretion is substantially increased in Rotor syndrome, in contrast to the normal levels seen in DJS. Although the fraction of coproporphyrin I in urine is elevated, it is usually <70% of the total, as compared to ≥80% in DJS. The disorders also can be distinguished by their patterns of BSP excretion. Although clearance of BSP from plasma is delayed in Rotor syndrome, there is

no reflux of conjugated BSP back into the circulation as seen in DJS. Kinetic analysis of plasma BSP infusion studies suggests the presence of a defect in intrahepatocellular storage of this compound. This has never been demonstrated directly, and the molecular basis of Rotor syndrome remains unknown.

Benign Recurrent Intrahepatic Cholestasis (BRIC)

This rare disorder is characterized by recurrent attacks of pruritus and jaundice. The typical episode begins with mild malaise and elevations in serum aminotransferase levels, followed rapidly by rises in alkaline phosphatase and conjugated bilirubin and onset of jaundice and itching. The first one or two episodes may be misdiagnosed as acute viral hepatitis. The cholestatic episodes, which may begin in childhood or adulthood, can vary in duration from several weeks to months, following which there is complete clinical and biochemical resolution. Intervals between attacks may vary from several months to years. Between episodes, physical examination is normal, as are serum levels of bile acids, bilirubin, transaminases, and alkaline phosphatase. The disorder is familial and has an autosomal recessive pattern of inheritance. BRIC is considered a benign disorder in that it does not lead to cirrhosis or end-stage liver disease. However, the episodes of jaundice and pruritus can be prolonged and debilitating, and some patients have undergone liver transplantation to relieve the intractable and disabling symptoms. Treatment during the cholestatic episodes is symptomatic; there is no specific treatment to prevent or shorten the occurrence of episodes.

A gene termed *FIC1* was recently identified and found to be mutated in patients with BRIC. Curiously, this gene is expressed strongly in the small intestine but only weakly in the liver. The protein encoded by *FIC1* shows little similarity to genes that have been shown to play a role in bile canalicular excretion of various compounds. Rather, it appears to be a member of a P-type ATPase family that transports aminophospholipids from the outer to the inner leaflet of a variety of cell membranes. Its relationship to the pathobiology of this disorder remains unclear. A second phenotypically identical form of BRIC, termed BRIC type 2, has been described resulting from mutations in the bile salt excretory protein (BSEP), the protein that is defective in progressive familial intrahepatic cholestasis type 2 (Table 36-2). How some mutations in this protein result in the episodic BRIC phenotype is unknown.

Progressive Familial Intrahepatic Cholestasis (FIC)

This name is applied to three phenotypically related syndromes (Table 36-2). Progressive FIC type 1 (Byler disease) presents in early infancy as cholestasis that may be initially episodic. However, in contrast to BRIC, Byler disease progresses to malnutrition, growth retardation, and end-stage liver disease during childhood. This disorder is also a consequence of a *FIC1* mutation. The functional relationship of the FIC1 protein to the pathogenesis of cholestasis in these disorders is unknown. Two other types of progressive FIC (types 2 and 3) have been described. Progressive FIC type 2 is associated with a mutation in the protein named *sister of p-glycoprotein*, which is the major bile canalicular exporter of bile acids and is also known as *bile salt excretory protein* (BSEP). As noted above, some mutations of this protein are associated with BRIC type 2, rather than the progressive FIC type 2 phenotype. Progressive FIC type 3 has been associated with a mutation of MDR3, a protein that is essential for normal hepatocellular excretion of phospholipids across the bile canaliculus. Although all three types of progressive FIC have similar clinical phenotypes, only type 3 is associated with high serum levels of γ-glutamyltransferase activity. In contrast, activity of this enzyme is normal or only mildly elevated in symptomatic BRIC and progressive FIC types 1 and 2.

FURTHER READINGS

Bosma P et al: The genetic basis of the reduced expression of bilirubin-UDP-glucuronosyltransferase 1 in Gilbert's syndrome. N Engl J Med 333:1171, 1995

———: Inherited disorders of bilirubin metabolism. J Hepatol 38:107, 2003

Burchell B: Genetic variation of human UDP-glucuronosyltransferase: Implications in disease and drug glucuronidation. Am J Pharmacogenomics 3:37, 2003

Fabris L et al: The patient presenting with isolated hyperbilirubinemia. Dig Liver Dis 41:375, 2009

Harris MJ et al: Progressive familial intrahepatic cholestasis: Genetic disorders of biliary transporters. J Gastroenterol Hepatol 20:807, 2005

Jansen PL: Diagnosis and management of Crigler-Najjar syndrome. Eur J Pediatr 158:S89, 1999

——— et al: Genes and cholestasis. Hepatology 34:1067, 2001

Klomp LW et al: Characterization of mutations in ATP8B1 associated with hereditary cholestasis. Hepatology 40:27, 2004

Korenblat KM et al: Hyperbilirubinemia in the setting of antiviral therapy. Clin Gastroenterol Hepatol 3:303, 2005

Miners JO et al: Genetic polymorphisms of UDP-glucuronosyltransferases and their functional significance. Toxicology 181:453, 2002

Mor-Cohen R et al: Identification and functional analysis of two novel mutations in the multidrug resistance protein 2 gene in Israeli patients with Dubin-Johnson syndrome. J Biol Chem 276:36923, 2001

Servedio V et al: Spectrum of UGT1A1 mutations in Crigler-Najjar (CN) syndrome patients: Identification of twelve novel alleles and genotype-phenotype correlation. Hum Mutat 25:325, 2005

Van Mil SW et al: Benign recurrent intrahepatic cholestasis type 2 is caused by mutations in ABCB11. Gastroenterology 127:379, 2004

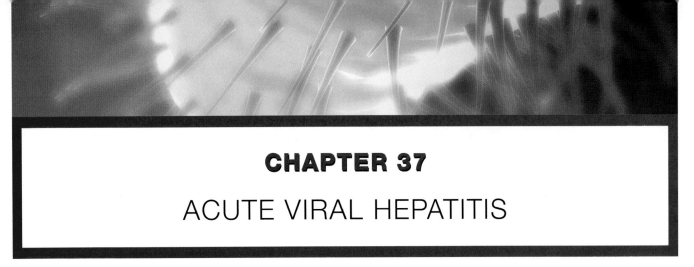

CHAPTER 37

ACUTE VIRAL HEPATITIS

Jules L. Dienstag

Acute viral hepatitis is a systemic infection affecting the liver predominantly. Almost all cases of acute viral hepatitis are caused by one of five viral agents: hepatitis A virus (HAV), hepatitis B virus (HBV), hepatitis C virus (HCV), the HBV-associated delta agent or hepatitis D virus (HDV), and hepatitis E virus (HEV). Other transfusion-transmitted agents, e.g., "hepatitis G" virus and "TT" virus, have been identified but do not cause hepatitis. All these human hepatitis viruses are RNA viruses, except for hepatitis B, which is a DNA virus. Although these agents can be distinguished by their molecular and antigenic properties, all types of viral hepatitis produce clinically similar illnesses. These range from asymptomatic and inapparent to fulminant and fatal acute infections common to all types, on the one hand, and from subclinical persistent infections to rapidly progressive chronic liver disease with cirrhosis and even hepatocellular carcinoma, common to the bloodborne types (HBV, HCV, and HDV), on the other.

VIROLOGY AND ETIOLOGY

Hepatitis A

Hepatitis A virus is a nonenveloped 27-nm, heat-, acid-, and ether-resistant RNA virus in the hepatovirus genus of the picornavirus family (Fig. 37-1). Its virion contains four capsid polypeptides, designated VP1 to VP4, which are cleaved posttranslationally from the polyprotein product of a 7500-nucleotide genome. Inactivation of viral activity can be achieved by boiling for 1 min, by contact with formaldehyde and chlorine, or by ultraviolet irradiation. Despite nucleotide sequence variation of up to 20% among isolates of HAV, all strains of this virus are immunologically indistinguishable and belong to one serotype. Hepatitis A has an incubation period of ~4 weeks. Its replication is limited to the liver, but the virus is present in the liver, bile, stools, and blood during the late incubation period and acute preicteric phase of illness. Despite persistence of virus in the liver, viral shedding in feces, viremia, and infectivity diminish rapidly once jaundice becomes apparent. HAV can be cultivated reproducibly in vitro.

Antibodies to HAV (anti-HAV) can be detected during acute illness when serum aminotransferase activity is elevated and fecal HAV shedding is still occurring. This early antibody response is predominantly of the IgM class and persists for several months, rarely for 6–12 months. During convalescence, however, anti-HAV of the IgG class becomes the predominant antibody (Fig. 37-2). Therefore, the diagnosis of hepatitis A is made during acute illness by demonstrating anti-HAV of the IgM class. After acute illness, anti-HAV of the IgG class remains detectable indefinitely, and patients with serum

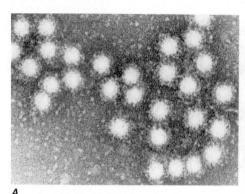 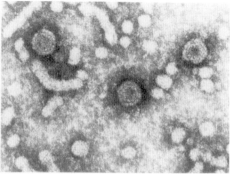

A　　　　　　　　　　　　　　　*B*

FIGURE 37-1

Electron micrographs of hepatitis A virus particles and serum from a patient with hepatitis B. *A.* 27-nm hepatitis A virus particles purified from stool of a patient with acute hepatitis A and aggregated by antibody to hepatitis A virus. ***B.*** Concentrated serum from a patient with hepatitis B, demonstrating the 42-nm virions, tubular forms, and spherical 22-nm particles of hepatitis B surface antigen. 132,000×. (Hepatitis D resembles 42-nm virions of hepatitis B but is smaller, 35–37 nm; hepatitis E resembles hepatitis A virus but is slightly larger, 32–34 nm; hepatitis C has been visualized as a 55-nm particle.)

anti-HAV are immune to reinfection. Neutralizing antibody activity parallels the appearance of anti-HAV, and the IgG anti-HAV present in immune globulin accounts for the protection it affords against HAV infection.

Hepatitis B

Hepatitis B virus is a DNA virus with a remarkably compact genomic structure; despite its small, circular, 3200-bp size, HBV DNA codes for four sets of viral products with a complex, multiparticle structure. HBV achieves its genomic economy by relying on an efficient strategy of encoding proteins from four overlapping genes: S, C, P, and X (Fig. 37-3), as detailed below. Once thought to be unique among viruses, HBV is now recognized as one of a family of animal viruses, hepadnaviruses (hepatotropic DNA viruses), and is classified as hepadnavirus type 1. Similar viruses infect certain species of woodchucks, ground and tree squirrels, and Pekin ducks, to mention the most carefully characterized. Like

HBV, all have the same distinctive three morphologic forms, have counterparts to the envelope and nucleocapsid virus antigens of HBV, replicate in the liver but exist in extrahepatic sites, contain their own endogenous DNA polymerase, have partially double-strand

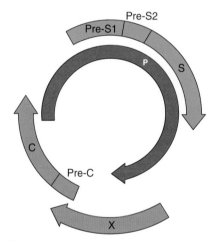

FIGURE 37-3

Compact genomic structure of HBV. This structure, with overlapping genes, permits HBV to code for multiple proteins. The S gene codes for the "major" envelope protein, HBsAg. Pre-S1 and pre-S2, upstream of S, combine with S to code for two larger proteins, "middle" protein, the product of pre-S2 + S, and "large" protein, the product of pre-S1 + pre-S2 + S. The largest gene, P, codes for DNA polymerase. The C gene codes for two nucleocapsid proteins, HBeAg, a soluble, secreted protein (initiation from the pre-C region of the gene) and HBcAg, the intracellular core protein (initiation after pre-C). The X gene codes for HBxAg, which can transactivate the transcription of cellular and viral genes; its clinical relevance is not known, but it may contribute to carcinogenesis by binding to p53.

FIGURE 37-2

Scheme of typical clinical and laboratory features of hepatitis A.

and partially single-strand genomes, are associated with acute and chronic hepatitis and hepatocellular carcinoma, and rely on a replicative strategy unique among DNA viruses but typical of retroviruses. Instead of DNA replication directly from a DNA template, hepadnaviruses rely on reverse transcription (effected by the DNA polymerase) of minus-strand DNA from a "pregenomic" RNA intermediate. Then plus-strand DNA is transcribed from the minus-strand DNA template by the DNA-dependent DNA polymerase and converted in the hepatocyte nucleus to a covalently closed circular DNA, which serves as a template for messenger RNA and pregenomic RNA. Viral proteins are translated by the messenger RNA, and the proteins and genome are packaged into virions and secreted from the hepatocyte. Although HBV is difficult to cultivate in vitro in the conventional sense from clinical material, several cell lines have been transfected with HBV DNA. Such transfected cells support in vitro replication of the intact virus and its component proteins.

Viral Proteins and Particles

Of the three particulate forms of HBV (Table 37-1), the most numerous are the 22-nm particles, which appear as spherical or long filamentous forms; these are antigenically indistinguishable from the outer surface or envelope protein of HBV and are thought to represent excess viral envelope protein. Outnumbered in serum by a factor of 100 or 1000 to 1 compared with the spheres and tubules are large, 42-nm, double-shelled spherical particles, which represent the intact hepatitis B virion (Fig. 37-1). The envelope protein expressed on the outer surface of the virion and on the smaller spherical and tubular structures is referred to as *hepatitis B surface antigen* (HBsAg). The concentration of HBsAg and virus particles in the blood may reach 500 μg/mL and 10 trillion particles per milliliter, respectively. The envelope protein, HBsAg, is the product of the S gene of HBV.

A number of different HBsAg subdeterminants have been identified. There is a common group-reactive antigen, *a*, shared by all HBsAg isolates. In addition, HBsAg may contain one of several subtype-specific antigens, namely, *d* or *y*, *w* or *r*, as well as other more recently characterized specificities. Hepatitis B isolates fall into one of at least eight subtypes and eight genotypes (A–H). Geographic distribution of genotypes and subtypes varies; genotypes A (corresponding to subtype *adw*) and D (*ayw*) predominate in the United States and Europe, while genotypes B (*adw*) and C (*adr*) predominate in Asia. Clinical course and outcome are independent of subtype, but preliminary reports suggest that genotype B is associated with less rapidly progressive liver disease and a lower likelihood, or delayed appearance, of hepatocellular carcinoma than genotype C. Patients with genotype A appear to be more likely to clear circulating viremia and to achieve HBsAg

seroconversion, both spontaneously and in response to antiviral therapy. In addition, "precore" mutations are favored by certain genotypes (see below).

Upstream of the S gene are the pre-S genes (Fig. 37-3), which code for pre-S gene products, including receptors on the HBV surface for polymerized human serum albumin and for hepatocyte membrane proteins. The pre-S region actually consists of both pre-S1 and pre-S2. Depending on where translation is initiated, three potential HBsAg gene products are synthesized. The protein product of the S gene is HBsAg (*major protein*), the product of the S region plus the adjacent pre-S2 region is the *middle protein*, and the product of the pre-S1 plus pre-S2 plus S regions is the *large protein*. Compared with the smaller spherical and tubular particles of HBV, complete 42-nm virions are enriched in the large protein. Both pre-S proteins and their respective antibodies can be detected during HBV infection, and the period of pre-S antigenemia appears to coincide with other markers of virus replication, as detailed below.

The intact 42-nm virion contains a 27-nm nucleocapsid core particle. Nucleocapsid proteins are coded for by the C gene. The antigen expressed on the surface of the nucleocapsid core is referred to as *hepatitis B core antigen* (HBcAg), and its corresponding antibody is anti-HBc. A third HBV antigen is *hepatitis B e antigen* (HBeAg), a soluble, nonparticulate, nucleocapsid protein that is immunologically distinct from intact HBcAg but is a product of the same C gene. The C gene has two initiation codons, a precore and a core region (Fig. 37-3). If translation is initiated at the precore region, the protein product is HBeAg, which has a signal peptide that binds it to the smooth endoplasmic reticulum and leads to its secretion into the circulation. If translation begins with the core region, HBcAg is the protein product; it has no signal peptide, it is not secreted, but it assembles into nucleocapsid particles, which bind to and incorporate RNA and which, ultimately, contain HBV DNA. Also packaged within the nucleocapsid core is a DNA polymerase, which directs replication and repair of HBV DNA. When packaging within viral proteins is complete, synthesis of the incomplete plus strand stops; this accounts for the single-strand gap and for differences in the size of the gap. HBcAg particles remain in the hepatocyte, where they are readily detectable by immunohistochemical staining, and are exported after encapsidation by an envelope of HBsAg. Therefore, naked core particles do not circulate in the serum. The secreted nucleocapsid protein, HBeAg, provides a convenient, readily detectable, qualitative marker of HBV replication and relative infectivity.

HBsAg-positive serum containing HBeAg is more likely to be highly infectious and to be associated with the presence of hepatitis B virions (and detectable HBV DNA, see later) than HBeAg-negative or anti-HBe-positive serum. For example, HBsAg carrier mothers

TABLE 37-1

NOMENCLATURE AND FEATURES OF HEPATITIS VIRUSES

HEPATITIS TYPE	VIRUS PARTICLE, nm	MORPHOLOGY	GENOME[a]	CLASSIFICATION	ANTIGEN(S)	ANTIBODIES	REMARKS
HAV	27	Icosahedral non-enveloped	7.5-kb RNA, linear, ss, +	Hepatovirus	HAV	Anti-HAV	Early fecal shedding Diagnosis: IgM anti-HAV Previous infection: IgG anti-HAV
HBV	42	Double-shelled virion (surface and core) spherical	3.2-kb DNA, circular, ss/ds	Hepadnavirus	HBsAg HBcAg HBeAg	Anti-HBs Anti-HBc Anti-HBe	Bloodborne virus; carrier state Acute diagnosis: HBsAg, IgM anti-HBc Chronic diagnosis IgG anti-HBc, HBsAg Markers of replication: HBeAg, HBV DNA Liver, lymphocytes, other organs
	27	Nucleocapsid core			HBcAg HBeAg	Anti-HBc Anti-HBe	Nucleocapsid contains DNA and DNA polymerase; present in hepatocyte nucleus; HBcAg does not circulate; HBeAg (soluble, nonparticulate) and HBV DNA circulate—correlate with infectivity and complete virions
	22	Spherical and filamentous; represents excess virus coat material			HBsAg	Anti-HBs	HBsAg detectable in >95% of patients with acute hepatitis B; found in serum, body fluids, hepatocyte cytoplasm; anti-HBs appears following infection—protective antibody
HCV	Approx. 40–60	Enveloped	9.4-kb RNA, linear, ss, +	Hepacivirus	HCV C100-3 C33c C22-3 NS5	Anti-HCV	Bloodborne agent, formerly labeled non-A, non-B hepatitis Acute diagnosis: anti-HCV (C33c, C22-3, NS5), HCV RNA Chronic diagnosis: anti-HCV (C100-3, C33c, C22-3, NS5) and HCV RNA; cytoplasmic location in hepatocytes
HDV	35–37	Enveloped hybrid particle with HBsAg coat and HDV core	1.7-kb RNA, circular, ss, −	Resembles viroids and plant satellite viruses	HBsAg HDV antigen	Anti-HBs Anti-HDV	Defective RNA virus, requires helper function of HBV (hepadnaviruses); HDV antigen present in hepatocyte nucleus Diagnosis: anti-HDV, HDV RNA; HBV/HDV coinfection—IgM anti-HBc and anti-HDV; HDV superinfection—IgG anti-HBc and anti-HDV
HEV	32–34	Nonenveloped icosahedral	7.6-kb RNA, linear, ss, +	Hepevirus	HEV antigen	Anti-HEV	Agent of enterically transmitted hepatitis; rare in USA; occurs in Asia, Mediterranean countries, Central America Diagnosis: IgM/IgG anti-HEV (assays being developed); virus in stool, bile, hepatocyte cytoplasm

[a]ss, single-strand; ss/ds, partially single-strand, partially double-strand; −, minus-strand; +, plus-strand.

who are HBeAg-positive almost invariably (>90%) transmit hepatitis B infection to their offspring, whereas HBsAg carrier mothers with anti-HBe rarely (10–15%) infect their offspring.

Early during the course of acute hepatitis B, HBeAg appears transiently; its disappearance may be a harbinger of clinical improvement and resolution of infection. Persistence of HBeAg in serum beyond the first 3 months of acute infection may be predictive of the development of chronic infection, and the presence of HBeAg during chronic hepatitis B is associated with ongoing viral replication, infectivity, and inflammatory liver injury.

The third of the HBV genes is the largest, the P gene (Fig. 37-3), which codes for the DNA polymerase; as noted above, this enzyme has both DNA-dependent DNA polymerase and RNA-dependent reverse transcriptase activities. The fourth gene, X, codes for a small, nonparticulate protein, *hepatitis B x antigen* (HBxAg), that is capable of transactivating the transcription of both viral and cellular genes (Fig. 37-3). In the cytoplasm, HBxAg effects calcium release (possibly from mitochrondria), which activates signal-transduction pathways that lead to stimulation of HBV reverse transcription and HBV DNA replication. Such transactivation may enhance the replication of HBV, leading to the clinical association observed between the expression of HBxAg and antibodies to it in patients with severe chronic hepatitis and hepatocellular carcinoma. The transactivating activity can enhance the transcription and replication of other viruses besides HBV, such as HIV. Cellular processes transactivated by X include the human interferon γ gene and class 1 major histocompatibility genes; potentially, these effects could contribute to enhanced susceptibility of HBV-infected hepatocytes to cytolytic T cells. The expression of X can also induce programmed cell death (apoptosis).

▮ Serologic and Virologic Markers

After a person is infected with HBV, the first virologic marker detectable in serum within 1–12 weeks, usually between 8 and 12 weeks, is HBsAg (**Fig. 37-4**). Circulating HBsAg precedes elevations of serum aminotransferase activity and clinical symptoms by 2–6 weeks and remains detectable during the entire icteric or symptomatic phase of acute hepatitis B and beyond. In typical cases, HBsAg becomes undetectable 1–2 months after the onset of jaundice and rarely persists beyond 6 months. After HBsAg disappears, antibody to HBsAg (anti-HBs) becomes detectable in serum and remains detectable indefinitely thereafter. Because HBcAg is intracellular and, when in the serum, sequestered within an HBsAg coat, naked core particles do not circulate in serum and, therefore, HBcAg is not detectable routinely in the serum of patients with HBV infection. By contrast, anti-HBc is readily demonstrable in serum, beginning within the first 1–2 weeks after the appearance of HBsAg and

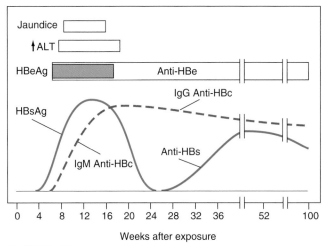

FIGURE 37-4
Scheme of typical clinical and laboratory features of acute hepatitis B.

preceding detectable levels of anti-HBs by weeks to months. Because variability exists in the time of appearance of anti-HBs after HBV infection, occasionally a gap of several weeks or longer may separate the disappearance of HBsAg and the appearance of anti-HBs. During this "gap" or "window" period, anti-HBc may represent the only serologic evidence of current or recent HBV infection, and blood containing anti-HBc in the absence of HBsAg and anti-HBs has been implicated in the development of transfusion-associated hepatitis B. In part because the sensitivity of immunoassays for HBsAg and anti-HBs has increased, however, this window period is rarely encountered. In some persons, years after HBV infection, anti-HBc may persist in the circulation longer than anti-HBs. Therefore, isolated anti-HBc does not necessarily indicate active virus replication; most instances of isolated anti-HBc represent hepatitis B infection in the remote past. Rarely, however, isolated anti-HBc represents low-level hepatitis B viremia, with HBsAg below the detection threshold; occasionally, isolated anti-HBc represents a cross-reacting or false-positive immunologic specificity. Recent and remote HBV infections can be distinguished by determination of the immunoglobulin class of anti-HBc. Anti-HBc of the IgM class (IgM anti-HBc) predominates during the first 6 months after acute infection, whereas IgG anti-HBc is the predominant class of anti-HBc beyond 6 months. Therefore, patients with current or recent acute hepatitis B, including those in the anti-HBc window, have IgM anti-HBc in their serum. In patients who have recovered from hepatitis B in the remote past as well as those with chronic HBV infection, anti-HBc is predominantly of the IgG class. Infrequently, in ≤1–5% of patients with acute HBV infection, levels of HBsAg are too low to be detected; in such cases, the presence of IgM anti-HBc establishes the diagnosis of acute hepatitis B. When isolated anti-HBc occurs in the rare patient with chronic hepatitis B whose HBsAg level is below the sensitivity threshold of contemporary immunoassays (a low-level carrier), the anti-HBc is of the IgG class. Generally, in persons who have recovered from hepatitis B, anti-HBs and anti-HBc persist indefinitely.

The temporal association between the appearance of anti-HBs and resolution of HBV infection as well as the observation that persons with anti-HBs in serum are protected against reinfection with HBV suggests that *anti-HBs are the protective antibody*. Therefore, strategies for prevention of HBV infection are based on providing susceptible persons with circulating anti-HBs (see later). Occasionally, in 10–20% of patients with chronic hepatitis B, low-level, low-affinity anti-HBs can be detected. This antibody is directed against a subtype determinant different from that represented by the patient's HBsAg; its presence is thought to reflect the stimulation of a related clone of antibody-forming cells, but it has no clinical relevance and does not signal imminent clearance of hepatitis B. These patients with HBsAg and such nonneutralizing anti-HBs should be categorized as having chronic HBV infection.

The other readily detectable serologic marker of HBV infection, HBeAg, appears concurrently with or shortly after HBsAg. Its appearance coincides temporally with high levels of virus replication and reflects the presence of circulating intact virions and detectable HBV DNA (with the notable exception of patients with precore mutations who cannot synthesize HBeAg—see the next section, "Molecular Variants"). Pre-S1 and pre-S2 proteins are also expressed during periods of peak replication, but assays for these gene products are not routinely available. In self-limited HBV infections, HBeAg becomes undetectable shortly after peak elevations in aminotransferase activity, before the disappearance of HBsAg, and anti-HBe then becomes detectable, coinciding with a period of relatively lower infectivity (Fig. 37-4). Because markers of HBV replication appear transiently during acute infection, testing for such markers is of little clinical utility in typical cases of acute HBV infection. In contrast, markers of HBV replication provide valuable information in patients with protracted infections.

Departing from the pattern typical of acute HBV infections, in chronic HBV infection, HBsAg remains detectable beyond 6 months, anti-HBc is primarily of the IgG class, and anti-HBs is either undetectable or detectable at low levels (see "Laboratory Features" later in the chapter) (Fig. 37-5). During early chronic HBV infection, HBV DNA can be detected both in serum and in hepatocyte nuclei, where it is present in free or episomal form. This *replicative stage* of HBV infection is the time of maximal infectivity and liver injury; HBeAg is a qualitative marker and HBV DNA a quantitative

marker of this replicative phase, during which all three forms of HBV circulate, including intact virions. Over time, the replicative phase of chronic HBV infection gives way to a relatively *nonreplicative phase*. This occurs at a rate of ~10% per year and is accompanied by seroconversion from HBeAg-positive to anti-HBe-positive. In most cases, this seroconversion coincides with a transient, acute hepatitis-like elevation in aminotransferase activity, believed to reflect cell-mediated immune clearance of virus-infected hepatocytes. In the nonreplicative phase of chronic infection, when HBV DNA is demonstrable in hepatocyte nuclei, it tends to be integrated into the host genome. In this phase, only spherical and tubular forms of HBV, *not intact virions*, circulate, and liver injury tends to subside. Most such patients would be characterized as *inactive HBV carriers*. In reality, the designations *replicative* and *nonreplicative* are only relative; even in the so-called nonreplicative phase, HBV replication can be detected at levels of ~$\leq 10^3$ virions with highly sensitive amplification probes such as the polymerase chain reaction (PCR); below this replication threshold, liver injury and infectivity of HBV are limited to negligible. Still, the distinctions are pathophysiologically and clinically meaningful. Occasionally, nonreplicative HBV infection converts back to replicative infection. Such spontaneous reactivations are accompanied by reexpression of HBeAg and HBV DNA, and sometimes of IgM

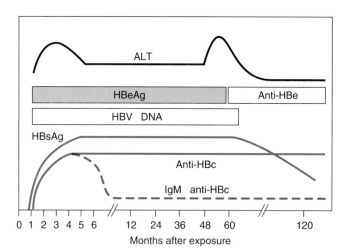

FIGURE 37-5

Scheme of typical laboratory features of wild-type chronic hepatitis B. HBeAg and HBV DNA can be detected in serum during the *replicative phase* of chronic infection, which is associated with infectivity and liver injury. Seroconversion from the replicative phase to the *nonreplicative phase* occurs at a rate of ~10% per year and is heralded by an acute hepatitis–like elevation of ALT activity; during the nonreplicative phase, infectivity and liver injury are limited. In HBeAg-negative chronic hepatitis B associated with mutations in the precore region of the HBV genome, replicative chronic hepatitis B occurs in the absence of HBeAg.

anti-HBc, as well as by exacerbations of liver injury. Because high-titer IgM anti-HBc can reappear during acute exacerbations of chronic hepatitis B, relying on IgM anti-HBc versus IgG anti-HBc to distinguish between acute and chronic hepatitis B infection, respectively, may not always be reliable; in such cases, patient history is invaluable in helping to distinguish de novo acute hepatitis B infection from acute exacerbation of chronic hepatitis B infection.

Molecular Variants

Variation occurs throughout the HBV genome, and clinical isolates of HBV that do not express typical viral proteins have been attributed to mutations in individual or even multiple gene locations. For example, variants have been described that lack nucleocapsid proteins, envelope proteins, or both. Two categories of naturally occurring HBV variants have attracted the most attention. One of these was identified initially in Mediterranean countries among patients with an unusual serologic-clinical profile. They have severe chronic HBV infection and detectable HBV DNA but with anti-HBe instead of HBeAg. These patients were found to be infected with an HBV mutant that contained an alteration in the precore region rendering the virus incapable of encoding HBeAg. Although several potential mutation sites exist in the pre-C region, the region of the C gene necessary for the expression of HBeAg (see "Virology and Etiology" earlier in the chapter), the most commonly encountered in such patients is a single base substitution, from G to A, which occurs in the second to last codon of the pre-C gene at nucleotide 1896. This substitution results in the replacement of the TGG tryptophan codon by a stop codon (TAG), which prevents the translation of HBeAg. Another mutation, in the core-promoter region, prevents transcription of the coding region for HBeAg and yields an HBeAg-negative phenotype. Patients with such mutations in the precore region and who are unable to secrete HBeAg tend to have severe liver disease that progresses more rapidly to cirrhosis. Both "wild-type" HBV and precore-mutant HBV can coexist in the same patient, or mutant HBV may arise late during wild-type HBV infection. In addition, clusters of fulminant hepatitis B in Israel and Japan have been attributed to common-source infection with a precore mutant. Fulminant hepatitis B in North America and western Europe, however, occurs in patients infected with wild-type HBV, in the absence of precore mutants, and both precore mutants and other mutations throughout the HBV genome occur commonly even in patients with typical, self-limited, milder forms of HBV infection. HBeAg-negative chronic hepatitis with mutations in the precore region is now the most frequently encountered form of hepatitis B in Mediterranean countries and in Europe. In the United States, where HBV genotype A (less prone to G1896A mutation) is prevalent, precore-mutant HBV is much less common; however, as a result of immigration from Asia and Europe, the proportion of HBeAg-negative hepatitis B–infected individuals has increased in the United States, and they now represent approximately a third of patients with chronic hepatitis B. Characteristic of such HBeAg-negative chronic hepatitis B are lower levels of HBV DNA (usually $\leq 10^5$ copies/mL) and one of several patterns of aminotransferase activity—persistent elevations, periodic fluctuations above the normal range, and periodic fluctuations between the normal and elevated range.

The second important category of HBV mutants consists of escape *mutants,* in which a single amino acid substitution, from glycine to arginine, occurs at position 145 of the immunodominant *a* determinant common to all subtypes of HBsAg. This change in HBsAg leads to a critical conformational change that results in a loss of neutralizing activity by anti-HBs. This specific HBV/*a* mutant has been observed in two situations, active and passive immunization, in which humoral immunologic pressure may favor evolutionary change ("escape") in the virus—in a small number of hepatitis B vaccine recipients who acquired HBV infection despite the prior appearance of neutralizing anti-HBs and in liver transplant recipients who underwent the procedure for hepatitis B and who were treated with a high-potency human monoclonal anti-HBs preparation. Although such mutants have not been recognized frequently, their existence raises a concern that may complicate vaccination strategies and serologic diagnosis. Different types of mutations emerge during antiviral therapy of chronic hepatitis B with nucleoside analogues; such "YMDD" and similar mutations in the polymerase motif of HBV are described in Chap. 39.

Extrahepatic Sites

Hepatitis B antigens and HBV DNA have been identified in extrahepatic sites, including lymph nodes, bone marrow, circulating lymphocytes, spleen, and pancreas. Although the virus does not appear to be associated with tissue injury in any of these extrahepatic sites, its presence in these "remote" reservoirs has been invoked to explain the recurrence of HBV infection after orthotopic liver transplantation. A more complete understanding of the clinical relevance of extrahepatic HBV remains to be defined.

Hepatitis D

The delta hepatitis agent, or HDV, is a defective RNA virus that coinfects with and requires the helper function of HBV (or other hepadnaviruses) for its replication and expression. Slightly smaller than HBV, delta is a formalin-sensitive, 35- to 37-nm virus with a hybrid structure. Its nucleocapsid expresses delta antigen, which bears no antigenic homology with any of the HBV antigens, and contains the virus genome. The delta core is "encapsidated" by an outer envelope of HBsAg, indistinguishable from that of HBV except in its relative compositions of major, middle, and large HBsAg component proteins. The genome is a small, 1700-nucleotide, circular, single-strand RNA (minus strand) that is nonhomologous with HBV DNA (except for a small area of the polymerase gene) but that has features and the rolling circle model of replication common to genomes of plant satellite viruses or viroids. HDV RNA contains many areas of internal complementarity; therefore, it can fold on itself by internal base pairing to form an unusual, very stable, rodlike structure. HDV RNA requires host RNA polymerase II for its replication via RNA-directed RNA synthesis by transcription of genomic RNA to a complementary antigenomic (plus strand) RNA; the antigenomic RNA, in turn, serves as a template for subsequent genomic RNA synthesis. Between the genomic and antigenomic RNAs of HDV, there are coding regions for nine proteins. Delta antigen, which is a product of the antigenomic strand, exists in two forms, a small, 195-amino-acid species, which plays a role in facilitating HDV RNA replication, and a large, 214-amino-acid species, which appears to suppress replication but is required for assembly of the antigen into virions. Delta antigens have been shown to bind directly to RNA polymerase II, resulting in stimulation of transcription. Although complete hepatitis D virions and liver injury require the cooperative helper function of HBV, intracellular replication of HDV RNA can occur without HBV. Genomic heterogeneity among HDV isolates has been described; however, pathophysiologic and clinical consequences of this genetic diversity have not been recognized.

HDV can either infect a person simultaneously with HBV (*co-infection*) or superinfect a person already infected with HBV (*superinfection*); when HDV infection is transmitted from a donor with one HBsAg subtype to an HBsAg-positive recipient with a different subtype, the HDV agent assumes the HBsAg subtype of the recipient, rather than the donor. Because HDV relies absolutely on HBV, the duration of HDV infection is determined by the duration of (and cannot outlast) HBV infection. HDV antigen is expressed primarily in hepatocyte nuclei and is occasionally detectable in serum. During acute HDV infection, anti-HDV of the IgM class predominates, and 30–40 days may elapse after symptoms appear before anti-HDV can be detected. In self-limited infection, anti-HDV is low titer and transient, rarely remaining detectable beyond the clearance of HBsAg and HDV antigen. In chronic HDV infection, anti-HDV circulates in high titer, and both IgM and IgG anti-HDV can be detected. HDV antigen in the liver and HDV RNA in serum and liver can be detected during HDV replication.

Hepatitis C

Hepatitis C virus, which, before its identification was labeled "non-A, non-B hepatitis," is a linear, single-strand, positive-sense, 9600-nucleotide RNA virus, the genome of which is similar in organization to that of flaviviruses and pestiviruses; HCV is the only member of the genus *Hepacivirus* in the family Flaviviridae. The HCV genome contains a single large open reading frame (gene) that codes for a virus polyprotein of ~3000 amino acids, which is cleaved after translation to yield 10 viral proteins. The 5′end of the genome consists of an untranslated region (containing an internal ribosomal entry site) adjacent to the genes for four structural proteins; the nucleocapsid core protein, C; two envelope glycoproteins, E1 and E2; and a membrane protein p7. The 5′ untranslated region and core gene are highly conserved among genotypes, but the envelope proteins are coded for by the hypervariable region, which varies from isolate to isolate and may allow the virus to evade host immunologic containment directed at accessible virus-envelope proteins. The 3′ end of the genome also includes an untranslated region and contains the genes for six nonstructural (NS) proteins: NS2, NS3, NS4A, NS4B, NS5A, and NS5B. The NS2 cysteine protease cleaves NS3 from NS2, and the NS3-4A serine protease cleaves all the downstream proteins from the polyprotein. Important NS proteins involved in virus replication include the NS3 helicase, NS3-NS4A serine protease, and the NS5B RNA-dependent RNA polymerase (**Fig. 37-6**). Because HCV does not replicate via a DNA intermediate, it does not integrate into the host genome. Because HCV tends to circulate in relatively low titer, 10^3–10^7 virions/mL, visualization of virus particles, estimated to be 40–60 nm in diameter, remains difficult. Still, the replication rate of HCV is very high, 10^{12} virions per day; its half-life is 2.7 h. The chimpanzee is a helpful but cumbersome animal model. Although a robust, reproducible, small-animal model is lacking, HCV replication has been documented in an immunodeficient-mouse model containing explants of human liver and in transgenic mouse and rat models. Although in vitro replication has been difficult, hepatocellular carcinoma–derived cell lines have been described (replicon systems) that support replication of genetically manipulated, truncated or full-length HCV RNA (but not intact virions). Recently, complete replication of HCV and intact 55-nm virions has been described in cell culture systems. Preliminary data suggest that HCV gains entry into the hepatocyte via the CD81 receptor.

At least six distinct genotypes, as well as >50 subtypes within genotypes, of HCV have been identified by nucleotide sequencing. Genotypes differ one from another in sequence homology by ≥30%. Because divergence of HCV isolates within a genotype or

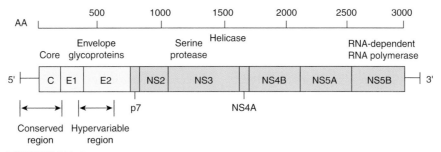

FIGURE 37-6

Organization of the hepatitis C virus genome and its associated, 3000-amino-acid (AA) proteins. The three structural genes at the 5′ end are the core region, C, which codes for the nucleocapsid, and the envelope regions, E1 and E2, which code for envelope glycoproteins. The 5′ untranslated region and the C region are highly conserved among isolates, while the envelope domain E2 contains the hypervariable region. Adjacent to the structural proteins is p7, a membrane protein that appears to function as an ion channel. At the 3′ end are six nonstructural (NS) regions, NS2, which codes for a cysteine protease; NS3, which codes for a serine protease and an RNA helicase; NS4 and NS4B; NS5A; and NS5B, which codes for an RNA-dependent RNA polymerase. After translation of the entire polyprotein, individual proteins are cleaved by both host and viral proteases.

subtype, and within the same host, may vary insufficiently to define a distinct genotype, these intragenotypic differences are referred to as *quasispecies* and differ in sequence homology by only a few percent. The genotypic and quasispecies diversity of HCV, resulting from its high mutation rate, interferes with effective humoral immunity. Neutralizing antibodies to HCV have been demonstrated, but they tend to be short-lived, and HCV infection does not induce lasting immunity against reinfection with different virus isolates or even the same virus isolate. Thus, neither *heterologous* nor *homologous* immunity appears to develop commonly after acute HCV infection. Some HCV genotypes are distributed worldwide, while others are more geographically confined (see "Epidemiology and Global Features" later in the chapter). In addition, differences exist among genotypes in responsiveness to antiviral therapy; however, early reports of differences in pathogenicity among genotypes have not been corroborated.

Currently available, third-generation immunoassays, which incorporate proteins from the core, NS3, and NS5 regions, detect anti-HCV antibodies during acute infection. The most sensitive indicator of HCV infection is the presence of HCV RNA, which requires molecular amplification by PCR or transcription-mediated amplification (TMA) (Fig. 37-7). To allow standardization of the quantification of HCV RNA among laboratories and commercial assays, HCV RNA is reported as international units (IU) per milliliter; quantitative assays are available that allow detection of HCV RNA with a sensitivity as low as 5 IU/mL. HCV RNA can be detected within a few days of exposure to HCV, well before the appearance of anti-HCV, and tends to persist for the duration of HCV infection; however, occasionally in patients with chronic HCV infection, HCV RNA may be detectable only intermittently. Application of sensitive molecular probes for HCV RNA has revealed the presence of replicative HCV in peripheral blood lymphocytes of infected persons; however, as is the case for HBV in lymphocytes, the clinical relevance of HCV lymphocyte infection is not known.

Hepatitis E

Previously labeled *epidemic* or *enterically transmitted non-A, non-B hepatitis*, HEV is an enterically transmitted virus that occurs primarily in India, Asia, Africa, and Central America; in those geographic areas, HEV is the most

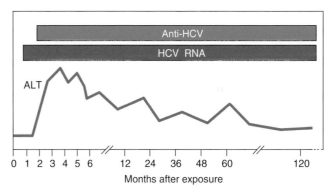

FIGURE 37-7

Scheme of typical laboratory features during acute hepatitis C progressing to chronicity. HCV RNA is the first detectable event, preceding ALT elevation and the appearance of anti-HCV.

common cause of acute hepatitis. This agent, with epidemiologic features resembling those of hepatitis A, is a 32- to 34-nm, nonenveloped, HAV-like virus with a 7600-nucleotide, single-strand, positive-sense RNA genome. HEV has three open reading frames (ORF) (genes), the largest of which, *ORF1*, encodes nonstructural proteins involved in virus replication. A middle-sized gene, *ORF2*, encodes the nucleocapsid protein, and the smallest, *ORF3*, encodes a structural protein whose function remains undetermined. All HEV isolates appear to belong to a single serotype, despite genomic heterogeneity of up to 25% and the existence of five genotypes, only four of which have been detected in humans; genotypes 1 and 2 appear to be more virulent, while genotypes 3 and 4 are more attenuated and account for subclinical infections. Contributing to the perpetuation of this virus are animal reservoirs, most notably in swine. There is no genomic or antigenic homology, however, between HEV and HAV or other picornaviruses; and HEV, although resembling caliciviruses, is sufficiently distinct from any known agent to merit a new classification of its own as a unique genus, *Hepevirus*, within the Hepeviridae family. The virus has been detected in stool, bile, and liver and is excreted in the stool during the late incubation period; immune responses to viral antigens occur very early during the course of acute infection. Both IgM anti-HEV and IgG anti-HEV can be detected, but both fall rapidly after acute infection, reaching low levels within 9–12 months. Currently, serologic testing for HEV infection is not available routinely.

PATHOGENESIS

Under ordinary circumstances, none of the hepatitis viruses is known to be directly cytopathic to hepatocytes. Evidence suggests that the clinical manifestations and outcomes after acute liver injury associated with viral hepatitis are determined by the immunologic responses of the host. Among the viral hepatitides, the immunopathogenesis of hepatitis B and C have been studied most extensively.

Hepatitis B

For HBV, the existence of inactive hepatitis B carriers with normal liver histology and function suggests that the virus is not directly cytopathic. The fact that patients with defects in cellular immune competence are more likely to remain chronically infected rather than to clear HBV is cited to support the role of cellular immune responses in the pathogenesis of hepatitis B–related liver injury. The model that has the most experimental support involves cytolytic T cells sensitized specifically to recognize host and hepatitis B viral antigens on the liver cell surface. Laboratory observations

suggest that nucleocapsid proteins (HBcAg and possibly HBeAg), present on the cell membrane in minute quantities, are the viral target antigens that, with host antigens, invite cytolytic T cells to destroy HBV-infected hepatocytes. Differences in the robustness of CD8+ cytolytic T cell responsiveness and in the elaboration of antiviral cytokines by T cells have been invoked to explain differences in outcomes between those who recover after acute hepatitis and those who progress to chronic hepatitis or between those with mild and those with severe (fulminant) acute HBV infection.

Although a robust cytolytic T cell response occurs and eliminates virus-infected liver cells during acute hepatitis B, >90% of HBV DNA has been found in experimentally infected chimpanzees to disappear from the liver and blood before maximal T cell infiltration of the liver and before most of the biochemical and histologic evidence of liver injury. This observation suggests that components of the innate immune system and inflammatory cytokines, independent of cytopathic antiviral mechanisms, participate in the early immune response to HBV infection; this effect has been shown to represent elimination of HBV replicative intermediates from the cytoplasm and covalently closed circular viral DNA from the nucleus of infected hepatocytes. Ultimately, HBV-HLA-specific cytolytic T cell responses of the adaptive immune system are felt to be responsible for recovery from HBV infection.

Debate continues over the relative importance of viral and host factors in the pathogenesis of HBV-associated liver injury and its outcome. As noted above, precore genetic mutants of HBV have been associated with the more severe outcomes of HBV infection (severe chronic and fulminant hepatitis), suggesting that, under certain circumstances, relative pathogenicity is a property of the virus, not the host. The fact that concomitant HDV and HBV infections are associated with more severe liver injury than HBV infection alone and the fact that cells transfected in vitro with the gene for HDV (delta) antigen express HDV antigen and then become necrotic in the absence of any immunologic influences are also consistent with a viral effect on pathogenicity. Similarly, in patients who undergo liver transplantation for end-stage chronic hepatitis B, occasionally, rapidly progressive liver injury appears in the new liver. This clinical pattern is associated with an unusual histologic pattern in the new liver, *fibrosing cholestatic hepatitis*, which, ultrastructurally, appears to represent a choking of the cell with overwhelming quantities of HBsAg. This observation suggests that under the influence of the potent immunosuppressive agents required to prevent allograft rejection, HBV may have a direct cytopathic effect on liver cells, independent of the immune system.

Although the precise mechanism of liver injury in HBV infection remains elusive, studies of nucleocapsid proteins have shed light on the profound immunologic tolerance to HBV of babies born to mothers with highly replicative (HBeAg-positive), chronic HBV infection. In HBeAg-expressing transgenic mice, in utero exposure to HBeAg, which is sufficiently small to traverse the placenta, induces T cell tolerance to both nucleocapsid proteins. This, in turn, may explain why, when infection occurs so early in life, immunologic clearance does not occur, and protracted, lifelong infection ensues.

An important distinction should be drawn between HBV infection acquired at birth, common in endemic areas, such as the Far East, and infection acquired in adulthood, common in the west. Infection in the neonatal period is associated with the acquisition of immunologic tolerance to HBV, absence of an acute-hepatitis illness, but the almost invariable establishment of chronic, often lifelong infection. Neonatally acquired HBV infection can culminate decades later in cirrhosis and hepatocellular carcinoma (see "Complications and Sequelae" later in the chapter.) In contrast, when HBV infection is acquired during adolescence or early adulthood, the host-immune response to HBV-infected hepatocytes tends to be robust, an acute hepatitis-like illness is the rule, and failure to recover is the exception. After adulthood-acquired infection, chronicity is uncommon, and the risk of hepatocellular carcinoma is very low. Based on these observations, some authorities categorize HBV infection into an "immunotolerant" phase, an "immunoreactive" phase, and an inactive phase. This somewhat simplistic formulation does not apply at all to the typical adult in the west with self-limited acute hepatitis B, in whom no period of immunologic tolerance occurs. Even among those with neonatally acquired HBV infection, in whom immunologic tolerance is established definitively, intermittent bursts of hepatic necroinflammatory activity punctuate the period during the early decades of life during which liver injury appears to be quiescent (labeled by some as the "immunotolerant" phase). In addition, even when clinically apparent liver injury and progressive fibrosis emerge during later decades (the so-called immunoreactive, or immunointolerant, phase), the level of immunologic tolerance to HBV remains substantial. More accurately, in patients with neonatally acquired HBV infection, a dynamic equilibrium exists between tolerance and intolerance, the outcome of which determines the clinical expression of chronic infection.

Hepatitis C

Cell-mediated immune responses and elaboration by T cells of antiviral cytokines contribute to the containment of infection and pathogenesis of liver injury associated with hepatitis C. Perhaps HCV infection of lymphoid cells plays a role in moderating immune responsiveness to the virus, as well. Intrahepatic HLA class I–restricted cytolytic T cells directed at nucleocapsid, envelope, and nonstructural viral protein antigens have been demonstrated in patients with chronic hepatitis C: however, such virus-specific cytolytic T cell responses do not correlate adequately with the degree of liver injury or with recovery. Yet, a consensus has emerged supporting a role in the pathogenesis of HCV-associated liver injury of virus-activated CD4 helper T cells that stimulate, via the cytokines they elaborate, HCV-specific CD8 cytotoxic T cells. These responses appear to be more robust (higher in number, more diverse in viral antigen specificity, more functionally effective, and more long-lasting) in those who recover from HCV than in those who have chronic infection. Several HLA alleles have been linked with self-limited hepatitis C, but such associations do not apply universally. Attention has been focused as well on adaptive immunity; the establishment of persistent infection correlates with failure of adaptive immune responses to HCV. Furthermore, HCV proteins have been shown to interfere with innate immunity by resulting in blocking of type 1 interferon responses and inhibition of interferon signaling and effector molecules in the interferon signaling cascade. Also shown to contribute to limiting HCV infection are natural killer cells of the innate immune system, which function when HLA class 1 molecules required for successful adaptive immunity are underexpressed. Of note, the emergence of substantial viral quasispecies diversity allows the virus to evade attempts by the host to contain HCV infection immunologically.

Finally, cross-reactivity between viral antigens (HCV NS3 and NS5A) and host autoantigens (cytochrome P450 2D6) has been invoked to explain the association between hepatitis C and a subset of patients with autoimmune hepatitis and antibodies to liver-kidney microsomal (LKM) antigen (anti-LKM) (Chap. 39).

EXTRAHEPATIC MANIFESTATIONS

Immune complex–mediated tissue damage appears to play a pathogenetic role in the extrahepatic manifestations of acute hepatitis B. The occasional prodromal serum sickness–like syndrome observed in acute hepatitis B appears to be related to the deposition in tissue blood vessel walls of HBsAg-anti-HBs circulating immune complexes, leading to activation of the complement system and depressed serum complement levels.

In patients with chronic hepatitis B, other types of immune-complex disease may be seen. Glomerulonephritis with the nephritic syndrome is occasionally observed; HBsAg, immunoglobulin, and C3 deposition has been found in the glomerular basement membrane. While polyarteritis nodosa develops in considerably fewer than 1% of patients with chronic HBV infection, 20–30% of patients with polyarteritis nodosa have

HBsAg in serum. In these patients, the affected small and medium-size arterioles have been shown to contain HBsAg, immunoglobulins, and complement components. Another extrahepatic manifestation of viral hepatitis, essential mixed cryoglobulinemia (EMC), was reported initially to be associated with hepatitis B. The disorder is characterized clinically by arthritis, cutaneous vasculitis (palpable purpura), and occasionally with glomerulonephritis and serologically by the presence of circulating cryoprecipitable immune complexes of more than one immunoglobulin class. Many patients with this syndrome have chronic liver disease, but the association with HBV infection is limited; instead, a substantial proportion has chronic HCV infection, with circulating immune complexes containing HCV RNA. Immune-complex glomerulonephritis is another recognized extrahepatic manifestation of chronic hepatitis C.

PATHOLOGY

The typical morphologic lesions of all types of viral hepatitis are similar and consist of panlobular infiltration with mononuclear cells, hepatic cell necrosis, hyperplasia of Kupffer cells, and variable degrees of cholestasis. Hepatic cell regeneration is present, as evidenced by numerous mitotic figures, multinucleated cells, and "rosette" or "pseudoacinar" formation. The mononuclear infiltration consists primarily of small lymphocytes, although plasma cells and eosinophils occasionally are present. Liver cell damage consists of hepatic cell degeneration and necrosis, cell dropout, ballooning of cells, and acidophilic degeneration of hepatocytes (forming so-called Councilman or apoptotic bodies). Large hepatocytes with a ground-glass appearance of the cytoplasm may be seen in chronic but not in acute HBV infection; these cells contain HBsAg and can be identified histochemically with orcein or aldehyde fuchsin. In uncomplicated viral hepatitis, the reticulin framework is preserved.

In hepatitis C, the histologic lesion is often remarkable for a relative paucity of inflammation, a marked increase in activation of sinusoidal lining cells, lymphoid aggregates, the presence of fat (more frequent in genotype 3 and linked to increased fibrosis), and, occasionally, bile duct lesions in which biliary epithelial cells appear to be piled up without interruption of the basement membrane. Occasionally, microvesicular steatosis occurs in hepatitis D. In hepatitis E, a common histologic feature is marked cholestasis. A cholestatic variant of slowly resolving acute hepatitis A also has been described.

A more severe histologic lesion, *bridging hepatic necrosis*, also termed *subacute* or *confluent necrosis* or *interface hepatitis*, is occasionally observed in some patients with acute hepatitis. "Bridging" between lobules results from large areas of hepatic cell dropout, with collapse of the reticulin framework. Characteristically, the bridge consists of condensed reticulum, inflammatory debris, and degenerating liver cells that span adjacent portal areas, portal to central veins, or central vein to central vein. This lesion had been thought to have prognostic significance; in many of the originally described patients with this lesion, a subacute course terminated in death within several weeks to months, or severe chronic hepatitis and postnecrotic cirrhosis developed. Subsequent investigations have failed to uphold the association between bridging necrosis and such a poor prognosis in patients with acute hepatitis. Therefore, although demonstration of this lesion in patients with chronic hepatitis has prognostic significance (Chap. 39), its demonstration during acute hepatitis is less meaningful, and liver biopsies to identify this lesion are no longer undertaken routinely in patients with acute hepatitis. In *massive hepatic necrosis* (fulminant hepatitis, "acute yellow atrophy"), the striking feature at postmortem examination is the finding of a small, shrunken, soft liver. Histologic examination reveals massive necrosis and dropout of liver cells of most lobules with extensive collapse and condensation of the reticulin framework. When histologic documentation is required in the management of fulminant or very severe hepatitis, a biopsy can be done by the angiographically guided transjugular route, which permits the performance of this invasive procedure in the presence of severe coagulopathy.

Immunohistochemical and electron-microscopic studies have localized HBsAg to the cytoplasm and plasma membrane of infected liver cells. In contrast, HBcAg predominates in the nucleus, but occasionally, scant amounts are also seen in the cytoplasm and on the cell membrane. HDV antigen is localized to the hepatocyte nucleus, while HAV, HCV, and HEV antigens are localized to the cytoplasm.

EPIDEMIOLOGY AND GLOBAL FEATURES

Before the availability of serologic tests for hepatitis viruses, all viral hepatitis cases were labeled either as "infectious" or "serum" hepatitis. Modes of transmission overlap, however, and *a clear distinction among the different types of viral hepatitis cannot be made solely on the basis of clinical or epidemiologic features* (Table 37-2). The most accurate means to distinguish the various types of viral hepatitis involves specific serologic testing.

Hepatitis A

This agent is transmitted almost exclusively by the fecal-oral route. Person-to-person spread of HAV is enhanced by poor personal hygiene and overcrowding; large outbreaks as well as sporadic cases have been traced to contaminated food, water, milk, frozen raspberries and strawberries, green onions imported from Mexico, and

TABLE 37-2

361

CLINICAL AND EPIDEMIOLOGIC FEATURES OF VIRAL HEPATITIS

FEATURE	HAV	HBV	HCV	HDV	HEV
Incubation (days)	15–45, mean 30	30–180, mean 60–90	15–160, mean 50	30–180, mean 60–90	14–60, mean 40
Onset	Acute	Insidious or acute	Insidious	Insidious or acute	Acute
Age preference	Children, young adults	Young adults (sexual and percutaneous), babies, toddlers	Any age, but more common in adults	Any age (similar to HBV)	Young adults (20–40 years)
Transmission					
Fecal-oral	+++	−	−	−	+++
Percutaneous	Unusual	+++	+++	+++	−
Perinatal	−	+++	±[a]	+	−
Sexual	±	++	±[a]	++	−
Clinical					
Severity	Mild	Occasionally severe	Moderate	Occasionally severe	Mild
Fulminant	0.1%	0.1–1%	0.1%	5–20%[b]	1–2%[e]
Progression to chronicity	None	Occasional (1–10%) (90% of neonates)	Common (85%)	Common[d]	None
Carrier	None	0.1–30%[c]	1.5–3.2%	Variable[f]	None
Cancer	None	+ (neonatal infection)	+	±	None
Prognosis	Excellent	Worse with age, debility	Moderate	Acute, good Chronic, poor	Good
Prophylaxis	IG Inactivated vaccine	HBIG Recombinant vaccine	None	HBV vaccine (none for HBV carriers)	Vaccine
Therapy	None	Interferon Lamivudine Adefovir Pegylated interferon Entecavir Telbivudine	Pegylated interferon plus ribavirin	Interferon ±	None

[a]Primarily with HIV co-infection and high-level viremia in index case; risk ~5%.
[b]Up to 5% in acute HBV/HDV co-infection; up to 20% in HDV superinfection of chronic HBV infection.
[c]Varies considerably throughout the world and in subpopulations within countries; see text.
[d]In acute HBV/HDV co-infection, the frequency of chronicity is the same as that for HBV; in HDV superinfection, chronicity is invariable.
[e]10–20% in pregnant women.
[f]Common in Mediterranean countries, rare in North America and western Europe.

shellfish. Intrafamily and intrainstitutional spread are also common. Early epidemiologic observations supported a predilection for hepatitis A to occur in late fall and early winter. In temperate zones, epidemic waves have been recorded every 5–20 years as new segments of nonimmune population appeared; however, in developed countries, the incidence of hepatitis A has been declining, presumably as a function of improved sanitation, and these cyclic patterns are no longer observed. No HAV carrier state has been identified after acute hepatitis A; perpetuation of the virus in nature depends presumably on nonepidemic, inapparent subclinical infection and/or contamination linked to environmental reservoirs.

In the general population, anti-HAV, a marker for previous HAV infection, increases in prevalence as a function of increasing age and of decreasing socioeconomic status. In the 1970s, serologic evidence of prior hepatitis A infection occurred in ~40% of urban populations in the United States, most of whose members never recalled having had a symptomatic case of hepatitis. In subsequent decades, however, the prevalence of anti-HAV has been declining in the United States. In developing countries, exposure, infection, and subsequent immunity are almost universal in childhood. As the frequency of subclinical childhood infections declines in developed countries, a susceptible cohort of adults emerges. Hepatitis A tends to be more symptomatic in adults; therefore, paradoxically, as the frequency of HAV infection declines, the likelihood of clinically apparent, even severe, HAV illnesses increases in the susceptible adult population. Travel to endemic areas is a common source of infection for adults from nonendemic areas. More recently recognized epidemiologic foci of HAV infection include child-care centers, neonatal intensive care units, promiscuous men who have sex with men, and injection drug users. Although hepatitis A is rarely bloodborne, several outbreaks have been recognized in recipients of clotting factor concentrates. In the United States, the introduction of hepatitis A vaccination programs among children from high-incidence states has resulted in >70% reduction in the annual incidence of new HAV infections and has shifted the burden of new infections from children to young adults.

Hepatitis B

Percutaneous inoculation has long been recognized as a major route of hepatitis B transmission, but the outmoded designation "serum hepatitis" is an inaccurate label for the epidemiologic spectrum of HBV infection recognized today. As detailed below, most of the hepatitis transmitted by blood transfusion is not caused by HBV; moreover, in approximately two-thirds of patients with acute type B hepatitis, no history of an identifiable percutaneous exposure can be elicited. We now recognize that many cases of hepatitis B result from less obvious modes of nonpercutaneous or covert percutaneous transmission. HBsAg has been identified in almost every body fluid from infected persons, and at least some of these body fluids—most notably semen and saliva—are infectious, albeit less so than serum, when administered percutaneously or nonpercutaneously to experimental animals. Among the nonpercutaneous modes of HBV transmission, oral ingestion has been documented as a potential but inefficient route of exposure. By contrast, the two nonpercutaneous routes considered to have the greatest impact are intimate (especially sexual) contact and perinatal transmission.

In sub-Saharan Africa, intimate contact among toddlers is considered instrumental in contributing to the maintenance of the high frequency of hepatitis B in the population. Perinatal transmission occurs primarily in infants born to HBsAg carrier mothers or mothers with acute hepatitis B during the third trimester of pregnancy or during the early postpartum period. Perinatal transmission is uncommon in North America and western Europe but occurs with great frequency and is the most important mode of HBV perpetuation in the Far East and developing countries. Although the precise mode of perinatal transmission is unknown, and although ~10% of infections may be acquired in utero, epidemiologic evidence suggests that most infections occur approximately at the time of delivery and are not related to breast feeding. The likelihood of perinatal transmission of HBV correlates with the presence of HBeAg; 90% of HBeAg-positive mothers but only 10–15% of anti-HBe-positive mothers transmit HBV infection to their offspring. In most cases, acute infection in the neonate is clinically asymptomatic, but the child is very likely to become an HBsAg carrier.

The >350 million HBsAg carriers in the world constitute the main reservoir of hepatitis B in human beings. Serum HBsAg is infrequent (0.1–0.5%) in normal populations in the United States and western Europe. However, a prevalence of up to 5–20% has been found in the Far East and in some tropical countries; in persons with Down's syndrome, lepromatous leprosy, leukemia, Hodgkin's disease, polyarteritis nodosa; in patients with chronic renal disease on hemodialysis; and in injection drug users.

Other groups with high rates of HBV infection include spouses of acutely infected persons, sexually promiscuous persons (especially promiscuous men who have sex with men), health care workers exposed to blood, persons who require repeated transfusions especially with pooled blood product concentrates (e.g., hemophiliacs), residents and staff of custodial institutions for the developmentally handicapped, prisoners, and, to a lesser extent, family members of chronically infected patients. In volunteer blood donors, the prevalence of anti-HBs, a reflection of previous HBV infection, ranges from 5–10%, but the prevalence is higher in lower socioeconomic strata, older age groups, and persons—including those mentioned above—exposed to blood products. Because of highly sensitive virologic screening of donor blood, the risk of acquiring HBV infection from a blood transfusion is 1 in 230,000.

Prevalence of infection, modes of transmission, and human behavior conspire to mold geographically different epidemiologic patterns of HBV infection. In the Far East and Africa, hepatitis B, a disease of the newborn and young children, is perpetuated by a cycle of maternal-neonatal spread. In North America and western Europe, hepatitis B is primarily a disease of adolescence and early adulthood, the time of life when intimate sexual contact as well as recreational and occupational percutaneous exposures tend to occur. The introduction of hepatitis B vaccine in the early 1980s and adoption of universal childhood vaccination policies in many countries resulted in a dramatic, ~90%, decline in the incidence of new HBV infections in those countries as well as in the dire consequences of chronic infection.

Hepatitis D

Infection with HDV has a worldwide distribution, but two epidemiologic patterns exist. In Mediterranean countries (northern Africa, southern Europe, the Middle East), HDV infection is endemic among those with hepatitis B, and the disease is transmitted predominantly by nonpercutaneous means, especially close personal contact. In nonendemic areas, such as the United States and northern Europe, HDV infection is confined to persons exposed frequently to blood and blood products, primarily injection drug users and hemophiliacs. HDV infection can be introduced into a population through drug users or by migration of persons from endemic to nonendemic areas. Thus, patterns of population migration and human behavior facilitating percutaneous contact play important roles in the introduction and amplification of HDV infection. Occasionally, the migrating epidemiology of hepatitis D is expressed in explosive outbreaks of severe hepatitis, such as those that have occurred in remote South American villages as well as in urban centers in the United States. Ultimately, such outbreaks of hepatitis D—either of co-infections with acute hepatitis B or of superinfections in those already infected with HBV—may blur the distinctions between endemic and nonendemic areas. On a global scale, HDV infection is declining. Even in Italy, an HDV-endemic area, public health measures introduced to control HBV infection resulted during the 1990s in a 1.5%/year reduction in the prevalence of HDV infection.

Hepatitis C

Routine screening of blood donors for HBsAg and the elimination of commercial blood sources in the early 1970s reduced the frequency of, but did not eliminate, transfusion-associated hepatitis. During the 1970s, the likelihood of acquiring hepatitis after transfusion of voluntarily donated, HBsAg-screened blood was ~10% per patient (up to 0.9% per unit transfused); 90–95% of these cases were classified, based on serologic exclusion of hepatitis A and B, as "non-A, non-B" hepatitis. For patients requiring transfusion of pooled products, such as clotting factor concentrates, the risk was even higher, up to 20–30%.

During the 1980s, voluntary self-exclusion of blood donors with risk factors for AIDS and then the introduction of donor screening for anti-HIV reduced further the likelihood of transfusion-associated hepatitis to <5%. During the late 1980s and early 1990s, the introduction first of "surrogate" screening tests for non-A, non-B hepatitis [alanine aminotransferase (ALT) and anti-HBc, both shown to identify blood donors with a higher likelihood of transmitting non-A, non-B hepatitis to recipients] and, subsequently, after the discovery of HCV, first-generation immunoassays for anti-HCV reduced the frequency of transfusion-associated hepatitis even further. A prospective analysis of transfusion-associated hepatitis conducted between 1986 and 1990 showed that the incidence of transfusion-associated hepatitis at one urban university hospital fell from a baseline of 3.8% per patient (0.45% per unit transfused) to 1.5% per patient (0.19% per unit) after the introduction of surrogate testing and to 0.6% per patient (0.03% per unit) after the introduction of first-generation anti-HCV assays. The introduction of second-generation anti-HCV assays reduced the frequency of transfusion-associated

hepatitis C to almost imperceptible levels, 1 in 100,000, and these gains were reinforced by the application of automated PCR testing of donated blood for HCV RNA, which has resulted in a reduction in the risk of transfusion-associated HCV infection to 1 in 2.3 million transfusions.

In addition to being transmitted by transfusion, hepatitis C can be transmitted by other percutaneous routes, such as injection drug use. In addition, this virus can be transmitted by occupational exposure to blood, and the likelihood of infection is increased in hemodialysis units. Although the frequency of transfusion-associated hepatitis C fell as a result of blood donor screening, the overall frequency of hepatitis C remained the same until the early 1990s, when the overall frequency fell by 80%, in parallel with a reduction in the number of new cases in injection drug users. After the exclusion of anti-HCV-positive plasma units from the donor pool, rare, sporadic instances have occurred of hepatitis C among recipients of immunoglobulin (IG) preparations for intravenous (but not intramuscular) use.

Serologic evidence for HCV infection occurs in 90% of patients with a history of transfusion-associated hepatitis (almost all occurring before 1992, when second-generation HCV-screening tests were introduced); hemophiliacs and others treated with clotting factors; injection drug users; 60–70% of patients with sporadic "non-A, non-B" hepatitis who lack identifiable risk factors; 0.5% of volunteer blood donors; and, in the most recent survey conducted in the United States between 1999 and 2000, 1.6% of the general population in the United States, which translates into 4.1 million persons (3.2 million with viremia). Comparable frequencies of HCV infection occur in most countries around the world, with 170 million persons infected worldwide, but extraordinarily high prevalences of HCV infection occur in certain countries, such as Egypt, where >20% of the population in some cities is infected. The high frequency in Egypt is attributable to contaminated equipment used for medical procedures and unsafe injection practices. In the United States, African Americans and Mexican Americans have higher frequencies of HCV infection than whites. Between 1988 and 1994, 30- to 40-year-old adult males had the highest prevalence of HCV infection; however, in a survey conducted between 1999 and 2000, the peak age decile had shifted to those age 40–49 years. Thus, despite an 80% reduction in new HCV infections during the 1990s, the prevalence of HCV infection in the population was sustained by an aging cohort that had acquired their infections two to three decades earlier, during the 1960s and 1970s, as a result predominantly of self inoculation with recreational drugs. Hepatitis C accounts for 40% of chronic liver disease, is the most frequent indication for liver transplantation, and is estimated to account for 8000–10,000 deaths per year in the United States.

The distribution of HCV genotypes varies in different parts of the world. World-wide, genotype 1 is the most common. In the United States, genotype 1 accounts for 70% of HCV infections, while genotypes 2 and 3 account for the remaining 30%; among African Americans, the frequency of genotype 1 is even higher, i.e., 90%. Genotype 4 predominates in Egypt; genotype 5 is localized to South Africa and genotype 6 to Hong Kong.

Most asymptomatic blood donors found to have anti-HCV and ~20–30% of persons with reported cases of acute hepatitis C do not fall into a recognized risk group; however, many such blood donors do recall risk-associated behaviors when questioned carefully.

As a bloodborne infection, HCV potentially can be transmitted sexually and perinatally; however, both of these modes of transmission are inefficient for hepatitis C. Although 10–15% of patients with acute hepatitis C report having potential sexual sources of infection, most studies have failed to identify sexual transmission of this agent. The chances of sexual and perinatal transmission have been estimated to be ~5%, well below comparable rates for HIV and HBV infections. Moreover, sexual transmission appears to be confined to such subgroups as persons with multiple sexual partners and sexually transmitted diseases; transmission of HCV infection is rare between stable, monogamous sexual partners. Breast feeding does not increase the risk of HCV infection between an infected mother and her infant. Infection of health workers is not dramatically higher than among the general population; however, health workers are more likely to acquire HCV infection through accidental needle punctures, the efficiency of which is ~3%. Infection of household contacts is rare as well.

Other groups with an increased frequency of HCV infection include patients who require hemodialysis and organ transplantation and those who require transfusions in the setting of cancer chemotherapy. In immunosuppressed individuals, levels of anti-HCV may be undetectable, and a diagnosis may require testing for HCV RNA. Although new acute cases of hepatitis C are rare, newly diagnosed cases are common among otherwise healthy persons who experimented briefly with injection drugs, as noted above, two or three decades earlier. Such instances usually remain unrecognized for years, until unearthed by laboratory screening for routine medical examinations, insurance applications, and attempted blood donation.

Hepatitis E

This type of hepatitis, identified in India, Asia, Africa, the Middle East, and Central America, resembles hepatitis A in its primarily enteric mode of spread. The commonly recognized cases occur after contamination of water supplies such as after monsoon flooding, but sporadic, isolated cases occur. An epidemiologic feature that distinguishes HEV from other enteric agents is the rarity of secondary person-to-person spread from infected persons to their close contacts. Infections arise in populations that are immune to HAV and favor young adults. In endemic areas, the prevalence of antibodies to HEV is ≤40%. In nonendemic areas of the world, such as the United States, clinically apparent acute hepatitis E is extremely rare; however, the prevalence of antibodies to HEV can be as high as 20% in such areas. In nonendemic areas, HEV does not account for any of the sporadic "non-A, non-B" cases of hepatitis; however, cases imported from endemic areas have been found in the United States. Several reports suggest a zoonotic reservoir for HEV in swine.

CLINICAL AND LABORATORY FEATURES

Symptoms and Signs

Acute viral hepatitis occurs after an incubation period that varies according to the responsible agent. Generally, incubation periods for hepatitis A range from 15–45 days (mean, 4 weeks), for hepatitis B and D from 30–180 days (mean, 8–12 weeks), for hepatitis C from 15–160 days (mean, 7 weeks), and for hepatitis E from 14–60 days (mean, 5–6 weeks). The *prodromal symptoms* of acute viral hepatitis are systemic and quite variable. Constitutional symptoms of anorexia, nausea and vomiting, fatigue, malaise, arthralgias, myalgias, headache, photophobia, pharyngitis, cough, and coryza may precede the onset of jaundice by 1–2 weeks. The nausea, vomiting, and anorexia are frequently associated with alterations in olfaction and taste. A low-grade fever between 38° and 39°C (100°–102°F) is more often present in hepatitis A and E than in hepatitis B or C, except when hepatitis B is heralded by a serum sickness–like syndrome; rarely, a fever of 39.5°–40°C (103°–104°F) may accompany the constitutional symptoms. Dark urine and clay-colored stools may be noticed by the patient from 1–5 days before the onset of clinical jaundice.

With the onset of *clinical jaundice*, the constitutional prodromal symptoms usually diminish, but in some patients mild weight loss (2.5–5 kg) is common and may continue during the entire icteric phase. The liver becomes enlarged and tender and may be associated with right upper quadrant pain and discomfort. Infrequently, patients present with a cholestatic picture, suggesting extrahepatic biliary obstruction. Splenomegaly and cervical adenopathy are present in 10–20% of patients with acute hepatitis. Rarely, a few spider angiomas appear during the icteric phase and disappear during convalescence. During the *recovery phase*, constitutional symptoms disappear, but usually some liver enlargement and abnormalities in liver biochemical tests are still evident. The duration of the posticteric phase is variable, ranging 2–12 weeks, and is usually more prolonged in acute hepatitis B and C. Complete clinical and biochemical recovery is to be expected 1–2 months after all cases of hepatitis A and E and 3–4 months after the onset of jaundice in three-quarters of uncomplicated, self-limited cases of hepatitis B and C (among healthy adults, acute hepatitis B is self-limited in 95–99% while hepatitis C is self-limited in only ~15%). In the remainder, biochemical recovery may be delayed. A substantial proportion of patients with viral hepatitis never become icteric.

Infection with HDV can occur in the presence of acute or chronic HBV infection; the duration of HBV infection determines the duration of HDV infection. When acute HDV and HBV infection occur simultaneously, clinical and biochemical features may be indistinguishable from those of HBV infection alone, although occasionally they are more severe. As opposed to patients with *acute* HBV infection, patients with *chronic* HBV infection can support HDV replication indefinitely. This can happen when acute HDV infection occurs in the presence of a nonresolving acute HBV infection. More commonly, acute HDV infection becomes chronic when it is superimposed on an underlying chronic HBV infection. In such cases, the HDV superinfection appears as a clinical exacerbation or an episode resembling acute viral hepatitis in someone already chronically infected with HBV. Superinfection with HDV in a patient with chronic hepatitis B often leads to clinical deterioration (see below).

In addition to superinfections with other hepatitis agents, acute hepatitis–like clinical events in persons with chronic hepatitis B may accompany spontaneous HBeAg-to–anti-HBe seroconversion or spontaneous reactivation, i.e., reversion from nonreplicative to replicative infection. Such reactivations can occur as well in therapeutically immunosuppressed patients with chronic HBV infection when cytotoxic/immunosuppressive drugs are withdrawn; in these cases, restoration of immune competence is thought to allow resumption of previously checked cell-mediated immune cytolysis of HBV-infected hepatocytes. Occasionally, acute clinical exacerbations of chronic hepatitis B may represent the emergence of a precore mutant (see "Virology and Etiology" near the start of the chapter), and the subsequent course in such patients may be characterized by periodic exacerbations.

Laboratory Features

The serum aminotransferases aspartate aminotransferase (AST) and ALT (previously designated SGOT and SGPT) show a variable increase during the prodromal phase of acute viral hepatitis and precede the rise in bilirubin level (Figs. 37-2 and 37-4). The acute level of these enzymes, however, does not correlate well with the degree of liver cell damage. Peak levels vary from 400–4000 IU or more; these levels are usually reached at the time the patient is clinically icteric and diminish progressively during the recovery phase of acute hepatitis. The diagnosis of anicteric hepatitis is based on clinical features and on aminotransferase elevations.

Jaundice is usually visible in the sclera or skin when the serum bilirubin value is >43 μmol/L (2.5 mg/dL). When jaundice appears, the serum bilirubin typically rises to levels ranging from 85–340 μmol/L (5–20 mg/dL). The serum bilirubin may continue to rise despite falling serum aminotransferase levels. In most instances, the total bilirubin is equally divided between the conjugated and unconjugated fractions. Bilirubin levels >340 μmol/L (20 mg/dL) extending and persisting late into the course of viral hepatitis are more likely to be associated with severe disease. In certain patients with underlying hemolytic anemia, however, such as glucose-6-phosphate dehydrogenase deficiency and sickle cell anemia, a high serum bilirubin level is common, resulting from superimposed hemolysis. In such patients, bilirubin levels >513 μmol/L (30 mg/dL) have been observed and are not necessarily associated with a poor prognosis.

Neutropenia and lymphopenia are transient and are followed by a relative lymphocytosis. Atypical lymphocytes (varying between 2 and 20%) are common during the acute phase. Measurement of the prothrombin time (PT) is important in patients with acute viral hepatitis, for a prolonged value may reflect a severe hepatic synthetic defect, signify extensive hepatocellular necrosis, and indicate a worse prognosis. Occasionally, a prolonged PT may occur with only mild increases in the serum bilirubin and aminotransferase levels. Prolonged nausea and vomiting, inadequate carbohydrate intake, and poor hepatic glycogen reserves may contribute to hypoglycemia noted occasionally in patients with severe viral hepatitis. Serum alkaline phosphatase may be normal or only mildly elevated, while a fall in serum albumin is uncommon in uncomplicated acute viral hepatitis. In some patients, mild and transient steatorrhea has been noted as well as slight microscopic hematuria and minimal proteinuria.

A diffuse but mild elevation of the γ globulin fraction is common during acute viral hepatitis. Serum IgG and IgM levels are elevated in about one-third of patients during the acute phase of viral hepatitis, but the serum IgM level is elevated more characteristically during acute hepatitis A. During the acute phase of viral hepatitis, antibodies to smooth muscle and other cell constituents may be present, and low titers of rheumatoid factor, nuclear antibody, and heterophil antibody can also be found occasionally. In hepatitis C and D, antibodies to LKM may occur; however, the species of LKM antibodies in the two types of hepatitis are different from each other as well as from the LKM antibody species characteristic of autoimmune hepatitis type 2 (Chap. 39). The autoantibodies in viral hepatitis are nonspecific and can also be associated with other viral and systemic diseases. In contrast, virus-specific antibodies, which appear during and after hepatitis virus infection, are serologic markers of diagnostic importance.

As described above, serologic tests are available with which to establish a diagnosis of hepatitis A, B, D, and C. Tests for fecal or serum HAV are not routinely available. Therefore, a diagnosis of hepatitis A is based on detection of IgM anti-HAV during acute illness (Fig. 37-2). Rheumatoid factor can give rise to false-positive results in this test.

A diagnosis of HBV infection can usually be made by detection of HBsAg in serum. Infrequently, levels of HBsAg are too low to be detected during acute HBV infection, even with contemporary, highly sensitive immunoassays. In such cases, the diagnosis can be established by the presence of IgM anti-HBc.

The titer of HBsAg bears little relation to the severity of clinical disease. Indeed, an inverse correlation exists between the serum concentration of HBsAg and the degree of liver cell damage. For example, titers are highest in immunosuppressed patients, lower in patients with chronic liver disease (but higher in mild chronic than in severe chronic hepatitis), and very low in patients with acute fulminant hepatitis. These observations suggest that, in hepatitis B, the degree of liver cell damage and the clinical course are related to variations in the patient's immune response to HBV rather than to the amount of circulating HBsAg. In immunocompetent persons, however, there is a correlation between markers of HBV *replication* and liver injury (see later).

Another serologic marker that may be of value in patients with hepatitis B is HBeAg. Its principal clinical usefulness is as an indicator of relative infectivity. Because HBeAg is invariably present during early acute hepatitis B, HBeAg testing is indicated primarily during follow-up of chronic infection.

In patients with hepatitis B surface antigenemia of unknown duration, e.g., blood donors found to be HBsAg-positive and referred to a physician for evaluation, testing for IgM anti-HBc may be useful to distinguish between acute or recent infection (IgM anti-HBc-positive) and chronic HBV infection (IgM anti-HBc-negative, IgG anti-HBc-positive). A false-positive test for IgM anti-HBc may be encountered in patients with high-titer rheumatoid factor.

Anti-HBs is rarely detectable in the presence of HBsAg in patients with *acute* hepatitis B, but 10–20% of persons with *chronic* HBV infection may harbor low-level anti-HBs. This antibody is directed not against the common group determinant, *a*, but against the heterotypic subtype determinant (e.g., HBsAg of subtype *ad* with anti-HBs of subtype *y*). In most cases, this serologic pattern cannot be attributed to infection with two different HBV subtypes, and the presence of this antibody is not a harbinger of imminent HBsAg clearance. When such antibody is detected, its presence is of no recognized clinical significance (see "Virology and Etiology" earlier in the chapter).

After immunization with hepatitis B vaccine, which consists of HBsAg alone, anti-HBs is the only serologic marker to appear. The commonly encountered serologic patterns of hepatitis B and their interpretations are summarized in **Table 37-3**. Tests for the detection of HBV

TABLE 37-3

COMMONLY ENCOUNTERED SEROLOGIC PATTERNS OF HEPATITIS B INFECTION

HBsAg	ANTI-HBs	ANTI-HBc	HBeAg	ANTI-HBe	INTERPRETATION
+	–	IgM	+	–	Acute hepatitis B, high infectivity
+	–	IgG	+	–	Chronic hepatitis B, high infectivity
+	–	IgG	–	+	1. Late acute or chronic hepatitis B, low infectivity 2. HBeAg-negative ("precoremutant") hepatitis B (chronic or, rarely, acute)
+	+	+	+/–	+/–	1. HBsAg of one subtype and heterotypic anti-HBs (common) 2. Process of seroconversion from HBsAg to anti-HBs (rare)
–	–	IgM	+/–	+/–	1. Acute hepatitis B 2. Anti-HBc "window"
–	–	IgG	–	+/–	1. Low-level hepatitis B carrier 2. Hepatitis B in remote past
–	+	IgG	–	+/–	Recovery from hepatitis B
–	+	–	–	–	1. Immunization with HBsAg (after vaccination) 2. Hepatitis B in the remote past (?) 3. False-positive

DNA in liver and serum are now available. Like HBeAg, serum HBV DNA is an indicator of HBV replication, but tests for HBV DNA are more sensitive and quantitative. First-generation hybridization assays for HBV DNA had a sensitivity of 10^5-10^6 virions/mL, a relative threshold below which infectivity and liver injury are limited and HBeAg is usually undetectable. Currently, testing for HBV DNA has shifted from insensitive hybridization assays to amplification assays, e.g., the PCR-based assay, which can detect as few as 10 or 100 virions/mL; among the commercially available PCR assays, the most useful are those with the highest sensitivity (5–10 IU/mL) and the largest dynamic range (10^0-10^9 IU/mL). With increased sensitivity, amplification assays remain reactive well below the threshold for infectivity and liver injury. These markers are useful in following the course of HBV replication in patients with chronic hepatitis B receiving antiviral chemotherapy, e.g., with interferon or nucleoside analogues (Chap. 39). In immunocompetent persons, a general correlation does appear to exist between the level of HBV replication, as reflected by the level of HBV DNA in serum, and the degree of liver injury. High serum HBV DNA levels, increased expression of viral antigens, and necroinflammatory activity in the liver go hand in hand unless immunosuppression interferes with cytolytic T cell responses to virus-infected cells; reduction of HBV replication with antiviral drugs tends to be accompanied by an improvement in liver histology. Among patients with chronic hepatitis B, high levels of HBV DNA increase the risk of cirrhosis, hepatic decompensation, and hepatocellular carcinoma (see "Complications and Sequelae" later in the chapter).

In patients with hepatitis C, an episodic pattern of aminotransferase elevation is common. A specific serologic diagnosis of hepatitis C can be made by demonstrating the presence in serum of anti-HCV. When contemporary immunoassays are used, anti-HCV can be detected in acute hepatitis C during the initial phase of elevated aminotransferase activity. This antibody may never become detectable in 5–10% of patients with acute hepatitis C, and levels of anti-HCV may become undetectable after recovery (albeit rare) from acute hepatitis C. In patients with chronic hepatitis C, anti-HCV is detectable in >95% of cases. Nonspecificity can confound immunoassays for anti-HCV, especially in persons with a low prior probability of infection, such as volunteer blood donors, or in persons with circulating rheumatoid factor, which can bind nonspecifically to assay reagents; testing for HCV RNA can be used in such settings to distinguish between true-positive and false-positive anti-HCV determinations. Assays for HCV RNA are the most sensitive tests for HCV infection and represent the "gold standard" in establishing a diagnosis of hepatitis C. HCV RNA can be detected even before acute elevation of aminotransferase activity and before the appearance of anti-HCV in patients with acute

hepatitis C. In addition, HCV RNA remains detectable indefinitely, continuously in most but intermittently in some, in patients with chronic hepatitis C (detectable as well in some persons with normal liver tests, i.e., inactive carriers). In the small minority of patients with hepatitis C who lack anti-HCV, a diagnosis can be supported by detection of HCV RNA. If all these tests are negative and the patient has a well-characterized case of hepatitis after percutaneous exposure to blood or blood products, a diagnosis of hepatitis caused by another agent, as yet unidentified, can be entertained.

Amplification techniques are required to detect HCV RNA, and two types are available. One is a branched-chain complementary DNA (bDNA) assay, in which the detection signal (a colorimetrically detectable enzyme bound to a complementary DNA probe) is amplified. The other involves target amplification, i.e., synthesis of multiple copies of the viral genome. This can be done by PCR or TMA, in which the viral RNA is reverse transcribed to complementary DNA and then amplified by repeated cycles of DNA synthesis. Both can be used as quantitative assays and a measurement of relative "viral load"; PCR and TMA, with a sensitivity of $10-10^2$ IU/mL, are more sensitive than bDNA, with a sensitivity of 10^3 IU/mL; assays are available with a wide dynamic range ($10-10^7$ IU/mL). Determination of HCV RNA level is not a reliable marker of disease severity or prognosis but is helpful in predicting relative responsiveness to antiviral therapy. The same is true for determinations of HCV genotype (Chap. 39).

A proportion of patients with hepatitis C have isolated anti-HBc in their blood, a reflection of a common risk in certain populations of exposure to multiple bloodborne hepatitis agents. The anti-HBc in such cases is almost invariably of the IgG class and usually represents HBV infection in the remote past (HBV DNA undetectable), rarely current HBV infection with low-level virus carriage.

The presence of HDV infection can be identified by demonstrating intrahepatic HDV antigen or, more practically, an anti-HDV seroconversion (a rise in titer of anti-HDV or de novo appearance of anti-HDV). Circulating HDV antigen, also diagnostic of acute infection, is detectable only briefly, if at all. Because anti-HDV is often undetectable once HBsAg disappears, retrospective serodiagnosis of acute self-limited, simultaneous HBV and HDV infection is difficult. Early diagnosis of acute infection may be hampered by a delay of up to 30–40 days in the appearance of anti-HDV.

When a patient presents with acute hepatitis and has HBsAg and anti-HDV in serum, determination of the class of anti-HBc is helpful in establishing the relationship between infection with HBV and HDV. Although IgM anti-HBc does not distinguish *absolutely* between acute and chronic HBV infection, its presence is a reliable indicator of recent infection and its absence a reliable indicator of infection in the remote past. In simultaneous acute HBV and HDV infections, IgM anti-HBc will be detectable, while in acute HDV infection superimposed on chronic HBV infection, anti-HBc will be of the IgG class.

Tests for the presence of HDV RNA are useful for determining the presence of ongoing HDV replication and relative infectivity. Diagnostic tests for hepatitis E are commercially available in several countries outside the United States; in the United States, diagnostic assays can be performed at the Centers for Disease Control and Prevention.

Liver biopsy is rarely necessary or indicated in acute viral hepatitis, except when the diagnosis is questionable or when clinical evidence suggests a diagnosis of chronic hepatitis.

A diagnostic algorithm can be applied in the evaluation of cases of acute viral hepatitis. A patient with acute hepatitis should undergo four serologic tests: HBsAg, IgM anti-HAV, IgM anti-HBc, and anti-HCV (Table 37-4). The presence of HBsAg, with or without IgM anti-HBc, represents HBV infection. If IgM anti-HBc is present, the HBV infection is considered acute; if IgM anti-HBc is absent, the HBV infection is considered chronic. A diagnosis of acute hepatitis B can be made in the absence of HBsAg when IgM anti-HBc is detectable. A diagnosis of acute hepatitis A is based on the presence of IgM anti-HAV. If IgM anti-HAV coexists with HBsAg, a diagnosis of simultaneous HAV and HBV infections can be made; if IgM anti-HBc (with or without HBsAg) is detectable, the patient has simultaneous acute hepatitis A and B, and if IgM anti-HBc is undetectable, the patient has acute hepatitis A

superimposed on chronic HBV infection. The presence of anti-HCV supports a diagnosis of acute hepatitis C. Occasionally, testing for HCV RNA or repeat anti-HCV testing later during the illness is necessary to establish the diagnosis. Absence of all serologic markers is consistent with a diagnosis of "non-A, non-B, non-C" hepatitis, if the epidemiologic setting is appropriate.

In patients with chronic hepatitis, initial testing should consist of HBsAg and anti-HCV. Anti-HCV supports and HCV RNA testing establishes the diagnosis of chronic hepatitis C. If a serologic diagnosis of chronic hepatitis B is made, testing for HBeAg and anti-HBe is indicated to evaluate relative infectivity. Testing for HBV DNA in such patients provides a more quantitative and sensitive measure of the level of virus replication and, therefore, is very helpful during antiviral therapy (Chap. 39). In patients with chronic hepatitis B and normal aminotransferase activity in the absence of HBeAg, serial testing over time is often required to distinguish between inactive carriage and HBeAg-negative chronic hepatitis B with fluctuating virologic and necroinflammatory activity. In patients with hepatitis B, testing for anti-HDV is useful under the following circumstances: patients with severe and fulminant disease, patients with severe chronic disease, patients with chronic hepatitis B who have acute hepatitis-like exacerbations, persons with frequent percutaneous exposures, and persons from areas where HDV infection is endemic.

PROGNOSIS

Virtually all previously healthy patients with hepatitis A recover completely from their illness with no clinical sequelae. Similarly, in acute hepatitis B, 95–99% of

TABLE 37-4

SIMPLIFIED DIAGNOSTIC APPROACH IN PATIENTS PRESENTING WITH ACUTE HEPATITIS

SEROLOGIC TESTS OF PATIENT'S SERUM				
HBsAg	IgM ANTI-HAV	IgM ANTI-HBc	ANTI-HCV	DIAGNOSTIC INTERPRETATION
+	−	+	−	Acute hepatitis B
+	−	−	−	Chronic hepatitis B
+	+	−	−	Acute hepatitis A superimposed on chronic hepatitis B
+	+	+	−	Acute hepatitis A and B
−	+	−	−	Acute hepatitis A
−	+	+	−	Acute hepatitis A and B (HBsAg below detection threshold)
−	−	+	−	Acute hepatitis B (HBsAg below detection threshold)
−	−	−	+	Acute hepatitis C

previously healthy adults have a favorable course and recover completely. Certain clinical and laboratory features, however, suggest a more complicated and protracted course. Patients of advanced age and with serious underlying medical disorders may have a prolonged course and are more likely to experience severe hepatitis. Initial presenting features such as ascites, peripheral edema, and symptoms of hepatic encephalopathy suggest a poorer prognosis. In addition, a prolonged PT, low serum albumin level, hypoglycemia, and very high serum bilirubin values suggest severe hepatocellular disease. Patients with these clinical and laboratory features deserve prompt hospital admission. The case-fatality rate in hepatitis A and B is very low (~0.1%) but is increased by advanced age and underlying debilitating disorders. Among patients ill enough to be hospitalized for acute hepatitis B, the fatality rate is 1%. Hepatitis C is less severe during the acute phase than hepatitis B and is more likely to be anicteric; fatalities are rare, but the precise case-fatality rate is not known. In outbreaks of waterborne hepatitis E in India and Asia, the case-fatality rate is 1–2% and up to 10–20% in pregnant women. Patients with simultaneous acute hepatitis B and hepatitis D do not necessarily experience a higher mortality rate than do patients with acute hepatitis B alone; however, in several recent outbreaks of acute simultaneous HBV and HDV infection among injection drug users, the case-fatality rate has been ~5%. In the case of HDV superinfection of a person with chronic hepatitis B, the likelihood of fulminant hepatitis and death is increased substantially. Although the case-fatality rate for hepatitis D has not been defined adequately, in outbreaks of severe HDV superinfection in isolated populations with a high hepatitis B carrier rate, the mortality rate has been recorded in excess of 20%.

COMPLICATIONS AND SEQUELAE

A small proportion of patients with hepatitis A experience *relapsing hepatitis* weeks to months after apparent recovery from acute hepatitis. Relapses are characterized by recurrence of symptoms, aminotransferase elevations, occasionally jaundice, and fecal excretion of HAV. Another unusual variant of acute hepatitis A is *cholestatic hepatitis*, characterized by protracted cholestatic jaundice and pruritus. Rarely, liver test abnormalities persist for many months, even up to a year. Even when these complications occur, hepatitis A remains self-limited and does not progress to chronic liver disease. During the prodromal phase of acute hepatitis B, a serum sickness–like syndrome characterized by arthralgia or arthritis, rash, angioedema, and rarely hematuria and proteinuria may develop in 5–10% of patients. This syndrome occurs before the onset of clinical jaundice, and these patients are often diagnosed erroneously as having

rheumatologic diseases. The diagnosis can be established by measuring serum aminotransferase levels, which are almost invariably elevated, and serum HBsAg. As noted above, EMC is an immune-complex disease that can complicate chronic hepatitis C and is part of a spectrum of B cell lymphoproliferative disorders, which, in rare instances, can evolve to B cell lymphoma. Attention has been drawn as well to associations between hepatitis C and such cutaneous disorders as porphyria cutanea tarda and lichen planus. A mechanism for these associations is unknown.

The most feared complication of viral hepatitis is *fulminant hepatitis* (massive hepatic necrosis); fortunately, this is a rare event. Fulminant hepatitis is primarily seen in hepatitis B and D, as well as hepatitis E, but rare fulminant cases of hepatitis A occur primarily in older adults and in persons with underlying chronic liver disease, including, according to some reports, chronic hepatitis B and C. Hepatitis B accounts for >50% of fulminant cases of viral hepatitis, a sizable proportion of which are associated with HDV infection and another proportion with underlying chronic hepatitis C. Fulminant hepatitis is hardly ever seen in hepatitis C, but hepatitis E, as noted above, can be complicated by fatal fulminant hepatitis in 1–2% of all cases and in up to 20% of cases occurring in pregnant women. Patients usually present with signs and symptoms of encephalopathy that may evolve to deep coma. The liver is usually small and the PT excessively prolonged. The combination of rapidly shrinking liver size, rapidly rising bilirubin level, and marked prolongation of the PT, even as aminotransferase levels fall, together with clinical signs of confusion, disorientation, somnolence, ascites, and edema, indicates that the patient has hepatic failure with encephalopathy. Cerebral edema is common; brainstem compression, gastrointestinal bleeding, sepsis, respiratory failure, cardiovascular collapse, and renal failure are terminal events. The mortality rate is exceedingly high (>80% in patients with deep coma), but patients who survive may have a complete biochemical and histologic recovery. If a donor liver can be located in time, liver transplantation may be life-saving in patients with fulminant hepatitis (Chap. 44).

Documenting the disappearance of HBsAg after apparent clinical recovery from acute hepatitis B is particularly important. Before laboratory methods were available to distinguish between acute hepatitis and acute hepatitis–like exacerbations (*spontaneous reactivations*) of chronic hepatitis B, observations suggested that ~10% of previously healthy patients remained HBsAg-positive for >6 months after the onset of clinically apparent acute hepatitis B. Half of these persons cleared the antigen from their circulations during the next several years, but the other 5% remained chronically HBsAg-positive. More recent observations suggest that the true rate of chronic infection after clinically apparent acute hepatitis B is as low as 1% in normal, immunocompetent, young adults. Earlier, higher estimates may have been confounded by inadvertent inclusion of acute exacerbations in chronically infected patients; these patients, chronically HBsAg-positive before exacerbation, were unlikely to seroconvert to HBsAg-negative thereafter. Whether the rate of chronicity is 10 or 1%, such patients have anti-HBc in serum; anti-HBs is either undetected or detected at low titer against the opposite subtype specificity of the antigen (see "Laboratory Features" earlier in the chapter). These patients may (1) be inactive carriers; (2) have low-grade, mild chronic hepatitis; or (3) have moderate to severe chronic hepatitis with or without cirrhosis. The likelihood of remaining chronically infected after acute HBV infection is especially high among neonates, persons with Down's syndrome, chronically hemodialyzed patients, and immunosuppressed patients, including persons with HIV infection.

Chronic hepatitis is an important late complication of acute hepatitis B occurring in a small proportion of patients with acute disease but more common in those who present with chronic infection without having experienced an acute illness, as occurs typically after neonatal infection or after infection in an immunosuppressed host (Chap. 39). Certain clinical and laboratory features suggest progression of acute hepatitis to chronic hepatitis: (1) lack of complete resolution of clinical symptoms of anorexia, weight loss, and fatigue and the persistence of hepatomegaly; (2) the presence of bridging/interface or multilobular hepatic necrosis on liver biopsy during protracted, severe acute viral hepatitis; (3) failure of the serum aminotransferase, bilirubin, and globulin levels to return to normal within 6–12 months after the acute illness; and (4) the persistence of HBeAg for >3 months or HBsAg for >6 months after acute hepatitis.

Although acute hepatitis D infection does not increase the likelihood of chronicity of simultaneous acute hepatitis B, hepatitis D has the potential for contributing to the severity of chronic hepatitis B. Hepatitis D superinfection can transform inactive or mild chronic hepatitis B into severe, progressive chronic hepatitis and cirrhosis; it also can accelerate the course of chronic hepatitis B. Some HDV superinfections in patients with chronic hepatitis B lead to fulminant hepatitis. Although HDV and HBV infections are associated with severe liver disease, mild hepatitis and even inactive carriage have been identified in some patients, and the disease may become indolent beyond the early years of infection. After acute HCV infection, the likelihood of remaining chronically *infected* approaches 85–90%. Although many patients with chronic hepatitis C have no symptoms, cirrhosis may develop in as many as 20% within 10–20 years of acute illness; in some series of cases reported by referral centers, cirrhosis has been reported in as many as 50% of patients with chronic hepatitis C. Although chronic hepatitis C accounts for at least 40% of cases of chronic liver disease and of patients undergoing liver transplantation for end-stage liver disease in the United States and Europe, in the majority of patients with chronic hepatitis C, morbidity and mortality are limited during the initial 20 years after the onset of infection. Progression of chronic hepatitis C may be influenced by age of acquisition, duration of infection, immunosuppression, coexisting excessive alcohol use, concomitant hepatic steatosis, other hepatitis virus infection, or HIV co-infection. In fact, instances of severe and rapidly progressive chronic hepatitis B and C are being recognized with increasing frequency in patients with HIV infection. In contrast, neither HAV nor HEV causes chronic liver disease.

Rare complications of viral hepatitis include pancreatitis, myocarditis, atypical pneumonia, aplastic anemia, transverse myelitis, and peripheral neuropathy. Persons with chronic hepatitis B, particularly those infected in infancy or early childhood and especially those with HBeAg and/or high-level HBV DNA, have an enhanced risk of hepatocellular carcinoma. The risk of hepatocellular carcinoma is increased as well in patients with chronic hepatitis C, almost exclusively in patients with cirrhosis, and almost always after at least several decades, usually after three decades of disease. In children, hepatitis B may present rarely with anicteric hepatitis, a nonpruritic papular rash of the face, buttocks, and limbs, and lymphadenopathy (papular acrodermatitis of childhood, or Gianotti-Crosti syndrome).

Rarely, autoimmune hepatitis (Chap. 39) can be triggered by a bout of otherwise self-limited acute hepatitis, as reported after acute hepatitis A, B, and C.

DIFFERENTIAL DIAGNOSIS

Viral diseases such as infectious mononucleosis; those due to cytomegalovirus, herpes simplex, and coxsackieviruses; and toxoplasmosis may share certain clinical features with viral hepatitis and cause elevations in serum aminotransferase and less commonly in serum bilirubin levels. Tests such as the differential heterophile and serologic tests for these agents may be helpful in the differential diagnosis if HBsAg, anti-HBc, IgM anti-HAV, and anti-HCV determinations are negative. Aminotransferase elevations can accompany almost any systemic viral infection; other rare causes of liver injury confused with viral hepatitis are infections with *Leptospira*, *Candida*, *Brucella*, *Mycobacteria*, and *Pneumocystis*. A complete drug history is particularly important, for many drugs and certain anesthetic agents can produce a picture of either acute hepatitis or cholestasis (Chap. 38). Equally important is a past history of unexplained "repeated episodes" of acute hepatitis. This history should alert the physician to the possibility that the underlying disorder is chronic hepatitis. Alcoholic hepatitis must also be considered, but usually the serum aminotransferase levels are not as markedly elevated and other stigmata of alcoholism may be present. The finding on liver biopsy of fatty infiltration, a neutrophilic inflammatory reaction, and "alcoholic hyaline" would be consistent with alcohol-induced rather than viral liver injury. Because acute hepatitis may present with right upper quadrant abdominal pain, nausea and vomiting, fever, and icterus, it is often confused with acute cholecystitis, common duct stone, or ascending cholangitis. Patients with acute viral hepatitis may tolerate surgery poorly; therefore, it is important to exclude this diagnosis, and in confusing cases, a percutaneous liver biopsy may be necessary before laparotomy. Viral hepatitis in the elderly is often misdiagnosed as obstructive jaundice resulting from a common duct stone or carcinoma of the pancreas. Because acute hepatitis in the elderly may be quite severe and the operative mortality high, a thorough evaluation including biochemical tests, radiographic studies of the biliary tree, and even liver biopsy may be necessary to exclude primary parenchymal liver disease. Another clinical constellation that may mimic acute hepatitis is right ventricular failure with passive hepatic congestion or hypoperfusion syndromes, such as those associated with shock, severe hypotension, and severe left ventricular failure. Also included in this general category is any disorder that interferes with venous return to the heart, such as right atrial myxoma, constrictive pericarditis, hepatic vein occlusion (Budd-Chiari syndrome), or venoocclusive disease. Clinical features are usually sufficient to distinguish between these vascular disorders and viral hepatitis. Acute fatty liver of pregnancy, cholestasis of pregnancy, eclampsia, and the HELLP syndrome (*h*emolysis, *e*levated *l*iver tests, and *l*ow *p*latelets) can be confused with viral hepatitis during pregnancy. Very rarely, malignancies metastatic to the liver can mimic acute or even fulminant viral hepatitis. Occasionally, genetic or metabolic liver disorders (e.g., Wilson's disease, α_1-antitrypsin deficiency) as well as nonalcoholic fatty liver disease are confused with viral hepatitis.

R_X Treatment: ACUTE VIRAL HEPATITIS

In hepatitis B, among previously healthy adults who present with clinically apparent acute hepatitis, recovery occurs in ~99%; therefore, antiviral therapy is not likely to improve the rate of recovery and is not required. In rare instances of severe acute hepatitis B, treatment with a nucleoside analogue, such as lamivudine, at the 100-mg/d oral dose used to treat chronic hepatitis B (Chap. 39), has been attempted successfully.

Although clinical trials have not been done to establish the efficacy of this approach, although severe acute hepatitis B is not an approved indication for therapy, and although the duration of therapy has not been determined, nonetheless, most authorities would recommend institution of antiviral therapy for severe, but not mild-moderate, acute hepatitis B. In typical cases of acute hepatitis C, recovery is rare, progression to chronic hepatitis is the rule, and meta-analyses of small clinical trials suggest that antiviral therapy with interferon α monotherapy (3 million units SC three times a week) is beneficial, reducing the rate of chronicity considerably by inducing sustained responses in 30–70% of patients. In a German multicenter study of 44 patients with acute symptomatic hepatitis C, initiation of intensive interferon α therapy (5 million units SC daily for 4 weeks, then three times a week for another 20 weeks) within an average of 3 months after infection resulted in a sustained virologic response rate of 98%. Although treatment of acute hepatitis C is recommended, the optimum regimen, duration of therapy, and time to initiate therapy remain to be determined. Many authorities now opt for a 24-week course (beginning within 2–3 months after onset) of the best regimen identified for the treatment of chronic hepatitis C, long-acting pegylated interferon plus the nucleoside analogue ribavirin, the efficacy of which is superior to that of standard interferon monotherapy regimens (see Chap. 39 for doses). Because of the marked reduction over the past two decades in the frequency of acute hepatitis C, opportunities to identify and treat patients with acute hepatitis C are rare indeed, except in injection drug users. Hospital epidemiologists, however, will encounter health workers who sustain hepatitis C–contaminated needle sticks; when monitoring for ALT elevations and HCV RNA after these accidents identifies acute hepatitis C (risk only ~3%), therapy should be initiated.

Notwithstanding these specific therapeutic considerations, in most cases of typical acute viral hepatitis, specific treatment generally is not necessary. Although hospitalization may be required for clinically severe illness, most patients do not require hospital care. Forced and prolonged bed rest is not essential for full recovery, but many patients will feel better with restricted physical activity. A high-calorie diet is desirable, and because many patients may experience nausea late in the day, the major caloric intake is best tolerated in the morning. Intravenous feeding is necessary in the acute stage if the patient has persistent vomiting and cannot maintain oral intake. Drugs capable of producing adverse reactions such as cholestasis and drugs metabolized by the liver should be avoided. If severe pruritus is present, the use of the bile salt–sequestering resin cholestyramine is helpful. Glucocorticoid therapy has no value in acute viral hepatitis, even in severe cases associated with *bridging necrosis*, and may be deleterious, even increasing the risk of chronicity (e.g., of acute hepatitis B).

Physical isolation of patients with hepatitis to a single room and bathroom is rarely necessary except in the case of fecal incontinence for hepatitis A and E or uncontrolled, voluminous bleeding for hepatitis B (with or without concomitant hepatitis D) and hepatitis C. Because most patients hospitalized with hepatitis A excrete little if any HAV, the likelihood of HAV transmission from these patients during their hospitalization is low. Therefore, burdensome *enteric precautions are no longer recommended*. Although gloves should be worn when the bedpans or fecal material of patients with hepatitis A are handled, these precautions do not represent a departure from sensible procedure and contemporary universal precautions for all hospitalized patients. For patients with hepatitis B and hepatitis C, emphasis should be placed on blood precautions, i.e., avoiding direct, ungloved hand contact with blood and other body fluids. Enteric precautions are unnecessary. The importance of simple hygienic precautions, such as hand washing, cannot be overemphasized. Universal precautions that have been adopted for all patients apply to patients with viral hepatitis.

Hospitalized patients may be discharged following substantial symptomatic improvement, a significant downward trend in the serum aminotransferase and bilirubin values, and a return to normal of the PT. Mild aminotransferase elevations should not be considered contraindications to the gradual resumption of normal activity.

In *fulminant hepatitis*, the goal of therapy is to support the patient by maintenance of fluid balance, support of circulation and respiration, control of bleeding, correction of hypoglycemia, and treatment of other complications of the comatose state in anticipation of liver regeneration and repair. Protein intake should be restricted, and oral lactulose or neomycin administered. Glucocorticoid therapy has been shown in controlled trials to be ineffective. Likewise, exchange transfusion, plasmapheresis, human cross-circulation, porcine liver cross-perfusion, hemoperfusion, and extracorporeal liver-assist devices have not been proved to enhance survival. Meticulous intensive care that includes prophylactic antibiotic coverage is the one factor that does appear to improve survival. Orthotopic liver transplantation is resorted to with increasing frequency, with excellent results, in patients with fulminant hepatitis (Chap. 44).

PROPHYLAXIS

Because application of therapy for acute viral hepatitis is limited, and because antiviral therapy for chronic viral hepatitis is cumbersome and costly but effective in only a proportion of patients (Chap. 39), emphasis is placed on prevention through immunization. The prophylactic approach differs for each of the types of viral hepatitis. In the past, immunoprophylaxis relied exclusively on passive immunization with antibody-containing globulin preparations purified by cold ethanol fractionation from the plasma of hundreds of normal donors. Currently, for hepatitis A and B, active immunization with vaccines is the preferable approach to prevention.

Hepatitis A

Both passive immunization with IG and active immunization with killed vaccines are available. All preparations of IG contain anti-HAV concentrations sufficient to be protective. When administered before exposure or during the early incubation period, IG is effective in preventing clinically apparent hepatitis A. For postexposure prophylaxis of intimate contacts (household, sexual, institutional) of persons with hepatitis A, the administration of 0.02 mL/kg is recommended as early after exposure as possible; it may be effective even when administered as late as 2 weeks after exposure. Prophylaxis is not necessary for those who have already received hepatitis A vaccine, casual contacts (office, factory, school, or hospital), for most elderly persons, who are very likely to be immune, or for those known to have anti-HAV in their serum. In day-care centers, recognition of hepatitis A in children or staff should provide a stimulus for immunoprophylaxis in the center and in the children's family members. By the time most common-source outbreaks of hepatitis A are recognized, it is usually too late in the incubation period for IG to be effective; however, prophylaxis may limit the frequency of secondary cases. For travelers to tropical countries, developing countries, and other areas outside standard tourist routes, IG prophylaxis had been recommended, before a vaccine became available. When such travel lasted <3 months, 0.02 mL/kg was given; for longer travel or residence in these areas, a dose of 0.06 mL/kg every 4–6 months was recommended. Administration of plasma-derived globulin is safe; all contemporary lots of IG are subjected to viral inactivation steps and must be free of HCV RNA as determined by PCR testing. Administration of IM lots of IG has not been associated with transmission of HBV, HCV, or HIV.

Formalin-inactivated vaccines made from strains of HAV attenuated in tissue culture have been shown to be safe, immunogenic, and effective in preventing hepatitis A. Hepatitis A vaccines are approved for use in persons who are at least 1 year old and appear to provide adequate protection beginning 4 weeks after a primary inoculation. If it can be given within 4 weeks of an expected exposure, such as by travel to an endemic area, hepatitis A vaccine is the preferred approach to *preexposure* immunoprophylaxis. If travel is more imminent, IG (0.02 mL/kg) should be administered at a different injection site, along with the first dose of vaccine. Because vaccination provides long-lasting protection (protective levels of anti–HAV should last 20 years after vaccination), persons whose risk will be sustained (e.g., frequent travelers or those remaining in endemic areas for prolonged periods) should be vaccinated, and vaccine should supplant the need for repeated IG injections. Shortly after its introduction, hepatitis A vaccine was recommended for children living in communities with a high incidence of HAV infection; in 1999, this recommendation was extended to include all children living in states, counties, and communities with high rates of HAV infection. As of 2006, the Advisory Committee on Immunization Practices of the U.S. Public Health Service recommended *routine hepatitis A vaccination of all children*. Other groups considered to be at increased risk for HAV infection and who are candidates for hepatitis A vaccination include military personnel, populations with cyclic outbreaks of hepatitis A (e.g., Alaskan natives), employees of day-care centers, primate handlers, laboratory workers exposed to hepatitis A or fecal specimens, and patients with chronic liver disease. Because of an increased risk of fulminant hepatitis A—observed in some experiences but not confirmed in others—among patients with chronic hepatitis C, patients with chronic hepatitis C have been singled out as candidates for hepatitis A vaccination. Other populations whose recognized risk of hepatitis A is increased should be vaccinated, including men who have sex with men, injection drug users, and persons with clotting disorders who require frequent administration of clotting-factor concentrates. Recommendations for dose and frequency differ for the two approved vaccine preparations (Table 37-5); all injections are IM. Hepatitis A vaccine has been reported to

be effective in preventing secondary household cases of acute hepatitis A, but its role in other instances of postexposure prophylaxis remains to be demonstrated.

Hepatitis B

Until 1982, prevention of hepatitis B was based on *passive* immunoprophylaxis either with standard IG, containing modest levels of anti-HBs, or hepatitis B immune globulin (HBIG), containing high-titer anti-HBs. The efficacy of standard IG has never been established and remains questionable; even the efficacy of HBIG, demonstrated in several clinical trials, has been challenged, and its contribution appears to be in reducing the frequency of clinical *illness*, not in preventing *infection*. The first vaccine for *active* immunization, introduced in 1982, was prepared from purified, noninfectious 22-nm spherical forms of HBsAg derived from the plasma of healthy HBsAg carriers. In 1987, the plasma-derived vaccine was supplanted by a genetically engineered vaccine derived from recombinant yeast. The latter vaccine consists of HBsAg particles that are nonglycosylated but are otherwise indistinguishable from natural HBsAg; two recombinant vaccines are licensed for use in the United States. Current recommendations can be divided into those for preexposure and postexposure prophylaxis.

For *preexposure* prophylaxis against hepatitis B in settings of frequent exposure (health workers exposed to blood; hemodialysis patients and staff; residents and staff of custodial institutions for the developmentally handicapped; injection drug users; inmates of long-term correctional facilities; persons with multiple sexual partners; persons such as hemophiliacs who require long-term, high-volume therapy with blood derivatives; household and sexual contacts of HBsAg carriers; persons living in or traveling extensively in endemic areas; unvaccinated children under the age of 18; and unvaccinated children who are Alaskan natives, Pacific Islanders, or residents in households of first-generation immigrants from endemic countries), three IM (deltoid, not gluteal) injections of hepatitis B vaccine are recommended at 0, 1, and 6 months (other, optional schedules are summarized in Table 37-6). Pregnancy is *not* a contraindication to vaccination. In areas of low HBV endemicity such as the United States, despite the availability of safe and effective hepatitis B vaccines, a strategy of vaccinating persons in high-risk groups has not been effective. The incidence of new hepatitis B cases continued to increase in the United States after introduction of vaccines; <10% of all targeted persons in high-risk groups have actually been vaccinated, and ~30% of persons with sporadic acute hepatitis B do not fall into any high-risk-group category. Therefore, to have an impact on the frequency of HBV infection in an area of low endemicity such as the United States,

TABLE 37-5

HEPATITIS A VACCINATION SCHEDULES			
AGE, YEARS	NO. OF DOSES	DOSE	SCHEDULE, MONTHS
HAVRIX (GlaxoSmithKline)[a]			
1–18	2	720 ELU[b] (0.5 mL)	0, 6–12
≥19	2	1440 ELU (1.0 mL)	0, 6–12
VAQTA (Merck)			
1–18	2	25 units (0.5 mL)	0, 6–18
≥19	2	50 units (1.0 mL)	0, 6–18

[a]A combination of this hepatitis A vaccine and hepatitis B vaccine, TWINRIX, is licensed for simultaneous protection against both of these viruses among adults (age ≥18 years). Each 1.0-mL dose contains 720 ELU[b] of hepatitis A vaccine and 20 μg of hepatitis B vaccine. These doses are recommended at months 0, 1, and 6.
[b]Enzyme-linked immunoassay units.

TABLE 37-6

PREEXPOSURE HEPATITIS B VACCINATION SCHEDULES

TARGET GROUP	NO. OF DOSES	DOSE	SCHEDULE, MONTHS
Recombivax-HB (Merck)[a]			
Infants, children (<1–10 years)	3	5 μg (0.5 mL)	0, 1–2, 4–6
Adolescents (11–19 years)	3 or 4	5 μg (0.5 mL)	0–2, 1–4, 4–6 *or* 0, 12, 24 *or* 0, 1, 2, 12
or			
	2	10 μg (1.0 mL)	0, 4–6 (age 11–15)
Adults (≥20 years)	3	10 μg (1.0 mL)	0–2, 1–4, 4–6
Hemodialysis patients[b]			
<20 years	3	5 μg (0.5 mL)	0, 1, 6
≥20 years	3	40 μg (4.0 mL)	0, 1, 6
Engerix-B (GlaxoSmithKline)[c]			
Infants, children (<1–10 years)	3 or 4	10 μg (0.5 mL)	0, 1–2, 4–6 *or* 0, 1, 2,12
Adolescents (10–19 years)	3 or 4	10 μg (0.5 mL)	0, 1–2, 4–6 *or* 0, 12, 24 *or* 0, 1, 2, 12
Adults (≥20 years)	3 or 4	20 μg (1.0 mL)	0–2, 1–4, 4–6 0, 1, 2, 12
Hemodialysis patients[b]			
<20 years	4	10 μg (0.5 mL)	0, 1, 2, 6
≥20 years	4	40 μg (2.0 mL)	0, 1, 2, 6

[a]This manufacturer produces a licensed combination of hepatitis B vaccine and vaccines against *Haemophilus influenzae* type b and *Neisseria meningitides*, Comvax, for use in infants and young children. Please consult product insert for dose and schedule.
[b]This group also includes other immunocompromised persons.
[c]This manufacturer produces two licensed combination hepatitis B vaccines: (1) Twinrix, recombinant hepatitis B vaccine plus inactivated hepatitis A vaccine, is licensed for simultaneous protection against both of these viruses among adults (age ≥ 18 years). Each 1.0-mL dose contains 720 ELU[b] of hepatitis A vaccine and 20 μg of hepatitis B vaccine. These doses are recommended at months 0, 1, and 6. (2) Pediatrix, recombinant hepatitis B vaccine plus diphtheria and tetanus toxoid, pertussis, and inactivated poliovirus, is licensed for use in infants and young children. Please consult product insert for doses and schedules.

universal hepatitis B vaccination in childhood has been recommended. For unvaccinated children born after the implementation of universal infant vaccination, vaccination during early adolescence, at age 11–12 years, was recommended, and this recommendation has been extended to include all unvaccinated children age 0–19 years. In HBV-hyperendemic areas, e.g., Asia, universal vaccination of children has resulted in a marked 10- to 15-year decline in hepatitis B and its complications.

The two available recombinant hepatitis B vaccines are comparable, one containing 10 μg of HBsAg (Recombivax-HB) and the other containing 20 μg of HBsAg (Engerix-B), and recommended doses for each injection vary for the two preparations (Table 37-6). Combinations of hepatitis B vaccine with other childhood vaccines are available as well (Table 37-6).

For unvaccinated persons sustaining an exposure to HBV, *postexposure* prophylaxis with a combination of HBIG (for rapid achievement of high-titer circulating anti-HBs) and hepatitis B vaccine (for achievement of long-lasting immunity as well as its apparent efficacy in attenuating clinical illness after exposure) is recommended. For *perinatal* exposure of infants born to HBsAg-positive mothers, a single dose of HBIG, 0.5 mL, should be administered IM in the thigh *immediately after birth*, followed by a complete course of three injections of recombinant hepatitis B vaccine (see doses earlier) to be started within the first 12 h of life. For those experiencing a direct percutaneous inoculation or transmucosal exposure to HBsAg-positive blood or body fluids (e.g., accidental *needle stick*, other mucosal penetration, or ingestion), a single IM dose of HBIG,

0.06 mL/kg, administered as soon after exposure as possible, is followed by a complete course of hepatitis B vaccine to begin within the first week. For those exposed by *sexual* contact to a patient with acute hepatitis B, a single IM dose of HBIG, 0.06 mL/kg, should be given within 14 days of exposure, to be followed by a complete course of hepatitis B vaccine. When both HBIG and hepatitis B vaccine are recommended, they may be given at the same time but at separate sites.

The precise duration of protection afforded by hepatitis B vaccine is unknown; however, ~80–90% of immunocompetent vaccinees retain protective levels of anti-HBs for at least 5 years, and 60–80% for 10 years. Thereafter and even after anti-HBs becomes undetectable, protection persists against clinical hepatitis B, hepatitis B surface antigenemia, and chronic HBV infection. Currently, *booster* immunizations are not recommended routinely, except in immunosuppressed persons who have lost detectable anti-HBs or immunocompetent persons who sustain percutaneous HBsAg-positive inoculations after losing detectable antibody. Specifically, for hemodialysis patients, annual anti-HBs testing is recommended after vaccination; booster doses are recommended when anti-HBs levels fall to <10 mIU/mL. As noted above, for persons at risk of both hepatitis A and B, a combined vaccine is available containing 720 enzyme-linked immunoassay units of inactivated HAV and 20 μg of recombinant HBsAg (at 0, 1, and 6 months).

Hepatitis D

Infection with hepatitis D can be prevented by vaccinating susceptible persons with hepatitis B vaccine. No product is available for immunoprophylaxis to prevent HDV superinfection in HBsAg carriers; for them, avoidance of percutaneous exposures and limitation of intimate contact with persons who have HDV infection are recommended.

Hepatitis C

IG is ineffective in preventing hepatitis C and is no longer recommended for postexposure prophylaxis in cases of perinatal, needle stick, or sexual exposure. Although prototype vaccines that induce antibodies to HCV envelope proteins have been developed, currently hepatitis C vaccination is not feasible practically. Genotype and quasispecies viral heterogeneity, as well as rapid evasion of neutralizing antibodies by this rapidly mutating virus, conspire to render HCV a difficult target for immunoprophylaxis with a vaccine. Prevention of transfusion-associated hepatitis C has been accomplished by the following successively introduced measures: Exclusion of commercial blood donors and

reliance on a volunteer blood supply; screening donor blood with surrogate markers such as ALT (no longer recommended) and anti-HBc, markers that identify segments of the blood donor population with an increased risk of bloodborne infections; exclusion of blood donors in high-risk groups for AIDS and the introduction of anti-HIV screening tests; and progressively sensitive serologic and virologic screening tests for HCV infection.

In the absence of active or passive immunization, prevention of hepatitis C includes behavior changes and precautions to limit exposures to infected persons. Recommendations designed to identify patients with clinically inapparent hepatitis as candidates for medical management have as a secondary benefit the identification of persons whose contacts could be at risk of becoming infected. A so-called look-back program has been recommended to identify persons who were transfused before 1992 with blood from a donor found subsequently to have hepatitis C. In addition, anti-HCV testing is recommended for anyone who received a blood transfusion or a transplanted organ before the introduction of second-generation screening tests in 1992, those who ever used injection drugs, chronically hemodialyzed patients, persons with clotting disorders who received clotting factors made before 1987 from pooled blood products, persons with elevated aminotransferase levels, health workers exposed to HCV-positive blood or contaminated needles, and children born to HCV-positive mothers.

For stable, monogamous sexual partners, sexual transmission of hepatitis C is unlikely, and sexual barrier precautions are not recommended. For persons with multiple sexual partners or with sexually transmitted diseases, the risk of sexual transmission of hepatitis C is increased, and barrier precautions (latex condoms) are recommended. A person with hepatitis C should avoid sharing such items as razors, toothbrushes, and nail clippers with sexual partners and family members. No special precautions are recommended for babies born to mothers with hepatitis C, and breast feeding does not have to be restricted.

Hepatitis E

Whether IG prevents hepatitis E remains undetermined. A recombinant vaccine has been developed and is undergoing clinical testing.

FURTHER READINGS

AHN SH et al: Long-term clinical and histological outcomes in patients with spontaneous hepatitis B surface antigen seroclearance. J Hepatol 42:188, 2005

ARMSTRONG GL et al: The prevalence of hepatitis C virus infection in the United States, 1999 through 2002. Ann Intern Med 144:705, 2006

BELL BP et al: Hepatitis A virus infection in the United States: Serologic results from the Third National Health and Nutrition Examination Survey. Vaccine. 23:5798, 2005

BLUM HE, MARCELLIN P: EASL Consensus Conference on Hepatitis B. J Hepatol 39(Suppl 1):1, 2003

BOUCHARD MJ et al: Calcium signaling by HBx protein in hepatitis B virus DNA replication. Science 294:2376, 2001

BOWEN DG, WALKER CM: Adaptive immune responses in acute and chronic hepatitis C virus infection. Nature 436:946, 2005

CENTERS FOR DISEASE CONTROL AND PREVENTION: Recommendations for prevention and control of hepatitis C virus (HCV) infection and HCV-related chronic disease. MMWR 47:1, 1998

————: Updated U.S. Public Health Service guidelines for the management of occupational exposures to HBV, HCV, and HIV and recommendations for postexposure prophylaxis. MMWR 50(RR-11):1, 2001

————: General recommendations on immunization: Recommendations of the Advisory Committee on Immunization Practices and the American Academy of Family Physicians. MMWR 51(RR-2):1, 2002

————: A comprehensive strategy to eliminate transmission of hepatitis B virus infection in the United States: Recommendations of the Advisory Committee on Immunization Practices (ACIP); Part 1: Immunization of infants, children, and adolescents. MMWR 54 (RR-16):1, 2005

————: A comprehensive immunization strategy to eliminate transmission of hepatitis B virus infection in the United States: Recommendations of the Advisory Committee on Immunization Practices (ACIP); Part 2: Immunization of adults. MMWR 55(RR-16):1, 2006

————: Prevention of hepatitis A through active or passive immunization: Recommendations of the Advisory Committee on Immunization Practices (ACIP). MMWR 55(RR-7):1, 2006

CHEN CJ et al: Risk of hepatocellular carcinoma across a biological gradient of serum hepatitis B virus DNA level. JAMA 295:65, 2006

CHISARI FV: Unscrambling hepatitis C virus-host interactions. Nature 436:930, 2005

CHU C-J et al: Clinical significance of hepatitis B virus genotypes. Hepatology 35:1274, 2002

———— et al: Hepatitis B virus genotype B is associated with earlier HBeAg seroconversion compared with hepatitis B virus genotype C. Gastroenterology 122:1756, 2002

———— et al: Hepatitis B virus genotypes in the United States: Results of a nationwide study. Gastroenterology 126:333, 2003

———— et al: Prevalence of HBV precore/core promoter variants in the United States. Hepatology 35:619, 2003

CONSENSUS STATEMENT: EASL International Consensus Conference on Hepatitis C. J Hepatol 30:956, 1999

DIENSTAG JL: Hepatitis C: A bitter harvest. Ann Intern Med 144:770, 2006

————, MCHUTCHISON JG: American Gastroenterological Association technical review on the management of hepatitis C. Gastroenterology 130:231, 2006

DI GIAMMARINO L, DIENSTAG JL: Hepatitis A—the price of progress. N Engl J Med 353:944, 2005

FATTOVICH G: Natural history of hepatitis B. J Hepatology 39(Suppl 1):S50, 2003

FERRARI C et al: Immunopathogenesis of hepatitis B. J Hepatol 39(Suppl 1):S36, 2003

GAETA GB et al: Chronic hepatitis D: A vanishing disease? An Italian multicenter study. Hepatology 32:824, 2000

GALE MJ, FOY EM: Evasion of intracellular host defense by hepatitis C virus. Nature 436:939, 2005

GISH RG, LOCARNINI SA: Chronic hepatitis B: Current testing strategies. Clin Gastroenterol Hepatol 4:666, 2006

GUIDOTTI LG et al: Viral clearance without destruction of infected cells during acute HBV infection. Science 284:825, 1999

HADZIYANNIS SJ, VASSILOPOULOS D: Hepatitis B e antigen-negative chronic hepatitis B. Hepatology 34:617, 2001

ILOEJE UH et al: Predicting cirrhosis risk based on the level of circulating hepatitis B viral load. Gastroenterology 130:678, 2006

JAECKEL E et al: Treatment of acute hepatitis C with interferon alfa-2b. N Engl J Med 345:1452, 2001

KIM WR et al: Changing epidemiology of hepatitis B in a U.S. community. Hepatology 39:811, 2004

KRAWCZYNSKI K: Hepatitis E. Hepatology 17:932, 1993

LAUER GM, WALKER BD: Medical progress: Hepatitis C virus infection. N Engl J Med 345:41, 2001

LAVANCHY D: Hepatitis B virus epidemiology, disease burden, treatment, and current and emerging prevention and control measures. J Viral Hepatitis 11:97, 2004

LINDENBACH BD, RICE CM: Unravelling hepatitis C virus replication from genome to function. Nature 436:933, 2005

———— et al: Complete replication of hepatitis C virus in cell culture. Science. 309:623, 2005

LOK ASF, MCMAHON BJ: Chronic hepatitis B. Hepatology 34:1225, 2001

MARGOLIS HS et al (eds): *Viral Hepatitis and Liver Disease.* Atlanta/London, International Medical Press, 2002

MARINOS G et al: Hepatitis B virus variants with core gene deletions in the evolution of chronic hepatitis B infection. Gastroenterology 111:183, 1996

MILLER RH et al: Compact organization of the hepatitis B virus genome. Hepatology 9:322, 1989

NATIONAL INSTITUTES OF HEALTH CONSENSUS DEVELOPMENT CONFERENCE: Management of hepatitis C. Hepatology 26(Suppl 1):1S, 1997

————: Management of hepatitis C. Hepatology 36(Suppl 1):1S, 2002

NI Y-H et al: Hepatitis B virus infection in children and adolescents in a hyperendemic area: 15 years after mass hepatitis B vaccination. Ann Intern Med 135:796, 2001

OHATA K et al: High viral load is a risk factor for hepatocellular carcinoma in patients with chronic hepatitis B virus infection. J Gastroenterol Hepatol 19:670, 2004

PAWLOTSKY J-M: Molecular diagnosis of viral hepatitis. Gastroenterology 122:1554, 2002

PURCELL RH: Hepatitis viruses: Changing patterns of human disease. Proc Natl Acad Sci USA 91:2401, 1994

REHERMANN B: Immune response in hepatitis B virus infection. Semin Liver Dis 23:21, 2003

ROSINA F et al: Changing pattern of chronic hepatitis D in southern Europe. Gastroenterology 117:161, 1999

SCHREIBER GB et al: The risk of transfusion-transmitted viral infection. N Engl J Med 334:1685, 1996

SEEFF LB: Natural history of chronic hepatitis C. Hepatology 36(Suppl 1):S35, 2002

———— et al: A serologic follow-up of the 1942 epidemic of postvaccination hepatitis in the United States Army. N Engl J Med 316:965, 1987

SEEGER C et al: Biochemical and genetic evidence for the hepatitis B virus replication strategy. Science 232:477, 1986

SHEPARD CW et al: Global epidemiology of hepatitis C virus infection. Lancet Infect Dis 5:558, 2005

SIMMONDS P: Variability of hepatitis C virus. Hepatology 21:570, 1995

STRADER DB et al: Diagnosis, management, and treatment of hepatitis C (AASLD practice guidelines). Hepatology 39:1147, 2004

SUMI H et al. Influence of hepatitis B virus genotypes on the progression of chronic heptitis B liver disease. Hepatology 37:19, 2003

TANAKA Y et al: Molecular tracing of the global hepatitis C virus epidemic predicts regional patterns of hepatocellular carcinoma mortality. Gastroenterology 130:703, 2006

THIMME R et al: Viral and immunological determinants of hepatitis C virus clearance, persistence, and disease. Proc Natl Acad Sci USA 99:15661, 2002

WASLEY A et al: Incidence of hepatitis A in the United States in the era of vaccination. JAMA 294:194, 2005

WEDEMEYER H et al: Impaired effector function of hepatitis C virus–specific CD8+ T cells in chronic hepatitis C virus infection. J Immunol 169:3447, 2002

WILNER IR et al: Serious hepatitis A: An analysis of patients hospitalized during an urban epidemic in the United States. Ann Intern Med 128:111, 1998

YANG H-I et al: Hepatitis B e antigen and the risk of hepatocellular carcinoma. N Engl J Med 347:168, 2002

ZHONG J et al: Robust hepatitis C virus infection in vitro. Proc Natl Acad Sci USA. 102:9294, 2005

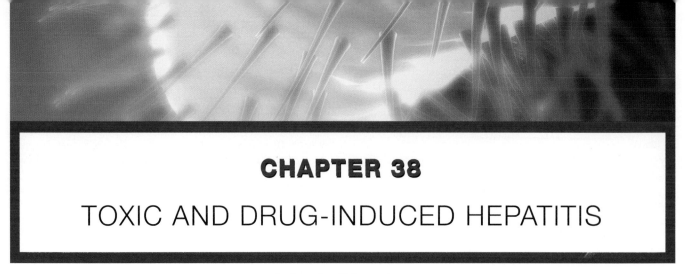

CHAPTER 38

TOXIC AND DRUG-INDUCED HEPATITIS

Jules L. Dienstag

Liver injury may follow the inhalation, ingestion, or parenteral administration of a number of pharmacologic and chemical agents. These include industrial toxins (e.g., carbon tetrachloride, trichloroethylene, and yellow phosphorus), the heat-stable toxic bicyclic octapeptides of certain species of *Amanita* and *Galerina* (hepatotoxic mushroom poisoning), and, more commonly, pharmacologic agents used in medical therapy. It is essential that any patient presenting with jaundice or altered biochemical liver tests be questioned carefully about exposure to chemicals used in work or at home, drugs taken by prescription or bought "over the counter," and herbal or alternative medicines. Hepatotoxic drugs can injure the hepatocyte directly, e.g., via a free-radical or metabolic intermediate that causes peroxidation of membrane lipids and that results in liver cell injury. Alternatively, the drug or its metabolite can distort cell membranes or other cellular molecules, bind covalently to intracellular proteins, activate apoptotic pathways, interfere with bile salt export proteins, or block biochemical pathways or cellular integrity. Interference with bile canalicular pumps can allow endogenous bile acids, which can injure the liver, to accumulate. Such injuries, in turn, may lead to necrosis of hepatocytes; injure bile ducts, producing cholestasis; or block pathways of lipid movement, inhibit protein synthesis, or impair mitochondrial oxidation of fatty acids, resulting in lactic acidosis and intracellular triglyceride accumulation (expressed histologically as microvesicular steatosis). In some cases, drug metabolites sensitize hepatocytes to toxic cytokines, and differences between susceptible and nonsusceptible drug recipients may be attributable to polymorphisms in elaboration of competing, protective cytokines, as has been suggested for acetaminophen hepatotoxicity (discussed later in the chapter). Immunologically mediated liver injury has been postulated to represent another mechanism of drug hepatotoxicity (see below). In addition, a role has been shown for activation of nuclear transporters, such as the constitutive androstane receptor (CAR), in the induction of drug hepatotoxicity. In general, two major types of chemical hepatotoxicity have been recognized: (1) direct toxic type and (2) idiosyncratic type.

Most drugs, which are water-insoluble, undergo a series of hepatic metabolic transformation steps, culminating in a water-soluble form appropriate for renal or biliary excretion. This process begins with oxidation or methylation initially mediated by the microsomal

TABLE 38-1

379

SOME FEATURES OF TOXIC AND DRUG-INDUCED HEPATIC INJURY

FEATURES	DIRECT TOXIC EFFECT[a]		IDIOSYNCRATIC[a]			OTHER[a]
	CARBON TETRA-CHLORIDE	ACETAMIN-OPHEN	HALOTHANE	ISONIAZID	CHLORPROMAZINE	ORAL CONTRA-CEPTIVE AGENTS
Predictable and dose-related toxicity	+	+	0	0	0	+
Latent period	Short	Short	Variable	Variable	Variable	Variable
Arthralgia, fever, rash, eosinophilia	0	0	+	0	+	0
Liver morphology	Necrosis, fatty infiltration	Centrilobular necrosis	Similar to viral hepatitis	Similar to viral hepatitis	Cholestasis *with* portal inflammation	Cholestasis *without* portal inflammation, vascular lesions

[a]The drugs listed are typical examples.

mixed-function oxygenases cytochrome P450 (phase I reaction), followed by glucuronidation or sulfation (phase II reaction) or inactivation by glutathione. Most drug hepatotoxicity is mediated by a phase I toxic metabolite, but glutathione depletion, precluding inactivation of harmful compounds by glutathione S-transferase, can contribute as well.

As shown in **Table 38-1**, direct toxic hepatitis occurs with predictable regularity in individuals exposed to the offending agent and is dose-dependent. The latent period between exposure and liver injury is usually short (often several hours), although clinical manifestations may be delayed for 24–48 h. Agents producing toxic hepatitis are generally systemic poisons or are converted in the liver to toxic metabolites. The direct hepatotoxins result in morphologic abnormalities that are reasonably characteristic and reproducible for each toxin. For example, carbon tetrachloride and trichloroethylene characteristically produce a centrilobular zonal necrosis, whereas yellow phosphorus poisoning typically results in periportal injury. The hepatotoxic octapeptides of *Amanita phalloides* usually produce massive hepatic necrosis; the lethal dose of the toxin is ~10 mg, the amount found in a single deathcap mushroom. Tetracycline, when administered in IV doses >1.5 g daily, leads to microvesicular fat deposits in the liver. Liver injury, which is often only one facet of the toxicity produced by the direct hepatotoxins, may go unrecognized until jaundice appears.

In idiosyncratic drug reactions, the occurrence of hepatitis is usually infrequent (1 in 10^3–10^5 patients) and unpredictable, the response is not dose-dependent, and liver injury may occur at any time during or shortly after exposure to the drug. Adding to the difficulty of predicting or identifying idiosyncratic drug hepatotoxicity is the occurrence of mild, transient, nonprogressive serum aminotransferase elevations that resolve with continued drug use. Such "adaptation," the mechanism of which is unknown, occurs in such drugs as isoniazid, valproate, phenytoin, and HMG-CoA reductase inhibitors (statins). Extrahepatic manifestations of hypersensitivity, such as rash, arthralgias, fever, leukocytosis, and eosinophilia, occur in about one-quarter of patients with idiosyncratic hepatotoxic drug reactions; this observation and the unpredictability of idiosyncratic drug hepatotoxicity contributed to the hypothesis that this category of drug reactions is immunologically mediated. More recent evidence, however, suggests that, in most cases, even idiosyncratic reactions represent direct hepatotoxicity but are caused by drug metabolites rather than by the intact compound. Even the prototypes of idiosyncratic hepatotoxicity reactions, halothane hepatitis and isoniazid hepatotoxicity, associated frequently with hypersensitivity manifestations, are now recognized to be mediated by toxic metabolites that damage liver cells directly. Currently, most idiosyncratic reactions are thought to result from differences in metabolic reactivity to specific agents; host susceptibility is mediated by the kinetics of toxic metabolite generation, which differs among individuals, probably mediated by genetic polymorphisms in drug-metabolizing pathways. Occasionally, however, the clinical features of an allergic reaction (prominent tissue eosinophilia, autoantibodies, etc.) are difficult to ignore. In vitro models have been described in which lymphocyte cytotoxicity can be demonstrated against rabbit hepatocytes altered by incubation with the potential offending drug. Furthermore, several instances of drug hepatotoxicity are associated with the appearance of autoantibodies, including a class of antibodies to liver-kidney microsomes, anti-LKM2, directed against a cytochrome P450 enzyme. Similarly, in selected cases, a drug or its metabolite has been shown to bind to a host cellular component forming a hapten; the immune response to this "neoantigen" is postulated to play a role in the pathogenesis of liver injury. Therefore, some authorities subdivide idiosyncratic drug hepatotoxicity into hypersensitivity (allergic) and "metabolic" categories. Several unusual exceptions notwithstanding, true drug allergy is difficult to support in most cases of idiosyncratic drug-induced liver injury.

Idiosyncratic reactions lead to a morphologic pattern that is more variable than those produced by direct toxins; a single agent is often capable of causing a variety of lesions, although certain patterns tend to predominate. Depending on the agent involved, idiosyncratic hepatitis may result in a clinical and morphologic picture indistinguishable from that of viral hepatitis (e.g., halothane) or may simulate extrahepatic bile duct obstruction clinically with morphologic evidence of cholestasis. Drug-induced cholestasis ranges from mild to increasingly severe: (1) bland cholestasis with limited hepatocellular injury (e.g., estrogens, 17, α–substituted androgens); (2) inflammatory cholestasis (e.g., phenothiazines, amoxicillin–clavulanic acid, oxacillin, erythromycin estolate); (3) sclerosing cholangitis (e.g., after intrahepatic infusion of the chemotherapeutic agent floxuridine for hepatic metastases from a primary colonic carcinoma); (4) disappearance of bile ducts, "ductopenic" cholestasis, similar to that observed in chronic rejection following liver transplantation (e.g., carbamazepine, chlorpromazine, tricyclic antidepressant agents). Cholestasis may result from binding of drugs to canalicular membrane transporters, accumulation of toxic bile acids resulting from canalicular pump failure, or genetic defects in canalicular transporter proteins. Morphologic alterations may also include bridging hepatic necrosis (e.g., methyldopa), or, infrequently, hepatic granulomas (e.g., sulfonamides). Some drugs result in macrovesicular or microvesicular steatosis or steatohepatitis, which in some cases has been linked to mitochondrial dysfunction and lipid peroxidation. Severe hepatotoxicity associated with steatohepatitis, most likely a result of mitochondrial toxicity, is being recognized with increasing frequency among patients receiving antiretroviral therapy with reverse transcriptase inhibitors (e.g., zidovudine, didanosine) or protease inhibitors (e.g., indinavir, ritonavir) for HIV infection. Generally, such mitochondrial hepatotoxicity of these antiretroviral agents is reversible, but dramatic, nonreversible hepatotoxicity associated with mitochondrial injury (inhibition of DNA polymerase γ) was the cause of acute liver failure encountered during early clinical trials of now-abandoned fialuridine, a fluorinated pyrimidine analogue with potent antiviral activity against hepatitis B virus. Another potential target for idiosyncratic drug hepato-

toxicity is sinusoidal lining cells; when these are injured, such as by high-dose chemotherapeutic agents (e.g., cyclophosphamide, melphalan, busulfan) administered prior to bone marrow transplantation, venoocclusive disease can result.

Not all adverse hepatic drug reactions can be classified as either toxic or idiosyncratic in type. For example, oral contraceptives, which combine estrogenic and progestational compounds, may result in impairment of hepatic tests and occasionally in jaundice; however, they do not produce necrosis or fatty change, manifestations of hypersensitivity are generally absent, and susceptibility to the development of oral contraceptive–induced cholestasis appears to be genetically determined. Such estrogen-induced cholestasis is more common in women with cholestasis of pregnancy, a disorder linked to genetic defects in multidrug resistance–associated canalicular transporter proteins. Other instances of genetically determined drug hepatotoxicity have been identified. For example, ~10% of the population have an autosomally recessive trait associated with the absence of cytochrome P450 enzyme 2D6 and have impaired debrisoquine-4-hydroxylase enzyme activity. As a result, they cannot metabolize, and are at increased risk of hepatotoxicity resulting from, certain compounds such as desipramine, propranolol, and quinidine.

Some forms of drug hepatotoxicity are so rare, e.g., occurring in <1:10,000 recipients, that they do not become apparent during clinical trials, involving only several thousand recipients, conducted to obtain drug registration. An example of such rare, but serious, idiosyncratic drug hepatotoxicity followed the approval and generalized use of troglitazone, a peroxisomal, proliferator activator–receptor γ agonist, the first-introduced example of a thiazolidinedione insulin-sensitizing agent. This instance of drug hepatotoxicity was not recognized until well after the drug was introduced, underlining the importance of postmarketing surveillance in identifying toxic drugs and in leading to their withdrawal from use. Fortunately, such hepatotoxicity is not characteristic of the second-generation thiazolidinedione insulin-sensitizing agents rosiglitazone and pioglitazone; in clinical trials, the frequency of aminotransferase elevations in patients treated with these medications did not differ from that in placebo recipients, and isolated reports of liver injury among recipients are extremely rare.

Because drug-induced hepatitis is often a presumptive diagnosis and many other disorders produce a similar clinicopathologic picture, evidence of a causal relationship between the use of a drug and subsequent liver injury may be difficult to establish. The relationship is most convincing for the direct hepatotoxins, which lead to a high frequency of hepatic impairment after a short latent period. Idiosyncratic reactions may be reproduced, in some instances, when rechallenge, after an asymptomatic period, results in a recurrence of signs, symptoms, and morphologic and biochemical abnormalities. Rechallenge, however, is often ethically unfeasible, because severe reactions may occur.

Generally, drug hepatotoxicity is not more frequent in persons with underlying chronic liver disease. Reported exceptions include hepatotoxicity of aspirin, methotrexate, isoniazid (only in certain experiences), and antiretroviral therapy for HIV infection.

℞ **Treatment:**
TOXIC AND DRUG-INDUCED HEPATIC DISEASE

Treatment is largely supportive, except in acetaminophen hepatotoxicity (described in the next section). In patients with fulminant hepatitis resulting from drug hepatotoxicity, liver transplantation may be life-saving (Chap. 44). Withdrawal of the suspected agent is indicated at the first sign of an adverse reaction. In the case of the direct toxins, liver involvement should not divert attention from renal or other organ involvement, which may also threaten survival. Glucocorticoids for drug hepatotoxicity with allergic features, silibinin for hepatotoxic mushroom poisoning, and ursodeoxycholic acid for cholestatic drug hepatotoxicity have never been shown to be effective and are not recommended.

In **Table 38-2**, classes of chemical agents are listed, together with examples of the pattern of liver injury produced by them. Certain drugs appear to be responsible for the development of chronic as well as acute hepatic injury. For example, oxyphenisatin, methyldopa, and isoniazid have been associated with moderate to severe chronic hepatitis, and halothane and methotrexate have been implicated in the development of cirrhosis. A syndrome resembling primary biliary cirrhosis has been described following treatment with chlorpromazine, methyl testosterone, tolbutamide, and other drugs. Portal hypertension in the absence of cirrhosis may result from alterations in hepatic architecture produced by vitamin A or arsenic intoxication, industrial exposure to vinyl chloride, or administration of thorium dioxide. The latter three agents have also been associated with angiosarcoma of the liver. Oral contraceptives have been implicated in the development of hepatic adenoma and, rarely, hepatocellular carcinoma and hepatic vein occlusion (Budd-Chiari syndrome). Another unusual lesion, peliosis hepatis (blood cysts of the liver), has been observed in some patients treated with anabolic steroids. The existence of these hepatic disorders expands the spectrum of liver injury induced by chemical agents and emphasizes the need for a thorough drug history in all patients with liver dysfunction.

The next sections describe the patterns of adverse hepatic reactions for some prototypic agents.

ACETAMINOPHEN HEPATOTOXICITY (DIRECT TOXIN)

Acetaminophen can cause severe centrilobular hepatic necrosis when ingested in large amounts in suicide attempts or accidentally by children; in the United States and England, acetaminophen hepatotoxicity is the most common culprit among patients presenting with acute liver failure. A single dose of 10–15 g, occasionally less, may produce clinical evidence of liver injury. Fatal fulminant disease is usually (although not invariably) associated with ingestion of ≥25 g. Blood levels of acetaminophen correlate with the severity of hepatic injury (levels > 300 μg/mL 4 h after ingestion are predictive of the development of severe damage; levels <150 μg/mL suggest that hepatic injury is highly unlikely). Nausea, vomiting, diarrhea, abdominal pain, and shock are early manifestations occurring 4–12 h after ingestion. Then 24–48 h later, when these features are abating, hepatic injury becomes apparent. Maximal abnormalities and hepatic failure may not be evident until 4–6 days after ingestion, and aminotransferase levels approaching 10,000 units are not uncommon, i.e., levels far exceeding those in patients with viral hepatitis. Renal failure and myocardial injury may be present.

Acetaminophen is metabolized predominantly by a phase II reaction to innocuous sulfate and glucuronide metabolites; however, a small proportion of acetaminophen is metabolized by a phase I reaction to a hepatotoxic metabolite formed from the parent compound by the cytochrome P450 CYP2E1. This metabolite, N-acetyl-benzoquinone-imine (NAPQI), is detoxified by binding to "hepatoprotective" glutathione to become harmless, water-soluble mercapturic acid, which undergoes renal excretion. When excessive amounts of NAPQI are formed, or when glutathione levels are low, glutathione levels are depleted and overwhelmed, permitting covalent binding to nucleophilic hepatocyte macromolecules forming acetaminophen-protein "adducts." These adducts, which can be measured in serum by high-performance liquid chromatography, hold promise as diagnostic markers of acetaminophen hepatotoxicity. The binding of acetaminophen to hepatocyte macromolecules is believed to lead to hepatocyte necrosis; the precise sequence and mechanism are unknown. Hepatic injury may be potentiated by prior administration of alcohol, phenobarbital, isoniazid, or other drugs; by conditions that stimulate the mixed-function oxidase system; or by conditions such as starvation that reduce hepatic glutathione levels. The xenobiotic (environmental, exogenous substance) receptor CAR has been shown in a mouse model of acetaminophen hepatotoxicity to induce acetaminophen-metabolizing

TABLE 38-2

PRINCIPAL ALTERATIONS OF HEPATIC MORPHOLOGY PRODUCED BY SOME COMMONLY USED DRUGS AND CHEMICALS[a]

PRINCIPAL MORPHOLOGIC CHANGE	CLASS OF AGENT	EXAMPLE
Cholestasis	Anabolic steroid	Methyl testosterone
	Antibiotic	Erythromycin estolate, nitrofurantoin, rifampin, amoxicillin-clavulanic acid, oxacillin
	Anticonvulsant	Carbamazine
	Antidepressant	Duloxetine, mirtazapine, tricyclic antidepressants
	Anti-inflammatory	Sulindac
	Antiplatelet	Clopidogrel
	Antihypertensive	Irbesartan
	Antithyroid	Methimazole
	Calcium channel blocker	Nifedipine, verapamil
	Immunosuppressive	Cyclosporine
	Lipid-lowering	Ezetimibe
	Oncotherapeutic	Anabolic steroids, busulfan, tamoxifen, irinotecan
	Oral contraceptive	Norethynodrel with mestranol
	Oral hypoglycemic	Chlorpropamide
	Tranquilizer	Chlorpromazine[b]
Fatty liver	Antiarrhythmic	Amiodarone
	Antibiotic	Tetracycline (high-dose, intravenous)
	Anticonvulsant	Valproic acid
	Antiviral	Dideoxynucleosides (e.g., zidovudine), protease inhibitors (e.g., indinavir, ritonavir)
	Oncotherapeutic	Asparaginase, methotrexate
Hepatitis	Anesthetic	Halothane[c]
	Antiandrogen	Flutamide
	Antibiotic	Isoniazid,[c] rifampicin, nitrofurantoin, telithromycin, minocycline, pyrazinamide, trovafloxacin[d]
	Anticonvulsant	Phenytoin, carbamazine
	Antidepressant	Iproniazid, amitriptyline, imipramine, trazodone, venlafaxine, fluoxetine, paroxetine, duloxetine, sertraline, nefazodone[d]
	Antifungal	Ketoconazole, fluconazole, itraconazole
	Antihypertensive	Methyldopa,[c] captopril, enalapril, lisinopril, losartan
	Anti-inflammatory	Ibuprofen, indomethacin, diclofenac, sulindac, bromfenac
	Antipsychotic	Risperidone
	Antiviral	Zidovudine, didanosine, stavudine, nevirapine, ritonavir, idinavir
	Calcium channel blocker	Nifedipine, verapamil, diltiazem
	Cholinesterase inhibitor	Tacrine
	Diuretic	Chlorothiazide
	Laxative	Oxyphenisatin[c,d]
	Norepinephrine-reuptake inhibitor	Atomoxetine
	Oral hypoglycemic	Troglitazone,[d] acarbose
Mixed hepatitis/ cholestatic	Antibiotic	Amoxicillin-clavulanic acid, trimethoprim-sulfamethoxazole
	Antifungal	Terbinafine
	Immunosuppressive	Azathioprine
	Lipid-lowering	Nicotinic acid, lovastatin, ezetimibe
Toxic (necrosis)	Analgesic	Acetaminophen
	Hydrocarbon	Carbon tetrachloride
	Metal	Yellow phosphorus
	Mushroom	*Amanita phalloides*
	Solvent	Dimethylformamide
Granulomas	Antiarrhythmic	Quinidine, diltiazem
	Antibiotic	Sulfonamides
	Anticonvulsant	Carbamazine
	Anti-inflammatory	Phenylbutazone
	Xanthine oxidase inhibitor	Allopurinol

[a]Several agents cause more than one type of liver lesion and appear under more than one category.
[b]Rarely associated with primary biliary cirrhosis-like lesion.
[c]Occasionally associated with chronic hepatitis or bridging hepatic necrosis or cirrhosis.
[d]Withdrawn from use because of severe hepatotoxicity.

enzymes and, thereby, regulate and increase hepatotoxicity. Cimetidine, which inhibits P450 enzymes, has the potential to reduce generation of the toxic metabolite. Alcohol induces cytochrome P450 CYP2E1; consequently, increased levels of the toxic metabolite NAPQI are produced in chronic alcoholics after acetaminophen ingestion. In addition, alcohol suppresses hepatic glutathione production. Therefore, in chronic alcoholics, the toxic dose of acetaminophen may be as low as 2 g, and alcoholic patients should be warned specifically about the dangers of even standard doses of this commonly used drug. Such "therapeutic misadventures" also occur occasionally in patients with severe, febrile illnesses or pain syndromes; in such a setting, several days of anorexia and near-fasting coupled with regular administration of extra-strength acetaminophen formulations result in a combination of glutathione depletion and relatively high NAPQI levels in the absence of a history of recognized acetaminophen overdose. Recently, aminotransferase elevations were identified in 31–44% of normal subjects treated for 14 days with the maximal recommended dose of acetaminophen, 4 g daily (administered alone or as part of an acetaminophen/opioid combination). Ironically, in patients with nonalcoholic liver disease, acetaminophen taken in recommended doses may be the safest analgesic/antipyretic.

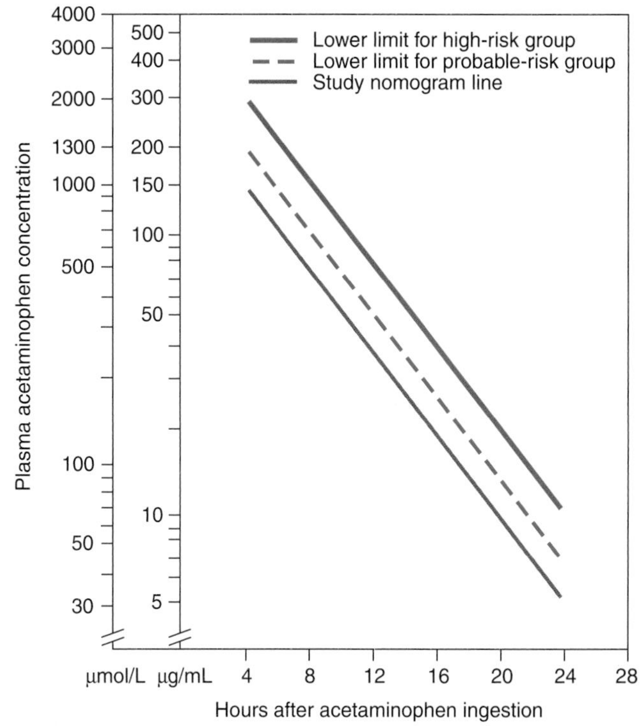

FIGURE 38-1

Nomogram to define risk of acetaminophen hepatotoxicity according to initial plasma acetaminophen concentration. *(After BH Rumack, H Matthew, Pediatrics 55:871, 1975.)*

℞ **Treatment:**
ACETAMINOPHEN OVERDOSAGE

Treatment includes gastric lavage, supportive measures, and oral administration of activated charcoal or cholestyramine to prevent absorption of residual drug. Neither of these agents appears to be effective if given >30 min after acetaminophen ingestion; if they are used, the stomach lavage should be done before other agents are administered orally. The chances of possible-, probable-, and high-risk hepatotoxicity can be derived from a nomogram plot (**Fig. 38-1**), readily available in emergency departments, of acetaminophen plasma levels as a function of hours after ingestion. In patients with high acetaminophen blood levels (>200 μg/mL measured at 4 h or >100 μg/mL at 8 h after ingestion), the administration of sulfhydryl compounds (e.g., cysteamine, cysteine, or N-acetylcysteine) reduces the severity of hepatic necrosis. These agents appear to act by providing a reservoir of sulfhydryl groups to bind the toxic metabolites or by stimulating synthesis and repletion of hepatic glutathione. Therapy should be begun within 8 h of ingestion but may be effective even if given as late as 24–36 h after overdose. Later administration of

sulfhydryl compounds is of uncertain value. Routine use of N-acetylcysteine has substantially reduced the occurrence of fatal acetaminophen hepatotoxicity. When given orally, N-acetylcysteine is diluted to yield a 5% solution. A loading dose of 140 mg/kg is given, followed by 70 mg/kg every 4 h for 15–20 doses. Whenever a patient with potential acetaminophen hepatotoxicity is encountered, a local poison control center should be contacted. Treatment can be stopped when plasma acetaminophen levels indicate that the risk of liver damage is low. If signs of hepatic failure (e.g., progressive jaundice, coagulopathy, confusion) occur despite N-acetylcysteine therapy for acetaminophen hepatotoxicity, liver transplantation may be the only option. Preliminary data suggest that early arterial blood lactate levels among such patients with acute liver failure may distinguish patients highly likely to require liver transplantation (lactate levels > 3.5 mmol/L) from those likely to survive without liver replacement.

Survivors of acute acetaminophen overdose usually have no evidence of hepatic sequelae. In a few patients, prolonged or repeated administration of acetaminophen in therapeutic doses appears to have led to the development of chronic hepatitis and cirrhosis.

HALOTHANE HEPATOTOXICITY (IDIOSYNCRATIC REACTION)

Although, currently, halothane anesthesia is administered in only rare situations, halothane hepatotoxicity was one of the prototypical, and most intensively studied, examples of idiosyncratic drug hepatotoxicity. Administration of halothane, a nonexplosive fluorinated hydrocarbon anesthetic agent that is structurally similar to chloroform, results in severe hepatic necrosis in a small number of individuals, many of whom have previously been exposed to this agent. The failure to produce similar hepatic lesions reliably in animals, the rarity of hepatic impairment in human beings, and the delayed appearance of hepatic injury suggest that halothane is not a direct hepatotoxin but rather a sensitizing agent; however, manifestations of hypersensitivity are seen in <25% of cases. A genetic predisposition leading to an idiosyncratic metabolic reactivity has been postulated and appears to be the most likely mechanism of halothane hepatotoxicity. Adults (rather than children), obese people, and women appear to be particularly susceptible. Fever, moderate leukocytosis, and eosinophilia may occur in the first week following halothane administration. Jaundice is usually noted 7–10 days after exposure but may occur earlier in previously exposed patients. Nausea and vomiting may precede the onset of jaundice. Hepatomegaly is often mild, but liver tenderness is common, and serum aminotransferase levels are elevated. The pathologic changes at autopsy are indistinguishable from massive hepatic necrosis resulting from viral hepatitis. The case-fatality rate of halothane hepatitis is not known but may vary from 20–40% in cases with severe liver involvement. Patients in whom unexplained spiking fever, especially delayed fever, or jaundice develops after halothane anesthesia should not receive this agent again. Because cross-reactions between halothane and methoxyflurane have been reported, the latter agent should not be used after halothane reactions. Later-generation halogenated hydrocarbon anesthetics, which have supplanted halothane except in rare instances (e.g., certain types of thoracic surgery), are felt to be associated with a lower risk of hepatotoxicity.

METHYLDOPA HEPATOTOXICITY (TOXIC AND IDIOSYNCRATIC REACTION)

Minor alterations in liver tests are reported in ~5% of patients treated with this antihypertensive agent. These trivial abnormalities typically resolve despite continued drug administration. In <1% of patients, acute liver injury resembling viral or chronic hepatitis or, rarely, a cholestatic reaction is seen 1–20 weeks after methyldopa is started. In 50% of cases the interval is <4 weeks. A prodrome of fever, anorexia, and malaise may be noted for a few days before the onset of jaundice. Rash, lymphadenopathy, arthralgia, and eosinophilia are rare. Serologic markers of autoimmunity are detected infrequently, and <5% of patients have a Coombs-positive hemolytic anemia. In ~15% of patients with methyldopa hepatotoxicity, the clinical, biochemical, and histologic features are those of moderate to severe chronic hepatitis, with or without bridging necrosis and macronodular cirrhosis. With discontinuation of the drug, the disorder usually resolves. Although methyldopa is currently used infrequently, its hepatotoxicity is very well characterized. Among the currently popular antihypertensive agents, angiotensin-converting enzyme (ACE) inhibitors, such as captopril and enalapril, have been blamed, albeit rarely, for hepatotoxicity (primarily cholestasis and cholestatic hepatitis, but also hepatocellular injury). Angiotensin-II receptor antagonists, such as losartan, are unlikely hepatotoxins, although rare reports of liver injury in their recipients have appeared.

ISONIAZID HEPATOTOXICITY (TOXIC AND IDIOSYNCRATIC REACTION)

In ~10% of adults treated with the antituberculosis agent isoniazid, elevated serum aminotransferase levels develop during the first few weeks of therapy; this appears to represent an adaptive response to a toxic metabolite of the drug. Whether or not isoniazid is continued, these values (usually <200 units) return to normal in a few weeks. In ~1% of treated patients, an illness develops that is indistinguishable from viral hepatitis; approximately half of these cases occur within the first 2 months of treatment, while in the remainder, clinical disease may be delayed for many months. Liver biopsy reveals morphologic changes similar to those of viral hepatitis or bridging hepatic necrosis. The disease may be severe, with a case-fatality rate of 10%. Important liver injury appears to be age-related, increasing substantially after age 35; the highest frequency is in patients over age 50, the lowest under the age of 20. Even for patients >50 years monitored carefully during therapy, hepatotoxicity occurs in only ~2%, well below the risk estimate derived from earlier experiences. Isoniazid hepatotoxicity is enhanced by alcohol, rifampin, and pyrazinamide. Fever, rash, eosinophilia, and other manifestations of drug allergy are distinctly unusual. A reactive metabolite of acetylhydrazine, a metabolite of isoniazid, may be responsible for liver injury, and patients who are rapid acetylators would be more prone to such injury. Counterintuitively, in some reports, the opposite is true; slow acetylators are more likely to experience hepatotoxicity and more severe hepatotoxicity than rapid acetylators. Contrary to past reports, more recent studies suggest that hepatotoxicity due to isoniazid as well as to combination antituberculous therapy that includes isoniazid is more likely in patients with underlying chronic hepatitis B. A picture resembling chronic hepatitis has been observed in a few patients. Careful liver-test monitoring is advisable in patients being treated with isoniazid.

SODIUM VALPROATE HEPATOTOXICITY (TOXIC AND IDIOSYNCRATIC REACTION)

Sodium valproate, an anticonvulsant useful in the treatment of petit mal and other seizure disorders, has been associated with the development of severe hepatic toxicity and, rarely, fatalities, predominantly in children but also in adults. Asymptomatic elevations of serum aminotransferase levels have been recognized in as many as 45% of treated patients. These "adaptive" changes, however, appear to have no clinical importance, for major hepatotoxicity is not seen in the majority of patients despite continuation of drug therapy. In those rare patients in whom jaundice, encephalopathy, and evidence of hepatic failure are found, examination of liver tissue reveals microvesicular fat and bridging hepatic necrosis, predominantly in the centrilobular zone. Bile duct injury may also be apparent. Most likely, sodium valproate is not directly hepatotoxic, but its metabolite, 4-pentenoic acid, may be responsible for hepatic injury. Valproate hepatotoxicity is more common in persons with mitochondrial enzyme deficiencies and may be ameliorated by IV administration of carnitine, which valproate therapy can deplete.

PHENYTOIN HEPATOTOXICITY (IDIOSYNCRATIC REACTION)

Phenytoin, formerly diphenylhydantoin, a mainstay in the treatment of seizure disorders, has been associated in rare instances with the development of severe hepatitis-like liver injury leading to fulminant hepatic failure. In many patients the hepatitis is associated with striking fever, lymphadenopathy, rash (Stevens-Johnson syndrome or exfoliative dermatitis), leukocytosis, and eosinophilia, suggesting an immunologically mediated hypersensitivity mechanism. Despite these observations, evidence suggests that metabolic idiosyncrasy may be responsible for hepatic injury. In the liver, phenytoin is converted by the cytochrome P450 system to metabolites, which include the highly reactive electrophilic arene oxides. These metabolites are

normally metabolized further by epoxide hydrolases. A defect (genetic or acquired) in epoxide hydrolase activity could permit covalent binding of arene oxides to hepatic macromolecules, thereby leading to hepatic injury. Regardless of the mechanism, hepatic injury is usually manifested within the first 2 months after beginning phenytoin therapy. With the exception of an abundance of eosinophils in the liver, the clinical, biochemical, and histologic picture resembles that of viral hepatitis. In rare instances, bile duct injury may be the salient feature of phenytoin hepatotoxicity, with striking features of intrahepatic cholestasis. Asymptomatic elevations of aminotransferase and alkaline phosphatase levels have been observed in a sizable proportion of patients receiving long-term phenytoin therapy. These liver changes are believed by some authorities to represent the potent hepatic enzyme– inducing properties of phenytoin and are accompanied histologically by swelling of hepatocytes in the absence of necroinflammatory activity or evidence of chronic liver disease.

AMIODARONE HEPATOTOXICITY (TOXIC AND IDIOSYNCRATIC REACTION)

Therapy with this potent antiarrhythmic drug is accompanied in 15–50% of patients by modest elevations of serum aminotransferase levels that may remain stable or diminish despite continuation of the drug. Such abnormalities may appear days to many months after beginning therapy. A proportion of those with elevated aminotransferase levels have detectable hepatomegaly, and clinically important liver disease develops in <5% of patients. Features that represent a direct effect of the drug on the liver and that are common to the majority of long-term recipients are ultrastructural phospholipidosis, unaccompanied by clinical liver disease, and interference with hepatic mixed-function oxidase metabolism of other drugs. The cationic amphiphilic drug and its major metabolite desethylamiodarone accumulate in hepatocyte lysosomes and mitochondria and in bile duct epithelium. The relatively common elevations in aminotransferase levels are also considered a predictable, dose-dependent, direct hepatotoxic effect. On the other hand, in the rare patient with clinically apparent, symptomatic liver disease, liver injury resembling that seen in alcoholic liver disease is observed. The so-called pseudoalcoholic liver injury can range from steatosis, to alcoholic hepatitis-like neutrophilic infiltration and Mallory's hyaline, to cirrhosis. Electron-microscopic demonstration of phospholipid-laden lysosomal lamellar bodies can help to distinguish amiodarone hepatotoxicity from typical alcoholic hepatitis. This category of liver injury appears to be a metabolic idiosyncrasy that allows hepatotoxic metabolites to be generated. Rarely, an acute idiosyncratic hepatocellular injury resembling viral hepatitis or cholestatic hepatitis occurs. Hepatic granulomas have occasionally been observed. Because amiodarone has a long half-life, liver injury may persist for months after the drug is stopped.

ERYTHROMYCIN HEPATOTOXICITY (CHOLESTATIC IDIOSYNCRATIC REACTION)

The most important adverse effect associated with erythromycin, more common in children than adults, is the infrequent occurrence of a cholestatic reaction. Although most of these reactions have been associated with erythromycin estolate, other erythromycins may also be responsible. The reaction usually begins during the first 2 or 3 weeks of therapy and includes nausea, vomiting, fever, right upper quadrant abdominal pain, jaundice, leukocytosis, and moderately elevated aminotransferase levels. The clinical picture can resemble acute cholecystitis or bacterial cholangitis. Liver biopsy reveals variable cholestasis; portal inflammation comprising lymphocytes, polymorphonuclear leukocytes, and eosinophils; and scattered foci of hepatocyte necrosis. Symptoms and laboratory findings usually subside within a few days of drug withdrawal, and evidence of chronic liver disease has not been found on follow-up. The precise mechanism remains ill-defined.

ORAL CONTRACEPTIVE HEPATOTOXICITY (CHOLESTATIC REACTION)

The administration of oral contraceptive combinations of estrogenic and progestational steroids leads to intrahepatic cholestasis with pruritus and jaundice in a small number of patients weeks to months after taking these agents. Especially susceptible seem to be patients with recurrent idiopathic jaundice of pregnancy, severe pruritus of pregnancy, or a family history of these disorders. With the exception of liver biochemical tests, laboratory studies are normal, and extrahepatic manifestations of hypersensitivity are absent. Liver biopsy reveals cholestasis with bile plugs in dilated canaliculi and striking bilirubin staining of liver cells. In contrast to chlorpromazine-induced cholestasis, portal inflammation is absent. The lesion is reversible on withdrawal of the agent. The two steroid components appear to act synergistically on hepatic function, although the estrogen may be primarily responsible. Oral contraceptives are contraindicated in patients with a history of recurrent jaundice of pregnancy. Primarily benign, but rarely malignant, neoplasms of the liver, hepatic vein occlusion, and peripheral sinusoidal dilatation have also been associated with oral contraceptive therapy. Focal nodular hyperplasia of the liver is not more frequent among users of oral contraceptives.

17, α-ALKYL-SUBSTITUTED ANABOLIC STEROIDS (CHOLESTATIC REACTION)

In the majority of patients receiving these agents, used therapeutically mainly in the treatment of bone marrow failure but used surreptitiously and without medical indication by athletes to improve their performance, mild hepatic dysfunction develops. Impaired excretory function is the predominant defect, but the precise mechanism is uncertain. Jaundice, which appears to be dose-related, develops in only a minority of patients and may be the sole clinical manifestation of hepatotoxicity, although anorexia, nausea, and malaise may occur. Pruritus is not a prominent feature. Serum aminotransferase levels are usually <100 units, and serum alkaline phosphatase levels are normal, mildly elevated, or, in <5% of patients, three or more times the upper limit of normal. Examination of liver tissue reveals cholestasis without inflammation or necrosis. Hepatic sinusoidal dilatation and peliosis hepatis have been found in a few patients. The cholestatic disorder is usually reversible on cessation of treatment, although fatalities have been linked to peliosis. An association with hepatic adenoma and hepatocellular carcinoma has been reported.

TRIMETHOPRIM-SULFAMETHOXAZOLE HEPATOTOXICITY (IDIOSYNCRATIC REACTION)

This antibiotic combination is used routinely for urinary tract infections in immunocompetent persons and for prophylaxis against and therapy of *Pneumocystis carinii* pneumonia in immunosuppressed persons (transplant recipients, patients with AIDS). With its increasing use, its occasional hepatotoxicity is being recognized with growing frequency. Its likelihood is unpredictable, but when it occurs, trimethoprim-sulfamethoxazole hepatotoxicity follows a relatively uniform latency period of several weeks and is often accompanied by eosinophilia, rash, and other features of a hypersensitivity reaction. Biochemically and histologically, acute hepatocellular necrosis predominates, but cholestatic features are quite frequent. Occasionally, cholestasis without necrosis occurs, and very rarely, a severe cholangiolytic pattern of liver injury is observed. In most cases, liver injury is self-limited, but rare fatalities have been recorded. The hepatotoxicity is attributable to the sulfamethoxazole component of the drug and is similar in features to that seen with other sulfonamides; tissue eosinophilia and granulomas may be seen. The risk of trimethoprim-sulfamethoxazole hepatotoxicity is increased in persons with HIV infection.

HMG-CoA REDUCTASE INHIBITORS (STATINS) (IDIOSYNCRATIC MIXED HEPATOCELLULAR AND CHOLESTATIC REACTION)

Between 1 and 2% of patients taking lovastatin, simvastatin, pravastatin, fluvastatin, or one of the newer statin drugs for the treatment of hypercholesterolemia experience asymptomatic, reversible elevations (>threefold) of aminotransferase activity. Acute hepatitis-like histologic changes, centrilobular necrosis, and centrilobular cholestasis have been described in several cases. In a larger proportion, minor aminotransferase elevations appear during the first several weeks of therapy. Careful laboratory monitoring can distinguish between patients with minor transitory changes, who may continue therapy, and those with more profound and sustained abnormalities, who should discontinue therapy. Because clinically meaningful aminotransferase elevations are so rare after statin use, a panel of liver experts recommended to the National Lipid Association's Safety Task Force that liver-test monitoring was not necessary in patients treated with statins and that statin therapy need not be discontinued in patients found to have asymptomatic isolated aminotransferase elevations during therapy. Statin hepatotoxicity is not increased in patients with chronic hepatitis C or hepatic steatosis, and statins can be used safely in these patients.

TOTAL PARENTERAL NUTRITION (STEATOSIS, CHOLESTASIS)

Total parenteral nutrition (TPN) is often complicated by cholestatic hepatitis attributable to either steatosis, cholestasis, or gallstones (or gallbladder sludge). Steatosis or steatohepatitis may result from the excess carbohydrate calories in these nutritional supplements and is the predominant form of TPN-associated liver disorder in adults. The frequency of this complication has been reduced substantially by the introduction of balanced TPN formulas that rely on lipid as an alternative caloric source. Cholestasis and cholelithiasis, caused by the absence of stimulation of bile flow and secretion resulting from the lack of oral intake, is the predominant form of TPN-associated liver disease in infants, especially in premature neonates. Often, cholestasis in such neonates is multifactorial, contributed to by other factors such as sepsis, hypoxemia, and hypotension; occasionally, TPN-induced cholestasis in neonates culminates in chronic liver disease and liver failure. When TPN-associated liver test abnormalities occur in adults, balancing the TPN formula with more lipid is the intervention of first recourse. In infants with TPN-associated cholestasis, the addition of oral feeding may ameliorate the problem. Therapeutic interventions suggested, but not shown to be of proven benefit, include cholecystokinin, ursodeoxycholic acid, *S*-adenosyl methionine, and taurine.

ALTERNATIVE AND COMPLEMENTARY MEDICINES (IDIOSYNCRATIC HEPATITIS, STEATOSIS)

The misguided popularity of herbal medications that are of scientifically unproven efficacy and that lack prospective safety oversight by regulatory agencies has resulted in occasional instances of hepatotoxicity. Included among the herbal remedies associated with toxic hepatitis are Jin Bu Huan, xiao-chai-hu-tang, germander, chaparral, senna, mistletoe, skullcap, gentian, comfrey (containing pyrrolizidine alkaloids), Ma huang, bee pollen, valerian root, pennyroyal oil, kava, celandine, Impila (*Callilepsis laureaola*), LipoKinetix, Hyroxycut, and herbal teas. Well characterized are the acute hepatitis-like histologic lesions following Jin Bu Huan use: focal hepatocellular necrosis, mixed mononuclear portal tract infiltration, coagulative necrosis, apoptotic hepatocyte degeneration, tissue eosinophilia, and microvesicular steatosis. Megadoses of vitamin A can injure the liver, as can pyrrolizidine alkaloids, which often contaminate Chinese herbal preparations and can cause a venoocclusive injury leading to sinusoidal hepatic vein obstruction. Because some alternative medicines induce toxicity via active metabolites, alcohol and drugs that stimulate cytochrome P450 enzymes may enhance the toxicity of some of these products. Conversely, some alternative medicines also stimulate cytochrome P450 and may result in or amplify the toxicity of recognized drug hepatotoxins. Given the widespread use of such poorly defined herbal preparations, hepatotoxicity is likely to be encountered with increasing frequency; therefore, a drug history in patients with acute and chronic liver disease should include use of alternative medicines and other nonprescription preparations sold in so-called health food stores.

HIGHLY ACTIVE ANTIRETROVIRAL THERAPY (HAART) FOR HIV INFECTION (MITOCHONDRIAL TOXIC, IDIOSYNCRATIC, STEATOSIS; HEPATOCELLULAR, CHOLESTATIC, AND MIXED)

The recognition of drug hepatotoxicity in persons with HIV infection is complicated in this population by the many alternative causes of liver injury (chronic viral hepatitis, fatty infiltration, infiltrative disorders, mycobacterial infection, etc.), but drug hepatotoxicity associated with HAART is an emerging and common type of liver injury in HIV-infected persons. Although no one antiviral agent is recognized as a potent hepatotoxin, combination regimens including reverse transcriptase and protease inhibitors cause hepatotoxicity in ~10% of treated patients. Implicated most frequently are combinations including nucleoside analogue reverse transcriptase inhibitors zidovudine, didanosine, and, to a lesser extent, stavudine; protease inhibitors ritonavir and indinavir (and amprenivir when used together with ritonavir); and nonnucleoside reverse transcriptase inhibitors nevirapine and, to a lesser extent, efavirenz. These drugs cause predominantly hepatocellular injury but cholestatic injury as well, and prolonged (>6 months) use of reverse transcriptase inhibitors has been associated with mitochondrial injury, steatosis, and lactic acidosis. Indirect hyperbilirubinemia, resulting from direct inhibition of bilirubin-conjugating activity by UDP-glucuronosyltransferase, usually without elevation of aminotransferase or alkaline phosphatase activities, occurs in ~10% of patients treated with the protease inhibitor indinavir. Distinguishing the impact of HAART hepatotoxicity in patients with HIV and hepatitis virus co-infection is made challenging by the following: (1) both chronic hepatitis B and hepatitis C can affect the natural history of HIV infection and the response to HAART, and (2) HAART can have an impact on chronic viral hepatitis. For example, immunologic reconstitution with HAART can result in immunologically mediated liver-cell injury in patients with chronic hepatitis B co-infection if treatment with an antiviral agent for hepatitis B, e.g., the nucleoside analogue lamivudine, is withdrawn or if nucleoside analogue resistance emerges. Infection with HIV, especially with low CD4+ T cell counts, has been reported to increase the rate of hepatic fibrosis associated with chronic hepatitis C, and HAART therapy can increase levels of serum aminotransferases and hepatitis C virus RNA in patients with hepatitis C co-infection.

ACKNOWLEDGMENT

Kurt J. Isselbacher, MD, contributed to this chapter in previous editions of Harrison's Principles of Internal Medicine.

FURTHER READINGS

ANDRADE RJ et al: Drug-induced liver injury: An analysis of 461 incidences submitted to the Spanish registry over a 10-year period. Gastroenterology 129:512, 2005

BERSON A et al: Steatohepatitis-inducing drugs cause mitochondrial dysfunction and lipid peroxidation in rat hepatocytes. Gastroenterology 114:764, 1998

BISSELL DM et al: Drug-induced liver injury: Mechanisms and test systems. Hepatology 33:1009, 2001

BJÖRNSSON E, OLSSON R: Outcome and prognostic markers in severe drug-induced liver disease. Hepatology 42:481:2005

BROWNING JD: Statins and hepatic steatosis: Perspectives from the Dallas Heart Study. Hepatology 44:466, 2006

CHALASANI N et al: Patients with elevated liver enzymes are not at higher risk for statin hepatotoxicity. Gastroenterology 126:1287, 2004

CHARIOT P et al: Zidovudine-induced mitochondrial disorder with massive liver steatosis, myopathy, lactic acidosis, and mitochondrial DNA depletion. J Hepatol 30:156, 1999

CHUNG RT et al: Immune recovery is associated with persistent rise in HCV RNA, infrequent liver test flares, and is not impaired by HCV in co-infected subjects. AIDS 16:1915, 2002

COHEN DE et al: An assessment of statin safety by hepatologists. Am J Cardiol 97(Suppl):77C, 2006

DAVERN TJ II et al: Measurement of serum acetaminophen-protein adducts in patients with acute liver failure. Gastroenterology 130:687, 2006

FARRELL GC, LIDDLE C (guest eds.): Hepatotoxicity in the twenty-first century. Semin Liver Dis 22:109, 2002

FONTANA RJ: Acute liver failure due to drugs. Semin Liver Dis 28:175, 2008

HUANG Y-S et al: Polymorphism of the N-acetyltransferase 2 gene as a susceptibility risk factor for antituberculous drug–induced hepatitis. Hepatology 35:883, 2002

KAPLOWITZ N: Biochemical and cellular mechanisms of toxic liver injury. Semin Liver Dis 22:137, 2002

———, DELEVE LD (eds): Drug-Induced Liver Disease. New York, Marcel Dekker, 2002

KHORASHADI S et al: Incidence of statin hepatotoxicity in patients with hepatitis C. Clin Gastroenterol Hepatol 4:902, 2006

LARSON AM: Acetaminophen hepatotoxicity. Clin Liver Dis 11:525, 2007

——— et al: Acetaminophen-induced acute liver failure: Results of a United States multicenter prospective study. Hepatology 42:1364, 2005

LEE WM: Drug-induced hepatotoxicity. N Engl J Med 349:474, 2003

MADDREY WC: Drug-induced hepatotoxicity. J Clin Gastroenterol 39(Suppl 2):S83, 2005

NAVARRO VJ, SENIOR JR: Drug-related hepatotoxicity. N Engl J Med 354:731, 2006

NOLAN CM et al: Hepatotoxicity associated with isoniazid preventive therapy. JAMA 281:1014, 1999

NORRIS W et al: Drug-induced liver injury in 2007. Curr Opin Gastroenterol 24:287, 2008

NUNEZ M: Hepatotoxicity of antiretrovirals: Incidence, mechanisms and management. J Hepatol 44(Suppl):S132, 2006

RAMACHANDRAN R, KAKAR S: Histological patterns in drug-induced liver disease. J Clin Pathol 62:481, 2009

RUSSO MW, WATKINS PB: Are patients with elevated liver tests at increased risk of drug-induced liver injury? Gastroenterology 126:1477, 2004

SALPETER SR et al: Monitored isoniazid prophylaxis for low-risk tuberculin reactors older than 35 years of age. Ann Intern Med 127:1051, 1997

SCHIODT FV et al: Acetaminophen toxicity in an urban county hospital. N Engl J Med 337:1112, 1997

SCHMIDT LE et al: Acute versus chronic alcohol consumption in acetaminophen-induced hepatotoxicity. Hepatology 35:876, 2002

SEEFF LB et al: Complementary and alternative medicine in chronic liver disease. Hepatology 34:595, 2001

STICKEL F et al: Herbal hepatotoxicity. J Hepatol 43:901, 2005

STRAVITZ RT: Critical management decisions in patients with acute liver failure. Chest 134:1092, 2008

SULKOWSKI MS et al: Hepatotoxicity associated with antiretroviral therapy in adults infected with human immunodeficiency virus and the role of hepatitis C or B virus infection. JAMA 283:74, 2000

WATKINS PB et al: Aminotransferase elevations in healthy adults receiving 4 grams of acetaminophen daily: A randomized controlled trial. JAMA 296:87, 2006

———, Seeff LB: Drug-induced liver injury: Summary of a single-topic clinical research conference. Hepatology 43:618, 2006

Wilkinson GR: Drug metabolism and variability among patients in drug response. N Engl J Med 352:2211, 2005

Zhang J et al: Modulation of acetaminophen-induced hepatotoxicity by the xenobiotic receptor CAR. Science 298:422, 2002

Zimmerman HJ: *Hepatotoxicity: The Adverse Effects of Drugs and Other Chemicals on the Liver,* 2d ed. Philadelphia, Lippincott Williams & Wilkins, 1999

———, Maddrey WC: Acetaminophen (paracetamol) hepatotoxicity with regular intake of alcohol: Analysis of instances of therapeutic misadventure. Hepatology 22:767, 1995

——— et al: Drug-induced liver disease, in *Schiff's Diseases of the Liver,* 8th ed, E Schiff et al (eds). Philadelphia, Lippincott-Raven, 1999, p 973

Zucker SD et al: Mechanism of idinavir-induced hyperbilirubinemia. Proc Natl Acad Sci USA 98:12671, 2001

CHAPTER 38

Toxic and Drug-Induced Hepatitis

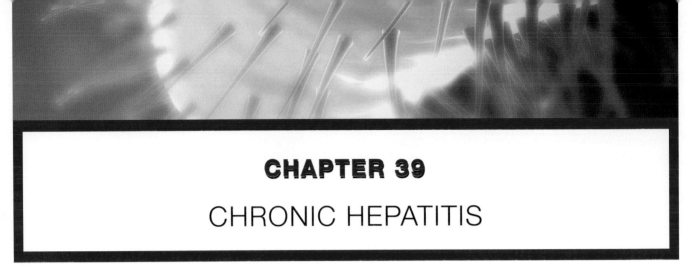

CHAPTER 39

CHRONIC HEPATITIS

Jules L. Dienstag

Chronic hepatitis represents a series of liver disorders of varying causes and severity in which hepatic inflammation and necrosis continue for at least 6 months. Milder forms are nonprogressive or only slowly progressive, while more severe forms may be associated with scarring and architectural reorganization, which, when advanced, lead ultimately to cirrhosis. Several categories of chronic hepatitis have been recognized. These include chronic viral hepatitis, drug-induced chronic hepatitis (Chap. 38), and autoimmune chronic hepatitis. In many cases, clinical and laboratory features are insufficient to allow assignment into one of these three categories; these "idiopathic" cases are also believed to represent autoimmune chronic hepatitis. Finally, clinical and laboratory features of chronic hepatitis are observed occasionally in patients with such hereditary/metabolic disorders as Wilson's disease (copper overload) and even occasionally in patients with alcoholic liver injury (Chap. 40). Although all types of chronic hepatitis share certain clinical, laboratory, and histopathologic features, chronic viral and chronic autoimmune hepatitis are sufficiently distinct to merit separate discussions. For discussion of acute hepatitis, see Chap. 37.

CLASSIFICATION OF CHRONIC HEPATITIS

Common to all forms of chronic hepatitis are histopathologic distinctions based on localization and extent of liver injury. These vary from the milder forms, previously labeled *chronic persistent hepatitis* and *chronic lobular hepatitis*, to the more severe form, formerly called *chronic active hepatitis*. When first defined, these designations were felt to have prognostic implications, which have been challenged by more recent observations. Categorization of chronic hepatitis based primarily on histopathologic features has been replaced by a more informative classification based on a combination of clinical, serologic, and histologic variables. Classification of chronic hepatitis is based on (1) its *cause*; (2) its histologic activity, or *grade*; and (3) its degree of progression, or *stage*. Thus, neither clinical features alone nor histologic features—requiring liver biopsy—alone are sufficient to characterize and distinguish among the several categories of chronic hepatitis.

TABLE 39-1

CLINICAL AND LABORATORY FEATURES OF CHRONIC HEPATITIS

TYPE OF HEPATITIS	DIAGNOSTIC TEST(S)	AUTOANTIBODIES	THERAPY
Chronic hepatitis B	HBsAg, IgG anti-HBc, HBeAg, HBV DNA	Uncommon	IFN-α, PEG IFN-α, lamivudine, adefovir, entecavir
Chronic hepatitis C	Anti-HCV, HCV RNA	Anti-LKM1[a]	PEG IFN-α plus ribavirin
Chronic hepatitis D	Anti-HDV, HDV RNA, HBsAg, IgG anti-HBc	Anti-LKM3	IFN-α, PEG IFN-α[b]
Autoimmune hepatitis	ANA[c] (homogeneous), anti-LKM1(±), hyperglobulinemia	ANA, anti-LKM1, anti-SLA[d]	Prednisone, azathioprine
Drug-associated	—	Uncommon	Withdraw drug
Cryptogenic	All negative	None	Prednisone (?), azathioprine (?)

[a]Antibodies to liver-kidney microsomes type 1 (autoimmune hepatitis type II and some cases of hepatitis C).
[b]Clinical trials suggest benefit of IFN-α therapy or PEG IFN-α.
[c]Antinuclear antibody (autoimmune hepatitis type I).
[d]Antibodies to soluble liver antigen (autoimmune hepatitis type III).
Note: HBc, hepatitis B core; HBeAg, hepatitis B e antigen; HBsAg, hepatitis B surface antigen; HBV, hepatitis B virus; HCV, hepatitis C virus; HDV, hepatitis D virus; IFN-α, interferon α; IgG, immunoglobulin G; LKM, liver-kidney microsome; PEG-IFN-α, pegylated interferon α; SLA, soluble liver antigen.

CHAPTER 39

Chronic Hepatitis

CLASSIFICATION BY CAUSE

Clinical and serologic features allow the establishment of a diagnosis of *chronic viral hepatitis*, caused by hepatitis B, hepatitis B plus D, or hepatitis C; *autoimmune hepatitis*, including several subcategories, I and II (perhaps III), based on serologic distinctions; *drug-associated chronic hepatitis*; and a category of unknown cause, or *cryptogenic chronic hepatitis* (Table 39-1). These are addressed in more detail below.

CLASSIFICATION BY GRADE

Grade, a histologic assessment of necroinflammatory activity, is based on examination of the liver biopsy. An assessment of important histologic features includes the degree of *periportal necrosis* and the disruption of the limiting plate of periportal hepatocytes by inflammatory cells (so-called *piecemeal necrosis* or *interface hepatitis*); the degree of confluent necrosis that links or forms bridges between vascular structures—between portal tract and portal tract or even more important bridges between portal tract and central vein—referred to as *bridging necrosis*; the degree of hepatocyte degeneration and focal necrosis within the lobule; and the degree of *portal inflammation*. Several scoring systems that take these histologic features into account have been devised, and the most popular are the histologic activity index (HAI) and the METAVIR score (Table 39-2). Based on the presence and degree of these features of histologic activity, chronic hepatitis can be graded as mild, moderate, or severe.

CLASSIFICATION BY STAGE

The stage of chronic hepatitis, which reflects the level of progression of the disease, is based on the degree of hepatic fibrosis. When fibrosis is so extensive that fibrous septa surround parenchymal nodules and alter the normal architecture of the liver lobule, the histologic lesion is defined as *cirrhosis*. Staging is based on the degree of fibrosis as categorized on a numerical scale from 0–6 (HAI) or 0–4 (METAVIR) (Table 39-2).

CHRONIC VIRAL HEPATITIS

Both the enterically transmitted forms of viral hepatitis, hepatitis A and E, are self-limited and do not cause chronic hepatitis (rare reports notwithstanding in which acute hepatitis A serves as a trigger for the onset of autoimmune hepatitis in genetically susceptible patients). In contrast, the entire clinicopathologic spectrum of chronic hepatitis occurs in patients with chronic viral hepatitis B and C as well as in patients with chronic hepatitis D superimposed on chronic hepatitis B.

CHRONIC HEPATITIS B

The likelihood of chronicity after acute hepatitis B varies as a function of age. Infection at birth is associated with clinically silent acute infection but a 90% chance of chronic infection, while infection in young adulthood in immunocompetent persons is typically associated with clinically apparent acute hepatitis but a risk of chronicity of only approximately 1%. Most cases of chronic hepatitis B among adults, however, occur in patients who never had a recognized episode of clinically apparent acute viral hepatitis. The degree of liver injury (grade) in patients with chronic hepatitis B is variable, ranging from none in inactive carriers to mild to moderate to severe. Among adults with chronic hepatitis B, histologic features are of prognostic importance. In one long-term

TABLE 39-2

HISTOLOGIC GRADING AND STAGING IN CHRONIC HEPATITIS

HISTOLOGIC FEATURE	HISTOLOGIC ACTIVITY INDEX (HAI)[a]			METAVIR[b]	
		SEVERITY	SCORE	SEVERITY	SCORE
Necroinflammatory Activity (Grade)					
Perioportal necrosis, including piecemeal necrosis (PN) and/or bridging necrosis (BN)		None	0	None	0
		Mild	1	Mild	1
		Mild/Moderate	2	Moderate	2
		Moderate	3	Severe	3
		Severe	4		
				Bridging necrosis	Yes
					No
Intralobular necrosis	Confluent	—None	0	None or mild	0
		—Focal	1	Moderate	1
		—Zone 3 some	2	Severe	2
		—Zone 3 most	3		
		—Zone 3 + BN few	4		
		—Zone 3 + BN multiple	5		
		—Panacinar/multiacinar	6		
	Focal	—None	0		
		—≤1 Focus/10× field	1		
		—2–4 Foci/10× field	2		
		—5–10 Foci/10× field	3		
		—>10 Foci/10× field	4		
Portal inflammation		None	0		
		Mild	1		
		Moderate	2		
		Moderate/marked	3		
		Marked	4		
		Total	0–18		A0–A3[c]
Fibrosis (Stage)					
None			0		F0
Portal fibrosis—some			1		F1
Portal fibrosis—most			2		F1
Bridging fibrosis—few			3		F2
Bridging fibrosis—many			4		F3
Incomplete cirrhosis			5		F4
Cirrhosis			6		F4
		Total	6		4

[a]J Hepatol 22:696, 1995.
[b]Hepatology 24:289, 1996.
[c]Necroinflammatory grade: A0 = none; A1 = mild; A2 = moderate; A3 = severe.

study of patients with chronic hepatitis B, investigators found a 5-year survival rate of 97% for patients with mild chronic hepatitis, 86% for patients with moderate to severe chronic hepatitis, and only 55% for patients with chronic hepatitis and postnecrotic cirrhosis. The 15-year survival in these cohorts was 77, 66, and 40%, respectively. On the other hand, more recent observations do not allow us to be so sanguine about the prognosis in patients with mild chronic hepatitis; among such patients followed for 1–13 years, progression to more severe chronic hepatitis and cirrhosis has been observed in more than a quarter of cases.

More important to consider than histology alone in patients with chronic hepatitis B is the degree of hepatitis B virus (HBV) replication. As reviewed in Chap. 37, chronic HBV infection can occur in the presence or absence of serum hepatitis B e antigen (HBeAg); and generally, for both HBeAg-reactive and HBeAg-negative chronic hepatitis B, the level of HBV DNA correlates with the level of liver injury and risk of progression. In *HBeAg-reactive chronic hepatitis B*, two phases have been recognized based on the relative level of HBV replication. The relatively *replicative phase* is characterized by the presence in the serum of HBeAg and HBV DNA levels well in excess of 10^5–10^6 virions/mL, by the presence in the liver of detectable intrahepatocyte nucleocapsid antigens [primarily hepatitis B core antigen (HBcAg)], by high infectivity, and by accompanying liver injury. In contrast, the relatively *nonreplicative phase* is characterized by the absence of the conventional serum marker of HBV replication (HBeAg), the appearance of anti-HBe, levels of HBV DNA below a threshold of ~10^3 virions/mL, the absence of intrahepatocytic HBcAg, limited infectivity, and minimal liver injury. Those patients in the replicative phase tend to have more severe chronic hepatitis, while those in the nonreplicative phase tend to have minimal or mild chronic hepatitis or to be inactive hepatitis B carriers; however, distinctions in HBV replication and in histologic category do not always coincide. The likelihood in a patient with HBeAg-reactive chronic hepatitis B of converting spontaneously from relatively replicative to nonreplicative infection is approximately 10–15% per year. In patients with HBeAg-reactive chronic HBV infection, especially when acquired at birth or in early childhood, as recognized commonly in Asian countries, a dichotomy is common between very high levels of HBV replication and negligible levels of liver injury. Yet despite the relatively immediate, apparently benign nature of liver disease for many decades in this population, patients with childhood-acquired HBV infection are the ones at ultimately increased risk later in life of cirrhosis and hepatocellular carcinoma (HCC). A discussion of the pathogenesis of liver injury in patients with chronic hepatitis B appears in Chap. 37.

HBeAg-negative chronic hepatitis B, i.e., chronic HBV infection with active virus replication, readily detectable HBV DNA but without HBeAg (anti-HBe-reactive), is more common than HBeAg-reactive chronic hepatitis B in Mediterranean and European countries and in Asia (and, correspondingly, in HBV genotypes other than A). Compared to patients with HBeAg-reactive chronic hepatitis B, patients with HBeAg-negative chronic hepatitis B have levels of HBV DNA that are several orders of magnitude lower (no more than 10^5–10^6 virions/mL) than those observed in the HBeAg-reactive subset. Most such cases represent precore or core-promoter mutations acquired late in the natural history of the disease (mostly early-life onset; age range 40–55 years, older than that for HBeAg-reactive chronic hepatitis B); these mutations prevent translation of HBeAg from the precore component of the HBV genome (precore mutants) or are characterized by down-regulated transcription of precore mRNA (core-promoter mutants; Chap. 37). Although their levels of HBV DNA tend to be lower than among patients with HBeAg-reactive chronic hepatitis B, patients with HBeAg-negative chronic hepatitis B can have progressive liver injury (complicated by cirrhosis and HCC) and experience episodic reactivation of liver disease reflected in fluctuating levels of aminotransferase activity ("flares"). The biochemical and histologic activity of HBeAg-negative disease tends to correlate closely with levels of HBV replication, unlike the case mentioned above of Asian patients with HBeAg-reactive chronic hepatitis B during the early decades of their HBV infection. An important point worth reiterating is the observation that the level of HBV replication is the most important risk factor for the ultimate development of cirrhosis and HCC in both HBeAg-reactive and HBeAg-negative patients. Although levels of HBV DNA are lower and more readily suppressed to undetectable levels in HBeAg-negative (compared to HBeAg-reactive) chronic hepatitis B, achieving sustained responses that permit discontinuation of antiviral therapy is less likely in HBeAg-negative patients (see below). Inactive carriers are patients with circulating hepatitis B surface antigen (HBsAg), normal serum aminotransferase levels, undetectable HBeAg, and levels of HBV DNA that are either undetectable or present at levels ≤10^3 virions/mL. This serologic profile can occur not only in inactive carriers but also in patients with HBeAg-negative chronic hepatitis B during periods of relative inactivity; distinguishing between the two requires sequential biochemical and virologic monitoring over many months.

The spectrum of *clinical features* of chronic hepatitis B is broad, ranging from asymptomatic infection to debilitating disease or even end-stage, fatal hepatic failure. As noted above, the onset of the disease tends to be insidious in most patients, with the exception of the very few in whom chronic disease follows failure of resolution of clinically apparent acute hepatitis B. The clinical and laboratory features associated with progression from acute to chronic hepatitis B are discussed in Chap. 37.

Fatigue is a common symptom, and persistent or intermittent *jaundice* is a common feature in severe or advanced cases. Intermittent deepening of jaundice and recurrence of malaise and anorexia, as well as worsening fatigue, are reminiscent of acute hepatitis; such exacerbations may occur spontaneously, often coinciding with evidence of virologic reactivation; may lead to progressive liver injury; and, when superimposed on well-established cirrhosis, may cause hepatic decompensation. Complications of cirrhosis occur in end-stage chronic hepatitis and include ascites, edema, bleeding gastroesophageal varices, hepatic encephalopathy, coagulopathy, or hypersplenism. Occasionally these complications bring the patient to initial clinical attention. Extrahepatic complications of chronic hepatitis B, similar to those seen during the prodromal phase of acute hepatitis B, are associated with deposition of circulating hepatitis B antigen–antibody immune complexes (Chap. 37). These include arthralgias and arthritis, which are common, and the more rare purpuric cutaneous lesions (leukocytoclastic vasculitis), immune-complex glomerulonephritis, and generalized vasculitis (polyarteritis nodosa).

Laboratory features of chronic hepatitis B do not distinguish adequately between histologically mild and severe hepatitis. Aminotransferase elevations tend to be modest for chronic hepatitis B but may fluctuate in the range of 100–1000 units. As is true for acute viral hepatitis B, alanine aminotransferase (ALT) tends to be more elevated than aspartate aminotransferase (AST); however, once cirrhosis is established, AST tends to exceed ALT. Levels of alkaline phosphatase activity tend to be normal or only marginally elevated. In severe cases, moderate elevations in serum bilirubin [51.3–171 μmol/L (3–10 mg/dL)] occur. Hypoalbuminemia and prolongation of the prothrombin time occur in severe or end-stage cases. Hyperglobulinemia and detectable circulating autoantibodies are distinctly absent in chronic hepatitis B (in contrast to autoimmune hepatitis). Viral markers of chronic HBV infection are discussed in Chap. 37.

R̠x Treatment:
CHRONIC HEPATITIS B

Although progression to cirrhosis is more likely in severe than in mild or moderate chronic hepatitis B, all forms of chronic hepatitis B can be progressive, and progression occurs primarily in patients with active HBV replication. Moreover, in populations of patients with chronic hepatitis B who are at risk for HCC, the risk is highest for those with continued, high-level HBV replication. Therefore, management of chronic hepatitis B is directed at suppressing the level of virus replication. To date, five drugs have been approved for treatment of chronic hepatitis B: injectable interferon (INF) α; pegylated interferon [long-acting IFN bound to polyethylene glycol (PEG), known as *PEG IFN*]; and the oral agents lamivudine, adefovir dipivoxil, and entecavir. Several other drugs, including emtricitabine, tenofovir, telbivudine, pradefovir, and clevudine, are in the process of efficacy testing in clinical trials.

Antiviral therapy for hepatitis B has evolved rapidly since the mid-1990s, as has the sensitivity of tests for HBV DNA. When IFN and lamivudine were evaluated in clinical trials, HBV DNA was measured by insensitive hybridization assays with detection thresholds of 10^5–10^6 virions/mL; when adefovir, entecavir, and PEG IFN were studied in clinical trials, HBV DNA was measured by sensitive amplification assays (polymerase chain reaction [PCR]) with detection thresholds of 10^2–10^3 virions/mL. Recognition of these distinctions is helpful when comparing results of clinical trials that established the efficacy of these therapies (reviewed below in chronological order of publication of these efficacy trials).

INTERFERON IFN-α was the first approved therapy for chronic hepatitis B. For immunocompetent adults with HBeAg-reactive chronic hepatitis B (who tend to have high-level HBV DNA [>10^5–10^6 virions/mL] and histologic evidence of chronic hepatitis on liver biopsy), a 16-week course of IFN given subcutaneously at a daily dose of 5 million units, or three times a week at a dose of 10 million units, results in a loss of HBeAg and hybridization-detectable HBV DNA (i.e., a reduction to levels below 10^5–10^6 virions/mL) in ~30% of patients, with a concomitant improvement in liver histology. Seroconversion from HBeAg to anti-HBe occurs in approximately 20%, and, in early trials, approximately 8% lost HBsAg. Successful INF therapy and seroconversion are often accompanied by an acute hepatitis-like elevation in aminotransferase activity, which has been postulated to result from enhanced cytolytic T cell clearance of HBV-infected hepatocytes. Relapse after successful therapy is rare (1 or 2%). The likelihood of responding to IFN is higher in patients with lower levels of HBV DNA and substantial elevations of ALT. Although children can respond as well as adults, IFN therapy has not been effective in very young children infected at birth. Similarly, IFN therapy has not been effective in immunosuppressed persons, Asian patients with minimal-to-mild ALT elevations, or patients with decompensated chronic hepatitis B (in whom such therapy can actually be detrimental, sometimes precipitating decompensation, often associated with severe adverse effects). Among patients with HBeAg loss during therapy, long-term follow-up has demonstrated that 80% experience eventual loss of HBsAg, i.e., all serologic markers of infection, and normalization of ALT over a 9-year posttreatment period. In addition, improved long-term and complication-free survival as well as a reduction in the frequency of HCC have been documented among interferon responders, supporting the conclusion that successful interferon therapy improves the natural history of chronic hepatitis B.

Retreatment of IFN nonresponders with another course of IFN may enhance response rates somewhat; currently, however, most would opt to address IFN nonresponders by offering them one of the newer, oral therapies.

Initial trials of brief-duration IFN therapy in patients with *HBeAg-negative chronic hepatitis B* were disappointing, suppressing HBV replication transiently during therapy but almost never resulting in sustained antiviral responses. In subsequent IFN trials among patients with HBeAg-negative chronic hepatitis B, however, more protracted courses, lasting up to a year and a half, have been reported to result in sustained remissions, with suppressed HBV DNA and aminotransferase activity, in ~20%.

Complications of IFN therapy include systemic "flu-like" symptoms; marrow suppression; emotional lability (irritability commonly, depression/anxiety less frequently); autoimmune reactions (especially autoimmune thyroiditis); and miscellaneous side effects such as alopecia, rashes, diarrhea, and numbness and tingling of the extremities. With the possible exception of autoimmune thyroiditis, all these side effects are reversible upon dose lowering or cessation of therapy.

Whether or not IFN remains competitive with the newer generation of antivirals, it did represent the first successful antiviral approach, and it set the standard against which subsequent drugs are measured—the achievement of durable virologic, serologic, biochemical, and histologic responses; consolidation of virologic and biochemical benefit in the ensuing years after therapy; and improvement in the natural history of chronic hepatitis B. For all practical purposes, standard IFN has been supplanted by long-acting PEG IFN (see later).

LAMIVUDINE The first of the nucleoside analogues to be approved, the dideoxynucleoside lamivudine, inhibits reverse transcriptase activity of both HIV and HBV and is a potent and effective agent for patients with chronic hepatitis B. In clinical trials among patients with HBeAg-reactive chronic hepatitis B, lamivudine therapy at daily doses of 100 mg for 48–52 weeks suppressed HBV DNA by a median of approximately 5.5 $\log_{10}$ copies/mL and to undetectable levels, as measured by PCR amplification assays, in approximately 40% of patients. Therapy was associated with HBeAg loss in 32–33%; HBeAg seroconversion (i.e., conversion from HBeAg-reactive to anti-HBe-reactive) in 16–21%; normalization of ALT in 40%–75%; improvement in histology in 50%–60%; retardation in fibrosis in 20–30%; and prevention of progression to cirrhosis. HBeAg responses can occur even in subgroups who are resistant to IFN (e.g., those with high-level HBV DNA) or who failed in the past to respond to it. As is true for IFN therapy of chronic hepatitis B, patients with near-normal ALT activity tend not to experience HBeAg responses (despite suppression of HBV DNA), and those with ALT levels exceeding five times the upper limit of normal can expect 1-year HBeAg seroconversion rates of 50–60%. Generally, HBeAg seroconversions are confined to patients who achieve suppression of HBV DNA to $<10^4$ genomes/mL. Among patients who undergo HBeAg responses during a year-long course of therapy and in whom the response is sustained for 4–6 months after cessation of therapy, the response is durable thereafter in the vast majority, >80%; therefore, the achievement of an HBeAg response represents a viable stopping point in therapy. Reduced durability has been reported in some Asian experiences; however, in most western and Asian patient study populations, long-term durability of HBeAg responses is the rule, which, at least in Western patients, is accompanied by a posttreatment HBsAg seroconversion rate comparable to that seen after IFN-induced HBeAg responses. If HBeAg is unaffected by lamivudine therapy, the current approach is to continue therapy until an HBeAg response occurs, but long-term therapy may be required to suppress HBV replication

and, in turn, limit liver injury; HBeAg seroconversions can increase to a level of 50% after 5 years of therapy. Histologic improvement continues to accrue with therapy beyond the first year; after a cumulative course of 3 years of lamivudine therapy, necroinflammatory activity is reduced in the majority of patients, and even cirrhosis has been shown to regress to precirrhotic stages.

Losses of HBsAg have been few during the first year of lamivudine therapy, and this observation had been cited as an advantage of IFN over lamivudine; however, in head-to-head comparisons between standard IFN and lamivudine monotherapy, HBsAg losses were rare in both groups. Trials in which lamivudine and interferon were administered in combination failed to show a benefit of combination therapy over lamivudine monotherapy for either treatment-naïve patients or prior interferon nonresponders.

In patients with *HBeAg-negative chronic hepatitis B*, i.e., in those with precore and core-promoter HBV mutations, 1 year of lamivudine therapy results in HBV DNA suppression and normalization of ALT in three-quarters of patients and in histologic improvement in approximately two-thirds. Therapy has been shown to suppress HBV DNA by approximately 4.5 $\log_{10}$ copies/mL (baseline HBV DNA levels are lower than in patients with HBeAg-reactive hepatitis B) and to undetectable levels in 70%, as measured by sensitive PCR amplification assays. Lacking HBeAg at the outset, patients with HBeAg-negative chronic hepatitis B cannot achieve an HBeAg response—a stopping point in HBeAg-reactive patients; invariably, when therapy is discontinued, reactivation is the rule. Therefore, these patients require long-term therapy; with successive years, the proportion with suppressed HBV DNA and normal ALT increases.

Clinical and laboratory side effects of lamivudine are negligible, indistinguishable from those observed in placebo recipients. During lamivudine therapy, transient ALT elevations, resembling those seen during IFN therapy and during spontaneous HBeAg-to-anti-HBe seroconversions, occur in a quarter of patients. These ALT elevations may result from restored cytolytic T cell activation permitted by suppression of HBV replication. Similar ALT elevations, however, occur at an identical frequency in placebo recipients, but ALT elevations associated with HBeAg seroconversion are confined to lamivudine-treated patients. When therapy is stopped after a year of therapy, two- to threefold ALT elevations occur in 20–30% of lamivudine-treated patients, representing renewed liver-cell injury as HBV replication returns. Although these posttreatment flares are almost always transient and mild, rare severe exacerbations, especially in cirrhotic patients, have been observed, mandating close and careful clinical and virologic monitoring after discontinuation of treatment. Many authorities caution against discontinuing therapy in patients with cirrhosis, in whom posttreatment flares could pre-cipitate decompensation.

Long-term monotherapy with lamivudine is associated with methionine-to-valine (M204V) or methionine-to-isoleucine (M204I) mutations, primarily at amino acid 204 in the tyrosine-methionine-aspartate-aspartate (YMDD) motif of HBV DNA polymerase, analogous to mutations that occur in HIV-infected patients treated with this drug. During a year of therapy, YMDD mutations occur in 15–30% of patients; the frequency increases with each year of therapy, reaching 70% at year 5. Although resis-tance to lamivudine may not lead to immediate loss of antiviral effect, patients with YMDD mutants ultimately experience degradation of clinical, biochemical, and histo-logic responses. Therefore, if treatment is begun with lamivudine monotherapy, the emergence of lamivudine resistance, reflected clinically by a breakthrough from sup-pressed levels of HBV DNA and ALT, is managed by adding another antiviral to which YMDD variants are sensitive (e.g., adefovir; see later).

Currently, although lamivudine is very safe and still used widely in other parts of the world, in the United States and Europe lamivudine has been eclipsed by more potent antivirals that have superior resistance profiles (see later). Still, as the first successful oral antiviral agent for use in hepatitis B, lamivudine has pro-vided proof of the concept that polymerase inhibitors can achieve both virologic, serologic, biochemical, and histologic benefit. In addition, lamivudine has been shown to be effective in the treatment of patients with decompensated hepatitis B (for whom IFN is contraindi-cated), in some of whom decompensation can be reversed. Moreover, among patients with cirrhosis or advanced fibrosis, lamivudine has been shown to be effective in reducing the risk of progression to hepatic decompensation and, marginally, the risk of HCC.

Because lamivudine monotherapy can result univer-sally in the rapid emergence of YMDD variants in per-sons with HIV infection, patients with chronic hepatitis B should be tested for anti-HIV prior to therapy; if HIV infection is identified, lamivudine monotherapy at the HBV daily dose of 100 mg is contraindicated. These patients should be treated with triple-drug antiretrovi-ral therapy, including a lamivudine daily dose of 6 mg. The safety of lamivudine during pregnancy has not been established; however, the drug is not teratogenic in rodents and has been used safely in pregnant women with HIV infection and with HBV infection. Limited data even suggest that administration of lamivudine during the last month of pregnancy to mothers with high-level hepatitis B viremia can reduce the likelihood of perina-tal transmission of hepatitis B.

ADEFOVIR DIPIVOXIL The acyclic nucleotide ana-logue adefovir dipivoxil, the prodrug of adevovir, is a potent antiviral that, at an oral daily dose of 10 mg, reduces HBV DNA by approximately 3.5–4 $\log_{10}$ copies/mL and is equally effective in treatment-naïve patients and IFN nonresponders. In HBeAg-reactive chronic hepatitis B, a 48-week course of adefovir dipivoxil was shown to achieve histologic improvement (and reduce the progression of fibrosis) and normalization of ALT in half of patients, HBeAg seroconversion in 12%, HBeAg loss in 23%, and suppression to an undetectable level of HBV DNA in 20–30%, as measured by PCR. Similar to IFN and lamivudine, adefovir dipivoxil is more likely to achieve an HBeAg response in patients with high base-line ALT; for example, among adefovir-treated patients with ALT level >5 times the upper limit of normal, HBeAg seroconversions occurred in 25%. The durability of ade-fovir-induced HBeAg responses is high (91% in one study); therefore, HBeAg response can be relied upon as a stopping point for adefovir therapy. Although data on the impact of additional therapy beyond one year are limited, biochemical, serologic, and virologic outcomes improve progressively as therapy is continued.

In patients with *HBeAg-negative chronic hepatitis B*, a 48-week course of 10 mg/d of adefovir dipivoxil resulted in histologic improvement in two-thirds, nor-malization of ALT in three-quarters, and suppression of HBV DNA to PCR-undetectable levels in half. As was true for lamivudine, because HBeAg responses—a potential stopping point—cannot be achieved in this group, reac-tivation is the rule when adefovir therapy is discontin-ued, and indefinite, long-term therapy is required. Treat-ment beyond the first year consolidates the gain of the first year; after 5 years of therapy, improvement in hepatic inflammation and regression of fibrosis was observed in three-quarters of patients, ALT was normal in 70%, and HBV DNA was undetectable in almost 70%.

Adefovir contains a flexible acyclic linker instead of the L-nucleoside ring of lamivudine, avoiding steric hindrance by mutated amino acids. In addition, the molecular struc-ture of phosphorylated adefovir is very similar to that of its natural substrate; therefore mutations to adefovir would also affect binding of the natural substrate, dATP. Hypothetically, these are among the reasons that resis-tance to adefovir dipivoxil is much less likely than resis-tance to lamivudine; no resistance was encountered in 1 year of clinical-trial therapy. In subsequent years, how-ever, adefovir resistance begins to emerge [asparagine to threonine at amino acid 236 (N236T) and alanine to valine or threonine at amino acid 181 (A181V/T) primarily], occur-ring in 2.5% after 2 years, but in 29% after 5 years of ther-apy. Among patients co-infected with HBV and HIV and who have normal CD4+ T cell counts, adefovir dipivoxil is effective in suppressing HBV dramatically (by 5 $\log_{10}$ in one study). Moreover, adefovir dipivoxil is effective in lamivudine-resistant, YMDD-mutant HBV and can be used when such lamivudine-induced variants emerge. When lamivudine resistance occurs, authorities have debated whether to add adefovir or switch to adefovir; however, adding adefovir, i.e., maintaining lamivudine to preempt the emergence of adefovir resistance, appears to be the favored approach. In this vein, almost invariably, patients with adefovir-mutant HBV respond to lamivudine. When, in the past, adefovir had been evaluated as therapy for HIV infection, doses of 60–120 mg were required to suppress HIV, and at these doses the drug was nephrotoxic. Even at 30 mg/d, creatinine elevations of 44 μmol/L (0.5 mg/dL) occur in 10% of patients; however, at the HBV-effective dose of 10 mg, such elevations of creatinine are rarely encountered. If any nephrotoxicity does occur, it rarely appears before 6–8 months of therapy. Although renal tubular injury is a rare potential side effect, and although creatinine monitoring is recommended during treatment, the therapeutic index of adefovir dipivoxil is high, and the nephrotoxicity observed in clinical trials at higher doses was reversible. For patients with underlying renal disease, adefovir dipivoxil dose reductions are recommended: administration reduced to every 48 h for creatinine clearances of 20–49 mL/min, to every 72 h for creatinine clearances of 10–19 mL/min, and once a week, following dialysis, for patients undergoing hemodialysis. Adefovir dipivoxil is very well tolerated, and ALT elevations during and after withdrawal of therapy are similar to those observed and described above in clinical trials of lamivudine. An advantage of adefovir is its relatively favorable resistance profile; however, it is not as potent as the other approved oral agents, it does not suppress HBV DNA as rapidly or as uniformly as the others, and a small proportion of patients have no demonstrable response to the drug ("primary nonresponders").

PEGYLATED INTERFERON After long-acting PEG IFN was shown to be effective in the treatment of hepatitis C (see below), this more convenient drug was evaluated in the treatment of chronic hepatitis B. Preliminary trials documented that once-a-week PEG IFN was more effective than the more frequently administered, standard IFN, following which several large-scale trials were conducted among patients with HBeAg-reactive and HBeAg-negative chronic hepatitis B.

In HBeAg-reactive chronic hepatitis B, two large-scale studies were done, one with PEG IFN-α2b (100 μg weekly for 32 weeks, then 50 μg weekly for another 20 weeks for a total of 52 weeks, with a comparison arm of combination PEG IFN with oral lamivudine) in 307 subjects; the other involved PEG IFN-α2a (180 μg weekly for 48 weeks) in 814 primarily Asian patients confined to those with ALT ≥2 × the upper limit of normal, with comparison arms of lamivudine monotherapy and combination PEG IFN plus lamivudine. At the end of therapy (48–52 weeks) in the PEG IFN monotherapy arms, HBeAg loss occurred in approximately 30%, HBeAg seroconversion in 22–27%,

undetectable HBV DNA (<400 copies/mL by PCR) in 10–25%, normal ALT in 34–39%, and a mean reduction in HBV DNA of 2 $\log_{10}$ copies/mL (PEG IFN-α2b) to 4.5 $\log_{10}$ copies/mL (PEG IFN-α2a). Six months after completing PEG IFN monotherapy in these trials, HBeAg losses were present in approximately 35%, HBeAg seroconversion in approximately 30%, undetectable HBV DNA in 7–14%, normal ALT in 32–41%, and a mean reduction in HBV DNA of 2–2.4 $\log_{10}$ copies/mL. Although the combination of PEG IFN and lamivudine was superior at the end of therapy in one or more serologic, virologic, or biochemical outcomes, neither the combination arm (in both studies) nor the lamivudine monotherapy arm (in the PEG IFN-α2a trial) demonstrated any benefit compared to the PEG IFN monotherapy arms 6 months after therapy. Moreover, HBsAg seroconversion occurred in 3%–7% of PEG IFN recipients (with or without lamivudine); some of these seroconversions were identified by the end of therapy, but many were identified during the posttreatment follow-up period. The likelihood of HBeAg loss in PEG IFN–treated HBeAg-reactive patients is associated with HBV genotype A > B > C > D.

Based on these results, some authorities concluded that PEG IFN monotherapy should be the first-line therapy of choice in HBeAg-reactive chronic hepatitis B; however, this conclusion has been challenged. Although a finite, 1-year course of PEG IFN results in a higher rate of sustained response (6 months after treatment) than is achieved with oral nucleoside/nucleotide analogue therapy, the comparison is confounded by the fact that oral agents are not discontinued at the end of a year. Instead, taken orally and free of side effects, therapy with oral agents is extended indefinitely or until after the occurrence of an HBeAg response. The rate of HBeAg responses after 2 years of oral-agent therapy is at least as high as, if not higher than, that achieved with PEG IFN after 1 year; favoring oral agents is the absence of injections and difficult-to-tolerate side effects as well as lower direct and indirect medical costs and inconvenience. The association of HBsAg responses with PEG IFN therapy occurs in such a small proportion of patients that subjecting everyone to PEG IFN for the marginal gain of HBsAg responses during or immediately after therapy in such a very small minority is questionable. Moreover, HBsAg responses occur in a comparable proportion of nucleoside/nucleotide-treated patients in the years after therapy. Of course, resistance is not an issue during PEG IFN therapy, but the risk of resistance is much lower with new agents (none recorded after 2 years in previously treatment-naïve entecavir-treated patients; see later). Finally, the level of HBV DNA inhibition that can be achieved with the newer agents, and even with lamivudine, exceeds that which can be achieved with PEG IFN, in some cases by several orders of magnitude.

In HBeAg-negative chronic hepatitis B, a trial of PEG IFN-α2a (180 μg weekly for 48 weeks versus comparison arms of lamivudine monotherapy and of combination therapy) in 564 patients showed that PEG IFN monotherapy resulted at the end of therapy in suppression of HBV DNA by a mean of 4.1 $\log_{10}$ copies/mL, undetectable HBV DNA (<400 copies/mL by PCR) in 63%, and normal ALT in 38%. Although lamivudine monotherapy and combination lamivudine–PEG IFN therapy were both superior to PEG IFN at the end of therapy, no advantage of lamivudine monotherapy or combination therapy was apparent over PEG IFN monotherapy 6 months after therapy—suppression of HBV DNA by a mean of 2.3 $\log_{10}$ copies/mL, undetectable HBV DNA in 19%, and normal ALT in 59%. As was the case for standard IFN therapy in HBeAg-negative patients, after longer periods of post-PEG IFN treatment observation, sustained response rates fell substantially, raising questions about the value of a finite period of PEG IFN in these patients.

ENTECAVIR Entecavir, an oral guanosine analogue polymerase inhibitor, appears to be the most potent of the HBV antivirals and is just as well tolerated as lamivudine. In a 709-subject clinical trial among HBeAg-reactive patients, oral entecavir, 0.5 mg daily, was compared to lamivudine, 100 mg daily. At 48 weeks, entecavir was superior to lamivudine in suppression of HBV DNA, mean 6.9 versus 5.5 $\log_{10}$ copies/mL and in percent with undetectable HBV DNA (<6 copies/mL by PCR), 67% versus 36%; histologic improvement (≥2-point improvement in necroinflammatory HAI score), 72% versus 62%; and normal ALT (68% versus 60%). The two treatments were indistinguishable in percent with HBeAg loss (22% versus 20%) and seroconversion (21% versus 18%). Among patients treated with entecavir for 96 weeks, HBV DNA was undetectable cumulatively in 80% (versus 39% for lamivudine), and HBeAg seroconversions had occurred in 31% (versus 26% for lamivudine). Similarly, in a 638-subject clinical trial among HBeAg-negative patients, at week 48, oral entecavir, 0.5 mg daily, was superior to lamivudine, 100 mg daily, in suppression of HBV DNA, mean 5.0 versus 4.5 $\log_{10}$ copies/mL and in percent with undetectable HBV DNA, 90% versus 72%; histologic improvement, 78% versus 71% and normal ALT, 68% versus 60%. No resistance mutations were encountered in previously treatment-naïve entecavir-treated patients during 96 weeks of therapy.

Entecavir is also effective against lamivudine-resistant HBV infection. In a trial of 286 lamivudine-resistant patients, entecavir, at a higher daily dose of 1.0 mg, was superior to lamivudine, as measured at week 48, in achieving suppression of HBV DNA (mean 5.1 versus 0.48 $\log_{10}$ copies/mL); undetectable HBV DNA, in 72% versus 19%; normal ALT, in 61% versus 15%; HBeAg loss, in 10% versus 3%; and HBeAg seroconversion, in 8% versus

3%. In this population of lamivudine-experienced patients, however, entecavir resistance did emerge in 7% at 48 weeks and in 9% at 96 weeks. Therefore, entecavir is not as attractive a choice as adefovir (or off-label tenofovir) for patients with lamivudine-resistant hepatitis B.

At the end of 2 years of entecavir therapy in clinical trials among HBeAg-reactive patients, HBsAg seroconversion were observed in 5% (≤2% during the first year). In addition, on-treatment and posttreatment ALT flares are relatively uncommon and relatively mild in entecavir-treated patients.

A comparison of the four antiviral therapies in current use appears in **Table 39-3**.

COMBINATION THERAPY Although the combination of lamivudine and PEG IFN suppresses HBV DNA more profoundly during therapy than does monotherapy with either drug alone (and is much less likely to be associated with lamivudine resistance), this combination used for a year is no better than a year of PEG IFN in achieving sustained responses. To date, combinations of oral nucleoside/nucleotide agents have not achieved an enhancement in virologic, serologic, or biochemical efficacy over that achieved by the more potent of the combined drugs given individually. On the other hand, combining agents that are not cross-resistant (e.g., lamivudine and adefovir) has the potential to reduce the risk or perhaps even to preempt entirely the emergence of drug resistance. In the future, the treatment paradigm is likely to shift from the current approach of sequential monotherapy to preemptive combination therapy; clinical trials are warranted.

TREATMENT RECOMMENDATIONS Several learned societies and groups of expert physicians have issued treatment recommendations for patients with chronic hepatitis B. Although the recommendations differ slightly, a consensus has emerged on most of the important points (**Table 39-4**). No treatment is recommended or available for inactive "nonreplicative" hepatitis B carriers (undetectable HBeAg with normal ALT and HBV DNA <10^4 copies/mL documented serially over time). In patients with detectable HBeAg and HBV DNA levels ≥10^5 copies/mL, treatment is recommended for those with elevated ALT levels (some authorities require the elevation to be at least twice the upper limit of normal). For those patients with normal ALT (or ≤2 × the upper limit of normal), in whom sustained responses are not likely and who would require multiyear therapy, antiviral therapy is not recommended currently. For patients with HBeAg-negative chronic hepatitis B, elevated ALT (≥2 × the upper limit of normal according to some authorities), and HBV DNA ≥10^4 (or 10^5 according to some authorities) copies/mL, antiviral therapy is recommended. If HBV DNA is <10^4–10^5 and ALT is normal (or near normal), treatment is not recommended; however, if HBV DNA is

TABLE 39-3

COMPARISON OF INTERFERON (PEG IFN), LAMIVUDINE, ADEFOVIR, AND ENTECAVIR THERAPY FOR CHRONIC HEPATITIS B[a]

FEATURE	PEG IFN[b]	LAMIVUDINE	ADEFOVIR	ENTECAVIR
Route of administration	Subcutaneous injection	Oral	Oral	Oral
Duration of therapy[c]	48–52 weeks	≥52 weeks	≥48 weeks	≥48 weeks
Tolerability	Poorly tolerated	Well tolerated	Well tolerated; creatinine monitoring recommended	Well tolerated
HBeAg loss 1 year	29–30%	20–33%	23%	22%
HBeAg seroconversion				
1 year Rx	18–20%	16–21%	12%	21%
>1 year Rx	NA	Up to 50% @ 5 years	43% @ 3 years[d]	31% @ 2 years
HBeAg seroconversion if ALT > 5× normal	Not reported	>50%	21%	Not reported
Log$_{10}$ HBV DNA reduction (mean copies/mL)				
HBeAg-reactive	4.5	5.5	Median 3.5–5	6.9
HBeAg-negative	4.1	4.4–4.7	Median 3.5–3.9	5.0
HBV DNA PCR negative (<6–400 copies/mL; <1000 copies/mL for adefovir) end of year 1				
HBeAg-reactive	10–25%	36–40%	12–21%	69% (80% @ 2 years)
HBeAg-negative	63%	39–73%	51% (79% @ 3 years)	90%
ALT normalization at end of year 1				
HBeAg-reactive	39%	41–75%	58% (81% @ year 3)	78%
HBeAg-negative	34–38%	62–79%	48% (69% @ year 3)	78%
HBsAg loss during year 1	0–7%	0–4%	0% (1–2% @ 2 years)	2% (5% @ 2 years)
HBsAg loss after therapy	3–7% after 6 months	23% after 2 years	Not reported	Not reported
Histologic improvement (≥2 point reduction in HAI) at year 1				
HBeAg-reactive	38% 6 months after	51–62%	53%	62%
HBeAg-negative	48% 6 months after	61–66%	64%	70%
Viral resistance	None	15–30% @ 1 year	None @ 1 year	None @ 2 years[e]
		70% @ 5 years	29% @ 5 years	
Durability of response 4–6 months after therapy[f]				
HBeAg-reactive	Limited data	70–80%	91%	82%
HBeAg-negative	36%	23–35%	Low	48%
Cost (U.S. $) for 1 year	~$18,000	~$2500	~$6500	~$8700[g]

[a]Generally, these comparisons are based on data on each drug tested individually versus placebo in registration clinical trials. With rare exception, these comparisons are not based on head-to-head testing of these drugs, hence relative advantages and disadvantages should be interpreted cautiously.

[b]Although standard interferon α administered daily or three times a week is approved as therapy for chronic hepatitis B, it has been supplanted by pegylated interferon (PEG IFN),which is administered once a week and is more effective. Standard interferon has no advantages over PEG IFN.

[c]Duration of therapy in clinical efficacy trials; use in clinical practice may vary.

[d]Because of a computer-generated randomization error that resulted in misallocation of drug versus placebo during the second year of clinical-trial treatment, the frequency of HBeAg serconversion beyond the first year is an estimate (Kaplan-Meier analysis) based on the small subset in whom adefovir was administered correctly.

[e]7% during a year of therapy (9% during two years) in lamivudine-resistant patients.

[f]In HBeAg-reactive patients, durability of HBeAg seroconversion; in HBeAg-negative patients, durability of virologic (HBV DNA undetectable by PCR) and biochemical (normal ALT) response.

[g]~17,400 for lamivudine-refractory patients.

Note: ALT, alanine aminotransferase; HAI, histologic activity index; HBeAg, hepatitis B e antigen; HBsAg, hepatitis B surface antigen; HBV, hepatitis B virus; NA, not applicable; Rx, therapy; PCR, polymerase chain reaction.

TABLE 39-4

RECOMMENDATIONS FOR TREATMENT OF CHRONIC HEPATITIS B

HBeAg STATUS	CLINICAL	HBV DNA (COPIES/mL)	ALT	RECOMMENDATION
HBeAg-reactive [a]		<10⁵	Normal (≤2 × ULN)[b]	No treatment; monitor
	Chronic hepatitis	≥10⁵	Normal (≤2 × ULN)[b, c]	No treatment; current treatment of limited benefit (Some suggest liver biopsy and treating if abnormal)
	Chronic hepatitis	≥10⁵	Elevated (>2 × ULN)[b]	Treat[d]
	Cirrhosis compensated	+ or –[e]	Normal or elevated	Treat[e] with oral agents,[f] not PEG IFN
	Cirrhosis decompensated	+ or –[e]	Normal or elevated	Treat[e] with oral agents,[g] not PEG IFN; refer for liver transplantation
HBeAg-negative [a]		<10⁴ or 10⁵ʰ	Normal (≤2 × ULN)[b]	Inactive carrier; treatment not necessary
	Chronic hepatitis	≥10⁴ or 10⁵ʰ	Normal	Consider liver biopsy; treat if biopsy abnormal
	Chronic hepatitis	≥10⁴ or 10⁵ʰ	Elevated (>2 × ULN)[b]	Treat[i]
	Cirrhosis compensated	+ or –	Elevated or normal	Treat with oral agents,[j] not PEG IFN (some authorites recommend either following or treating for HBV DNA <10⁴ copies/mL)
	Cirrhosis decompensated	+ or –	Elevated or normal	Treat with oral agents,[j] not PEG IFN (some authorities would follow without therapy for undetectable HBV DNA; refer for liver transplantation)

[a]Liver disease tends to be mild or inactive clinically; most such patients do not undergo liver biopsy.

[b]In some guidelines, ALT categories are normal and elevated; in others, ALT categories are ≤ or >2 times the upper limit of normal.

[c]Typical pattern in childhood-acquired infection, common in Asian populations.

[d]Any of the oral drugs (lamivudine, adefovir, entecavir) or PEG IFN can be used as first-line therapy (see text); although still used extensively in some parts of the world, lamivudine has been supplanted in some countries as first-line therapy because of its resistance profile. The oral agents, but not PEG IFN, should be used for interferon-refractory/intolerant and immunocompromised patients. PEG IFN is administered weekly by subcutaneous injection for a year; the oral agents are administered daily for at least a year and continued indefinitely or until at least 6 months after HBeAg seroconversion.

[e]Treating or monitoring without therapy are options for patients with HBV DNA <10⁴ or <10⁵ copies/mL.

[f]Some authorities would observe without treatment if HBV DNA is undetectable (<10⁴ copies/mL), while others would treat regardless of the HBV DNA status. Lamivudine monotherapy is not an attractive choice because of its resistance profile.

[g]Some authorities recommend treating regardless of HBV DNA status, while others suggest referring for liver transplantation, without treatment, for those with undetectable HBV DNA (<10⁵ copies/mL). Lamivudine is a less attractive choice because of its resistance profile. Because the emergence of resistance can lead to loss of antiviral benefit and further deterioration in decompensated cirrhosis, some authorities recommend combination therapy (e.g., lamivudine or entecavir plus adefovir) for patients with decompensated cirrhosis.

[h]Some authorities rely on a cutoff of 10⁴ copies/mL, while others choose 10⁵ copies/mL.

[i]Because HBeAg seroconversion is not an option, the goal of therapy is to suppress HBV DNA and maintain a normal ALT. Although any of the oral agents or PEG IFN can be used as first-line therapy, lamivudine is less favored because of its resistance profile and the need, in the vast majority of cases, for long-term therapy. PEG IFN is administered by subcutaneous injection weekly for a year (caution is warranted in relying on a 6-month posttreatment interval to define a sustained response; the majority of such responses are lost thereafter). Adefovir and entecavir are administered daily, usually indefinitely or, until, as occurs very rarely, virologic and biochemical responses are accompanied by an HBsAg seroconversion.

[j]Low-resistance regimen favored (i.e., adefovir or entecavir, not lamivudine) indefinitely.

Note: ALT, alanine aminotransferase; HBeAg, hepatitis B e antigen; HBsAg, hepatitis B surface antigen; HBV, hepatitis B virus; ULN, upper limits of normal; PEG IFN, pegylated interferon.

≥10⁴ copies/mL but ALT is normal or near normal, some would recommend considering liver biopsy and basing a decision to treat on the presence of substantial liver injury.

For patients with compensated cirrhosis, because antiviral therapy has been shown to retard clinical progression, many authorities would choose to treat regardless of HBeAg status, HBV DNA level and ALT; however, some authorities favor monitoring without therapy for those with HBV DNA levels <10⁴ copies/mL. For patients with decompensated cirrhosis, treatment is recommended by some authorities regardless of serologic, virologic, and biochemical status; however, other experts do not recommend therapy if HBV DNA is undetectable or low (<10⁵ copies/mL). At the same time, patients with decompensated cirrhosis should be evaluated as candidates for liver transplantation.

Among the five available drugs for hepatitis B, PEG IFN has supplanted standard IFN. Because entecavir has been proved superior to lamivudine in clinical trials, entecavir has supplanted lamivudine in some countries.

PEG IFN, lamivudine, adefovir, and entecavir can each be used as first-line therapy (Table 39-3). PEG IFN requires finite-duration therapy, achieves the highest rate of HBeAg responses after a year of therapy, and does not support viral mutations, but it requires subcutaneous injections and is associated with inconvenience and intolerability. Lamivudine, adefovir, and entecavir require long-term therapy in most patients, and when used alone, lamivudine fosters the emergence of viral mutations, adefovir much less so, and entecavir rarely at all, except in lamivudine-experienced patients. These oral agents do not require injections, are very well tolerated, lead to improved histology in 50–90% of patients, for the most part suppress HBV DNA more profoundly than does PEG IFN, and are effective even in patients who fail to respond to IFN-based therapy. Although these oral agents are less likely to result in HBeAg responses during the first year of therapy, as compared to PEG IFN, treatment with oral agents tends to be extended beyond the first year and, by the end of the second year, yields HBeAg responses (and even HBsAg responses) comparable in frequency to those achieved after 1 year of PEG IFN (and without the associated side effects). Although adefovir is safe, creatinine monitoring is recommended. Substantial experience with lamivudine during pregnancy (see earlier) has identified no teratogenicity. Standard IFN does not appear to cause congenital anomalies, and data on the safety of PEG IFN during pregnancy are not available. Adefovir during pregnancy has not been associated with birth defects; however, there may be an increased risk of spontaneous abortion. Data on the safety of entecavir during pregnancy have not been published. In general, except perhaps for lamivudine, and until additional data become available, the other antivirals for hepatitis B should be avoided or used with extreme caution during pregnancy.

As noted above, some physicians prefer to begin with PEG IFN, while other physicians and patients prefer oral agents as first-line therapy. For patients with decompensated cirrhosis, the emergence of resistance can result in further deterioration and loss of antiviral effectiveness. Therefore, in this patient subset, the threshold for relying on therapy with a very favorable resistance profile (e.g., entecavir) or on combination therapy (e.g., lamivudine or entecavir along with adefovir or the yet-to-be-approved tenofovir) is low. PEG IFN should not be used in patients with compensated or decompensated cirrhosis.

For patients with end-stage chronic hepatitis B who undergo liver transplantation, reinfection of the new liver is almost universal in the absence of antiviral therapy. The majority of patients become high-level viremic carriers with minimal liver injury. Before the availability of antiviral therapy, an unpredictable proportion experienced severe hepatitis B–related liver injury, sometimes a fulminant-like hepatitis, sometimes a rapid recapitulation of the original severe chronic hepatitis B (Chap. 44). Currently, however, prevention of recurrent hepatitis B after liver transplantation has been achieved definitively by combining hepatitis B immune globulin with one of the oral nucleoside or nucleotide analogues (lamivudine, adefovir, or entecavir) (Chap. 44).

Patients with HBV-HIV co-infection can have progressive HBV-associated liver disease and, occasionally, a severe exacerbation of hepatitis B resulting from immunologic reconstitution following highly active antiretroviral therapy. Lamivudine should never be used as monotherapy in patients with HBV-HIV infection, because HIV resistance emerges rapidly to both viruses. Adefovir and entecavir have been used successfully to treat chronic hepatitis B in HBV-HIV co-infected patients. Tenofovir and the combination of tenofovir and emtricitabine in one pill are approved therapies for HIV and represent excellent choices for treating HBV infection in HBV-HIV co-infected patients.

Patients with chronic hepatitis B who undergo cytotoxic chemotherapy for treatment of malignancies experience enhanced HBV replication and viral expression on hepatocyte membranes during chemotherapy coupled with suppression of cellular immunity. When chemotherapy is withdrawn, such patients are at risk for reactivation of hepatitis B, often severe and occasionally fatal. Such rebound reactivation represents restoration of cytolytic T-cell function against a target organ enriched in HBV expression. Preemptive treatment with lamivudine prior to the initiation of chemotherapy has been shown to reduce the risk of such reactivation. In all likelihood, the newer, more potent oral antiviral agents will work as well and with a lower risk of antiviral drug resistance. The optimal duration of antiviral therapy after completion of chemotherapy is not known, but some authorities have suggested 3 months.

NOVEL ANTIVIRALS AND STRATEGIES In addition to the five approved antiviral drugs for hepatitis B, several others are being evaluated in clinical trials, as listed in Table 39-5. Telbivudine, a cytosine analogue, appears to be similar in efficacy to entecavir but slightly less potent in suppressing HBV DNA, and it is associated with low-level resistance (M204I, not M204V mutations). This drug was

TABLE 39-5

NEW ANTIVIRAL DRUGS BEING DEVELOPED FOR THE TREATMENT OF CHRONIC HEPATITIS B	
Telbivudine[a]	Emtricitabine (FTC)
Tenofovir[b]	Clevudine (L-MFAU)

[a]Approved in October 2006.
[b]Active against lamivudine-associated YMDD-mutant HBV. (YMDD, tyrosine-methionine-aspartate-aspartate.)

approved in October 2006. Resistance mutations after 2 years of treatment occur in ~20%. Tenofovir, a nucleotide analogue, is similar to adefovir but more potent in suppressing HBV DNA and inducing HBeAg responses; it is highly active against both wild-type and lamivudine-resistant HBV and active in patients with primary nonresponse to adefovir. Its safety and resistance profile are very favorable as well; in all likelihood, it will supplant adefovir once comparisons in clinical trials are complete. Emtricitabine is a fluorinated cytosine analogue very similar to lamivudine in structure, efficacy, and resistance profile. A combination of emtricitabine and tenofovir is approved for the treatment of HIV infection and is an appealing combination therapy for hepatitis B; however, neither emtricitabine nor the combination are approved yet for hepatitis B. Clevudine is a pyrimidine nucleoside analogue whose potency in the woodchuck model of hepatitis B is higher than that of any other antiviral agent; however, in human trials, maximal HBV DNA suppression has been 5 $\log_{10}$ copies/mL; after clevudine therapy, HBV DNA is much slower to rebound than after withdrawal of other agents. Because direct-acting antivirals have been so successful in the management of chronic hepatitis B, more unconventional approaches—e.g., immunologic or genetic manipulation—are not likely to be competitive. Finally, initial emphasis in the development of antiviral therapy for hepatitis B was placed on monotherapy; however, in the future, with or without additive or synergistic efficacy, combination therapy regimens that prevent resistance are likely to become the norm.

CHRONIC HEPATITIS D (DELTA HEPATITIS)

Chronic hepatitis D (HDV) may follow acute co-infection with HBV but at a rate no higher than the rate of chronicity of acute hepatitis B. That is, although HDV co-infection can increase the severity of acute hepatitis B, HDV does not increase the likelihood of progression to chronic hepatitis B. When, however, HDV superinfection occurs in a person who is already chronically infected with HBV, long-term HDV infection is the rule and a worsening of the liver disease the expected consequence. Except for severity, chronic hepatitis B plus D has similar clinical and laboratory features to those seen in chronic hepatitis B alone. Relatively severe chronic hepatitis, with or without cirrhosis, is the rule, and mild chronic hepatitis is the exception. Occasionally, mild hepatitis or even, rarely, inactive carriage occurs in patients with chronic hepatitis B plus D, and the disease may become indolent after several years of infection. A distinguishing serologic feature of chronic hepatitis D is the presence in the circulation of antibodies to liver-kidney microsomes (anti-LKM); however, the anti-LKM seen in hepatitis D,

anti-LKM3, are directed against uridine diphosphate glucuronosyltransferase and are distinct from anti-LKM1 seen in patients with autoimmune hepatitis and in a subset of patients with chronic hepatitis C (see below). The clinical and laboratory features of chronic HDV infection are summarized in Chap. 37.

℞ **Treatment:**
CHRONIC HEPATITIS D

Management is not well defined. Glucocorticoids are ineffective and are not used. Preliminary experimental trials of IFN-α suggested that conventional doses and durations of therapy lower levels of HDV RNA and aminotransferase activity only transiently during treatment but have no impact on the natural history of the disease. In contrast, high-dose IFN-α (9 million units three times a week) for 12 months may be associated with a sustained loss of HDV replication and clinical improvement in up to 50% of patients. Moreover, the beneficial impact of treatment has been observed to persist for 15 years and to be associated with a reduction in grade of hepatic necrosis and inflammation, reversion of advanced fibrosis (improved stage), and clearance of HDV RNA in some patients. A suggested approach to therapy has been high-dose, long-term IFN for at least a year and, in responders, extension of therapy until HDV RNA and HBsAg clearance. Although experience with PEG IFN in the treatment of chronic hepatitis D is limited, if future studies confirm its equivalence to, or superiority over, standard IFN, PEG IFN is likely to become a more convenient replacement for standard IFN. None of the new antiviral agents for hepatitis B—lamivudine, adefovir, entecavir—are effective in hepatitis D; however, preliminary indications in the woodchuck model of hepatitis B are that clevudine may be. In patients with end-stage liver disease secondary to chronic hepatitis D, liver transplantation has been effective. If hepatitis D recurs in the new liver without the expression of hepatitis B (an unusual serologic profile in immunocompetent persons but common in transplant patients), liver injury is limited. In fact, the outcome of transplantation for chronic hepatitis D is superior to that for chronic hepatitis B (Chap. 44).

CHRONIC HEPATITIS C

Regardless of the epidemiologic mode of acquisition of hepatitis C virus (HCV) infection, chronic hepatitis follows acute hepatitis C in 50–70% of cases; chronic infection is common even in those with a return to normal in aminotransferase levels after acute hepatitis C, adding up to an 85% likelihood of chronic HCV infection after acute hepatitis C. Furthermore, in patients with chronic transfusion–associated hepatitis followed for 10–20 years, progression to cirrhosis occurs in about 20%. Such is the case even for patients with relatively clinically mild chronic hepatitis, including those without symptoms, with only modest elevations of aminotransferase activity and with mild chronic hepatitis on liver biopsy. Even in cohorts of well-compensated patients with chronic hepatitis C referred for clinical research trials (no complications of chronic liver disease and with normal hepatic synthetic function), the prevalence of cirrhosis may be as high as 50%. Most cases of hepatitis C are identified initially in asymptomatic patients who have no history of acute hepatitis C, e.g., those discovered while attempting to donate blood, while undergoing lab testing as part of an application for life insurance, or as a result of routine laboratory tests. The source of HCV infection in many of these cases is not defined, although a long-forgotten percutaneous exposure in the remote past can be elicited in a substantial proportion and probably accounts for most infections; most of these infections were acquired in the 1960s and 1970s, coming to clinical attention decades later.

Approximately a third of patients with chronic hepatitis C have normal or near-normal aminotransferase activity; although a third to a half of these patients have chronic hepatitis on liver biopsy, the grade of liver injury and stage of fibrosis tend to be mild in the vast majority. In some cases, more severe liver injury has been reported—even, rarely, cirrhosis, most likely the result of previous histologic activity. Among patients with persistent normal aminotransferase activity sustained over ≥5–10 years, histologic progression has been shown not to occur; however, approximately a quarter of patients with normal aminotransferase activity experience subsequent aminotransferase elevations, and histologic injury can be progressive once abnormal biochemical activity resumes. Therefore, continued clinical monitoring is indicated, even for patients with normal aminotransferase activity.

Despite this substantial rate of progression of chronic hepatitis C, and despite the fact that liver failure can result from end-stage chronic hepatitis C, the long-term prognosis for chronic hepatitis C in a majority of patients is relatively benign. Mortality over 10–20 years among patients with transfusion-associated chronic hepatitis C has been shown not to differ from mortality in a matched population of transfused patients in whom hepatitis C did not develop. Although death in the hepatitis group is more likely to result from liver failure, and although hepatic decompensation may occur in ~15% of such patients over the course of a decade, the majority (almost 60%) of patients remain asymptomatic and well compensated, with no clinical sequelae of chronic liver disease. Overall, then, chronic hepatitis C tends to be very slowly and insidiously progressive, if at all, in the vast majority of patients, while in approximately a quarter of cases, chronic hepatitis C will progress eventually to end-stage cirrhosis. In fact, because HCV infection is so prevalent, and

because a proportion of patients progress inexorably to end-stage liver disease, hepatitis C is the most frequent indication for liver transplantation (Chap. 44). Referral bias may account for the more severe outcomes described in cohorts of patients reported from tertiary care centers (20-year progression of 20%) versus the more benign outcomes in cohorts of patients monitored from initial blood-product-associated acute hepatitis or identified in community settings (20-year progression of only 4–7%). Still unexplained, however, are the wide ranges in reported progression to cirrhosis, from 2% over 17 years in a population of women with hepatitis C infection acquired from contaminated anti-D immune globulin to 30% over ≤11 years in recipients of contaminated intravenous immune globulin.

Progression of liver disease in patients with chronic hepatitis C has been reported to be more likely in patients with older age, longer duration of infection, advanced histologic stage and grade, genotype 1, more complex quasispecies diversity, increased hepatic iron, concomitant other liver disorders (alcoholic liver disease, chronic hepatitis B, hemochromatosis, α_1-antitrypsin deficiency, and steatohepatitis), HIV infection, and obesity. Among these variables, however, duration of infection appears to be the most important, and some of the others probably reflect disease duration to some extent (e.g., quasispecies diversity, hepatic iron accumulation). No other epidemiologic or clinical features of chronic hepatitis C (e.g., severity of acute hepatitis, level of aminotransferase activity, level of HCV RNA, presence or absence of jaundice during acute hepatitis) are predictive of eventual outcome. Despite the relatively benign nature of chronic hepatitis C over time in many patients, cirrhosis following chronic hepatitis C has been associated with the late development, after several decades, of HCC; the annual rate of HCC in cirrhotic patients with hepatitis C is 1–4%, occurring primarily in patients who have had HCV infection for 30 or more years.

Perhaps the best prognostic indicator in chronic hepatitis C is liver histology; the rate of hepatic fibrosis may be slow, moderate, or rapid. Patients with mild necrosis and inflammation as well as those with limited fibrosis have an excellent prognosis and limited progression to cirrhosis. In contrast, among patients with moderate to severe necroinflammatory activity or fibrosis, including septal or bridging fibrosis, progression to cirrhosis is highly likely over the course of 10–20 years. Among patients with compensated cirrhosis associated with hepatitis C, the 10-year survival is close to 80%; mortality occurs at a rate of 2–6% per year, decompensation at a rate of 4–5% per year, and, as noted above, HCC at a rate of 1–4% per year.

Clinical features of chronic hepatitis C are similar to those described above for chronic hepatitis B. Generally, *fatigue* is the most common symptom; jaundice is rare. Immune complex–mediated extrahepatic complications of chronic hepatitis C are less common than in chronic hepatitis B (despite the fact that assays for immune complexes are often positive in patients with chronic hepatitis C), with the exception of essential mixed cryoglobulinemia (Chap. 37). In addition, chronic hepatitis C has been associated with extrahepatic complications unrelated to immune-complex injury. These include Sjögren's syndrome, lichen planus, and porphyria cutanea tarda.

Laboratory features of chronic hepatitis C are similar to those in patients with chronic hepatitis B, but aminotransferase levels tend to fluctuate more (the characteristic episodic pattern of aminotransferase activity) and to be lower, especially in patients with long-standing disease. An interesting and occasionally confusing finding in patients with chronic hepatitis C is the presence of autoantibodies. Rarely, patients with autoimmune hepatitis (see below) and hyperglobulinemia have false-positive immunoassays for anti-HCV. On the other hand, some patients with serologically confirmable chronic hepatitis C have circulating anti-LKM. These antibodies are anti-LKM1, as seen in patients with autoimmune hepatitis type II (see below), and are directed against a 33-amino-acid sequence of cytochrome P450 IID6. The occurrence of anti-LKM1 in some patients with chronic hepatitis C may result from the partial sequence homology between the epitope recognized by anti-LKM1 and two segments of the HCV polyprotein. In addition, the presence of this autoantibody in some patients with chronic hepatitis C suggests that autoimmunity may be playing a role in the pathogenesis of chronic hepatitis C.

Histopathologic features of chronic hepatitis C, especially those that distinguish hepatitis C from hepatitis B, are described in Chap. 37.

℞ Treatment:
CHRONIC HEPATITIS C

Therapy for chronic hepatitis C has evolved substantially in the decade and a half since IFN-α was introduced for this indication. When first approved, IFN-α was administered via subcutaneous injection three times a week for 6 months but achieved a sustained virologic response (a reduction of HCV RNA to undetectable levels by PCR when measured ≥6 months after completion of therapy) below 10%. Doubling the duration of therapy—but not increasing the dose or changing IFN preparations—increased the sustained virologic response rate to ~20%, and addition to the regimen of daily ribavirin, an oral guanosine nucleoside, increased sustained virologic responses to 40%. When used alone, ribavirin is ineffective and does not reduce HCV RNA levels, but ribavirin enhances the efficacy of IFN by reducing the likelihood of virologic relapse after the achievement of an end-treatment response (response measured during, and maintained to the end of, treatment). Proposed mechanisms to

explain the role of ribavirin include subtle direct reduction of HCV replication, inhibition of host inosine monophosphate dehydrogenase activity (and associated depletion of guanosine pools), immune modulation, and induction of virologic mutational catastrophe.

Many important lessons about antiviral therapy for chronic hepatitis C were learned from the experience with IFN monotherapy and combination IFN-ribavirin therapy. Even in the absence of biochemical and virologic responses, histologic improvement occurs in approximately three-quarters of all treated patients. In chronic hepatitis C, unlike the case in hepatitis B, responses to therapy are not accompanied by transient, acute hepatitis–like aminotransferase elevations. Instead, ALT levels fall precipitously during therapy. Up to 90% of virologic responses are achieved within the first 12 weeks of therapy; responses thereafter are rare. Most relapses occur within the first 12 weeks after treatment. Sustained virologic responses are very durable; normal ALT, improved histology, and absence of HCV RNA in serum and liver have been documented 5–6 years after successful therapy, and "relapses" 2 years after sustained responses are almost unheard of. Thus, sustained virologic responses to antiviral therapy of chronic hepatitis C are tantamount to cures.

Patient variables that tend to correlate with sustained virologic responsiveness to IFN include favorable genotype (genotypes 2 and 3 as opposed to genotypes 1 and 4), low baseline HCV RNA level (<2 million copies/mL, which is equivalent to ~800,000 international units/mL, the current convention of quantitation), histologically mild hepatitis and minimal fibrosis, age <40, absence of obesity, and female gender. Patients with cirrhosis can respond, but they are less likely to do so. Studies of combination IFN-ribavirin therapy showed conclusively that in patients with genotype 1, therapy should last a full year, while in those with genotypes 2 and 3, a 6-month course of therapy suffices. The response rate in African Americans is disappointingly low for reasons that remain obscure. Finally, the likelihood of a sustained response is best if adherence to the treatment regimen is high, i.e., if patients receive ≥80% of the IFN and ribavirin doses and if they continue treatment for ≥80% of the anticipated duration of therapy. Other variables reported to correlate with increased responsiveness include brief duration of infection, low HCV quasispecies diversity, immunocompetence, and low liver iron levels. High levels of HCV RNA, more histologically advanced liver disease, and high quasispecies diversity all go hand in hand with advanced duration of infection, which may be the single most important variable determining IFN responsiveness. The ironic fact, then, is that patients whose disease is least likely to progress are the ones *most* likely to respond to interferon and vice versa. Finally, among patients with genotype 1b, responsiveness to IFN is enhanced in those with amino-acid-substitution mutations in the nonstructural protein 5A gene.

Side effects of IFN therapy are described above in the section on treatment of chronic hepatitis B. The most pronounced side effect of ribavirin therapy is hemolysis; a reduction in hemoglobin of up to 2–3 g or in hematocrit of 5–10% can be anticipated. A small, unpredictable proportion of patients experience profound, brisk hemolysis, resulting in symptomatic anemia; therefore, close monitoring of blood counts is crucial, and ribavirin should be avoided in patients with anemia or hemoglobinopathies and in patients with coronary artery disease or cerebrovascular disease, in whom anemia can precipitate an ischemic event. When symptomatic anemia occurs, ribavirin dose reductions or addition of erythropoietin to boost red blood cell levels may be required. In addition, ribavirin, which is renally excreted, should not be used in patients with renal insufficiency; the drug is teratogenic, precluding its use during pregnancy and mandating the scrupulous use of efficient contraception during therapy.

Ribavirin can also cause nasal and chest congestion, pruritus, and precipitation of gout. Combination IFN-ribavirin therapy is more difficult to tolerate than IFN monotherapy. In one large clinical trial of combination therapy versus monotherapy, among those in the 1-year treatment group, 21% of the combination group (but only 14% of the monotherapy group) had to discontinue treatment, while 26% of the combination group (but only 9% of the monotherapy group) required dose reductions.

Studies of viral kinetics have shown that despite a virion half-life in serum of only 2–3 h, the level of HCV is maintained by a high replication rate of 10^{12} hepatitis C virions per day. IFN-α blocks virion production or release with an efficacy that increases with increasing drug doses; moreover, the calculated death rate for infected cells during IFN therapy is inversely related to viral load; patients with the most rapid death rate of infected hepatocytes are more likely to achieve undetectable HCV RNA at 3 months; achieving this landmark is predictive of a subsequent sustained response. Therefore, to achieve rapid viral clearance from serum and the liver, *high-dose induction therapy* has been advocated. In practice, however, high-dose induction therapy has not yielded higher sustained response rates.

TREATMENT OF CHOICE For the treatment of chronic hepatitis C, standard IFNs have now been supplanted by PEG IFNs. These have elimination times up to sevenfold longer than standard IFNs, i.e., a substantially longer half-life, and achieve prolonged concentrations, permitting administration once (rather than three times) a week. Instead of the frequent drug peaks (linked to side effects) and troughs (when drug is absent) associated

with frequent administration of short-acting IFNs, administration of PEG IFNs results in drug concentrations that are more stable and sustained over time. Once-a-week PEG IFN monotherapy is twice as effective as monotherapy with its standard IFN counterpart, approaches the efficacy of combination standard IFN plus ribavirin, and is as well tolerated as standard IFNs, without more difficult-to-manage thrombocytopenia and leukopenia than standard IFNs. The current standard of care, however, is a combination of PEG IFN plus ribavirin.

Two PEG IFNs are available: PEG IFN-α2b and α2a. In the registration trial for PEG IFN-α2b plus ribavirin, the best regimen was 48 weeks of 1.5 μg/kg of PEG IFN once a week plus 800 mg of ribavirin daily. A post hoc analysis suggested that weight-based dosing of ribavirin would have been more effective than the fixed 800-mg dose used in the study. In the first registration trial for PEG IFN-α2a plus ribavirin, the best regimen was 48 weeks of 180 μg of PEG IFN plus 1000 mg (for patients <75 kg) to 1200 mg (for patients ≥75 kg) of ribavirin. Sustained virologic responses of 54 and 56% were reported in these two studies, respectively. A subsequent study of PEG IFN-α2a plus ribavirin showed that, for patients with genotypes 2 and 3, a duration of 6 months and a ribavirin dose of 800 mg was sufficient. Among the three studies, for patients in the optimal treatment arm, sustained response rates for patients with genotype 1 were 42–51% and for patients with genotypes 2 and 3 rates were 76–82%. Subsequent studies have shown that, in patients with genotypes 2 and 3, if HCV RNA is undetectable at 4 weeks ("rapid virologic response"), the total duration of therapy required to achieve a sustained virologic response can be as short as 12–16 weeks, especially for patients with genotype 2 (less so for those with genotype 3). These clinical trials of abbreviated treatment, however, were conducted with full, weight-based ribavirin doses rather than the current convention of uniform, 800-mg flat dosing; studies of abbreviated-duration therapy with flat ribavirin dosing in patients with genotypes 2 and 3 are awaited. Between genotypes 2 and 3, genotype 3 is somewhat more refractory, and some authorities would extend therapy for a full 48 weeks in patients with genotype 3, especially if they have advanced hepatic fibrosis or cirrhosis and/or high-level HCV RNA.

In the initial registration trials for combination PEG IFN plus ribavirin, both combination PEG IFN regimens were compared to standard IFN-α2b plus ribavirin. Side effects of the combination PEG IFN-α2b regimen were comparable to those for the combination standard IFN regimen; however, when the combination PEG IFN-α2a regimen was compared to the combination standard IFN-α2b regimen, flulike symptoms and depression were less common in the combination PEG IFN group. Although the two combination PEG IFN regimens were not tested head-to-head, and although ascertainment of side effects differed between studies of the two drugs, when each was tested against standard IFN-α2b plus ribavirin, combination PEG IFN-α2a plus ribavirin appeared to be better tolerated. Recommended doses for the two PEG IFNs plus ribavirin and other comparisons between the two therapies are shown in **Table 39-6**.

TABLE 39-6

PEGYLATED INTERFERON-α-2A AND α-2B FOR CHRONIC HEPATITIS C

	PEG IFN-α2B	PEG IFN-α2A
PEG size	12 kD linear	40 kD branched
Elimination half-life	54 h	65 h
Clearance	725 mL/h	60 mL/h
Best dose monotherapy[a]	1.0 µg/kg (weight-based)	180 µg
Best dose combination therapy	1.5 µg/kg (weight-based)	180 µg
Storage	Room temperature	Refrigerated
Ribavirin dose		
Genotype 1	800 mg[b]	1000–1200 mg[c]
Genotype 2/3	800 mg	800 mg
Duration of therapy		
Genotype 1	48 weeks	48 weeks
Genotype 2/3	48 weeks[d]	24 weeks
Efficacy of combination Rx[e]	54%	56%
Genotype 1	42%	46–51%
Genotype 2/3	82%	76–78%

[a]Reserved for patients in whom ribavirin is contraindicated or not tolerated.

[b]In the registration trial for PEG IFN-α2b plus ribavirin, the optimal regimen was 1.5 µg of PEG IFN plus 800 mg of ribavirin; however, a post hoc analysis of this study suggested that higher ribavirin doses are better. In addition, data from the study of PEG IFN-α2a supported weight-based dosing, 1000 mg (for patients weighing <75 kg) and 1200 mg (for patients weighing ≥75 kg) for genotype 1. Therefore, the higher ribavirin doses are recommended for both types of PEG IFN in patients with genotype 1.

[c]1000 mg for patients weighing <75 kg; 1200 mg for patients weighing ≥75 kg.

[d]In the registration trial for PEG IFN-α2b plus ribavirin, all patients were treated for 48 weeks; however, data from other trials of standard interferons and the other PEG IFN demonstrated that 24 weeks suffices for patients with genotypes 2 and 3. For patients with genotype 3 who have advanced fibrosis/cirrhosis and/or high-level HCV RNA, a full 48 weeks is preferable.

[e]To date, direct, head-to-head comparisons of the two PEG IFNs have not been reported. Attempts to compare the two PEG IFN preparations based on the results of registration clinical trials are confounded by differences between trials of the two agents in methodological details (different ribavirin doses, different methods for recording depression and other side effects) and study-population composition (different proportion with bridging fibrosis/cirrhosis, proportion from the United States versus international, mean weight, proportion with genotype 1, and proportion with high-level HCV RNA).

Note: HCV RNA, hepatitis C virus RNA; PEG, polyethylene glycol; PEG IFN, pegylated interferon.

Unless ribavirin is contraindicated (see earlier), combination PEG IFN plus ribavirin is the recommended course of therapy—24 weeks for genotypes 2 and 3 and 48 weeks for genotype 1. Measurement of quantitative HCV RNA levels at 12 weeks is helpful in guiding therapy; if a 2-$\log_{10}$ drop in HCV RNA has not been achieved by this time, chances for a sustained virologic response are negligible. If the 12-week HCV RNA has fallen by two $\log_{10}$ ("early virologic response"), the chances for a sustained virologic response at the end of therapy are approximately two-thirds; if the 12-week HCV RNA is undetectable, the chances for a sustained virologic response exceed 80%. If the goal of therapy is sustained virologic response, failure to achieve a 12-week 2-$\log_{10}$ drop in HCV RNA may be used as a signal to discontinue therapy, especially in those who do not tolerate the drugs well. Still, conceivably, some may achieve histologic benefit in the absence of a virologic response, and some clinicians choose to continue therapy even in the absence of a 2-$\log_{10}$ HCV RNA reduction at 12 weeks. Studies are underway to determine whether, even in the absence of a virologic response, maintenance therapy with PEG IFN can slow histologic and clinical progression of hepatitis C.

Studies have suggested that the frequency of sustained virologic responses to PEG IFN/ribavirin therapy can be increased by raising the dose of ribavirin (if tolerated or supplemented by erythropoietin) or by tailoring treatment based on viral response to prolong the duration of viral clearance before discontinuing therapy, i.e., extending therapy from 48 to 72 weeks for patients with genotype 1 and a slow virologic response, i.e., those whose HCV RNA has not fallen rapidly to undetectable levels within 4 weeks (absence of "rapid virologic response"). Confirmatory studies are awaited. Tailoring therapy based on the kinetics of HCV RNA reduction has also been applied to abbreviating the duration of therapy in patients with genotype 1. The results of several clinical trials suggest that, in genotype 1 patients with a 4-week rapid virologic response, but only in the subset with a baseline low level of HCV RNA, 24 weeks of therapy with PEG IFN and weight-based ribavirin suffices, yielding sustained response rates comparable to those achieved with 48 weeks of therapy. Again, although regulatory agencies in Europe have adopted this treatment approach, broad adoption of this approach awaits confirmatory studies.

INDICATIONS FOR ANTIVIRAL THERAPY
Patients with chronic hepatitis C who have detectable HCV RNA in serum and chronic hepatitis of at least moderate grade and stage (portal or bridging fibrosis) are candidates for antiviral therapy with PEG IFN plus ribavirin. Most authorities recommend 800 mg of ribavirin for patients with genotypes 2 and 3 and weight-based 1000–1200 mg for patients with genotype 1 (and 4) for both types of PEG IFN, unless ribavirin is contraindicated

(Table 39-7). Although patients with persistently normal ALT activity tend not to progress histologically, they respond to antiviral therapy just as well as do patients with elevated ALT levels; therefore, while observation without therapy is an option, such patients are potential candidates for antiviral therapy. Therapy with IFN has been shown to improve survival and complication-free survival and to slow progression of fibrosis.

Prior to therapy, HCV genotype should be determined, and the genotype dictates the duration of therapy: 1 year (48 weeks) for patients with genotype 1; 6 months (24 weeks) for those with genotypes 2 and 3; and potentially only 12–16 weeks for patients with genotype 2 whose HCV RNA becomes undetectable within 4 weeks. As noted above, the absence of a 2-$\log_{10}$ drop in HCV RNA at week 12 (an *early virologic response*) weighs heavily against the likelihood of a sustained virologic response even if therapy is continued for the remainder of the planned full year. Therefore, measuring HCV RNA at baseline and at 12 weeks is recommended routinely, especially for patients with genotype 1. The consensus view is that therapy can be discontinued if an early virologic response is not achieved; however, histologic benefit may occur even in the absence of a virologic response. In addition, if current trials show that maintenance therapy can slow the progression of chronic hepatitis C, early virologic nonresponders may be identified as candidates for maintenance therapy; the results of these trials are awaited. Although response rates are lower in patients with certain pretreatment variables, selection for treatment should not be based on symptoms, genotype, HCV RNA level, mode of acquisition of hepatitis C, or advanced hepatic fibrosis. Patients with cirrhosis can respond and should not be excluded as candidates for therapy.

Patients who have relapsed after a course of IFN monotherapy are candidates for retreatment with PEG IFN plus ribavirin (i.e., a more effective treatment regimen is required). For nonresponders to a prior course of IFN monotherapy, retreatment with IFN monotherapy or combination IFN plus ribavirin therapy is unlikely to achieve a sustained virologic response; however, a trial of combination PEG IFN plus ribavirin may be worthwhile. End-treatment virologic responses as high as 40% can occur in this setting, but a sustained virologic response is the outcome in <15–20% of patients. Sustained virologic responses to retreatment of nonresponders are more frequent in those who had never received ribavirin in the past, those with genotypes 2 and 3, those with low pretreatment HCV RNA levels, and noncirrhotics, but less frequent in African Americans, those who failed to achieve a substantial reduction in HCV RNA during their previous course of therapy, and those who required ribavirin-dose reductions. Potential approaches to improving responsiveness to PEG IFN/ribavirin in prior nonresponders include longer duration of treatment; higher doses of either PEG IFN, ribavirin, or both; and switching to a different IFN preparation. However, none of these approaches is of proven efficacy.

Early treatment is indicated for persons with acute hepatitis C (Chap. 37). In patients with biochemically and histologically mild chronic hepatitis C, the rate of progression is slow, and monitoring without therapy is an option; however, such patients respond just as well to combination PEG IFN plus ribavirin therapy as those with elevated ALT and more histologically severe hepatitis. Therefore, therapy for these patients should be considered and the decision made based on such factors as patient motivation, genotype, stage of fibrosis, age, and comorbid conditions. A pretreatment liver biopsy to assess histologic grade and stage provides substantial information about progression of hepatitis C in the past and has prognostic value for future progression. As therapy has improved for patients with a broad range of histologic severity, and as noninvasive laboratory markers of fibrosis have gained popularity, some authorities have placed less value on pretreatment liver biopsies. On the other hand, serum markers of fibrosis are not considered sufficiently accurate, and histologic findings provide important prognostic information to physician and patient. Therefore, a pretreatment liver biopsy is still recommended in most cases.

Patients with compensated cirrhosis can respond to therapy, although their likelihood of a sustained response is lower than in noncirrhotics. Whether survival is improved after successful antiviral therapy in cirrhotics is controversial. Similarly, although several retrospective studies have suggested that antiviral therapy in cirrhotics with chronic hepatitis C reduces the frequency of HCC, less advanced disease in the treated cirrhotics, not treatment itself, may have accounted for the reduced frequency of HCC observed in the treated cohort; prospective studies to address this question are in progress. Patients with decompensated cirrhosis are not candidates for IFN-based antiviral therapy but should be referred for liver transplantation. Some liver transplantation centers have evaluated progressively escalated, low-dose antiviral therapy in an attempt to eradicate hepatitis C viremia prior to transplantation; however, data supporting this approach are limited. After liver transplantation, recurrent hepatitis C is the rule, and the pace of disease progression is more accelerated than in immunocompetent patients (Chap. 44). Current therapy with PEG IFN and ribavirin is unsatisfactory in most patients, but attempts to minimize immunosuppression are beneficial. The cutaneous and renal vasculitis of HCV-associated essential mixed cryoglobulinemia (Chap. 37) may respond to antiviral therapy, but sustained responses are rare after discontinuation of therapy; therefore, prolonged, perhaps indefinite, therapy is recommended in

TABLE 39-7

INDICATIONS AND RECOMMENDATIONS FOR ANTIVIRAL THERAPY OF CHRONIC HEPATITIS C

Standard Indications for Therapy

Detectable HCV RNA (with or without elevated ALT)
Portal/bridging fibrosis or moderate to severe hepatitis on liver biopsy

Retreatment Recommended

Relapsers after a previous course of standard interferon monotherapy or combination standard interferon/ribavirin therapy
   A course of PEG IFN plus ribavirin
Nonresponders to a previous course of standard IFN monotherapy or combination standard IFN/ribavirin therapy
   A course of PEG IFN plus ribavirin—more likely to achieve a sustained virologic response in Caucasian patients without
    previous ribavirin therapy, with low baseline HCV RNA levels, with a 2-$\log_{10}$ reduction in HCV RNA during previous
    therapy, with genotypes 2 and 3, and without reduction in ribavirin dose.

Antiviral Therapy Not Recommended Routinely But Management Decisions Made on an Individual Basis

Children (age <18 years)
Age >60
Mild hepatitis on liver biopsy

Long-Term Maintenance Therapy Recommended

Cutaneous vasculitis and glomerulonephritis associated with chronic hepatitis C

Long-Term Maintenance Therapy Being Assessed in Clinical Trials

Relapsers
Nonresponders

Antiviral Therapy Not Recommended

Decompensated cirrhosis
Pregnancy (teratogenicity of ribavirin)

Therapeutic Regimens

First-line treatment: PEG IFN subcutaneously once a week plus daily ribavirin orally
   <u>HCV genotypes 1 and 4</u>–48 weeks of therapy
   PEG IFN-α2a 180 μg weekly plus ribavirin 1000 mg/d (weight <75 kg) to 1200 mg/d (weight ≥75 kg) or
   PEG IFN-α2b 1.5 μg/kg weekly plus ribavirin 800 mg/d (the dose used in registration clinical trials, but the higher,
    weight-based ribavirin doses above are recommended for both types of PEG IFN)
   <u>HCV genotypes 2 and 3</u>–24 weeks of therapy
   PEG IFN-α2a 180 μg weekly plus ribavirin 800 mg/d or PEG IFN-α2b 1.5 μg/kg weekly plus ribavirin 800 mg/d (for patients
    with genotype 3 who have advanced fibrosis and/or high-level HCV RNA, a full 48 weeks of therapy may be preferable)
Alternative regimen: PEG IFN (α2a 180 μg or α2b 1.0 μg/kg) subcutaneously once a week (primarily for patients in whom
   ribavirin is contraindicated or not tolerated) for 24 (genotypes 2 and 3) or 48 (genotypes 1 and 4) weeks
For HCV-HIV co-infected patients: 48 weeks, regardless of genotype, of weekly PEG IFN-α2a (180 μg) or PEG IFN-α2b
  (1.5 μg/kg) plus a daily ribavirin dose of at least 600–800 mg, up to full weight-based 1000–1200 mg dosing if tolerated

Features Associated with Reduced Responsiveness

Genotype 1
High-level HCV RNA (>2 million copies/mL or >800,000 IU/mL)
Advanced fibrosis (bridging fibrosis, cirrhosis)
Long-duration disease
Age >40
High HCV quasispecies diversity
Immunosuppression
African American
Obesity
Hepatic steatosis
Reduced adherence (lower drug doses and reduced duration of therapy)

Note: ALT, alanine aminotransferase; HCV, hepatitis C virus; IFN, interferon; PEG IFN, pegylated interferon; IU, international units (1 IU/mL is equivalent to ~2.5 copies/mL).

this group. Anecdotal reports suggest that antiviral therapy may be effective in porphyria cutanea tarda or lichen planus associated with hepatitis C.

In patients with HCV/HIV co-infection, hepatitis C is more progressive and severe than in HCV-monoinfected patients. Although patients with HCV/HIV co-infection respond to antiviral therapy for hepatitis C, they do not respond as well as patients with HCV infection alone. Four large national and international trials of antiviral therapy among patients with HCV/HIV co-infection have shown that PEG IFN (both α2a and α2b) plus ribavirin (daily doses ranging from flat-dosed 600–800 mg to weight-based 1000/1200 mg) is superior to standard IFN regimens; however, sustained response rates were lower than in HCV-monoinfected patients, ranging from 14 to 38% for patients with genotypes 1 and 4 and from 44 to 73% for patients with genotypes 2 and 3. In the three largest trials, all patients, including those with genotypes 2 and 3, were treated for a full 48 weeks. In addition, tolerability of therapy was lower than in HCV-monoinfected patients; therapy was discontinued because of side effects in 12–39% of patients in these clinical trials. Based on these trials, weekly PEG IFN plus daily ribavirin at a daily dose of at least 600–800 mg, up to full weight-based doses if tolerated, is recommended for a full 48 weeks, regardless of genotype. An alternative recommendation for ribavirin doses was issued by a European Consensus Conference and consisted of standard, weight-based 1000–1200 mg for genotypes 1 and 4, but 800 mg for genotypes 2 and 3. In HCV/HIV-infected patients, ribavirin can potentiate the toxicity of—and should not be used together with—didanosine.

Persons with a history of injection-drug use and alcoholism can be treated successfully for chronic hepatitis C, preferably in conjunction with drug and alcohol treatment programs. Because ribavirin is excreted renally, patients with end-stage renal disease, including those undergoing dialysis (which does not clear ribavirin), are not candidates for ribavirin therapy. Rare reports suggest that reduced-dose ribavirin can be used, but the frequency of anemia is very high and data on efficacy are limited. In addition, the manufacturer of PEG IFN-α2a recommends a dose reduction from 180 to 135 μg daily in patients with renal failure. Neither the optimal regimen nor the efficacy of therapy is established in this population.

NOVEL ANTIVIRALS Among the new approaches to antiviral therapy are direct antivirals (so-called specifically targeted antiviral therapy), including orally administered polymerase and protease inhibitors. For example, in preliminary studies among small numbers of subjects, one of the protease inhibitors being investigated has been shown to suppress HCV RNA by 4 $logs_{10}$ in 14 days when used as monotherapy, to suppress HCV RNA by 5.5 $logs_{10}$ in 14 days when combined with PEG IFN injections, and to suppress HCV RNA to undetectable levels in 12 of 12 subjects treated for 28 days when combined with PEG IFN and ribavirin. Because resistance to these oral agents used alone has been both anticipated and observed, polymerase and protease inhibitors are being evaluated in combinations with PEG IFN (± ribavirin) to preempt the emergence of resistance. Potentially, in the future, combinations of specifically targeted antiviral agents will be used in drug cocktails that may replace IFN-based regimens entirely.

AUTOIMMUNE HEPATITIS

DEFINITION

Autoimmune hepatitis is a chronic disorder characterized by continuing hepatocellular necrosis and inflammation, usually with fibrosis, which can progress to cirrhosis and liver failure. When fulfilling criteria of severity, this type of chronic hepatitis, when untreated, may have a 6-month mortality of as high as 40%. Based on contemporary estimates of the natural history of treated autoimmune hepatitis, the 10-year survival is 80–90%. The prominence of extrahepatic features of autoimmunity as well as seroimmunologic abnormalities in this disorder supports an autoimmune process in its pathogenesis; this concept is reflected in the labels *lupoid*, *plasma cell*, or *autoimmune hepatitis*. Autoantibodies and other typical features of autoimmunity, however, do not occur in all cases; among the broader categories of "idiopathic" or cryptogenic chronic hepatitis, many, perhaps the majority, are probably autoimmune in origin. Cases in which hepatotropic viruses, metabolic/genetic derangements, and hepatotoxic drugs have been excluded represent a spectrum of heterogeneous liver disorders of unknown cause, a proportion of which are most likely autoimmune hepatitis.

IMMUNOPATHOGENESIS

The weight of evidence suggests that the progressive liver injury in patients with autoimmune hepatitis is the result of a cell-mediated immunologic attack directed against liver cells. In all likelihood, predisposition to autoimmunity is inherited, while the liver specificity of this injury is triggered by environmental (e.g., chemical or viral) factors. For example, patients have been described in whom apparently self-limited cases of acute hepatitis A, B, or C led to autoimmune hepatitis, presumably because of genetic susceptibility or predisposition. Evidence to support an autoimmune pathogenesis in this type of hepatitis includes the following: (1) In the liver, the histopathologic lesions are composed predominantly of cytotoxic T cells and plasma cells; (2) circulating autoantibodies (nuclear, smooth muscle, thyroid, etc.; see below), rheumatoid factor, and hyperglobulinemia are common; (3) other autoimmune disorders—such as thyroiditis, rheumatoid arthritis, autoimmune hemolytic anemia, ulcerative colitis, membranoproliferative glomerulonephritis, juvenile diabetes mellitus, celiac disease, and Sjögren's syndrome—occur with increased frequency in patients who have autoimmune hepatitis and in their relatives; (4) histocompatibility haplotypes associated with autoimmune diseases, such as HLA-B1, -B8, -DR3, and -DR4 as well as extended haplotype DRB1 alleles, are common in patients with autoimmune hepatitis; and (5) this type of chronic hepatitis is responsive to glucocorticoid/immunosuppressive therapy, effective in a variety of autoimmune disorders.

Cellular immune mechanisms appear to be important in the pathogenesis of autoimmune hepatitis. In vitro studies have suggested that in patients with this disorder, lymphocytes are capable of becoming sensitized to hepatocyte membrane proteins and of destroying liver cells. Abnormalities of immunoregulatory control over cytotoxic lymphocytes (impaired regulatory CD4+CD25+ T cell influences) may play a role as well. Studies of genetic predisposition to autoimmune hepatitis demonstrate that certain haplotypes are associated with the disorder, as enumerated above. The precise triggering factors, genetic influences, and cytotoxic and immunoregulatory mechanisms involved in this type of liver injury remain poorly defined.

Intriguing clues into the pathogenesis of autoimmune hepatitis come from the observation that circulating autoantibodies are prevalent in patients with this disorder. Among the autoantibodies described in these patients are antibodies to nuclei [so-called antinuclear antibodies (ANAs), primarily in a homogeneous pattern] and smooth muscle (so-called anti-smooth-muscle antibodies, directed at actin), anti-LKM (see below), antibodies to "soluble liver antigen/liver pancreas antigen" (directed against a uracil-guanine-adenine transfer RNA suppressor protein), as well as antibodies to the liver-specific asialoglycoprotein receptor (or "hepatic lectin") and other hepatocyte membrane proteins. Although some of these provide helpful diagnostic markers, their involvement in the pathogenesis of autoimmune hepatitis has not been established.

Humoral immune mechanisms have been shown to play a role in the extrahepatic manifestations of autoimmune and idiopathic hepatitis. Arthralgias, arthritis, cutaneous vasculitis, and glomerulonephritis occurring in patients with autoimmune hepatitis appear to be mediated by the deposition of circulating immune complexes in affected tissue vessels, followed by complement activation, inflammation, and tissue injury. While specific viral antigen-antibody complexes can be identified in acute and chronic viral hepatitis, the nature of the immune complexes in autoimmune hepatitis has not been defined.

Many of the *clinical features* of autoimmune hepatitis are similar to those described for chronic viral hepatitis. The onset of disease may be insidious or abrupt; the disease may present initially like, and be confused with, acute viral hepatitis; a history of recurrent bouts of what had been labeled *acute hepatitis* is not uncommon. A subset of patients with autoimmune hepatitis has distinct features. Such patients are predominantly young to middle-aged women with marked hyperglobulinemia and high-titer circulating ANAs. This is the group with positive lupus erythematosus (LE) preparations (initially labeled "lupoid" hepatitis) in whom other autoimmune features are common. Fatigue, malaise, anorexia, amenorrhea, acne, arthralgias, and jaundice are common. Occasionally arthritis, maculopapular eruptions (including cutaneous vasculitis), erythema nodosum, colitis, pleurisy, pericarditis, anemia, azotemia, and sicca syndrome (keratoconjunctivitis, xerostomia) occur. In some patients, complications of cirrhosis, such as ascites and edema (associated with hypoalbuminemia), encephalopathy, hypersplenism, coagulopathy, or variceal bleeding may bring the patient to initial medical attention.

The course of autoimmune hepatitis may be variable. In those with mild disease or limited histologic lesions (e.g., piecemeal necrosis without bridging), progression to cirrhosis is limited. In those with severe symptomatic autoimmune hepatitis (aminotransferase levels >10 times normal, marked hyperglobulinemia, "aggressive" histologic lesions—bridging necrosis or multilobular collapse, cirrhosis), the 6-month mortality without therapy may be as high as 40%. Such severe disease accounts for only 20% of cases; the natural history of milder disease is variable, often accentuated by spontaneous remissions and exacerbations. Especially poor prognostic signs include the presence histologically of multilobular collapse at the time of initial presentation and failure of the bilirubin to improve after 2 weeks of therapy. Death may result from hepatic failure, hepatic coma, other complications of cirrhosis (e.g., variceal hemorrhage), and intercurrent infection. In patients with established cirrhosis, HCC may be a late complication but occurs less frequently than in cirrhosis associated with viral hepatitis.

Laboratory features of autoimmune hepatitis are similar to those seen in chronic viral hepatitis. Liver biochemical tests are invariably abnormal but may not correlate with the clinical severity or histopathologic features in individual cases. Many patients with autoimmune hepatitis have normal serum bilirubin, alkaline phosphatase, and globulin levels with only minimal aminotransferase elevations. Serum AST and ALT levels are increased and fluctuate in the range of 100–1000 units. In severe cases, the serum bilirubin level is moderately elevated [51–171 μmol/L (3–10 mg/dL)]. Hypoalbuminemia occurs in patients with very active or advanced disease. Serum alkaline phosphatase levels may be moderately elevated or near normal. In a small proportion of patients, marked elevations of alkaline phosphatase activity occur; in such patients, clinical and laboratory features overlap with those of primary biliary cirrhosis (Chap. 41). The prothrombin time is often prolonged, particularly late in the disease or during active phases.

Hypergammaglobulinemia (>2.5 g/dL) is common in autoimmune hepatitis. Rheumatoid factor is common as well. As noted above, circulating autoantibodies are also prevalent. The most characteristic are ANAs in a homogeneous staining pattern. Smooth-muscle antibodies are less specific, seen just as frequently in chronic viral hepatitis. Because of the high levels of globulins achieved in the circulation of some patients with autoimmune hepatitis, occasionally the globulins may bind nonspecifically in solid-phase binding immunoassays for viral antibodies. This has been recognized most commonly in tests for antibodies to hepatitis C virus, as noted above. In fact, studies of autoantibodies in autoimmune hepatitis have led to the recognition of new categories of autoimmune hepatitis. *Type I autoimmune hepatitis* is the classic syndrome occurring in young women, associated with marked hyperglobulinemia, lupoid features, circulating ANAs, and HLA-DR3 or HLA-DR4. Also associated with type I autoimmune hepatitis are autoantibodies against actin as well as atypical perinuclear antineutrophilic cytoplasmic antibodies (pANCA).

Type II autoimmune hepatitis, often seen in children, more common in Mediterranean populations, and linked to HLA-DRB1 and HLA-DQB1 haplotypes, is associated not with ANA but with anti-LKM. Actually, anti-LKM represent a heterogeneous group of antibodies. In type II autoimmune hepatitis, the antibody is anti-LKM1, directed against cytochrome P450 2D6. This is the same anti-LKM seen in some patients with chronic hepatitis C. Anti-LKM2 is seen in drug-induced hepatitis, and anti-LKM3 is seen in patients with chronic hepatitis D. Another autoantibody observed in type II autoimmune hepatitis is directed against liver cytosol formiminotransferase cyclodeaminase (anti-liver cytosol 1). Another type of autoimmune hepatitis has been recognized, *type III autoimmune hepatitis*. These patients lack ANA and anti-LKM1 but have circulating antibodies to soluble liver antigen/liver pancreas antigen. Most of these patients are women and have clinical features similar to, perhaps more severe than, those of patients with type I autoimmune hepatitis. Whether type III autoimmune hepatitis actually represents a distinct category or is part of the spectrum of type I autoimmune hepatitis remains controversial, and this subcategory has not been adopted by a consensus of international experts.

Liver biopsy abnormalities are similar to those described for chronic viral hepatitis. Expanding portal tracts and extending beyond the plate of periportal hepatocytes into the parenchyma (designated *interface hepatitis* or *piecemeal necrosis*) is a mononuclear cell infiltrate that, in autoimmune hepatitis, may include the presence of plasma cells. Necroinflammatory activity characterizes the lobular parenchyma, and evidence of hepatocellular regeneration is reflected by "rosette" formation, the occurrence of thickened liver cell plates, and regenerative "pseudolobules." Septal fibrosis, bridging fibrosis, and cirrhosis are frequent. Bile duct injury and granulomas are uncommon; however, a subgroup of patients with autoimmune hepatitis have histologic, biochemical, and serologic features overlapping those of primary biliary cirrhosis (Chap. 41).

DIAGNOSTIC CRITERIA

An international group has suggested a set of criteria for establishing a diagnosis of autoimmune hepatitis. Exclusion of liver disease caused by genetic disorders, viral hepatitis, drug hepatotoxicity, and alcohol are linked with such inclusive diagnostic criteria as hyperglobulinemia, autoantibodies, and characteristic histologic features. This international group has also suggested a comprehensive diagnostic scoring system that, rarely required for typical cases, may be helpful when typical features are not present. Factors that weigh in favor of the diagnosis include female gender; predominant aminotransferase elevation; presence and level of globulin elevation; presence of nuclear, smooth muscle, LKM1, and other autoantibodies; concurrent other autoimmune diseases; characteristic histologic features (interface hepatitis, plasma cells, rosettes); HLA DR3 or DR4 markers; and response to treatment (see later). Weighing against the diagnosis are predominant alkaline phosphatase elevation, mitochondrial antibodies, markers of viral hepatitis, history of hepatotoxic drugs or excessive alcohol, histologic evidence of bile duct injury, or such atypical histologic features as fatty infiltration, iron overload, and viral inclusions.

DIFFERENTIAL DIAGNOSIS

Early during the course of chronic hepatitis, autoimmune hepatitis may resemble typical *acute viral hepatitis*. Without histologic assessment, severe chronic hepatitis cannot be readily distinguished based on clinical or biochemical criteria from mild chronic hepatitis. In adolescence, *Wilson's disease* may present with features of chronic hepatitis long before neurologic manifestations become apparent and before the formation of Kayser-Fleischer rings. In this age group, serum ceruloplasmin and serum and urinary copper determinations plus measurement of liver copper levels will establish the correct diagnosis. *Postnecrotic* or *cryptogenic cirrhosis* and *primary biliary cirrhosis* share clinical features with autoimmune hepatitis, and both alcoholic hepatitis and nonalcoholic steatohepatitis may present with many features common to autoimmune hepatitis; historic, biochemical, serologic, and histologic assessments are usually sufficient to allow these entities to be distinguished from autoimmune hepatitis. Of course, the distinction between autoimmune and chronic viral hepatitis is not always straightforward, especially when viral antibodies occur in patients with autoimmune disease or when autoantibodies occur in patients with viral disease. Furthermore, the presence of extrahepatic features such as arthritis, cutaneous vasculitis, or pleuritis—not to mention the presence of circulating autoantibodies—may cause confusion with *rheumatologic disorders* such as rheumatoid arthritis and systemic lupus erythematosus. The existence of clinical and biochemical features of progressive necroinflammatory liver disease distinguishes chronic hepatitis from these other disorders, which are not associated with severe liver disease.

Finally, occasionally, features of autoimmune hepatitis overlap with features of autoimmune biliary disorders such as primary biliary cirrhosis, primary sclerosing cholangitis, or, even more rarely, mitochondrial antibody-negative autoimmune cholangitis. Such overlap syndromes are difficult to categorize, and often response to therapy may be the distinguishing factor that establishes the diagnosis.

℞ Treatment:
AUTOIMMUNE HEPATITIS

The mainstay of management in autoimmune hepatitis is glucocorticoid therapy. Several controlled clinical trials have documented that such therapy leads to symptomatic, clinical, biochemical, and histologic improvement as well as increased survival. A therapeutic response can be expected in up to 80% of patients. Unfortunately, therapy has not been shown to prevent ultimate progression to cirrhosis; however, instances of reversal of fibrosis and cirrhosis have been reported in patients responding to treatment. Although some advocate the use of prednisolone (the hepatic metabolite of prednisone), prednisone is just as effective and is favored by most authorities. Therapy may be initiated at 20 mg/d, but a popular regimen in the United States relies on an initiation dose of 60 mg/d. This high dose is tapered successively over the course of a month down to a maintenance level of 20 mg/d. An alternative but equally effective approach is to begin with half the prednisone dose (30 mg/d) along with azathioprine (50 mg/d). With azathioprine maintained at 50 mg/d, the prednisone dose is tapered over the course of a month down to a maintenance level of 10 mg/d. The advantage of the combination approach is a reduction, over the span of an 18-month course of therapy, in serious, life-threatening complications of steroid therapy from 66% down to under 20%. In combination regimens, 6-mercaptopurine may be substituted for its prodrug azathioprine, but this is rarely required. Azathioprine alone, however, is not effective in achieving remission, nor is alternate-day glucocorticoid therapy. Although therapy has been shown to be effective for severe autoimmune hepatitis (AST ≥10

times the upper limit of normal or ≥5 times the upper limit of normal in conjunction with serum globulin ≥ twice normal; bridging necrosis or multilobular necrosis on liver biopsy; presence of symptoms), therapy is not indicated for mild forms of chronic hepatitis, and the efficacy of therapy in mild or asymptomatic autoimmune hepatitis has not been established.

Improvement of fatigue, anorexia, malaise, and jaundice tends to occur within days to several weeks; biochemical improvement occurs over the course of several weeks to months, with a fall in serum bilirubin and globulin levels and an increase in serum albumin. Serum aminotransferase levels usually drop promptly, but improvements in AST and ALT alone do not appear to be a reliable marker of recovery in individual patients; histologic improvement, characterized by a decrease in mononuclear infiltration and in hepatocellular necrosis, may be delayed for 6–24 months. Still, if interpreted cautiously, aminotransferase levels are valuable indicators of relative disease activity, and many authorities do *not* advocate serial liver biopsies to assess therapeutic success or to guide decisions to alter or stop therapy. Therapy should continue for at least 12–18 months. After tapering and cessation of therapy, the likelihood of relapse is at least 50%, even if posttreatment histology has improved to show mild chronic hepatitis, and the majority of patients require therapy at maintenance doses indefinitely. Continuing azathioprine alone (2 mg/kg body weight daily) after cessation of prednisone therapy may reduce the frequency of relapse.

In medically refractory cases, an attempt should be made to intensify treatment with high-dose glucocorticoid monotherapy (60 mg daily) or combination glucocorticoid (30 mg daily) plus high-dose azathioprine (150 mg daily) therapy. After a month, doses of prednisone can be reduced by 10 mg a month, and doses of azathioprine can be reduced by 50 mg a month toward ultimate, conventional maintenance doses. Patients refractory to this regimen may be treated with cyclosporine, tacrolimus, or mycophenolate mofetil; however, to date only limited anecdotal reports support these approaches. If medical therapy fails, or when chronic hepatitis progresses to cirrhosis and is associated with life-threatening complications of liver decompensation, liver transplantation is the only recourse (Chap. 44); failure of the bilirubin to improve after 2 weeks of therapy should prompt early consideration of the patient for liver transplantation. Recurrence of autoimmune hepatitis in the new liver occurs rarely in most experiences but in as many as 35–40% of cases in others.

ACKNOWLEDGMENT

Kurt J. Isselbacher, MD, contributed to this chapter in previous editions of Harrison's Principles of Internal Medicine.

FURTHER READINGS

ALVAREZ F et al: International Autoimmune Hepatitis Group report: review of criteria for diagnosis of autoimmune hepatitis. J Hepatol 31:929, 1999

BENHAMOU Y, SALMON D (guest ed): Proceedings of the 1st European consensus conference on the treatment of chronic hepatitis B and C in HIV co-infected patients. J Hepatol 44(Suppl 1):S1, 2006

BERG T et al: Extended treatment duration for hepatitis C virus type 1: Comparing 48 versus 72 weeks of peginterferon-alfa-2a plus ribavirin. Gastroenterology 130:1086, 2006

CACOUB P, TERRIER B: Hepatitis B-related autoimmune manifestations. Rheum Dis Clin North Am 35:125, 2009

CAMMÀ C et al: Effect of peginterferon alfa-2a on liver histology in chronic hepatitis C: A meta-analysis of individual patient data. Hepatology 39:333, 2004

CHANG T-T et al: A comparison of entecavir and lamivudine for HBeAg-positive chronic hepatitis B. N Engl J Med 354:1001, 2006

CONJEEVARAM HS, LOK AS-F: Management of chronic hepatitis B. J Hepatol 38:S90, 2003

CZAJA AJ, FREESE DK: AASLD practice guidelines: Diagnosis and treatment of autoimmune hepatitis. Hepatology 36:479, 2002

——— et al: Treatment challenges and investigational opportunities in autoimmune hepatitis. Hepatology 41:207, 2005

DE FRANCESCO R, MIGLIACCIO G: Challenges and successes in developing new therapies for hepatitis C. Nature 436:953, 2005

DIENSTAG JL: American Gastroenterological Association technical review on the management of hepatitis C. Gastroenterology 130:231, 2006

———, MCHUTCHISON JG: American Gastroenterological Association medical position statement on the management of hepatitis C. Gastroenterology 130:225, 2006

——— et al: Histologic outcome during long-term lamivudine therapy. Gastroenterology 124:105, 2003

EUROPEAN ASSOCIATION FOR THE STUDY OF THE LIVER: Consensus Statement: EASL International Consensus Conference on Hepatitis C. J Hepatol 30:956, 1999

———: Consensus Statement: EASL International Consensus Conference on hepatitis B 13-14 September, 2002. J Hepatol 39(Suppl 1):S3, 2003

———: EASL Consensus Conference on Hepatitis B. J Hepatol 39(Suppl 1):S1, 2003

FARCI P et al: Long-term benefit of interferon a therapy of chronic hepatitis D: Regression of advanced hepatic fibrosis. Gastroenterology 126:1740, 2004

FELD JJ, HOOFNAGLE JH: Mechanism of action of interferon and ribavirin in treatment of hepatitis C. Nature 436:967, 2005

FRIED MV et al: Peginterferon alfa-2a plus ribavirin for chronic hepatitis C virus infection. N Engl J Med 347:975, 2002

FUNG SK, LOK ASF: Treatment of chronic hepatitis B: Who to treat, what to use, and for how long? Clin Gastroenterol Hepatol 2:839, 2004

GANEM D, PRINCE AM: Mechanisms of disease: Hepatitis B virus infection—natural history and clinical consequences. N Engl J Med 350:1118, 2004

GHANY MG et al: Progression of fibrosis in chronic hepatitis C. Gastroenterology 124:97, 2003

HADZIYANNIS SJ: Long-term therapy with adefovir dipivoxil for HBeAg-negative chronic hepatitis B. N Engl J Med 352:2673, 2005

——— et al: Peginterferon-α2a and ribavirin combination therapy in chronic hepatitis C: A randomized study of treatment duration and ribavirin dose. Ann Intern Med 140:346, 2004

HENNES EM et al: Simplified criteria for the diagnosis of autoimmune hepatitis. Hepatology 48:169, 2008

JANSSEN HL et al: Pegylated interferon alfa-2b alone or in combination with lamivudine for HBeAg-positive chronic hepatitis B: A randomized trial. Lancet 365:123, 2005

KEEFE EB et al: A treatment algorithm for the management of chronic hepatitis B virus infection in the United States: an update. Clin Gastroenterol Hepatol 4:936, 2006

KENNY-WALSH E et al: Clinical outcomes after hepatitis C infection from contaminated anti-D immune globulin. N Engl J Med 340:1228, 1999

KRAWITT EL: Autoimmune hepatitis. N Engl J Med 354:54, 2006

LAI C-L et al: Entecavir versus lamivudine for patients with HBeAg-negative chronic hepatitis B. N Engl J Med 354:1011, 2006

LAU DT-Y et al: Long-term follow up of patients with chronic hepatitis B treated with interferon alfa. Gastroenterology 113:1660, 1997

LAU GKK et al: Peginterferon alfa-2a, lamivudine, and the combination for HBeAg-positive chronic hepatitis B. N Engl J Med 352:2682, 2005

LAUER GM, WALKER BD: Medical progress: Hepatitis C virus infection. N Engl J Med 345:41, 2001

LIANG TJ: Hepatitis B: the virus and disease. Hepatology 49:S13, 2009

LIAW Y-F: Asian-Pacific consensus statement on the management of chronic hepatitis B: A 2005 update. Liver International 25:472, 2005

——— et al: Lamivudine for patients with chronic hepatitis B and advanced liver disease. N Engl J Med 351:1521, 2004

LIN S-M et al: Long-term beneficial effect of interferon therapy in patients with chronic hepatitis B virus infection. Hepatology 29:971, 1999

LOCARNINI SA (guest ed): The control of hepatitis B: The role for chemoprevention. Semin Liver Dis 26:1, 2006

LOK ASF: AASLD practice guidelines: Chronic hepatitis B: Update of recommendations. Hepatology 39:857, 2004

———, MCMAHON BJ: AASLD practice guidelines: Chronic hepatitis B. Hepatology 34:1225, 2001

——— et al: Management of hepatitis B: 2000—Summary of a workshop. Gastroenterology 120:1828, 2001

LONGHI MS et al: Functional study of CD4+CD25+ regulatory T cells in health and autoimmune hepatitis. J Immunol 176:4484, 2006

MANGIA A et al: Peginterferon alfa-2b and ribavirin for 12 vs. 24 weeks in HCV genotype 2 or 3. N Engl J Med 352:2609, 2005

MANNS MP (guest ed): Autoimmune hepatitis. Semin Liver Dis 22:1, 2002

———, STRASSBURG CP: Autoimmune hepatitis: Clinical challenges. Gastroenterology 120:1502, 2001

———, VOGEL AL: Autoimmune hepatitis, from mechanisms to therapy. Hepatology 43:S132, 2006

——— et al: Peginterferon alfa-2b plus ribavirin compared with interferon alfa-2b plus ribavirin for initial treatment of chronic hepatitis C: A randomised trial. Lancet 358:958, 2001

MARCEAU G et al: LKM1 autoantibodies in chronic hepatitis C infection: A case of molecular mimicry? Hepatology 42:675, 2005

MARCELLIN P et al: Long-term histologic improvement and loss of detectable intrahepatic HCV RNA in patients with chronic hepatitis C and sustained response to interferon alpha therapy. Ann Intern Med 127:875, 1997

——— et al: Adefovir dipivoxil for the treatment of hepatitis B e antigen–positive chronic hepatitis B. N Engl J Med 348:808, 2003

——— et al: Peginterferon alfa-2a alone, lamivudine alone, and the two in combination in patients with HBeAg-negative chronic hepatitis B. N Engl J Med 351:1206, 2004

414 McHutchison JG et al: The face of future hepatitis C antiviral drug development: Recent biological and virology advances and their translation to drug development and clinical practice. J Hepatol 44:411, 2006

———— et al: Peginterferon alfa-2b or alfa-2a with ribavirin for treatment of hepatitis C infection. N Engl J Med 361:580, 2009

———— et al: Telaprevir with peginterferon and ribavirin for chronic HCV genotype 1 infection. N Engl J Med 360:1827, 2009

National Institutes of Health Consensus Development Conference: Management of hepatitis C. Hepatology 36(Suppl 1): 1S, 2002

————: Management of hepatitis C. Hepatology 26(Suppl 1):1S, 1997

Neumann AU et al: Hepatitis C viral dynamics in vivo and the antiviral efficacy of interferon-a therapy. Science 282:103, 1998

Niederau C et al: Long-term follow-up of HBeAg-positive patients treated with interferon alfa for chronic hepatitis B. N Engl J Med 334:1422, 1996

———— et al: Prognosis of chronic hepatitis C: Results of a large, prospective cohort study. Hepatology 28:1687, 1998

Pawlotsky J-M: Therapy of hepatitis C: From empiricism to eradication. Hepatology 43:S207, 2006

Pearlman BL: Chronic hepatitis C therapy: Changing the rules of duration. Clin Gastroenterol Hepatol 4:963, 2006

Sánchez-Tapias JM et al: Peginterferon-alfa2a plus ribavirin for 48 versus 72 weeks in patients with detectable hepatitis C virus RNA at week 4 of treatment. Gastroenterology 131:451, 2006

Sorrell MF et al: National Institutes of Health consensus development conference statement: management of hepatitis B. Hepatology 49:S4-S12, 2009

Strader DB et al: AASLD practice guideline: Diagnosis, management, and treatment of hepatitis C. Hepatology 39:1147, 2004

Summerskill WHJ et al: Prednisone for chronic active liver disease: Dose titration, standard dose, and combination with azathioprine compared. Gut 16:876, 1975

Taliani G et al: Pegylated interferon alfa-2b plus ribavirin in the retreatment of interferon-ribavirin nonresponder patients. Gastroenterology 130:1098, 2006

Thimme R et al: Hepatitis B or hepatitis C and human immunodeficiency virus infection. J Hepatol 42:S37, 2005

Von Wagner M et al: Peginterferon-α-2a (40KD) and ribavirin for 16 or 24 weeks in patients with genotype 2 or 3 chronic hepatitis C. Gastroenterology 129:522, 2005

Wong W, Terrault N: Update on chronic hepatitis C. Clin Gastroenterol Hepatol 3:507, 2005

Yoshida H et al: Interferon therapy prolonged life expectancy among chronic hepatitis C patients. Gastroenterology 123:483, 2002

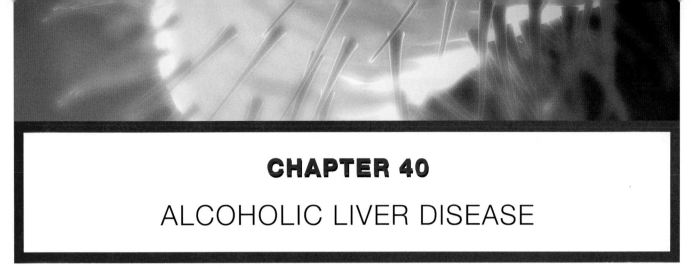

CHAPTER 40

ALCOHOLIC LIVER DISEASE

Mark E. Mailliard ■ Michael F. Sorrell

Chronic and excessive alcohol ingestion is one of the major causes of liver disease. The pathology of alcoholic liver disease comprises three major lesions, with the injury rarely existing in a pure form: (1) fatty liver, (2) alcoholic hepatitis, and (3) cirrhosis. Fatty liver is present in >90% of binge and chronic drinkers. A much smaller percentage of heavy drinkers will progress to alcoholic hepatitis, thought to be a precursor to cirrhosis. The prognosis of severe alcoholic liver disease is dismal; the mortality of patients with alcoholic hepatitis concurrent with cirrhosis is nearly 60% at 4 years. Although alcohol is considered a direct hepatotoxin, only between 10 and 20% of alcoholics will develop alcoholic hepatitis. The explanation for this apparent paradox is unclear but involves the complex interaction of facilitating and comorbid factors such as gender, heredity, and immunity.

ETIOLOGY AND PATHOGENESIS

Quantity and duration of alcohol intake are the most important risk factors involved in the development of alcoholic liver disease (Table 40-1). The roles of beverage type(s), i.e., wine, beer, or spirits, and pattern of drinking are less clear. Progress of the hepatic injury beyond the fatty liver stage seems to require additional risk factors that remain incompletely defined. Women are more susceptible to alcoholic liver injury when compared to men. They develop advanced liver disease with substantially less alcohol intake. Hispanic men have a much higher age-adjusted death rate in the United States from alcoholic cirrhosis than do non-Hispanic whites and blacks. In general, the time it takes to develop liver disease is directly related to the amount of alcohol consumed. It is useful in estimating alcohol consumption to understand that one beer, four ounces of wine, or one ounce of 80% spirits all contain ~12 g of alcohol. The threshold for developing alcoholic liver disease in men is an intake of >60–80 g/d of alcohol for 10 years, while women are at increased risk for developing similar degrees of liver injury by consuming 20–40 g/d. Ingestion of 160 g/d is associated with 25–fold increased risk of developing alcoholic cirrhosis. Gender-dependent differences result from poorly understood effects of estrogen and the metabolism of alcohol. Social, immunologic, and heritable factors have all been postulated to play a part in the development of the pathogenic process.

Chronic infection with hepatitis C (HCV) (Chap. 39) is an important comorbidity in the progression of alcoholic liver disease to cirrhosis in chronic and excessive drinkers. Even moderate alcohol intake of 20–50 g/d increases the risk of cirrhosis and hepatocellular cancer in HCV-infected individuals. Patients with both alcoholic liver injury and HCV infection develop decompensated liver disease at a younger age and have poorer overall survival. Increased liver iron stores and, rarely, porphyria cutanea tarda can occur as a consequence of the overlapping injurious processes secondary to alcohol abuse and HCV infection. In addition, alcohol intake of

TABLE 40-1

RISK FACTORS FOR ALCOHOLIC LIVER DISEASE

RISK FACTOR	COMMENT
Quantity	In men, 40–80 g/d of ethanol produces fatty liver; 160 g/d for 10–20 years causes hepatitis or cirrhosis. Only 15% of alcoholics develop alcoholic liver disease.
Gender	Women exhibit increased susceptibility to alcoholic liver disease at amounts >20 g/d; two drinks per day probably safe.
Hepatitis C	HCV infection concurrent with alcoholic liver disease is associated with younger age for severity, more advanced histology, decreased survival.
Genetics	Gene polymorphisms may include alcohol dehydrogenase, cytochrome P4502E1, and those associated with alcoholism (twin studies).
Malnutrition	Alcohol injury does not require malnutrition, but obesity and fatty liver from the effect of carbohydrate on the transcriptional control of lipid synthesis and transport may be factors. Patients should receive vigorous attention to nutritional support.

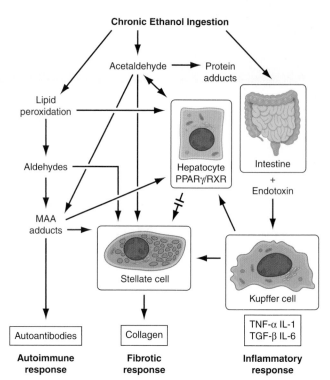

FIGURE 40-1

Biomedical and cellular pathogenesis of liver injury secondary to chronic ethanol ingestion. MAA, malondialdehyde-acetaldehyde; TNF, tumor necrosis factor; TGF, transforming growth factor; IL, interleukin; PPAR, peroxisome proliferator-activated receptor; RXR, retinoid X receptor.

>50 g/d by HCV-infected patients decreases the efficacy of interferon-based antiviral therapy.

Our understanding of the pathogenesis of alcoholic liver injury is incomplete. Alcohol is a direct hepatotoxin, but ingestion of alcohol initiates a variety of metabolic responses that influence the final hepatotoxic response. The initial concept of malnutrition as the major pathogenic mechanism has been replaced by the understanding that the hepatic metabolism of alcohol initiates a pathogenic process involving production of toxic protein-aldehyde adducts, endotoxins, oxidative stress, immunologic activity, and pro-inflammatory cytokine release (Fig. 40-1). The complex interaction of intestinal and hepatic cells is crucial to alcohol-mediated liver injury. Tumor necrosis factor α (TNF-α) and intestine-derived endotoxemia facilitate hepatocyte apoptosis and necrosis. Stellate cell activation and collagen production are key events in hepatic fibrogenesis. The resulting fibrosis determines the architectural derangement of the liver following chronic alcohol ingestion.

PATHOLOGY

The liver has a limited repertoire in response to injury. Fatty liver is the initial and most common histologic response to hepatotoxic stimuli, including excessive alcohol ingestion. The accumulation of fat within the perivenular hepatocytes coincides with the location of alcohol dehydrogenase, the major enzyme responsible for

alcohol metabolism. Continuing alcohol ingestion results in fat accumulation throughout the entire hepatic lobule. Despite extensive fatty change and distortion of the hepatocytes with macrovesicular fat, the cessation of drinking results in normalization of hepatic architecture and fat content within the liver. Alcoholic fatty liver has traditionally been regarded as entirely benign, but similar to the spectrum of nonalcoholic fatty liver disease (Chap. 42), the appearance of steatohepatitis and certain pathologic features such as giant mitochondria, perivenular fibrosis, and macrovesicular fat may be associated with progressive liver injury.

The transition between fatty liver and the development of alcoholic hepatitis is blurred. The hallmark of alcoholic hepatitis is hepatocyte injury characterized by ballooning degeneration, spotty necrosis, polymorphonuclear infiltrate, and fibrosis in the perivenular and perisinusoidal space of Disse. Mallory bodies are often present in florid cases but are neither specific nor necessary to establishing the diagnosis. Alcoholic hepatitis is thought to be a precursor to the development of cirrhosis. However, like fatty liver, it is potentially reversible with cessation of drinking. Cirrhosis is present in up to 50% of patients with biopsy-proven alcoholic hepatitis and its regression is uncertain, even with abstention.

CLINICAL FEATURES

The clinical manifestations of alcoholic fatty liver are subtle and characteristically detected as a consequence of the patient's visit for a seemingly unrelated matter. Previously unsuspected hepatomegaly is often the only clinical finding. Occasionally, patients with fatty liver will present with right upper quadrant discomfort, tender hepatomegaly, nausea, and jaundice. Differentiation of alcoholic fatty liver from nonalcoholic fatty liver is difficult unless an accurate drinking history is ascertained. In every instance where liver disease is present, a thoughtful and sensitive drinking history should be obtained. Standard, validated questions accurately detect alcohol-related problems. Alcoholic hepatitis is associated with a wide gamut of clinical features. Cytokine production is thought to be responsible for the systemic manifestations of alcoholic hepatitis. Fever, spider nevi, jaundice, and abdominal pain simulating an acute abdomen represent the extreme end of the spectrum, while many patients will be entirely asymptomatic. Portal hypertension, ascites, or variceal bleeding can occur in the absence of cirrhosis. Recognition of the clinical features of alcoholic hepatitis is central to the initiation of an effective and appropriate diagnostic and therapeutic strategy. It is important to recognize that patients with alcoholic cirrhosis often exhibit clinical features identical to other causes of cirrhosis.

LABORATORY FEATURES

Patients with alcoholic liver disease are often identified through routine screening tests. The typical laboratory abnormalities seen in fatty liver are nonspecific and include modest elevations of the aspartate aminotransferase (AST), alanine aminotransferase (ALT), and γ-glutamyl transpeptidase (GGTP), accompanied by hypertriglyceridemia, hypercholesterolemia, and occasionally hyperbilirubinemia. In alcoholic hepatitis and in contrast to other causes of fatty liver, the AST and ALT are usually elevated two- to sevenfold. They are rarely >400 IU, and the AST/ALT ratio >1 (Table 40-2). Hyperbilirubinemia is common and is accompanied by modest increases in the alkaline phosphatase level. Derangement in hepatocyte synthetic function indicates more serious disease. Hypoalbuminemia and coagulopathy are common in advanced liver injury. Ultrasonography is useful in detecting fatty infiltration of the liver and determining liver size. The demonstration by ultrasound of portal vein flow reversal, ascites, and intraabdominal collaterals indicates serious liver injury with less potential for complete reversal of liver disease.

PROGNOSIS

Critically ill patients with alcoholic hepatitis have short-term (30 day) mortality rates >50%. Severe alcoholic hepatitis is heralded by coagulopathy (prothrombin

TABLE 40-2

LABORATORY DIAGNOSIS OF ALCOHOLIC FATTY LIVER AND ALCOHOLIC HEPATITIS	
TEST	**COMMENT**
AST	Increased two- to sevenfold, <400 U/L, greater than ALT
ALT	Increased two- to sevenfold, <400 U/L
AST/ALT	Usually >1
GGTP	Not specific to alcohol, easily inducible, elevated in all forms of fatty liver
Bilirubin	May be markedly increased in alcoholic hepatitis despite modest elevation in alkaline phosphatase
PMN	If >5500/μL, predicts severe alcoholic hepatitis when discriminant function > 32

Note: AST, aspartate aminotransferase; ALT, alanine aminotransferase; GGTP, gamma-glutamyl transpeptidase; PMN, polymorphonuclear cells.

time >5 s), anemia, serum albumin concentrations <25 g/L (2.5 mg/dL), serum bilirubin levels >137 μmol/L (8 mg/dL), renal failure, and ascites. A discriminant function calculated as 4.6 × [prothrombin time − control (s)] + serum bilirubin (mg/dL) can identify patients with a poor prognosis (discriminant function >32). The presence of ascites, variceal hemorrhage, deep encephalopathy, or hepatorenal syndrome predicts a dismal prognosis. The pathologic stage of the injury can be helpful in predicting prognosis. Liver biopsy should be performed whenever possible to confirm the diagnosis, to establish potential reversibility of the liver disease, and to guide the therapeutic decisions.

℞ Treatment:
ALCOHOLIC LIVER DISEASE

Complete abstinence from alcohol is the cornerstone in the treatment of alcoholic liver disease. Improved survival and the potential for reversal of histologic injury regardless of the initial clinical presentation are associated with total avoidance of alcohol ingestion. Referral of patients to experienced alcohol counselors and/or alcohol treatment programs should be routine in the management of patients with alcoholic liver disease. Attention should be directed to the nutritional and psychosocial states during the evaluation and treatment periods. Because of data suggesting that the pathogenic mechanisms in alcoholic hepatitis involve cytokine release and the perpetuation of injury by immunologic processes, glucocorticoids have been extensively evaluated in the treatment of alcoholic hepatitis. Patients with severe alcoholic hepatitis, defined as a discriminant function >32, were given prednisone, 40 mg/d, or prednisolone, 32 mg/d, for 4 weeks followed by a

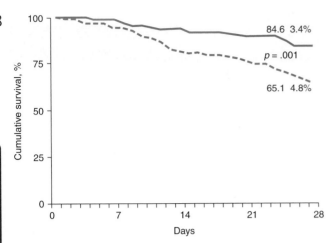

FIGURE 40-2

Effect of glucocorticoid therapy of severe alcoholic hepatitis on short-term survival: the result of a meta-analysis of individual data from three studies. Prednisolone, solid line; placebo, dotted line. (*Adapted from Mathurin et al.; with permission from Elsevier Science.*)

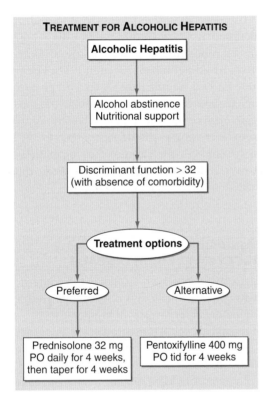

FIGURE 40-3

Treatment algorithm for alcoholic hepatitis. As identified by a calculated discriminant function >32 (see text), patients with severe alcoholic hepatitis, without the presence of gastrointestinal bleeding or infection, would be candidates for either glucocorticoids or pentoxifylline administration.

steroid taper (**Fig. 40-2**). Exclusion criteria included active gastrointestinal bleeding, sepsis, renal failure, or pancreatitis. Women with encephalopathy from severe alcoholic hepatitis may be particularly good candidates for glucocorticoids.

Newer understanding of the role of TNF-α expression and receptor activity in alcoholic liver injury has led to an examination of TNF inhibition as an alternative to glucocorticoids for severe alcoholic hepatitis. The nonspecific TNF inhibitor, pentoxifylline, recently demonstrated improved survival in the therapy of severe alcoholic hepatitis (**Fig. 40-3**). Preliminary trials of neutralizing monoclonal antibody specific for TNF have been disappointing because of increased deaths secondary to infection. Because of inordinate surgical mortality and the high rates of recidivism following transplantation, patients with alcoholic hepatitis are not candidates for immediate liver transplantation. The transplant candidacy of these patients should be reevaluated after a defined period of sobriety.

FURTHER READINGS

AKRIVIADIS E et al: Pentoxifylline improves short-term survival in severe acute alcoholic hepatitis: A double blind placebo controlled trial. Gastroenterology 119:1637, 2000

BELL H et al: Long-term prognosis of patients with alcoholic liver cirrhosis: A 15-year follow-up study of 100 Norwegian patients admitted to one unit. Scand J Gastroenterol 9: 858, 2004

LEVITSKY J, MAILLIARD ME: Diagnosis and therapy of alcoholic liver disease. Semin Liver Dis 24: 233, 2004

LUCEY MR et al. Alcoholic hepatitis. N Engl J Med 360:2758, 2009

MATHURIN P et al: Corticosteroids improve short-term survival in patients with severe alcoholic hepatitis (AH): Individual data analysis of the last three randomized placebo controlled double blind trials of corticosteroids in severe AH. J Hepatol 36:480, 2002

REUBEN A: Alcohol and the liver. Curr Opin Gastroenterol 24:328, 2008

SAFDAR K, SCHIFF ER: Alcohol and hepatitis C. Semin Liver Dis 24: 305, 2004

ZAKHARI S, LI TK: Determinants of alcohol use and abuse: Impact of quantity and frequency patterns on liver disease. Hepatology 46:2032, 2007

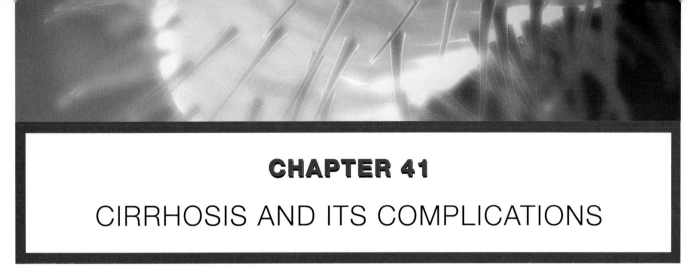

CHAPTER 41

CIRRHOSIS AND ITS COMPLICATIONS

Bruce R. Bacon

Cirrhosis is a condition that is defined histopathologically and has a variety of clinical manifestations and complications, some of which can be life-threatening. In the past, it has been thought that cirrhosis was never reversible; however, it has become apparent that when the underlying insult that has caused the cirrhosis has been removed, there can be reversal of fibrosis. This is most apparent with the successful treatment of chronic hepatitis C; however, reversal of fibrosis is also seen in patients with hemochromatosis who have been successfully treated and in patients with alcoholic liver disease who have discontinued alcohol use.

Regardless of the cause of cirrhosis, the pathologic features consist of the development of fibrosis to the point that there is architectural distortion with the formation of regenerative nodules. This results in a decrease in hepatocellular mass, and thus function, and an alteration of blood flow. The induction of fibrosis occurs with activation of hepatic stellate cells, resulting in the formation of increased amounts of collagen and other components of the extracellular matrix.

Clinical features of cirrhosis are the result of pathologic changes and mirror the severity of the liver disease. Most hepatic pathologists provide an assessment of grading and staging when evaluating liver biopsy samples.

These grading and staging schemes vary between disease states and have been developed for most conditions, including chronic viral hepatitis, nonalcoholic fatty liver disease, and primary biliary cirrhosis. Advanced fibrosis usually includes bridging fibrosis with nodularity designated as stage 3 and cirrhosis designated as stage 4. Patients who have cirrhosis have varying degrees of compensated liver function, and clinicians need to differentiate between those who have stable, compensated cirrhosis and those who have decompensated cirrhosis. Patients who have developed complications of their liver disease and have become decompensated should be considered for liver transplantation. Many of the complications of cirrhosis will require specific therapy. *Portal hypertension* is a significant complicating feature of decompensated cirrhosis and is responsible for the development of ascites and bleeding from esophagogastric varices, two complications that signify decompensated cirrhosis. Loss of hepatocellular function results in jaundice, coagulation disorders, and hypoalbuminemia and contributes to the causes of portosystemic encephalopathy. The complications of cirrhosis are basically the same regardless of the etiology. Nonetheless, it is useful to classify patients by the cause of their liver disease (Table 41-1); patients can be divided into broad groups

TABLE 41-1

CAUSES OF CIRRHOSIS	
Alcoholism	Cardiac cirrhosis
Chronic viral hepatitis	Inherited metabolic liver
Hepatitis B	disease
Hepatitis C	Hemochromatosis
Autoimmune hepatitis	Wilson's disease
Nonalcoholic	α_1 Antitrypsin deficiency
steatohepatitis	Cystic fibrosis
Biliary cirrhosis	Cryptogenic cirrhosis
Primary biliary cirrhosis	
Primary sclerosing	
cholangitis	
Autoimmune	
cholangiopathy	

with alcoholic cirrhosis, cirrhosis due to chronic viral hepatitis, biliary cirrhosis, and other less-common causes such as cardiac cirrhosis, cryptogenic cirrhosis, and other miscellaneous causes.

ALCOHOLIC CIRRHOSIS

Excessive chronic alcohol use can cause several different types of chronic liver disease, including alcoholic fatty liver, alcoholic hepatitis, and alcoholic cirrhosis. Furthermore, use of excessive alcohol can contribute to liver damage in patients with other liver diseases, such as hepatitis C, hemochromatosis, and those patients who have fatty liver disease related to obesity. Chronic alcohol use can produce fibrosis in the absence of accompanying inflammation and/or necrosis. Fibrosis can be centrilobular, pericellular, or periportal. When fibrosis reaches a certain degree, there is disruption of the normal liver architecture and replacement of liver cells by regenerative nodules. In alcoholic cirrhosis, the nodules are usually <3 mm in diameter; this form of cirrhosis is referred to as *micronodular*. With cessation of alcohol use, larger nodules may form, resulting in a mixed micronodular and macronodular cirrhosis.

Pathogenesis

Alcohol is the most commonly used drug in the United States, and more than two-thirds of adults drink alcohol each year. Thirty percent have had a binge within the past month, and over 7% of adults regularly consume more than two drinks per day. Unfortunately, more than 14 million adults in the United States meet the diagnostic criteria for alcohol abuse or dependence. In the United States, chronic liver disease is the tenth most common cause of death in adults, and alcoholic cirrhosis accounts for approximately 40% of deaths due to cirrhosis.

Ethanol is mainly absorbed by the small intestine and, to a lesser degree, through the stomach. Gastric alcohol dehydrogenase (ADH) initiates alcohol metabolism.

Three enzyme systems account for metabolism of alcohol in the liver. These include cytosolic ADH, the microsomal-oxidizing system (MEOS), and peroxisomal catalase. The majority of ethanol oxidation occurs via ADH to form acetaldehyde, which is a highly reactive molecule that may have multiple effects. Ultimately, acetaldehyde is metabolized to acetate by aldehyde dehydrogenase (ALDH). Intake of ethanol increases intracellular accumulation of triglycerides by increasing fatty acid uptake and by reducing fatty acid oxidation and lipoprotein secretion. Protein synthesis, glycosylation, and secretion are impaired. Oxidative damage to hepatocyte membranes occurs due to the formation of reactive oxygen species; acetaldehyde is a highly reactive molecule that combines with proteins to form protein-acetaldehyde adducts. These adducts may interfere with specific enzyme activities, including microtubular formation and hepatic protein trafficking. With acetaldehyde-mediated hepatocyte damage, certain reactive oxygen species can result in Kupffer cell activation. As a result, profibrogenic cytokines are produced that initiate and perpetuate stellate cell activation, with the resultant production of excess collagen and extracellular matrix. Connective tissue appears in both periportal and pericentral zones and eventually connects portal triads with central veins forming regenerative nodules. Hepatocyte loss occurs, and with increased collagen production and deposition, together with continuing hepatocyte destruction, the liver contracts and shrinks in size. This process generally takes from years to decades to occur and requires repeated insults.

Clinical Features

The diagnosis of alcoholic liver disease requires an accurate history regarding both amount and duration of alcohol consumption. Patients with alcoholic liver disease can present with nonspecific symptoms such as vague right upper quadrant pain, fever, nausea and vomiting, diarrhea, anorexia, and malaise. Alternatively, they may present with more specific complications of chronic liver disease, including ascites, edema, or upper gastrointestinal (GI) hemorrhage. Many cases present incidentally at the time of autopsy or elective surgery. Other clinical manifestations include the development of jaundice or encephalopathy. The abrupt onset of any of these complications may be the first event prompting the patient to seek medical attention. Other patients may be identified in the course of an evaluation of routine laboratory studies that are found to be abnormal. On physical examination, the liver and spleen may be enlarged, with the liver edge being firm and nodular. Other frequent findings include scleral icterus, palmar erythema, spider angiomas, parotid gland enlargement, digital clubbing, muscle wasting, or the development of edema and ascites. Men may have decreased body hair and gynecomastia as well as testicular atrophy, which may be a consequence of hormonal abnormalities or a direct toxic effect of alcohol on the testes. In women with advanced alcoholic cirrhosis, menstrual irregularities usually occur, and some women may be amenorrheic. These changes are often reversible following cessation of alcohol.

Laboratory tests may be completely normal in patients with early compensated alcoholic cirrhosis. Alternatively, in advanced liver disease, many abnormalities usually are present. Patients may be anemic either from chronic GI blood loss, nutritional deficiencies, or hypersplenism related to portal hypertension, or as a direct suppressive effect of alcohol on the bone marrow. A unique form of hemolytic anemia (with spur cells and acanthocytes) called *Zieve's syndrome* can occur in patients with severe alcoholic hepatitis. Platelet counts are often reduced early in the disease, reflective of portal hypertension with hypersplenism. Serum total bilirubin can be normal or elevated with advanced disease. Direct bilirubin is frequently mildly elevated in patients with a normal total bilirubin, but the abnormality typically progresses as the disease worsens. Prothrombin times are often prolonged and usually do not respond to administration of parenteral vitamin K. Serum sodium levels are usually normal unless patients have ascites and then can be depressed, largely due to ingestion of excess free water. Serum aminotransferases (ALT, AST) are typically elevated, particularly in patients who continue to drink, with AST levels being higher than ALT levels, usually by a 2:1 ratio.

Diagnosis

Patients who have any of the above-mentioned clinical features, physical examination findings, or laboratory studies should be considered to have alcoholic liver disease. The diagnosis, however, requires accurate knowledge that the patient is continuing to use and abuse alcohol. Furthermore, other forms of chronic liver disease (e.g., chronic viral hepatitis, metabolic or autoimmune liver diseases) must be considered or ruled out or, if present, an estimate of relative causality along with the alcohol use should be determined. Liver biopsy can be helpful to confirm a diagnosis, but generally when patients present with alcoholic hepatitis and are still drinking, liver biopsy is withheld until abstinence has been maintained for at least 6 months in order to determine residual, nonreversible disease.

In patients who have had complications of cirrhosis and who continue to drink, there is a <50% 5-year survival. In contrast, in those patients who are able to remain abstinent, the prognosis is significantly improved. In patients with advanced liver disease, the prognosis remains poor; however, in those individuals who are able to remain abstinent, liver transplantation is a viable option.

℞ Treatment: ALCOHOLIC CIRRHOSIS

Abstinence is the cornerstone of therapy for patients with alcoholic liver disease. In addition, patients require good nutrition and long-term medical supervision in order to manage underlying complications that may develop. Complications such as the development of ascites and edema, variceal hemorrhage, or portosystemic encephalopathy all require specific management and treatment. Glucocorticoids are occasionally used in patients with severe alcoholic hepatitis in the absence of infection. Survival has been shown to improve in certain studies. Treatment is restricted to patients with a discriminant function (DF) value of >32. The DF is calculated as the serum total bilirubin plus the difference in the patient's prothrombin time compared to control (in seconds) multiplied by 4.6. In patients for whom this value is >32, there is improved survival at 28 days with the use of glucocorticoids.

Other therapies that have been used include oral pentoxifylline, which decreases the production of tumor necrosis factor a (TNF-α) and other proinflammatory cytokines. In contrast to glucocorticoids, with which complications can occur, pentoxifylline is relatively easy to administer and has few if any side effects. A variety of nutritional therapies have been tried with either parenteral or enteral feedings; however, it is unclear whether any of these modalities have significantly improved survival.

Recent studies have used parenterally administered inhibitors of TNF-α such as infliximab or etanercept. Early results have shown no adverse events; however, there was no clear-cut improvement in survival. Anabolic steroids, propylthiouracil, antioxidants, colchicine, and penicillamine have all been used but do not show clear-cut benefit and are not recommended.

As mentioned above, the cornerstone to treatment is cessation of alcohol use. Recent experience with medications that reduce craving for alcohol such as acamprosate calcium has been favorable. Patients may take other necessary medications even in the presence of cirrhosis. Acetaminophen use is often discouraged in patients with liver disease; however, if no more than 2 g of acetaminophen per day are consumed, there generally are no problems.

CIRRHOSIS DUE TO CHRONIC VIRAL HEPATITIS B OR C

Of patients exposed to the hepatitis C virus (HCV), approximately 80% develop chronic hepatitis C, and of those, about 20–30% will develop cirrhosis over 20–30 years. Many of these patients have had concomitant alcohol use, and the true incidence of cirrhosis due to hepatitis C alone is unknown.

Nonetheless, this represents a significant number of patients. It is expected that an even higher percentage will go on to develop cirrhosis over longer periods of time. In the United States, approximately 5 million people have been exposed to the hepatitis C virus, with about $3^{1/2}$–4 million who are chronically viremic. Worldwide, about 170 million individuals have hepatitis C, with some areas of the world (e.g., Egypt) having up to 15% of the population infected. HCV is a noncytopathic virus, and liver damage is probably immune-mediated. Progression of liver disease due to chronic hepatitis C is characterized by portal-based fibrosis with bridging fibrosis and nodularity developing, ultimately culminating in the development of cirrhosis. In cirrhosis due to chronic hepatitis C, the liver is small and shrunken with characteristic features of a mixed micro- and macronodular cirrhosis seen on liver biopsy. In addition to the increased fibrosis that is seen in cirrhosis due to hepatitis C, an inflammatory infiltrate is found in portal areas with interface hepatitis and occasionally some lobular hepatocellular injury and inflammation. In patients with HCV genotype 3, steatosis is often present.

Similar findings are seen in patients with cirrhosis due to chronic hepatitis B. Of patients exposed to hepatitis B, about 5% develop chronic hepatitis B, and about 20% of those patients will go on to develop cirrhosis. Special stains for HBc (hepatitis B core) and HBs (hepatitis B surface) antigen will be positive, and ground glass hepatocytes signifying HBsAg (hepatitis B surface antigen) may be present. In the United States, there are about 1.25 million carriers of hepatitis B, whereas in other parts of the world where hepatitis B virus (HBV) is endemic (i.e., Southeast Asia, sub-Saharan Africa), up to 15% of the population may be infected having acquired the infection vertically at the time of birth. Thus, over 300–400 million individuals are thought to have hepatitis B worldwide. Approximately 25% of these individuals may ultimately develop cirrhosis.

Clinical Features and Diagnosis

Patients with cirrhosis due to either chronic hepatitis C or B can present with the usual symptoms and signs of chronic liver disease. Fatigue, malaise, vague right upper quadrant pain, and laboratory abnormalities are frequent presenting features. Diagnosis requires a thorough laboratory evaluation, including quantitative HCV RNA testing and analysis for HCV genotype, or hepatitis B serologies to include HBsAg, anti-HBs, HBeAg (hepatitis B e antigen), anti-HBe, and quantitative HBV DNA levels.

Treatment:
℞ CIRRHOSIS DUE TO CHRONIC VIRAL HEPATITIS B OR C

Management of complications of cirrhosis revolves around specific therapy for treatment of whatever complications occur, whether they be esophageal variceal hemorrhage, development of ascites and edema, or encephalopathy. In patients with chronic hepatitis B, numerous studies have shown beneficial effects of antiviral therapy, which is effective at viral suppression, as evidenced by reducing aminotransferase levels and HBV DNA levels, and improving histology by reducing inflammation and fibrosis. Several clinical trials and case series have demonstrated that patients with decompensated liver disease can become compensated with the use of antiviral therapy directed against hepatitis B. Currently available therapy includes lamivudine, adefovir, entecavir, and tenofovir. Interferon α can also be used for treating hepatitis B, but it should not be used in cirrhotics.

Treatment of patients with cirrhosis due to hepatitis C is a little more difficult because the side effects of pegylated interferon and ribavirin therapy are oftentimes difficult to manage in patients with cirrhosis. Dose-limiting cytopenias (platelets, white blood cells, red blood cells) or severe side effects can result in discontinuation of treatment. Nonetheless, if patients can tolerate treatment, and if it is successful, the benefit is great and disease progression is reduced.

CIRRHOSIS FROM AUTOIMMUNE HEPATITIS AND NONALCOHOLIC FATTY LIVER DISEASE

Other causes of posthepatitic cirrhosis include autoimmune hepatitis and cirrhosis due to nonalcoholic steatohepatitis. Many patients with autoimmune hepatitis (AIH) present with cirrhosis that is already established. Typically, these patients will not benefit from immunosuppressive therapy with glucocorticoids or azathioprine since the AIH is "burned out." In this situation, liver biopsy does not show a significant inflammatory infiltrate. Diagnosis in this setting requires positive autoimmune markers such as antinuclear antibody (ANA) or anti–smooth-muscle antibody (ASMA). When patients with AIH present with cirrhosis and active inflammation accompanied by elevated liver enzymes, there can be considerable benefit from the use of immunosuppressive therapy.

Patients with nonalcoholic steatohepatitis are increasingly being found to have progressed to cirrhosis. With the epidemic of obesity that continues in Western countries, more and more patients are identified with nonalcoholic fatty liver disease. Of these, a significant subset have nonalcoholic steatohepatitis and can progress to increased fibrosis and cirrhosis. Over the past several years, it has been increasingly recognized that many patients who were thought to have cryptogenic cirrhosis in fact have nonalcoholic steatohepatitis. As their cirrhosis progresses, they become catabolic and then lose the telltale signs of steatosis seen on biopsy. Management of complications of cirrhosis due to either AIH or nonalcoholic steatohepatitis is similar to that for other forms of cirrhosis.

BILIARY CIRRHOSIS

Biliary cirrhosis has pathologic features that are different from either alcoholic cirrhosis or posthepatitic cirrhosis, yet the manifestations of end-stage liver disease are the same. Cholestatic liver disease may result from necroinflammatory lesions, congenital or metabolic processes, or external bile duct compression. Thus, two broad categories reflect the anatomic sites of abnormal bile retention: *intrahepatic* and *extrahepatic*. The distinction is important for obvious therapeutic reasons. Extrahepatic obstruction may benefit from surgical or endoscopic biliary tract decompression, whereas intrahepatic cholestatic processes will not improve with such interventions and require a different approach.

The major causes of chronic cholestatic syndromes are primary biliary cirrhosis (PBC), autoimmune cholangitis, primary sclerosing cholangitis (PSC), and idiopathic adulthood ductopenia. These syndromes are usually clinically distinguished from each other by antibody testing, cholangiographic findings, and clinical presentation. However, they all share the histopathologic features of chronic cholestasis, such as cholate stasis, copper deposition, xanthomatous transformation of hepatocytes, and irregular so-called biliary fibrosis. In addition, there may be chronic portal inflammation, interface activity, and chronic lobular inflammation. Ductopenia is a result of this progressive disease as patients develop cirrhosis.

PRIMARY BILIARY CIRRHOSIS

PBC is seen in about 100–200 individuals per million, with a strong female preponderance and a median age of around 50 years at the time of diagnosis. The cause of PBC is unknown; it is characterized by portal inflammation and necrosis of cholangiocytes in small and medium-sized bile ducts. Cholestatic features prevail, and biliary cirrhosis is characterized by an elevated bilirubin level and progressive liver failure. Liver transplantation is the treatment of choice for patients with decompensated cirrhosis due to PBC. A variety of therapies have been proposed, but ursodeoxycholic acid (UDCA) is the only approved treatment that has some degree of efficacy by slowing the rate of progression of the disease.

Antimitochondrial antibodies (AMA) are present in about 90% of patients with PBC. These autoantibodies recognize intermitochondrial membrane proteins that are enzymes of the pyruvate dehydrogenase complex (PDC), the branched chain–2-oxoacid dehydrogenase complex, and the 2-oxogluterate dehydrogenase complex.

Most relate to pyruvate dehydrogenase. These autoantibodies are not pathogenic but rather are useful markers for making a diagnosis of PBC.

Pathology

Histopathologic analyses of liver biopsies of patients with PBC have resulted in identifying four distinct stages of the disease as it progresses. The earliest lesion is termed *chronic nonsuppurative destructive cholangitis* and is a necrotizing inflammatory process of the portal tracts. Medium and small bile ducts are infiltrated with lymphocytes and undergo duct destruction. Mild fibrosis and sometimes bile stasis can occur. With progression, the inflammatory infiltrate becomes less prominent, but the number of bile ducts is reduced and there is proliferation of smaller bile ductules. Increased fibrosis ensues with the expansion of periportal fibrosis to bridging fibrosis. Finally, cirrhosis, which may be micronodular or macronodular, develops.

Clinical Features

Currently most patients with PBC are diagnosed well before the end-stage manifestations of the disease are present, and, as such, most patients are actually asymptomatic. When symptoms are present, they most prominently include a significant degree of fatigue out of proportion to what would be expected for either the severity of the liver disease or the age of the patient. Pruritus is seen in approximately 50% of patients at the time of diagnosis and can be debilitating. It may be intermittent and usually is most bothersome in the evening. In some patients, pruritus can develop toward the end of pregnancy, and there are examples of patients having been diagnosed with cholestasis of pregnancy rather than PBC. Pruritus that presents prior to the development of jaundice indicates severe disease and a poor prognosis.

Physical examination can show jaundice and other complications of chronic liver disease including hepatomegaly, splenomegaly, ascites, and edema. Other features that are unique to PBC include hyperpigmentation, xanthelasma, and xanthomata, which are related to the altered cholesterol metabolism seen in this disease. Hyperpigmentation is evident on the trunk and the arms and is seen in areas of exfoliation and lichenification associated with progressive scratching related to the pruritus. Bone pain resulting from osteopenia or osteoporosis is occasionally seen at the time of diagnosis.

Laboratory Findings

Laboratory findings in PBC show cholestatic liver enzyme abnormalities with an elevation in γ-glutamyl transpeptidase and alkaline phosphatase (ALP) along with mild elevations in aminotransferases (ALT and AST). Immunoglobulins, particularly IgM, are typically increased. Hyperbilirubinemia usually is seen once cirrhosis has developed. Thrombocytopenia, leukopenia, and anemia may be seen in patients with portal hypertension and hypersplenism. Liver biopsy shows characteristic features as described above and should be evident to any experienced hepatopathologist. Up to 10% of patients with characteristic PBC will have features of AIH as well and are defined as having "overlap" syndrome. These patients are treated as PBC patients and may progress to cirrhosis with the same frequency as typical PBC patients.

Diagnosis

PBC should be considered in patients with chronic cholestatic liver enzyme abnormalities. It is most often seen in middle-aged women. AMA testing may be negative, and it should be remembered that as many as 10% of patients with PBC may be AMA-negative. Liver biopsy is most important in this setting of AMA-negative PBC. In patients who are AMA-negative with cholestatic liver enzymes, PSC should be ruled out by way of cholangiography.

℞ Treatment: PRIMARY BILIARY CIRRHOSIS

Treatment of the typical manifestations of cirrhosis are no different for PBC than for other forms of cirrhosis. UDCA has been shown to improve both biochemical and histologic features of the disease. Improvement is greatest when therapy is initiated early; the likelihood of significant improvement with UDCA is low in patients with PBC who present with manifestations of cirrhosis. UDCA is given in doses of 13–15 mg/kg per day; the medication is usually well-tolerated, although some patients have worsening pruritus with initiation of therapy. A small proportion of patients may have diarrhea or headache as a side effect of the drug. UDCA has been shown to slow the rate of progression of PBC, but it does not reverse or cure the disease. Patients with PBC require long-term follow-up by a physician experienced with the disease. Certain patients may need to be considered for liver transplantation should their liver disease decompensate.

The main symptoms of PBC are fatigue and pruritus, and symptom management is important. Several therapies have been tried for treatment of fatigue, but none of them have been successful; frequent naps should be encouraged. Pruritus is treated with antihistamines, narcotic receptor antagonists (naltrexone), and rifampin. Cholestyramine, a bile salt sequestering agent, has been helpful in some patients but is somewhat tedious and difficult to take. Plasmapheresis has been utilized rarely in patients with severe intractable pruritus. There is an increased incidence of osteopenia and osteoporosis in patients with cholestatic liver disease, and bone density testing should be performed. Treatment with a bisphosphonate should be instituted when bone disease is identified.

PRIMARY SCLEROSING CHOLANGITIS

As in PBC, the cause of PSC remains unknown. PSC is a chronic cholestatic syndrome that is characterized by diffuse inflammation and fibrosis involving the entire biliary tree, resulting in chronic cholestasis. This pathologic process ultimately results in obliteration of both the intra- and extrahepatic biliary tree, leading to biliary cirrhosis, portal hypertension, and liver failure. The cause of PSC remains unknown despite extensive investigation into various mechanisms related to bacterial and viral infections, toxins, genetic predisposition, and immunologic mechanisms, all of which have been postulated to contribute to the pathogenesis and progression of this syndrome.

Pathologic changes that can occur in PSC show bile duct proliferation as well as ductopenia and fibrous cholangitis (pericholangitis). Oftentimes, liver biopsy changes in PSC are not pathognomonic, and establishing the diagnosis of PSC must involve imaging of the biliary tree. Periductal fibrosis is occasionally seen on biopsy specimens and can be quite helpful in making the diagnosis. As the disease progresses, biliary cirrhosis is the final end-stage manifestation of PSC.

Clinical Features

The usual clinical features of PSC are those found in cholestatic liver disease, with fatigue, pruritus, steatorrhea, deficiencies of fat-soluble vitamins, and the associated consequences. As in PBC, the fatigue is profound and nonspecific. Pruritus can oftentimes be debilitating and is related to the cholestasis. The severity of pruritus does not correlate with the severity of the disease. Metabolic bone disease, as seen in PBC, can occur with PSC and should be treated (see "Primary Biliary Cirrhosis" earlier in the chapter).

Laboratory Findings

Patients with PSC typically are identified in the course of an evaluation of abnormal liver enzymes. Most patients have at least a twofold increase in ALP and may have elevated aminotransferases as well. Albumin levels may be decreased, and prothrombin times are prolonged in a substantial proportion of patients at the time of diagnosis. Some degree of correction of a prolonged prothrombin time may occur with parenteral vitamin K.

A small subset of patients have aminotransferase elevations greater than five times the upper limit of normal and may have features of AIH on biopsy. These individuals are thought to have an overlap syndrome between PSC and AIH. Autoantibodies are frequently positive in patients with the overlap syndrome but are typically negative in patients who only have PSC. One autoantibody, the perinuclear antineutrophil cytoplasmic antibody (P-ANCA) is positive in about 65% of patients with PSC. Over 50% of patients with PSC also have ulcerative colitis (UC); accordingly, once a diagnosis of PSC is established, colonoscopy should be performed looking for evidence of UC.

Diagnosis

The definitive diagnosis of PSC requires cholangiographic imaging. Over the last several years, MRI with magnetic resonance cholangiopancreatography (MRCP) has been utilized as the imaging technique of choice for initial evaluation. Once patients are screened in this manner, some investigators feel that endoscopic retrograde cholangiopancreatography (ERCP) should also be performed to be certain whether or not a dominant stricture is present. Typical cholangiographic findings in PSC are multifocal stricturing and beading involving both the intrahepatic and extrahepatic biliary tree. However, though involvement may be of the intrahepatic bile ducts alone or of the extrahepatic bile ducts alone, more commonly both are involved. These strictures are typically short and with intervening segments of normal or slightly dilated bile ducts that are distributed diffusely, producing the classic beaded appearance. The gallbladder and cystic duct can be involved in up to 15% of cases. Patients with high-grade, diffuse stricturing of the intrahepatic bile ducts have an overall poor prognosis. Gradually, biliary cirrhosis develops, and patients will progress to decompensated liver disease with all the manifestations of ascites, esophageal variceal hemorrhage, and encephalopathy.

℞ Treatment:
PRIMARY SCLEROSING CHOLANGITIS

There is no specific proven treatment for PSC, although studies are currently ongoing using high-dose (20 mg/kg per day) UDCA to determine its benefit. Endoscopic dilatation of dominant strictures can be helpful, but the ultimate treatment is liver transplantation. A dreaded complication of PSC is the development of cholangiocarcinoma, which is a relative contraindication to liver transplantation. Symptoms of pruritus are common, and the approach is as mentioned previously for this problem in patients with PBC (see "Primary Biliary Cirrhosis" earlier in the chapter).

CARDIAC CIRRHOSIS

Definition

Patients with long-standing right-sided congestive heart failure may develop chronic liver injury and cardiac cirrhosis. This is an increasingly uncommon, if not rare, cause of chronic liver disease given the advances made in the care of patients with heart failure.

Etiology and Pathology

In the case of long-term right-sided heart failure, there is an elevated venous pressure transmitted via the inferior vena cava and hepatic veins to the sinusoids of the liver, which become dilated and engorged with blood. The liver becomes enlarged and swollen, and with long-term passive congestion and relative ischemia due to poor circulation, centrilobular hepatocytes can become necrotic, leading to pericentral fibrosis. This fibrotic pattern can extend to the periphery of the lobule outward until a unique pattern of fibrosis causing cirrhosis can occur.

Clinical Features

Patients typically have signs of congestive heart failure and will manifest an enlarged firm liver on physical examination. ALP levels are characteristically elevated, and aminotransferases may be normal or slightly increased with AST usually higher than ALT. It is unlikely that patients will develop variceal hemorrhage or encephalopathy.

Diagnosis

The diagnosis is usually made in someone with clear-cut cardiac disease who has an elevated ALP and an enlarged liver. Liver biopsy shows a pattern of fibrosis that can be recognized by an experienced hepatopathologist. Differentiation from Budd-Chiari syndrome (BCS) can be made by seeing extravasation of red blood cells in BCS, but not in cardiac hepatopathy. Venoocclusive disease can also affect hepatic outflow and has characteristic features on liver biopsy. Venoocclusive disease can be seen under the circumstances of conditioning for bone marrow transplant with radiation and chemotherapy; it can also be seen with the ingestion of certain herbal teas as well as pyrrolizidine alkaloids. This is typically seen in Caribbean countries and rarely in the United States. Treatment is based on management of the underlying cardiac disease.

OTHER TYPES OF CIRRHOSIS

There are several other less common causes of chronic liver disease that can progress to cirrhosis. These include inherited metabolic liver diseases such as hemochromatosis,

Wilson's disease, α_1 antitrypsin (α_1AT) deficiency, and cystic fibrosis. For all of these disorders, the manifestations of cirrhosis are similar, with some minor variations, to those seen in other patients with other causes of cirrhosis.

Hemochromatosis is an inherited disorder of iron metabolism that results in a progressive increase in hepatic iron deposition which, over time, can lead to a portal-based fibrosis progressing to cirrhosis, liver failure, and hepatocellular cancer. While the frequency of hemochromatosis is relatively common, with genetic susceptibility occurring in 1 in 250 individuals, the frequency of end-stage manifestations due to the disease is relatively low, and fewer than 5% of those patients who are genotypically susceptible will go on to develop severe liver disease from hemochromatosis. Diagnosis is made with serum iron studies showing an elevated transferrin saturation and an elevated ferritin level, along with abnormalities identified by *HFE* mutation analysis. Treatment is straightforward, with regular therapeutic phlebotomy.

Wilson's disease is an inherited disorder of copper homeostasis with failure to excrete excess amounts of copper, leading to an accumulation in the liver. This disorder is relatively uncommon, affecting 1 in 30,000 individuals. Wilson's disease typically affects adolescents and young adults. Prompt diagnosis before end-stage manifestations become irreversible can lead to significant clinical improvement. Diagnosis requires determination of ceruloplasmin levels, which are low; 24-hour urine copper levels, which are elevated; typical physical examination findings, including Kayser-Fleischer corneal rings, and characteristic liver biopsy findings. Treatment consists of copper chelating medications.

α_1AT deficiency results from an inherited disorder that causes abnormal folding of the α_1AT protein, resulting in failure of secretion of that protein from the liver. It is unknown how the retained protein leads to liver disease. Patients with α_1AT deficiency at greatest risk for developing chronic liver disease have the ZZ genotype, but only about 10–20% of such individuals will develop chronic liver disease. Diagnosis is made by determining α_1AT levels and genotype. Characteristic PAS-positive, diastase-resistant globules are seen on liver biopsy. The only effective treatment is liver transplantation, which is curative.

Cystic fibrosis is an uncommon inherited disorder affecting Caucasians of Northern European descent. A biliary-type cirrhosis can occur, and some patients derive benefit from the chronic use of UDCA.

MAJOR COMPLICATIONS OF CIRRHOSIS

The clinical course of patients with advanced cirrhosis is often complicated by a number of important sequelae that can occur regardless of the underlying cause of the liver disease. These include portal hypertension and its

TABLE 41-2

COMPLICATIONS OF CIRRHOSIS

Portal hypertension	Coagulopathy
Gastroesophageal varices	Factor deficiency
Portal hypertensive gastropathy	Fibrinolysis
Splenomegaly, hypersplenism	Thrombocytopenia
Ascites	Bone disease
Spontaneous bacterial peritonitis	Osteopenia
Hepatorenal syndrome	Osteoporosis
Type 1	Osteomalacia
Type 2	Hematologic abnormalities
Hepatic encephalopathy	Anemia
Hepatopulmonary syndrome	Hemolysis
Portopulmonary hypertension	Thrombocytopenia
Malnutrition	Neutropenia

consequences of gastroesophageal variceal hemorrhage, splenomegaly, ascites, hepatic encephalopathy, spontaneous bacterial peritonitis (SBP), hepatorenal syndrome, and hepatocellular carcinoma (**Table 41-2**).

PORTAL HYPERTENSION

Portal hypertension is defined as the elevation of the hepatic venous pressure gradient (HVPG) to >5 mmHg. Portal hypertension is caused by a combination of two simultaneously occurring hemodynamic processes: (1) increased intrahepatic resistance to the passage of blood flow through the liver due to cirrhosis and regenerative nodules, and (2) increased splanchnic blood flow secondary to vasodilatation within the splanchnic vascular bed. Portal hypertension is directly responsible for the two major complications of cirrhosis, variceal hemorrhage and ascites. *Variceal hemorrhage* is an immediate life-threatening problem with a 20–30% mortality associated with each episode of bleeding. The portal venous system normally drains blood from the stomach, intestines, spleen, pancreas, and gallbladder, and the portal vein is formed by the confluence of the superior mesenteric and splenic veins. Deoxygenated blood from the small bowel drains into the superior mesenteric vein along with blood from the head of the pancreas, the ascending colon, and part of the transverse colon. Conversely, the splenic vein drains the spleen and the pancreas and is joined by the inferior mesenteric vein, which brings blood from the transverse and descending colon as well as from the superior two-thirds of the rectum. Thus, the portal vein normally receives blood from almost the entire GI tract.

The causes of portal hypertension are usually subcategorized as prehepatic, intrahepatic, and posthepatic

TABLE 41-3

CLASSIFICATION OF PORTAL HYPERTENSION

Prehepatic
    Portal vein thrombosis
    Splenic vein thrombosis
    Massive splenomegaly (Banti's syndrome)
Hepatic
    Presinusoidal
        Schistosomiasis
        Congenital hepatic fibrosis
    Sinusoidal
        Cirrhosis—many causes
        Alcoholic hepatitis
    Postsinusoidal
        Hepatic sinusoidal obstruction (venoocclusive
        syndrome)
Posthepatic
    Budd-Chiari syndrome
    Inferior vena caval webs
    Cardiac causes
        Restrictive cardiomyopathy
        Constrictive pericarditis
        Severe congestive heart failure

(Table 41-3). Prehepatic causes of portal hypertension are those affecting the portal venous system before it enters the liver; they include portal vein thrombosis and splenic vein thrombosis. Posthepatic causes encompass those affecting the hepatic veins and venous drainage to the heart; they include BCS, venoocclusive disease, and chronic right-sided cardiac congestion. Intrahepatic causes account for over 95% of cases of portal hypertension and are represented by the major forms of cirrhosis. Intrahepatic causes of portal hypertension can be further subdivided into presinusoidal, sinusoidal, and postsinusoidal causes. Postsinusoidal causes include venoocclusive disease, while presinusoidal causes include congenital hepatic fibrosis and schistosomiasis. Sinusoidal causes are related to cirrhosis from various causes.

Cirrhosis is the most common cause of portal hypertension in the United States, and clinically significant portal hypertension is present in >60% of patients with cirrhosis. Portal vein obstruction may be idiopathic or can occur in association with cirrhosis or with infection, pancreatitis, or abdominal trauma.

Coagulation disorders that can lead to the development of portal vein thrombosis include polycythemia vera; essential thrombocytosis; deficiencies in protein C, protein S, antithrombin 3, and factor V Leiden; and abnormalities in the gene regulating prothrombin production. Some patients may have a subclinical myeloproliferative disorder.

Clinical Features

The three primary complications of portal hypertension are gastroesophageal varices with hemorrhage, ascites,

and hypersplenism. Thus, patients may present with upper GI bleeding, which on endoscopy is found to be due to esophageal or gastric varices, with the development of ascites along with peripheral edema, or with an enlarged spleen with associated reduction in platelets and white blood cells on routine laboratory testing.

Esophageal Varices

Over the last decade, it has become common practice to screen known cirrhotics with endoscopy to look for esophageal varices. Such screening studies have shown that approximately one-third of patients with histologically confirmed cirrhosis have varices. Approximately 5–15% of cirrhotics per year develop varices, and it is estimated that the majority of patients with cirrhosis will develop varices over their lifetime. Furthermore, it is anticipated that roughly one-third of patients with varices will develop bleeding. Several factors predict the risk of bleeding, including the severity of cirrhosis (Child's class); the height of wedged-hepatic vein pressure; the size of the varix; the location of the varix; and certain endoscopic stigmata, including red wale signs, hematocystic spots, diffuse erythema, bluish color, cherry-red spots, or white-nipple spots. Patients with tense ascites are also at increased risk for bleeding from varices.

Diagnosis

In patients with cirrhosis who are being followed chronically, the development of portal hypertension is usually revealed by the presence of thrombocytopenia; the appearance of an enlarged spleen; or the development of ascites, encephalopathy and/or esophageal varices with or without bleeding. In previously undiagnosed patients, any of these features should prompt further evaluation to determine the presence of portal hypertension and liver disease. Varices should be identified by endoscopy. Abdominal imaging, either by CT or MRI, can be helpful in demonstrating a nodular liver and in finding changes of portal hypertension with intraabdominal collateral circulation. If necessary, interventional radiologic procedures can be performed to determine wedged and free hepatic vein pressures that will allow for the calculation of a wedged-to-free gradient, which is equivalent to the portal pressure. The average normal wedged-to-free gradient is 5 mmHg, and patients with a gradient >12 mmHg are at risk for variceal hemorrhage.

℞ Treatment:
VARICEAL HEMORRHAGE

Treatment for variceal hemorrhage as a complication of portal hypertension is divided into two main categories: (1) primary prophylaxis and (2) prevention of re-bleeding once there has been an initial variceal hemorrhage. Primary prophylaxis requires routine screening by endoscopy of all patients with cirrhosis. Once varices that are at increased risk for bleeding are identified, then primary prophylaxis can be achieved either through nonselective beta blockade or by variceal band ligation. Numerous placebo-controlled clinical trials of either propranolol or nadolol have been reported in the literature. The most rigorous studies were those that only included patients with significantly enlarged varices or with hepatic vein pressure gradients >12 mmHg. Patients treated with beta blockers have a lower risk of variceal hemorrhage than those treated with placebo over 1 and 2 years of follow-up. There is also a decrease in mortality related to variceal hemorrhage. Unfortunately, overall survival was improved in only one study. Further studies have demonstrated that the degree of reduction of portal pressure is a significant feature to determine success of therapy. Therefore, it is has been suggested that repeat measurements of hepatic vein pressure gradients may be used to guide pharmacologic therapy; however, this may be cost prohibitive. Several studies have evaluated variceal band ligation and variceal sclerotherapy as methods for providing primary prophylaxis.

Endoscopic variceal ligation (EVL) has achieved a level of success and comfort with most gastroenterologists who see patients with these complications of portal hypertension. Thus, in patients with cirrhosis who are screened for portal hypertension and are found to have large varices, it is recommended that they receive either beta blockade or primary prophylaxis with EVL.

The approach to patients once they have had a variceal bleed is first to treat the acute bleed, which can be life-threatening, and then to prevent further bleeding. Prevention of further bleeding is usually accomplished with repeated variceal band ligation until varices are obliterated. Treatment of acute bleeding requires both fluid and blood product replacement as well as prevention of subsequent bleeding with EVL.

The medical management of acute variceal hemorrhage includes the use of vasoconstricting agents, usually somatostatin or Octreotide. Vasopressin was used in the past but is no longer commonly used. Balloon tamponade (Sengstaken-Blakemore tube or Minnesota tube) can be used in patients who cannot get endoscopic therapy immediately or who need stabilization prior to endoscopic therapy. Control of bleeding can be achieved in the vast majority of cases; however, bleeding recurs in the majority of patients if definitive endoscopic therapy has not been instituted. Octreotide, a direct splanchnic vasoconstrictor, is given at dosages of 50–100 μg/h by continuous infusion. Endoscopic intervention is employed as first-line treatment to control bleeding acutely. Some endoscopists will use variceal injection therapy (sclerotherapy) as initial therapy, particularly when bleeding is vigorous. Variceal band ligation is used to control acute bleeding in over 90% of cases and should be repeated until obliteration of all varices is accomplished. When esophageal varices extend into the proximal stomach, band ligation is less successful. In these situations, when bleeding continues from gastric varices, consideration for transjugular intrahepatic portosystemic shunt (TIPS) should be made. This technique creates a portosystemic shunt by a percutaneous approach using an expandable metal stent, which is advanced under angiographic guidance to the hepatic veins and then through the substance of the liver to create a direct portocaval shunt. This offers an alternative to surgery for acute decompression of portal hypertension. Encephalopathy can occur in as many as 20% of patients after TIPS and is particularly problematic in elderly patients and in those patients with preexisting encephalopathy. TIPS should be reserved for those individuals who fail endoscopic or medical management or who are poor surgical risks. TIPS can sometimes be used as a bridge to transplantation. Surgical esophageal transection is a procedure that is rarely used and generally is associated with a poor outcome.

PREVENTION OF RECURRENT BLEEDING (Fig. 41-1) Once patients have had an acute bleed and have been managed successfully, attention should be paid to prevent recurrent bleeding. This usually requires repeated variceal band ligation until varices are obliterated. Beta blockade may be of adjunctive benefit in patients who are having recurrent variceal band ligation; however, once varices have been obliterated, the need for beta blockade is lessened. Despite successful variceal obliteration, many patients will still have portal hypertensive gastropathy from which bleeding can occur. Nonselective beta blockade may be helpful to prevent further bleeding from portal hypertensive gastropathy once varices have been obliterated.

Portosystemic shunt surgery is less commonly performed with the advent of TIPS; nonetheless, this procedure should be considered for patients with good hepatic synthetic function who could benefit by having portal decompressive surgery.

SPLENOMEGALY AND HYPERSPLENISM

Congestive splenomegaly is common in patients with portal hypertension. Clinical features include the presence of an enlarged spleen on physical examination and the development of thrombocytopenia and leukopenia in patients who have cirrhosis. Some patients will have fairly significant left-sided and left-upper quadrant abdominal pain related to an enlarged and engorged spleen. Splenomegaly itself usually requires no specific

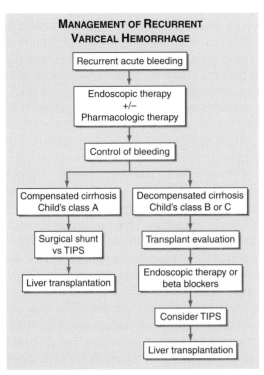

FIGURE 41-1

Management of recurrent variceal hemorrhage. This algorithm describes an approach to management of patients who have recurrent bleeding from esophageal varices. Initial therapy is generally with endoscopic therapy often supplemented by pharmacologic therapy. With control of bleeding, a decision needs to be made as to whether patients should go on to a surgical shunt or TIPS (if they are Child's class A) and be considered for transplant, or if they should have TIPS and be considered for transplant (if they are Child's class B or C). TIPS, transjugular intrahepatic portosystemic shunt.

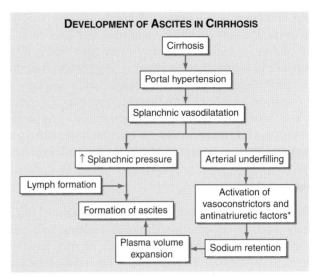

FIGURE 41-2

Development of ascites in cirrhosis. This flow diagram illustrates the importance of portal hypertension with splanchnic vasodilatation in the development of ascites. *Antinatriuretic factors include the renin-angiotensin-aldosterone system and the sympathetic nervous system.

treatment, although splenectomy can be successfully performed under very special circumstances.

Hypersplenism with the development of thrombocytopenia is a common feature of patients with cirrhosis and is usually the first indication of portal hypertension.

ASCITES

Definition

Ascites is the accumulation of fluid within the peritoneal cavity. Overwhelmingly, the most common cause of ascites is portal hypertension related to cirrhosis; however, clinicians should remember that malignant or infectious causes of ascites can be present as well, and careful differentiation of these other causes are obviously important for patient care.

Pathogenesis

The presence of portal hypertension contributes to the development of ascites in patients who have cirrhosis

(Fig. 41-2). There is an increase in intrahepatic resistance, causing increased portal pressure, but there is also vasodilatation of the splanchnic arterial system, which in turn results in an increase in portal venous inflow. Both of these abnormalities result in increased production of splanchnic lymph. Vasodilating factors such as nitric oxide are responsible for the vasodilatory effect. These hemodynamic changes result in sodium retention by causing activation of the renin-angiotensin-aldosterone system with the development of hyperaldosteronism. The renal effects of increased aldosterone leading to sodium retention also contribute to the development of ascites. Sodium retention causes fluid accumulation and expansion of the extracellular fluid volume, which results in the formation of peripheral edema and ascites. Sodium retention is the consequence of a homeostatic response caused by underfilling of the arterial circulation secondary to arterial vasodilatation in the splanchnic vascular bed. Because the retained fluid is constantly leaking out of the intravascular compartment into the peritoneal cavity, the sensation of vascular filling is not achieved, and the process continues. Hypoalbuminemia and reduced plasma oncotic pressure also contribute to the loss of fluid from the vascular compartment into the peritoneal cavity. Hypoalbuminemia is due to decreased synthetic function in a cirrhotic liver.

Clinical Features

Patients typically note an increase in abdominal girth that is often accompanied by the development of peripheral edema. The development of ascites is often insidious, and it is surprising that some patients wait so long and become so distended before seeking medical attention. Patients usually have at least 1–2 L of fluid in the abdomen before they are aware that there is an increase. If ascitic fluid is massive, respiratory function can be compromised, and patients will complain of shortness of breath. Hepatic hydrothorax may also occur in this setting, contributing to respiratory symptoms. Patients with massive ascites are often malnourished and have muscle wasting and excessive fatigue and weakness.

Diagnosis

Diagnosis of ascites is by physical examination and is often aided by abdominal imaging. Patients will have bulging flanks, may have a fluid wave, or may have the presence of shifting dullness. This is determined by taking patients from a supine position to lying on either their left or right side and noting the movement of the dullness to percussion. Subtle amounts of ascites can be detected by ultrasound or CT scanning. Hepatic hydrothorax is more common on the right side and implicates a rent in the diaphragm with free flow of ascitic fluid into the thoracic cavity.

When patients present with ascites for the first time, it is recommended that a diagnostic paracentesis be performed to characterize the fluid. This should include the determination of total protein and albumin content, blood cell counts with differential, and cultures. In the appropriate setting, amylase may be measured and cytology performed. In patients with cirrhosis, the protein concentration of the ascitic fluid is quite low, with the majority of patients having an ascitic fluid protein concentration <1 g/dL. The development of the serum ascites-to-albumin gradient (SAAG) has replaced the description of exudative or transudative fluid. When the gradient between the serum albumin level and the ascitic fluid albumin level is >1.1 g/dL, then the cause of the ascites is most likely due to portal hypertension; this is most often in the setting of cirrhosis. When the gradient is <1.1 g/dL, infectious or malignant causes of ascites should be considered. When levels of ascitic fluid proteins are very low, patients are at increased risk for developing SBP. A high level of red blood cells in the ascitic fluid signifies a traumatic tap, or perhaps a hepatocellular cancer, or a ruptured omental varix. When the absolute level of polymorphonuclear leukocytes is >250 mm^3, then the question of ascitic fluid infection should be strongly considered. Ascitic fluid cultures should be obtained using bedside inoculation of culture media.

℞ Treatment: ASCITES

Patients with small amounts of ascites can usually be managed with dietary sodium restriction alone. Most average diets in the United States contain 6–8 g of

sodium per day and if patients eat at restaurants or fast food outlets, the amount of sodium in their diet can exceed this amount. Thus, it is often extremely difficult to get patients to change their dietary habits to ingest < 2 g of sodium per day, which is the amount that is recommended. Patients are frequently surprised to realize how much sodium is in the standard U.S. diet and thus it is important to make educational pamphlets available to the patient. Often, a simple recommendation is to eat fresh or frozen foods, avoiding canned or processed foods, which are usually preserved with sodium. When a moderate amount of ascites is present, diuretic therapy is usually necessary. Traditionally, spironolactone at 100–200 mg/d as a single dose is started, and furosemide may be added at 40–80 mg/d, particularly in patients who have peripheral edema. In patients who have never received diuretics before, the failure of the above-mentioned dosages suggests that they are not being compliant with a low-sodium diet. If compliance is confirmed and ascitic fluid is not being mobilized, spironolactone can be increased to 400–600 mg/d and furosemide increased to 120–160 mg/d. If ascites is still present with these dosages of diuretics in patients who are compliant with a low-sodium diet, then they are defined as having *refractory ascites*, and alternative treatment modalities including repeated large-volume paracentesis, or a TIPS procedure should be considered (**Fig. 41-3**). Recent studies have shown that TIPS, while managing the ascites, does not improve survival in these patients. Unfortunately, TIPS is often associated with an increased frequency of hepatic encephalopathy and must be considered carefully on a case-by-case basis. The prognosis for patients with cirrhosis with

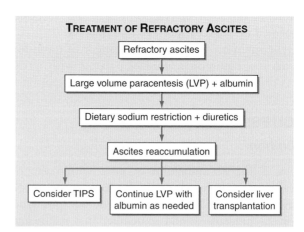

FIGURE 41-3

Treatment of refractory ascites. In patients who develop azotemia in the course of receiving diuretics in the management of their ascites, some will require repeated large-volume paracentesis (LVP), some may be considered for transjugular intrahepatic portosystemic shunt (TIPS), and some would be good candidates for liver transplantation. These decisions are all individualized.

ascites is poor, and some studies have shown that <50% of patients survive 2 years after the onset of ascites. Thus, there should be consideration for liver transplantation in patients with the onset of ascites.

SPONTANEOUS BACTERIAL PERITONITIS

SBP is a common and severe complication of ascites characterized by spontaneous infection of the ascitic fluid without an intraabdominal source. In patients with cirrhosis and ascites severe enough for hospitalization, SBP can occur in up to 30% of individuals and can have a 25% in-hospital mortality rate. Bacterial translocation is the presumed mechanism for development of SBP, with gut flora traversing the intestine into mesenteric lymph nodes, leading to bacteremia and seeding of the ascitic fluid. The most common organisms are *Escherichia coli* and other gut bacteria; however, gram-positive bacteria, including *Streptococcus viridans, Staphococcus aureus,* and *Enterococcus* sp., can also be found. If more than two organisms are identified, secondary bacterial peritonitis due to a perforated viscus should be considered. The diagnosis of SBP is made when the fluid sample has an absolute neutrophil count >250/mm^3. Bedside cultures should be obtained when ascitic fluid is tapped. Patients with ascites may present with fever, altered mental status, elevated white blood cell count, and abdominal pain or discomfort, or they may present without any of these features. Therefore, it is necessary to have a high degree of clinical suspicion, and peritoneal taps are important for making the diagnosis. Treatment is with a second-generation cephalosporin, with cefotaxime being the most commonly used antibiotic. In patients with variceal hemorrhage, the frequency of SBP is significantly increased, and prophylaxis against SBP is recommended when a patient presents with upper GI bleeding. Furthermore, in patients who have had an episode(s) of SBP and recovered, once-weekly administration of antibiotics is used as prophylaxis for recurrent SBP.

HEPATORENAL SYNDROME

The hepatorenal syndrome (HRS) is a form of functional renal failure without renal pathology that occurs in about 10% of patients with advanced cirrhosis or acute liver failure. There are marked disturbances in the arterial renal circulation in patients with HRS; these include an increase in vascular resistance accompanied by a reduction in systemic vascular resistance. The reason for renal vasoconstriction is most likely multifactorial and is poorly understood. The diagnosis is made usually in the presence of a large amount of ascites in patients who have a step-wise progressive increase in creatinine. Type 1 HRS is characterized by a progressive impairment in renal function and a significant reduction in creatinine clearance within 1–2 weeks of presentation. Type 2 HRS is characterized by a reduction in glomerular filtration rate with an elevation of serum creatinine level, but it is fairly stable and is associated with a better outcome than that of type 1 HRS.

HRS is often seen in patients with refractory ascites and requires exclusion of other causes of acute renal failure. Treatment has unfortunately been difficult, and in the past, dopamine or prostaglandin analogs were used as renal vasodilating medications. Carefully performed studies have failed to show clear-cut benefit from these therapeutic approaches. Currently, patients are treated with midodrine, an α-agonist, along with octreotide and intravenous albumin. The best therapy for HRS is liver transplantation; recovery of renal function is typical in this setting. In patients with either type 1 or type 2 HRS, the prognosis is poor unless transplant can be achieved within a short period of time.

HEPATIC ENCEPHALOPATHY

Portosystemic encephalopathy is a serious complication of chronic liver disease and is broadly defined as an alteration in mental status and cognitive function occurring in the presence of liver failure. In acute liver injury with fulminant hepatic failure, the development of encephalopathy is a requirement for a diagnosis of fulminant failure. Encephalopathy is much more commonly seen in patients with chronic liver disease. Gut-derived neurotoxins that are not removed by the liver because of vascular shunting and decreased hepatic mass get to the brain and cause the symptoms that we know of as hepatic encephalopathy. Ammonia levels are typically elevated in patients with hepatic encephalopathy, but the correlation between severity of liver disease and height of ammonia levels is often poor, and most hepatologists do not rely on ammonia levels to make a diagnosis. Other compounds and metabolites that may contribute to the development of encephalopathy include certain false neurotransmitters and mercaptans.

Clinical Features

In acute liver failure, changes in mental status can occur within weeks to months. Brain edema can be seen in these patients, with severe encephalopathy associated with swelling of the gray matter. Cerebral herniation is a feared complication of brain edema in acute liver failure, and treatment is meant to decrease edema with mannitol and judicious use of intravenous fluids.

In patients with cirrhosis, encephalopathy is often found as a result of certain precipitating events such as hypokalemia, infection, an increased dietary protein load, or electrolyte disturbances. Patients may be confused or exhibit a change in personality. They may actually be quite violent and difficult to manage; alternatively, patients may be very sleepy and difficult to arouse. Because precipitating events are so commonly found, they should be sought carefully. If patients have ascites, this should be tapped to rule out infection. Evidence of GI bleeding should be sought, and patients should be appropriately hydrated. Electrolytes should be measured and abnormalities corrected. In patients presenting with encephalopathy, asterixis is often present. Asterixis can be elicited by having patients extend their arms and bend their wrists back. In this maneuver, patients who are encephalopathic have a "liver flap"—i.e., a sudden forward movement of the wrist. This requires patients to be able to cooperate with the examiner and obviously cannot be elicited in patients who are severely encephalopathic or in hepatic coma.

The diagnosis of hepatic encephalopathy is clinical and requires an experienced clinician to recognize and put together all of the various features. Often when patients have encephalopathy for the first time, they are unaware of what is transpiring, but once they have been through the experience for the first time, they can identify when this is developing in subsequent situations and can often self-medicate to impair the development or worsening of encephalopathy.

℞ Treatment:
HEPATIC ENCEPHALOPATHY

Treatment is multifactorial and includes management of the above-mentioned precipitating factors. Sometimes hydration and correction of electrolyte imbalance is all that is necessary. In the past, restriction of dietary protein was considered for patients with encephalopathy; however, the negative impact of that maneuver on overall nutrition is thought to outweigh the benefit when treating encephalopathy, and it is thus discouraged. There may be some benefit to replacing animal-based protein with vegetable-based protein in some patients with encephalopathy that is difficult to manage. The mainstay of treatment for encephalopathy, in addition to correcting precipitating factors, is to use lactulose, a nonabsorbable disaccharide, which results in colonic acidification. Catharsis ensues, contributing to the elimination of nitrogenous products in the gut that are responsible for the development of encephalopathy. The goal of lactulose therapy is to promote 2–3 soft stools per day. Patients are asked to titrate their amount of ingested lactulose to achieve the desired effect. Poorly absorbed antibiotics are often used as adjunctive therapies for patients who have had a difficult time with lactulose. The alternating administration of neomycin and metronidazole has commonly been employed to reduce the individual side effects of each: neomycin for renal insufficiency and ototoxicity and metronidazole for peripheral neuropathy. More recently, rifaximin has been very

effective in treating encephalopathy without the known side effects of neomycin or metronidazole. Zinc supplementation is sometimes helpful in patients with encephalopathy and is relatively harmless. The development of encephalopathy in patients with chronic liver disease is a poor prognostic sign, but this complication can be managed in the vast majority of patients.

MALNUTRITION IN CIRRHOSIS

Because the liver is principally involved in the regulation of protein and energy metabolism in the body, it is not surprising that patients with advanced liver disease are commonly malnourished. Once patients become cirrhotic, they are more catabolic, and muscle protein is metabolized. There are multiple factors that contribute to the malnutrition of cirrhosis, including poor dietary intake, alterations in gut nutrient absorption, and alterations in protein metabolism. Dietary supplementation for patients with cirrhosis is helpful in preventing patients from becoming catabolic.

ABNORMALITIES IN COAGULATION

Coagulopathy is almost universal in patients with cirrhosis. There is decreased synthesis of clotting factors and impaired clearance of anticoagulants. In addition, patients may have thrombocytopenia from hypersplenism due to portal hypertension. Vitamin K–dependent clotting factors are Factors II, VII, IX, and X. Vitamin K requires biliary excretion for its subsequent absorption; thus, in patients with chronic cholestatic syndromes, vitamin K absorption is frequently diminished. Intravenous or intramuscular vitamin K can quickly correct this abnormality. More commonly, the synthesis of vitamin K–dependent clotting factors is diminished because of a decrease in hepatic mass, and under these circumstances administration of parenteral vitamin K does not improve the clotting factors or the prothrombin time. Platelet function is often abnormal in patients with chronic liver disease, in addition to decreases in platelet levels due to hypersplenism.

BONE DISEASE IN CIRRHOSIS

Osteoporosis is common in patients with chronic cholestatic liver disease because of malabsorption of vitamin D and decreased calcium ingestion. The rate of bone resorption exceeds that of new bone formation in patients with cirrhosis resulting in bone loss. Dual x-ray absorptiometry (DEXA) is a useful method for determining osteoporosis or osteopenia in patients with chronic liver disease. When a DEXA scan shows decreased bone mass, treatment should be administered with bisphosphonates that are effective at inhibiting resorption of bone and efficacious in the treatment of osteoporosis.

HEMATOLOGIC ABNORMALITIES IN CIRRHOSIS

Numerous hematologic manifestations of cirrhosis are present, including anemia from a variety of causes including hypersplenism, hemolysis, iron deficiency, and perhaps folate deficiency from malnutrition. Macrocytosis is a common abnormality in red blood cell morphology seen in patients with chronic liver disease, and neutropenia may be seen as a result of hypersplenism.

FURTHER READINGS

ARROYO V, COLMENERO J: Ascites and hepatorenal syndrome in cirrhosis: Pathophysiological basis of therapy and current management. J Hepatol 38:S69, 2003

BLEI AT, CORDOBA J: Hepatic encephalopathy. Am J Gastroenterol 96:1968, 2001

CÁRDENAS A, ARROYO V: Mechanisms of water and sodium retention in cirrhosis and the pathogenesis of ascites. Best Pract Res Clin Endocrinol Metab 17:607, 2003

DE FRANCHIS R: Updating consensus in portal hypertension: Report of the Baveno III Consensus Workshop on definitions, methodology, and therapeutic strategies in portal hypertension. J Hepatol 33:846, 2000

FERNANDEZ J et al: Diagnosis, treatment, and prevention of spontaneous bacterial peritonitis. Baillieres Best Pract Res Clin Gastroenterol 14:975, 2000

GARCIA-TSAO G et al: Management and treatment of patients with cirrhosis and portal hypertension: recommendations from the Department of Veterans Affairs Hepatitis C Resource Center Program and the National Hepatitis C Program. Am J Gastroenterol 104:1802, 2009

GINES P et al: Management of cirrhosis and ascites. N Engl J Med 350:1646, 2004

——— et al: Hyponatremia in cirrhosis: From pathogenesis to treatment. Hepatology 28:851, 1998

HALSTED CH: Nutrition and alcoholic liver disease. Semin Liver Dis 24:289, 2004

HOU W, SANYAL AJ: Ascites: diagnosis and management. Med Clin North Am 93:801, 2009

KAPLAN MM, GERSHWIN ME: Primary biliary cirrhosis. N Engl J Med 353:1261, 2005

KROWKA MJ et al: Hepatopulmonary syndrome and portopulmonary hypertension: A report of the multicenter liver transplant database. Liver Transpl 10:174, 2004

LINDOR K: Ursodeoxycholic acid for the treatment of primary biliary cirrhosis. N Engl J Med. 357:1524, 2007

SASS DA, CHOPRA KB: Portal hypertension and variceal hemorrhage. Med Clin North Am 93:837, 2009

CHAPTER 42

GENETIC, METABOLIC, AND INFILTRATIVE DISEASES AFFECTING THE LIVER

Bruce R. Bacon

There are a number of disorders of the liver that fit within the categories of genetic, metabolic, and infiltrative disorders. Inherited disorders include hemochromatosis, Wilson disease, α_1 antitrypsin (α_1AT) deficiency, and cystic fibrosis. Hemochromatosis is the most common disorder affecting Caucasian populations, with the genetic susceptibility for the disease being identified in 1 in 250 individuals. Over the past 10 years, it has become increasingly apparent that nonalcoholic fatty liver disease (NAFLD) is the most common cause of elevated liver enzymes found in the U.S. population. With the obesity epidemic in the United States, it is estimated that 20% of the population may have abnormal liver enzymes on the basis of NAFLD and 3% may have nonalcoholic steatohepatitis (NASH). Infiltrative disorders of the liver are relatively rare.

GENETIC LIVER DISEASES

Hereditary Hemochromatosis

Hereditary hemochromatosis (HH) is a common inherited disorder of iron metabolism. Our knowledge of the disease and its phenotypic expression has changed since 1996 when the gene for HH, called *HFE,* was identified, allowing for genetic testing for the two major mutations (C282Y, H63D) that are responsible for *HFE*-related HH. Subsequently, several additional genes/proteins involved in the regulation of iron homeostasis have been identified, contributing to a better understanding of cellular iron uptake and release and the characterization of additional causes of inherited iron overload (Table 42–1). All

of these inherited syndromes result in the inappropriately high absorption of iron by the gastrointestinal mucosa, leading to the pathologic deposition of excess iron in the parenchymal cells of the liver, heart, pancreas, and other organs. Ultimately, parenchymal iron deposition leads to cell and tissue damage with the development of

TABLE 42-1

CLASSIFICATION OF IRON OVERLOAD SYNDROMES

Hereditary hemochromatosis (HH)
   HFE-related (type 1)
     C282Y/C282Y
     C282Y/H63D
     Other *HFE* mutations
   Non-*HFE*-related
     Juvenile HH
       HJV—hemojuvelin (type 2a)
       HAMP—hepcidin (type 2b)
     TfR2-related HH (type 3)
     Ferroportin-related HH (type 4)
     African iron overload

Secondary iron overload
   Iron-loading anemias
   Parenteral iron overload
   Chronic liver disease

Miscellaneous
   Neonatal iron overload
   Aceruloplasminemia
   Congenital atransferrinemia

Note: HJV, hemojuvelin; HAMP, hepcidin; TfR2, transferrin receptor 2.

fibrosis and functional insufficiency. The liver is always the principal site of deposition of the majority of the excess absorbed iron, and the liver is always involved in symptomatic hemochromatosis. Recent studies have shown a central role for hepcidin, a 25-amino-acid peptide that is involved in the regulation of iron uptake by enterocytes and iron released by reticuloendothelial cells.

Most patients with HH are asymptomatic; however, when patients present with symptoms, they are frequently nonspecific and include weakness, fatigue, lethargy, and weight loss. Specific organ-related symptoms include abdominal pain, arthralgias, and symptoms and signs of chronic liver disease. Increasingly, most patients are now identified before they have symptoms, either through family studies or from the performance of screening iron studies. Several prospective population studies have shown that C282Y homozygosity is found in about 1 in 250 individuals of northern European descent, with the heterozygote frequency seen in approximately 1 in 10 individuals (Table 42-2). When systematic studies of either arthritis or diabetes clinics have looked specifically for HH, previously undiagnosed cases have been identified, often to the surprise of the clinician. These studies illustrate the need to consider HH in patients who present with the symptoms and signs known to occur in established HH. In older series of patients with HH, when patients were identified by symptoms or objective findings of the disease, women typically presented about 10 years later than men and there were about 10 times the number of men presenting as women, presumably because of the "protective" effect of menstrual blood loss and iron loss during pregnancy. More recently, when greater proportions of patients have been identified by screening blood tests or by family screening studies, the age of diagnosis for women was found to be approximately equivalent to that for men and the number of men identified was roughly equivalent to that of women.

When confronted with abnormal serum iron studies, clinicians should not wait for typical symptoms or findings of HH to appear before considering the diagnosis. However, once the diagnosis of HH is considered, either by an evaluation of abnormal screening iron studies, in the context of family studies, in a patient with an abnormal genetic test, or in the evaluation of a patient with any of the typical symptoms or clinical findings, definitive diagnosis is relatively straightforward. Fasting transferrin saturation [serum iron divided by total iron-binding capacity (TIBC) or transferrin, times 100%] and ferritin levels should be obtained. Both of these will be elevated in a symptomatic patient. It must be remembered that ferritin is an acute-phase reactant and can be elevated in a number of other inflammatory disorders, such as rheumatoid arthritis, or in various neoplastic diseases, such as lymphoma or other cancers. Also, serum ferritin is elevated in a majority of patients with NASH, in the absence of iron overload.

At present, if patients have an elevated transferrin saturation or ferritin level, then genetic testing should be performed; if they are a C282Y homozygote or a compound heterozygote (C282Y/H63D), the diagnosis is confirmed. If the ferritin is >1000 µg/L, the patient should be considered for liver biopsy since there is an increased frequency of advanced fibrosis in these individuals. If liver biopsy is performed, iron deposition is found in a periportal distribution with a periportal to pericentral gradient; iron is found predominantly in parenchymal cells, and Kupffer cells are spared.

R_x Treatment:
HEREDITARY HEMOCHROMATOSIS

Treatment of HH is relatively straightforward with weekly phlebotomy aimed to reduce iron stores, recognizing that each unit of blood contains 250 mg of iron. If patients are diagnosed and treated before the development of hepatic fibrosis, all complications of the disease can be avoided. Maintenance phlebotomy is required in most patients and usually can be achieved with 1 unit of blood removed every 2–3 months. Family studies should be performed with transferrin saturation, ferritin, and genetic testing offered to all first-degree relatives.

Wilson's Disease

Wilson's disease is an inherited disorder of copper homeostasis first described in 1912. The Wilson's disease gene

TABLE 42-2

PREVALENCE OF C282Y HOMOZYGOTES WITHOUT IRON OVERLOAD IN POPULATION SCREENING STUDIES

POPULATION SAMPLE	COUNTRY	n	PREVALENCE OF HOMOZYGOTES	C282Y HOMOZYGOTES WITH A NORMAL FERRITIN, %
Electoral roll	New Zealand	1064	1 in 213	40
Primary care	United States	1653	1 in 276	50
Epidemiologic survey	Australia	3011	1 in 188	25
Blood donors	Canada	4211	1 in 327	81
General public	United States	41,038	1 in 270	33
Primary care	North America	44,082	1 in 227	25
		Total: 95,059	Average: 1 in 250	42

was identified in 1993 with the identification of *ATP7B*. This P-type ATPase is involved in copper transport and is necessary for the export of copper from the hepatocyte. Thus, in patients with mutations in *ATP7B*, copper is retained in the liver, leading to increased copper storage and ultimately liver disease as a result. Whereas hemochromatosis is found in 1 in 250 individuals, Wilson's disease is much less common, being seen in 1 in 30,000 individuals.

The clinical presentation of Wilson's disease is variable and includes chronic hepatitis, hepatic steatosis, and cirrhosis in adolescents and young adults. Neurologic manifestations indicate that liver disease is present and include speech disorders and various movement disorders. Diagnosis includes the demonstration of a reduced ceruloplasmin level, increased urinary excretion of copper, the presence of Kayser-Fleischer rings in the cornea of the eyes, and an elevated hepatic copper level, in the appropriate clinical setting. Whereas genetic testing is valuable in establishing the diagnosis of hemochromatosis, the genetic diagnosis of Wilson's disease is difficult because >200 mutations in *ATP7B* have been described with different degrees of frequency and penetration in certain populations.

℞ Treatment: WILSON'S DISEASE

Treatment consists of copper chelating medications such as D-penicillamine and trientine. A role for zinc has also been established; zinc competes with copper absorption in the gut and induces metallothionein in the intestine, which then sequesters copper. Medical treatment is lifelong, and severe relapses leading to liver failure and death can occur with cessation of therapy. Liver transplantation is curative with respect to the underlying metabolic defect and restores the normal phenotype with respect to copper homeostasis.

α_1 *Antitrypsin Deficiency*

α_1AT deficiency was first described in the late 1960s in patients with severe pulmonary disease. Shortly thereafter it was discovered to be a cause of neonatal liver disease, and now it is known to be a cause of liver disease in infancy, early childhood, adolescence, and in adults. The natural history of liver disease in α_1AT deficiency is quite variable. Many individuals with the ZZ genotype never develop disease throughout their entire lives. α_1AT deficiency becomes apparent in adults because of screening for liver disease in individuals who have liver function test abnormalities. The only hint to diagnosis may be coexistent lung disease at a relatively young age or a family history of liver and/or lung disease. Diagnosis is established by determining a reduced serum level of α_1AT as well as the performance of α_1AT genotyping. The ZZ genotype is found in about 1 in 2000 individuals; however, it should

be remembered that liver disease can be found in individuals with the SZ genotype and occasionally in those with the MZ genotype. Liver biopsy in α_1AT disease shows characteristic PAS-positive diastase-resistant globules in the periphery of the hepatic lobule.

℞ Treatment: α_1 ANTITRYPSIN DEFICIENCY

Treatment of α_1AT is nonspecific and supportive. Liver transplantation is curative. Recombinant AT administered IV has been used in patients with chronic lung disease due to α_1AT deficiency but is of no benefit in patients with α_1AT liver disease.

Cystic Fibrosis

Cystic fibrosis (CF) should also be considered as an inherited form of chronic liver disease, although the principal manifestations of CF include chronic lung disease and pancreatic insufficiency. A small percentage of patients with CF who survive to adulthood have a form of biliary cirrhosis characterized by cholestatic liver enzyme abnormalities and the development of chronic liver disease. Ursodeoxycholic acid is occasionally helpful in improving liver test abnormalities and in reducing symptoms. The disease is slowly progressive.

METABOLIC LIVER DISEASES

Nonalcoholic Fatty Liver Disease

NAFLD was first described in the 1950s when fatty liver was characterized in a group of obese patients. In 1980, Ludwig and colleagues at the Mayo Clinic described 20 obese, diabetic, nonalcoholic patients who had similar findings on liver biopsy to patients with alcoholic liver disease, and the term nonalcoholic steatohepatitis was introduced. The prevalence of NAFLD in the United States and Europe ranges from 14–20%. This increased prevalence relates directly to the obesity epidemic seen in these populations. In the United States, NASH is thought to occur in ~3% of the general population, with fibrosis due to NASH being seen in >40% of significantly obese patients. The spectrum of NAFLD includes simple hepatic steatosis, which over time can progress to NASH, with the subsequent development of fibrosis and cirrhosis. Causes of macrovesicular steatosis are listed in **Table 42-3**. It is now known that many patients with hitherto identified "cryptogenic" cirrhosis in fact have liver disease on the basis of NASH, with the resolution of the steatosis once patients become catabolic due to cirrhosis.

Most patients who come to medical attention with NAFLD are identified as a result of incidentally discovered elevated liver enzymes (ALT, AST). When patients are symptomatic, symptoms include fatigue or a vague right upper quadrant discomfort. ALT is generally higher

TABLE 42-3

CAUSES OF MACROVESICULAR STEATOSIS

Insulin resistance, hyperinsulinemia
  Centripetal obesity
  Type 2 diabetes

Medications
  Glucocorticoids
  Estrogens
  Tamoxifen
  Amiodarone

Nutritional
  Starvation
  Protein deficiency (Kwashiorkor)
  Choline deficiency

Liver disease
  Wilson disease
  Chronic hepatitis C—genotype 3
  Indian childhood cirrhosis
  Jejunoileal bypass

than AST, and aminotransferases are only mildly (1.5–2 times the upper limit of normal) elevated. Recent studies have shown that many patients can have advanced NASH and even cirrhosis due to NASH with normal liver enzymes indicating that the prevalence of the disease may be even greater than was previously suspected. NASH is frequently seen in conjunction with other components of the metabolic syndrome (hypertension, diabetes mellitus, elevated lipids, and obesity), with NAFLD being considered the hepatic manifestation of this syndrome. Insulin resistance is the underlying link between these various disorders and numerous studies have shown that virtually all patients with NASH have insulin resistance. Abnormal ferritin values are seen in ~50% of patients with NASH, and an elevated ferritin level may be a marker of insulin resistance in NASH.

The diagnosis of NAFLD requires a careful history to determine the amount of alcohol used. Most investigators in the field of fatty liver disease require that <20 g/d of alcohol be consumed to exclude alcoholic liver disease. Laboratory testing for hepatitis B and C, iron studies, and autoimmune serologies should also be determined. Imaging studies can show characteristic features of a fatty liver, but the ultimate diagnosis of either hepatic steatosis or NASH requires liver biopsy. Liver biopsy shows characteristic macrovesicular steatosis with occasional microvesicular fat being identified. A mixed inflammatory infiltrate is found in a lobular distribution. The histologic features of NASH are very similar to those seen in alcoholic liver disease; Mallory's hyaline can be seen in both disorders, although the number of hepatocytes containing Mallory's hyaline is frequently greater in alcoholic liver disease than in NASH. The fibrosis that occurs in NASH has a characteristic perivenular and perisinusoidal distribution. Most studies show that up to 30–40% of NASH patients can develop advanced fibrosis, with cirrhosis being identified in 10–15% of individuals. Increasingly, patients are being identified with cryptogenic cirrhosis who have most likely had NASH for decades. These patients can develop liver failure and require liver transplantation, and some patients can progress to the development of hepatocellular cancer.

℞ **Treatment:**
NONALCOHOLIC FATTY LIVER DISEASE

The mainstay of treatment of fatty liver disease is weight loss and exercise, which is often difficult to achieve in this population. As an aid to weight loss, orlistat, which is a reversible inhibitor of gastric and pancreatic lipase, has been shown to result in a small decrease in body weight and is usually fairly well tolerated. Bariatric surgery has been utilized and shows striking success, but is obviously a fairly drastic maneuver for induction of weight loss. Recent studies have focused on the presence of insulin resistance at the center of the pathophysiologic mechanisms of NAFLD. The thiazolidinedione medications are PPAR gamma inhibitors, which improve insulin sensitivity within the adipocyte and skeletal muscle by upregulating specific protein kinases involved in decreasing fatty acid synthesis. Two drugs—pioglitizone and rosiglitizone—are currently available and are being evaluated as potential therapeutic options in the treatment of NASH. Antioxidants have also been utilized, and small studies have shown benefit from vitamin E supplementation. Treatment of hyperlipidemia with statin-type agents has shown improvement in liver enzymes, but they have not been assessed for effects on histology. Ursodeoxycholic acid has been utilized and improves liver enzymes in patients with many liver diseases, but it has not been definitely helpful for fatty liver disease. At present, efforts should be directed to encouraging patients with NAFLD to lose weight.

Lipid Storage Diseases

There are a number of rare lipid storage diseases that involve the liver, including the inherited disorders of Gaucher's and Niemann-Pick disease. Other rare disorders include abetalipoproteinemia, Tangier disease, Fabray's disease, and types I and V hyperlipoproteinemia. Hepatomegaly is present due to increased fat deposition and increased glycogen found in the liver.

Porphyrias

The porphyrias are a group of metabolic disorders in which there are defects in the biosynthesis of heme necessary for incorporation into numerous hemoproteins such as hemoglobin, myoglobin, catalase, and the cytochromes. Porphyrias can present as either acute or chronic diseases, with the acute disorder causing recurring bouts of abdominal pain, and the chronic disorders characterized by painful skin lesions. Porphyria cutanea tarda (PCT) is the most commonly encountered porphyria. Patients present with characteristic vesicular lesions on sun-exposed areas of the skin, principally the dorsum of the hands, the tips of the ears, or the cheeks. About 40% of patients with PCT have mutations in the gene for hemochromatosis (*HFE*), and ~50% have hepatitis C; thus, iron studies and *HFE* mutation analysis as well as hepatitis C testing should be considered in all patients who present with PCT. PCT is also associated with excess alcohol use and some medications, most notably estrogens.

℞ **Treatment:**
PORPHYRIAS

The mainstay of treatment of PCT is iron reduction by therapeutic phlebotomy, which is successful in reversing the skin lesions in the majority of patients. If hepatitis C is present, this should be treated as well. Acute intermittent porphyria presents with abdominal pain, with the diagnosis made by avoidance of certain precipitating factors such as starvation or certain diets. Intravenous heme as hematin has been used for treatment.

INFILTRATIVE DISORDERS

Amyloidosis

Amyloidosis is a metabolic storage disease that results from deposition of insoluble proteins that are aberrantly folded and assembled and then deposited in a variety of tissues. Amyloidosis is divided into two types, primary and secondary, based on the broad concepts of association with myeloma (primary) or chronic inflammatory illnesses (secondary). The disease is generally considered rare, although in certain disease states or in certain populations, it can be more common. For example, when associated with familial Mediterranean fever, it is seen in high frequency in Sephardic Jews and Armenians living in Armenia and less frequently in Ashkenazi Jews, Turks, and Arabs. Amyloidosis frequently affects patients suffering from tuberculosis and leprosy and can be seen in upwards of 10–15% of patients with ankylosing spondylitis, rheumatoid arthritis, or Crohn's disease. In one surgical pathology series, amyloid was found in <1% of cases. The liver is commonly involved in cases of systemic amyloidosis, but it is frequently inapparent clinically and only documented at autopsy. Pathologic findings in the liver include positive staining with the Congo red histochemical stain where there is an apple-green birefringence noted under polarizing light.

Granulomas

Granulomas are frequently found in the liver when patients are being evaluated for cholestatic liver enzyme abnormalities. Granulomas can be seen in primary biliary cirrhosis, but there are other characteristic clinical and laboratory findings that allow for a definitive diagnosis of that disorder. Granulomatous infiltration can also be seen as the principal hepatic manifestation of sarcoidosis, and this is the most common presentation of hepatic granulomas. The vast majority of these patients do not require any specific treatment, other than what would normally be used for treatment of their sarcoidosis. A small subset, however, can develop a particularly bothersome desmoplastic reaction with a significant increase in fibrosis, which can progress to cirrhosis and liver failure. These patients may require treatment with immunosuppressive therapy and may require liver transplantation. In patients who have granulomas in the liver not associated with sarcoidosis, treatment is rarely needed.

Diagnosis requires liver biopsy, and it is important to establish a diagnosis so that a cause for the elevated liver enzymes is carefully identified. Some medications can cause granulomatous infiltration of the liver, the most notable of which is allopurinol.

Lymphoma

Involvement of the liver with lymphoma can sometimes be with bulky mass lesions but can also be as a difficult-to-diagnose infiltrative disorder that does not show any characteristic findings on abdominal imaging studies. Patients may present with severe liver disease, jaundice, hypoalbuminemia, mild to moderately elevated aminotransferases, and an elevated alkaline phosphatase.

A liver biopsy is required for diagnosis and should be considered when routine blood testing does not lead to a diagnosis of the liver dysfunction.

FURTHER READINGS

ALA A, SCHILSKY ML: Wilson disease: Pathophysiology, diagnosis, treatment, and screening. Clin Liver Dis 8:787, 2004
———— et al: Wilson's disease. Lancet 369:397, 2007
FINK S, SCHILSKY ML: Inherited metabolic disease of the liver. Curr Opin Gastroenterol 23:237, 2007
FLEMING R, BACON BR: Orchestration of iron homeostasis. N Eng J Med 352:1741, 2005
HARRISON SA, NEUSCHWANDER-TETRI BA: Nonalcoholic fatty liver disease and nonalcoholic steatohepatitis. Clin Liver Dis 8:861, 2004
O'NEILL J, POWELL L: Clinical aspects of hemochromatosis. Semin Liver Dis 25:381, 2005
PERLMUTTER DH: Alpha-1-antitrypsin deficiency: Diagnosis and treatment. Clin Liver Dis 8:839, 2004
PIETRANGELO A: Hemochromatosis: an endocrine liver disease. Hepatology 46:1291, 2007
SILVERMAN EK, SANDHAUS RA. Clinical practice. Alpha1-antitrypsin deficiency. N Engl J Med 360:2749, 2009
WIECKOWSKA A et al: Noninvasive diagnosis and monitoring of nonalcoholic steatohepatitis: present and future. Hepatology 46:582, 2007
WOOD MJ et al: Environmental and genetic modifiers of the progression to fibrosis and cirrhosis in hemochromatosis. Blood 111:4456, 2008

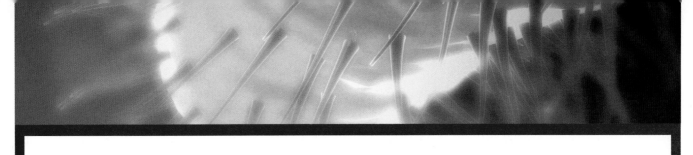

CHAPTER 43

DISEASES OF THE GALLBLADDER AND BILE DUCTS

Norton J. Greenberger ■ Gustav Paumgartner

PHYSIOLOGY OF BILE PRODUCTION AND FLOW

BILE SECRETION AND COMPOSITION

Bile formed in the hepatic lobules is secreted into a complex network of canaliculi, small bile ductules, and larger bile ducts that run with lymphatics and branches of the portal vein and hepatic artery in portal tracts situated between hepatic lobules. These interlobular bile ducts coalesce to form larger septal bile ducts that join to form the right and left hepatic ducts, which in turn unite to form the common hepatic duct. The common hepatic duct is joined by the cystic duct of the gallbladder to form the common bile duct (CBD), which enters the duodenum (often after joining the main pancreatic duct) through the ampulla of Vater.

Hepatic bile is an isotonic fluid with an electrolyte composition resembling blood plasma. The electrolyte composition of gallbladder bile differs from that of hepatic bile because most of the inorganic anions, chloride and bicarbonate, have been removed by reabsorption across the gallbladder epithelium. As a result of water reabsorption, total solute concentration of bile increases from 3–4 g/dL in hepatic bile and 10–15 g/dL in gallbladder bile.

Major solute components of bile by moles percent include bile acids (80%), lecithin and traces of other phospholipids (16%), and unesterified cholesterol (4.0%). In the lithogenic state the cholesterol value can be as high as 8–10%. Other constituents include conjugated bilirubin, proteins (all immunoglobulins, albumin, metabolites of hormones, and other proteins metabolized in the liver), electrolytes, mucus, and, often, drugs and their metabolites.

The total daily basal secretion of hepatic bile is ~500–600 mL. Many substances taken up or synthesized by the hepatocyte are secreted into the bile canaliculi. The canalicular membrane forms microvilli and is associated with microfilaments of actin, microtubules, and other contractile elements. Prior to their secretion into the bile, many substances are taken up into the hepatocyte, while others such as phospholipids, a portion of primary bile acids, and some cholesterol are synthesized de novo in the hepatocyte. Three mechanisms are important in regulating bile flow: (1) active transport of bile acids from hepatocytes into the bile canaliculi, (2) active transport of other organic anions, and (3) cholangiocellular secretion. The last is a secretin-mediated and cyclic AMP–dependent mechanism that results in the secretion of a sodium- and bicarbonate-rich fluid into the bile ducts.

Active vectorial secretion of biliary constituents from the portal blood into the bile canaliculi is driven by a distinct set of polarized transport systems at the basolateral (sinusoidal) and the canalicular apical plasma membrane domains of the hepatocyte. Two sinusoidal bile salt uptake systems have been cloned in humans, the Na^+/taurocholate cotransporter (NTCP) and the organic anion transporting proteins (OATPs), which also transport a large variety of non–bile salt organic anions. Several ATP-dependent canalicular transport systems ("export pumps") have been identified, the most important of which are: the bile salt export pump (BSEP); the anionic conjugate export pump (MRP2), which mediates the canalicular excretion of various amphiphilic conjugates formed by phase II conjugation (e.g., bilirubin mono- and diglucuronides and drugs); the multidrug export pump (MDR1) for hydrophobic cationic compounds; and the phospholipid export pump (MDR3). Two hemitransporters ABCG5/G8, functioning as a couple, constitute the principal canalicular cholesterol and phytosterol transporter. F1C1 (ATP8B1) is an aminophospholipid transferase ("flippase") essential for maintaining the lipid asymmetry of the canalicular membrane. The canalicular membrane also contains ATP-independent transport systems such as the Cl/HCO_3 anion exchanger isoform 2 for canalicular bicarbonate secretion. For most of these transporters, genetic defects have been identified that are associated with various forms of cholestasis or defects of biliary excretion. F1C1 is defective in Byler's disease and results in ablation of all other ATP-dependent transporter functions. BSEP is defective in progressive familial intrahepatic cholestasis (PFIC) and benign recurrent intrahepatic cholestasis (BRIC) type 2 which can also be secondary to minor F1C1 (ATP8B1) mutations. Mutations of MRP2 cause the Dubin-Johnson syndrome, an inherited form of conjugated hyperbilirubinemia (Chap. 36). A defective MDR3 results in PFIC-3. ABCG5/G8, the canalicular half transporters for cholesterol and other neutral sterols, are defective in sitosterolemia. The cystic fibrosis transmembrane regulator (CFTR) located on bile duct epithelial cells but not on canalicular membranes is defective in cystic fibrosis, which is associated with impaired cholangiocellular pH regulation during ductular bile formation and chronic cholestatic liver disease, occasionally resulting in biliary cirrhosis.

THE BILE ACIDS

The primary bile acids, cholic acid and chenodeoxycholic acid (CDCA), are synthesized from cholesterol in the liver, conjugated with glycine or taurine, and secreted into the bile. Secondary bile acids, including deoxycholate and lithocholate, are formed in the colon as bacterial metabolites of the primary bile acids. However, lithocholic acid is much less efficiently absorbed from the colon than deoxycholic acid. Another secondary bile acid, found in low concentration, is ursodeoxycholic acid (UDCA), a stereoisomer of CDCA. In healthy subjects, the ratio of glycine to taurine conjugates in bile is ~3:1.

Bile acids are detergent-like molecules that in aqueous solutions and above a critical concentration of about 2 mM form molecular aggregates called *micelles*. Cholesterol alone is sparingly soluble in aqueous environments, and its solubility in bile depends on both the total lipid concentration and the relative molar percentages of bile acids and lecithin. Normal ratios of these constituents favor the formation of solubilizing *mixed micelles*, while abnormal ratios promote the precipitation of cholesterol crystals in bile via an intermediate liquid crystal phase.

In addition to facilitating the biliary excretion of cholesterol, bile acids facilitate the normal intestinal absorption of dietary fats, mainly cholesterol and fat-soluble vitamins, via a micellar transport mechanism (Chap. 15). Bile acids also serve as a major physiologic driving force for hepatic bile flow and aid in water and electrolyte transport in the small bowel and colon.

ENTEROHEPATIC CIRCULATION

Bile acids are efficiently conserved under normal conditions. Unconjugated, and to a lesser degree also conjugated, bile acids are absorbed by *passive diffusion* along the entire gut. Quantitatively much more important for bile salt recirculation, however, is the *active transport* mechanism for conjugated bile acids in the distal ileum (Chap. 15). The reabsorbed bile acids enter the portal bloodstream and are taken up rapidly by hepatocytes, reconjugated, and resecreted into bile (enterohepatic circulation).

The normal bile acid pool size is approximately 2–4 g. During digestion of a meal, the bile acid pool undergoes at least one or more enterohepatic cycles, depending on the size and composition of the meal. Normally, the bile acid pool circulates ~5–10 times daily. Intestinal absorption of the pool is about 95% efficient; therefore, fecal loss of bile acids is in the range of 0.2–0.4 g/d. In the steady state this fecal loss is compensated by an equal daily synthesis of bile acids by the liver, and thus the size of the bile acid pool is maintained. Bile acids returning to the liver suppress de novo hepatic synthesis of primary bile acids from cholesterol by inhibiting the rate-limiting enzyme cholesterol 7-hydroxylase. While the loss of bile salts in stool is usually matched by increased hepatic synthesis, the maximum rate of synthesis is ~5 g/d, which may be insufficient to replete the bile acid pool size when there is pronounced impairment of intestinal bile salt reabsorption.

GALLBLADDER AND SPHINCTERIC FUNCTIONS

In the fasting state, the sphincter of Oddi offers a high-pressure zone of resistance to bile flow from the CBD into the duodenum. This tonic contraction serves to (1) prevent reflux of duodenal contents into the pancreatic and bile ducts and (2) promote filling of the gallbladder. The major factor controlling the evacuation of the gallbladder is the peptide hormone cholecystokinin (CCK), which is released from the duodenal mucosa in response to the ingestion of fats and amino acids. CCK produces (1) powerful contraction of the gallbladder, (2) decreased resistance of the sphincter of Oddi, and (3) enhanced flow of biliary contents into the duodenum.

Hepatic bile is "concentrated" within the gallbladder by energy-dependent transmucosal absorption of water and electrolytes. Almost the entire bile acid pool may be sequestered in the gallbladder following an overnight fast for delivery into the duodenum with the first meal of the day. The normal capacity of the gallbladder is ~30 mL of bile.

DISEASES OF THE GALLBLADDER

CONGENITAL ANOMALIES

Anomalies of the biliary tract are not uncommon and include abnormalities in number, size, and shape (e.g., agenesis of the gallbladder, duplications, rudimentary or oversized "giant" gallbladders, and diverticula). *Phrygian cap* is a clinically innocuous entity in which a partial or complete septum (or fold) separates the fundus from the body. Anomalies of position or suspension are not uncommon and include left-sided gallbladder, intrahepatic gallbladder, retrodisplacement of the gallbladder, and "floating" gallbladder. The latter condition predisposes to acute torsion, volvulus, or herniation of the gallbladder.

GALLSTONES

Pathogenesis

Gallstones are quite prevalent in most western countries. In the United States, several series have shown gallstones in at least 20% of women and in 8% of men over the age of 40 and in up to 40% of women over the age of 65 years. It is estimated that at least 25 million persons in the United States have gallstones and that ~1 million new cases of cholelithiasis develop each year.

Gallstones are formed because of abnormal bile constituents. They are divided into two major types: cholesterol stones account for 80% of the total, with pigment stones comprising the remaining 20%. Cholesterol gallstones usually contain >50% cholesterol monohydrate plus an admixture of calcium salts, bile pigments, proteins, and fatty acids, the latter in "brown" pigment stones. Pigment stones are composed primarily of calcium bilirubinate; they contain <20% cholesterol and are classified into "black" and "brown" types, the latter forming secondary to chronic biliary infection.

Cholesterol is essentially water insoluble and requires aqueous dispersion into either micelles or vesicles, both of which require the presence of a second lipid to solubilize the cholesterol. Cholesterol and phospholipids are secreted into bile as unilamellar bilayered vesicles, which are converted into mixed micelles consisting of bile acids, phospholipids, and cholesterol by the action of bile acids. If there is an excess of cholesterol in relation to phospholipids and bile acids, unstable cholesterol-rich vesicles remain, which aggregate into large multilamellar vesicles from which cholesterol crystals precipitate (Fig. 43-1).

There are several important mechanisms in the formation of lithogenic (stone-forming) bile. The most important is increased biliary secretion of cholesterol. This may occur in association with obesity, high-caloric and cholesterol-rich diets, or drugs (e.g., clofibrate) and may result from increased activity of HMG-CoA reductase, the

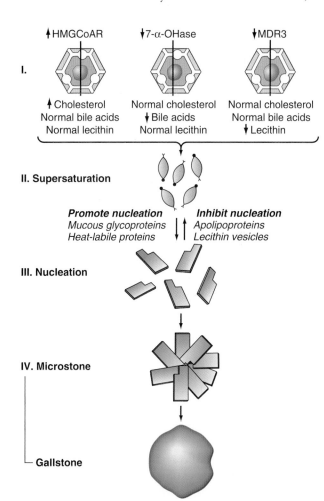

FIGURE 43-1

Scheme showing pathogenesis of cholesterol gallstone formation. Conditions or factors that increase the ratio of cholesterol to bile acids and phospholipids (lecithin) favor gallstone formation. HMG-CoAR, hydroxymethylglutaryl–coenzyme A reductase; 7-α-OHase, cholesterol, 7α-hydroxylase; MDR3, multidrug resistance–associated protein 3, also called phospholipid export pump.

rate-limiting enzyme of hepatic cholesterol synthesis, and increased hepatic uptake of cholesterol from blood. In patients with gallstones, dietary cholesterol *increases* biliary cholesterol secretion. This does not occur in non-gallstone patients on high-cholesterol diets. In addition to environmental factors such as high-caloric and cholesterol-rich diets, genetic factors play an important role in gallstone disease. A large study of symptomatic gallstones in Swedish twins provided strong evidence for a role of genetic factors in gallstone pathogenesis. Genetic factors accounted for 25%, shared environmental factors for 13%, and individual environmental factors for 62% of the phenotypic variation among monozygotic twins. A high prevalence of gallstones is found among first-degree relatives of gallstone carriers and in certain ethnic populations such as American Indians as well as Chilean Indians and Chilean Hispanics. A common genetic trait has been identified for some of these populations by mitochondrial DNA analysis. In some patients, impaired hepatic conversion of cholesterol to bile acids may also occur, resulting in an increase of the lithogenic cholesterol/bile acid ratio. Although most cholesterol stones have a polygenic basis, there are rare monogenic (mendelian) causes. Recently, a mutation in the *CYP7A1* gene has been described that results in a deficiency of the enzyme cholesterol 7-hydroxylase, which catalyzes the initial step in cholesterol catabolism and bile acid synthesis. The homozygous state is associated with hypercholesterolemia and gallstones. Because the phenotype is expressed in the heterozygote state, mutations in the *CYP7A1* gene may contribute to the susceptibility to cholesterol gallstone disease in the population. Mutations in the *MDR3* gene, which encodes the phospholipid export pump in the canalicular membrane of the hepatocyte, may cause defective phospholipid secretion into bile, resulting in cholesterol supersaturation of bile and formation of cholesterol gallstones in the gallbladder and in the bile ducts. Thus an excess of biliary cholesterol in relation to bile acids and phospholipids is primarily due to hypersecretion of cholesterol, but hyposecretion of bile acids or phospholipids may contribute. An additional disturbance of bile acid metabolism that is likely to contribute to supersaturation of bile with cholesterol is enhanced conversion of cholic acid to deoxycholic acid, with replacement of the cholic acid pool by an expanded deoxycholic acid pool. It may result from enhanced dehydroxylation of cholic acid and increased absorption of newly formed deoxycholic acid. An increased deoxycholate secretion is associated with hypersecretion of cholesterol into bile.

While supersaturation of bile with cholesterol is an important prerequisite for gallstone formation, it is generally not sufficient by itself to produce cholesterol precipitation in vivo. Most individuals with supersaturated bile do not develop stones because the time required for cholesterol crystals to nucleate and grow is longer than the time bile spends in the gallbladder.

An important mechanism is *nucleation* of cholesterol monohydrate crystals, which is greatly accelerated in human lithogenic bile. Accelerated nucleation of cholesterol monohydrate in bile may be due to either an *excess of pronucleating factors* or a *deficiency of antinucleating factors*. Mucin and certain non-mucin glycoproteins, principally immunoglobulins, appear to be pronucleating factors, while apolipoproteins AI and AII and other glycoproteins appear to be antinucleating factors. Cholesterol monohydrate crystal nucleation and crystal growth probably occur within the mucin gel layer. Vesicle fusion leads to liquid crystals, which, in turn, nucleate into solid cholesterol monohydrate crystals. Continued growth of the crystals occurs by direct nucleation of cholesterol molecules from supersaturated unilamellar or multilamellar biliary vesicles.

A third important mechanism in cholesterol gallstone formation is *gallbladder hypomotility*. If the gallbladder emptied all supersaturated or crystal-containing bile completely, stones would not be able to grow. A high percentage of patients with gallstones exhibits abnormalities of gallbladder emptying. Ultrasonographic studies show that gallstone patients display an increased gallbladder volume during fasting and also after a test meal (residual volume) and that fractional emptying after gallbladder stimulation is decreased. Gallbladder emptying is a major determinant of gallstone recurrence in patients who underwent biliary lithotripsy.

Biliary sludge is a thick mucous material that upon microscopic examination reveals lecithin-cholesterol crystals, cholesterol monohydrate crystals, calcium bilirubinate, and mucin gels. Biliary sludge typically forms a crescent-like layer in the most dependent portion of the gallbladder and is recognized by characteristic echoes on ultrasonography (see below). The presence of biliary sludge implies two abnormalities: (1) the normal balance between gallbladder mucin secretion and elimination has become deranged and (2) nucleation of biliary solutes has occurred. That biliary sludge may be a precursor form of gallstone disease is evident from several observations. In one study, 96 patients with gallbladder sludge were followed prospectively by serial ultrasound studies. In 18%, biliary sludge disappeared and did not recur for at least 2 years. In 60%, biliary sludge disappeared and reappeared; in 14%, gallstones (8% asymptomatic, 6% symptomatic) developed, and in 6%, severe biliary pain with or without acute pancreatitis occurred. In 12 patients, cholecystectomies were performed, 6 for gallstone-associated biliary pain and 3 in symptomatic patients with sludge but without gallstones who had prior attacks of pancreatitis; the latter did not recur after cholecystectomy. It should be emphasized that biliary sludge can develop with disorders that cause gallbladder hypomotility, i.e., surgery, burns, total parenteral nutrition, pregnancy, and oral contraceptives—all of which are associated with gallstone formation. However, the presence of biliary sludge implies supersaturation of bile with either cholesterol or calcium bilirubinate.

Two other conditions are associated with cholesterol stone or biliary sludge formation: pregnancy and very low calorie diet. There appear to be two key changes during pregnancy that contribute to a "cholelithogenic state": (1) a marked increase in cholesterol saturation during the third trimester and (2) sluggish gallbladder contraction in response to a standard meal, resulting in impaired gallbladder emptying. That these changes are related to pregnancy per se is supported by several studies that show reversal of these abnormalities quite rapidly after delivery. During pregnancy, gallbladder sludge develops in 20–30% of women and gallstones in 5–12%. Although biliary sludge is a common finding during pregnancy, it is usually asymptomatic and often resolves spontaneously after delivery. Gallstones, which are less common than sludge and frequently associated with biliary colic, may also disappear after delivery because of spontaneous dissolution related to bile becoming unsaturated with cholesterol post-partum.

Approximately 10–20% of persons with rapid weight reduction achieved through very low calorie dieting develop gallstones. In a study involving 600 patients who completed a 16-week, 520-kcal/d diet, UDCA in a dosage of 600 mg/d proved highly effective in preventing gallstone formation; gallstones developed in only 3% of UDCA recipients, compared to 28% of placebo-treated patients.

To summarize, cholesterol gallstone disease occurs because of several defects, which include (1) bile supersaturation with cholesterol, (2) nucleation of cholesterol monohydrate with subsequent crystal retention and stone growth, and (3) abnormal gallbladder motor function with delayed emptying and stasis. Other important factors known to predispose to cholesterol stone formation are summarized in Table 43-1.

▬ Pigment Stones

Black pigment stones are composed of either pure calcium bilirubinate or polymer-like complexes with calcium and mucin glycoproteins. They are more common in patients who have chronic hemolytic states (with increased conjugated bilirubin in bile), liver cirrhosis, Gilbert's syndrome, or cystic fibrosis. Gallbladder stones in patients with ileal diseases, ileal resection, or ileal bypass generally are also black pigment stones. Enterohepatic recycling of bilirubin in ileal disease states contributes to their pathogenesis. Brown pigment stones are composed of calcium salts of unconjugated bilirubin with varying amounts of cholesterol and protein. They are caused by the presence of increased amounts of unconjugated, insoluble bilirubin in bile that precipitates to form stones. Deconjugation of an excess of soluble bilirubin mono- and diglucuronides may be mediated by endogenous β-glucuronidase but may also occur by spontaneous hydrolysis. Sometimes, the enzyme is also produced when bile is chronically infected by bacteria, and such stones are brown. Pigment stone formation is especially prominent in Asians and is often associated with infections in the gallbladder and biliary tree (Table 43-1).

TABLE 43-1

PREDISPOSING FACTORS FOR CHOLESTEROL AND PIGMENT GALLSTONE FORMATION

Cholesterol Stones

1. Demographic/genetic factors: Prevalence highest in North American Indians, Chilean Indians, and Chilean Hispanics, greater in Northern Europe and North America than in Asia, lowest in Japan; familial disposition; hereditary aspects
2. Obesity: Normal bile acid pool and secretion but increased biliary secretion of cholesterol
3. Weight loss: Mobilization of tissue cholesterol leads to increased biliary cholesterol secretion while enterohepatic circulation of bile acids is decreased
4. Female sex hormones
   a. Estrogens stimulate hepatic lipoprotein receptors, increase uptake of dietary cholesterol, and increase biliary cholesterol secretion
   b. Natural estrogens, other estrogens, and oral contraceptives lead to decreased bile salt secretion and decreased conversion of cholesterol to cholesteryl esters
5. Increasing age: Increased biliary secretion of cholesterol, decreased size of bile acid pool, decreased secretion of bile salts
6. Gallbladder hypomotility leading to stasis and formation of sludge
   a. Prolonged parenteral nutrition
   b. Fasting
   c. Pregnancy
   d. Drugs such as octreotide
7. Clofibrate therapy: Increased biliary secretion of cholesterol
8. Decreased bile acid secretion
   a. Primary biliary cirrhosis
   b. Genetic defect of the *CYP7A1* gene
9. Decreased phospholipid secretion: Genetic defect of the *MDR3* gene
10. Miscellaneous
    a. High-calorie, high-fat diet
    b. Spinal cord injury

Pigment Stones

1. Demographic/genetic factors: Asia, rural setting
2. Chronic hemolysis
3. Alcoholic cirrhosis
4. Pernicious anemia
5. Cystic fibrosis
6. Chronic biliary tract infection, parasite infections
7. Increasing age
8. Ileal disease, ileal resection or bypass

Diagnosis

Procedures of potential use in the diagnosis of cholelithiasis and other diseases of the gallbladder are detailed in Table 43-2. Ultrasonography of the gallbladder is very accurate in the identification of cholelithiasis and has replaced oral cholecystography (Fig. 43-2A). Stones as

TABLE 43-2

DIAGNOSTIC EVALUATION OF THE GALLBLADDER

DIAGNOSTIC ADVANTAGES	DIAGNOSTIC LIMITATIONS	COMMENT
Gallbladder Ultrasound		
Rapid Accurate identification of gallstones (>95%) Simultaneous scanning of GB, liver, bile ducts, pancreas "Real-time" scanning allows assessment of GB volume, contractility Not limited by jaundice, pregnancy May detect very small stones	Bowel gas Massive obesity Ascites	Procedure of choice for detection of stones
Plain Abdominal X-Ray		
Low cost Readily available	Relatively low yield ? Contraindicated in pregnancy	Pathognomonic findings in: calcified gallstones Limey bile, porcelain GB Emphysematous cholecystitis Gallstone ileus
Oral Cholecystogram: Replaced by GBUS		
Radioisotope Scans (HIDA, DIDA, etc.)		
Accurate identification of cystic duct obstruction Simultaneous assessment of bile ducts	? Contraindicated in pregnancy Serum bilirubin >103–205 µmol/L (6–12 mg/dL) Cholecystogram of low resolution	Indicated for confirmation of suspected acute cholecystitis; less sensitive and less specific in chronic cholecystitis; useful in diagnosis of acalculous cholecystopathy, especially if given with CCK to assess gallbladder emptying

Note: GB, gallbladder; CCK, cholecystokinin; GBUS, gallbladder ultrasound.

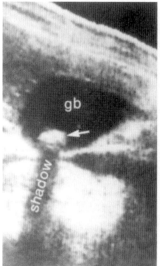 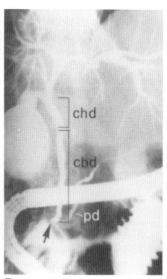 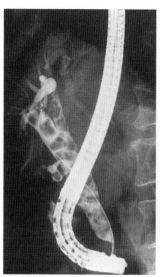 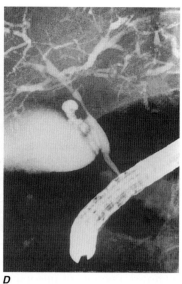

A   B   C   D

FIGURE 43-2

Examples of ultrasound and radiologic studies of the biliary tract. A. An ultrasound study showing a distended gallbladder containing a single large stone (*arrow*) which casts an acoustic shadow. **B.** Endoscopic retrograde cholangiopancreatogram (ERCP) showing normal biliary tract anatomy. In addition to the endoscope and large vertical gallbladder filled with contrast dye, the common hepatic duct (chd), common bile duct (cbd), and pancreatic duct (pd) are shown. The arrow points to the ampulla of Vater. **C.** Endoscopic retrograde cholangiogram (ERC) showing choledocholithiasis. The biliary tract is dilatated and contains multiple radiolucent calculi. **D.** ERCP showing sclerosing cholangitis. The common bile duct shows areas that are strictured and narrowed.

small as 2 mm in diameter may be confidently identified provided that firm criteria are used [e.g., acoustic "shadowing" of opacities that are within the gallbladder lumen and that change with the patient's position (by gravity)]. In major medical centers, the false-negative and false-positive rates for ultrasound in gallstone patients are ~2–4%. Biliary sludge is material of low echogenic activity that typically forms a layer in the most dependent position of the gallbladder. This layer shifts with postural changes but fails to produce acoustic shadowing; these two characteristics distinguish sludges from gallstones. Ultrasound can also be used to assess the emptying function of the gallbladder.

The plain abdominal film may detect gallstones containing sufficient calcium to be radiopaque (10–15% of cholesterol and ~50% of pigment stones). Plain radiography may also be of use in the diagnosis of emphysematous cholecystitis, porcelain gallbladder, limey bile, and gallstone ileus.

Oral cholecystography (OCG) has historically been a useful procedure for the diagnosis of gallstones but has been replaced by ultrasound. It may be used to assess the patency of the cystic duct and gallbladder emptying function. Further, OCG can also delineate the size and number of gallstones and determine whether they are calcified.

Radiopharmaceuticals such as ^{99m}Tc-labeled *N*-substituted iminodiacetic acids (HIDA, DIDA, DISIDA, etc.) are rapidly extracted from the blood and are excreted into the biliary tree in high concentration even in the presence of mild to moderate serum bilirubin elevations. Failure to image the gallbladder in the presence of biliary ductal visualization may indicate cystic duct obstruction, acute or chronic cholecystitis, or surgical absence of the organ. Such scans have some application in the diagnosis of acute cholecystitis.

Symptoms of Gallstone Disease

Gallstones usually produce symptoms by causing inflammation or obstruction following their migration into the cystic duct or CBD. The most specific and characteristic symptom of gallstone disease is biliary colic that is a constant and often long-lasting pain (see below). Obstruction of the cystic duct or CBD by a stone produces increased intraluminal pressure and distention of the viscus that cannot be relieved by repetitive biliary contractions. The resultant visceral pain is characteristically a severe, steady ache or fullness in the epigastrium or right upper quadrant (RUQ) of the abdomen with frequent radiation to the interscapular area, right scapula, or shoulder.

Biliary colic begins quite suddenly and may persist with severe intensity for 30 min to 5 h, subsiding gradually or rapidly. It is steady rather than intermittent as would be suggested by the word *colic*, which must be regarded as a misnomer, although in widespread use. An episode of biliary pain persisting beyond 5 h should raise the suspicion of acute cholecystitis (see below). Nausea and vomiting frequently accompany episodes of biliary pain. An elevated level of serum bilirubin and/or alkaline phosphatase suggests a common duct stone. Fever or chills (rigors) with biliary pain usually imply a complication, i.e., cholecystitis, pancreatitis, or cholangitis. Complaints of vague epigastric fullness, dyspepsia, eructation, or flatulence, especially following a fatty meal, should not be confused with biliary pain. Such symptoms are frequently elicited from patients with or without gallstone disease but are not specific for biliary calculi. Biliary colic may be precipitated by eating a fatty meal, by consumption of a large meal following a period of prolonged fasting, or by eating a normal meal; it is frequently nocturnal, occurring within a few hours of retiring.

Natural History

Gallstone disease discovered in an asymptomatic patient or in a patient whose symptoms are not referable to cholelithiasis is a common clinical problem. The natural history of "silent," or asymptomatic, gallstones has occasioned much debate. A study of predominantly male silent gallstone patients suggests that the cumulative risk for the development of symptoms or complications is relatively low—10% at 5 years, 15% at 10 years, and 18% at 15 years. Patients remaining asymptomatic for 15 years were found to be unlikely to develop symptoms during further follow-up, and most patients who did develop complications from their gallstones experienced *prior* warning symptoms. Similar conclusions apply to diabetic patients with silent gallstones. Decision analysis has suggested that (1) the cumulative risk of death due to gallstone disease while on expectant management is small, and (2) prophylactic cholecystectomy is not warranted.

Complications requiring cholecystectomy are much more common in gallstone patients who have developed symptoms of biliary pain. Patients found to have gallstones at a young age are more likely to develop symptoms from cholelithiasis than are patients >60 years at the time of initial diagnosis. Patients with diabetes mellitus and gallstones may be somewhat more susceptible to septic complications, but the magnitude of risk of septic biliary complications in diabetic patients is incompletely defined.

℞ Treatment: GALLSTONES

SURGICAL THERAPY In asymptomatic gallstone patients, the risk of developing symptoms or complications requiring surgery is quite small (in the range of 1–2% per year). Thus a recommendation for cholecystectomy in a patient with gallstones should probably be based on assessment of three factors: (1) the presence of symptoms that are frequent enough or severe enough to interfere with the patient's general routine;

(2) the presence of a prior complication of gallstone disease, i.e., history of acute cholecystitis, pancreatitis, gallstone fistula, etc.; or (3) the presence of an underlying condition predisposing the patient to increased risk of gallstone complications (e.g., calcified or porcelain gallbladder and/or a previous attack of acute cholecystitis regardless of current symptomatic status). Patients with very large gallstones (>3 cm in diameter) and patients having gallstones in a congenitally anomalous gallbladder might also be considered for prophylactic cholecystectomy. Although young age is a worrisome factor in asymptomatic gallstone patients, few authorities would now recommend routine cholecystectomy in all young patients with silent stones. Laparoscopic cholecystectomy is a minimal-access approach for the removal of the gallbladder together with its stones. Its advantages include a markedly shortened hospital stay, minimal disability, as well as decreased cost, and it is the procedure of choice for most patients referred for elective cholecystectomy.

From several studies involving >4000 patients undergoing laparoscopic cholecystectomy, the following key points emerge: (1) complications develop in ~4% of patients, (2) conversion to laparotomy occurs in 5%, (3) the death rate is remarkably low (i.e., <0.1%), and (4) bile duct injuries are unusual (i.e., 0.2–0.5%) but more frequent than with open cholecystectomy. These data indicate why laparoscopic cholecystectomy has become the "gold standard" for treating symptomatic cholelithiasis.

MEDICAL THERAPY—GALLSTONE DISSOLUTION Ursodeoxycholic acid (UDCA) decreases cholesterol saturation of bile and also appears to produce a lamellar liquid crystalline phase in bile that allows a dispersion of cholesterol from stones by physical-chemical means. UDCA may also retard cholesterol crystal nucleation. In carefully selected patients with a functioning gallbladder and with radiolucent stones <10 mm in diameter, complete dissolution can be achieved in ~50% of patients within 6 months to 2 years with UDCA at a dose of 8–10 mg/kg per day. The highest success rate (i.e., >70%) occurs in patients with small (<5 mm) floating radiolucent gallstones. Probably ≤10% of patients with *symptomatic* cholelithiasis are candidates for such treatment. However, in addition to the vexing problem of recurrent stones (30–50% over 3–5 years of follow-up), there is also the factor of taking an expensive drug for up to 2 years. The advantages and success of laparoscopic cholecystectomy have largely reduced the role of gallstone dissolution to patients who wish to avoid or are not candidates for elective cholecystectomy.

However, patients with cholesterol gallstone disease who develop recurrent choledocholithiasis after cholecystectomy should be on long-term treatment with ursodeoxycholic acid.

ACUTE AND CHRONIC CHOLECYSTITIS

Acute Cholecystitis

Acute inflammation of the gallbladder wall usually follows obstruction of the cystic duct by a stone. Inflammatory response can be evoked by three factors: (1) *mechanical inflammation* produced by increased intraluminal pressure and distention with resulting ischemia of the gallbladder mucosa and wall, (2) *chemical inflammation* caused by the release of lysolecithin (due to the action of phospholipase on lecithin in bile) and other local tissue factors, and (3) *bacterial inflammation*, which may play a role in 50–85% of patients with acute cholecystitis. The organisms most frequently isolated by culture of gallbladder bile in these patients include *Escherichia coli*, *Klebsiella* spp., *Streptococcus* spp., and *Clostridium* spp.

Acute cholecystitis often begins as an attack of biliary pain that progressively worsens. Approximately 60–70% of patients report having experienced prior attacks that resolved spontaneously. As the episode progresses, however, the pain of acute cholecystitis becomes more generalized in the right upper abdomen. As with biliary colic, the pain of cholecystitis may radiate to the interscapular area, right scapula, or shoulder. Peritoneal signs of inflammation such as increased pain with jarring or on deep respiration may be apparent. The patient is anorectic and often nauseated. Vomiting is relatively common and may produce symptoms and signs of vascular and extracellular volume depletion. Jaundice is unusually early in the course of acute cholecystitis but may occur when edematous inflammatory changes involve the bile ducts and surrounding lymph nodes.

A low-grade fever is characteristically present, but shaking chills or rigors are not uncommon. The RUQ of the abdomen is almost invariably tender to palpation. An enlarged, tense gallbladder is palpable in 25–50% of patients. Deep inspiration or cough during subcostal palpation of the RUQ usually produces increased pain and inspiratory arrest (Murphy's sign). Localized rebound tenderness in the RUQ is common, as are abdominal distention and hypoactive bowel sounds from paralytic ileus, but generalized peritoneal signs and abdominal rigidity are usually lacking, in the absence of perforation.

The diagnosis of acute cholecystitis is usually made on the basis of a characteristic history and physical examination. The triad of sudden onset of RUQ tenderness, fever, and leukocytosis is highly suggestive. Typically, leukocytosis in the range of 10,000–15,000 cells per microliter with a left shift on differential count is found. The serum bilirubin is mildly elevated [<85.5 μmol/L (5 mg/dL)] in fewer than half of patients, while about one-fourth have modest elevations in serum aminotransferases (usually less than a fivefold elevation). Ultrasound will demonstrate calculi in 90–95% of cases and is useful for detection of signs of gallbladder inflammation including thickening of the wall, pericholecystic fluid, and dilation of the bile duct. The radionuclide (e.g., HIDA) biliary scan may be confirmatory if bile duct imaging is seen without visualization of the gallbladder.

Approximately 75% of patients treated medically have remission of acute symptoms within 2–7 days following hospitalization. In 25%, however, a complication of acute cholecystitis will occur despite conservative treatment (see below). In this setting, prompt surgical intervention is required. Of the 75% of patients with acute cholecystitis who undergo remission of symptoms, ~25% will experience a recurrence of cholecystitis within 1 year, and 60% will have at least one recurrent bout within 6 years. In view of the natural history of the disease, acute cholecystitis is best treated by early surgery whenever possible.

Mirizzi's syndrome is a rare complication in which a gallstone becomes impacted in the cystic duct or neck of the gallbladder causing compression of the CBD, resulting in CBD obstruction and jaundice. Ultrasound shows gallstone(s) lying outside the hepatic duct. Endoscopic retrograde cholangiopancreatography (ERCP) or percutaneous transhepatic cholangiography (PTC) or MRCP will usually demonstrate the characteristic extrinsic compression of the CBD. Surgery consists of removing the cystic duct, diseased gallbladder, and the impacted stone. The preoperative diagnosis of Mirizzi's syndrome is important to avoid CBD injury.

Acalculous Cholecystitis

In 5–10% of patients with acute cholecystitis, calculi obstructing the cystic duct are not found at surgery. In >50% of such cases, an underlying explanation for acalculous inflammation is not found. An increased risk for the development of acalculous cholecystitis is especially associated with serious trauma or burns, with the postpartum period following prolonged labor, and with orthopedic and other nonbiliary major surgical operations in the postoperative period. It may possibly complicate periods of prolonged parenteral hyperalimentation. For some of these cases, biliary sludge in the cystic duct may be responsible. Other precipitating factors include vasculitis, obstructing adenocarcinoma of the gallbladder, diabetes mellitus, torsion of the gallbladder, "unusual" bacterial infections of the gallbladder (e.g., *Leptospira, Streptococcus, Salmonella,* or *Vibrio cholerae*), and parasitic infestation of the gallbladder. Acalculous cholecystitis may also be seen with a variety of other systemic disease processes (sarcoidosis, cardiovascular disease, tuberculosis, syphilis, actinomycosis, etc.).

Although the clinical manifestations of acalculous cholecystitis are indistinguishable from those of calculous cholecystitis, the setting of acute gallbladder inflammation complicating severe underlying illness is characteristic of acalculous disease. Ultrasound, CT, or radionuclide examinations demonstrating a large, tense, static gallbladder without stones and with evidence of poor emptying over a prolonged period may be diagnostically useful in some cases. The complication rate for acalculous cholecystitis exceeds that for calculous cholecystitis. Successful management of acute acalculous cholecystitis appears to depend primarily on early diagnosis and surgical intervention, with meticulous attention to postoperative care.

Acalculous Cholecystopathy

Disordered motility of the gallbladder can produce recurrent biliary pain in patients without gallstones. Infusion of an octapeptide of CCK can be used to measure the gallbladder ejection fraction during cholescintigraphy. The surgical findings have included abnormalities such as chronic cholecystitis, gallbladder muscle hypertrophy, and/or a markedly narrowed cystic duct. Some of these patients may well have had antecedent gallbladder disease. The following criteria can be used to identify patients with acalculous cholecystopathy: (1) recurrent episodes of typical RUQ pain characteristic of biliary tract pain, (2) abnormal CCK cholescintigraphy demonstrating a gallbladder ejection fraction of <40%, and (3) infusion of CCK reproduces the patient's pain. An additional clue would be the identification of a large gallbladder on ultrasound examination. Finally, it should be noted that sphincter of Oddi dysfunction can also give rise to recurrent RUQ pain and CCK-scintigraphic abnormalities.

Emphysematous Cholecystitis

So-called emphysematous cholecystitis is thought to begin with acute cholecystitis (calculous or acalculous) followed by ischemia or gangrene of the gallbladder wall and infection by gas-producing organisms. Bacteria most frequently cultured in this setting include anaerobes, such as *C. welchii* or *C. perfringens,* and aerobes, such as *E. coli.* This condition occurs most frequently in elderly men and in patients with diabetes mellitus. The clinical manifestations are essentially indistinguishable from those of nongaseous cholecystitis. The diagnosis is usually made on plain abdominal film by finding gas within the gallbladder lumen, dissecting within the gallbladder wall to form a gaseous ring, or in the pericholecystic tissues. The morbidity and mortality rates with emphysematous cholecystitis are considerable. Prompt surgical intervention coupled with appropriate antibiotics is mandatory.

Chronic Cholecystitis

Chronic inflammation of the gallbladder wall is almost always associated with the presence of gallstones and is thought to result from repeated bouts of subacute or acute cholecystitis or from persistent mechanical irritation of the gallbladder wall by gallstones. The presence of bacteria in the bile occurs in >25% of patients with chronic cholecystitis. The presence of infected bile in a patient with *chronic* cholecystitis undergoing elective cholecystectomy probably adds little to the operative risk. Chronic cholecystitis may be asymptomatic for years, may progress to symptomatic gallbladder disease or to acute cholecystitis, or may present with complications (see the next section).

Complications of Cholecystitis

Empyema and Hydrops

Empyema of the gallbladder usually results from progression of acute cholecystitis with persistent cystic duct obstruction to superinfection of the stagnant bile with a pus-forming bacterial organism. The clinical picture resembles that of cholangitis with high fever, severe RUQ pain, marked leukocytosis, and often, prostration. Empyema of the gallbladder carries a high risk of gram-negative sepsis and/or perforation. Emergency surgical intervention with proper antibiotic coverage is required as soon as the diagnosis is suspected.

Hydrops or mucocele of the gallbladder may also result from prolonged obstruction of the cystic duct, usually by a large solitary calculus. In this instance, the obstructed gallbladder lumen is progressively distended, over a period of time, by mucus (mucocele) or by a clear transudate (hydrops) produced by mucosal epithelial cells. A visible, easily palpable, nontender mass sometimes extending from the RUQ into the right iliac fossa may be found on physical examination. The patient with hydrops of the gallbladder frequently remains asymptomatic, although chronic RUQ pain may also occur. Cholecystectomy is indicated, since empyema, perforation, or gangrene may complicate the condition.

Gangrene and Perforation

Gangrene of the gallbladder results from ischemia of the wall and patchy or complete tissue necrosis. Underlying conditions often include marked distention of the gallbladder, vasculitis, diabetes mellitus, empyema, or torsion resulting in arterial occlusion. Gangrene usually predisposes to perforation of the gallbladder, but perforation may also occur in chronic cholecystitis without premonitory warning symptoms. *Localized perforations* are usually contained by the omentum or by adhesions produced by recurrent inflammation of the gallbladder. Bacterial superinfection of the walled-off gallbladder contents results in abscess formation. Most patients are best treated with cholecystectomy, but some seriously ill patients may be managed with cholecystostomy and drainage of the abscess. *Free perforation* is less common but is associated with a mortality rate of ~30%. Such patients may experience a sudden transient relief of RUQ pain as the distended gallbladder decompresses; this is followed by signs of generalized peritonitis.

Fistula Formation and Gallstone Ileus

Fistulization into an adjacent organ adherent to the gallbladder wall may result from inflammation and adhesion formation. Fistulas into the duodenum are most common, followed in frequency by those involving the hepatic flexure of the colon, stomach or jejunum, abdominal wall, and renal pelvis. Clinically "silent" biliary-enteric fistulas occurring as a complication of acute cholecystitis have been found in up to 5% of patients undergoing cholecystectomy. Asymptomatic cholecystoenteric fistulas may sometimes be diagnosed by finding gas in the biliary tree on plain abdominal films. Barium contrast studies or endoscopy of the upper gastrointestinal tract or colon may demonstrate the fistula. Treatment in the symptomatic patient usually consists of cholecystectomy, CBD exploration, and closure of the fistulous tract.

Gallstone ileus refers to mechanical intestinal obstruction resulting from the passage of a large gallstone into the bowel lumen. The stone customarily enters the duodenum through a cholecystoenteric fistula at that level. The site of obstruction by the impacted gallstone is usually at the ileocecal valve, provided that the more proximal small bowel is of normal caliber. The majority of patients do not give a history of either prior biliary tract symptoms or complaints suggestive of acute cholecystitis or fistulization. Large stones, >2.5 cm in diameter, are thought to predispose to fistula formation by gradual erosion through the gallbladder fundus. Diagnostic confirmation may occasionally be found on the plain abdominal film (e.g., small-intestinal obstruction with gas in the biliary tree and a calcified, ectopic gallstone) or following an upper gastrointestinal series (cholecystoduodenal fistula with small-bowel obstruction at the ileocecal valve). Laparotomy with stone extraction (or propulsion into the colon) remains the procedure of choice to relieve obstruction. Evacuation of large stones within the gallbladder should also be performed. In general, the gallbladder and its attachment to the intestines should be left alone.

Limey (Milk of Calcium) Bile and Porcelain Gallbladder

Calcium salts may be secreted into the lumen of the gallbladder in sufficient concentration to produce calcium precipitation and diffuse, hazy opacification of bile or a layering effect on plain abdominal roentgenography. This so-called limey bile, or milk of calcium bile, is usually clinically innocuous, but cholecystectomy is recommended, especially when it occurs in a hydropic gallbladder. In the entity called *porcelain gallbladder*, calcium salt deposition within the wall of a chronically inflamed gallbladder may be detected on the plain abdominal film. Cholecystectomy is advised in all patients with porcelain gallbladder because in a high percentage of cases this finding appears to be associated with the development of carcinoma of the gallbladder.

℞ Treatment:
ACUTE CHOLECYSTITIS

MEDICAL THERAPY Although surgical intervention remains the mainstay of therapy for acute cholecystitis and its complications, a period of in-hospital stabilization may be required before cholecystectomy. Oral intake is eliminated, nasogastric suction may be indicated, and extracellular volume depletion and electrolyte abnormalities are repaired. Meperidine or nonsteroidal anti-inflammatory drugs (NSAIDs) are usually employed for analgesia because they may produce less spasm of the sphincter of Oddi than drugs such as morphine. Intravenous antibiotic therapy is usually indicated in patients with severe acute cholecystitis, even though bacterial superinfection of bile may not have occurred in the early stages of the inflammatory process. Antibiotic therapy is guided by the most common organisms likely to be present, which are *E. coli*, *Klebsiella* spp., and *Streptococcus* spp. Effective antibiotics include ureidopenicillins such as piperacillin or mezlocillin, ampicillin sulbactam, ciprofloxacin, moxifloxacin, and third-generation cephalosporins. Anaerobic coverage by a drug such as metronidazole should be added if gangrenous or emphysematous cholecystitis is suspected. Imipenem/meropenem represent potent parenteral antibiotics that cover the whole spectrum of bacteria causing ascending cholangitis. They should, however, be reserved for the most severe, life-threatening infections when other regimens have failed. Postoperative complications of wound infection, abscess formation, or sepsis are reduced in antibiotic-treated patients.

SURGICAL THERAPY The optimal timing of surgical intervention in patients with acute cholecystitis depends on stabilization of the patient. The clear trend is toward earlier surgery, and this is due in part to requirements for shorter hospital stays. Urgent (emergency) cholecystectomy or cholecystostomy is probably appropriate in most patients in whom a complication of acute cholecystitis such as empyema, emphysematous cholecystitis, or perforation is suspected or confirmed. In uncomplicated cases of acute cholecystitis, up to 30% of patients fail to resolve their symptoms on appropriate medical therapy, and progression of the attack or a supervening complication leads to the performance of early operation (within 24–72 h). The technical complications of surgery are not increased in patients undergoing early as opposed to delayed cholecystectomy. Delayed surgical intervention is probably best reserved for (1) patients in whom the overall medical condition imposes an unacceptable risk for early surgery and (2) patients in whom the diagnosis of acute cholecystitis is in doubt. Early cholecystectomy is the treatment of choice for most patients with acute cholecystitis. Mortality figures for emergency cholecystectomy in most centers approach 3%, while the mortality risk for elective or early cholecystectomy ~0.5% in patients under age 60. Of course, the operative risks increase with age-related diseases of other organ systems and with the presence of long- or short-term complications of gallbladder disease. Seriously ill or debilitated patients with cholecystitis may be managed with cholecystostomy and tube drainage of the gallbladder. Elective cholecystectomy may then be done at a later date.

Early complications following cholecystectomy include atelectasis and other pulmonary disorders, abscess formation (often subphrenic), external or internal hemorrhage, biliary-enteric fistula, and bile leaks. Jaundice may indicate absorption of bile from an intraabdominal collection following a biliary leak or mechanical obstruction of the CBD by retained calculi, intraductal blood clots, or extrinsic compression. Routine performance of intraoperative cholangiography during cholecystectomy has helped to reduce the incidence of these early complications.

Overall, cholecystectomy is a very successful operation that provides total or near-total relief of preoperative symptoms in 75–90% of patients. The most common cause of persistent postcholecystectomy symptoms is an overlooked symptomatic nonbiliary disorder (e.g., reflux esophagitis, peptic ulceration, pancreatitis, or—most often—irritable bowel syndrome). In a small percentage of patients, however, a disorder of the extrahepatic bile ducts may result in persistent symptomatology. These so-called postcholecystectomy syndromes may be due to (1) biliary strictures, (2) retained biliary calculi, (3) cystic duct stump syndrome, (4) stenosis or dyskinesia of the sphincter of Oddi, or (5) bile salt–induced diarrhea or gastritis.

Cystic Duct Stump Syndrome

In the absence of cholangiographically demonstrable retained stones, symptoms resembling biliary pain or cholecystitis in the postcholecystectomy patient have frequently been attributed to disease in a long (>1 cm) cystic duct remnant (cystic duct stump syndrome). Careful analysis, however, reveals that postcholecystectomy complaints are attributable to other causes in almost all patients in whom the symptom complex was originally thought to result from the existence of a long cystic duct stump. Accordingly, considerable care should be taken to investigate the possible role of other factors in the production of postcholecystectomy symptoms before attributing them to cystic duct stump syndrome.

Papillary Dysfunction, Papillary Stenosis, Spasm of the Sphincter of Oddi, and Biliary Dyskinesia

Symptoms of biliary colic accompanied by signs of recurrent, intermittent biliary obstruction may be produced by papillary stenosis, papillary dysfunction, spasm of the sphincter of Oddi, and biliary dyskinesia. Papillary stenosis is thought to result from acute or chronic inflammation of the papilla of Vater or from glandular hyperplasia of the papillary segment. Five criteria have been used to define papillary stenosis: (1) upper abdominal pain, usually RUQ or epigastric; (2) abnormal liver tests; (3) dilatation of the common bile duct upon ERCP examination; (4) delayed (>45 min) drainage of contrast material from the duct; and (5) increased basal pressure of the sphincter of Oddi, a finding that may be of only minor significance. An alternative to ERCP is magnetic resonance cholangiography (MRC) if ERCP and/or biliary manometry are either unavailable or not feasible. In patients with papillary stenosis, quantitative hepatobiliary scintigraphy has revealed delayed transit from the common bile duct to the bowel, ductal dilatation, and abnormal time-activity dynamics. This technique can also be used before and after sphincterotomy to document improvement in biliary emptying. Treatment consists of endoscopic or surgical sphincteroplasty to ensure wide patency of the distal portions of both the bile and pancreatic ducts. The greater the number of the preceding criteria present, the greater the likelihood that a patient does have a degree of papillary stenosis sufficient to justify correction. The factors usually considered as indications for sphincterotomy include (1) prolonged duration of symptoms, (2) lack of response to symptomatic treatment, (3) presence of severe disability, and (4) the patient's choice of sphincterotomy over surgery (given a clear understanding on his or her part of the risks involved in both procedures).

Criteria for diagnosing dyskinesia of the sphincter of Oddi are even more controversial than those for papillary stenosis. Proposed mechanisms include spasm of the sphincter, denervation sensitivity resulting in hypertonicity, and abnormalities of the sequencing or frequency rates of sphincteric contraction waves. When thorough evaluation has failed to demonstrate another cause for the pain, and when cholangiographic and manometric criteria suggest a diagnosis of biliary dyskinesia, medical treatment with nitrites or anticholinergics to attempt pharmacologic relaxation of the sphincter has been proposed. Endoscopic biliary sphincterotomy (EBS) or surgical sphincteroplasty may be indicated in patients who fail to respond to a 2- to 3-month trial of medical therapy, especially if basal sphincter of Oddi pressures are elevated. EBS has become the procedure of choice for removing bile duct stones and for other biliary and pancreatic problems.

Bile Salt–Induced Diarrhea and Gastritis

Postcholecystectomy patients may develop symptoms of dyspepsia, which have been attributed to duodenogastric reflux of bile. However, firm data linking these symptoms to bile gastritis after surgical removal of the gallbladder are lacking. Cholecystectomy induces persistent changes in gut transit, and these changes effect a noticeable modification of bowel habits. Cholecystectomy shortens gut transit time by accelerating passage of the fecal bolus through the colon with marked acceleration in the right colon, thus causing an increase in colonic bile acid output and a shift in bile acid composition toward the more diarrheagenic secondary bile acids. Diarrhea that is severe enough, i.e., three or more watery movements per day, can be classified as postcholecystectomy diarrhea, and this occurs in 5–10% of patients undergoing elective

cholecystectomy. Treatment with bile acid sequestering agents such as cholestyramine or colestipol is often effective in ameliorating troublesome diarrhea.

THE HYPERPLASTIC CHOLECYSTOSES

The term *hyperplastic cholecystoses* is used to denote a group of disorders of the gallbladder characterized by excessive proliferation of normal tissue components.

Adenomyomatosis is characterized by a benign proliferation of gallbladder surface epithelium with glandlike formations, extramural sinuses, transverse strictures, and/or fundal nodule ("adenoma" or "adenomyoma") formation. Outpouchings of mucosa termed *Rokitansky-Aschoff sinuses* may be seen on oral cholecystography in conjunction with hyperconcentration of contrast medium. Characteristic dimpled filling defects also may be seen.

Cholesterolosis is characterized by abnormal deposition of lipid, especially cholesteryl esters within macrophages in the lamina propria of the gallbladder wall. In its diffuse form ("strawberry gallbladder"), the gallbladder mucosa is brick red and speckled with bright yellow flecks of lipid. The localized form shows solitary or multiple "cholesterol polyps" studding the gallbladder wall. Cholesterol stones of the gallbladder are found in nearly half the cases. Cholecystectomy is indicated in both adenomyomatosis and cholesterolosis when symptomatic or when cholelithiasis is present.

The prevalence of gallbladder polyps in the adult population is ~5%, with a marked male predominance. Few significant changes have been found over a 5-year period in asymptomatic patients with gallbladder polyps <10 mm in diameter. Cholecystectomy is recommended in symptomatic patients, as well as in asymptomatic patients >50 years of age, or in those whose polyps are >10 mm in diameter or associated with gallstones or polyp growth on serial ultrasonography.

DISEASES OF THE BILE DUCTS

CONGENITAL ANOMALIES

Biliary Atresia and Hypoplasia

Atretic and hypoplastic lesions of the extrahepatic and large intrahepatic bile ducts are the most common biliary anomalies of clinical relevance encountered in infancy. The clinical picture is one of severe obstructive jaundice during the first month of life, with pale stools. When biliary atresia is suspected on the basis of clinical, laboratory, and imaging findings the diagnosis is confirmed by surgical exploration and operative cholangiography. Approximately 10% of cases of biliary atresia are treatable with roux-en-Y choledochojejunostomy, with the Kasai procedure (hepatic portoenterostomy) being attempted in the remainder in an effort to restore some bile flow. Most patients, even those having successful biliary-enteric anastomoses, eventually develop chronic cholangitis, extensive hepatic fibrosis, and portal hypertension.

Choledochal Cysts

Cystic dilatation may involve the free portion of the CBD, i.e., choledochal cyst, or may present as diverticulum formation in the intraduodenal segment. In the latter situation, chronic reflux of pancreatic juice into the biliary tree can produce inflammation and stenosis of the extrahepatic bile ducts leading to cholangitis or biliary obstruction. Because the process may be gradual, ~50% of patients present with onset of symptoms after age 10. The diagnosis may be made by ultrasound, abdominal CT, MRC, or cholangiography. Only one-third of patients show the classic triad of abdominal pain, jaundice, and an abdominal mass. Ultrasonographic detection of a cyst separate from the gallbladder should suggest the diagnosis of choledochal cyst, which can be confirmed by demonstrating the entrance of extrahepatic bile ducts into the cyst. Surgical treatment involves excision of the "cyst" and biliary-enteric anastomosis. Patients with choledochal cysts are at increased risk for the subsequent development of cholangiocarcinoma.

Congenital Biliary Ectasia

Dilatation of intrahepatic bile ducts may involve either the major intrahepatic radicles (Caroli's disease), the inter- and intralobular ducts (congenital hepatic fibrosis), or both. In Caroli's disease, clinical manifestations include recurrent cholangitis, abscess formation in and around the affected ducts, and, often, gallstone formation within portions of ectatic intrahepatic biliary radicles. Ultrasound, MRC, and CT are of great diagnostic value in demonstrating cystic dilatation of the intrahepatic bile ducts. Treatment with ongoing antibiotic therapy is usually undertaken in an effort to limit the frequency and severity of recurrent bouts of cholangitis. Progression to secondary biliary cirrhosis with portal hypertension, extrahepatic biliary obstruction, cholangiocarcinoma, or recurrent episodes of sepsis with hepatic abscess formation is common.

CHOLEDOCHOLITHIASIS

Pathophysiology and Clinical Manifestations

Passage of gallstones into the CBD occurs in ~10–15% of patients with cholelithiasis. The incidence of common duct stones increases with increasing age of the patient, so that up to 25% of elderly patients may have calculi in the common duct at the time of cholecystectomy. Undetected duct stones are left behind in ~1–5% of cholecystectomy patients. The overwhelming majority of bile duct stones are cholesterol stones formed in the gallbladder, which then migrate into the extrahepatic

biliary tree through the cystic duct. Primary calculi arising de novo in the ducts are usually pigment stones developing in patients with (1) hepatobiliary parasitism or chronic, recurrent cholangitis; (2) congenital anomalies of the bile ducts (especially Caroli's disease); (3) dilated, sclerosed, or strictured ducts; or (4) an *MDR3* gene defect leading to impaired biliary phospholipids secretion. Common duct stones may remain asymptomatic for years, may pass spontaneously into the duodenum, or (most often) may present with biliary colic or a complication.

Complications

Cholangitis

Cholangitis may be acute or chronic, and symptoms result from inflammation, which usually is caused by at least partial obstruction to the flow of bile. Bacteria are present on bile culture in ~75% of patients with acute cholangitis early in the symptomatic course. The characteristic presentation of acute cholangitis involves biliary pain, jaundice, and spiking fevers with chills (Charcot's triad). Blood cultures are frequently positive, and leukocytosis is typical. *Nonsuppurative acute cholangitis* is most common and may respond relatively rapidly to supportive measures and to treatment with antibiotics. In *suppurative acute cholangitis*, however, the presence of pus under pressure in a completely obstructed ductal system leads to symptoms of severe toxicity—mental confusion, bacteremia, and septic shock. Response to antibiotics alone in this setting is relatively poor, multiple hepatic abscesses are often present, and the mortality rate approaches 100% unless prompt endoscopic or surgical relief of the obstruction and drainage of infected bile are carried out. Endoscopic management of bacterial cholangitis is as effective as surgical intervention. ERCP with endoscopic sphincterotomy is safe and the preferred initial procedure for both establishing a definitive diagnosis and providing effective therapy.

Obstructive Jaundice

Gradual obstruction of the CBD over a period of weeks or months usually leads to initial manifestations of jaundice or pruritus without associated symptoms of biliary colic or cholangitis. Painless jaundice may occur in patients with choledocholithiasis, but is much more characteristic of biliary obstruction secondary to malignancy of the head of the pancreas, bile ducts, or ampulla of Vater.

In patients whose obstruction is secondary to choledocholithiasis, associated chronic calculous cholecystitis is very common, and the gallbladder in this setting may be relatively indistensible. The absence of a palpable gallbladder in most patients with biliary obstruction from duct stones is the basis for *Courvoisier's law*, i.e., that the presence of a palpably enlarged gallbladder suggests that the biliary obstruction is secondary to an underlying malignancy rather than to calculous disease. Biliary obstruction causes progressive dilatation of the intrahepatic bile ducts as intrabiliary pressures rise. Hepatic bile flow is suppressed, and reabsorption and regurgitation of conjugated bilirubin into the bloodstream lead to jaundice accompanied by dark urine (bilirubinuria) and light-colored (acholic) stools.

CBD stones should be suspected in any patient with cholecystitis whose serum bilirubin level is >85.5 μmol/L (5 mg/dL). The maximum bilirubin level is seldom >256.5 μmol/L (15.0 mg/dL) in patients with choledocholithiasis unless concomitant hepatic disease or another factor leading to marked hyperbilirubinemia exists. Serum bilirubin levels ≥ 342.0 μmol/L (20 mg/dL) should suggest the possibility of neoplastic obstruction. The serum alkaline phosphatase level is almost always elevated in biliary obstruction. A rise in alkaline phosphatase often precedes clinical jaundice and may be the only abnormality in routine liver function tests. There may be a two- to tenfold elevation of serum aminotransferases, especially in association with acute obstruction. Following relief of the obstructing process, serum aminotransferase elevations usually return rapidly to normal, while the serum bilirubin level may take 1–2 weeks to return to normal. The alkaline phosphatase level usually falls slowly, lagging behind the decrease in serum bilirubin.

Pancreatitis

The most common associated entity discovered in patients with nonalcoholic acute pancreatitis is biliary tract disease. Biochemical evidence of pancreatic inflammation complicates acute cholecystitis in 15% of cases and choledocholithiasis in >30%, and the common factor appears to be the passage of gallstones through the common duct. Coexisting pancreatitis should be suspected in patients with symptoms of cholecystitis who develop (1) back pain or pain to the left of the abdominal midline, (2) prolonged vomiting with paralytic ileus, or (3) a pleural effusion, especially on the left side. Surgical treatment of gallstone disease is usually associated with resolution of the pancreatitis.

Secondary Biliary Cirrhosis

Secondary biliary cirrhosis may complicate prolonged or intermittent duct obstruction with or without recurrent cholangitis. Although this complication may be seen in patients with choledocholithiasis, it is more common in cases of prolonged obstruction from stricture or neoplasm. Once established, secondary biliary cirrhosis may be progressive even after correction of the obstructing process, and increasingly severe hepatic cirrhosis may lead to portal hypertension or to hepatic failure and death. Prolonged biliary obstruction may also be associated with clinically relevant deficiencies of the fat-soluble vitamins A, D, E, and K.

Diagnosis and Treatment

The diagnosis of choledocholithiasis is usually made by cholangiography (Table 43-3), either preoperatively by ERCP or intraoperatively at the time of cholecystectomy. As many as 15% of patients undergoing cholecystectomy will prove to have CBD stones. When CBD stones are suspected prior to laparoscopic cholecystectomy, preoperative ERCP with endoscopic papillotomy and stone extraction is the preferred approach. It not only provides stone clearance but also defines the anatomy of the biliary tree in relationship to the cystic duct. CBD stones should be suspected in gallstone patients who have any of the following risk factors: (1) a history of jaundice or pancreatitis, (2) abnormal tests of liver function, and (3) ultrasonographic evidence of a dilated CBD or stones in the duct. Alternatively, if intraoperative cholangiography reveals retained stones, postoperative ERCP can be carried out. The need for preoperative ERCP is expected to decrease further as laparoscopic techniques for bile duct exploration improve.

The widespread use of laparoscopic cholecystectomy and ERCP has decreased the incidence of complicated biliary tract disease and the need for choledocholithotomy and T-tube drainage of the bile ducts. EBS followed by spontaneous passage or stone extraction is the treatment of choice in the management of patients with common duct stones, especially in elderly or poor-risk patients.

TRAUMA, STRICTURES, AND HEMOBILIA

Most benign strictures of the extrahepatic bile ducts result from surgical trauma and occur in about 1 in 500 cholecystectomies. Strictures may present with bile leak or abscess formation in the immediate postoperative period or with biliary obstruction or cholangitis as long as 2 years or more following the inciting trauma. The diagnosis is established by percutaneous or endoscopic cholangiography. Endoscopic brushing of biliary strictures may be helpful in establishing the nature of the lesion and is more accurate than bile cytology alone. When positive exfoliative cytology is obtained, the diagnosis of a neoplastic stricture is established. This procedure is especially important in patients with primary sclerosing cholangitis (PSC) who are predisposed to the development of cholangiocarcinomas. Successful operative correction of non-PSC bile duct strictures by a skillful surgeon with duct-to-bowel anastomosis is usually possible, although mortality rates from surgical complications, recurrent cholangitis, or secondary biliary cirrhosis are high.

Hemobilia may follow traumatic or operative injury to the liver or bile ducts, intraductal rupture of a hepatic abscess or aneurysm of the hepatic artery, biliary or hepatic tumor hemorrhage, or mechanical complications of choledocholithiasis or hepatobiliary parasitism. Diagnostic procedures such as liver biopsy, PTC, and transhepatic biliary

TABLE 43-3

DIAGNOSTIC EVALUATION OF THE BILE DUCTS

	DIAGNOSTIC ADVANTAGES	DIAGNOSTIC LIMITATIONS	CONTRAINDICATIONS	COMPLICATIONS	COMMENT
Hepatobiliary Ultrasound	Rapid Simultaneous scanning of GB, liver, bile ducts, pancreas Accurate identification of dilated bile ducts Not limited by jaundice, pregnancy Guidance for fine-needle biopsy	Bowel gas Massive obesity Ascites Barium Partial bile duct obstruction Poor visualization of distal CBD	None	None	Initial procedure of choice in investigating possible biliary tract obstruction
Computed Tomography	Simultaneous scanning of GB, liver, bile ducts, pancreas Accurate identification of dilated bile ducts, masses Not limited by jaundice, gas, obesity, ascites High-resolution image Guidance for fine-needle biopsy	Extreme cachexia Movement artifact Ileus Partial bile duct obstruction	Pregnancy	Reaction to iodinated contrast, if used	Indicated for evaluation of hepatic or pancreatic masses Procedure of choice in investigating possible biliary obstruction if diagnostic limitations prevent HBUS
Magnetic Resonance Cholangiopancreatography	Useful modality for visualizing pancreatic and biliary ducts Has excellent sensitivity for bile duct dilatation, biliary stricture, and intraductal abnormalities Can identify pancreatic duct dilatation or stricture, pancreatic duct stenosis, and pancreas divisum	Cannot offer therapeutic intervention High cost	Claustrophobia Certain metals (iron)	None	
Endoscopic Retrograde Cholangiopancreatography	Simultaneous pancreatography Best visualization of distal biliary tract Bile or pancreatic cytology Endoscopic sphincterotomy and stone removal Biliary manometry	Gastroduodenal obstruction ? Roux en Y biliary-enteric anastomosis	Pregnancy ? Acute pancreatitis ? Severe cardiopulmonary disease	Pancreatitis Cholangitis, sepsis Infected pancreatic pseudocyst Perforation (rare) Hypoxemia, aspiration	Cholangiogram of choice in: Absence of dilated ducts ?Pancreatic, ampullary or gastroduodenal disease Prior biliary surgery Endoscopic sphincterotomy a treatment possibility
Percutaneous Transhepatic Cholangiogram	Extremely successful when bile ducts dilated Best visualization of proximal biliary tract Bile cytology/culture Percutaneous transhepatic drainage	Nondilated or sclerosed ducts	Pregnancy Uncorrectable coagulopathy Massive ascites ? Hepatic abscess	Bleeding Hemobilia Bile peritonitis Bacteremia, sepsis	Indicated when ERCP is contraindicated or failed
Endoscopic Ultrasound	Most sensitive method to detect ampullary stones				

drainage catheter placement may also be complicated by hemobilia. Patients often present with a classic triad of biliary pain, obstructive jaundice, and melena or occult blood in the stools. The diagnosis is sometimes made by cholangiographic evidence of blood clot in the biliary tree, but selective angiographic verification may be required. Although minor episodes of hemobilia may resolve without operative intervention, surgical ligation of the bleeding vessel is frequently required.

EXTRINSIC COMPRESSION OF THE BILE DUCTS

Partial or complete biliary obstruction may be produced by extrinsic compression of the ducts. The most common cause of this form of obstructive jaundice is carcinoma of the head of the pancreas. Biliary obstruction may also occur as a complication of either acute or chronic pancreatitis or involvement of lymph nodes in the porta hepatis by lymphoma or metastatic carcinoma. The latter should be distinguished from cholestasis resulting from massive replacement of the liver by tumor.

HEPATOBILIARY PARASITISM

Infestation of the biliary tract by adult helminths or their ova may produce a chronic, recurrent pyogenic cholangitis with or without multiple hepatic abscesses, ductal stones, or biliary obstruction. This condition is relatively rare but does occur in inhabitants of southern China and elsewhere in Southeast Asia. The organisms most commonly involved are trematodes or flukes, including *Clonorchis sinensis*, *Opisthorchis viverrini* or *O. felineus*, and *Fasciola hepatica*. The biliary tract also may be involved by intraductal migration of adult *Ascaris lumbricoides* from the duodenum or by intrabiliary rupture of hydatid cysts of the liver produced by *Echinococcus* spp. The diagnosis is made by cholangiography and the presence of characteristic ova on stool examination. When obstruction is present, the treatment of choice is laparotomy under antibiotic coverage, with common duct exploration and a biliary drainage procedure.

SCLEROSING CHOLANGITIS

Primary or idiopathic sclerosing cholangitis is characterized by a progressive, inflammatory, sclerosing, and obliterative process affecting the extrahepatic and/or the intrahepatic bile ducts. The disorder occurs up to 75% in association with inflammatory bowel disease, especially ulcerative colitis. It may also be associated with autoimmune pancreatitis; multifocal fibrosclerosis syndromes such as retroperitoneal, mediastinal, and/or periureteral fibrosis; Riedel's struma; or pseudotumor of the orbit.

Patients with primary sclerosing cholangitis often present with signs and symptoms of chronic or intermittent biliary obstruction: RUQ abdominal pain, pruritus, jaundice, or acute cholangitis. Late in the course, complete biliary obstruction, secondary biliary cirrhosis, hepatic failure, or portal hypertension with bleeding varices may occur. The diagnosis is usually established by finding multifocal, diffusely distributed strictures with intervening segments of normal or dilated ducts, producing a beaded appearance on cholangiography (Fig. 43-2*D*). The cholangiographic technique of choice in suspected cases is ERCP. When a diagnosis of sclerosing cholangitis has been established, a search for associated diseases, especially for chronic inflammatory bowel disease, should be carried out.

A recent study describes the natural history and outcome for 11 patients of Swedish descent with primary sclerosing cholangitis; 134 (44%) of the patients were asymptomatic at the time of diagnosis and, not surprisingly, had a significantly higher survival rate. The independent predictors of a bad prognosis were age, serum bilirubin concentration, and liver histologic changes. Cholangiocarcinoma was found in 24 patients (8%). Inflammatory bowel disease was closely associated with primary sclerosing cholangitis and had a prevalence of 81% in this study population.

Small duct PSC is defined by the presence of chronic cholestasis and hepatic histology consistent with PSC but with normal findings on cholangiography. Small duct PSC is found in ~5% of patients with PSC and may represent an earlier stage of PSC associated with a significantly better long-term prognosis. However, such patients may progress to classic PSC and/or end-stage liver disease with consequent necessity of liver transplantation.

In patients with AIDS, cholangiopancreatography may demonstrate a broad range of biliary tract changes as well as pancreatic duct obstruction and occasionally pancreatitis. Further, biliary tract lesions in AIDS include infection and cholangiopancreatographic changes similar to those of PSC. Changes noted include (1) diffuse involvement of intrahepatic bile ducts alone, (2) involvement of both intra- and extrahepatic bile ducts, (3) ampullary stenosis, (4) stricture of the intrapancreatic portion of the common bile duct, and (5) pancreatic duct involvement. Associated infectious organisms include *Cryptosporidium*, *Mycobacterium avium-intracellulare*, cytomegalovirus, *Microsporidia*, and *Isospora*. In addition, acalculous cholecystitis occurs in up to 10% of patients. ERCP sphincterotomy, while not without risk, provides significant pain reduction in patients with AIDS-associated papillary stenosis. Secondary sclerosing cholangitis may occur as a long-term complication of choledocholithiasis, cholangiocarcinoma, operative or traumatic biliary injury, or contiguous inflammatory processes.

℞ **Treatment:**
SCLEROSING CHOLANGITIS

Therapy with cholestyramine may help control symptoms of pruritus, and antibiotics are useful when cholangitis complicates the clinical picture. Vitamin D and calcium supplementation may help prevent the loss of bone mass frequently seen in patients with chronic cholestasis. Glucocorticoids, methotrexate, and cyclosporine have not been shown to be efficacious in PSC. UDCA in high dosage (20 mg/kg) improves serum liver tests, but an effect on survival has not been documented. In cases where high-grade biliary obstruction (dominant strictures) has occurred, balloon dilatation or stenting may be appropriate. Only rarely is surgical intervention indicated. Efforts at biliary-enteric anastomosis or stent placement may, however, be complicated by recurrent cholangitis and further progression of the stenosing process. The prognosis is unfavorable, with a median survival of 9–12 years following the diagnosis, regardless of therapy. Four variables (age, serum bilirubin level, histologic stage, and splenomegaly) predict survival in patients with PSC and serve as the basis for a risk score. PSC is one of the most common indications for liver transplantation.

FURTHER READINGS

APSTEIN MD, CAREY MC: Pathogenesis of cholesterol gallstones: A parsimonious hypothesis. Eur J Clin Invest 26:343, 1996

ATTASARANYA S et al: Choledocholithiasis, ascending cholangitis, and gallstone pancreatitis. Med Clin North Am 92:925, 2008

BERR F et al: 7-Alpha-dehydroxylating bacteria enhance deoxycholic acid input and cholesterol saturation of bile in patients with gallstones. Gastroenterology 111:1611, 1996

BROOME U et al: Natural history and outcome in 32 Swedish patients with small duct primary sclerosing cholangitis (PSC). J Hepatol 36:586, 2002

————— et al: Natural history and prognostic factors in 305 Swedish patients with primary sclerosing cholangitis. Gut 38:610, 1996

CAREY MC et al: Epidemiology of the American Indians' burden and its likely genetic origins. Hepatology 36:781, 2002

ELWOOD DR: Cholecystitis. Surg Clin North Am 88:1241, 2008

FARMAR J et al: AIDS-related cholangiopancreatic changes. Abdom Imaging 19:417, 1994

FORT JM et al: Bowel habit after cholecystectomy: Physiologic changes and clinical implications. Gastroenterology 111:617, 1996

FREEMAN ML et al: Complications of endoscopic biliary sphincterotomy. N Engl J Med 335:909, 1996

HOFMANN AF: Bile acids: trying to understand their chemistry and biology with the hope of helping patients. Hepatology 49:1403, 2009

HOLZKNECHT N et al: Breath-hold MR cholangiography using snapshot techniques: A prospective comparison with endoscopic cholangiography. Radiology 206:657, 1998

KOITSIKA D et al: Genetic and environmental influences on symptomatic gallstone disease: A Swedish study of 43,141 twin pairs. Hepatology 41: 1138, 2005

KULLOCK-UBLICK GA et al: Euterohepatic bile salt transporter in normal physiology and liver disease. Gastroenterology 126: 322, 2004

LAMMERT F, MIQUEL JF: Gallstone disease: from genes to evidence-based therapy. J Hepatol 48:S124, 2008

—————, SAUERBRUCH T: Mechanisms of disease: The genetic epidemiology of gallbladder stones. Nat Clin Pract Gastroenterol Hepatol 2: 423, 2005

MACFAYDEN BV JR et al: Bile duct injury after laparoscopic cholescystectomy. The United States experience. Surg Endosc 12:315, 1998

MARINGHINI A et al: Gallstones, gallbladder cancer, and other gastrointestinal malignancies: An epidemiologic study in Rochester, Minnesota. Ann Intern Med 107:30, 1987

MAY GR et al: Efficacy of bile acid therapy for gallstone dissolution: A meta-analysis of randomized trials. Aliment Pharmacol Ther 7:139, 1993

MYERS RP et al: Gallbladder polyps: Epidemiology, natural history and management. Can J Gastroenterol 16:187, 2002 (Review)

PAUMPARTNER G: Nonsurgical management of gallstone disease, in Sleisenger and Fordtran's Gastrointestinal and Liver Disease, 7th ed, M Feldman et al (eds). Philadelphia, Saunders, 2002, pp 1107–1115

PORTINCASA P et al: Cholesterol gallstone disease. Lancet 368:230, 2006

PULLINGER CR et al: Human cholesterol 7-hydroxylase (CYPA1) deficiency has a hypercholesterolemic phenotype. J Clin Invest 110:109, 2002

RANSOHOFF DF, GRACIE WA: Treatment of gallstones. Ann Intern Med 119:606, 1993

ROSMORDUC O et al: ABCB4 gene mutation-associated cholelithiasis in adults. Gastroenterology 125: 452, 2003

SARIN SK et al: High familial prevalence of gallstones in the first degree relatives of gallstone patients. Hepatology 22:138, 1995

SHIFFMAN M et al: Prophylaxis against gallstone formation with ursodeoxycholic acid in patients. Ann Intern Med 122:999, 1995

STRASBERG SM: Cholelithiasis and acute cholecystitis. Baillieres Clin Gastroenterol 22:643, 1997

TRAUNER M et al: Molecular pathogenesis of cholestasis. N Engl J Med 339:1217, 1998

VENNEMAN NG et al: Small gallstones, preferred gallbladder motility, and fast crystallization are associated with pancreatitis. Hepatology 41: 738, 2005

ZACKS SL et al: A population-based cohort study comparing laparoscopic cholecystectomy and open cholecystectomy. Ann J Gastroenterol 97:334, 2002

ZALIEKAS J, MUNSON JL: Complications of gallstones: the Mirizzi syndrome, gallstone ileus, gallstone pancreatitis, complications of "lost" gallstones. Surg Clin North Am 88:1345, 2008

LIVER TRANSPLANTATION

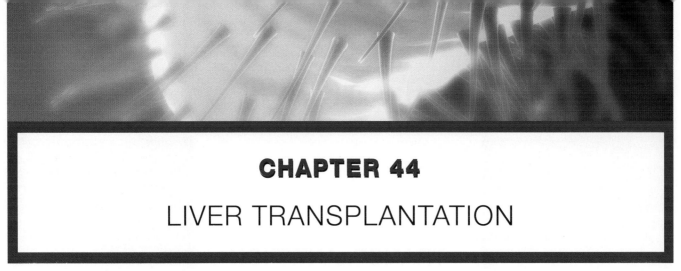

CHAPTER 44

LIVER TRANSPLANTATION

Jules L. Dienstag ■ Raymond T. Chung

Liver transplantation—the replacement of the native, diseased liver by a normal organ (allograft)—has matured from an experimental procedure reserved for desperately ill patients to an accepted, lifesaving operation applied more optimally in the natural history of end-stage liver disease. The preferred and technically most advanced approach is *orthotopic transplantation*, in which the native organ is removed and the donor organ is inserted in the same anatomic location. Pioneered in the 1960s by Starzl at the University of Colorado and, later, at the University of Pittsburgh and by Calne in Cambridge, England, liver transplantation is now performed routinely worldwide. Success measured as 1-year survival has improved from ~30% in the 1970s to about 90% today. These improved prospects for prolonged survival, dating back to the early 1980s, resulted from refinements in operative technique, improvements in organ procurement and preservation, advances in immunosuppressive therapy, and, perhaps most influentially, more enlightened patient selection and timing. Despite the perioperative morbidity and mortality, the technical and management challenges of the procedure, and its costs, liver transplantation has become the approach of choice for selected patients whose chronic or acute liver disease is progressive, life-threatening, and unresponsive to medical therapy. Based on the current level of success, the number of liver transplants has continued to grow each year; in 2005, approximately 6000 patients received liver allografts in the United States. Still, the demand for new livers continues to outpace availability; in the same period, >17,000 patients in the United States were on a waiting list for a donor liver. In response to this drastic shortage of donor organs, many transplantation centers have begun to supplement cadaver-organ liver transplantation with living-donor transplantation.

INDICATIONS

Potential candidates for liver transplantation are children and adults who, in the absence of contraindications (see later), suffer from severe, irreversible liver disease for which alternative medical or surgical treatments have been exhausted or are unavailable. *Timing of the operation is of critical importance.* Indeed, improved timing and better patient selection are felt to have contributed more to the increased success of liver transplantation in the 1980s and beyond than all the impressive technical and immunologic advances combined. Although the disease should be advanced, and although opportunities for spontaneous or medically induced stabilization or recovery should be allowed, the procedure should be done sufficiently early to give the surgical procedure a fair chance for success. Ideally, transplantation should be considered in patients with end-stage liver disease who are experiencing or have experienced a life-threatening complication of hepatic decompensation or whose quality of life has deteriorated to unacceptable levels. Although patients with well-compensated cirrhosis can survive for many years, many patients with quasi-stable chronic liver disease have much more advanced disease than may be apparent. As discussed below, the better the status of the patient prior to transplantation, the higher will be the anticipated success rate of transplantation. The decision about *when* to transplant is complex and requires the combined judgment of an experienced team of hepatologists, transplant surgeons, anesthesiologists, and specialists in support services, not to mention the well-informed consent of the patient and the patient's family.

TRANSPLANTATION IN CHILDREN

Indications for transplantation in children are listed in Table 44-1. The most common is *biliary atresia. Inherited or genetic disorders of metabolism* associated with liver failure constitute another major indication for transplantation in children and adolescents. In Crigler-Najjar disease type I and in certain hereditary disorders of the urea cycle and of amino acid or lactate-pyruvate

metabolism, transplantation may be the only way to prevent impending deterioration of CNS function, despite the fact that the native liver is structurally normal. Combined heart and liver transplantation has yielded dramatic improvement in cardiac function and in cholesterol levels in children with homozygous familial hypercholesterolemia; combined liver and kidney transplantation has been successful in patients with primary hyperoxaluria type I. In hemophiliacs with transfusion-associated hepatitis and liver failure, liver transplantation has been associated with recovery of normal Factor VIII synthesis.

TRANSPLANTATION IN ADULTS

Liver transplantation is indicated for end-stage *cirrhosis* of all causes (Table 44-1). In *sclerosing cholangitis* and *Caroli's disease* (multiple cystic dilatations of the intrahepatic biliary tree), recurrent infections and sepsis associated with inflammatory and fibrotic obstruction of the biliary tree may be an indication for transplantation. Because prior biliary surgery complicates, and is a relative contraindication for, liver transplantation, surgical diversion of the biliary tree has been all but abandoned for patients with sclerosing cholangitis. In patients who undergo transplantation for *hepatic vein thrombosis (Budd-Chiari syndrome)*, postoperative anticoagulation is essential; underlying myeloproliferative disorders may have to be treated but are not a contraindication to liver transplantation. If a donor organ can be located quickly, before life-threatening complications—including cerebral edema—set in, patients with acute liver failure are candidates for liver transplantation. Routine candidates for liver transplantation are patients with *alcoholic cirrhosis, chronic viral hepatitis,* and *primary hepatocellular malignancies.* Although all three of these categories are considered to be high risk, liver transplantation can be offered to carefully selected patients. Currently, chronic hepatitis C and alcoholic liver disease are the most common indications for liver transplantation, accounting for over 40% of all adult candidates who undergo the procedure. Patients with alcoholic cirrhosis can be considered as candidates for transplantation if they meet strict criteria for abstinence and reform; however, these criteria still do not prevent recidivism in up to a quarter of cases. Patients with chronic hepatitis C have early allograft and patient survival comparable to those of other subsets of patients after transplantation; however, reinfection in the donor organ is universal, recurrent hepatitis C is insidiously progressive, the impact of antiviral therapy is limited, allograft cirrhosis develops in 20–30% at 5 years, and cirrhosis and late organ failure are being recognized with increasing frequency beyond 5 years. In patients with chronic hepatitis B, in the absence of measures to prevent recurrent hepatitis B, survival after transplantation is reduced by approximately 10–20%; however,

TABLE 44-1

INDICATIONS FOR LIVER TRANSPLANTATION

CHILDREN	ADULTS
Biliary atresia	Primary biliary cirrhosis
Neonatal hepatitis	Secondary biliary cirrhosis
Congenital hepatic fibrosis	Primary sclerosing cholangitis
Alagille's disease[a]	
Byler's disease[b]	Autoimmune hepatitis
α_1-Antitrypsin deficiency	Caroli's disease[c]
Inherited disorders of metabolism	Cryptogenic cirrhosis
Wilson's disease	Chronic hepatitis with cirrhosis
Tyrosinemia	Hepatic vein thrombosis
Glycogen storage diseases	Fulminant hepatitis
Lysosomal storage diseases	Alcoholic cirrhosis
Protoporphyria	Chronic viral hepatitis
Crigler-Najjar disease type I	Primary hepatocellular malignancies
Familial hypercholesterolemia	Hepatic adenomas
Primary hyperoxaluria type I	Nonalcoholic steatohepatitis
Hemophilia	Familial amyloid polyneuropathy

[a]Arteriohepatic dysplasia, with paucity of bile ducts, and congenital malformations, including pulmonary stenosis.
[b]Intrahepatic cholestasis, progressive liver failure, mental and growth retardation.
[c]Multiple cystic dilatations of the intrahepatic biliary tree.

prophylactic use of hepatitis B immune globulin (HBIg) during and after transplantation increases the success of transplantation to a level comparable to that seen in patients with nonviral causes of liver decompensation. The specific oral antiviral drugs lamivudine, adefovir dipivoxil, and entecavir (Chap. 39) can be used both for prophylaxis against and for treatment of recurrent hepatitis B, facilitating further the management of patients undergoing liver transplantation for end-stage hepatitis B; most transplantation centers rely on a combination of HBIg and antiviral drugs to manage patients with hepatitis B. Issues of disease recurrence are discussed in more detail below. Patients with nonmetastatic primary hepatobiliary tumors—primary hepatocellular carcinoma (HCC), cholangiocarcinoma, hepatoblastoma, angiosarcoma, epithelioid hemangioendothelioma, and multiple or massive hepatic adenomata—have undergone liver transplantation; however, for some hepatobiliary malignancies, overall survival is significantly lower than that for other categories of liver disease. Most transplantation centers have reported 5-year recurrence-free survival rates in patients with unresectable HCC for single tumors <5 cm in diameter or for three or fewer lesions all <3 cm comparable to those seen in patients undergoing transplantation for nonmalignant indications. Consequently, liver transplantation is currently restricted to patients whose hepatic malignancies meet these criteria. Expanded criteria for patients with HCC are being evaluated. Because the likelihood of recurrent cholangiocarcinoma is very high, only highly selected patients with limited disease are being evaluated for transplantation after intensive chemotherapy and radiation.

CONTRAINDICATIONS

Absolute contraindications for transplantation include life-threatening systemic diseases, uncontrolled extrahepatic bacterial or fungal infections, preexisting advanced cardiovascular or pulmonary disease, multiple uncorrectable life-threatening congenital anomalies, metastatic malignancy, active drug or alcohol abuse (Table 44-2). Because carefully selected patients in their sixties and even seventies have undergone transplantation successfully, advanced age per se is no longer considered an absolute contraindication; however, in older patients a more thorough preoperative evaluation should be undertaken to exclude ischemic cardiac disease and other comorbid conditions. Advanced age (>70 years), however, should be considered a *relative contraindication*—that is, a factor to be taken into account with other relative contraindications. Other relative contraindications include portal vein thrombosis, HIV infection, preexisting renal disease not associated with liver disease, intrahepatic or biliary sepsis, severe hypoxemia (P_{O_2} <50 mmHg)

TABLE 44-2

CONTRAINDICATIONS TO LIVER TRANSPLANTATION

ABSOLUTE	RELATIVE
Uncontrolled extrahepatobiliary infection	Age >70
Active, untreated sepsis	Prior extensive hepatobiliary surgery
Uncorrectable, life-limiting congenital anomalies	Portal vein thrombosis
Active substance or alcohol abuse	Renal failure
Advanced cardiopulmonary disease	Previous extrahepatic malignancy (not including nonmelanoma skin cancer)
Extrahepatobiliary malignancy (not including nonmelanoma skin cancer)	Severe obesity
	Severe malnutrition/ wasting
	Medical noncompliance
Metastatic malignancy to the liver	HIV seropositivity
Cholangiocarcinoma	Intrahepatic sepsis
AIDS	Severe hypoxemia secondary to right-to-left intrapulmonary shunts (P_{O_2} < 50 mmHg)
Life-threatening systemic diseases	Severe pulmonary hypertension (mean PA pressure >35 mmHg)
	Uncontrolled psychiatric disorder

resulting from right-to-left intrapulmonary shunts, portopulmonary hypertension with high mean pulmonary artery pressures (>35 mmHg), previous extensive hepatobiliary surgery, any uncontrolled serious psychiatric disorder, and lack of sufficient social supports. Any one of these relative contraindications is insufficient in and of itself to preclude transplantation. For example, the problem of portal vein thrombosis can be overcome by constructing a graft from the donor liver portal vein to the recipient's superior mesenteric vein. Now that highly active antiretroviral therapy has dramatically improved the survival of persons with HIV infection, and because end-stage liver disease caused by chronic hepatitis C and B has emerged as a serious source of morbidity and mortality in the HIV-infected population, liver transplantation has now been performed successfully in selected HIV-positive persons who have excellent control of HIV infection. A multicenter National Institutes of Health (NIH) consortium is currently studying outcomes of liver transplantation in HIV-infected recipients.

TECHNICAL CONSIDERATIONS

CADAVER DONOR SELECTION

Cadaver donor livers for transplantation are procured primarily from victims of head trauma. Organs from brain-dead donors up to age 60 are acceptable if the following criteria are met: hemodynamic stability, adequate oxygenation, absence of bacterial or fungal infection, absence of abdominal trauma, absence of hepatic dysfunction, and serologic exclusion of hepatitis B and C viruses and HIV. Occasionally, organs from donors with hepatitis B and C are used, e.g., for recipients with prior hepatitis B and C, respectively. Donor organs with antibody to hepatitis B core antigen (anti-HBc) can also be used when the need is especially urgent, and recipients of these organs are treated prophylactically with HBIg and other antiviral drugs. Cardiovascular and respiratory functions are maintained artificially until the liver can be removed. Transplantation of organs procured from deceased donors who have succumbed to cardiac death can be performed successfully under selected circumstances, when ischemic time is minimized and liver histology preserved. Compatibility in ABO blood group and organ size between donor and recipient are important considerations in donor selection; however, ABO-incompatible, split liver, or reduced-donor-organ transplants can be performed in emergency or marked donor-scarcity situations. Tissue typing for HLA matching is not required, and preformed cytotoxic HLA antibodies do not preclude liver transplantation. Following perfusion with cold electrolyte solution, the donor liver is removed and packed in ice. The use of University of Wisconsin (UW) solution, rich in lactobionate and raffinose, has permitted the extension of cold ischemic time up to 20 h; however, 12 h may be a more reasonable limit. Improved techniques for harvesting multiple organs from the same donor have increased the availability of donor livers, but the availability of donor livers is far outstripped by the demand. Currently in the United States, all donor livers are distributed through a nationwide organ-sharing network [United Network of Organ Sharing (UNOS)] designed to allocate available organs based on regional considerations and recipient acuity. Recipients who have the highest disease severity generally have the highest priority, but allocation strategies that balance highest urgency against best outcomes continue to evolve to distribute cadaver organs most effectively. Allocation based on the Child-Turcotte-Pugh (CTP) score, which uses five clinical variables (encephalopathy stage, ascites, bilirubin, albumin, and prothrombin time) and waiting time, has been replaced by allocation based upon urgency alone, calculated by the Model for End-Stage Liver Disease (MELD) score. The MELD score is based upon a mathematical model that includes bilirubin, creatinine, and prothrombin time expressed as international normalized ratio (INR) (Table 44-3). Neither waiting time (except as a tie breaker between two potential recipients with the same MELD scores) nor posttransplantation outcome is taken into account, but the MELD score has been shown to be the best predictor of pretransplantation mortality, satisfies the prevailing view that medical need should be the decisive determinant, and eliminates both the subjectivity inherent in the CTP scoring system (presence and degree of ascites and hepatic encephalopathy) and the differences in waiting times among different regions of the country. Under the CTP or the MELD system, highest priority (status 1) continues to be reserved for those patients with fulminant hepatic failure. Because candidates for liver transplantation who have HCC may not be sufficiently decompensated to compete for donor organs based upon urgency criteria alone, and because protracted waiting for cadaver donor organs results often in tumor growth beyond acceptable limits for transplantation, such patients are assigned disease-specific MELD points (Table 44-3).

LIVING-DONOR TRANSPLANTATION

Occasionally, especially for liver transplantation in children, one cadaver organ can be split between two (one adult and one child) recipients. A more viable alternative, transplantation of the right lobe of the liver from a healthy adult into an adult recipient, has gained increased popularity. Living-donor transplantation of the left lobe (left lateral segment), introduced in the early 1990s to alleviate the extreme shortage of donor organs for small children, accounts currently for approximately a third of all liver transplantation procedures in children. Driven by the shortage of cadaver organs, living-donor transplantation involving the more sizable right lobe is being considered with increasing frequency in adults; however, living-donor liver transplantation cannot be expected to solve the donor organ shortage. About 300 such procedures were done in 2005, representing only about 5% of all liver transplant operations done in the United States.

Living-donor transplantation can reduce waiting time and cold-ischemia time; is done under elective, rather than emergency, circumstances; and may be lifesaving in recipients who cannot afford to wait for a cadaver donor. The downside, of course, is the risk to the healthy donor (a mean of 10 weeks of medical disability; biliary complications in ~5%; postoperative complications such as wound infection, small-bowel obstruction, and incisional hernias in 9–19%; and, even, in 0.2–0.4%, death) as well as the increased frequency of biliary (15–32%) and vascular (10%) complications in the recipient. Potential donors must participate voluntarily without coercion, and transplantation teams should go to great lengths to exclude subtle coercive or inappropriate psychological factors as well as outline carefully to both donor and recipient the potential benefits and risks of the procedure. Donors for the procedure should be 18–60 years old; have a compatible blood type with the recipient; have no chronic medical problems or history of major abdominal surgery; be related genetically or emotionally to the recipient; and pass an exhaustive

TABLE 44-3

| UNITED NETWORK FOR ORGAN SHARING (UNOS) LIVER TRANSPLANTATION WAITING LIST CRITERIA |

PREVIOUS ALLOCATION SCHEME (IN ORDER OF DESCENDING URGENCY)

Status 1	Fulminant hepatic failure (including primary graft nonfunction and hepatic artery thrombosis within 7 days after transplantation as well as acute decompensated Wilson's disease)[a]
Status 2A	Chronic liver disease with CTP[b] score ≥10, in intensive care unit, predicted <7 days to live, plus one of following: hepatic encephalopathy ≥stage III, unresponsive variceal bleeding, hepatorenal syndrome, refractory ascites or hepatic hydrothorax, coagulopathy with ongoing bleeding (cannot have extrahepatic sepsis, high-dose or double pressor dependency, or multiorgan failure)
Status 2B	Chronic liver disease with CTP score ≥10 or CTP score ≥7 plus one of following: variceal bleeding, hepatorenal syndrome, history of spontaneous bacterial peritonitis, refractory ascites or hepatic hydrothorax, refractory bleeding
Status 3	CTP score ≥7
Status 7	Inactive

CURRENT ALLOCATION SCHEME

The Model for End-Stage Liver Disease (MELD) score, on a continuous scale,[c] determines allocation of donor organs. This model is based upon the following calculation:

$3.78 \times \log_e$ bilirubin (mg/100 mL) $+ 11.2 \times \log_e$ international normalized ratio (INR) $+ 9.57 \times \log_e$ creatinine (mg/100 mL) $+ 6.43$ ($\times 0$ for alcoholic and cholestatic liver disease, $\times 1$ for all other types of liver disease).[d,e,f]

Online calculators to determine MELD scores are available, such as *www.mayoclinic.org/gi-rst/mayomodel6.htm*

[a]For children <18 years, status 1 includes acute or chronic liver failure plus hospitalization in an intensive care unit or inborn errors of metabolism.
[b]Child-Turcotte-Pugh (CTP) score components

Points	1	2	3
Encephalopathy	None	Stages I–II	Stages III–IV
Ascites	Absent	Slight, responsive	Moderate-severe
Bilirubin (mg/100 mL)	<2	2–3	>3
Albumin (g/100 mL)	>3.5	2.8–3.5	<2.8
Prothrombin time	<15 s	15–17 s	>17 s

The CTP score is calculated by assigning 1 point for any feature in column 1, 2 points for any feature in column 2, and 3 points for any feature in column 3. Class A = ≤6; class B = 7–9; class C = ≥10. For cholestatic disorders, such as primary biliary cirrhosis, primary sclerosing cholangitic, etc., the bilirubin categories are <4, 4–10, and >10.
[c]Instead of the 4 categories of severity in the previous system and 8 potential CTP scores between 7 and 15, the MELD scale is continuous, with 34 levels ranging between 6 and 40. The MELD scale replaces status 2A, 2B, and 3 (and 7), but status 1 is retained for those with the highest priority. Donor organs rarely become available unless the MELD score exceeds 20 to 30.
[d]Patients with hepatocellular carcinoma receive an extra 20 (for stage T1) or 24 (for stage T2) points. An α-fetoprotein level ≥500 ng/mL is considered as stage I hepatocellular carcinoma even without evidence for a tumor on imaging.
[e]Patients with stage T2 hepatocellular carcinoma receive 22 disease-specific points. An α fetoprotein level = 500 ng/mL is considered as stage I hepatocellular carcinoma even without evidence for a tumor on imaging.
[f]Creatinine is included, because renal function is a validated predictor of survival in patients with liver disease. For adults undergoing dialysis twice a week, the creatinine in the equation is set to 4 mg/100 mL.
[g]For children <18 years, the Pediatric End-Stage Liver Disease (PELD) scale is used. This scale is based upon albumin, bilirubin, INR, growth failure, and age. Status 1 is retained, but the PELD replaces status 2 and 3.

series of clinical, biochemical, and serologic evaluations to unearth disqualifying medical disorders. The recipient should meet the same UNOS criteria for liver transplantation as recipients of a cadaver donor allograft. The multicenter NIH A2ALL Study is collecting comprehensive data regarding outcomes of adult-to-adult living-donor liver transplantation (*http://www.nih-a2all.org/*).

SURGICAL TECHNIQUE

Removal of the recipient's native liver is technically difficult, particularly in the presence of portal hypertension with its associated collateral circulation and extensive varices. Further complicating removal is the presence of scarring from previous abdominal operations. The

combination of portal hypertension and coagulopathy (elevated prothrombin time and thrombocytopenia) may translate into large blood product transfusion requirements. After the portal vein and infrahepatic and suprahepatic inferior vena cavae are dissected, the hepatic artery and common bile duct are dissected. Then the native liver is removed and the donor organ inserted. During the anhepatic phase, coagulopathy, hypoglycemia, hypocalcemia, and hypothermia are encountered and must be managed by the anesthesiology team. Caval, portal vein, hepatic artery, and bile duct anastomoses are performed in succession, the last by end-to-end suturing of the donor and recipient common bile ducts or by choledochojejunostomy to a Roux-en-Y loop if the recipient common bile duct cannot be used for reconstruction (e.g., in sclerosing cholangitis). A typical transplant operation lasts 8 h, with a range of 6–18 h. Because of excessive bleeding, large volumes of blood, blood products, and volume expanders may be required during surgery; however, blood requirements have fallen sharply with improvements in surgical technique and experience.

As noted above, emerging alternatives to orthotopic liver transplantation include split-liver grafts, in which one donor organ is divided and inserted into two recipients; and living-donor procedures, in which the left (for children) or the right (for adults) lobe of the liver is harvested from a living donor for transplantation into the recipient. In the adult procedure, once the right lobe is removed from the donor, the donor right hepatic vein is anastomosed to the recipient right hepatic vein remnant, followed by donor-to-recipient anastomoses of the portal vein and then the hepatic artery. Finally, the biliary anastomosis is performed, duct-to-duct if practical or via Roux-en-Y anastomosis. Heterotopic liver transplantation, in which the donor liver is inserted without removal of the native liver, has met with very limited success and acceptance, except in a very small number of centers. In attempts to support desperately ill patients until a suitable donor organ can be identified, several transplantation centers are studying extracorporeal perfusion with bioartificial liver cartridges constructed from hepatocytes bound to hollow fiber systems and used as temporary hepatic-assist devices, but their efficacy remains to be established. Areas of research with the potential to overcome the shortage of donor organs include hepatocyte transplantation and xenotransplantation with genetically modified organs of nonhuman origin (e.g., swine).

POSTOPERATIVE COURSE AND MANAGEMENT

IMMUNOSUPPRESSIVE THERAPY

The introduction in 1980 of cyclosporine as an immunosuppressive agent contributed substantially to the improvement in survival after liver transplantation. Cyclosporine, a calcineurin inhibitor, blocks early activation of T cells and is specific for T cell functions that result from the interaction of the T cell with its receptor and that involve the calcium-dependent signal transduction pathway. As a result, the activity of cyclosporine leads to inhibition of lymphokine gene activation, blocking interleukins 2, 3, and 4, tumor necrosis factor α, and other lymphokines. Cyclosporine also inhibits B cell functions. This process occurs without affecting rapidly dividing cells in the bone marrow, which may account for the reduced frequency of posttransplantation systemic infections. The most common and important side effect of cyclosporine therapy is nephrotoxicity. Cyclosporine causes dose-dependent renal tubular injury and direct renal artery vasospasm. Following renal function, therefore,

is important in monitoring cyclosporine therapy, perhaps even a more reliable indicator than blood levels of the drug. Nephrotoxicity is reversible and can be managed by dose reduction. Other adverse effects of cyclosporine therapy include hypertension, hyperkalemia, tremor, hirsutism, glucose intolerance, and gum hyperplasia.

Tacrolimus (originally labeled *FK 506*) is a macrolide lactone antibiotic isolated from a Japanese soil fungus, *Streptomyces tsukubaensis*. It has the same mechanism of action as cyclosporine but is 10–100 times more potent. Initially applied as "rescue" therapy for patients in whom rejection occurred despite the use of cyclosporine, tacrolimus was shown in two large, multicenter, randomized trials to be associated with a reduced frequency of acute rejection, refractory rejection, and chronic rejection. Although patient and graft survival are the same with these two drugs, the advantage of tacrolimus in minimizing episodes of rejection, reducing the need for additional glucocorticoid doses, and reducing the likelihood of bacterial and cytomegalovirus (CMV) infection has simplified the management of patients undergoing liver transplantation. In addition, the oral absorption of tacrolimus is more predictable than that of cyclosporine, especially during the early postoperative period when T-tube drainage interferes with the enterohepatic circulation of cyclosporine. As a result, in most transplantation centers tacrolimus has now supplanted cyclosporine for primary immunosuppression, and many centers rely on oral rather than intravenous administration from the outset. For transplantation centers that prefer cyclosporine, a new, better-absorbed microemulsion preparation is now available.

Although tacrolimus is more potent than cyclosporine, it is also more toxic and more likely to be discontinued for adverse events. The toxicity of tacrolimus is similar to that of cyclosporine; nephrotoxicity and neurotoxicity are the most commonly encountered adverse effects, and neurotoxicity (tremor, seizures, hallucinations, psychoses, coma) is more likely and more severe in tacrolimus-treated patients. Both drugs can cause diabetes mellitus, but tacrolimus does not cause hirsutism or gingival hyperplasia. Because of overlapping toxicity between cyclosporine and tacrolimus, especially nephrotoxicity, and because tacrolimus reduces cyclosporine clearance, these two drugs should not be used together. Since 99% of tacrolimus is metabolized by the liver, hepatic dysfunction reduces its clearance; in primary graft nonfunction (when, for technical reasons or because of ischemic damage prior to its insertion, the allograft is defective and does not function normally from the outset), tacrolimus doses have to be reduced substantially, especially in children. Both cyclosporine and tacrolimus are metabolized by the cytochrome P450 IIIA system, and therefore drugs that induce cytochrome P450 (e.g., phenytoin, phenobarbital, carbamazepine, rifampin) reduce available levels of cyclosporine and tacrolimus; drugs that inhibit cytochrome P450 (e.g., erythromycin, fluconazole, ketoconazole, clotrimazole, itraconazole, verapamil, diltiazem, nicardipine, cimetidine, danazol, metoclopramide, bromocriptine, and the HIV protease inhibitor ritonavir) increase cyclosporine and tacrolimus blood levels. Indeed, itraconazole is commonly used to help boost tacrolimus levels. Like azathioprine, cyclosporine and tacrolimus appear to be associated with a risk of lymphoproliferative malignancies (see later), which may occur earlier after cyclosporine or tacrolimus than after azathioprine therapy. Because of these side effects, combinations of cyclosporine or tacrolimus with prednisone and azathioprine—all at reduced doses—are preferable regimens for immunosuppressive therapy.

In patients with pretransplantation renal dysfunction or renal deterioration that occurs intraoperatively or immediately postoperatively, tacrolimus or cyclosporine therapy may not be practical; under these circumstances, induction or maintenance of immunosuppression with monoclonal antibodies to T cells, OKT3, may be appropriate. Therapy with OKT3 has been especially effective in reversing acute rejection in the posttransplant period and is the standard treatment for acute rejection that fails to respond to methylprednisolone boluses. Intravenous infusions of OKT3 may be complicated by transient fever, chills, and diarrhea, or by pulmonary edema, which can be fatal. When this drug is used to induce immunosuppression initially or to provide "rescue" in those who reject despite "conventional" therapy, the incidence of bacterial, fungal, and especially CMV infections is increased during and after such therapy. In some centers, ganciclovir antiviral therapy is initiated prophylactically as a routine along with OKT3. Because OKT3 is such a potent immunosuppressive agent, its use is more likely to be complicated by opportunistic infection or lymphoproliferative disorders; therefore, and because of the availability of alternative immunosuppressive drugs, OKT3 is used less often nowadays. Another immunosuppressive drug being used for patients undergoing liver transplantation is mycophenolic acid, a nonnucleoside purine metabolism inhibitor derived as a fermentation product from several *Penicillium* species. Mycophenolate has been shown to be better than azathioprine, when used with other standard immunosuppressive drugs, in preventing rejection after renal transplantation and has been adopted as well for use in liver transplantation. The most common adverse effects of mycophenolate are leukopenia and gastrointestinal complaints. Rapamycin, an inhibitor of later events in T cell activation, is approved for use in kidney transplantation but is not approved for use in liver transplant recipients because of the association with an increased frequency of hepatic artery thrombosis in the first month posttransplantation. Studies to examine the safety and efficacy of conversion to rapamycin from calcineurin inhibitors are ongoing. Because of its profound antiproliferative effects, rapamycin has also been suggested to be a useful immunosuppressive agent in patients with a prior or current history of malignancy, such as HCC. Further evaluation is underway.

The most important principle of immunosuppression is that the ideal approach strikes a balance between immunosuppression and immunologic competence. In general, given sufficient immunosuppression, acute liver allograft rejection is nearly always reversible. On the one hand, incompletely treated acute rejection predisposes to the development of chronic rejection, which can threaten graft survival. On the other hand, if the cumulative dose of immunosuppressive therapy is too large, the patient may succumb to opportunistic infection. In hepatitis C, pulse glucocorticoids or OKT3 use accelerate recurrent allograft hepatitis. Further complicating matters, acute rejection can be difficult to distinguish histologically from recurrent hepatitis C. Therefore, immunosuppressive drugs must be used judiciously, with strict attention to the infectious consequences of such therapy and careful confirmation of the diagnosis of acute rejection. In this vein, efforts have been made to minimize the use of glucocorticoids, a mainstay of immunosuppressive regimens, and steroid-free immunosuppression can be achieved in some instances. In this regard, patients who undergo liver transplantation for autoimmune diseases such as primary biliary cirrhosis, autoimmune hepatitis, and primary sclerosing cholangitis, are less likely to achieve freedom from steroids.

POSTOPERATIVE COMPLICATIONS

Complications of liver transplantation can be divided into hepatic and nonhepatic categories (**Tables 44-4** and **44-5**). In addition, both immediately postoperative and late complications are encountered. Patients who undergo liver transplantation as a rule have been chronically ill for protracted periods and may be malnourished and wasted. The impact of such chronic illness and the multisystem failure that accompanies liver failure continue to require attention in the postoperative period. Because of the massive fluid losses and fluid shifts that occur during the operation, patients may remain fluid-overloaded during the immediate postoperative period, straining cardiovascular reserve; this effect can be amplified in the face of transient renal dysfunction and pulmonary capillary vascular permeability. Continuous monitoring of cardiovascular and pulmonary function, measures to maintain the integrity of the intravascular compartment and to treat extravascular volume overload, and scrupulous attention to potential sources and sites of infection are of paramount importance. Cardiovascular instability may also result from the electrolyte imbalance that may accompany reperfusion of the donor liver as well as from restoration of systemic vascular resistance following implantation. Pulmonary function may be compromised further by paralysis of the right

TABLE 44-4

NONHEPATIC COMPLICATIONS OF LIVER TRANSPLANTATION

Fluid overload	
Cardiovascular instability	Arrhythmias
	Congestive heart failure
	Cardiomyopathy
Pulmonary compromise	Pneumonia
	Pulmonary capillary vascular permeability
	Fluid overload
Renal dysfunction	Prerenal azotemia
	Hypoperfusion injury (acute tubular necrosis)
	Drug nephrotoxicity
	↓ Renal blood flow secondary to ↑ intraabdominal pressure
Hematologic	Anemia 2° to gastrointestinal and/or intraabdominal bleeding
	Hemolytic anemia, aplastic anemia
	Thrombocytopenia
Infection	Bacterial: early, common post-operative infections
	Fungal/parasitic: late, opportunistic infections
	Viral: late, opportunistic infections, recurrent hepatitis
Neuropsychiatric	Seizures
	Metabolic encephalopathy
	Depression
	Difficult psychosocial adjustment
Diseases of donor	Infectious
	Malignant
Malignancy	B-cell lymphoma (posttransplantation lymphoproliferative disorders)
	De novo neoplasms (particularly squamous cell skin carcinoma)

TABLE 44-5

HEPATIC COMPLICATIONS OF LIVER TRANSPLANTATION

Hepatic Dysfunction Common after Major Surgery

Prehepatic	Pigment load
	Hemolysis
	Blood collections (hematomas, abdominal collections)
Intrahepatic	
Early	Hepatotoxic drugs and anesthesia
	Hypoperfusion (hypotension, shock, sepsis)
	Benign postoperative cholestasis
Late	Transfusion-associated hepatitis
	Exacerbation of primary hepatic disease
Posthepatic	Biliary obstruction
	↓ Renal clearance of conjugated bilirubin (renal dysfunction)

Hepatic Dysfunction Unique to Liver Transplantation

Primary graft nonfunction	
Vascular compromise	Portal vein obstruction
	Hepatic artery thrombosis
	Anastomotic leak with intraabdominal bleeding
Bile duct disorder	Stenosis, obstruction, leak
Rejection	
Recurrent primary hepatic disease	

hemidiaphragm associated with phrenic nerve injury. The hyperdynamic state with increased cardiac output that is characteristic of patients with liver failure reverses rapidly after successful liver transplantation.

Other immediate management issues include renal dysfunction. Prerenal azotemia, acute kidney injury associated with hypoperfusion (acute tubular necrosis), and renal toxicity caused by antibiotics, tacrolimus, or cyclosporine are encountered frequently in the postoperative period, sometimes necessitating dialysis. Hemolytic uremic syndrome can be associated with cyclosporine, tacrolimus, or OKT3. Occasionally, postoperative intraperitoneal bleeding may be sufficient to increase intraabdominal pressure, which, in turn, may reduce renal blood flow; this effect is rapidly reversible when abdominal distention is relieved by exploratory laparotomy to identify and ligate the bleeding site and to remove intraperitoneal clot.

Anemia may also result from acute upper gastrointestinal bleeding or from transient hemolytic anemia, which may be autoimmune, especially when blood group O livers are transplanted into blood group A or B recipients. This autoimmune hemolytic anemia is mediated by donor intrahepatic lymphocytes that recognize red blood cell A or B antigens on recipient erythrocytes. Transient in nature, this process resolves once the donor liver is repopulated by recipient bone marrow–derived lymphocytes; the hemolysis can be treated by transfusing blood group O red blood cells and/or by administering higher doses of glucocorticoids. Transient thrombocytopenia is also commonly encountered. Aplastic anemia, a late occurrence, is rare but has been reported in almost 30% of patients who underwent liver transplantation for acute, severe hepatitis of unknown cause.

Bacterial, fungal, or viral infections are common and may be life-threatening postoperatively. Early after transplant surgery, common postoperative infections predominate—pneumonia, wound infections, infected intraabdominal collections, urinary tract infections, and intravenous line infections—rather than opportunistic infections; these infections may involve the biliary tree and liver as well. Beyond the first postoperative month, the toll of immunosuppression becomes evident, and opportunistic infections—CMV, herpes viruses, fungal infections (*Aspergillus*, *Candida*, cryptococcal disease), mycobacterial infections, parasitic infections (*Pneumocystis*, *Toxoplasma*), bacterial infections (*Nocardia*, *Legionella*, and *Listeria*)—predominate. Rarely, early infections represent those transmitted with the donor liver, either infections present in the donor or infections acquired during procurement processing. De novo viral hepatitis infections acquired from the donor organ or, almost unheard of nowadays, from transfused blood products occur after typical incubation periods for these agents (well beyond the first month). Obviously, infections in an immunosuppressed host demand early recognition and prompt management; prophylactic antibiotic therapy is administered routinely in the immediate postoperative period. Use of sulfamethoxazole with trimethoprim reduces the incidence of postoperative *Pneumocystis jiroveci* pneumonia. Antiviral prophylaxis for CMV with ganciclovir should be administered in patients at high risk (e.g., when a CMV-seropositive donor organ is implanted into a CMV-seronegative recipient).

Neuropsychiatric complications include seizures (commonly associated with cyclosporine and tacrolimus toxicity), metabolic encephalopathy, depression, and difficult psychosocial adjustment. Rarely, diseases are transmitted by the allograft from the donor to the recipient. In addition to viral and bacterial infections, malignancies of donor origin have occurred. Posttransplantation lymphoproliferative disorders, especially B cell lymphoma, are a recognized complication associated with immunosuppressive drugs such as azathioprine, tacrolimus, and cyclosporine (see earlier). Epstein-Barr virus has been shown to play a contributory role in some of these tumors, which may regress when immunosuppressive therapy is reduced. De novo neoplasms appear at increased frequency after liver transplantation, particularly squamous cell carcinomas of the skin. Routine screening should be performed.

Long-term complications after liver transplantation attributable primarily to immunosuppressive medications include diabetes mellitus (associated with glucocorticoids) as well as hypertension, hyperlipidemia, and chronic renal insufficiency (associated with cyclosporine and tacrolimus). Monitoring and treating these disorders is a routine component of posttransplantation care; in some cases, they respond to changes in immunosuppressive regimen, while in others, specific treatment of the disorder is introduced.

HEPATIC COMPLICATIONS

Hepatic dysfunction after liver transplantation is similar to the hepatic complications encountered after major abdominal and cardiothoracic surgery; however, in addition, there may be complications such as primary graft failure, vascular compromise, failure or stricture of the biliary anastomoses, and rejection. As in nontransplant surgery, postoperative jaundice may result from prehepatic, intrahepatic, and posthepatic sources. *Prehepatic* sources represent the massive hemoglobin pigment load from transfusions, hemolysis, hematomas, ecchymoses, and other collections of blood. *Early intrahepatic* liver injury includes effects of hepatotoxic drugs and anesthesia; hypoperfusion injury associated with hypotension, sepsis, and shock; and benign postoperative cholestasis. *Late intrahepatic* sources of liver injury include posttransfusion hepatitis and exacerbation of primary disease. *Posthepatic* sources of hepatic dysfunction include biliary obstruction and reduced renal clearance of conjugated bilirubin. Hepatic complications unique to liver transplantation include primary graft failure associated with ischemic injury to the organ during harvesting; vascular compromise associated with thrombosis or stenosis of the portal vein or hepatic artery anastomoses; vascular anastomotic leak; stenosis, obstruction, or leakage of the anastomosed common bile duct; recurrence of primary hepatic disorder (see later); and rejection.

TRANSPLANT REJECTION

Despite the use of immunosuppressive drugs, rejection of the transplanted liver still occurs in a proportion of patients, beginning 1–2 weeks after surgery. Clinical signs suggesting rejection are fever, right upper quadrant pain, and reduced bile pigment and volume. Leukocytosis may occur, but the most reliable indicators are increases in serum bilirubin and aminotransferase levels. Because these tests lack specificity, distinguishing among rejection and biliary obstruction, primary graft nonfunction, vascular compromise, viral hepatitis, CMV infection, drug hepatotoxicity, and recurrent primary disease may be difficult. Radiographic visualization of the biliary tree and/or percutaneous liver biopsy often helps to establish the correct diagnosis. Morphologic features of acute rejection include a mixed portal cellular infiltrate, bile duct injury, and/or endothelial inflammation ("endothelialitis"); some of these findings are reminiscent of graft-versus-host disease, primary biliary cirrhosis, or recurrent allograft hepatitis C. As soon as transplant rejection is suspected, treatment consists of intravenous methylprednisolone in repeated boluses; if this fails to abort rejection, many centers use antibodies to lymphocytes, such as OKT3, or polyclonal antilymphocyte globulin. Caution should be exercised when managing acute rejection with pulse glucocorticoids in patients with hepatitis C virus (HCV) infection, because of the high risk of triggering recurrent allograft hepatitis C.

Chronic rejection is a relatively rare outcome that can follow repeated bouts of acute rejection or that occurs unrelated to preceding rejection episodes. Morphologically, chronic rejection is characterized by progressive cholestasis, focal parenchymal necrosis, mononuclear infiltration, vascular lesions (intimal fibrosis, subintimal foam cells, fibrinoid necrosis), and fibrosis. This process may be reflected as ductopenia—the vanishing bile duct syndrome. Reversibility of chronic rejection is limited; in patients with therapy-resistant chronic rejection, retransplantation has yielded encouraging results.

OUTCOME

SURVIVAL

The survival rate for patients undergoing liver transplantation has improved steadily since 1983. One-year survival rates have increased from ~70% in the early 1980s to 85–90% from 2000 to 2006. Currently the 5-year survival rate exceeds 60%. An important observation is the relationship between clinical status before transplantation and outcome. For patients who undergo liver transplantation when their level of compensation is high (e.g., still working or only partially disabled), a 1-year survival rate of >85% is common. For those whose level of decompensation mandates continuous in-hospital care prior to transplantation, the 1-year survival rate is about 70%, while for those who are so decompensated that they require life support in an intensive care unit, the 1-year survival rate is ~50%. Since UNOS's adoption in 2002 of the MELD system for organ allocation, posttransplantation survival has been found to be affected adversely for candidates with MELD scores >25, considered high disease severity. Thus, irrespective of allocation scheme, high disease severity pretransplantation corresponds to diminished posttransplantation survival. Another important distinction in survival has been drawn between high-risk and low-risk patient categories. For patients who do not fit any "high-risk" designations, 1-year and 5-year survival rates of 85 and 80%, respectively, have been recorded. In contrast, among patients in high-risk categories—cancer, fulminant hepatitis, age >65, concurrent renal failure, respirator dependence, portal vein thrombosis, and history of a portacaval shunt or multiple right upper quadrant operations—survival statistics fall into the range of 60% at 1 year and 35% at 5 years. Survival after retransplantation for primary graft nonfunction is ~50%. Causes of failure of liver transplantation vary with time. Failures within the first 3 months result primarily from technical complications, postoperative infections, and hemorrhage. Transplant failures after the first 3 months are more likely to result from infection, rejection, or recurrent disease (such as malignancy or viral hepatitis).

RECURRENCE OF PRIMARY DISEASE

Features of autoimmune hepatitis, primary sclerosing cholangitis, and primary biliary cirrhosis overlap with those of rejection or posttransplantation bile-duct injury.

Whether autoimmune hepatitis and sclerosing cholangitis recur after liver transplantation is controversial; data supporting recurrent autoimmune hepatitis (in up to a third of patients in some series) are more convincing than those supporting recurrent sclerosing cholangitis. Similarly, reports of recurrent primary biliary cirrhosis after liver transplantation have appeared; however, the histologic features of primary biliary cirrhosis and chronic rejection are virtually indistinguishable and occur as frequently in patients with primary biliary cirrhosis as in patients undergoing transplantation for other reasons. The presence of a florid inflammatory bile duct lesion is highly suggestive of the recurrence of primary biliary cirrhosis, but even this lesion can be observed in acute rejection. Hereditary disorders such as Wilson's disease and α_1 antitrypsin deficiency have not recurred after liver transplantation; however, recurrence of disordered iron metabolism has been observed in some patients with hemochromatosis. Hepatic vein thrombosis (Budd-Chiari syndrome) may recur; this can be minimized by treating underlying myeloproliferative disorders and by anticoagulation. Because cholangiocarcinoma recurs almost invariably, few centers now offer transplantation to such patients; however, a few highly selected patients with operatively confirmed stage I or II cholangiocarcinoma who undergo liver transplantation combined with neoadjuvant chemoradiation may experience excellent outcomes. In patients with intrahepatic hepatocellular carcinoma who meet criteria for transplantation, 1- and 5-year survivals are similar to those observed in patients undergoing liver transplantation for nonmalignant disease. Finally, metabolic disorders such as nonalcoholic steatohepatitis recur frequently, especially if the underlying metabolic predisposition is not altered.

Hepatitis A can recur after transplantation for fulminant hepatitis A, but such acute reinfection has no serious clinical sequelae. In fulminant hepatitis B, recurrence is not the rule; however, in the absence of any prophylactic measures, hepatitis B usually recurs after transplantation for end-stage chronic hepatitis B. Before the introduction of prophylactic antiviral therapy, immunosuppressive therapy sufficient to prevent allograft rejection led inevitably to marked increases in hepatitis B viremia, regardless of pretransplantation values. Overall graft and patient survival were poor, and some patients experienced a rapid recapitulation of severe injury—severe chronic hepatitis or even fulminant hepatitis—after transplantation. Also recognized in the era before availability of antiviral regimens was *fibrosing cholestatic hepatitis*, rapidly progressive liver injury associated with marked hyperbilirubinemia, substantial prolongation of the prothrombin time (both out of proportion to relatively modest elevations of aminotransferase activity), and rapidly progressive liver failure. This lesion has been suggested to represent a "choking off" of the hepatocyte by an overwhelming density of hepatitis B virus (HBV) proteins. Complications such as sepsis and pancreatitis were also observed more frequently in patients undergoing liver transplantation for hepatitis B prior to the introduction of antiviral therapy. The introduction of long-term prophylaxis with HBIg revolutionized liver transplantation for chronic hepatitis B. Neither preoperative hepatitis B vaccination, preoperative or postoperative interferon therapy, nor short-term (≤2 months) HBIg prophylaxis has been shown to be effective, but a retrospective analysis of data from several hundred European patients followed for 3 years after transplantation has shown that long-term (≥6 months) prophylaxis with HBIg is associated with a lowering of the risk of HBV reinfection from ~75% to 35% and a reduction in mortality from ~50% to 20%.

As a result of long-term HBIg use following liver transplantation for chronic hepatitis B, similar improvements in outcome have been observed in the United States, with 1-year survival rates between 75 and 90%. Currently, with HBIg prophylaxis, the outcome of liver transplantation for chronic hepatitis B is indistinguishable from that for chronic liver disease unassociated with chronic hepatitis B; essentially, medical concerns regarding liver transplantation for chronic hepatitis B have been eliminated. Passive immunoprophylaxis with HBIg is begun during the anhepatic stage of surgery, repeated daily for the first 6 postoperative days, then continued with infusions that are given either at regular intervals of 4–6 weeks or, alternatively, when anti-HBs levels fall below a threshold of 100 mIU/mL. The current approach in most centers is to continue HBIg indefinitely, which can add approximately $20,000 per year to the cost of care; some centers are evaluating regimens that shift to less frequent administration or to intramuscular administration in the late posttransplantation period. Still, occasionally "breakthrough" HBV infection occurs.

Further improving the outcome of liver transplantation for chronic hepatitis B is the current availability of such antiviral drugs as lamivudine, adefovir dipivoxil, and entecavir (Chap. 39). When these drugs are administered to patients with decompensated liver disease, a proportion improve sufficiently to postpone imminent liver transplantation. In addition, lamivudine can be used to prevent recurrence of HBV infection when administered *prior* to transplantation; to treat hepatitis B that recurs *after* transplantation, including in patients who break through HBIg prophylaxis; and to reverse the course of otherwise fatal fibrosing cholestatic hepatitis. Clinical trials have shown that lamivudine antiviral therapy reduces the level of HBV replication substantially, sometimes even resulting in clearance of hepatitis B surface antigen (HBsAg); reduces alanine aminotransferase (ALT) levels; and improves histologic features of necrosis and inflammation. Long-term use of lamivudine is safe and effective, but after several months a proportion of patients become resistant to lamivudine, resulting from

YMDD (tyrosine-methionine-aspartate-aspartate) mutations in the HBV polymerase motif (Chap. 39). In approximately half of such resistant patients, hepatic deterioration may ensue. Fortunately, adefovir dipivoxil is available as well and can be used to treat lamivudine-associated YMDD variants, effectively "rescuing" patients experiencing hepatic decompensation after lamivudine breakthrough. Currently, most liver transplantation centers combine HBIg plus lamivudine or adefovir, and additional antivirals such as the more recently approved entecavir are being introduced as well. Clinical trials are underway to define the optimal application of these antiviral agents in the management of patients undergoing liver transplantation for chronic hepatitis B; conceivably, in the future, combinations of oral antiviral drugs may even supplant HBIg.

Prophylactic approaches applied to patients undergoing liver transplantation for chronic hepatitis B are being used as well for patients without hepatitis B who receive organs from donors with anti-HBc. Patients who undergo liver transplantation for chronic hepatitis B plus D are less likely to experience recurrent liver injury than patients undergoing liver transplantation for hepatitis B alone; still, such co-infected patients would also be offered standard posttransplantation prophylactic therapy for hepatitis B.

Accounting for up to 40% of all liver transplantation procedures, the most common indication for liver transplantation is end-stage liver disease resulting from chronic hepatitis C. Recurrence of HCV infection after liver transplantation can be documented in almost every patient if sufficiently sensitive virus markers are used. The clinical consequences of recurrent hepatitis C are limited during the first 5 years after transplantation. Nonetheless, despite the relative clinical benignity of recurrent hepatitis C in the early years after liver transplantation, and despite the negligible impact on patient survival during these early years, histologic studies have documented the presence of moderate to severe chronic hepatitis in more than half of all patients and bridging fibrosis or cirrhosis in ~10%. Moreover, progression to cirrhosis within 5 years is even more common, occurring in up to two-thirds of patients if moderate hepatitis is detected in a 1-year biopsy. Not surprisingly, then, for patients undergoing transplantation for hepatitis C, allograft and patient survival are diminished substantially between 5 and 10 years after transplantation. In a proportion of patients, even during the early posttransplantation period, recurrent hepatitis C may be sufficiently severe biochemically and histologically to merit antiviral therapy. Treatment with pegylated interferon can *suppress* HCV-associated liver injury but rarely leads to *sustained* benefit. Sustained virologic responses are the exception, and reduced tolerability is often dose-limiting. Preemptive combination antiviral therapy with pegylated interferon and the nucleoside analogue ribavirin immediately after transplantation does not appear to provide any advantage over therapy introduced after clinical hepatitis has occurred. Similarly, although interferon-based antiviral therapy is not recommended for patients with decompensated liver disease, some centers have experimented with pretransplantation antiviral therapy in an attempt to eradicate HCV replication prior to transplantation; preliminary results are promising, but interferon treatment of patients with end-stage liver disease can lead to worsening of hepatic decompensation, and HCV infection has recurred after transplantation in some of these recipients. Initial trials of hepatitis C immune globulin preparations to prevent recurrent hepatitis C after liver transplantation have not been successful.

A small number succumb to early HCV-associated liver injury, and a syndrome reminiscent of fibrosing cholestatic hepatitis (see above) has been observed rarely. Because patients with more episodes of rejection receive more immunosuppressive therapy, and because immunosuppressive therapy enhances HCV replication, patients with severe or multiple episodes of rejection are more likely to experience early recurrence of hepatitis C after transplantation. Both high viral load and older donor age have been linked to recurrent HCV-induced liver disease and to earlier disease recurrence after transplantation.

Patients who undergo liver transplantation for end-stage alcoholic cirrhosis are at risk of resorting to drinking again after transplantation, a potential source of recurrent alcoholic liver injury. Currently, alcoholic liver disease is one of the more common indications for liver transplantation, accounting for 20–25% of all liver transplantation procedures, and most transplantation centers screen candidates carefully for predictors of continued abstinence. Recidivism is more likely in patients whose sobriety prior to transplantation was <6 months. For abstinent patients with alcoholic cirrhosis, liver transplantation can be undertaken successfully, with outcomes comparable to those for other categories of patients with chronic liver disease, when coordinated by a team approach that includes substance abuse counseling.

POSTTRANSPLANTATION QUALITY OF LIFE

Full rehabilitation is achieved in the majority of patients who survive the early postoperative months and escape chronic rejection or unmanageable infection. Psychosocial maladjustment interferes with medical compliance in a small number of patients, but most manage to adhere to immunosuppressive regimens, which must be continued indefinitely. In one study, 85% of patients who survived their transplant operations returned to gainful activities. In fact, some women have conceived and carried pregnancies to term after transplantation without demonstrable injury to their infants.

FURTHER READINGS

BATTS KP: Acute and chronic hepatic allograft rejection: Pathology and classification. Liver Transpl Surg 5(Suppl 1):S21, 1999

BENLLOCH S et al: De novo internal neoplasms after liver transplantation: Increased risk and aggressive behavior in recent years? Am J Transplant 4:596, 2004

BERENGUER M: Treatment of hepatitis C after liver transplantation. Clin Liver Dis 9:579, 2005

——— et al: Contribution of donor age to the recent decrease in patient survival among HCV-infected liver transplant recipients. Hepatology 36:202, 2002

——— et al: Effect of calcineurin inhibitors on survival and histologic disease severity in HCV-infected liver transplant recipients. Liver Transpl 12:762, 2006

BROWN RS JR et al: A survey of liver transplantation from living adult donors in the United States. N Engl J Med 348:818, 2003

CARITHERS RL JR: Liver transplantation. Liver Transpl 6:122, 2000

DICKSON RC et al: Transmission of hepatitis B by transplantation of livers from donors positive for antibody to hepatitis B core antigen. Gastroenterology 113:1668, 1997

FÉRAY C et al: European collaborative study on factors influencing outcome after liver transplantation for hepatitis C. Gastroenterology 117:619, 1999

FISHMAN JA, RUBIN RH: Infection in organ-transplant recipients. N Engl J Med 338:1741, 1998

FORMAN LM et al: The association between hepatitis C infection and survival after orthotopic liver transplantation. Gastroenterology 122:889, 2002

GALLEGOS-OROZCO JF, VARGAS HE: Liver transplantation: from Child to MELD. Med Clin North Am 93:931, 2009

HABIB S et al: MELD and prediction of post-liver transplantation survival. Liver Transpl 12:440, 2006

HIRSCHFIELD GM et al: Adult liver transplantation: what non-specialists need to know. BMJ 338:1670, 2009

KAMATH PS et al: A model to predict survival in patients with end-stage liver disease. Hepatology 33:464, 2001

KEEFFE EB et al: Liver transplantation: Current status and novel approaches to liver replacement. Gastroenterology 120:749, 2001

LOK ASF et al (eds): Liver transplantation for viral hepatitis. Liver Transpl 8(Suppl 1):S1, 2002

KULKARNI S et al: Living donor liver transplantation for pediatric and adult recipients. Nat Clin Prac Gastro Hep 3:149, 2006

MAZZAFERRO V et al: Liver transplantation for the treatment of small hepatocellular carcinoma in patients with cirrhosis. N Engl J Med 334:693, 1996

PERRILLO R et al: A multicenter United States—Canadian trial to assess lamivudine monotherapy before and after liver transplantation for chronic hepatitis B. Hepatology 33:424, 2001

POST DJ et al: Immunosuppression in liver transplantation. Liver Transplant 11:1307, 2005

ROLAND ME, STOCK PG: Liver transplantation in HIV-infected recipients. Semin Liver Dis 26:273, 2006

ROSS A et al: Pegylated interferon alpha-2b plus ribavirin in the treatment of post-liver transplant recurrent hepatitis C. Clin Transplant 18:166, 2004

SCHREIBMAN IR, SCHIFF ER: Prevention and treatment of recurrent hepatitis B after liver transplantation: The current role of nucleoside and nucleotide analogues. Ann Clin Microbiol Antimicrob 5:8, 2006

SHARMA P, LOK AS: Viral hepatitis and liver transplantation. Semin Liver Dis 26:285, 2006

470

SORRELL MF (ed): Liver transplantation in the new millennium. Semin Liver Dis 20:409, 2000

TROTTER JF et al: Adult-to-adult transplantation of the right hepatic lobe from a living donor. N Engl J Med 346:1074, 2002

U.S. MULTICENTER FK506 LIVER STUDY GROUP: A comparison of tacrolimus (FK506) and cyclosporine for immunosuppression in liver transplantation. N Engl J Med 331:1110, 1994

VARGAS HE et al: A concise update on the status of liver transplantation for hepatitis B virus: The challenges in 2002. Liver Transpl 8:2, 2002

VIERLING JM, TEPERMAN LW (eds): Hepatitis B and liver transplantation. Semin Liver Dis 20(Suppl 1):1, 2000

WEBB K et al: Transplantation for alcoholic liver disease: Report of a consensus meeting. Liver Transplant 12:301, 2006

WIESNER R: Patient selection in an era of donor liver shortage: Current US policy. Nat Clin Prac Gastro Hep 2:24, 2005

——— et al: Model for end-stage liver disease (MELD) and allocation of donor livers. Gastroenterology 124:91, 2003

YAO FY et al: The impact of pre-operative loco-regional therapy on outcome after liver transplantation for hepatocellular carcinoma. Am J Transplant 5:795, 2005

——— et al. Liver transplantation for hepatocellular carcinoma: Comparison of the proposed UCSF criteria with the Milan criteria and the Pittsburgh modified TNM criteria. Liver Transpl 8:765, 2002

SECTION VII

Liver Transplantation

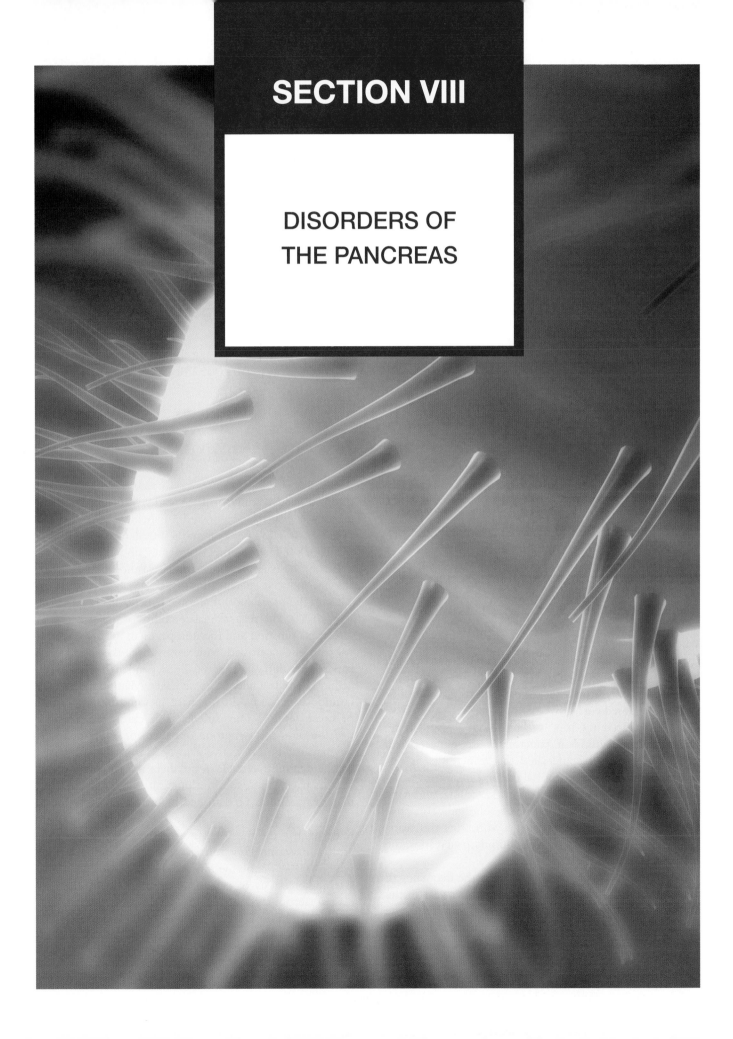

SECTION VIII

DISORDERS OF THE PANCREAS

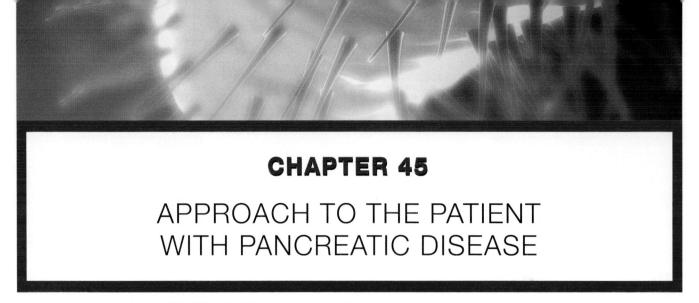

CHAPTER 45

APPROACH TO THE PATIENT WITH PANCREATIC DISEASE

Phillip P. Toskes ■ Norton J. Greenberger

GENERAL CONSIDERATIONS

The clinical manifestations of acute and chronic pancreatitis and pancreatic insufficiency are protean. Thus, patients may present with hypertriglyceridemia, vitamin B_{12} malabsorption, hypercalcemia, hypocalcemia, hyperglycemia, ascites, pleural effusions, and chronic abdominal pain with normal blood amylase levels. Indeed, if the clinician considers pancreatitis as a possible diagnosis only when presented with a patient having classic symptoms (i.e., severe, constant epigastric pain that radiates through to the back, along with an elevated blood amylase or lipase level), only a minority of patients with pancreatitis will be diagnosed correctly.

As emphasized in Chap. 46, the etiologies as well as the clinical manifestations of pancreatitis are quite varied. Although it is well appreciated that pancreatitis is frequently secondary to alcohol abuse and biliary tract disease, it can also be caused by drugs, trauma, and viral infections and is associated with metabolic and connective tissue disorders. In ~30% of patients with acute pancreatitis and 25–40% of patients with chronic pancreatitis, the etiology is obscure.

Although good data exist concerning the frequency of acute pancreatitis (about 5000 new cases per year in the United States, with a mortality rate of about 10%), the number of patients who suffer with recurrent acute pancreatitis or chronic pancreatitis is largely undefined. These statistics have not changed over the past 25 years. Only one prospective study on the incidence of chronic pancreatitis is available; it showed an incidence of 8.2 new cases per 100,000 per year and a prevalence of 26.4 cases per 100,000. These numbers probably underestimate considerably the true incidence and prevalence, because non-alcohol-induced pancreatitis was largely ignored. At autopsy, the prevalence of chronic pancreatitis ranges from 0.04 to 5%. The relative inaccessibility of the pancreas to direct examination and the nonspecificity of the abdominal pain associated with pancreatitis make the diagnosis of pancreatitis difficult and usually dependent on elevation of blood amylase and/or lipase levels. Many patients with chronic pancreatitis do not have elevated blood amylase or lipase levels. Some patients with chronic pancreatitis develop signs and symptoms of pancreatic exocrine insufficiency, and thus objective evidence for pancreatic disease can be demonstrated. However, there is a very large reservoir of pancreatic exocrine function. More than 90% of the pancreas must be damaged before maldigestion of fat and protein is manifested. Even the secretin stimulation test, which is the most sensitive method of assessing pancreatic exocrine function, is probably abnormal only when >60% of exocrine function has been lost. Noninvasive, indirect tests of pancreatic exocrine function (fecal elastase, serum trypsinogen) are much more likely to give abnormal results in patients with obvious pancreatic disease, i.e., pancreatic calcification, steatorrhea, or diabetes mellitus, than in patients with occult disease. Thus, the number of patients who have subclinical exocrine dysfunction (<90% loss of function) is unknown.

TESTS USEFUL IN THE DIAGNOSIS OF PANCREATIC DISEASE

Several tests have proved of value in the evaluation of pancreatic exocrine function. Examples of specific tests and their usefulness in the diagnosis of acute and chronic pancreatitis are summarized in Table 45-1 and Fig. 45-1. At most institutions, pancreatic function tests are performed if the diagnosis of pancreatic disease remains a possibility after noninvasive tests (ultrasound, CT) and invasive tests [endoscopic retrograde cholangiopancreatography (ERCP), endoscopic ultrasonography (EUS)] have given normal or inconclusive results. In this regard, tests employing *direct* stimulation of the pancreas are the most sensitive.

Pancreatic Enzymes in Body Fluids

The serum amylase and lipase levels are widely used as screening tests for acute pancreatitis in the patient with acute abdominal pain or back pain. Values greater than three times the upper limit of normal virtually clinch the diagnosis if gut perforation or infarction is excluded. In the absence of objective evidence of pancreatitis by abdominal ultrasound, CT scan, ERCP, or EUS, mild to moderate elevations of amylase and/or lipase are problematic in making a diagnosis of pancreatitis. In acute pancreatitis, the serum amylase is usually elevated within 24 h of onset and remains so for 1–3 days. Levels return to normal within 3–5 days unless there is extensive pancreatic necrosis, incomplete ductal obstruction, or pseudocyst formation. Approximately 85% of patients with acute pancreatitis have an elevated serum amylase level. This index may be normal, however, if (1) there is a delay (of 2–5 days) before blood samples are obtained, (2) the underlying disorder is chronic pancreatitis rather than acute pancreatitis, or (3) hypertriglyceridemia is present. Patients with hypertriglyceridemia and proven pancreatitis have been found to have spuriously low levels of amylase and perhaps lipase activity.

The serum amylase is often elevated in other conditions (Table 45-2), in part because the enzyme is found in many organs in addition to the pancreas (salivary glands, liver, small intestine, kidney, fallopian tube) and can be produced by various tumors (carcinomas of the lung, esophagus, breast, and ovary). An assay of serum trypsinogen (performed by several commercial laboratories) is quite helpful in this regard. Since this enzyme is secreted specifically by the pancreas, a normal serum trypsinogen level in a patient with minimal elevation of serum amylase essentially rules out acute pancreatitis. Urinary amylase measurements, including the amylase/creatinine clearance ratio, are no more sensitive or specific than

blood amylase levels. Isoamylase determinations do not accurately distinguish elevated blood amylase levels due to bona fide pancreatitis from elevated blood amylase levels due to a nonpancreatic source of amylase, especially when the blood amylase level is only moderately elevated.

Elevation of ascitic fluid amylase occurs in acute pancreatitis as well as in (1) pancreatogenous ascites due to disruption of the main pancreatic duct or a leaking pseudocyst and (2) other abdominal disorders that simulate pancreatitis (e.g., intestinal obstruction, intestinal infarction, and perforated peptic ulcer). Elevation of pleural fluid amylase occurs in acute pancreatitis, chronic pancreatitis, carcinoma of the lung, and esophageal perforation.

Lipase may now be the single best enzyme to measure for the diagnosis of acute pancreatitis. Improvements in substrates and technology offer clinicians improved options, especially when a turbidimetric assay is used. The newer lipase assays have colipase as a cofactor and are fully automated.

An assay for trypsinogen (or for trypsin-like immunoreactivity) has a theoretical advantage over amylase and lipase determinations in that the pancreas is the only organ that contains this enzyme. The test appears to be useful in the diagnosis of both acute and chronic pancreatitis. Sensitivity and specificity are comparable to those of amylase and lipase determinations. Since trypsinogen is also excreted by the kidney, elevated serum values are found in renal failure, as is the case with serum amylase and lipase levels. *No single blood test is reliable for the diagnosis of acute pancreatitis in patients with renal failure.* Determining whether a patient with renal failure and abdominal pain has pancreatitis remains a difficult clinical problem. A recent study found that serum amylase levels were elevated in patients with renal dysfunction only when creatinine clearance was <0.8 mL/s (<50 mL/min). In such patients, the serum amylase level was invariably <8.3 μkat/L (<500 IU/L) in the absence of objective evidence of acute pancreatitis. In that study, serum lipase and trypsin levels paralleled serum amylase values.

A recent study evaluated the sensitivity and specificity of five assays used to diagnose acute pancreatitis: two for amylase, one for lipase, one for trypsin-like immunoreactivity (TLI), and one for pancreatic isoamylase. The data obtained (1) show that, if the best cutoff level is used, all these assays have similar specificities and (2) suggest that total serum amylase is as good an indicator of acute pancreatitis as any of the alternatives. However, inherent in many such studies is the problem that the recognition and diagnosis of acute pancreatitis hinge on the finding of an elevated serum amylase level. The question arises as to whether any diagnostic test result can be proved superior to the total serum amylase level if hyperamylasemia is required for the diagnosis. In other studies, when "objective" confirmation of the clinical diagnosis of pancreatitis was required (ultrasonography, CT, laparotomy), the sensitivity of the serum amylase has

TABLE 45-1

TESTS USEFUL IN THE DIAGNOSIS OF ACUTE AND CHRONIC PANCREATITIS AND PANCREATIC TUMORS

TEST	PRINCIPLE	COMMENT
Pancreatic Enzymes in Body Fluids		
Amylase		
1. Serum	Pancreatic inflammation leads to increased enzyme levels	Simple; 20–40% false negatives and positives; reliable if test results are three times the upper limit of normal
2. Urine	Renal clearance of amylase is increased in acute pancreatitis	May be abnormal when serum levels normal; false negatives and positives
3. Ascitic fluid	Disruption of gland or main pancreatic duct leads to increased amylase concentration	Can establish diagnosis of pancreatitis; false positives occur with intestinal obstruction and perforated ulcer
4. Pleural fluid	Exudative pleural effusion with pancreatitis	False positives occur with carcinoma of the lung and esophageal perforation
5. Isoenzymes	P isoamylases arise from the pancreas; S isoamylases are from other sources	More specific than total serum amylase in diagnosis of acute pancreatitis; useful in identifying nonpancreatic causes of hyperamylasemia
Serum lipase	Pancreatic inflammation leads to increased enzyme levels	New methods have greatly simplified determination; positive in 70–85% of cases
Serum trypsinogen	Pancreatic inflammation leads to increased levels	*Elevated* in acute pancreatitis; *decreased* in chronic pancreatitis *with* steatorrhea; normal in chronic pancreatitis *without* steatorrhea and in steatorrhea with normal pancreatic function
Studies Pertaining to Pancreatic Structure		
Radiologic and radionuclide tests		
1. Plain film of the abdomen	Abnormal in acute and chronic pancreatitis	Simple; normal in >50% of cases of both acute and chronic pancreatitis
2. Upper gastrointestinal x-rays	Abnormally thickened duodenal folds; displacement of stomach or widening of duodenal loop suggests a pancreatic mass (inflammatory, neoplastic, cystic)	Simple; frequently normal; largely superseded by US and CT scanning
3. Ultrasonography (US)	Can provide information on edema, inflammation, calcification, pseudocysts, and mass lesions	Simple, noninvasive; sequential studies quite feasible; useful in diagnosis of pseudocyst
4. CT scan	Permits detailed visualization of pancreas and surrounding structures	Useful in the diagnosis of pancreatic calcification, dilated pancreatic ducts, and pancreatic tumors; may not be able to distinguish between inflammatory and neoplastic mass lesions
5. Selective angiography	Can identify pancreatic neoplasms (1) by sheathing of celiac or superior mesenteric branches by tumor or (2) by tumor staining; displacement of vessels by tumor	Indicated (1) in suspected islet cell tumors and (2) before pancreatic or duodenal resection; most reliable features reflect nonresectable pancreatic cancer
6. Endoscopic retrograde cholangiopancreatography (ERCP)	Cannulation of pancreatic and common bile duct permits visualization of pancreatic-biliary ductal system	Provides diagnostic data in 60–85% of cases; differentiation of chronic pancreatitis from pancreatic carcinoma may be difficult
7. Endoscopic ultrasonography (EUS)	High-frequency transducer employed with EUS can produce very high resolution images and depict changes in the pancreatic duct and parenchyma with better detail	Exact role of EUS versus ERCP and CT not yet fully defined; sensitivity and specificity under study
8. Magnetic resonance cholangiopancreatography	Three-dimensional rendering has been used to produce very good images of the pancreatic duct by a noninvasive technique	May be used to evaluate patients judged to be at high risk for ERCP, such as the elderly; may replace ERCP as a diagnostic test, although large controlled studies need to be done
Pancreatic biopsy with US or CT guidance	Percutaneous biopsy with skinny needle and localization of lesion by US	High diagnostic yield; laparotomy avoided; requires special technical skills

(Continued)

TABLE 45-1 (CONTINUED)

TESTS USEFUL IN THE DIAGNOSIS OF ACUTE AND CHRONIC PANCREATITIS AND PANCREATIC TUMORS

TEST	PRINCIPLE	COMMENT
Tests of Exocrine Pancreatic Function		
Direct stimulation of the pancreas with analysis of duodenal contents		
1. Secretin-pancreozymin (CCK) test	Secretin leads to increased output of pancreatic juice and HCO_3^-; CCK leads to increased output of pancreatic enzymes; pancreatic secretory response is related to the functional mass of pancreatic tissue	Sensitive enough to detect occult disease; involves duodenal intubation and fluoroscopy; poorly defined normal enzyme response; overlap in chronic pancreatitis; large secretory reserve capacity of the pancreas
Measurement of intraluminal digestion products		
1. Microscopic examination of stool for undigested meat fibers and fat	Lack of proteolytic and lipolytic enzymes causes decreased digestion of meat fibers and triglycerides	Simple, reliable; not sensitive enough to detect milder cases of pancreatic insufficiency
2. Quantitative stool fat determination	Lack of lipolytic enzymes brings about impaired fat digestion	Reliable, reference standard for defining severity of malabsorption; does not distinguish between maldigestion and malabsorption
3. Fecal nitrogen	Lack of proteolytic enzymes leads to impaired protein digestion, resulting in an increase in stool nitrogen	Does not distinguish between maldigestion and malabsorption; low sensitivity
Measurement of pancreatic enzymes in feces		
1. Elastase	Pancreatic secretion of proteolytic enzymes	Excellent specificity; sensitivity similar to that of serum trypsinogen
Miscellaneous tests		
1. Dual-labeled Schilling test	Intrinsic factor [^{57}Co]cobalamin and Hog R protein [^{58}Co]cobalamin are given together. Since proteases are necessary to cleave R protein, the ratio of labeled cobalamin excreted in urine is an index of exocrine dysfunction.	Time-consuming and expensive

been found to be as low as 68%. With these limitations in mind, the recommended screening tests for acute pancreatitis are *total serum amylase* and *serum lipase activities*. Serum amylase values greater than three times normal are highly specific.

Studies Pertaining to Pancreatic Structure

Radiologic Tests

Plain films of the abdomen may provide useful information in patients with acute pancreatitis. The most frequent abnormalities include (1) a localized ileus, usually involving the jejunum ("sentinel loop"); (2) a generalized ileus with air-fluid levels; (3) the "colon cutoff sign," which results from isolated distention of the transverse colon; (4) duodenal distention with air-fluid levels; and (5) a mass, which is frequently a pseudocyst. In chronic pancreatitis, an important radiographic finding is pancreatic calcification, which characteristically is localized adjacent to and superimposed on the second lumbar vertebra (Fig. 46-3A).

Upper gastrointestinal x-rays may reveal displacement of the stomach by the retroperitoneal mass (Fig. 46-2A) or widening and effacement of the duodenal C loop, which also suggest the presence of a pancreatic mass, which could be inflammatory, cystic, or neoplastic. However, the use of x-ray films has been largely superseded by ultrasound.

Ultrasonography can provide important information in patients with acute pancreatitis, chronic pancreatitis, pancreatic calcification, pseudocyst, and pancreatic carcinoma. Echographic appearances can indicate the presence of edema, inflammation, and calcification (not obvious on plain films of the abdomen), as well as

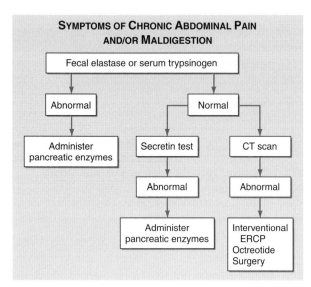

SYMPTOMS OF CHRONIC ABDOMINAL PAIN AND/OR MALDIGESTION

FIGURE 45-1

An approach to the patient with suspected chronic pancreatitis. Endoscopic ultrasonography and magnetic resonance cholangiopancreatography are appropriate diagnostic alternatives. ERCP, endoscopic retrograde cholangiopancreatography.

pseudocysts, mass lesions, and gallstones (Figs. 46-2*B* and 46-3*B*). In acute pancreatitis, the pancreas is characteristically enlarged. In pancreatic pseudocyst, the usual appearance is that of an echo-free, smooth, round fluid collection. Pancreatic carcinoma distorts the usual landmarks, and mass lesions >3.0 cm are usually detected as localized, echo-free solid lesions. Ultrasound is often the initial investigation for most patients with suspected pancreatic disease. However, obesity, excess small- and large-bowel gas, and recently performed barium contrast examinations can interfere with ultrasound studies.

CT is the best imaging study for initial evaluation of a suspected chronic pancreatic disorder and for the complications of acute and chronic pancreatitis. It is especially useful in the detection of pancreatic tumors, fluid-containing lesions such as pseudocysts and abscesses, and calcium deposits (Figs. 46-3*C* and 46-4*A*). Most lesions are characterized by (1) enlargement of the pancreatic outline, (2) distortion of the pancreatic contour, and/or (3) a fluid filling that has a different attenuation coefficient than normal pancreas. However, it is difficult to distinguish between inflammatory and neoplastic lesions. Oral water-soluble contrast agents may be used to opacify the stomach and duodenum during CT scans; this strategy permits more precise delineation of various organs as well as mass lesions. Dynamic CT (using rapid IV administration of contrast) is useful in estimating the degree of pancreatic necrosis and in predicting morbidity and mortality. Spiral (helical) CT provides clear images much more rapidly and essentially negates artifact caused by patient movement (Fig. 46-2*D*).

TABLE 45-2

CAUSES OF HYPERAMYLASEMIA AND HYPERAMYLASURIA

Pancreatic Disease

I. Pancreatitis	II. Pancreatic trauma
A. Acute	III. Pancreatic carcinoma
B. Chronic: ductal obstruction	
C. Complications of pancreatitis	
1. Pancreatic pseudocyst	
2. Pancreatogenous ascites	
3. Pancreatic abscess	
4. Pancreatic necrosis	

Nonpancreatic Disorders

I. Renal insufficiency	IV. Macroamylasemia
II. Salivary gland lesions	V. Burns
A. Mumps	VI. Diabetic ketoacidosis
B. Calculus	VII. Pregnancy
C. Irradiation sialadenitis	VIII. Renal transplantation
D. Maxillofacial surgery	IX. Cerebral trauma
III. "Tumor" hyperamylasemia	X. Drugs: morphine
A. Carcinoma of the lung	
B. Carcinoma of the esophagus	
C. Breast carcinoma, ovarian carcinoma	

Other Abdominal Disorders

I. Biliary tract disease: cholecystitis, choledocholithiasis
II. Intraabdominal disease
  A. Perforated or penetrating peptic ulcer
  B. Intestinal obstruction or infarction
  C. Ruptured ectopic pregnancy
  D. Peritonitis
  E. Aortic aneurysm
  F. Chronic liver disease
  G. Postoperative hyperamylasemia

Endoscopic ultrasonography (EUS) produces high-resolution images of the pancreatic parenchyma and pancreatic duct with a transducer fixed to an endoscope that can be directed onto the surface of the pancreas through the stomach or duodenum. EUS is replacing ERCP for diagnostic purposes in many centers. EUS allows one to obtain information about the pancreatic duct as well as the parenchyma and has no complications associated with it, in contrast to the 5–20% of post-ERCP pancreatitis observed. EUS is also very good in detecting common bile duct stones. Pancreatic masses can be biopsied via EUS and one can deliver nerve blocks through EUS. Although criteria for abnormalities on EUS in severe pancreatic disease have been developed, the true sensitivity and specificity of this procedure has yet to be determined.

TABLE 45-3

ENDOSCOPIC ULTRASONOGRAPHIC CRITERIA FOR CHRONIC PANCREATITIS

DUCTAL	PARENCHYMAL
Stones	Echogenic strands
Echogenic ductal walls	Echogenic foci
Irregular ductal walls	Calcifications
Stricture	Lobular contour
Visible side branches	Cyst
Ductular dilatation	

Currently chronic pancreatitis is diagnosed by EUS if three or more criteria listed in Table 45-3 are present. That concept has now been vigorously challenged since normal subjects and patients with nonulcer dyspepsia may have an abnormal EUS based on just three abnormalities. Many EUS experts are now requiring five or more abnormalities before chronic pancreatitis is diagnosed. Recent studies comparing EUS to the secretin test in patients with unexplained abdominal pain suspected of having chronic pancreatitis show a significantly better sensitivity and specificity for the secretin test over EUS in detecting early changes of chronic pancreatitis. The exact role of EUS versus CT, ERCP, or function testing has yet to be defined.

Magnetic resonance cholangiopancreatography (MRCP) is now being used to view both the bile duct and the pancreatic duct. Non-breath-holding and three-dimensional turbo spin-echo techniques are being utilized to produce superb MRCP images. The main pancreatic duct and common bile duct can be seen well, but there is still a question as to whether changes can be detected consistently in the secondary ducts. MRCP may be particularly useful to evaluate the pancreatic duct in high-risk patients such as the elderly because this is a noninvasive procedure.

Both EUS and MRCP may replace ERCP in some patients. As these techniques become more refined, they may well be the diagnostic tests of choice to evaluate the pancreatic duct. ERCP is still needed to perform therapy of bile duct and pancreatic duct lesions.

Selective catheterization of the celiac and superior mesenteric arteries combined with superselective catheterization of others arteries, such as the hepatic, splenic, and gastroduodenal arteries, permits visualization of the pancreas and detection of pancreatic neoplasms and pseudocysts. Pancreatic neoplasms can be identified by the sheathing of blood vessels by a mass lesion (Fig. 46-1D). Hormone-producing pancreatic tumors are especially likely to exhibit increased vascularity and tumor staining. Angiographic abnormalities are noted in many patients with pancreatic carcinoma but are uncommon in patients without pancreatic disease. Angiography complements ultrasonography and ERCP in the study of patients with a suspected pancreatic lesion and may be carried out if ERCP is either unsuccessful or nondiagnostic.

ERCP may provide useful information on the status of the pancreatic ductal system and thus aid in the differential diagnosis of pancreatic disease (Figs. 46-1C, 46-3D, and 46-4B). Pancreatic carcinoma is characterized by stenosis or obstruction of either the pancreatic duct or the common bile duct; both ductal systems are often abnormal. In chronic pancreatitis, ERCP abnormalities include (1) luminal narrowing; (2) irregularities in the ductal system with stenosis, dilation, sacculation, and ectasia; and (3) blockage of the pancreatic duct by calcium deposits. The presence of ductal stenosis and irregularity can make it difficult to distinguish chronic pancreatitis from carcinoma. It is important to be aware that ERCP changes interpreted as indicating chronic pancreatitis actually may be due to the effects of aging on the pancreatic duct or to the fact that the procedure was performed within several weeks of an attack of acute pancreatitis. Although aging may cause impressive ductal alterations, it does not affect the results of pancreatic function tests (i.e., the secretin test). Elevated serum and/or urine amylase levels after ERCP have been reported in 25–75% of patients, and clinical pancreatitis in 5–20% of patients. There are no satisfactory means to pharmacologically prevent ERCP-induced pancreatitis, despite many agents having been suggested and evaluated. The best way to prevent ERCP-induced pancreatitis is to not perform this procedure for diagnostic purposes in high-risk patients, who include women with acute relapsing pancreatitis in whom there is no evidence of biliary obstruction and patients with unexplained abdominal pain but no other abnormalities. If no lesion is found in the biliary and/or pancreatic ducts in a patient with repeated attacks of acute pancreatitis, manometric studies of the sphincter of Oddi may be indicated. Such studies, however, do increase the risk of post-ERCP/manometry acute pancreatitis. Such pancreatitis appears to be more common in patients with a nondilated pancreatic duct.

Pancreatic Biopsy with Radiologic Guidance

Percutaneous aspiration biopsy of a pancreatic mass often distinguishes a pancreatic inflammatory mass from a pancreatic neoplasm.

TESTS OF EXOCRINE PANCREATIC FUNCTION

Pancreatic function tests (Table 45-1) can be divided into the following:

1. *Direct stimulation of the pancreas* by IV infusion of secretin or secretin plus cholecystokinin (CCK) followed by collection and measurement of duodenal contents.

2. Study of *intraluminal digestion products*, such as undigested meat fibers, stool fat, and fecal nitrogen.
3. *Measurement of fecal pancreatic enzymes* such as elastase.

The secretin test, used to detect diffuse pancreatic disease, is based on the physiologic principle that the pancreatic secretory response is directly related to the functional mass of pancreatic tissue. In the standard assay, secretin is given IV in a dose of 0.2 μg/kg of synthetic human or synthetic porcine secretin as either a bolus or a continuous infusion. Normal values for the standard secretin test are (1) volume output > 2.0 mL/kg per hour, (2) bicarbonate (HCO_3^-) concentration > 80 mmol/L, and (3) HCO_3^- output > 10 mmol/L in 1 h. The most reproducible measurement, giving the highest level of discrimination between normal subjects and patients with chronic pancreatitis, appears to be the maximal bicarbonate concentration.

There may be a dissociation between the results of the secretin test and those of tests of absorptive function. For example, patients with chronic pancreatitis often have abnormally low outputs of HCO_3^- after secretin but have normal fecal fat excretion. Thus the secretin test measures the secretory capacity of ductular epithelium, while fecal fat excretion indirectly reflects intraluminal lipolytic activity. Steatorrhea does not occur until intraluminal levels of lipase are markedly reduced, underscoring the fact that only small amounts of enzymes are necessary for intraluminal digestive activities. An abnormal secretin test result suggests only that chronic pancreatic damage is present; it will not consistently distinguish between chronic pancreatitis and pancreatic carcinoma.

The *serum trypsinogen level*, which is determined by radioimmunoassay, also has excellent specificity but is not very sensitive. It is a simple blood test that can detect severe damage to the exocrine pancreas. The normal values are 28–58 ng/mL, and any value <20 ng/mL reflects pancreatic steatorrhea.

Measurement of *intraluminal digestion products*, i.e., undigested muscle fibers, stool fat, and fecal nitrogen, is discussed in Chap. 15. The amount of human elastase in stool reflects the pancreatic output of this proteolytic enzyme. Decreased elastase activity in stool is an excellent test to detect severe pancreatic exocrine insufficiency in patients with chronic pancreatitis and cystic fibrosis. Tests useful in the diagnosis of exocrine pancreatic insufficiency and the differential diagnosis of malabsorption are also discussed in Chaps. 15 and 46.

FURTHER READINGS

MAUREA S et al: Comparative diagnostic evaluation with MR cholangiopancreatography, ultrasonography and CT in patients with pancreatobiliary disease. Radiol Med 114:390, 2009

SCHÜTTE K, MALFERTHEINER P: Markers for predicting severity and progression of acute pancreatitis. Best Pract Res Clin Gastroenterol 22:75, 2008

SIDDIQI AJ, MILLER F: Chronic pancreatitis: ultrasound, computed tomography, and magnetic resonance imaging features. Semin Ultrasound CT MR 28:384, 2007

SUGIYAMA M et al: Magnetic resonance imaging for diagnosing chronic pancreatitis. J Gastroenterol. 42:108, 2007

YADAY Y et al: A critical evaluation of laboratory tests in acute pancreatitis. Am J Gastroenterol 97:1309, 2002

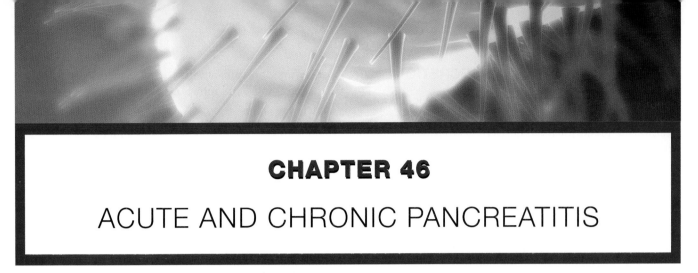

CHAPTER 46

ACUTE AND CHRONIC PANCREATITIS

Norton J. Greenberger ■ Phillip P. Toskes

BIOCHEMISTRY AND PHYSIOLOGY OF PANCREATIC EXOCRINE SECRETION

GENERAL CONSIDERATIONS

The pancreas secretes 1500–3000 mL of isosmotic alkaline (pH > 8.0) fluid per day containing about 20 enzymes and zymogens. The pancreatic secretions provide the enzymes needed to effect the major digestive activity of the gastrointestinal tract and provide an optimal pH for the function of these enzymes.

REGULATION OF PANCREATIC SECRETION

The exocrine pancreas is influenced by intimately interacting hormonal and neural systems. *Gastric acid* is the stimulus for the release of secretin, which stimulates the secretion of pancreatic juice rich in water and electrolytes. Release of cholecystokinin (CCK) from the duodenum and jejunum is largely triggered by long-chain fatty acids, certain essential amino acids (tryptophan, phenylalanine, valine, methionine), and gastric acid

itself. CCK evokes an enzyme-rich secretion from the pancreas. The *parasympathetic nervous system* (via the vagus nerve) exerts significant control over pancreatic secretion. Secretion evoked by secretin and CCK depends on permissive roles of vagal afferent and efferent pathways. This is particularly true for enzyme secretion, whereas water and bicarbonate secretions are heavily dependent on the hormonal effects of secretin and CCK. Also, vagal stimulation effects the release of vasoactive intestinal peptide (VIP), a secretin agonist. Bile salts also stimulate pancreatic secretion, thereby integrating the functions of the biliary tract, pancreas, and small intestine.

Pancreatic exocrine secretion is influenced by inhibitory neuropeptides such as somatostatin, pancreatic polypeptide, peptide YY, neuropeptide Y, enkephalin, pancreastatin, calcitonin gene-related peptides, glucagon, and galanin. Although pancreatic polypeptide and peptide YY may act primarily on nerves outside the pancreas, somatostatin acts at multiple sites. Nitric oxide is also an important neurotransmitter. The mechanism of action of these various factors has not been fully defined.

WATER AND ELECTROLYTE SECRETION

Bicarbonate is the ion of primary physiologic importance within pancreatic secretion. The ductal cells secrete bicarbonate predominantly derived from plasma (93%) rather than intracellular metabolism (7%). Bicarbonate enters through the sodium bicarbonate co-transporter with depolarization caused by chloride efflux through the cystic fibrosis transmembrane conductance regulator (CFTR). Secretin and VIP, both of which increase intracellular cyclic AMP, act on the ductal cells opening the CFTR in promoting secretion. CCK, acting as a neuromodulator, markedly potentiates the stimulatory effects of secretin. Acetylcholine also plays an important role in ductal cell secretion. Bicarbonate helps neutralize gastric acid and creates the appropriate pH for the activity of pancreatic enzymes.

ENZYME SECRETION

The acinar cell is highly compartmentalized and is concerned with the secretion of pancreatic enzymes. Proteins synthesized by the rough endoplasmic reticulum are processed in the Golgi and then targeted to the appropriate site, whether that be zymogen granules, lysosomes, or other cell compartments. The pancreas secretes amylolytic, lipolytic, and proteolytic enzymes. *Amylolytic enzymes*, such as amylase, hydrolyze starch to oligosaccharides and to the disaccharide maltose. The *lipolytic enzymes* include lipase, phospholipase A, and cholesterol esterase. Bile salts inhibit lipase in isolation; but colipase, another constituent of pancreatic secretion, binds to lipase and prevents this inhibition. Bile salts activate phospholipase A and cholesterol esterase. *Proteolytic enzymes* include endopeptidases (trypsin, chymotrypsin), which act on internal peptide bonds of proteins and polypeptides; exopeptidases (carboxypeptidases, aminopeptidases), which act on the free carboxyl- and amino-terminal ends of peptides, respectively; and elastase. The proteolytic enzymes are secreted as inactive precursors (zymogens). Ribonucleases (deoxyribonucleases, ribonuclease) are also secreted. *Enterokinase*, an enzyme found in the duodenal mucosa, cleaves the lysine-isoleucine bond of trypsinogen to form trypsin. Trypsin then activates the other proteolytic zymogens in a cascade phenomenon. All pancreatic enzymes have pH optima in the alkaline range. The nervous system initiates pancreatic enzyme secretion. The neurologic stimulation is cholinergic, involving extrinsic innervation by the vagus nerve and subsequent innervation by intrapancreatic cholinergic nerves. The stimulatory neurotransmitters are acetylcholine and gastrin-releasing peptides. These neurotransmitters activate calcium-dependent second messenger systems resulting in the release of zymogen granules. VIP is present in intrapancreatic nerves and potentiates the effect of acetylcholine. In contrast to other species, there are no CCK receptors on acinar cells in humans. CCK in physiologic concentrations stimulates pancreatic secretion by stimulating central vagal and intrapancreatic nerves.

AUTOPROTECTION OF THE PANCREAS

Autodigestion of the pancreas is prevented by the packaging of proteases in precursor form and by the synthesis of protease inhibitors, i.e., pancreatic secretory trypsin inhibitor (PSTI) and serine protease inhibitor, kazal type 1 (SPINK1). These protease inhibitors are found in the acinar cell, the pancreatic secretions, and the α_1- and α_2-globulin fractions of plasma. In addition, low calcium concentrations within the pancreas decrease trypsin activity. Loss of any of these protective mechanisms leads to zymogen activation, autodigestion, and acute pancreatitis.

EXOCRINE-ENDOCRINE RELATIONSHIPS

Insulin appears to be needed locally for secretin and CCK to promote exocrine secretion; thus, it acts in a permissive role for these two hormones.

ENTEROPANCREATIC AXIS AND FEEDBACK INHIBITION

Pancreatic enzyme secretion is controlled, at least in part, by a negative feedback mechanism induced by the presence of active serine proteases in the duodenum. To illustrate, perfusion of the duodenal lumen with phenylalanine causes a prompt increase in plasma CCK levels as well as increased secretion of chymotrypsin. However, simultaneous perfusion with trypsin blunts both responses. Conversely, perfusion of the duodenal lumen with protease inhibitors actually leads to enzyme hypersecretion. The available evidence supports the concept that the duodenum contains a peptide called *CCK-releasing factor* (CCK-RF) that is involved in stimulating CCK release. It appears that serine proteases inhibit pancreatic secretion by acting on a CCK-releasing peptide in the lumen of the small intestine. Thus the integrative result of both bicarbonate and enzyme secretion depends on a feedback process for both bicarbonate and pancreatic enzymes. Acidification of the duodenum releases secretin, which stimulates vagal-vagal and other neural pathways to activate pancreatic duct cells, which secrete bicarbonate. This bicarbonate then neutralizes the duodenal acid, and the feedback loop is completed. Duodenal proteins lead to a reduction in free proteases, thereby leading to an increase in free CCK-RF. CCK-RF is then released into the blood in physiologic concentrations, acting primarily through the neural pathways (vagal-vagal). This leads to acetylcholine-mediated pancreatic enzyme secretion. Proteases continue to be secreted from the pancreas until the protein within the duodenum and CCK-RF are digested. At this point, the free duodenal proteases rise again, thus completing this step in the feedback process.

ACUTE PANCREATITIS

GENERAL CONSIDERATIONS

Pancreatic inflammatory disease may be classified as (1) acute pancreatitis or (2) chronic pancreatitis. The pathologic spectrum of acute pancreatitis varies from *interstitial pancreatitis*, which is usually a mild and self-limited disorder, to *necrotizing pancreatitis*, in which the degree of pancreatic necrosis correlates with the severity of the attack and its systemic manifestations.

The incidence of pancreatitis varies in different countries and depends on cause, e.g., alcohol, gallstones, metabolic factors, and drugs (Table 46-1). The estimated incidence in England is 5.4/100,000 per year; in the United States it is 79.8/100,000 per year, thus resulting in >200,000 new cases of acute pancreatitis annually.

ETIOLOGY AND PATHOGENESIS

There are many causes of acute pancreatitis (Table 46-1), but the mechanisms by which these conditions trigger pancreatic inflammation have not been identified. Gallstones continue to be the leading cause of acute pancreatitis in most series (30–60%). Alcohol is the second most common cause, responsible for 15–30% of cases in the United States. The incidence of pancreatitis in alcoholics is surprisingly low (5/100,000), indicating that in addition to the amount of alcohol ingested unknown factors affect a person's susceptibility to pancreatic injury. The mechanism of injury is not well understood. Hypertriglyceridemia is the cause of acute pancreatitis in 1.3–3.8% of cases; serum triglyceride levels are usually >11.3 mmol/L (>1000 mg/dL). Most patients with hypertriglyceridemia, when subsequently examined, show evidence of an underlying derangement in lipid metabolism, probably unrelated to pancreatitis. Patients with diabetes mellitus who have developed ketoacidosis or who are on certain medications may also develop high triglyceride levels. Acute pancreatitis occurs in 5–20% of patients following endoscopic retrograde cholangiopancreatography (ERCP). Approximately 2–5% of cases of acute pancreatitis are drug-related. Drugs cause pancreatitis either by a hypersensitivity reaction or by the generation of a toxic metabolite, although in some cases it is not clear which of these mechanisms is operative (Table 46-1).

Autodigestion is one pathogenic theory, according to which pancreatitis results when proteolytic enzymes (e.g., trypsinogen, chymotrypsinogen, proelastase, and phospholipase A) are activated in the pancreas rather than in the intestinal lumen. A number of factors (e.g., endotoxins, exotoxins, viral infections, ischemia, anoxia, and direct trauma) are believed to activate these proenzymes.

TABLE 46-1

CAUSES OF ACUTE PANCREATITIS

Common Causes

Gallstones (including microlithiasis)
Alcohol (acute and chronic alcoholism)
Hypertriglyceridemia
Endoscopic retrograde cholangiopancreatography (ERCP), especially after biliary manometry
Trauma (especially blunt abdominal trauma)
Postoperative (abdominal and nonabdominal operations)
Drugs (azathioprine, 6-mercaptopurine, sulfonamides, estrogens, tetracycline, valproic acid, anti-HIV medications)
Sphincter of Oddi dysfunction

Uncommon Causes

Vascular causes and vasculitis (ischemic-hypoperfusion states after cardiac surgery)
Connective tissue disorders and thrombotic thrombocytopenic purpura (TTP)
Cancer of the pancreas
Hypercalcemia
Periampullary diverticulum
Pancreas divisum
Hereditary pancreatitis
Cystic fibrosis
Renal failure

Rare Causes

Infections (mumps, coxsackievirus, cytomegalovirus, echovirus, parasites)
Autoimmune (e.g., Sjögren's syndrome)

Causes to Consider in Patients with Recurrent Bouts of Acute Pancreatitis without an Obvious Etiology

Occult disease of the biliary tree or pancreatic ducts, especially microlithiasis, sludge
Drugs
Hypertriglyceridemia
Pancreas divisum
Pancreatic cancer
Sphincter of Oddi dysfunction
Cystic fibrosis
Idiopathic

Activated proteolytic enzymes, especially trypsin, not only digest pancreatic and peripancreatic tissues but also can activate other enzymes, such as elastase and phospholipase.

ACTIVATION OF PANCREATIC ENZYMES IN THE PATHOGENESIS OF ACUTE PANCREATITIS

Several recent studies have suggested that pancreatitis is a disease that evolves in three phases. The initial phase is characterized by intrapancreatic digestive enzyme activation and acinar cell injury. Zymogen activation appears to be mediated by lysosomal hydrolases such as cathepsin B which become co-localized with digestive enzymes in intracellular organelles; it is currently believed that acinar cell injury is the consequence of zymogen activation. The second phase of pancreatitis involves the activation, chemoattraction, and sequestration of neutrophils in the pancreas, resulting in an intrapancreatic inflammatory reaction of variable severity. Neutrophil depletion induced by prior administration of an antineutrophil serum has been shown to reduce the severity of experimentally induced pancreatitis. There is also evidence to support the concept that neutrophil sequestration can activate trypsinogen. Thus, intrapancreatic acinar cell activation of trypsinogen could be a two-step process, i.e., with a neutrophil-independent and a neutrophil-dependent phase. The third phase of pancreatitis is due to the effects of activated proteolytic enzymes and cytokines, released by the inflamed pancreas, on distant organs. Activated proteolytic enzymes, especially trypsin, not only digest pancreatic and peripancreatic tissues but also activate other enzymes such as elastase and phospholipase. The active enzymes then digest cellular membranes and cause proteolysis, edema, interstitial hemorrhage, vascular damage, coagulation necrosis, fat necrosis, and parenchymal cell necrosis. Cellular injury and death result in the liberation of bradykinin peptides, vasoactive substances, and histamine that can produce vasodilation, increased vascular permeability, and edema with profound effects on many organs, most notably the lung. The systemic inflammatory response syndrome (SIRS) and acute respiratory distress syndrome (ARDS) as well as multiorgan failure may occur as result of this cascade of local as well as distant effects.

The course of acute pancreatitis appears to be modified by genetic factors that can increase the susceptibility and/or modify the severity of pancreatic injury. Four susceptibility genes have been identified: (1) cationic trypsinogen mutations (PRSS1m, R122Hm, and N291), (2) pancreatic secretory trypsin inhibitor (SPINK1), (3) cystic fibrosis transmembrane conductance regulator (CFTR), and (4) monocyte chemotactic protein (MCP-1). Experimental and clinical data indicate that MCP-1 may be an important inflammatory mediator in the early pathologic process of acute pancreatitis, a determinant of the severity of the inflammatory response, and a promoter of organ failure. MCP-1 helps drive the inflammatory response after pancreatic injury. The MCP-1 2518 G allele polymorphism is a gain-of-function promoter that increases MCP-1 expression. In a recent study, 14 patients with severe pancreatitis all had elevated MCP-1 levels, with the mean value being eightfold greater than 116 controls and also eightfold greater than 63 patients with mild pancreatitis; 5 of the 14 died. The MCP-1 2518 G allele is a risk factor for severe acute pancreatitis. MCP-1 levels measured early in the course of acute pancreatitis appear to be an accurate predictor of severity and death.

Approach to the Patient:
ABDOMINAL PAIN

Abdominal pain is the major symptom of acute pancreatitis. Pain may vary from a mild and tolerable discomfort to severe, constant, and incapacitating distress. Characteristically, the pain, which is steady and boring in character, is located in the epigastrium and periumbilical region and often radiates to the back as well as to the chest, flanks, and lower abdomen. The pain is frequently more intense when the patient is supine, and patients often obtain relief by sitting with the trunk flexed and knees drawn up. Nausea, vomiting, and abdominal distention due to gastric and intestinal hypomotility and chemical peritonitis are also frequent complaints.

Physical examination frequently reveals a distressed and anxious patient. Low-grade fever, tachycardia, and hypotension are fairly common. Shock is not unusual and may result from (1) hypovolemia secondary to exudation of blood and plasma proteins into the retroperitoneal space (a "retroperitoneal burn"); (2) increased formation and release of kinin peptides, which cause vasodilation and increased vascular permeability; and (3) systemic effects of proteolytic and lipolytic enzymes released into the circulation. Jaundice occurs infrequently; when present, it usually is due to edema of the head of the pancreas with compression of the intrapancreatic portion of the common bile duct. Erythematous skin nodules due to subcutaneous fat necrosis may occur. In 10–20% of patients, there are pulmonary findings, including basilar rales, atelectasis, and pleural effusion, the latter most frequently left-sided. Abdominal tenderness and muscle rigidity are present to a variable degree, but, compared with the intense pain, these signs may be unimpressive. Bowel sounds are usually diminished or absent. An enlarged pancreas with organized necrosis or a pseudocyst may be palpable in the upper abdomen. A faint blue discoloration around the umbilicus (Cullen's sign) may occur as the result of hemoperitoneum, and a blue-red-purple or green-brown discoloration of the flanks (Turner's sign) reflects tissue catabolism of hemoglobin. The latter two findings, which are uncommon, indicate the presence of a severe necrotizing pancreatitis.

LABORATORY DATA

The diagnosis of acute pancreatitis is usually established by the detection of an increased level of serum amylase. Values threefold or more above normal virtually clinch the diagnosis if overt salivary gland disease and gut perforation or infarction are excluded. However, there appears to be no definite correlation between the severity of pancreatitis and the degree of serum amylase elevation. After 48–72 h, even with continuing evidence of pancreatitis, total serum amylase values tend to return to normal. However, pancreatic isoamylase and lipase levels may remain elevated for 7–14 days. It will be recalled that amylase elevations in serum and urine occur in many conditions other than pancreatitis (Table 45-2). Importantly, patients with *acidemia* (arterial pH ≤7.32) may have spurious elevations in serum amylase. In one study, 12 of 33 patients with acidemia had elevated serum amylase, but only 1 had an elevated lipase value; in 9, salivary-type amylase was the predominant serum isoamylase. This finding explains why patients with diabetic ketoacidosis may have marked elevations in serum amylase without any other evidence of acute pancreatitis. Serum lipase activity increases in parallel with amylase activity. Measurement of both enzymes is important as serum amylase tends to be higher in gallstone pancreatitis and serum lipase higher in alcohol-associated pancreatitis. A threefold elevated serum lipase value is usually diagnostic of acute pancreatitis; these tests are especially helpful in patients with nonpancreatic causes of hyperamylasemia (Table 46-2). Markedly increased levels of peritoneal or pleural fluid amylase [>1500 nmol/L (>5000 U/dL)] are also helpful, if present, in establishing the diagnosis.

Leukocytosis (15,000–20,000 leukocytes per μL) occurs frequently. Patients with more severe disease may show hemoconcentration with hematocrit values >44% because of loss of plasma into the retroperitoneal space and peritoneal cavity. Hemoconcentration may be the harbinger of more severe disease, i.e., pancreatic necrosis. *Hyperglycemia* is common and is due to multiple factors, including decreased insulin release, increased glucagon release, and an increased output of adrenal glucocorticoids and catecholamines. *Hypocalcemia* occurs in ~25%

of patients, and its pathogenesis is incompletely understood. Although earlier studies suggested that the response of the parathyroid gland to a decrease in serum calcium is impaired, subsequent observations have failed to confirm this idea. Intraperitoneal saponification of calcium by fatty acids in areas of fat necrosis occurs occasionally, with large amounts (up to 6.0 g) dissolved or suspended in ascitic fluid. Such "soap formation" may also be significant in patients with pancreatitis, mild hypocalcemia, and little or no obvious ascites. *Hyperbilirubinemia* [serum bilirubin >68 μmol/L (>4.0 mg/dL)] occurs in ~10% of patients. However, jaundice is transient, and serum bilirubin levels return to normal in 4–7 days. Serum alkaline phosphatase and aspartate aminotransferase (AST) levels are also transiently elevated and parallel serum bilirubin values. Markedly elevated serum lactic dehydrogenase (LDH) levels [>8.5 μmol/L (>500 U/dL)] suggest a poor prognosis. Serum albumin is decreased to 30 g/L (3.0 g/dL) in ~10% of patients; this finding is associated with more severe pancreatitis and a higher mortality rate (Table 46-2). *Hypertriglyceridemia* occurs in 15–20% of patients, and serum amylase and lipase levels in these individuals are often spuriously normal (Chap. 45). Approximately 25% of patients have *hypoxemia* (arterial P_{O_2} ≤60 mmHg), which may herald the onset of ARDS. Finally, the electrocardiogram is occasionally abnormal in acute pancreatitis with ST-segment and T-wave abnormalities simulating myocardial ischemia.

A CT scan can confirm the clinical impression of acute pancreatitis even in the face of normal serum amylase levels. Importantly, CT is quite helpful in indicating the severity of acute pancreatitis and the risk of morbidity and mortality and in evaluating the complications of acute pancreatitis (see later). Sonography is useful in acute pancreatitis to evaluate the gallbladder. Radiologic studies useful in the diagnosis of acute pancreatitis are discussed in Chap. 45 and listed in Table 45-1.

DIAGNOSIS

Any severe acute pain in the abdomen or back should suggest acute pancreatitis. The diagnosis is usually entertained when a patient with a possible predisposition to pancreatitis presents with severe and constant abdominal pain, nausea, emesis, fever, tachycardia, and abnormal findings on abdominal examination. Laboratory studies frequently reveal leukocytosis, hypocalcemia, and hyperglycemia. The diagnosis is usually confirmed by the finding of a threefold or greater elevated level of serum amylase and/or lipase. Not all the above features have to be present for the diagnosis to be established. Strong indicators include hemoconcentration (hematocrit > 44%) and signs of organ failure (Table 46-2).

TABLE 46-2

RISK FACTORS THAT ADVERSELY AFFECT SURVIVAL IN ACUTE PANCREATITIS
Severe Acute Pancreatitis
1. Associated with organ failure and/or local complications such as necrosis
2. Clinical manifestations
a. Obesity BMI >30
b. Hemoconcentration (hematocrit >44%)
c. Age >70
3. Organ failure[a]
a. Shock
b. Pulmonary insufficiency (P_{O_2} <60)
c. Renal failure (CR >2.0 mg%)
d. GI bleeding
4. ≥3 Ranson criteria (not fully utilizable until 48 h)
5. Apache II score >8 (cumbersome)

[a]Usually declares itself shortly after onset.

484

The *differential diagnosis* should include the following disorders: (1) perforated viscus, especially peptic ulcer; (2) acute cholecystitis and biliary colic; (3) acute intestinal obstruction; (4) mesenteric vascular occlusion; (5) renal colic; (6) myocardial infarction; (7) dissecting aortic aneurysm; (8) connective tissue disorders with vasculitis; (9) pneumonia; and (10) diabetic ketoacidosis. A penetrating duodenal ulcer can usually be identified by imaging studies or endoscopy. A perforated duodenal ulcer is readily diagnosed by the presence of free intraperitoneal air. It may be difficult to differentiate acute cholecystitis from acute pancreatitis, since an elevated serum amylase may be found in both disorders. Pain of biliary tract origin is more right-sided or epigastric than periumbilical and is gradual in onset; ileus is usually absent. Sonography and radionuclide scanning are helpful in establishing the diagnosis of cholelithiasis and cholecystitis. Intestinal obstruction due to mechanical factors can be differentiated from pancreatitis by the history of colicky pain, findings on abdominal examination, and x-rays of the abdomen showing changes characteristic of mechanical obstruction. Acute mesenteric vascular occlusion is usually evident in elderly debilitated patients with brisk leukocytosis, abdominal distention, and bloody diarrhea, in whom paracentesis shows sanguineous fluid and angiography shows vascular occlusion. Serum as well as peritoneal fluid amylase levels are increased, however, in patients with intestinal infarction. Systemic lupus erythematosus and polyarteritis nodosa may be confused with pancreatitis, especially since pancreatitis may develop as a complication of these diseases. Diabetic ketoacidosis is often accompanied by abdominal pain and elevated total serum amylase levels, thus closely mimicking acute pancreatitis. However, the serum lipase level is not elevated in diabetic ketoacidosis.

COURSE OF THE DISEASE AND COMPLICATIONS

It is important to identify patients with acute pancreatitis who have an increased risk of dying. Multiple factor scoring systems (Ranson, Imrie, Apache II) are difficult to use, show poor predictive powers, and have not been uniformly embraced by clinicians. The key indicators of a severe attack of pancreatitis are listed in Table 46-2 and include age >70 years, body mass index (BMI) >30, hematocrit >44%, and admission C-reactive protein >150 mg/L. However, it is organ failure, in which respiratory failure (PO_2 <60 mmHg) dominates, that determines outcome in the majority of difficult to manage cases. The presence of shock (systolic blood pressure <90 mmHg or tachycardia >130), renal failure [serum creatinine >177 μmol/L (>2.0 mg/dL)], and gastrointestinal bleeding (>500 mL/24 h) are also key factors. The high mortality rate of such severely ill patients is due in large part to multiorgan failure, especially during the first week, and warrants intensive monitoring and/or a combination of radiologic and surgical means, as discussed in detail below.

The local and systemic complications of acute pancreatitis are listed in **Table 46-3**. In the first 2–3 weeks after pancreatitis, patients frequently develop an inflammatory mass, which may be due to organized pancreatic necrosis (with or without infection) or a pseudocyst. Pancreatic abscess develops later, i.e., usually after

TABLE 46-3

COMPLICATIONS OF ACUTE PANCREATITIS

Local

Necrosis	Pancreatic ascites
Sterile	Disruption of main
Infected	pancreatic duct
Organized	Leaking pseudocyst
Pancreatic fluid collections	Involvement of contiguous
Pancreatic abscess	organs by necrotizing
Pancreatic pseudocyst	pancreatitis
Pain	Massive intraperitoneal
Rupture	hemorrhage
Hemorrhage	Thrombosis of blood
Infection	vessels (splenic vein,
Obstruction of	portal vein)
gastrointestinal tract	Bowel infarction
(stomach, duodenum,	Obstructive jaundice
colon)	

Systemic

Pulmonary	Renal
Pleural effusion	Oliguria
Atelectasis	Azotemia
Mediastinal abscess	Renal artery and/or renal
Pneumonitis	vein thrombosis
Adult respiratory	Acute tubular necrosis
distress syndrome	Metabolic
Cardiovascular	Hyperglycemia
Hypotension	Hypertriglyceridemia
Hypovolemia	Hypocalcemia
Sudden death	Encephalopathy
Nonspecific ST-T changes	Sudden blindness
in electrocardiogram	(Purtscher's retinopathy)
simulating myocardial	Central nervous system
infarction	Psychosis
Pericardial effusion	Fat emboli
Hematologic	Fat necrosis
Disseminated intravascular	Subcutaneous tissues
coagulation	(erythematous nodules)
Gastrointestinal hemorrhage	Bone
Peptic ulcer disease	Miscellaneous
Erosive gastritis	(mediastinum, pleura,
Hemorrhagic pancreatic	nervous system)
necrosis with erosion	
into major blood vessels	
Portal vein thrombosis,	
variceal hemorrhage	

SECTION VIII

Disorders of the Pancreas

6 weeks. Systemic complications include pulmonary, cardiovascular, hematologic, renal, metabolic, and central nervous system abnormalities. Pancreatitis and hypertriglyceridemia constitute an association in which cause and effect remain incompletely understood. However, several reasonable conclusions can be drawn. First, hypertriglyceridemia can precede and apparently cause pancreatitis. Second, the vast majority (>80%) of patients with acute pancreatitis do not have hypertriglyceridemia. Third, almost all patients with pancreatitis and hypertriglyceridemia have preexisting abnormalities in lipoprotein metabolism. Fourth, many of the patients with this association have persistent hypertriglyceridemia after recovery from pancreatitis and are prone to recurrent episodes of pancreatitis. Fifth, any factor (e.g., drugs or alcohol) that causes an abrupt increase in serum triglycerides to levels >11 mmol/L (1000 mg/dL) can precipitate a bout of pancreatitis that can be associated with significant complications and even become fulminant. To avert the risk of triggering pancreatitis, a fasting serum triglyceride measurement should be obtained before estrogen replacement therapy is begun in postmenopausal women. Fasting levels <3.4 mmol/L (300 mg/dL) pose no risk, whereas levels >8.5 mmol/L (750 mg/dL) are associated with a high probability of developing pancreatitis. Finally, patients with a deficiency of apolipoprotein CII have an increased incidence of pancreatitis; apolipoprotein CII activates lipoprotein lipase, which is important in clearing chylomicrons from the bloodstream.

Purtscher's retinopathy, a relatively unusual complication, is manifested by a sudden and severe loss of vision in a patient with acute pancreatitis. It is characterized by a peculiar funduscopic appearance with cotton-wool spots and hemorrhages confined to an area limited by the optic disk and macula; it is believed to be due to occlusion of the posterior retinal artery with aggregated granulocytes.

The two most common causes of acute pancreatitis are biliary tract disease and alcoholism; other causes are listed in Table 46-1. The risk of acute pancreatitis in patients with at least one gallstone <5 mm in diameter is fourfold greater than that in patients with larger stones. However, after a conventional workup, a specific cause is not identified in ~30% of patients.

In one series of 31 patients diagnosed initially as having idiopathic acute pancreatitis, 23 were found to have occult gallstone disease. Thus, approximately two-thirds of patients with recurrent acute pancreatitis without an obvious cause actually have occult gallstone disease due to microlithiasis. Other diseases of the biliary tree and pancreatic ducts that can cause acute pancreatitis include choledochocele; ampullary tumors; pancreas divisum; and pancreatic duct stones, stricture, and tumor. Approximately 2–4% of patients with pancreatic carcinoma present with acute pancreatitis.

Recurrent Pancreatitis

Approximately 25% of patients who have had an attack of acute pancreatitis have a recurrence. The two most common etiologic factors are alcohol and cholelithiasis. In patients with recurrent pancreatitis without an obvious cause the differential diagnosis should encompass occult biliary tract disease including microlithiasis, hypertriglyceridemia, drugs, pancreatic cancer, sphincter of Oddi dysfunction, pancreas divisum, cystic fibrosis, and pancreatic cancer (Table 46-1).

Pancreatitis in Patients with AIDS

The incidence of acute pancreatitis is increased in patients with AIDS for two reasons: (1) the high incidence of infections involving the pancreas, such as infections with cytomegalovirus, *Cryptosporidium*, and the *Mycobacterium avium* complex; and (2) the frequent use by patients with AIDS of medications such as didanosine, pentamidine, trimethoprim-sulfamethoxazole, and protease inhibitors.

℞ **Treatment:**
ACUTE PANCREATITIS

In most patients (85–90%) with acute pancreatitis, the disease is self-limited and subsides spontaneously, usually within 3–7 days after treatment is instituted. Conventional measures include (1) analgesics for pain, (2) IV fluids and colloids to maintain normal intravascular volume, and (3) no oral alimentation. Controlled trials have shown that nasogastric suction offers no clear-cut advantages in the treatment of mild to moderately severe acute pancreatitis. Its use, therefore, must be considered elective rather than mandatory.

It has been demonstrated that CCK-stimulated pancreatic secretion is almost abolished in four different experimental models of acute pancreatitis. This finding probably explains why drugs to block pancreatic secretion in acute pancreatitis have failed to have any therapeutic benefit. For this and other reasons, anticholinergic drugs are not indicated in acute pancreatitis. In addition to nasogastric suction and anticholinergic drugs, other therapies designed to "rest the pancreas" by inhibiting pancreatic secretion have not changed the course of the disease.

ROLE OF ANTIBIOTICS The benefit of antibiotic prophylaxis in the treatment of necrotizing acute pancreatitis remains controversial. A Cochrane database review of four randomized controlled trials (218 patients) compared antibiotic therapy with supportive medical treatment. Antibiotic prophylaxis reduced all-cause mortality from 17% to 6% and pancreatic sepsis from 32% to

21%, but did not differ from supportive therapy for rates of extrapancreatic infection, operative treatment, fungal infection, or length of hospital stay. However, none of the four studies were double blind and they varied in case mix and in choice and duration of antibiotic treatment.

A recent double-blind placebo-controlled trial investigated the effect of ciprofloxacin and metronidazole on the course and outcome of 114 patients with predicted severe acute pancreatitis. Although there were fewer multiorgan failure and extrapancreatic infections in the antibiotic treated group, this study detected no benefit of antibiotic prophylaxis with regard to the risk of developing infected pancreatic necrosis. However, the high crossover rate to antibiotic therapy in 21 of 56 patients in the placebo group may have contributed to the negative results.

Although the optimal drugs and duration of therapy remain incompletely defined, the current recommendation in patients with necrotizing acute pancreatitis is the use of a systemic antibiotic such as imipenem cilastin, 500 mg thrice daily for 7 days.

Intraabdominal *Candida* infection during acute necrotizing pancreatitis is increasing in frequency and is associated with increased use of antibiotics. In one representative trial, intraabdominal *Candida* infection was found in 13 of 37 cases and was associated with a

mortality rate fourfold greater than that associated with intraabdominal bacterial infection alone. Given the impact of *Candida* infection on the mortality rate in acute necrotizing pancreatitis and the apparent benefit of prophylactic antibiotics, these data suggest earlier use of fungicides.

Several other drugs have been evaluated by prospective controlled trials and found ineffective in the treatment of acute pancreatitis. The list, by no means complete, includes glucagon, H_2 blockers, protease inhibitors such as aprotinin, glucocorticoids, calcitonin, nonsteroidal anti-inflammatory drugs (NSAIDs), and lexipafant, a platelet-activating factor inhibitor. A recent meta-analysis of somatostatin, octreotide, and the antiprotease gabexate mesylate in therapy of acute pancreatitis suggested (1) a reduced mortality rate but no change in complications with octreotide, and (2) no effect on the mortality rate but reduced pancreatic damage with gabexate.

A CT scan, especially a dynamic contrast-enhanced CT (CECT) scan, provides valuable information on the severity and prognosis of acute pancreatitis (**Fig. 46-1**). In particular, a CECT scan allows estimation of the presence and extent of pancreatic necrosis. Recent studies suggest that the likelihood of prolonged pancreatitis or a serious complication is negligible when the CT severity index is 1 or 2 and low with scores of 3–6. However,

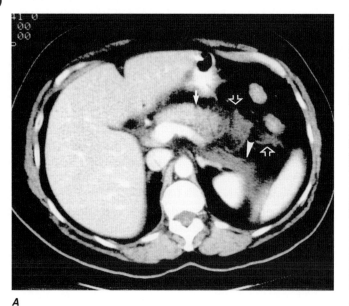
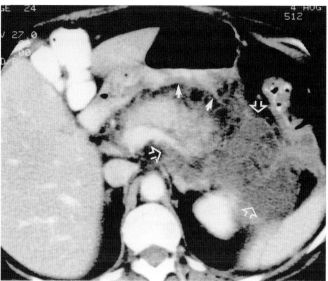

A   *B*

FIGURE 46-1

Acute pancreatitis: CT evolution. *A.* Contrast-enhanced CT scan of the abdomen performed on admission of a patient with clinical evidence of acute pancreatitis. Note the mildly decreased density of the body of the pancreas to the left of the midline (*arrow*). There are a few linear strands in the peripancreatic fat, suggesting inflammation (*open arrows*). A small amount of fluid is seen in the anterior pararenal space (*arrowhead*). ***B.*** Nine days after admission, there is a marked worsening with severe inflammation of the pancreas evidenced by anterior displacement of the posterior gastric wall (*arrows*), increased inflammation of the peripancreatic fat, and increased pancreatic effusion in the anterior perirenal space and around the splenic vein (*open arrows*). (*Courtesy of Dr. PR Ros, University of Florida College of Medicine; with permission.*)

patients with scores of 7–10 had a 92% morbidity rate and a 17% mortality rate. Necrosis is present in 12–20% of patients with acute pancreatitis. Those with necrosis have a morbidity rate of 50% and mortality rate of 20%, whereas those without necrosis have a morbidity rate <10% and a negligible mortality rate. A few retrospective studies have raised concern that the use of IV contrast early in the course of acute pancreatitis might intensify pancreatic necrosis. However, since prospective human studies are not available, it is reasonable to reserve CECT scans for patients with severe pancreatitis or suspected local septic complications.

The patient with mild to moderate pancreatitis usually requires treatment with IV fluids and fasting. A clear liquid diet is frequently started on the third to sixth day and a regular diet by the fifth to seventh day. The decision to reintroduce oral intake is usually based on the following criteria: (1) a decrease in or resolution of abdominal pain; (2) the patient is hungry; and (3) organ dysfunction, if present, has resolved. Elevation of serum amylase/lipase or persistent inflammatory changes seen on CT scans should not discourage feeding a hungry asymptomatic patient. In this regard, persistence of inflammatory changes on CT scans or persistent elevations in serum amylase/lipase may not resolve for weeks to months. The patient with unremitting *fulminant pancreatitis* usually requires inordinate amounts of fluid and close attention to complications such as cardiovascular collapse, respiratory insufficiency, and pancreatic infection. The latter should be managed by a combination of radiologic and surgical means (see below). While earlier uncontrolled studies suggested that *peritoneal lavage* through a percutaneous dialysis catheter was helpful in severe pancreatitis, subsequent studies indicate that this treatment does not influence the outcome of such attacks. Aggressive surgical pancreatic debridement (necrosectomy) should be undertaken soon after confirmation of the presence of infected necrosis, and multiple operations may be required. Since the mortality rate from sterile acute necrotizing pancreatitis is ~10%, laparotomy with adequate drainage and removal of necrotic tissue should be considered if conventional therapy does not halt the patient's deterioration. The use of total parenteral nutrition (TPN) makes it possible to give nutritional support to patients with severe, acute, or protracted pancreatitis who are unable to eat normally. It has been suggested that enteral feeding with a nasojejunal tube may be preferred over TPN because of decreased infection. Less expensive enteral feeds meet approximately only 50% of nutritional needs, whereas TPN meets 90% of those needs. There are no large, well-controlled trials comparing enteral feeds to TPN in patients with severe acute pancreatitis. Only a small percentage of patients with acute pancreatitis need hyperalimentation.

Patients with severe gallstone-induced pancreatitis may improve dramatically if papillotomy is carried out within the first 36–72 h of the attack. Studies indicate that only those patients with gallstone pancreatitis who are in the very severe group should be considered for urgent ERCP. Finally, the treatment for patients with hypertriglyceridemia-associated pancreatitis includes (1) weight loss to ideal weight, (2) a lipid-restricted diet, (3) exercise, (4) avoidance of alcohol and of drugs that can elevate serum triglycerides (i.e., estrogens, vitamin A, thiazides, and propanolol), and (5) control of diabetes.

INFECTED PANCREATIC NECROSIS, ABSCESS, AND PSEUDOCYST

Infected pancreatic necrosis should be differentiated from pancreatic abscess. The former is a diffuse infection of an acutely inflamed, necrotic pancreas occurring most often in the first 2–4 weeks after the onset of pancreatitis. In contrast, a pancreatic abscess is an ill-defined, liquid collection of pus that evolves over a longer period, often 4–6 weeks. It tends to be less life-threatening and is associated with a lower rate of surgical mortality. Infected pancreatic necrosis should be treated by surgical debridement because the solid component of the infected pancreas is not amenable to effective radiologically guided percutaneous evacuation. Pancreatic abscess can be treated surgically or, in selected cases, by percutaneous drainage. The necrotic pancreas becomes secondarily infected in 20–35% of patients, most frequently with gram-negative bacteria of alimentary origin. Whether infection occurs depends on several factors, including the extent of pancreatic and peripancreatic necrosis, the degree of pancreatic ischemia and hypoperfusion, and the presence of organ or multiorgan failure.

The early diagnosis of pancreatic infection can be accomplished by CT-guided needle aspiration. In one study, 60 patients, representing 5% of all admissions for acute pancreatitis, were suspected of harboring a pancreatic infection on the basis of fever, leukocytosis, and an abnormal CT scan (pseudocyst or extrapancreatic fluid collection). Importantly, 60% of these patients had a pancreatic infection, and 55% of these infections developed in the first 3 weeks. These findings suggest that only guided aspiration can reliably distinguish sterile from infected pancreatic necrosis. The following are guidelines for patients meeting the above selection criteria: (1) Pseudocysts should be aspirated promptly in seriously ill patients because more than half may be infected, whereas asymptomatic pseudocysts need not be; (2) extrapancreatic fluid collections need not be aspirated promptly, because most are sterile; (3) if a necrotic pancreas is found initially to be sterile but fever and leukocytosis persist, 5–7 days of observation should be allowed to pass before reaspiration is considered, as clinical improvement frequently occurs; and (4) if fever and leukocytosis recur after an interval of well-being, reaspiration should be considered.

Severe pancreatitis with the presence of key risk factors, postoperative pancreatitis, early oral feeding, early laparotomy, and perhaps injudicious use of antibiotics predispose to the development of pancreatic abscess, which occurs in 3–4% of patients with acute pancreatitis. Pancreatic abscess may also develop because of a communication between a pseudocyst and the colon, inadequate surgical drainage of a pseudocyst, or needling of a pseudocyst. The characteristic signs of abscess are fever, leukocytosis, ileus, and rapid deterioration in a patient previously recovering from pancreatitis. Sometimes, however, the only manifestations are persistent fever and signs of continuing pancreatic inflammation. Drainage of pancreatic abscesses (now seen less frequently) by percutaneous techniques, using CT guidance, has been frequently successful with resolution in 50–60% of patients. Laparotomy with radical sump drainage and possibly resection of necrotic tissue are occasionally required.

Pseudocysts of the pancreas are collections of tissue, fluid, debris, pancreatic enzymes, and blood that develop over a period of 4–6 weeks after the onset of acute pancreatitis; they form in ~15% of patients with acute pancreatitis. In contrast to true cysts, pseudocysts do not have an epithelial lining; their walls consist of necrotic tissue, granulation tissue, and fibrous tissue. Many lesions that have the imaging appearance of a pseudocyst are actually organized necrosis. Disruption of the pancreatic ductal system is common. However, the subsequent course of this disruption varies widely, ranging from spontaneous healing to continuous leakage of pancreatic juice, which results in tense ascites. Pseudocysts are preceded by pancreatitis in 90% of cases and by trauma in 10%. Approximately 85% are located in the body or tail of the pancreas and 15% in the head. Some patients have two or more pseudocysts. Abdominal pain, with or without radiation to the back, is the usual presenting complaint. A palpable, tender mass may be found in the middle or left upper abdomen. The serum amylase level is elevated in 75% of patients at some point during their illness and may fluctuate markedly.

On x-ray examination, 75% of pseudocysts can be seen to displace some portion of the gastrointestinal tract (**Fig. 46-2**). Sonography, however, is reliable in detecting pseudocysts. Sonography also permits differentiation between an edematous, inflamed pancreas, which can give rise to a palpable mass, and an actual pseudocyst. Furthermore, serial ultrasound studies will indicate whether a pseudocyst has resolved. CT complements ultrasonography in the diagnosis of pancreatic pseudocyst (Fig. 46-2), especially when the pseudocyst is infected.

In earlier studies with sonography, pseudocysts were seen to resolve in 25–40% of patients. Pseudocysts that are >5 cm in diameter may persist for >6 weeks. Recent natural history studies have suggested that noninterventional, expectant management is the best course in selected patients with minimal symptoms and no evidence of active alcohol use in whom the pseudocyst appears mature by radiography and does not resemble a cystic neoplasm. A significant number of these pseudocysts resolve spontaneously >6 weeks after their formation. Also, these studies demonstrate that large pseudocyst size is not an absolute indication for interventional therapy and that many peripancreatic fluid collections detected on CT in cases of acute pancreatitis resolve spontaneously. A pseudocyst that does not resolve spontaneously may lead to serious complications, such as (1) pain caused by expansion of the lesion and pressure on other viscera, (2) rupture, (3) hemorrhage, and (4) abscess. Rupture of a pancreatic pseudocyst is a particularly serious complication. Shock almost always supervenes, and mortality rates range from 14% if the rupture is not associated with hemorrhage to >60% if hemorrhage has occurred. Rupture and hemorrhage are the prime causes of death from pancreatic pseudocyst. A triad of findings—an increase in the size of the mass, a localized bruit over the mass, and a sudden decrease in hemoglobin level and hematocrit without obvious external blood loss—should alert one to the possibility of hemorrhage from a pseudocyst. Thus, in patients who are stable and free of complications and in whom serial ultrasound studies show that the pseudocyst is shrinking, conservative therapy is indicated. Conversely, if the pseudocyst is expanding and is complicated by rupture, hemorrhage, or abscess, the patient should be operated on. With ultrasound or CT guidance, sterile chronic pseudocysts can be treated safely with single or repeated needle aspiration or more prolonged catheter drainage with a success rate of 45–75%. The success rate of these techniques for infected pseudocysts is considerably less (40–50%). Patients who do not respond to drainage require surgical therapy for internal or external drainage of the cyst.

Pseudoaneurysms develop in up to 10% of patients with acute pancreatitis at sites reflecting the distribution of pseudocysts and fluid collections (Fig. 46-2D). The splenic artery is most frequently involved, followed by the inferior and superior pancreatic duodenal arteries. This diagnosis should be suspected in patients with pancreatitis who develop upper gastrointestinal bleeding without an obvious cause or in whom thin-cut CT scanning reveals a contrast-enhanced lesion within or adjacent to a suspected pseudocyst. Arteriography is necessary to confirm the diagnosis and allow treatment.

PANCREATIC ASCITES AND PANCREATIC PLEURAL EFFUSIONS

Pancreatic ascites is usually due to disruption of the main pancreatic duct, often by an internal fistula between the duct and the peritoneal cavity or a leaking

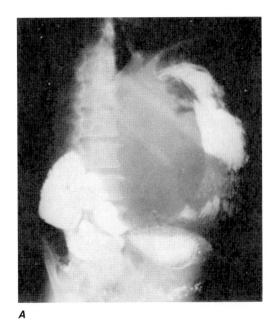

A

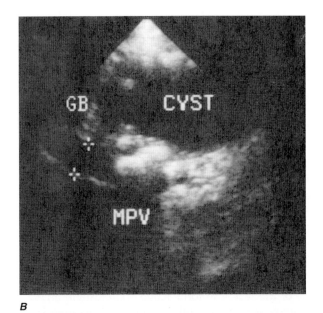

B

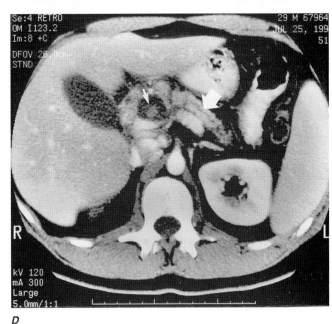

C

D

FIGURE 46-2

Pseudocyst of pancreas. A. Upper gastrointestinal x-ray showing displacement of stomach by pseudocyst. **B.** Sonogram showing pseudocyst (*cyst*). GB, gallbladder; MPV, portal vein. Behind the large pseudocyst is seen the calcified head of the pancreas. A dilated common bile duct (*asterisk*) is noted. **C.** CT scan showing pseudocyst. Note the large, lobulated fluid collection (*arrows*) surrounding the tail of the pancreas (*arrowheads*). Note also the dense, thin rim in the periphery representing the fibrous capsule of the pseudocyst. **D.** Spiral CT showing a pseudocyst (*small arrow*) with a pseudoaneurysm (light area in pseudocyst). Note the demonstration of the main pancreatic duct (*big arrow*), even though this duct is minimally dilated by ERCP. (*A, B, courtesy of Dr. CE Forsmark, University of Florida College of Medicine; C, D, courtesy of Dr. PR Ros, University of Florida College of Medicine; with permission.*)

pseudocyst (Chap. 10). This diagnosis is suggested in a patient with an elevated serum amylase level in whom the ascites fluid has both increased levels of albumin [>30 g/L (>3.0 g/dL)] and a markedly elevated level of amylase. The fluid in true pancreatic ascites usually has an amylase concentration of >20,000 U/L as a result of the ruptured duct or leaking pseudocyst. Lower amylase elevations may be found in the peritoneal fluid of patients with acute pancreatitis. In addition, ERCP often demonstrates passage of contrast material from a major pancreatic duct or a pseudocyst into the peritoneal cavity. As many as 15% of patients with pseudocysts have concurrent pancreatic ascites. The differential diagnosis should include intraperitoneal carcinomatosis, tuberculous peritonitis, constrictive pericarditis, and Budd-Chiari syndrome.

CHAPTER 46 Acute and Chronic Pancreatitis

Treatment:
R_X PANCREATIC ASCITES AND PANCREATIC PLEURAL EFFUSIONS

If the pancreatic duct disruption is posterior, an internal fistula may develop between the pancreatic duct and the pleural space, producing a pleural effusion, which is usually left-sided and often massive. This complication is best treated by ERCP and stent placement and infrequently requires thoracentesis or chest tube drainage. If the pancreatic duct disruption is anterior, amylase- and lipase-rich peritoneal fluid accumulate. ERCP and stenting are the preferred initial approach.

Treatment may require nasogastric suction and parenteral alimentation to decrease pancreatic secretion. In addition, paracentesis may be necessary to keep the peritoneal cavity free of fluid and, it is hoped, to effect sealing of the leak. The long-acting somatostatin analogue octreotide, which inhibits pancreatic secretion, is useful in cases of pancreatic ascites and pleural effusion. If ascites continues to recur after 2–3 weeks of medical management, the patient should be operated on after pancreatography to define the anatomy of the abnormal duct. Patients in whom ERCP identifies two or more sites of extravasation are unlikely to respond to conservative management and/or stenting.

CHRONIC PANCREATITIS AND PANCREATIC EXOCRINE INSUFFICIENCY

PATHOPHYSIOLOGY

Chronic pancreatitis is a disease process characterized by irreversible damage to the pancreas as distinct from the reversible changes noted in acute pancreatitis. The condition is best defined by the presence of histologic abnormalities, including chronic inflammation, fibrosis, and progressive destruction of both exocrine and eventually endocrine tissue. A number of etiologies may result in chronic pancreatitis, but all may ultimately lead to irreversible morphologic damage to the pancreas, and these etiologies may produce the cardinal complications of chronic pancreatitis such as abdominal pain, steatorrhea, and diabetes mellitus.

The events that initiate the inflammatory process in the pancreas are still not well understood. Current experimental and clinical observations have shown that alcohol has a direct toxic effect on the pancreas. While patients with alcohol-induced pancreatitis generally consume large amounts of alcohol, some consume very little, as little as ≤50 g/d. Prolonged consumption of socially acceptable amounts of alcohol is compatible with the development of chronic pancreatitis. Findings of extensive pancreatic fibrosis in patients who died during their first attack of clinical acute alcohol-induced pancreatitis support the concept that such patients already have chronic pancreatitis.

The biochemical and molecular mechanisms that may be important to the pathogenesis of chronic pancreatitis continue to be explored. Overexpression of fibroblasts and growth factors in tissue in patients with chronic pancreatitis has been reported. High levels of transforming growth factor α and its receptor protein epidermal growth factor have been documented in patients with chronic pancreatitis. It is yet to be determined whether these observations are truly relevant in the pathogenesis of chronic pancreatitis.

ETIOLOGIC CONSIDERATIONS

Among adults in the United States, alcoholism is the most common cause of clinically apparent chronic pancreatitis, while cystic fibrosis is the most frequent cause in children. In up to 25% of adults in the United States with chronic pancreatitis, the cause is not known. That is, they are labeled as *idiopathic chronic pancreatitis*. Recent investigations have indicated that up to 15% of patients with idiopathic pancreatitis may have pancreatitis due to genetic defects (**Table 46-4**).

Whitcomb and associates studied several large families with hereditary chronic pancreatitis and were able to identify a genetic defect that affects the gene encoding for trypsinogen. Several additional defects of this gene have also been described. The defect allows trypsinogen to be resistant to the effect of trypsin inhibitor, become spontaneously activated, and to remain activated. It is hypothesized that this continual activation of digestive enzymes within the gland leads to acute injury and, finally, chronic pancreatitis. This group of investigators has also reported that a second form of hereditary chronic pancreatitis tends to present later, has a female predominance, and frequently leads to chronic pancreatitis.

Several other groups of investigators have documented mutations of *CFTR*. This gene functions as a cyclic AMP-regulated chloride channel. In patients with cystic fibrosis, the high concentration of macromolecules can block the pancreatic ducts. It must be appreciated, however, that there is a great deal of heterogeneity in relationship to the *CFTR* gene defect. More than 1000 putative mutations of the *CFTR* gene have been identified. Attempts to elucidate the relationship between the genotype and pancreatic manifestations have been hampered by the number of mutations. The ability to detect *CFTR* mutations has led to the recognition that the clinical spectrum of the disease is broader than previously thought. Two recent studies have clarified the association between mutations of the *CFTR* gene and another monosymptomatic form of cystic fibrosis, i.e., chronic pancreatitis. It is estimated that in patients with idiopathic pancreatitis, the frequency of a single *CFTR* mutation is 11 times the expected

TABLE 46-4

CHRONIC PANCREATITIS AND PANCREATIC EXOCRINE INSUFFICIENCY: TIGAR-O CLASSIFICATION SYSTEM

Toxic-metabolic
  Alcoholic
  Tobacco smoking
  Hypercalcemia
  Hyperlipidemia
  Chronic renal failure
  Medications—phenacetin abuse
  Toxins—organotin compounds
    (e.g., DBTC)

Idiopathic
  Early onset
  Late onset
  Tropical

Genetic
  Hereditary pancreatitis
  Cationic trypsinogen
  CFTR mutations
  SPINK1 mutations

Autoimmune
  Isolated autoimmune CP
  Autoimmune CP associated with
    Sjögren's syndrome
    Inflammatory bowel disease
    Primary biliary cirrhosis

Recurrent and severe acute pancreatitis
  Postnecrotic (severe acute pancreatitis)
  Recurrent acute pancreatitis
  Vascular diseases/ischemia
  Postirradiation

Obstructive
  Pancreas divisum
  Sphincter of Oddi disorders
    (controversial)
  Duct obstruction (e.g., tumor)
  Preampullary duodenal wall cysts
  Posttraumatic pancreatic duct scars

CP, chronic pancreatitis; TIGAR-O, toxic-metabolic, idiopathic, genetic, autoimmune, recurrent and severe acute pancreatitis, obstructive.

frequency and the frequency of two mutant alleles is 80 times the expected frequency. In these studies, the patients were adults when the diagnosis of pancreatitis was made; none had any clinical evidence of pulmonary disease, and sweat test results were not diagnostic of cystic fibrosis. The prevalence of such mutations is unclear, and further studies are certainly needed. In addition, the therapeutic and prognostic implication of these findings with respect to managing pancreatitis remains to be determined. Long-term follow-up of affected patients is needed. *CFTR* mutations are common in the general population. It is unclear whether the *CFTR* mutation alone can lead to pancreatitis as an autosomal recessive disease. A recent study evaluated 39 patients with idiopathic chronic pancreatitis to assess the risk associated with these mutations. Patients with two *CFTR* mutations (compound heterozygotes) demonstrated *CFTR* function at a level between that seen in typical cystic fibrosis and cystic fibrosis carriers and had a 40-fold increased risk of pancreatitis. The presence of an *N34S SPINK1* mutation increased the risk 20-fold. A combination of two *CFTR* mutations and an *N34S SPINK1* mutation increased the risk of pancreatitis 900-fold. Table 46-4 lists recognized causes of chronic pancreatitis and pancreatic exocrine insufficiency.

AUTOIMMUNE PANCREATITIS

Autoimmune pancreatitis (AIP) is an increasingly recognized disorder of presumed autoimmune etiology that is associated with characteristic clinical, histologic, and morphologic findings (Table 46-5). It has been referred to by a variety of names including *sclerosing pancreatitis*, *tumefactive pancreatitis*, and *nonalcoholic destructive pancreatitis* depending, in part, upon the specific pathologic findings and the presence of extrapancreatic manifestations. However, it is generally believed that the pathologic heterogeneity may reflect different stages or manifestations of the same disease.

Clinical Features of Chronic Pancreatitis

Patients with chronic pancreatitis seek medical attention predominantly because of two symptoms: abdominal pain or maldigestion. The abdominal pain may be quite variable in location, severity, and frequency. The pain can be constant or intermittent with frequent pain-free intervals. Eating may exacerbate the pain, leading to a fear of eating with consequent weight loss. The spectrum of abdominal pain ranges from mild to quite severe with narcotic dependence as a frequent consequence. Maldigestion is manifested as chronic diarrhea, steatorrhea, weight loss, and fatigue. Patients with abdominal pain may or may not progress to maldigestion, and ~20% of patients will present with symptoms of maldigestion without a history of abdominal pain. Patients with chronic pancreatitis have significant morbidity and mortality and utilize appreciable amounts of societal resources. Despite the steatorrhea, clinically apparent deficiencies of fat-soluble vitamins are surprisingly uncommon. Physical findings in these patients are usually unimpressive

TABLE 46-5

CLINICAL FEATURES OF AUTOIMMUNE PANCREATITIS (AIP)

- Mild symptoms usually abdominal pain, but without frequent attacks of pancreatitis, which are unusual
- Presentation with obstructive jaundice
- Diffuse swelling and enlargement of the pancreas, especially the head, the latter mimicking carcinoma of the pancreas
- Diffuse irregular narrowing of the pancreatic duct in ERCP
- Increased levels of serum gamma globulins especially IgG$_4$
- Presence of other auto-antibodies (ANA), rheumatoid factor (RF)
- Can occur with other autoimmune diseases Sjögren's syndrome, PSC, UC, rheumatoid arthritis
- Extra pancreatic bile duct changes such as stricture of the common bile duct and intrahepatic ducts
- Absence of pancreatic calcifications or cysts
- Pancreatic biopsies reveal extensive fibrosis and lymphoplasmacytic infiltration
- Glucocorticoids are effective in alleviating symptoms, decreasing size of the pancreas, and reversing histopathologic changes
- $^2/_3$ of patients present with either obstructive jaundice or a "mass" in the head of the pancreas mimicking carcinoma

so that there is a disparity between the severity of abdominal pain and the physical signs, which usually consist of some mild tenderness and mild temperature elevation.

It is helpful to differentiate chronic pancreatitis into its different forms. One obvious demarcation is whether the patient has small-duct or large-duct disease. Table 46-6 describes features that distinguish between these two kinds of pancreatitis. The pathogenesis, diagnostic approach, clinical course, and treatment results vary greatly between these two forms of chronic pancreatitis. In contrast to

acute pancreatitis, the serum amylase and lipase levels are usually not elevated in chronic pancreatitis. Elevation of serum bilirubin and alkaline phosphatase may indicate cholestasis secondary to chronic inflammation and/or stricture around the common bile duct. Many patients have impaired glucose tolerance with elevated fasting blood glucose levels. The diagnostic test with the best sensitivity and specificity is the hormone stimulation test utilizing secretin. It becomes abnormal when ≥60% of the pancreatic exocrine function has been lost. This usually correlates well with the onset of chronic abdominal pain. Approximately 40% of patients with chronic pancreatitis have cobalamin (vitamin B$_{12}$) malabsorption. This can be corrected by the administration of oral pancreatic enzymes. The serum trypsinogen and D-xylose excretion tests are useful in patients with pancreatic steatorrhea. The trypsinogen level will be abnormal and the D-xylose excretion usually normal in such patients. A decrease of serum trypsinogen level to <20 mg/mL strongly suggests severe pancreatic exocrine insufficiency, as does a fecal elastase of <100 μg per gram of stool.

Utilizing radiographic techniques (Figs. 46-3 and 46-4), it can be shown that diffuse calcifications noted on plain film of the abdomen usually indicate ~80% damage to the pancreas. While alcohol is by far the most common cause of pancreatic calcification, such calcification may also be noted in severe protein-calorie malnutrition, hereditary pancreatitis, posttraumatic pancreatitis, hypercalcemic pancreatitis, islet cell tumors, and idiopathic chronic pancreatitis. Abdominal ultrasonography, CT scanning, and ERCP greatly aid in the diagnosis of pancreatic disease (Fig. 46-3). In addition to excluding a pseudocyst and pancreatic cancer, sonography and CT may show calcification, dilated ducts, or an atrophic pancreas. ERCP or magnetic resonance cholangiopancreatography (MRCP) provides a direct view of the pancreatic duct and may show a pseudocyst missed by

TABLE 46-6

LARGE DUCT VERSUS SMALL DUCT CHRONIC PANCREATITIS

	LARGE DUCT	SMALL DUCT
Sex Predominance	Male	Female
Diagnostic Tests		
Secretin test	Abnormal	Abnormal
Serum trypsinogen	Often abnormal	Usually normal
Fecal elastase	Often abnormal	Usually normal
Pancreatic calcification on plain film of the abdomen	Frequent	Infrequent
ERCP	Often markedly abnormal	Minimally abnormal to normal
Natural History		
Progression to steatorrhea	Frequent	Rare
Therapy of pain		
Pancreatic enzymes	Poor response	Good to excellent response
Surgical procedures	Sometimes helpful	Not usually indicated

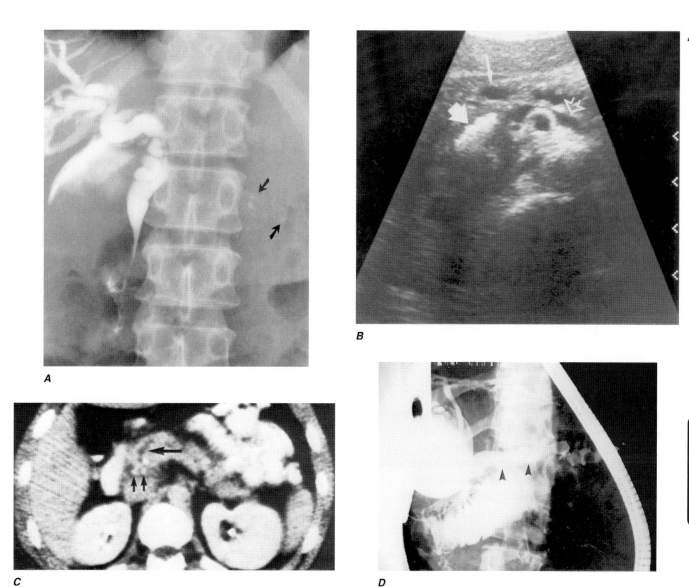

FIGURE 46-3

Radiologic abnormalities in chronic pancreatitis. *A.* Pancreatic calcification (*arrows*) and stenosis (tapering) of the intrahepatic portion of the common bile duct demonstrated by percutaneous transhepatic cholangiography. ***B.*** Pancreatic calcification (*large white arrow*) demonstrated by sonography. Note dilated pancreatic duct (*thin white arrow*) and splenic vein (*open arrow*). ***C.*** Pancreatic calcification (*vertical arrows*) and dilated pancreatic duct (*horizontal arrow*) demonstrated by CT scan. ***D.*** Endoscopic retrograde cholangiogram shows grossly dilated pancreatic ducts (*arrows*) in a patient with long-standing pancreatitis.

sonography or CT. The role of endoscopic ultrasonography (EUS) in diagnosing early chronic pancreatitis is still being defined. EUS complements pancreatic function tests, and a combination of a hormone-stimulation function test and EUS is the most complete way to evaluate the presence or extent of chronic pancreatitis (Chap. 45). Whether EUS can detect early chronic pancreatitis, i.e., small-duct disease, with the same degree of accuracy as the hormone-stimulation test is controversial. Recent data comparing these modalities head-to-head would indicate that EUS is not a sensitive test for detecting early chronic pancreatitis (Chap. 45) and may lead to

false-positive tests in patients who have dyspepsia or even in normal controls.

Complications of Chronic Pancreatitis

The complications of chronic pancreatitis are protean and are listed in Table 46-7. Although most patients have impaired glucose tolerance, diabetic ketoacidosis and coma are uncommon. Likewise, end-organ damage (retinopathy, neuropathy, nephropathy) is also uncommon. A nondiabetic retinopathy may be due to either vitamin A and/or zinc deficiency. Gastrointestinal bleeding may

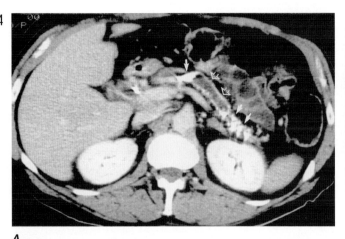
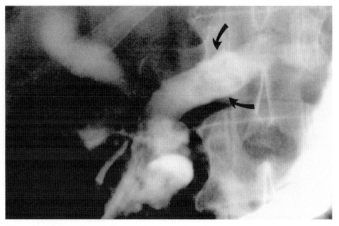

A   *B*

FIGURE 46-4

Chronic pancreatitis and pancreatic calculi: CT scan and ERCP appearance. **A.** In this contrast-enhanced CT scan of the abdomen, there is evidence of an atrophic pancreas with multiple calcifications (*arrows*). Note the markedly dilated pancreatic duct seen in this section through the body and tail (*open arrows*). **B.** ERCP in the same patient demonstrates the dilated pancreatic duct as well as an intrapancreatic duct calculus (*arrows*). These findings correlate nicely with the CT scan appearance.

occur from peptic ulceration, gastritis, a pseudocyst eroding into the duodenum, or ruptured varices secondary to splenic vein thrombosis due to inflammation of the tail of the pancreas. Jaundice, cholestasis, and biliary cirrhosis may occur from the chronic inflammatory reaction around the intrapancreatic portion of the common bile duct. Twenty years after the diagnosis of chronic pancreatitis, the cumulative risk of pancreatic carcinoma is 4%. Patients with hereditary pancreatitis are at a tenfold higher risk for pancreatic cancer.

℞ Treatment:
CHRONIC PANCREATITIS

The treatment of steatorrhea with pancreatic enzymes is straightforward even though complete correction of steatorrhea is unusual. Enzyme therapy usually brings diarrhea under control and restores absorption of fat to an acceptable level. Thus, pancreatic enzymes, largely from porcine sources, have been the cornerstone of pancreatic therapy. In treating steatorrhea, it is important to use a potent pancreatic formulation that will

TABLE 46-7

COMPLICATIONS OF CHRONIC PANCREATITIS	
Narcotic addiction	Gastrointestinal bleeding
Impaired glucose tolerance	Jaundice
Gastroparesis	Cholangitis and/or biliary
Cobalamin malabsorption	cirrhosis
Nondiabetic retinopathy	Subcutaneous fat necrosis
Effusions with high	Bone pain
amylase content	Pancreatic cancer

deliver sufficient lipase into the duodenum to correct maldigestion and decrease steatorrhea (Table 46-8).

The management of pain in patients with chronic pancreatitis is problematic. In patients with large-duct disease usually from alcohol-induced chronic pancreatitis, ductal decompression has been the therapy of choice. Among such patients, 80% seem to obtain immediate relief; however, at the end of 3 years, half the patients have recurrence of pain. Preliminary data suggest that large doses of octreotide may decrease the pain in patients with large-duct disease.

Octreotide was initially selected and evaluated for the treatment of abdominal pain associated with large-duct chronic pancreatitis. It is a somatostatin analogue that inhibits pancreatic secretion and lowers blood CCK levels. A multicenter, double-blinded, placebo-controlled, dose-ranging study showed that 200 µg of octreotide given SC three times daily was superior to placebo and decreased the abdominal pain of patients. Octreotide significantly relieves pain in some patients with severe chronic pancreatitis refractory to other forms of therapy, including surgery.

In patients with small-duct disease, conventional nonenteric coated enzyme preparations containing high concentrations of serine proteases relieve pain. The patients who respond best to these proteases are those with an abnormal hormone stimulation test or minimal changes on ERCP and normal fat absorption. It appears that these serum proteases relieve pain by catabolizing a CCK-releasing peptide that ultimately leads to a lower CCK level in the blood and, thus, less stimulation to the pancreas. This feedback inhibition mechanism appears to be operative in the upper small intestine. Nonenteric

TABLE 46-8

FREQUENTLY UTILIZED PANCREATIC ENZYME PREPARATIONS

	PROTEASE[a] (×1000)	LIPASE[a] (×1000)
Nonenteric Coated		
Viokase 8 (Axcan Scandipharm, Birmingham, AL)	30	8
Viokase 16 (Axcan Scandipharm)	60	16
Kuzyme HP (Schwartz, Milwaukee, WI)	30	8
Cotazym (Organon, East Orange, NJ)	30	8
Enteric Coated		
Creon 5 (Solvay, Marietta, GA)	18.75	5
Creon 10 (Solvay)	37.5	10
Creon 20 (Solvay)	75	20
Pancrease MT4 (McNeil Pharmaceuticals, Ft. Washington, PA)	12	4
Pancrease MT10 (McNeil Pharmaceuticals)	30	10
Pancrease MT16 (McNeil Pharmaceuticals)	48	16
Ultrase 12 (Scandipharm, Birmingham, AL)	39	12
Ultrase 18 (Scandipharm)	58.5	18
Ultrase 20 (Scandipharm)	65	20
Cotazym-S (Organon)	20	5

[a]United States Pharmacopea units per tablet or capsule.
Manufacturers and their locations follow names of drugs.
For pain 4 to 8 nonenteric coated tablets four times daily.
For maldigestion 1–2 enteric coated capsules with each meal.

coated enzymes are preferable because when given with a proton pump inhibitor, those enzymes that escape acid destruction within the stomach are delivered directly into the duodenum, where the feedback principle is operative. Enteric-coated enzymes, although appropriate for treating steatorrhea, are not the enzymes of choice for treating abdominal pain because the enteric-coated compounds have been demonstrated to open their enteric coat when they pass beyond the duodenum and into the mid small intestine. This feedback principle is not operative in that part of the intestine. The ideal pancreatic enzyme preparation will be one that has enteric-coated lipase and free proteases. The free proteases would enter into the duodenum and evoke a positive feedback control mechanism, and the enteric-coated lipase would open beyond the duodenum and enhance fat absorption. Table 46-8 lists the frequently utilized pancreatic enzyme preparations in the United States.

Gastroparesis is also quite common in patients with chronic pancreatitis, particularly those who have small-duct painful chronic pancreatitis. It is important to recognize this because treatment with enzymes may fail simply because gastroparesis is preventing the appropriate delivery of enzymes into the upper intestine where the enzymes can then act via a feedback inhibition process. In patients with small-duct disease and painful chronic pancreatitis, it is important to evaluate gastric emptying and if gastric emptying is impaired, to effect proper emptying with prokinetic agents. In this setting enzyme therapy is more apt to be successful.

Endoscopic treatment of chronic pancreatitis pain may involve sphincterotomy, stenting, stone extraction, and drainage of a pancreatic pseudocyst. Therapy directed to the pancreatic duct would seem to be most appropriate in the setting of a dominant stricture, if a ductal stone has led to obstruction. The use of endoscopic stenting for patients with chronic pain, but without a dominant stricture, has not been proven in any controlled trials. It is now appreciated that significant complications can occur from stenting, i.e., bleeding, cholangitis, stent migration, and stent clogging. All of these may lead to pancreatitis. Importantly, damage to the pancreatic duct and the pancreatic parenchyma can occur following stenting.

Total pancreatectomy and autologous islet cell transplantation have been used in selected patients with chronic pancreatitis and abdominal pain refractory to conventional therapy. The patients who have benefited the most to date have chronic pancreatitis without prior pancreatic surgery or evidence of islet cell insufficiency. The role of this procedure remains to be fully defined but may be an option in lieu of ductal decompression surgery or pancreatic resection in patients with intractable, painful small-duct disease, particularly as the standard surgical procedures tend to decrease islet cell yield.

CHAPTER 46 Acute and Chronic Pancreatitis

HEREDITARY PANCREATITIS

Hereditary pancreatitis is a rare disease that is similar to chronic pancreatitis except for an early age of onset and evidence of hereditary factors (involving an autosomal dominant gene with incomplete penetrance). A genome-wide search using genetic linkage analysis identified the hereditary pancreatitis gene on chromosome 7. Mutations in ion codons 29 (exon 2) and 122 (exon 3) of the cationic trypsinogen gene cause autosomal dominant forms of hereditary pancreatitis. The codon 122 mutations lead to a substitution of the corresponding arginine with another amino acid, usually histidine. This substitution, when it occurs, eliminates a fail-safe trypsin self-destruction site necessary to eliminate trypsin that is prematurely activated within the acinar cell. These patients have recurring attacks of severe abdominal pain that may last from a few days to a few weeks. The serum amylase and lipase levels may be elevated during acute attacks but are usually normal. Patients frequently develop pancreatic calcification, diabetes mellitus, and steatorrhea; in addition, they have an increased incidence of pancreatic carcinoma, with the cumulative incidence being as high as 40% by age 70. Such patients often require ductal decompression for pain relief. Abdominal complaints in relatives of patients with hereditary pancreatitis should raise the question of pancreatic disease.

Pancreatic Secretory Trypsin Inhibitor (PSTI) Gene Mutations

PSTI, or SPINK1, is a 56-amino-acid peptide that specifically inhibits trypsin by physically blocking its active site. SPINK1 acts as the first line of defense against prematurely activated trypsinogen in the acinar cell. Recently, it has been shown that the frequency of SPINK1 mutations in patients with idiopathic chronic pancreatitis is markedly increased, suggesting that these mutations may be associated with pancreatitis.

PANCREATIC ENDOCRINE TUMORS

Pancreatic endocrine tumors are discussed in Chap. 50.

OTHER CONDITIONS

ANNULAR PANCREAS

When the ventral pancreatic anlage fails to migrate correctly to make contact with the dorsal anlage, the result may be a ring of pancreatic tissue encircling the duodenum. Such an annular pancreas may cause intestinal obstruction in the neonate or the adult. Symptoms of postprandial fullness, epigastric pain, nausea, and vomiting may be present for years before the diagnosis is entertained. The radiographic findings are symmetric dilation of the proximal duodenum with bulging of the recesses on either side of the annular band, effacement but not destruction of the duodenal mucosa, accentuation of the findings in the right anterior oblique position, and lack of change on repeated examinations. The differential diagnosis should include duodenal webs, tumors of the pancreas or duodenum, postbulbar peptic ulcer, regional enteritis, and adhesions. Patients with annular pancreas have an increased incidence of pancreatitis and peptic ulcer. Because of these and other potential complications, the treatment is surgical even if the condition has been present for years. Retrocolic duodenojejunostomy is the procedure of choice, although some surgeons advocate Billroth II gastrectomy, gastroenterostomy, and vagotomy.

PANCREAS DIVISUM

Pancreas divisum occurs when the embryologic ventral and dorsal pancreatic anlagen fail to fuse, so that pancreatic drainage is accomplished mainly through the accessory papilla. Pancreas divisum is the most common congenital anatomic variant of the human pancreas. Current evidence indicates that this anomaly does not predispose to the development of pancreatitis in the great majority of patients who harbor it. However, the combination of pancreas divisum and a small accessory orifice could result in dorsal duct obstruction. The challenge is to identify this subset of patients with dorsal duct pathology. Cannulation of the dorsal duct by ERCP is not as easily done as is cannulation of the ventral duct. Patients with pancreatitis and pancreas divisum demonstrated by ERCP should be treated with conservative measures. In many of these patients, pancreatitis is idiopathic and unrelated to the pancreas divisum. Endoscopic or surgical intervention is indicated only when the above methods fail. If marked dilation of the dorsal duct can be demonstrated, surgical ductal decompression should be performed. The appropriate therapy for patients without dilation of the dorsal duct is not yet defined. It should be stressed that the ERCP appearance of pancreas divisum-i.e., a small-caliber ventral duct with an arborizing pattern-may be mistaken as representing an obstructed main pancreatic duct secondary to a mass lesion.

MACROAMYLASEMIA

In macroamylasemia, amylase circulates in the blood in a polymer form too large to be easily excreted by the kidney. Patients with this condition demonstrate an elevated serum amylase value, a low urinary amylase value, and a C_{am}/C_{cr} ratio of <1%. The presence of macroamylase can be documented by chromatography of the serum. The prevalence of macroamylasemia is 1.5% of the nonalcoholic general adult hospital population. Usually macroamylasemia is an incidental finding and is not related to disease of the pancreas or other organs.

Macrolipasemia has now been documented in a few patients with cirrhosis or non-Hodgkin's lymphoma. In these patients, the pancreas appeared normal on ultrasound and CT examination. Lipase was shown to be complexed with immunoglobulin A. Thus, the possibility of *both* macroamylasemia and macrolipasemia should be considered in patients with elevated blood levels of these enzymes.

ACKNOWLEDGMENT

This chapter represents a revised version of the chapter by Dr. Norton J. Greenberger, Dr. Phillip P. Toskes, and Dr. Kurt J. Isselbacher that was in the previous editions of Harrison's Principles of Internal Medicine.

FURTHER READINGS

CAPPELL MS: Acute pancreatitis: etiology, clinical presentation, diagnosis, and therapy. Med Clin North Am 92:889, 2008

CHOWDHURY R et al: Prevalence of gastroparesis in patients with small duct chronic pancreatitis. Pancreas 26:235, 2003

—— et al: Comparative analysis of direct pancreatic function testing versus morphological assessment by endoscopic ultrasonography for the evaluation of chronic unexplained abdominal pain of presumed pancreatic origin. Pancreas 31:63, 2005

COCHRANE DATABASE: System Review 2004; (2) CD 002941

CONWELL DL, BANKS PA: Chronic pancreatitis. Curr Opin Gastroenterol 24:586, 2008

DRAGANOV P et al: Is a 15 minute collection of duodenal secretions after secretin stimulation sufficient to diagnose chronic pancreatitis? Pancreas 28:89, 2004

DURIE PR: Pancreatic aspects of cystic fibrosis and other inherited causes of pancreatic dysfunction. Med Clin North Am 84:609, 2000

ENTEMAD B, WHITCOMB DC: Chronic pancreatitis: Diagnosis, classification, and new genetic developments. Gastroenterology 120:682, 2001

FREEMAN ML et al: Risk factors for post-ERCP pancreatitis: A prospective, multicenter study. Gastrointest Endosc 54:425, 2001

FROSSARD JL et al: Acute pancreatitis. Lancet 371:143, 2008

GELTECK CJ: Severe hypertriglyceridemia and pancreatitis when estrogen replacement therapy is given to hypertriglyceridemic women. J Lab Clin Med 123:59, 1994

GRESS F et al: Endoscopic ultrasound-guided celiac plexus block for managing abdominal pain associated with chronic pancreatitis: A prospective single center experience. Am J Gastroenterol 96:409, 2001

GUPTA V, TOSKES PP: Diagnosis and management of chronic pancreatitis. Postgrad Med J 81:491, 2005

ISENMAN R et al: Prophylactic antibiotic treatment in patients with predicted severe acute pancreatitis: A placebo controlled, double-blinded trial. Gastroenterology 126:997, 2004

JAFRI NS et al: Antibiotic prophylaxis is not protective in severe acute pancreatitis: a systematic review and meta-analysis. Am J Surg 197:806, 2009

LOWENFELS AB et al: Prognosis of chronic pancreatitis: An international multicenter study. Am J Gastroenterol 89:1467, 1994

—— et al: The changing character of acute pancreatitis: epidemiology, etiology, and prognosis. Curr Gastroenterol Rep 11:97, 2009

NOONE PG et al: Cystic fibrosis gene mutations and pancreatitis risk: Relation to epithelial ion transport and trypsin gene mutations. Gastroenterology 121:1310, 2001

PAPACHRISTOU GI, WHITCOMB DC: Predictors of severity and necrosis in acute pancreatitis. Clin Gastroenterol North Am 33:871, 2004

—— et al: Is the monocyte-chemotactic protein J-2518G allele a factor for severe acute pancreatitis. Clin Gastroenterol Hepatol 3:425, 2005

PEARSON RK et al: Autoimmune pancreatitis: Does it exist? Pancreas 27:1, 2003

SOMOGYI L et al: Recurrent acute pancreatitis: An algorithmic approach to identification and elimination of inciting factors. Gastroenterology 120:708, 2001

STEER M: Pancreatitis severity: Who calls the shots? Gastroenterology 122:1168, 2002

SUTTON R: Autoimmune pancreatitis—also a Western disease. Gut 54:581, 2005

THOMSON A: Enteral versus parenteral nutritional support in acute pancreatitis: A clinical review. J Gastroenterol Hepatol 21:22, 2006

WARSHAW AL et al: AGA technical review: Treatment of pain in chronic pancreatitis. Gastroenterology 115:765, 1998

YADAY Y et al: A critical evaluation of laboratory tests in acute pancreatitis. Am J Gastroenterol 97:1309, 2002

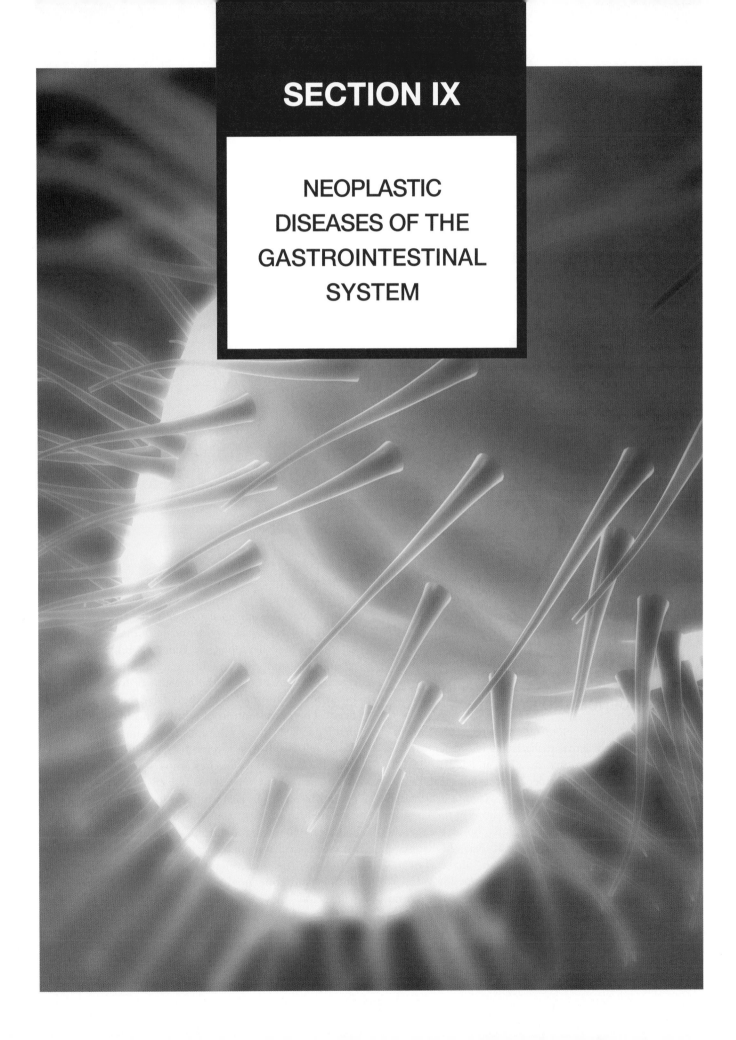

SECTION IX

NEOPLASTIC DISEASES OF THE GASTROINTESTINAL SYSTEM

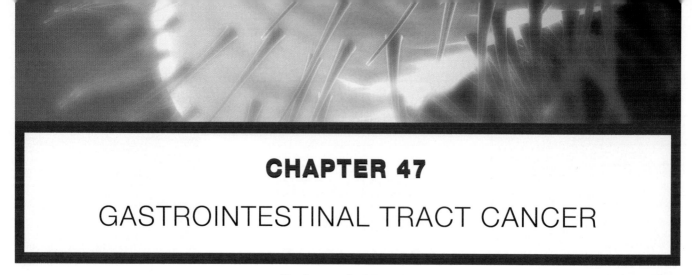

CHAPTER 47

GASTROINTESTINAL TRACT CANCER

Robert J. Mayer

The gastrointestinal tract is the second most common noncutaneous site for cancer and the second major cause of cancer-related mortality in the United States.

ESOPHAGEAL CANCER

INCIDENCE AND ETIOLOGY

Cancer of the esophagus is a relatively uncommon but extremely lethal malignancy. The diagnosis was made in 15,560 Americans in 2007 and led to 13,940 deaths. Worldwide, the incidence of esophageal cancer varies strikingly. It occurs frequently within a geographic region extending from the southern shore of the Caspian Sea on the west to northern China on the east and encompassing parts of Iran, Central Asia, Afghanistan, Siberia, and Mongolia. High-incidence "pockets" of the disease are also present in such disparate locations as Finland, Iceland, Curaçao, southeastern Africa, and northwestern France. In North America and western Europe, the disease is more common in blacks than whites and in males than females; it appears most often after age 50 and seems to be associated with a lower socioeconomic status.

A variety of causative factors have been implicated in the development of the disease (Table 47-1). In the United States, esophageal cancer cases are either squamous cell carcinomas or adenocarcinomas. The etiology of squamous cell esophageal cancer is related to excess alcohol consumption and/or cigarette smoking. The relative risk increases with the amount of tobacco smoked or alcohol consumed, with these factors acting synergistically. The consumption of whiskey is linked to a higher incidence than the consumption of wine or beer. Squamous cell esophageal carcinoma has also been associated with the ingestion of nitrites, smoked opiates, and fungal toxins in pickled vegetables, as well as mucosal damage caused by such physical insults as long-term exposure to extremely hot tea, the ingestion of lye, radiation-induced strictures, and chronic achalasia. The presence of an esophageal web in association with glossitis and iron deficiency (i.e., Plummer-Vinson or Paterson-Kelly syndrome) and congenital hyperkeratosis and pitting of the palms and soles (i.e., tylosis palmaris et plantaris) have each been linked with squamous cell esophageal cancer, as have dietary deficiencies of molybdenum, zinc, and vitamin A.

For unclear reasons, the incidence of squamous cell esophageal cancer has decreased somewhat in both the

TABLE 47-1

SOME ETIOLOGIC FACTORS BELIEVED TO BE ASSOCIATED WITH ESOPHAGEAL CANCER

Excess alcohol consumption
Cigarette smoking
Other ingested carcinogens
   Nitrates (converted to nitrites)
   Smoked opiates
   Fungal toxins in pickled vegetables
Mucosal damage from physical agents
   Hot tea
   Lye ingestion
   Radiation-induced strictures
   Chronic achalasia
Host susceptibility
   Esophageal web with glossitis and iron deficiency
      (i.e., Plummer-Vinson or Paterson-Kelly syndrome)
   Congenital hyperkeratosis and pitting of the palms and
      soles (i.e., tylosis palmaris et plantaris)
? Dietary deficiencies molybdenum, zinc, vitamin A
? Celiac sprue
Chronic gastric reflux (i.e., Barrett's esophagus) for
  adenocarcinoma

black and white population in the United States over the past 30 years, while the rate of adenocarcinoma has risen dramatically, particularly in white males. Adenocarcinomas arise in the distal esophagus in the presence of chronic gastric reflux and gastric metaplasia of the epithelium (Barrett's esophagus), which is more common in obese persons. Adenocarcinomas arise within dysplastic columnar epithelium in the distal esophagus. Even before frank neoplasia is detectable, aneuploidy and p53 mutations are found in the dysplastic epithelium. These adenocarcinomas behave clinically like gastric adenocarcinoma and now account for >60% of esophageal cancers.

CLINICAL FEATURES

About 10% of esophageal cancers occur in the upper third of the esophagus (cervical esophagus), 35% in the middle third, and 55% in the lower third. Squamous cell carcinomas and adenocarcinomas cannot be distinguished radiographically or endoscopically.

Progressive dysphagia and weight loss of short duration are the initial symptoms in the vast majority of patients. Dysphagia initially occurs with solid foods and gradually progresses to include semisolids and liquids. By the time these symptoms develop, the disease is usually incurable, since difficulty in swallowing does not occur until >60% of the esophageal circumference is infiltrated with cancer. Dysphagia may be associated with pain on swallowing (odynophagia), pain radiating to the chest and/or back, regurgitation or vomiting, and

aspiration pneumonia. The disease most commonly spreads to adjacent and supraclavicular lymph nodes, liver, lungs, pleura, and bone. Tracheoesophageal fistulas may develop as the disease advances, leading to severe suffering. As with other squamous cell carcinomas, hypercalcemia may occur in the absence of osseous metastases, probably from parathormone-related peptide secreted by tumor cells.

DIAGNOSIS

Attempts at endoscopic and cytologic screening for carcinoma in patients with Barrett's esophagus, while effective as a means of detecting high-grade dysplasia, have not yet been shown to improve the prognosis in individuals found to have a carcinoma. Routine contrast radiographs effectively identify esophageal lesions large enough to cause symptoms. In contrast to benign esophageal leiomyomas, which result in esophageal narrowing with preservation of a normal mucosal pattern, esophageal carcinomas show ragged, ulcerating changes in the mucosa in association with deeper infiltration, producing a picture resembling achalasia. Smaller, potentially resectable tumors are often poorly visualized despite technically adequate esophagograms. Because of this, esophagoscopy should be performed in all patients suspected of having an esophageal abnormality, to visualize the tumor and to obtain histopathologic confirmation of the diagnosis. Because the population of persons at risk for squamous cell carcinoma of the esophagus (i.e., smokers and drinkers) also has a high rate of cancers of the lung and the head and neck region, endoscopic inspection of the larynx, trachea, and bronchi should also be done. A thorough examination of the fundus of the stomach (by retroflexing the endoscope) is imperative as well. Endoscopic biopsies of esophageal tumors fail to recover malignant tissue in one-third of cases because the biopsy forceps cannot penetrate deeply enough through normal mucosa pushed in front of the carcinoma. Cytologic examination of tumor brushings complements standard biopsies and should be performed routinely. The extent of tumor spread to the mediastinum and para-aortic lymph nodes should be assessed by CT scans of the chest and abdomen and by endoscopic ultrasound. Positron emission tomography scanning provides a useful assessment of resectability, offering accurate information regarding spread to mediastinal lymph nodes.

℞ Treatment:
ESOPHAGEAL CANCER

The prognosis for patients with esophageal carcinoma is poor. Fewer than 5% of patients survive 5 years after the diagnosis; thus, management focuses on symptom control. Surgical resection of all gross tumor (i.e., total resection) is feasible in only 45% of cases, with residual tumor cells frequently present at the resection margins. Such esophagectomies have been associated with a postoperative mortality rate of 5–10% due to anastomotic fistulas, subphrenic abscesses, and respiratory complications. About 20% of patients who survive a total resection live 5 years. The efficacy of primary radiation therapy (5500–6000 cGy) for squamous cell carcinomas is similar to that of radical surgery, sparing patients perioperative morbidity but often resulting in less satisfactory palliation of obstructive symptoms. The evaluation of chemotherapeutic agents in patients with esophageal carcinoma has been hampered by ambiguity in the definition of "response" and the debilitated physical condition of many treated individuals. Nonetheless, significant reductions in the size of measurable tumor masses have been reported in 15–25% of patients given single-agent treatment and in 30–60% of patients treated with drug combinations that include cisplatin. Combination chemotherapy and radiation therapy as the initial therapeutic approach, either alone or followed by an attempt at operative resection, seems to be beneficial. When administered along with radiation therapy, chemotherapy produces a better survival outcome than radiation therapy alone. The use of preoperative chemotherapy and radiation therapy followed by esophageal resection appears to prolong survival as compared with controls in small, randomized trials, and some reports suggest that no additional benefit accrues when surgery is added if significant shrinkage of tumor has been achieved by the chemoradiation combination.

For the incurable, surgically unresectable patient with esophageal cancer, dysphagia, malnutrition, and the management of tracheoesophageal fistulas are major issues. Approaches to palliation include repeated endoscopic dilatation, the surgical placement of a gastrostomy or jejunostomy for hydration and feeding, and endoscopic placement of an expansive metal stent to bypass the tumor. Endoscopic fulguration of the obstructing tumor with lasers is the most promising of these techniques.

TUMORS OF THE STOMACH

GASTRIC ADENOCARCINOMA

Incidence and Epidemiology

For unclear reasons, the incidence and mortality rates for gastric cancer have decreased markedly during the past 75 years. The mortality rate from gastric cancer in the United States has dropped in men from 28 to 5.8 per 100,000 persons, while in women the rate has decreased from 27 to 2.8 per 100,000. Nonetheless,

21,260 new cases of stomach cancer were diagnosed in the United States, and 11,210 Americans died of the disease in 2007. Gastric cancer incidence has decreased worldwide but remains high in Japan, China, Chile, and Ireland.

The risk of gastric cancer is greater among lower socioeconomic classes. Migrants from high- to low-incidence nations maintain their susceptibility to gastric cancer, while the risk for their offspring approximates that of the new homeland. These findings suggest that an environmental exposure, probably beginning early in life, is related to the development of gastric cancer, with dietary carcinogens considered the most likely factor(s).

Pathology

About 85% of stomach cancers are adenocarcinomas, with 15% due to lymphomas and gastrointestinal stromal tumors (GIST) and leiomyosarcomas. Gastric adenocarcinomas may be subdivided into two categories: a *diffuse type*, in which cell cohesion is absent, so that individual cells infiltrate and thicken the stomach wall without forming a discrete mass; and an *intestinal type*, characterized by cohesive neoplastic cells that form glandlike tubular structures. The diffuse carcinomas occur more often in younger patients, develop throughout the stomach (including the cardia), result in a loss of distensibility of the gastric wall (so-called linitis plastica, or "leather bottle" appearance), and carry a poorer prognosis. Intestinal-type lesions are frequently ulcerative, more commonly appear in the antrum and lesser curvature of the stomach, and are often preceded by a prolonged precancerous process. While the incidence of diffuse carcinomas is similar in most populations, the intestinal type tends to predominate in the high-risk geographic regions and is less likely to be found in areas where the frequency of gastric cancer is declining. Thus, different etiologic factor(s) may be involved in these two subtypes. In the United States, ~30% of gastric cancers originate in the distal stomach, ~20% arise in the midportion of the stomach, and ~37% originate in the proximal third of the stomach. The remaining 13% involve the entire stomach.

Etiology

The long-term ingestion of high concentrations of nitrates in dried, smoked, and salted foods appears to be associated with a higher risk. The nitrates are thought to be converted to carcinogenic nitrites by bacteria (Table 47-2). Such bacteria may be introduced exogenously through the ingestion of partially decayed foods, which are consumed in abundance worldwide by the lower socioeconomic classes. Bacteria such as *Helicobacter pylori* may also contribute to this effect by causing

TABLE 47-2

NITRATE-CONVERTING BACTERIA AS A FACTOR IN THE CAUSATION OF GASTRIC CARCINOMA[a]

Exogenous sources of nitrate-converting bacteria:
  Bacterially contaminated food (common in lower socioeconomic classes, who have a higher incidence of the disease; diminished by improved food preservation and refrigeration)
  ? *Helicobacter pylori* infection
Endogenous factors favoring growth of nitrate-converting bacteria in the stomach:
  Decreased gastric acidity
  Prior gastric surgery (antrectomy) (15- to 20-year latency period)
  Atrophic gastritis and/or pernicious anemia
  ? Prolonged exposure to histamine H_2-receptor antagonists

[a]Hypothesis: Dietary nitrates are converted to carcinogenic nitrites by bacteria.

chronic gastritis, loss of gastric acidity, and bacterial growth in the stomach. The effect of *H. pylori* eradication on the subsequent risk for gastric cancer in high-incidence areas is under investigation. Loss of acidity may occur when acid-producing cells of the gastric antrum have been removed surgically to control benign peptic ulcer disease or when achlorhydria, atrophic gastritis, and even pernicious anemia develop in the elderly. Serial endoscopic examinations of the stomach in patients with atrophic gastritis have documented replacement of the usual gastric mucosa by intestinal-type cells. This process of intestinal metaplasia may lead to cellular atypia and eventual neoplasia. Since the declining incidence of gastric cancer in the United States primarily reflects a decline in distal, ulcerating, intestinal-type lesions, it is conceivable that better food preservation and the availability of refrigeration to all socioeconomic classes have decreased the dietary ingestion of exogenous bacteria. *H. pylori* has not been associated with the diffuse, more proximal form of gastric carcinoma.

Several additional etiologic factors have been associated with gastric carcinoma. Gastric ulcers and adenomatous polyps have occasionally been linked, but data on a cause-and-effect relationship are unconvincing. The inadequate clinical distinction between benign gastric ulcers and small ulcerating carcinomas may, in part, account for this presumed association. The presence of extreme hypertrophy of gastric rugal folds (i.e., Ménétrier's disease), giving the impression of polypoid lesions, has been associated with a striking frequency of malignant transformation; such hypertrophy, however, does not represent the presence of true adenomatous polyps. Individuals with blood group A have a higher incidence of gastric cancer than persons with blood group O; this observation may be related to differences in the mucous secretion, leading to

altered mucosal protection from carcinogens. A germline mutation in the E-cadherin gene, inherited in an autosomal dominant pattern and coding for a cell adhesion protein, has been linked to a high incidence of occult gastric cancers in young asymptomatic carriers. Duodenal ulcers are not associated with gastric cancer.

Clinical Features

Gastric cancers, when superficial and surgically curable, usually produce no symptoms. As the tumor becomes more extensive, patients may complain of an insidious upper abdominal discomfort varying in intensity from a vague, postprandial fullness to a severe, steady pain. Anorexia, often with slight nausea, is very common but is not the usual presenting complaint. Weight loss may eventually be observed, and nausea and vomiting are particularly prominent with tumors of the pylorus; dysphagia and early satiety may be the major symptoms caused by diffuse lesions originating in the cardia. There are no early physical signs. A palpable abdominal mass indicates long-standing growth and predicts regional extension.

Gastric carcinomas spread by direct extension through the gastric wall to the perigastric tissues, occasionally adhering to adjacent organs such as the pancreas, colon, or liver. The disease also spreads via lymphatics or by seeding of peritoneal surfaces. Metastases to intraabdominal and supraclavicular lymph nodes occur frequently, as do metastatic nodules to the ovary (Krukenberg's tumor), periumbilical region ("Sister Mary Joseph node"), or peritoneal cul-de-sac (Blumer's shelf palpable on rectal or vaginal examination); malignant ascites may also develop. The liver is the most common site for hematogenous spread of tumor.

The presence of iron-deficiency anemia in men and of occult blood in the stool in both sexes mandates a search for an occult gastrointestinal tract lesion. A careful assessment is of particular importance in patients with atrophic gastritis or pernicious anemia. Unusual clinical features associated with gastric adenocarcinomas include migratory thrombophlebitis, microangiopathic hemolytic anemia, and acanthosis nigricans.

Diagnosis

A double-contrast radiographic examination is the simplest diagnostic procedure for the evaluation of a patient with epigastric complaints. The use of double-contrast techniques helps to detect small lesions by improving mucosal detail. The stomach should be distended at some time during every radiographic examination, since decreased distensibility may be the only indication of a diffuse infiltrative carcinoma. Although gastric ulcers can be detected fairly early, distinguishing benign from malignant lesions radiographically is difficult. The anatomic location of an ulcer is not in itself an indication of the presence or absence of a cancer.

TABLE 47-3

STAGING SYSTEM FOR GASTRIC CARCINOMA

STAGE	TNM	FEATURES	DATA FROM ACS	
			NO. OF CASES, %	5-YEAR SURVIVAL, %
0	TisN0M0	Node negative; limited to mucosa	1	90
IA	T1N0M0	Node negative; invasion of lamina propria or submucosa	7	59
IB	T2N0M0	Node negative; invasion of muscularis propria	10	44
II	T1N2M0 T2N1M0	Node positive; invasion beyond mucosa but within wall	17	29
		or		
	T3N0M0	Node negative; extension through wall		
IIIA	T2N2M0 T3N1-2M0	Node positive; invasion of muscularis propria or through wall	21	15
IIIB	T4N0-1M0	Node negative; adherence to surrounding tissue	14	9
IV	T4N2M0	Node positive; adherence to surrounding tissue	30	3
		or		
	T1-4N0-2M1	Distant metastases		

Note: ACS, American Cancer Society.

Gastric ulcers that appear benign by radiography present special problems. Some physicians believe that gastroscopy is not mandatory if the radiographic features are typically benign, if complete healing can be visualized by x-ray within 6 weeks, and if a follow-up contrast radiograph obtained several months later shows a normal appearance. However, we recommend gastroscopic biopsy and brush cytology for all patients with a gastric ulcer in order to exclude a malignancy. Malignant gastric ulcers must be recognized before they penetrate into surrounding tissues, because the rate of cure of early lesions limited to the mucosa or submucosa is >80%. Since gastric carcinomas are difficult to distinguish clinically or radiographically from gastric lymphomas, endoscopic biopsies should be made as deeply as possible, due to the submucosal location of lymphoid tumors.

The staging system for gastric carcinoma is shown in Table 47-3.

℞ **Treatment:**
GASTRIC ADENOCARCINOMA

Complete surgical removal of the tumor with resection of adjacent lymph nodes offers the only chance for cure. However, this is possible in less than a third of patients. A subtotal gastrectomy is the treatment of choice for patients with distal carcinomas, while total or near-total gastrectomies are required for more proximal tumors. The inclusion of extended lymph node dissection in these procedures appears to confer an added risk for complications without enhancing survival. The prognosis following complete surgical resection depends on the degree of tumor penetration into the stomach wall and is adversely influenced by regional lymph node involvement, vascular invasion, and abnormal DNA content (i.e., aneuploidy), characteristics found in the vast majority of American patients. As a result, the probability of survival after 5 years for the 25–30% of patients able to undergo complete resection is ~20% for distal tumors and <10% for proximal tumors, with recurrences continuing for at least 8 years after surgery. In the absence of ascites or extensive hepatic or peritoneal metastases, even patients whose disease is believed to be incurable by surgery should be offered resection of the primary lesion. Reduction of tumor bulk is the best form of palliation and may enhance the probability of benefit from subsequent therapy.

Gastric adenocarcinoma is a relatively radioresistant tumor, and adequate control of the primary tumor requires doses of external beam irradiation that exceed the tolerance of surrounding structures, such as bowel mucosa and spinal cord. As a result, the major role of radiation therapy in patients has been palliation of pain. Radiation therapy alone after a complete resection does not prolong survival. In the setting of surgically unresectable disease limited to the epigastrium, patients treated with 3500–4000 cGy did not live longer than similar patients not receiving radiotherapy; however, survival was prolonged slightly when 5-fluorouracil (5-FU) was given in combination with radiation therapy. In this clinical setting, the 5-FU may be functioning as a radiosensitizer.

The administration of combinations of cytotoxic drugs to patients with advanced gastric carcinoma has been associated with partial responses in 30–50% of cases; responders appear to benefit from treatment. Such drug combinations have generally included cisplatin combined with either epirubicin and infusional 5-FU or with irinotecan. Despite this encouraging response rate, complete remissions are uncommon, the partial responses are transient, and the overall influence of multidrug therapy on survival has been unclear. The use of adjuvant chemotherapy alone following the complete resection of a gastric cancer has only minimally improved survival. However, combination chemotherapy administered before and after surgery (*perioperative treatment*) as well as postoperative chemotherapy combined with radiation therapy reduces the recurrence rate and prolongs survival.

PRIMARY GASTRIC LYMPHOMA

Primary lymphoma of the stomach is relatively uncommon, accounting for <15% of gastric malignancies and ~2% of all lymphomas. The stomach is, however, the most frequent extranodal site for lymphoma, and gastric lymphoma has increased in frequency during the past 30 years. The disease is difficult to distinguish clinically from gastric adenocarcinoma; both tumors are most often detected during the sixth decade of life; present with epigastric pain, early satiety, and generalized fatigue; and are usually characterized by ulcerations with a ragged, thickened mucosal pattern demonstrated by contrast radiographs. The diagnosis of lymphoma of the stomach may occasionally be made through cytologic brushings of the gastric mucosa but usually requires a biopsy at gastroscopy or laparotomy. Failure of gastroscopic biopsies to detect lymphoma in a given case should not be interpreted as being conclusive, since superficial biopsies may miss the deeper lymphoid infiltrate. The macroscopic pathology of gastric lymphoma may also mimic adenocarcinoma, consisting of either a bulky ulcerated lesion localized in the corpus or antrum or a diffuse process spreading throughout the entire gastric submucosa and even extending into the duodenum. Microscopically, the vast majority of gastric lymphoid tumors are non-Hodgkin's lymphomas of B cell origin; Hodgkin's disease involving the stomach is extremely uncommon. Histologically, these tumors may range from well-differentiated, superficial processes [mucosa-associated lymphoid tissue (MALT)] to high-grade, large-cell lymphomas. Like gastric adenocarcinoma, infection with *H. pylori* increases the risk for gastric lymphoma in general and MALT lymphomas in particular. Gastric lymphomas spread initially to regional lymph nodes (often to Waldeyer's ring) and may then disseminate. Gastric lymphomas are staged like other lymphomas.

℞ **Treatment:**
PRIMARY GASTRIC LYMPHOMA

Primary gastric lymphoma is a far more treatable disease than adenocarcinoma of the stomach, a fact that underscores the need for making the correct diagnosis. Antibiotic treatment to eradicate *H. pylori* infection has led to regression of about 75% of gastric MALT lymphomas and should be considered before surgery, radiation therapy, or chemotherapy are undertaken in patients having such tumors. A lack of response to such antimicrobial treatment has been linked to a specific chromosomal abnormality, i.e., t(11;18). Responding patients should undergo periodic endoscopic surveillance because it remains unclear whether the neoplastic clone is eliminated or merely suppressed, although the response to antimicrobial treatment is quite durable. Subtotal gastrectomy, usually followed by combination chemotherapy, has led to 5-year survival rates of 40–60% in patients with localized high-grade lymphomas. The need for a major surgical procedure has been questioned, particularly in patients with preoperative radiographic evidence of nodal involvement, for whom chemotherapy [CHOP (cyclophosphamide, doxorubicin, vincristine, and prednisone)] plus rituximab is effective therapy. A role for radiation therapy is not defined because most recurrences develop at distant sites.

GASTRIC (NONLYMPHOID) SARCOMA

Leiomyosarcomas and GISTs make up 1–3% of gastric neoplasms. They most frequently involve the anterior and posterior walls of the gastric fundus and often ulcerate and bleed. Even those lesions that appear benign on histologic examination may behave in a malignant fashion. These tumors rarely invade adjacent viscera and characteristically do not metastasize to lymph nodes, but they may spread to the liver and lungs. The treatment of choice is surgical resection. Combination chemotherapy should be reserved for patients with metastatic disease. All such tumors should be analyzed for a mutation in the *c-kit* receptor. GISTs are unresponsive to conventional chemotherapy; ~50% of patients experience objective response and prolonged survival when treated with imatinib mesylate (Gleevec) (400–800 mg PO daily), a selective inhibitor of the *c-kit* tyrosine kinase. Many patients with GIST whose tumors have become refractory to imatinib subsequently benefit from sunitinib (Sutent), another inhibitor of the *c-kit* tyrosine kinase.

COLORECTAL CANCER

INCIDENCE

Cancer of the large bowel is second only to lung cancer as a cause of cancer death in the United States: 153,760 new cases occurred in 2007, and 52,180 deaths were due to colorectal cancer. The incidence rate has remained relatively unchanged during the past 30 years, while the mortality rate has decreased, particularly in females. Colorectal cancer generally occurs in persons ≥50 years.

POLYPS AND MOLECULAR PATHOGENESIS

Most colorectal cancers, regardless of etiology, arise from adenomatous polyps. A polyp is a grossly visible protrusion from the mucosal surface and may be classified pathologically as a nonneoplastic hamartoma (*juvenile polyp*), a hyperplastic mucosal proliferation (*hyperplastic polyp*), or an adenomatous polyp. Only adenomas are clearly premalignant, and only a minority of such lesions becomes cancer. Adenomatous polyps may be found in the colons of ~30% of middle-aged and ~50% of elderly people; however, <1% of polyps ever become malignant. Most polyps produce no symptoms and remain clinically undetected. Occult blood in the stool is found in <5% of patients with polyps.

A number of molecular changes are noted in adenomatous polyps, dysplastic lesions, and polyps containing microscopic foci of tumor cells (carcinoma in situ), which are thought to reflect a multistep process in the evolution of normal colonic mucosa to life-threatening invasive carcinoma. These developmental steps toward carcinogenesis include, but are not restricted to, point mutations in the K-*ras* protooncogene; hypomethylation of DNA, leading to gene activation; loss of DNA (*allelic loss*) at the site of a tumor-suppressor gene [the adenomatous polyposis coli (*APC*) gene] on the long arm of chromosome 5 (5q21); allelic loss at the site of a tumor-suppressor gene located on chromosome 18q [the deleted in colorectal cancer (*DCC*) gene]; and allelic loss at chromosome 17p, associated with mutations in the p53 tumor-suppressor gene. Thus, the altered proliferative pattern of the colonic mucosa, which results in progression to a polyp and then to carcinoma, may involve the mutational activation of an oncogene followed by and coupled with the loss of genes that normally suppress tumorigenesis. It remains uncertain whether the genetic aberrations always occur in a defined order. Based on this model, however, cancer is believed to develop only in those polyps in which most (if not all) of these mutational events take place.

Clinically, the probability of an adenomatous polyp becoming a cancer depends on the gross appearance of the lesion, its histologic features, and its size. Adenomatous polyps may be pedunculated (stalked) or sessile (flat-based). Cancers develop more frequently in sessile polyps. Histologically, adenomatous polyps may be tubular, villous (i.e., papillary), or tubulovillous. Villous adenomas, most of which are sessile, become malignant more than three times as often as tubular adenomas. The likelihood that any polypoid lesion in the large bowel contains invasive cancer is related to the size of the polyp, being negligible (<2%) in lesions <1.5 cm, intermediate (2–10%) in lesions 1.5–2.5 cm in size, and substantial (10%) in lesions >2.5 cm.

Following the detection of an adenomatous polyp, the entire large bowel should be visualized endoscopically or radiographically, since synchronous lesions are noted in about one-third of cases. Colonoscopy should then be repeated periodically, even in the absence of a previously documented malignancy, since such patients have a 30–50% probability of developing another adenoma and are at a higher-than-average risk for developing a colorectal carcinoma. Adenomatous polyps are thought to require >5 years of growth before becoming clinically significant; colonoscopy need not be carried out more frequently than every 3 years.

ETIOLOGY AND RISK FACTORS

Risk factors for the development of colorectal cancer are listed in Table 47-4.

Diet

The etiology for most cases of large-bowel cancer appears to be related to environmental factors. The disease occurs more often in upper socioeconomic populations who live in urban areas. Mortality from colorectal cancer is directly correlated with per capita consumption of calories, meat protein, and dietary fat and oil as well as elevations in the serum cholesterol concentration and mortality from coronary artery disease. Geographic variations in incidence are unrelated to genetic differences, since migrant groups tend to assume the large-bowel cancer incidence rates of their adopted countries. Furthermore, population groups such as Mormons and Seventh Day Adventists, whose lifestyle and dietary habits differ somewhat from those of their neighbors, have significantly lower-than-expected incidence and mortality rates for colorectal cancer. Colorectal cancer has increased in Japan since that nation has adopted a more "western" diet. At least three hypotheses have been proposed to explain the relationship to diet, none of which is fully satisfactory.

Animal Fats

One hypothesis is that the ingestion of animal fats found in red meats and processed meat leads to an increased proportion of anaerobes in the gut microflora, resulting in the conversion of normal bile acids into carcinogens.

TABLE 47-4

RISK FACTORS FOR THE DEVELOPMENT OF COLORECTAL CANCER
Diet: Animal fat
Hereditary syndromes (autosomal dominant inheritance)
Polyposis coli
Nonpolyposis syndrome (Lynch syndrome)
Inflammatory bowel disease
Streptococcus bovis bacteremia
Ureterosigmoidostomy
? Tobacco use

This provocative hypothesis is supported by several reports of increased amounts of fecal anaerobes in the stools of patients with colorectal cancer. Diets high in animal (but not vegetable) fats are also associated with high serum cholesterol, which is also associated with enhanced risk for the development of colorectal adenomas and carcinomas.

Insulin Resistance

The large number of calories in "western" diets coupled with physical inactivity has been associated with a higher prevalence of obesity. Obese persons develop insulin resistance with increased circulating levels of insulin, leading to higher circulating concentrations of insulin-like growth factor type I (IGF-I). This growth factor appears to stimulate proliferation of the intestinal mucosa.

Fiber

Contrary to prior beliefs, the results of randomized trials and case-controlled studies have failed to show any value for dietary fiber or diets high in fruits and vegetables in preventing the recurrence of colorectal adenomas or the development of colorectal cancer. The weight of epidemiologic evidence, however, implicates diet as being the major etiologic factor for colorectal cancer, particularly diets high in animal fat and in calories.

HEREDITARY FACTORS AND SYNDROMES

Up to 25% of patients with colorectal cancer have a family history of the disease, suggesting a hereditary predisposition. Inherited large-bowel cancers can be divided into two main groups: the well-studied but uncommon polyposis syndromes and the more common nonpolyposis syndromes (**Table 47–5**).

Polyposis Coli

Polyposis coli (familial polyposis of the colon) is a rare condition characterized by the appearance of thousands of adenomatous polyps throughout the large bowel. It is transmitted as an autosomal dominant trait; the occasional patient with no family history probably developed the condition due to a spontaneous mutation. Polyposis coli is associated with a deletion in the long arm of chromosome 5 [including the *APC* (adenomatous polyposis coli) gene] in both neoplastic (somatic mutation) and normal (germline mutation) cells. The loss of this genetic material (i.e., allelic loss) results in the absence of tumor-suppressor genes whose protein products would normally inhibit neoplastic growth. The presence of soft tissue and bony tumors, congenital hypertrophy of the retinal pigment epithelium, mesenteric desmoid tumors, and ampullary cancers in addition to the colonic polyps characterizes a subset of polyposis coli known as *Gardner's syndrome*. The appearance of malignant tumors of the central nervous system accompanying polyposis coli defines *Turcot's syndrome*. The colonic polyps in all these conditions are rarely present before puberty but are generally evident in affected individuals by age 25. If the polyposis is not treated surgically, colorectal cancer will develop in almost all patients before age 40. Polyposis coli results from a defect in the colonic mucosa, leading to an abnormal proliferative pattern and impaired DNA repair mechanisms. Once the multiple polyps are detected, patients should undergo a total colectomy. The ileoanal anastomotic technique allows removal of the entire bowel while retaining the anal sphincter. Medical therapy with nonsteroidal anti-inflammatory drugs (NSAIDs) such as sulindac and cyclooxygenase-2 inhibitors such as celecoxib can decrease the number and size of polyps in

TABLE 47-5

HEREDITABLE (AUTOSOMAL DOMINANT) GASTROINTESTINAL POLYPOSIS SYNDROMES

SYNDROME	DISTRIBUTION OF POLYPS	HISTOLOGIC TYPE	MALIGNANT POTENTIAL	ASSOCIATED LESIONS
Familial adenomatous polyposis	Large intestine	Adenoma	Common	None
Gardner's syndrome	Large and small intestines	Adenoma	Common	Osteomas, fibromas, lipomas, epidermoid cysts, ampullary cancers, congenital hypertrophy of retinal pigment epithelium
Turcot's syndrome	Large intestine	Adenoma	Common	Brain tumors
Nonpolyposis syndrome (Lynch syndrome)	Large intestine (often proximal)	Adenoma	Common	Endometrial and ovarian tumors
Peutz-Jeghers syndrome	Small and large intestines, stomach	Hamartoma	Rare	Mucocutaneous pigmentation; tumors of the ovary, breast, pancreas, endometrium
Juvenile polyposis	Large and small intestines, stomach	Hamartoma, rarely progressing to adenoma	Rare	Various congenital abnormalities

patients with polyposis coli; however, this effect on polyps is only temporary, and NSAIDs are not proven to reduce the risk of cancer. Colectomy remains the primary therapy/prevention. The offspring of patients with polyposis coli, who often are prepubertal when the diagnosis is made in the parent, have a 50% risk for developing this premalignant disorder and should be carefully screened by annual flexible sigmoidoscopy until age 35. Proctosigmoidoscopy is a sufficient screening procedure because polyps tend to be evenly distributed from cecum to anus, making more-invasive and expensive techniques such as colonoscopy or barium enema unnecessary. Testing for occult blood in the stool is an inadequate screening maneuver. An alternative method for identifying carriers is testing DNA from peripheral blood mononuclear cells for the presence of a mutated *APC* gene. The detection of such a germline mutation can lead to a definitive diagnosis before the development of polyps.

Hereditary Nonpolyposis Colon Cancer

Hereditary nonpolyposis colon cancer (HNPCC), also known as *Lynch syndrome*, is another autosomal dominant trait. It is characterized by the presence of three or more relatives with histologically documented colorectal cancer, one of whom is a first-degree relative of the other two; one or more cases of colorectal cancer diagnosed before age 50 in the family; and colorectal cancer involving at least two generations. In contrast to polyposis coli, HNPCC is associated with an unusually high frequency of cancer arising in the proximal large bowel. The median age for the appearance of an adenocarcinoma is <50 years, 10–15 years younger than the median age for the general population. Despite having a poorly differentiated histologic appearance, the proximal colon tumors in HNPCC have a better prognosis than sporadic tumors from patients of similar age. Families with HNPCC often include individuals with multiple primary cancers; the association of colorectal cancer with either ovarian or endometrial carcinomas is especially strong in women. It has been recommended that members of such families undergo biennial colonoscopy beginning at age 25 years, with intermittent pelvic ultrasonography and endometrial biopsy for afflicted women; such a screening strategy has not yet been validated. HNPCC is associated with germline mutations of several genes, particularly *hMSH2* on chromosome 2 and *hMLH1* on chromosome 3. These mutations lead to errors in DNA replication and are thought to result in DNA instability because of defective repair of DNA mismatches, resulting in abnormal cell growth and tumor development. Testing tumor cells through molecular analysis of DNA or immunohistochemical staining of paraffin-fixed tissue for "microsatellite instability" (sequence changes reflecting defective mismatch repair) in patients under age 50 with colorectal cancer and a positive family history for colorectal or endometrial cancer may identify probands with HNPCC.

INFLAMMATORY BOWEL DISEASE

(Chap. 16) Large-bowel cancer is increased in incidence in patients with long-standing inflammatory bowel disease (IBD). Cancers develop more commonly in patients with ulcerative colitis than in those with granulomatous colitis, but this impression may result in part from the occasional difficulty of differentiating these two conditions. The risk of colorectal cancer in a patient with IBD is relatively small during the initial 10 years of the disease, but then it appears to increase at a rate of ~0.5–1% per year. Cancer may develop in 8–30% of patients after 25 years. The risk is higher in younger patients with pancolitis.

Cancer surveillance in patients with IBD is unsatisfactory. Symptoms such as bloody diarrhea, abdominal cramping, and obstruction, which may signal the appearance of a tumor, are similar to the complaints caused by a flare-up of the underlying disease. In patients with a history of IBD lasting ≥15 years who continue to experience exacerbations, the surgical removal of the colon can significantly reduce the risk for cancer and also eliminate the target organ for the underlying chronic gastrointestinal disorder. The value of such surveillance techniques as colonoscopy with mucosal biopsies and brushings for less-symptomatic individuals with chronic IBD is uncertain. The lack of uniformity regarding the pathologic criteria that characterize dysplasia and the absence of data that such surveillance reduces the development of lethal cancers have made this costly practice an area of controversy.

OTHER HIGH-RISK CONDITIONS
Streptococcus Bovis Bacteremia

For unknown reasons, individuals who develop endocarditis or septicemia from this fecal bacterium have a high incidence of occult colorectal tumors and, possibly, upper gastrointestinal cancers as well. Endoscopic or radiographic screening appears advisable.

Tobacco Use

Cigarette smoking is linked to the development of colorectal adenomas, particularly after >35 years of tobacco use. No biologic explanation for this association has yet been proposed.

PRIMARY PREVENTION

Several orally administered compounds have been assessed as possible inhibitors of colon cancer. The most effective class of chemopreventive agents is aspirin and other NSAIDs, which are thought to suppress cell proliferation by inhibiting prostaglandin synthesis. Regular aspirin use reduces the risk of colon adenomas and carcinomas as well as death from large-bowel cancer; such use also appears to diminish the likelihood for developing additional premalignant adenomas following treatment for a prior colon carcinoma. This effect of aspirin on colon carcinogenesis increases with the duration and dosage of drug use. Oral folic acid supplements and oral calcium supplements reduce the risk of adenomatous polyps and colorectal cancers in case-controlled studies. Antioxidant vitamins such as ascorbic acid, tocopherols, and β-carotene are ineffective at reducing the incidence of subsequent adenomas in patients who have undergone the removal of a colon adenoma. Estrogen-replacement therapy has been associated with a reduction in the risk of colorectal cancer in women, conceivably by an effect on bile acid synthesis and composition or by decreasing synthesis of IGF-I. The otherwise unexplained reduction in colorectal cancer mortality in women may be a result of the widespread use of estrogen replacement in postmenopausal individuals.

SCREENING

The rationale for colorectal cancer screening programs is that earlier detection of localized, superficial cancers in asymptomatic individuals will increase the surgical cure rate. Such screening programs are important for individuals having a family history of the disease in first-degree relatives. The relative risk for developing colorectal cancer increases to 1.75 in such individuals and may be even higher if the relative was afflicted before age 60. The prior use of proctosigmoidoscopy as a screening tool was based on the observation that 60% of early lesions are located in the rectosigmoid. For unexplained reasons, however, the proportion of large-bowel cancers arising in the rectum has been decreasing during the past several decades, with a corresponding increase in the proportion of cancers in the more proximal descending colon. As such, the potential for rigid proctosigmoidoscopy to detect a sufficient number of occult neoplasms to make the procedure cost-effective has been questioned. Flexible, fiberoptic sigmoidoscopes permit trained operators to visualize the colon for up to 60 cm, which enhances the capability for cancer detection. However, this technique still leaves the proximal half of the large bowel unscreened.

Most programs directed at the early detection of colorectal cancers have focused on digital rectal examinations and fecal occult blood testing. The digital examination should be part of any routine physical evaluation in adults older than age 40, serving as a screening test for prostate cancer in men, a component of the pelvic examination in women, and an inexpensive maneuver for the detection of masses in the rectum. The development of the Hemoccult test has greatly facilitated the detection of occult fecal blood. Unfortunately, even when performed optimally, the Hemoccult test has

major limitations as a screening technique. About 50% of patients with documented colorectal cancers have a negative fecal Hemoccult test, consistent with the intermittent bleeding pattern of these tumors. When random cohorts of asymptomatic persons have been tested, 2–4% have Hemoccult-positive stools. Colorectal cancers have been found in <10% of these "test-positive" cases, with benign polyps being detected in an additional 20–30%. Thus, a colorectal neoplasm will not be found in most asymptomatic individuals with occult blood in their stool. Nonetheless, persons found to have Hemoccult-positive stool routinely undergo further medical evaluation, including sigmoidoscopy, barium enema, and/or colonoscopy—procedures that are not only uncomfortable and expensive but also associated with a small risk for significant complications. The added cost of these studies would appear justifiable if the small number of patients found to have occult neoplasms because of Hemoccult screening could be shown to have an improved prognosis and prolonged survival. Prospectively controlled trials showed a statistically significant reduction in mortality from colorectal cancer for individuals undergoing annual screening. However, this benefit only emerged after >13 years of follow-up and was extremely expensive to achieve, since all positive tests (most of which were false-positive) were followed by colonoscopy. Moreover, these colonoscopic examinations quite likely provided the opportunity for cancer prevention through the removal of potentially premalignant adenomatous polyps since the eventual development of cancer was reduced by 20% in the cohort undergoing annual screening.

Screening techniques for large-bowel cancer in asymptomatic persons remain unsatisfactory. Compliance with any screening strategy within the general population is poor. At present, the American Cancer Society suggests fecal Hemoccult screening annually and flexible sigmoidoscopy every 5 years beginning at age 50 for asymptomatic individuals having no colorectal cancer risk factors. The American Cancer Society has also endorsed a "total colon examination" (i.e., colonoscopy or double-contrast barium enema) every 10 years as an alternative to Hemoccult testing with periodic flexible sigmoidoscopy. Colonoscopy has been shown to be superior to double-contrast barium enema and also to have a higher sensitivity for detecting villous or dysplastic adenomas or cancers than the strategy employing occult fecal blood testing and flexible sigmoidoscopy. Whether colonoscopy performed every 10 years beginning after age 50 will prove to be cost-effective and whether it may be supplanted as a screening maneuver by sophisticated radiographic techniques ("virtual colonoscopy") remains unclear. More effective techniques for screening are needed, perhaps taking advantage of the molecular changes that have been described in these tumors. Analysis of fecal DNA for multiple mutations associated with colorectal cancer is being tested.

CLINICAL FEATURES

Presenting Symptoms

Symptoms vary with the anatomic location of the tumor. Since stool is relatively liquid as it passes through the ileocecal valve into the right colon, cancers arising in the cecum and ascending colon may become quite large without resulting in any obstructive symptoms or noticeable alterations in bowel habits. Lesions of the right colon commonly ulcerate, leading to chronic, insidious blood loss without a change in the appearance of the stool. Consequently, patients with tumors of the ascending colon often present with symptoms such as fatigue, palpitations, and even angina pectoris and are found to have a hypochromic, microcytic anemia indicative of iron deficiency. Since the cancer may bleed intermittently, a random fecal occult blood test may be negative. As a result, the unexplained presence of iron-deficiency anemia in any adult (with the possible exception of a premenopausal, multiparous woman) mandates a thorough endoscopic and/or radiographic visualization of the entire large bowel (**Fig. 47-1**).

Since stool becomes more formed as it passes into the transverse and descending colon, tumors arising there tend to impede the passage of stool, resulting in the development of abdominal cramping, occasional obstruction, and even perforation. Radiographs of the abdomen often reveal characteristic annular, constricting lesions ("apple-core" or "napkin-ring") (**Fig. 47-2**).

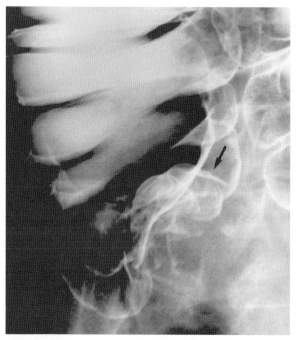

FIGURE 47-1
Double-contrast air-barium enema revealing a sessile tumor of the cecum in a patient with iron-deficiency anemia and guaiac-positive stool. The lesion at surgery was a stage II adenocarcinoma.

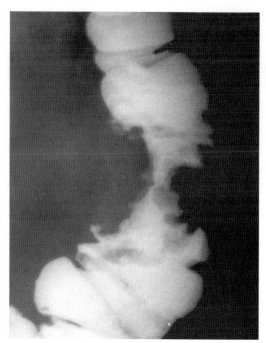

FIGURE 47-2
Annular, constricting adenocarcinoma of the descending colon. This radiographic appearance is referred to as an "apple-core" lesion and is always highly suggestive of malignancy.

Cancers arising in the rectosigmoid are often associated with hematochezia, tenesmus, and narrowing of the caliber of stool; anemia is an infrequent finding. While these symptoms may lead patients and their physicians to suspect the presence of hemorrhoids, the development of rectal bleeding and/or altered bowel habits demands a prompt digital rectal examination and proctosigmoidoscopy.

Staging, Prognostic Factors, and Patterns of Spread

The prognosis for individuals having colorectal cancer is related to the depth of tumor penetration into the bowel wall and the presence of both regional lymph node involvement and distant metastases. These variables are incorporated into the staging system introduced by Dukes and applied to a TNM classification method, in which T represents the depth of tumor penetration, N the presence of lymph node involvement, and M the presence or absence of distant metastases (**Fig. 47-3**). Superficial lesions that do not involve regional lymph nodes and do not penetrate through the submucosa (T_1) or the muscularis (T_2) are designated as *stage I* ($T_{1-2}N_0M_0$) disease; tumors that penetrate through the muscularis but have not spread to lymph nodes are *stage II* disease ($T_3N_0M_0$); regional lymph node involvement defines *stage III* ($T_xN_1M_0$) disease; and metastatic spread to sites such as liver, lung, or bone indicates *stage IV* ($T_xN_xM_1$) disease. Unless gross evidence of metastatic

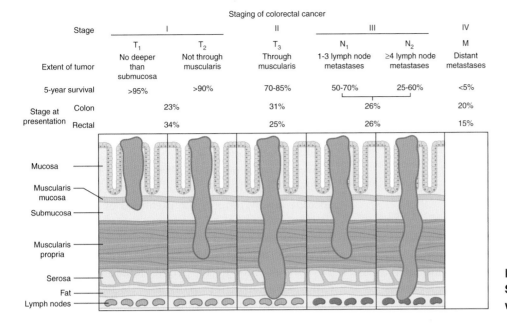

Staging of colorectal cancer						
Stage	I		II	III		IV
	T₁	T₂	T₃	N₁	N₂	M
Extent of tumor	No deeper than submucosa	Not through muscularis	Through muscularis	1-3 lymph node metastases	≥4 lymph node metastases	Distant metastases
5-year survival	>95%	>90%	70-85%	50-70%	25-60%	<5%

Stage at presentation		I	II	III	IV
	Colon	23%	31%	26%	20%
	Rectal	34%	25%	26%	15%

Mucosa
Muscularis mucosa
Submucosa
Muscularis propria
Serosa
Fat
Lymph nodes

FIGURE 47-3
Staging and prognosis for patients with colorectal cancer.

disease is present, disease stage cannot be determined accurately before surgical resection and pathologic analysis of the operative specimens. It is not clear whether the detection of nodal metastases by special immunohistochemical molecular techniques has the same prognostic implications as disease detected by routine light microscopy.

Most recurrences after a surgical resection of a large-bowel cancer occur within the first 4 years, making 5-year survival a fairly reliable indicator of cure. The likelihood for 5-year survival in patients with colorectal cancer is stage-related (Fig. 47-3). That likelihood has improved during the past several decades when similar surgical stages have been compared. The most plausible explanation for this improvement is more thorough intraoperative and pathologic staging. In particular, more exacting attention to pathologic detail has revealed that the prognosis following the resection of a colorectal cancer is not related merely to the presence or absence of regional lymph node involvement. Prognosis may be more precisely gauged by the number of involved lymph nodes (one to three lymph nodes versus four or more lymph nodes). A minimum of 12 sampled lymph nodes is thought necessary to accurately define tumor stage. Other predictors of a poor prognosis after a total surgical resection include tumor penetration through the bowel wall into pericolic fat, poorly differentiated histology, perforation and/or tumor adherence to adjacent organs (increasing the risk for an anatomically adjacent recurrence), and venous invasion by tumor (Table 47-6). Regardless of the clinicopathologic stage, a preoperative elevation of the plasma carcinoembryonic antigen (CEA) level predicts eventual tumor recurrence. The presence of aneuploidy and specific chromosomal deletions, such as allelic loss in chromosome 18q (involving the *DCC*

gene) in tumor cells, appears to predict a higher risk for metastatic spread, particularly in patients with stage II (T₃N₀M₀) disease. Conversely, the detection of microsatellite instability in tumor tissue indicates a more favorable outcome. In contrast to most other cancers, the prognosis in colorectal cancer is not influenced by the size of the primary lesion when adjusted for nodal involvement and histologic differentiation.

Cancers of the large bowel generally spread to regional lymph nodes or to the liver via the portal venous circulation. The liver represents the most frequent visceral site of metastasis; it is the initial site of distant spread in one-third of recurring colorectal cancers and is involved in more than two-thirds of such patients at the time of death. In general, colorectal cancer rarely spreads to the lungs, supraclavicular lymph nodes, bone, or brain without prior spread to the liver. A major exception to this rule occurs in patients having primary tumors in the distal rectum, from which tumor cells may

TABLE 47-6

PREDICTORS OF POOR OUTCOME FOLLOWING TOTAL SURGICAL RESECTION OF COLORECTAL CANCER

Tumor spread to regional lymph nodes
Number of regional lymph nodes involved
Tumor penetration through the bowel wall
Poorly differentiated histology
Perforation
Tumor adherence to adjacent organs
Venous invasion
Preoperative elevation of CEA titer (>5.0 ng/mL)
Aneuploidy
Specific chromosomal deletion (e.g., allelic loss on chromosome 18q)

Note: CEA, carcinoembryonic antigen.

spread through the paravertebral venous plexus, escaping the portal venous system and thereby reaching the lungs or supraclavicular lymph nodes without hepatic involvement. The median survival after the detection of distant metastases has ranged in the past from 6–9 months (hepatomegaly, abnormal liver chemistries) to 24–30 months (small liver nodule initially identified by elevated CEA level and subsequent CT scan), but effective systemic therapy is improving the prognosis.

R$_X$ Treatment: COLORECTAL CANCER

Total resection of tumor is the optimal treatment when a malignant lesion is detected in the large bowel. An evaluation for the presence of metastatic disease, including a thorough physical examination, chest radiograph, biochemical assessment of liver function, and measurement of the plasma CEA level, should be performed before surgery. When possible, a colonoscopy of the entire large bowel should be performed to identify synchronous neoplasms and/or polyps. The detection of metastases should not preclude surgery in patients with tumor-related symptoms such as gastrointestinal bleeding or obstruction, but it often prompts the use of a less radical operative procedure. At the time of laparotomy, the entire peritoneal cavity should be examined, with thorough inspection of the liver, pelvis, and hemidiaphragm and careful palpation of the full length of the large bowel. Following recovery from a complete resection, patients should be observed carefully for 5 years by semiannual physical examinations and yearly blood chemistry measurements. If a complete colonoscopy was not performed preoperatively, it should be carried out within the first several postoperative months. Some authorities favor measuring plasma CEA levels at 3-month intervals because of the sensitivity of this test as a marker for otherwise undetectable tumor recurrence. Subsequent endoscopic or radiographic surveillance of the large bowel, probably at triennial intervals, is indicated, since patients who have been cured of one colorectal cancer have a 3–5% probability of developing an additional bowel cancer during their lifetime and a >15% risk for the development of adenomatous polyps. Anastomotic ("suture-line") recurrences are infrequent in colorectal cancer patients provided the surgical resection margins are adequate and free of tumor. The value of periodic CT scans of the abdomen, assessing for an early, asymptomatic indication of tumor recurrence, is an area of uncertainty, with some experts recommending the test be performed annually for the first three postoperative years.

Radiation therapy to the pelvis is recommended for patients with rectal cancer because it reduces the 20–25% probability of regional recurrences following complete surgical resection of stage II or III tumors,

especially if they have penetrated through the serosa. This alarmingly high rate of local disease recurrence is believed to be due to the fact that the contained anatomic space within the pelvis limits the extent of the resection and because the rich lymphatic network of the pelvic side wall immediately adjacent to the rectum facilitates the early spread of malignant cells into surgically inaccessible tissue. The use of sharp rather than blunt dissection of rectal cancers (*total mesorectal excision*) appears to reduce the likelihood of local disease recurrence to ~10%. Radiation therapy, either pre- or postoperatively, reduces the likelihood of pelvic recurrences but does not appear to prolong survival. Preoperative radiotherapy is indicated for patients with large, potentially unresectable rectal cancers; such lesions may shrink enough to permit subsequent surgical removal. Radiation therapy is not effective in the primary treatment of colon cancer.

Systemic therapy for patients with colorectal cancer has become more effective. 5-FU remains the backbone of treatment for this disease. Partial responses are obtained in 15–20% of patients. The probability of tumor response appears to be somewhat greater for patients with liver metastases when chemotherapy is infused directly into the hepatic artery, but intraarterial treatment is costly and toxic and does not appear to appreciably prolong survival. The concomitant administration of folinic acid (leucovorin) improves the efficacy of 5-FU in patients with advanced colorectal cancer, presumably by enhancing the binding of 5-FU to its target enzyme, thymidylate synthase. A threefold improvement in the partial response rate is noted when folinic acid is combined with 5-FU; however, the effect on survival is marginal, and the optimal dose schedule remains to be defined. 5-FU is generally administered intravenously but may also be given orally in the form of capecitabine with seemingly similar efficacy.

Irinotecan (CPT-11), a topoisomerase 1 inhibitor, prolongs survival when compared to supportive care in patients whose disease has progressed on 5-FU. Furthermore, the addition of irinotecan to 5-FU and leucovorin (LV) improves response rates and survival of patients with metastatic disease. The *FOLFIRI regimen* is as follows: irinotecan, 180 mg/m^2 as a 90-min infusion day 1; LV, 400 mg/m^2 as a 2-h infusion during irinotecan, immediately followed by 5-FU bolus, 400 mg/m^2 and 46-h continuous infusion of 2.4–3 g/m^2 every 2 weeks. Diarrhea is the major side effect from irinotecan. Oxaliplatin, a platinum analogue, also improves the response rate when added to 5-FU and LV as initial treatment of patients with metastatic disease. The *FOLFOX regimen* is the following: 2-h infusion of LV (400 mg/m^2 per day) followed by a 5-FU bolus (400 mg/m^2 per day) and 22-h infusion (1200 mg/m^2) every 2 weeks, together with oxaliplatin, 85 mg/m^2 as a 2-h infusion on day 1. Oxaliplatin frequently causes a dose-dependent sensory neuropathy that usually resolves following the cessation of therapy. FOLFIRI and FOLFOX are equal in efficacy.

Monoclonal antibodies are also effective in patients with advanced colorectal cancer. Cetuximab (Erbitux) and panitumumab (Vectibix) are directed against the epidermal growth factor receptor (EGFR), a transmembrane glycoprotein involved in signaling pathways affecting growth and proliferation of tumor cells. Both cetuximab and panitumumab, when given alone, have been shown to benefit a small proportion of previously treated patients, and cetuximab appears to have therapeutic synergy with such chemotherapeutic agents as irinotecan, even in patients previously resistant to this drug; this suggests that cetuximab can reverse cellular resistance to cytotoxic chemotherapy. The use of both cetuximab and panitumumab can lead to an acne-like rash with the development and severity of the rash being correlated with the likelihood of antitumor efficacy. Inhibitors of the EGFR tyrosine kinase such as erlotinib (Tarceva) do not appear to be effective in colorectal cancer.

Bevacizumab (Avastin) is a monoclonal antibody directed against the vascular endothelial growth factor (VEGF) and is thought to act as an anti-angiogenesis agent. The addition of bevacizumab to irinotecan-containing combinations and to FOLFOX improves the outcome observed with the chemotherapy alone. The use of bevacizumab can lead to hypertension, proteinuria, and an increased likelihood of thromboembolic events.

Patients with solitary hepatic metastases without clinical or radiographic evidence of additional tumor involvement should be considered for partial liver resection, because such procedures are associated with 5-year survival rates of 25–30% when performed on selected individuals by experienced surgeons.

The administration of 5-FU and LV for 6 months after resection of tumor in patients with stage III disease leads to a 40% decrease in recurrence rates and 30% improvement in survival. The likelihood of recurrence has been further reduced when oxaliplatin has been combined with 5-FU and LV (e.g. FOLFOX); unexpectedly, the addition of irinotecan to 5-FU and LV did not enhance outcome. Patients with stage II tumors do not appear to benefit from adjuvant therapy. In rectal cancer, the delivery of preoperative or postoperative combined modality therapy (5-FU plus radiation therapy) reduces the risk of recurrence and increases the chance of cure for patients with stages II and III tumors, with the preoperative approach being better tolerated. The 5-FU acts as a radiosensitizer when delivered together with radiation therapy. Life-extending adjuvant therapy is used in only about half of patients over age 65 years. This age bias is completely inappropriate as the benefits and tolerance of adjuvant therapy in patients age 65+ appear similar to those seen in younger individuals.

Small-bowel tumors comprise <3% of gastrointestinal neoplasms. Because of their rarity, a correct diagnosis is often delayed. Abdominal symptoms are usually vague and poorly defined, and conventional radiographic studies of the upper and lower intestinal tract often appear normal. Small-bowel tumors should be considered in the differential diagnosis in the following situations: (1) recurrent, unexplained episodes of crampy abdominal pain; (2) intermittent bouts of intestinal obstruction, especially in the absence of IBD or prior abdominal surgery; (3) intussusception in the adult; and (4) evidence of chronic intestinal bleeding in the presence of negative conventional contrast radiographs. A careful small-bowel barium study is the diagnostic procedure of choice; the diagnostic accuracy may be improved by infusing barium through a nasogastric tube placed into the duodenum (enteroclysis).

BENIGN TUMORS

The histology of benign small-bowel tumors is difficult to predict on clinical and radiologic grounds alone. The symptomatology of benign tumors is not distinctive, with pain, obstruction, and hemorrhage being the most frequent symptoms. These tumors are usually discovered during the fifth and sixth decades of life, more often in the distal rather than the proximal small intestine. The most common benign tumors are adenomas, leiomyomas, lipomas, and angiomas.

Adenomas

These tumors include those of the islet cells and Brunner's glands as well as polypoid adenomas. *Islet cell adenomas* are occasionally located outside the pancreas; the associated syndromes are discussed in Chap. 50. *Brunner's gland adenomas* are not truly neoplastic but represent a hypertrophy or hyperplasia of submucosal duodenal glands. These appear as small nodules in the duodenal mucosa that secrete a highly viscous alkaline mucus. Most often, this is an incidental radiographic finding not associated with any specific clinical disorder.

Polypoid Adenomas

About 25% of benign small-bowel tumors are polypoid adenomas (Table 47-5). They may present as single polypoid lesions or, less commonly, as papillary villous adenomas. As in the colon, the sessile or papillary form of the tumor is sometimes associated with a coexisting carcinoma. Occasionally, patients with Gardner's syndrome develop premalignant adenomas in the small bowel; such lesions are generally in the duodenum. Multiple polypoid tumors may occur throughout the small bowel (and occasionally the stomach and colorectum) in the Peutz-Jeghers syndrome. The polyps are usually hamartomas (juvenile polyps) having a low potential for malignant degeneration. Mucocutaneous melanin deposits as well as tumors of the ovary, breast, pancreas, and endometrium are also associated with this autosomal dominant condition.

Leiomyomas

These neoplasms arise from smooth-muscle components of the intestine and are usually intramural, affecting the overlying mucosa. Ulceration of the mucosa may cause gastrointestinal hemorrhage of varying severity. Cramping or intermittent abdominal pain is frequently encountered.

Lipomas

These tumors occur with greatest frequency in the distal ileum and at the ileocecal valve. They have a characteristic radiolucent appearance, are usually intramural and asymptomatic, but on occasion cause bleeding.

Angiomas

While not true neoplasms, these lesions are important because they frequently cause intestinal bleeding. They may take the form of telangiectasia or hemangiomas. Multiple intestinal telangiectasias occur in a nonhereditary form confined to the gastrointestinal tract or as part of the hereditary Osler-Rendu-Weber syndrome. Vascular tumors may also take the form of isolated hemangiomas, most commonly in the jejunum. Angiography, especially during bleeding, is the best procedure for evaluating these lesions.

MALIGNANT TUMORS

While rare, small-bowel malignancies occur in patients with long-standing regional enteritis and celiac sprue as well as in individuals with AIDS. Malignant tumors of the small bowel are frequently associated with fever, weight loss, anorexia, bleeding, and a palpable abdominal mass. After ampullary carcinomas (many of which arise from biliary or pancreatic ducts), the most frequently occurring small-bowel malignancies are adenocarcinomas, lymphomas, carcinoid tumors, and leiomyosarcomas.

Adenocarcinomas

The most common primary cancers of the small bowel are adenocarcinomas, accounting for ~50% of malignant tumors. These cancers occur most often in the distal duodenum and proximal jejunum, where they tend to ulcerate and cause hemorrhage or obstruction. Radiologically, they may be confused with chronic duodenal ulcer disease or with Crohn's disease if the patient has long-standing regional enteritis. The diagnosis is best made by endoscopy and biopsy under direct vision. Surgical resection is the treatment of choice.

Lymphomas

Lymphoma in the small bowel may be primary or secondary. A diagnosis of a primary intestinal lymphoma requires histologic confirmation in a clinical setting in which palpable adenopathy and hepatosplenomegaly are absent and no evidence of lymphoma is seen on chest radiograph, CT scan, or peripheral blood smear or on bone marrow aspiration and biopsy. Symptoms referable to the small bowel are present, usually accompanied by an anatomically discernible lesion. Secondary lymphoma of the small bowel consists of involvement of the intestine by a lymphoid malignancy extending from involved retroperitoneal or mesenteric lymph nodes.

Primary intestinal lymphoma accounts for ~20% of malignancies of the small bowel. These neoplasms are non-Hodgkin's lymphomas; they usually have a diffuse, large-cell histology and are of T cell origin. Intestinal lymphoma involves the ileum, jejunum, and duodenum, in decreasing frequency, a pattern that mirrors the relative amount of normal lymphoid cells in these anatomic areas. The risk of small-bowel lymphoma is increased in patients with a prior history of malabsorptive conditions (e.g., celiac sprue), regional enteritis, and depressed immune function due to congenital immunodeficiency syndromes, prior organ transplantation, autoimmune disorders, or AIDS.

The development of localized or nodular masses that narrow the lumen results in periumbilical pain (made worse by eating) as well as weight loss, vomiting, and occasional intestinal obstruction. The diagnosis of small-bowel lymphoma may be suspected from the appearance on contrast radiographs of patterns such as infiltration and thickening of mucosal folds, mucosal nodules, areas of irregular ulceration, or stasis of contrast material. The diagnosis can be confirmed by surgical exploration and resection of involved segments. Intestinal lymphoma can occasionally be diagnosed by peroral intestinal mucosal biopsy, but since the disease mainly involves the lamina propria, full-thickness surgical biopsies are usually required.

Resection of the tumor constitutes the initial treatment modality. While postoperative radiation therapy has been given to some patients following a total resection, most authorities favor short-term (three cycles) systemic treatment with combination chemotherapy. The frequent presence of widespread intraabdominal disease at the time of diagnosis and the occasional multicentricity of the tumor often make a total resection impossible. The probability of sustained remission or cure is ~75% in patients with localized disease but is ~25% in individuals with unresectable lymphoma. In patients whose tumors are not resected, chemotherapy may lead to bowel perforation.

A unique form of small-bowel lymphoma, diffusely involving the entire intestine, was first described in oriental Jews and Arabs and is referred to as *immunoproliferative* small intestinal disease (IPSID), *Mediterranean lymphoma,* or α-*heavy chain disease.* This is a B cell tumor. The typical presentation includes chronic diarrhea and steatorrhea associated with vomiting and abdominal cramps; clubbing of the digits may be observed. A curious feature in many patients with IPSID is the presence in the blood and intestinal secretions of an abnormal IgA that contains a shortened α-heavy chain and is devoid of light chains. It is suspected that the abnormal α chains are produced by plasma cells infiltrating the small bowel. The clinical course of patients with IPSID is generally one of exacerbations and remissions, with death frequently resulting from either progressive malnutrition and wasting or the development of an aggressive lymphoma. The use of oral antibiotics such as tetracycline appears to be beneficial in the early phases of the disorder, suggesting a possible infectious etiology. Combination chemotherapy has been administered during later stages of the disease, with variable results. Results are better when antibiotics and chemotherapy are combined.

Carcinoid Tumors

Carcinoid tumors arise from argentaffin cells of the crypts of Lieberkühn and are found from the distal duodenum to the ascending colon, areas embryologically derived from the midgut. More than 50% of intestinal carcinoids are found in the distal ileum, with most congregating close to the ileocecal valve. Most intestinal carcinoids are asymptomatic and of low malignant potential, but invasion and metastases may occur, leading to the carcinoid syndrome (Chap. 50).

Leiomyosarcomas

Leiomyosarcomas often are >5 cm in diameter and may be palpable on abdominal examination. Bleeding, obstruction, and perforation are common. Such tumors should be analyzed for the expression of mutant *c-kit* receptor (defining GIST), and in the presence of metastatic disease, justifying treatment with imatinib mesylate (Gleevec) or, in imatinib refractory patients, sunitinib (Sutent).

CANCERS OF THE ANUS

Cancers of the anus account for 1–2% of the malignant tumors of the large bowel. Most such lesions arise in the anal canal, the anatomic area extending from the anorectal ring to a zone approximately halfway between the pectinate (or dentate) line and the anal verge. Carcinomas arising proximal to the pectinate line (i.e., in the transitional zone between the glandular mucosa of the rectum and the squamous epithelium of the distal anus) are known as *basaloid, cuboidal,* or *cloacogenic* tumors; about one-third of anal cancers have this histologic pattern. Malignancies arising distal to the pectinate line have

squamous histology, ulcerate more frequently, and constitute ~55% of anal cancers. The prognosis for patients with basaloid and squamous cell cancers of the anus is identical when corrected for tumor size and the presence or absence of nodal spread.

The development of anal cancer is associated with infection by human papillomavirus, the same organism etiologically linked to cervical cancer. The virus is sexually transmitted. The infection may lead to anal warts (condyloma accuminata), which may progress to anal intraepithelial neoplasia and on to squamous cell carcinoma. The risk for anal cancer is increased among homosexual males, presumably related to anal intercourse. Anal cancer risk is increased in both men and women with AIDS, possibly because their immunosuppressed state permits more severe papillomavirus infection. Anal cancers occur most commonly in middle-aged persons and are more frequent in women than men. At diagnosis, patients may experience bleeding, pain, sensation of a perianal mass, and pruritus.

Radical surgery (abdominal-perineal resection with lymph node sampling and a permanent colostomy) was once the treatment of choice for this tumor type. The 5-year survival rate after such a procedure was 55–70% in the absence of spread to regional lymph nodes and <20% if nodal involvement was present. An alternative therapeutic approach combining external beam radiation therapy with concomitant chemotherapy has resulted in biopsy-proven disappearance of all tumor in >80% of patients whose initial lesion was <3 cm in size. Tumor recurrences develop in <10% of these patients, meaning that ~70% of patients with anal cancers can be cured with nonoperative treatment. Surgery should be reserved for the minority of individuals who are found to have residual tumor after being managed initially with radiation therapy combined with chemotherapy.

FURTHER READINGS

BIRD-LIEBERMAN EL, FITZGERALD RC: Early diagnosis of oesophageal cancer. Br J Cancer 101:1, 2009

CRUMP W et al: Lymphoma of the gastrointestinal tract. Semin Oncol 26:324, 1999

DEMETRI GD et al: Efficacy and safety of imatinib mesylate in advanced gastrointestinal stromal tumors. N Engl J Med 347:472, 2002

ENZINGER PC, MAYER RJ: Esophageal cancer. N Engl J Med 349:2241, 2003

HOHENBERGER P, GRETSCHEL S: Gastric cancer. Lancet 362:305, 2003

KOHNE CH, LENZ HJ: Chemotherapy with targeted agents for the treatment of metastatic colorectal cancer. Oncologist 14:478, 2009

LYNCH HT, DE LA CHAPELLE A: Hereditary colorectal cancer. N Engl J Med 348:919, 2003

MCCOURT M et al: Rectal cancer. Surgeon 7:162, 2009

MEYERHARDT JA, MAYER RJ: Systemic therapy for colorectal cancer. N Engl J Med 352:476, 2005

516 ROSTRUM A et al: Nonsteroidal anti-inflammatory drugs and cyclooxygenase-2 inhibitors for primary prevention of colorectal cancer: A systematic review prepared for the US Preventive Services Task Force. Ann Intern Med 146:376, 2007

RYAN DP et al: Carcinoma of the anal canal. N Engl J Med 342:792, 2000

SPECHLER SJ: Barrett's esophagus. N Engl J Med 346:836, 2002

UEMURA N et al: *Helicobacter pylori* infection and the development of gastric cancer. N Engl J Med 345:784, 2001

WAGNER AD, MOEHLER M: Development of targeted therapies in advanced gastric cancer: promising exploratory steps in a new era. Curr Opin Oncol 21:381, 2009

WALSH JME, TERDIMAN JP: Colorectal cancer screening. JAMA 289:1288, 2003

WEITZ J et al: Colorectal cancer. Lancet 365:153, 2005

WOLAN BM et al: Adjuvant treatment of colorectal cancer. CA Cancer Clin J 57:168, 2007

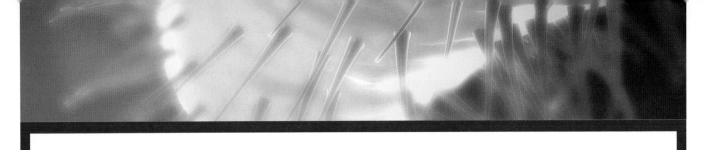

CHAPTER 48

TUMORS OF THE LIVER AND BILIARY TREE

Brian I. Carr

HEPATOCELLULAR CARCINOMA

INCIDENCE

Hepatocellular carcinoma (HCC) is one of the most common malignancies worldwide. The annual global incidence is about 1 million cases, with a male to female ratio of about 4:1. The incidence rate equals the death rate. In the United States, 19,160 new cases and 16,780 deaths were noted in 2007. The death rate in males in low-incidence countries such as the United States is 1.9 per 100,000 per year; in intermediate-incidence areas such as Austria and South Africa, annual death rates range from 5.1-20.0 per 100,000; and in high-incidence areas such as in Asia (China and Korea), death rates are as high as 23.1–150 per 100,000 per year (Table 48-1). The incidence of HCC in the United States is around 3 per 100,000 persons, with significant sex, ethnic, and geographic variations. These numbers are rapidly increasing and may be an underestimate. Around 4 million persons in the United States are chronic carriers of hepatitis C virus (HCV). About 10% of them, or 400,000, are likely to develop cirrhosis. Around 5% or 20,000 of these may develop HCC annually. Add to this the two other common predisposing factors—hepatitis B virus (HBV) and chronic alcohol consumption—and 60,000 new HCC cases annually seem possible. Future advances in HCC survival will likely depend on immunization strategies for HBV and HCV and earlier diagnosis by screening of patients at risk of HCC development.

EPIDEMIOLOGY

Endemic hot spots occur in areas of China and sub-Saharan Africa, which are associated with both high endemic hepatitis B carrier rates and mycotoxin contamination of foodstuffs, stored grains, drinking water, and soil. Environmental factors are important; Japanese in Japan have a higher incidence than those living in Hawaii, who in turn have a higher incidence than those living in California.

ETIOLOGIC FACTORS

Chemical Carcinogens

Probably the best-studied and most potent ubiquitous natural chemical carcinogen is a product of the *Aspergillus* fungus, called aflatoxin B_1. This mold and aflatoxin product can be found in stored grains in hot, humid places, where peanuts and rice are stored in unrefrigerated conditions. Aflatoxin contamination of foodstuffs correlates well with incidence rates in Africa and to some extent in China. In endemic areas of China, even farm animals such as ducks have HCC. The most potent carcinogens appear to be natural products of plants, fungi, and bacteria, such as bush trees containing

TABLE 48-1

AGE-ADJUSTED INCIDENCE RATES FOR HEPATOCELLULAR CARCINOMA

COUNTRY	PERSONS PER 100,000 PER YEAR	
	MALE	FEMALE
Argentina	6.0	2.5
Brazil, Recife	9.2	8.3
Brazil, Sao Paulo	3.8	2.6
Burma	25.5	8.8
China, Shanghai	34.4	11.6
France	6.9	1.2
Gambia	33.1	12.6
Great Britain	1.6	0.8
India, Mumbai	4.9	2.5
India, Chennai	2.1	0.7
Italy, Varese	7.1	2.7
Japan	7.2	2.2
Korea	13.8	3.2
Mozambique	112.9	30.8
Nigeria	15.4	3.2
Norway	1.8	1.1
South Africa, Cape: black	26.3	8.4
South Africa, Cape: white	1.2	0.6
Senegal	25.6	9.0
Spain, Navarra	7.9	4.7

pyrrolizidine alkaloids as well as tannic acid and safrole. Pollutants such as pesticides and insecticides are known rodent carcinogens.

Hepatitis

Both case-control and cohort studies have shown a strong association between chronic hepatitis B carrier rates and increased incidence of HCC. In Taiwanese male postal carriers who were hepatitis B surface antigen (HBsAg)-positive, a 98-fold greater risk for HCC was found compared to HBsAg-negative individuals. The incidence of HCC in Alaskan natives is markedly increased related to a high prevalence of HBV infection. HBV-based HCC may arise from rounds of hepatic destruction with subsequent proliferation and not necessarily from frank cirrhosis. The increase in Japanese HCC incidence rates in the past three decades is thought to be from hepatitis C. A large-scale intervention study sponsored by the World Health Organization (WHO) is currently underway in Asia involving HBV vaccination of the newborn. HCC in African blacks is not associated with severe cirrhosis but is poorly differentiated and very aggressive. Despite uniform HBV carrier rates among the South African Bantu, there is a ninefold difference in HCC incidence between Mozambicans living along the coast and inland. These differences are attributed to the additional exposure to dietary aflatoxin B_1 and other carcinogenic mycotoxins.

A typical interval between HCV-associated transfusion and subsequent HCC is ~30 years. HCV-associated HCC patients tend to have more frequent and advanced cirrhosis, but in HBV-associated HCC, only half the patients have cirrhosis; the remainder have chronic active hepatitis (Chap. 39).

Other Etiologic Conditions

The 75–85% association of HCC with underlying cirrhosis has long been recognized, more typically with macronodular cirrhosis in Southeast Asia but also with micronodular cirrhosis (alcohol) in Europe and the United States (Chap. 41). It is still not clear whether cirrhosis itself is a predisposing factor to the development of HCC or whether the underlying causes of the cirrhosis are actually the carcinogenic factors. However, ~20% of U.S. patients with HCC do not have underlying cirrhosis. Several underlying conditions are associated with an increased risk for cirrhosis-associated HCC (Table 48-2), including hepatitis, alcohol abuse, autoimmune chronic active hepatitis, cryptogenic cirrhosis, and nonalcoholic steatohepatitis (NASH). A less common association is with primary biliary cirrhosis and several metabolic diseases, including hemochromatosis, Wilson's disease, α_1-antitrypsin deficiency, tyrosinemia, porphyria cutanea tarda, glycogenesis types 1 and 3, citrullinemia, and orotic aciduria. The etiology of HCC in those 20% of patients who have no cirrhosis is unclear, and their HCC natural history not well-defined.

CLINICAL FEATURES

Symptoms in HCC patients include abdominal pain, weight loss, weakness, abdominal fullness and swelling, jaundice, and nausea (Table 48-3). Presenting signs and symptoms differ somewhat between high- and low-incidence areas. The most common symptom is abdominal pain in high-risk areas, especially in South African blacks; by contrast, only 40–50% of Chinese and Japanese patients present with abdominal pain. Abdominal

TABLE 48-2

RISK FACTORS FOR HEPATOCELLULAR CARCINOMA

COMMON	UNUSUAL
Cirrhosis from any cause	Primary biliary cirrhosis
Hepatitis B or C chronic infection	Hemochromatosis
	α_1-Antitrypsin deficiency
Ethanol chronic consumption	Glycogen storage diseases
Nonalcoholic steatohepatitis (NASH)	Citrullinemia
	Porphyria cutanea tarda
Aflatoxin B_1 or other mycotoxins	Hereditary tyrosinemia
	Wilson's disease

TABLE 48-3

HEPATOCELLULAR CARCINOMA: CLINICAL PRESENTATION AT THE UNIVERSITY OF PITTSBURGH LIVER CANCER CENTER (*n* = 547)	
	NUMBER OF PATIENTS (%)
Symptom	
No symptom	129 (24)
Abdominal pain	219 (40)
Other (workup of anemia and various diseases)	64 (12)
Routine physical exam finding, elevated LFTs	129 (24)
Weight loss	112 (20)
Appetite loss	59 (11)
Weakness/malaise	83 (15)
Jaundice	30 (5)
Routine CT scan screening of known cirrhosis	92 (17)
Cirrhosis symptoms (ankle swelling, abdominal bloating, increased girth, pruritus, GI bleed)	98 (18)
Diarrhea	7 (1)
Tumor rupture	1
Patient Characteristics	
Mean age (years)	56 ± 13
Male: Female	3:1
Ethnicity	
Caucasian	72%
Middle Eastern	10%
Asian	13%
African American	5%
Cirrhosis	81%
No cirrhosis	19%
Tumor Characteristics	
Hepatic tumor numbers	
1	20%
2	25%
3 or more	65%
Portal vein invasion	75%
Unilobar	25%
Bilobar	75%

Note: LFTs, liver function tests; GI, gastrointestinal.

swelling may occur as a consequence of ascites due to the underlying chronic liver disease or may be due to a rapidly expanding tumor. Occasionally, central necrosis or acute hemorrhage into the peritoneal cavity leads to death. In countries with an active surveillance program, HCC tends to be identified at an earlier stage when symptoms may be due only to the underlying disease. Jaundice is usually due to obstruction of the intrahepatic ducts by the underlying liver disease. Hematemesis may occur due to esophageal varices from the underlying portal hypertension. Bone pain is seen in 3–12% of patients, but necropsies show bone metastases in ~20% of patients. Patients may be asymptomatic.

Physical Signs

Hepatomegaly is the most common physical sign, occurring in 50–90% of patients. Abdominal bruits are noted in 6–25%, and ascites occurs in 30–60% of patients. Ascites should be examined by cytology. Splenomegaly is mainly due to portal hypertension. Weight loss and muscle wasting are common, particularly with rapidly growing or large tumors. Fever is found in 10–50% of patients, from unclear cause. The signs of chronic liver disease may be present, including jaundice, dilated abdominal veins, palmar erythema, gynecomastia, testicular atrophy, and peripheral edema. Budd-Chiari syndrome can occur due to HCC invasion of the hepatic veins; it should be suspected in patients with tense ascites and a large tender liver (Chap. 41).

Paraneoplastic Syndromes

Most paraneoplastic syndromes in HCC are biochemical abnormalities without associated clinical consequences. They include hypoglycemia (also caused by end-stage liver failure), erythrocytosis, hypercalcemia, hypercholesterolemia, dysfibrinogenemia, carcinoid syndrome, increased thyroxin-binding globulin, changes in secondary sex characteristics (gynecomastia, testicular atrophy, and precocious puberty), and porphyria cutanea tarda. Mild hypoglycemia occurs in rapidly growing HCC as part of terminal illness, and profound hypoglycemia may occur, although the cause is unclear. Erythrocytosis occurs in 3–12% of patients, and hypercholesterolemia in 10–40%. A high percentage of patients have thrombocytopenia or leukopenia not caused by cancer infiltration of bone marrow, as in other tumor types.

STAGING

Although the TNM (primary *t*umor, regional *n*odes, *m*etastasis) staging system set up by the American Joint Commission for Cancers (AJCC) is sometimes used, the newer Cancer of the Liver Italian Program (CLIP) system is now popular as it takes cirrhosis into account, as does the Okuda system (Table 48-4). Other staging systems have been proposed and a consensus is needed. The best prognosis is stage I, solitary tumor <2 cm in diameter without vascular invasion. Adverse prognostic features include ascites, vascular invasion, and lymph node spread. Vascular invasion, in particular, has profound effects on prognosis and may be microscopic or macroscopic (visible on CT). Most large tumors have microscopic vascular invasion, so full staging can usually be

made only after surgical resection. Stage III disease contains a mixture of lymph node–positive and –negative tumors. Stage III patients with positive lymph node disease have a poor prognosis, and few patients survive 1 year. The prognosis of stage IV is poor after either resection or transplantation, and 1-year survival is rare. A working staging system based entirely on clinical grounds that incorporates the contribution of the underlying liver disease was originally developed by Okuda et al. (Table 48-4). Patients with Okuda stage III have a dire prognosis, because they usually cannot be curatively resected and the condition of their liver typically precludes chemotherapy.

Approach to the Patient:
HEPATOCELLULAR CARCINOMA

History and Physical The history is important in evaluating putative predisposing factors, including a history of hepatitis or jaundice, blood transfusion, or use of intravenous drugs. A family history of HCC or hepatitis should be sought, and a detailed social history taken to include job descriptions for industrial exposure to possible carcinogenic drugs as well as contraceptive hormones. Physical examination should include assessing stigmata of underlying liver disease such as jaundice, ascites, peripheral edema, spider nevi, palmar erythema, and weight loss. Evaluation of the abdomen for hepatic size, masses or ascites,

TABLE 48-4

CLIP AND OKUDA STAGING SYSTEMS FOR HEPATOCELLULAR CARCINOMA

CLIP CLASSIFICATION

	Points		
Variables	**0**	**1**	**2**
i. Tumor number	Single	Multiple	—
Hepatic replacement by tumor (%)[a]	<50	<50	>50
ii. Child-Pugh score	A	B	C
iii. α-Fetoprotein level (ng/mL)	<400	≥400	—
iv. Portal vein thrombosis (CT)	No	Yes	—

CLIP stages (score = sum of points): CLIP 0, 0 points; CLIP 1, 1 point; CLIP 2, 2 points; CLIP 3, 3 points.

OKUDA CLASSIFICATION

Tumor Size[a]		Ascites		Albumin (g/L)		Bilirubin (mg/dL)	
≥50%	<50	+	−	≤3	>3	≥3	<3
(+)	(−)	(+)	(−)	(+)	(−)	(+)	(−)

Okuda stages: stage 1, all (−); stage 2, 1 or 2 (+); stage 3, 3 or 4 (+).

[a]Extent of liver occupied by tumor.
Note: CLIP, Cancer of the Liver Italian Program.

hepatic nodularity and tenderness, and splenomegaly is needed, as is assessment of overall clinical performance status and psychosocial evaluation.

Serologic Assays α–Fetoprotein (AFP) is a serum tumor marker in HCC; however, it is only increased in about half of U.S. patients. The other widely used assay is that for des-γ-carboxy prothrombin (DCP), a protein induced by vitamin K absence (PIVKA-2). This protein is increased in as many as 80% of HCC patients but may also be elevated in patients with vitamin K deficiency; it is always elevated after use of warfarin. It may predict for portal vein invasion. In a patient presenting with either a new hepatic mass or other indications of recent hepatic decompensation, carcinoembryonic antigen (CEA), vitamin B_{12}, AFP, ferritin, PIVKA-2, and antimitochondrial Ab should be measured, and standard liver function tests should be performed, including prothrombin time (PT), partial thromboplastin time (PTT), albumin, transaminases, γ-glutamyl transpeptidase, and alkaline phosphatase. Decreases in platelet count and white blood cell count may reflect portal hypertension and associated hypersplenism. Hepatitis A, B, and C serology should be measured. If HBV or HCV serology is positive, quantitative measurements of HBV DNA or HCV RNA are needed.

Radiology An ultrasound examination of the liver is an excellent screening tool. The two characteristic vascular abnormalities are hypervascularity of the tumor mass (neovascularization or abnormal tumor-feeding arterial vessels) and thrombosis by tumor invasion of otherwise normal portal veins. To determine tumor size and extent and the presence of portal vein invasion accurately, a helical/triphasic CT scan of the abdomen and pelvis with fast contrast bolus technique should be performed to detect the vascular lesions typical of HCC. Portal vein invasion is normally detected as an obstruction and expansion of the vessel. A chest CT is used to exclude metastases. MRI can also provide detailed information, especially with the newer contrast agents. Ethiodol (Lipiodol) is an ethiodized oil emulsion retained by liver tumors that can be delivered by hepatic artery injection (5–15 mL) for CT imaging 1 week later. For small tumors, ethiodol injection is very helpful before biopsy because its histologic presence constitutes proof that the needle biopsied the mass under suspicion. A prospective comparison of triphasic CT, gadolinium-enhanced MRI, ultrasound, and fluorodeoxyglucose positron emission tomography (FDG-PET) scans demonstrated similar results for CT, MRI, and ultrasound; PET imaging was unsuccessful.

Pathologic Diagnosis Histologic proof of the presence of HCC is obtained through a core liver biopsy of the mass under ultrasound guidance as well as random biopsy of the underlying liver. Bleeding risk is increased compared to other cancers because (1) the tumors are hypervascular, and (2) patients often have thrombocytopenia and decreased clotting factors. Bleeding risk is further increased in the presence of ascites. Tracking of tumor has been an uncommon problem. Fine-needle aspirates may provide sufficient material for diagnosis of cancer, but core biopsies are preferred. Tissue architecture must be examined to distinguish between HCC and metastatic adenocarcinoma; laparoscopic approaches can also be used. For patients suspected of having portal vein involvement, a core biopsy of the portal vein may be performed safely. If positive, this is regarded as an exclusion criterion for transplantation for HCC.

SCREENING HIGH-RISK POPULATIONS

Screening has not been shown to save lives. Prospective studies in high-risk populations showed that ultrasound was more sensitive than AFP elevations. An Italian study in patients with cirrhosis identified a yearly HCC incidence of 3% but showed no increase in the rate of detection of potentially curable tumors with aggressive screening. Prevention strategies including universal vaccination against hepatitis viruses are more likely to be effective than screening efforts. Despite absence of formal guidelines, most practitioners obtain 6-monthly AFP levels and perform CT (or ultrasound) when following high-risk patients (HBV carriers, HCV cirrhosis, family history of HCC).

℞ **Treatment:**
HEPATOCELLULAR CARCINOMA

Most HCC patients have two liver diseases, cirrhosis and HCC, each of which is an independent cause of death. The presence of cirrhosis usually places constraints on resection surgery, ablative therapies, and chemotherapy. Thus patient assessment and treatment planning have to take the severity of the nonmalignant liver disease into account. The clinical management choices for HCC can be complex (**Fig. 48-1**). The natural history of HCC is highly variable. Patients presenting with advanced tumors (vascular invasion, symptoms, extrahepatic spread) have a median survival of ~4 months, with or without treatment. Treatment results from the literature are difficult to interpret. Survival is not always a measure of the efficacy of therapy because of the adverse effects on survival of the underlying liver disease. A multidisciplinary team, including a hepatologist, interventional

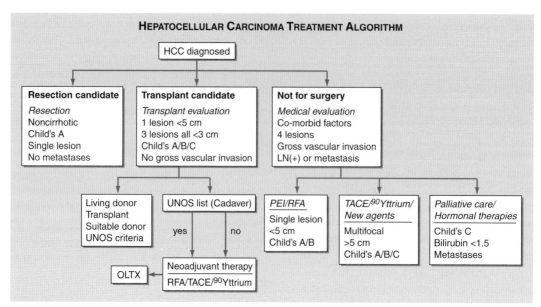

FIGURE 48-1

Treatment approach to patients with hepatocellular carcinoma. The initial clinical evaluation is aimed at assessing the extent of the tumor and the underlying functional compromise of the liver by cirrhosis. Patients are classified as having resectable disease, unresectable disease, or as transplantation candidates. Abbreviations: OLTX, orthotopic liver transplantation; TACE, transarterial chemoembolization; PEI, percutaneous ethanol injection; RFA, radiofrequency ablation; LN, lymph node. Child's A/B/C refers to the Child-Pugh classification of liver failure.

radiologist, surgical oncologist, transplant surgeon, and medical oncologist, is important for the comprehensive management of HCC patients.

STAGES I AND II HCC Early-stage tumors are successfully treated using various techniques, including surgical resection, local ablation (thermal or radiofrequency), and local injection therapies (ethanol or acetic acid). Because the majority of patients with HCC suffer from a field defect in the cirrhotic liver, they are at risk for subsequent multiple primary liver tumors. Many will also have significant underlying liver disease and may not tolerate major surgical loss of hepatic parenchyma; they may be eligible for orthotopic liver transplant (OLTX) in the future. An important principle in treating early-stage HCC is to use liver-sparing treatments and to focus on treatment of both the tumor and the cirrhosis.

Surgical Excision The risk of major hepatectomy is high (5–10% mortality) due to the underlying liver disease and the potential for liver failure. Preoperative portal vein occlusion can sometimes be performed to cause atrophy of the HCC-involved lobe and compensatory hypertrophy of the noninvolved liver, permitting safer resection. Intraoperative ultrasound is useful for planning the surgical approach. In cirrhotic patients, any major liver surgery can result in liver failure. The Child-Pugh classification of liver

failure (Chap. 34) is a reliable prognosticator for tolerance of hepatic surgery, and only Child A patients should be considered for surgical resection. Child B and C patients with stages I and II HCC should be referred for OLTX if appropriate, as should patients with ascites or a recent history of variceal bleeding. Although open surgical excision is the most reliable, the patient may be better served with a laparoscopic approach to resection, using RFA or percutaneous ethanol injection (PEI). No adequate comparisons of these different techniques have been undertaken, and the choice of treatment is usually based on physician skill.

Local Ablation Strategies Radiofrequency ablation (RFA) uses heat to ablate tumors. The maximum size of the probe arrays allows for a 7-cm zone of necrosis, which would be adequate for a 3- to 4-cm tumor. The heat reliably kills cells within the zone of necrosis. Treatment of tumors close to the main portal pedicles can lead to bile duct injury and obstruction. This limits the tumors that are anatomically suited for this technique. RFA can be performed percutaneously with CT or ultrasound guidance, or by laparoscopy with ultrasound guidance.

Local Injection Therapy Numerous agents have been used for local injection into tumors, most commonly, ethanol (PEI). The relatively soft HCC within the hard background of cirrhotic liver allows for injection of large volumes of ethanol into the tumor without diffusion into the hepatic parenchyma or leakage out of the liver. PEI causes direct destruction of cancer cells, but it is not selective for cancer cells and will destroy normal cells in the vicinity. It usually requires multiple injections (average of three), in contrast to one for RFA. The maximum size of tumor reliably treated is 3 cm, even with multiple injections.

Liver Transplantation A viable option for stages I and II tumors in the setting of cirrhosis is OLTX, with survival approaching that for noncancer cases. OLTX for patients with a single lesion ≤5 cm or three or fewer nodules, each ≤3 cm (Milan criteria), resulted in excellent tumor-free survival (≥70% at 5 years). For advanced HCC, OLTX has been abandoned due to high tumor recurrence rates. Priority scoring for OLTX previously led to HCC patients waiting too long for their OLTX, resulting in some tumors becoming too advanced during the patient's wait for a donated liver. A variety of therapies were used as a "bridge" to OLTX, including RFA, PEI, and transarterial chemoembolization (TACE). These pretransplant treatments allow patients to remain on the waiting list longer, giving them greater opportunities to be transplanted. What remains unclear is whether this translates into prolonged survival after transplant. Further, it is not known whether patients who have had their tumor(s) treated preoperatively follow the recurrence pattern predicted by their tumor status at the time of transplant (i.e., post local ablative therapy), or if they follow the course set by their tumor parameters present before such treatment. The United Network for Organ Sharing (UNOS) point system for priority scoring of OLTX recipients now includes additional points for patients with HCC. The success of living related donor liver transplantation programs has also led to patients receiving transplantation earlier for HCC and often with greater than minimal tumors.

Adjuvant Therapy The role of adjuvant chemotherapy for patients after resection or OLTX remains unclear. No clear advantage in disease-free or overall survival has been found for either adjuvant or neoadjuvant approaches, though a meta-analysis of several trials revealed a significant improvement in disease-free and overall survival. Analysis of postoperative adjuvant systemic chemotherapy trials demonstrated no disease-free or overall survival advantage, but single studies of TACE and neoadjuvant ^{131}I-ethiodol have shown enhanced survival after resection.

Stages III and IV HCC Fewer surgical options exist for stage III tumors. In patients without cirrhosis, a major hepatectomy is feasible, although prognosis is poor. Patients with Child's A cirrhosis may be resected, but a lobectomy is associated with significant morbidity and

mortality, and long-term prognosis is poor. Nevertheless, a small percentage of patients will achieve long-term survival, justifying an attempt at resection when feasible. Because of the advanced nature of these tumors, even successful resection can be followed by rapid recurrence. These patients are not considered candidates for transplantation because of the high tumor recurrence rates, unless their tumors can first be down-staged with neoadjuvant therapy. Decreasing the size of the primary tumor allows for less surgery, and the delay in surgery allows for extrahepatic disease to manifest on imaging studies and avoid unhelpful OLTX. The prognosis is poor for stage IV tumors, and no surgical treatment is recommended.

Systemic Chemotherapy A large number of controlled and uncontrolled clinical studies have been performed with most of the major classes of cancer chemotherapy. No single agent or combination of agents given systemically reproducibly leads to even a 25% response rate or has any effect on survival.

Regional Chemotherapy In contrast to the dismal results of systemic chemotherapy, a variety of agents given via the hepatic artery have activity in HCC confined to the liver (Table 48-5). Two randomized controlled trials have shown a survival advantage for TACE in a selected subset of patients. One used doxorubicin and the other used cisplatin. Despite the fact that increased hepatic extraction of chemotherapy has been shown for very few drugs, some drugs such as cisplatin, doxorubicin, mitomycin C, and possibly neocarzinostatin produce substantial objective responses when administered regionally. Few data are available on continuous hepatic arterial infusion for HCC, although pilot studies with cisplatin have shown encouraging responses. Because the reports have not usually stratified responses or survival based on TNM staging, it is difficult to know long-term prognosis in relation to tumor extent. Most of the studies on regional hepatic arterial chemotherapy also use an embolizing agent such as ethiodol, gelatin sponge particles (Gelfoam), starch (Spherex), or microspheres. Two products are composed of microspheres of defined size ranges–Embospheres (Biospheres) and Contour SE–using particles of 40–120, 100–300, 300–500, and 500–1000 μm in size. The optimal diameter of the particles for TACE has yet to be defined. Consistently higher objective response rates appear to be reported for arterial administration of drugs together with some form of hepatic artery occlusion compared with any form of systemic chemotherapy to date. The widespread use of some form of embolization in addition to chemotherapy has added to its toxicities. These include a frequent but transient fever, abdominal pain, and anorexia (all in >60% of patients). In addition, >20% of patients have increased ascites or transient elevation of transaminases. Cystic artery spasm and cholecystitis

TABLE 48-5

SOME RANDOMIZED CLINICAL TRIALS INVOLVING TRANSHEPATIC ARTERY CHEMOEMBOLIZATION (TACE) FOR HEPATOCELLULAR CARCINOMA				
AUTHOR	**YEAR**	**AGENTS 1**	**AGENTS 2**	**SURVIVAL EFFECT**
Kawaii	1992	Doxorubicin + embo	Embo	No
Chang	1994	Cisplatin + embo	Embo	No
Hatanaka	1995	Cisplatin, doxorubicin + embo	Same + ethiodol	No
Uchino	1993	Cisplatin, doxorubicin + oral FU	Same + tamoxifen	No
Lin	1988	Embo	Embo + IV FU	No
Yoshikawa	1994	Epirubicin + ethiodol (Lipiodol)	Epirubicin	No
Pelletier	1990	Doxorubicin + Gelfoam	None	No
Trinchet	1995	Cisplatin + Gelfoam	None	No
Bruix	1998	Coils and Gelfoam	None	No
Pelletier	1998	Cisplatin + ethiodol	None	No
Trinchet	1995	Cisplatin + Gelfoam	None	No
Pelletier	1998	Cisplatin + ethiodol	None	No
Lo	2002	Cisplatin + ethiodol	None	Yes
Llovet	2002	Doxorubicin + ethiodol	None	Yes

Note: embo, embolization; FU, fluorouracil.

are also not uncommon. However, higher responses have also been obtained. The hepatic toxicities associated with embolization may be ameliorated by the use of degradable starch microspheres, with 50–60% response rates. A major problem in showing a survival advantage in patients responding to TACE is that many patients die of their underlying cirrhosis, not the tumor. However, improving patient quality of life is a legitimate goal of regional therapies.

Experimental Therapies Several therapies are being evaluated (Table 48-6). Epidermal growth factor (EGF) receptor antibodies and EGF receptor kinase inhibitors are in clinical trials, as are various anti-angiogenesis therapies. No effects on survival are yet reported. Oral sorafenib increases median survival from 6 to 9 months in advanced, unresectable HCC. Several forms of *radiation therapy* have been used in the treatment of HCC, including external beam and conformal radiation therapy. Radiation hepatitis remains a significant dose-limiting problem. The pure beta emitter ^{90}yttrium attached to either glass or resin microspheres has been assessed in phase II trials of HCC and has encouraging survival effects with minimal toxicities. Randomized trials have yet to be performed. Vitamin K has been assessed in clinical trials at high dosage for its HCC-inhibitory actions. This idea is based on the characteristic biochemical defect in HCC of elevated plasma levels of immature prothrombin (DCP or PIVKA-2), due to a defect in the activity of prothrombin carboxylase, a vitamin K–dependent enzyme. Two vitamin K randomized controlled trials from Japan show decreased tumor occurrence. Patient participation in clinical trials aimed at assessing new therapies is encouraged.

TABLE 48-6

SOME NOVEL MEDICAL TREATMENTS FOR HEPATOCELLULAR CARCINOMA
EGF receptor antibody
Erlotinib, Gefitinib
Kinase antagonists, Sorafenib
Vitamin K
IL–2
^{131}I – ethiodol (Lipiodol)
^{131}I – Ferritin
^{90}Yttrium microspheres
^{166}Holmium
Three-dimensional conformal radiation
Proton beam high-dose radiotherapy
Anti-angiogenesis strategies, Bevacizumab

Note: EGF, epidermal growth factor; IL, interleukin.

SUMMARY

Most Common Modes of Patient Presentation

1. A patient with known history of hepatitis, jaundice, or cirrhosis, with an abnormality on ultrasound or CT scan, or rising AFP or DCP (PIVKA-2)
2. A patient with an abnormal liver function test as part of a routine examination
3. Radiologic workup for liver transplant for cirrhosis
4. Symptoms of HCC including cachexia, abdominal pain, or fever.

History and Physical Examination

1. Clinical jaundice, asthenia, itching (scratches), tremors, or disorientation

2. Hepatomegaly, splenomegaly, ascites, peripheral edema, skin signs of liver failure.

Clinical Evaluation

1. Blood tests: full blood count (splenomegaly), liver function tests, ammonia levels, electrolytes, α-fetoprotein and DCP (PIVKA-2), Ca^{2+} and Mg^{2+}; hepatitis B and C serology (and quantitative HBV DNA or HCV RNA, if either is positive); neurotensin (specific for fibrolamellar HCC)
2. Triphasic dynamic helical (spiral) CT scan of liver (if inadequate, then follow with an MRI); chest CT scan; upper and lower gastrointestinal endoscopy (for varices, bleeding, ulcers); and brain scan (only if symptoms suggest)
3. A core biopsy: of the tumor and separately of the underlying liver.

Therapy

(See also Fig. 48-1)

1. HCC <2 cm: RFA ablation, PEI, or resection
2. HCC >2 cm, no vascular invasion: liver resection, RFA, or OLTX
3. Multiple unilobar tumors or tumor with vascular invasion: TACE
4. Bilobar tumors, no vascular invasion: TACE with OLTX for patients whose tumors have a response
5. Extrahepatic HCC or elevated bilirubin: Phase I and II studies.

OTHER PRIMARY LIVER TUMORS

FIBROLAMELLAR HCC (FL-HCC)

This rarer variant of HCC has a different biology than adult-type HCC. None of the known HCC causative factors seem important here. It is typically a disease of younger adults, often teenagers and predominantly females. It is AFP negative, but patients typically have elevated blood neurotensin levels, normal liver function tests, and no cirrhosis. Radiology is similar for HCC, except that characteristic adult-type portal vein invasion is less common. Although it is often multifocal in the liver, and therefore not resectable, metastases are common, especially to lungs and locoregional lymph nodes, but survival is often much better than with adult-type HCC. Resectable tumors are associated with 5-year survival of ≥50%. Patients often present with a huge liver or unexplained weight loss, fever, or elevated liver function tests on routine evaluations. These huge masses suggest slow growth. Surgical resection is the best management option, even for metastases, since these tumors respond much less well to chemotherapy than adult-type HCC. Although several series of OLTX for FL-HCC have

been reported, the patients usually to die from tumor recurrences, with a 2- to 5-year lag compared with OLTX for adult-type HCC. Anecdotal responses to gemcitabine plus cisplatin-TACE are reported.

EPITHELIOID HEMANGIOENDOTHELIOMA (EHE)

This rare vascular tumor of adults is also usually multifocal and can also be associated with prolonged survival, even in the presence of metastases, which are commonly in the lung. There is usually no underlying cirrhosis. Histologically, these tumors are usually of borderline malignancy and express factor VIII antigen, confirming their endothelial origin. OLTX may be associated with prolonged survival.

CHOLANGIOCARCINOMA (CCC)

CCC typically refers to mucin-producing adenocarcinomas (different from HCC) that arise from the bile ducts. They are grouped by their anatomic site of origin as intrahepatic, hilar (central, ~65% of CCCs), and peripheral (or distal, ~30% of CCCs). They arise on the basis of cirrhosis less frequently than HCC, excepting primary biliary cirrhosis. Nodular tumors arising at the bifurcation of the common bile duct are called *Klatskin tumors* and are often associated with a collapsed gallbladder, a finding that mandates visualization of the entire biliary tree. The approach to management of central and peripheral CCC is quite different. The incidence seems to be increasing in the United States. Although most CCCs have no obvious cause, several predisposing factors have been identified, including primary sclerosing cholangitis, an autoimmune disease (10–20% of PSC patients), and liver fluke in Asians, especially *Opisthorchis viverrini* and *Clonorchis sinensis*. CCC seems also to be associated with any cause of chronic biliary inflammation and injury, with alcoholic liver disease, choledocholithiasis, choledochal cysts (10%), and Caroli's disease. CCC most typically presents as painless jaundice, often with pruritus or weight loss, and acholic stools. Diagnosis is made by biopsy, percutaneously for peripheral liver lesions or, more commonly, via endoscopic retrograde cholangiopancreatography (ERCP) under direct vision for central lesions. The tumors often stain positively for cytokeratins 7, 8, and 19 and negatively for cytokeratin 20. However, histology alone cannot usually distinguish CCC from metastases from primary tumors of the colon or pancreas. Serologic tumor markers appear to be nonspecific, but CEA, CA 19-9, and CA-125 are often elevated in CCC patients and are useful for following response to therapy. Radiologic evaluation typically starts with ultrasound, which is useful in visualizing dilated bile ducts, and then proceeds with either MRI or magnetic resonance cholangiopancreatography (MRCP) or helical

CT scans. Invasive ERCP is then needed to define the biliary tree and obtain a biopsy or is needed therapeutically to decompress an obstructed biliary tree with internal stent placement. If that fails, then percutaneous biliary drainage will be needed, with the biliary drainage flowing into an external bag. Central tumors often invade the porta hepatis, and locoregional lymph node involvement by tumor is frequent.

℞ Treatment: CHOLANGIOCARCINOMA

Hilar CCC is resectable in ~30% of patients and usually involves bile duct resection and lymphadenectomy. Typical survival is around 24 months, with recurrences being mainly in the operative bed but with ~30% in the lungs and liver. Distal CCC, which involves the main ducts, is normally treated by resection of the extrahepatic bile ducts, often with pancreaticoduodenectomy. Survival is similar. Due to the high rates of locoregional recurrences or positive surgical margins, many patients get treated with postoperative adjuvant radiotherapy. Its effect on survival has not been assessed. Intraluminal brachyradiotherapy has also shown some promise. However, photodynamic therapy enhanced survival in one study. In this technique, sodium porfimer is injected IV and then subjected to intraluminal red light laser photoactivation. OLTX has been assessed for treatment of unresectable CCC, but 5-year survival was previously ~20%, so enthusiasm waned. However, neoadjuvant radiotherapy with sensitizing chemotherapy has shown better survival rates for CCC treated by OLTX from one institution; confirmation is needed. Multiple chemotherapeutic agents have been assessed for activity and survival in unresectable CCC. Most have been inactive. However, both systemic and hepatic arterial gemcitabine have shown promising results. The combination of this drug with others and with radiotherapy is being explored.

GALLBLADDER CANCER (GB Ca)

GB Ca has an even worse prognosis than CCC, with typical survival ~6 months or less. Women are affected much more commonly than men (4:1), unlike in HCC or CCC, and GB Ca is more common than CCC. Most patients have a history of gallstones, but very few patients with gallstones develop GB Ca (~0.2%). It presents similarly to CCC and is often diagnosed unexpectedly during gallstone or cholecystitis surgery. Presentation is typically that of chronic cholecystitis, chronic right upper quadrant pain and weight loss. Useful but nonspecific serum markers include CEA and CA 19-9. CT scans or MRCP typically reveal a gallbladder mass. The mainstay of treatment is surgical, either simple or radical cholecystectomy for stages I or II disease, respectively. Survival is nearly 100% at 5 years for stage I, and ranges from 60–90% at 5 years for stage II. More advanced GB Ca has worse survival, and many are unresectable. Adjuvant radiotherapy, used in the presence of local lymph node disease, has not been shown to enhance survival. Similar to CCC, chemotherapy is not useful in advanced or metastatic GB Ca.

CARCINOMA OF THE AMPULLA OF VATER

This tumor arises within 2 cm of the distal end of the common bile duct, and is mainly (90%) an adenocarcinoma. Locoregional lymph nodes are commonly involved (50%), and the liver is the most frequent site for metastases. The commonest clinical presentation is jaundice, and many patients also have pruritus, weight loss, and epigastric pain. Initial evaluation is performed with an abdominal ultrasound to assess vascular involvement, biliary dilatation, and liver lesions. This is followed by a CT scan, or MRI and especially MRCP. The most effective therapy is resection by pylorus-sparing pancreaticoduodenectomy, an aggressive procedure resulting in better survival rates than local resection. Survival rates are ~25% at 5 years in operable patients with involved lymph nodes and ~50% in patients without involved nodes. Unlike CCC, ~80% of patients are thought to be resectable at diagnosis. Adjuvant chemotherapy or radiotherapy has not been shown to be useful in enhancing survival. For metastatic tumors, chemotherapy is currently experimental.

TUMORS METASTATIC TO THE LIVER

These are predominantly from colon, pancreas, and breast primary tumors but can originate from any organ primary. Ocular melanomas are prone to liver metastasis. Tumor spread to the liver normally carries a poor prognosis for that tumor type. Colorectal and breast hepatic metastases were previously treated with continuous hepatic arterial infusion chemotherapy. However, more effective systemic drugs for these cancers, especially the addition of oxaliplatin to colorectal cancer regimens, have reduced the use of hepatic artery infusion therapy. In a large randomized study of systemic versus infusional plus systemic chemotherapy for resected colorectal metastases to the liver, the patients receiving infusional therapy had no survival advantage, mainly due to extrahepatic tumor spread. ^{90}Yttrium resin beads are approved in the United States for treatment of colorectal hepatic metastases. The role of this modality, either alone or in combination with chemotherapy, is being evaluated in many centers. Palliation may be obtained from chemoembolization, PEI, or RFA.

BENIGN LIVER TUMORS

Three common benign tumors occur and all are found predominantly in women. They are *hemangiomas*, *adenomas*, and *focal nodular hyperplasia* (FNH). FNH is typically benign, and usually no treatment is needed. Hemangiomas are the commonest and are entirely benign. Treatment is unnecessary unless their expansion causes symptoms. Adenomas are associated with contraceptive hormone use. They can cause pain and can bleed or rupture, causing acute problems. Their main interest for the physician is a low potential for malignant change and a 30% risk of bleeding. For this reason, considerable effort has gone into differentiating these three entities radiologically. Upon discovery of a liver mass, patients are usually advised to stop taking sex steroids, since adenoma regression may then occasionally occur. Adenomas can often be large masses ranging from 8–15 cm. Due to their size and definite, but low, malignant potential and potential for bleeding, adenomas are typically resected. The most useful diagnostic differentiating tool is a triphasic CT scan performed with HCC fast bolus protocol for arterial-phase imaging, together with subsequent delayed venous-phase imaging. Adenomas usually do not appear on the basis of cirrhosis, although both adenomas and HCCs are intensely vascular on the CT arterial phase and both can exhibit hemorrhage (40% of adenomas). However, adenomas have smooth, well-defined edges and enhance homogeneously, especially in the portal venous phase on delayed images, when HCCs no longer enhance. FNHs exhibit a characteristic central scar that is hypovascular on the arterial-phase and hypervascular on the delayed-phase CT images. MRI is even more sensitive in depicting the characteristic central scar of FNH.

FURTHER READINGS

BARTLETT DL: Intrahepatic cholangiocarcinoma: a worthy challenge. Cancer J 15:255, 2009

FURUKAWA H et al: Living-donor liver transplantation for hepatocellular carcinoma. J Hepatobiliary Pancreat Surg 13:393, 2006

GOIN JE et al: Treatment of unresectable hepatocellular carcinoma with intrahepatic yttrium 90 microspheres. J Vasc Interv Radiol 16:161, 2005

LLOVET JM et al: A molecular signature to discriminate dysplastic nodules from early hepatocellular carcinoma. Gastroenterology 131:1758, 2006

MENDIZABAL M, REDDY KR: Current management of hepatocellular carcinoma. Med Clin North Am 93:885, 2009

PARIKH S, HYMAN D: Hepatocellular cancer: A guide for the internist. Am J Med 120:194, 2007

STEEL JL et al: Clinically meaningful changes in health-related quality of life in patients with hepatobiliary cancer. Ann Oncol 17:304, 2006

THORGEIRSSON S et al: Molecular prognostication of liver cancer: End of the beginning. J Hepatol 44:798, 2006

VERSLYPE C et al: The management of hepatocellular carcinoma. Current expert opinion and recommendations derived from the 10th World Congress on Gastrointestinal Cancer, Barcelona, 2008. Ann Oncol 20 (suppl 7):vii1, 2009

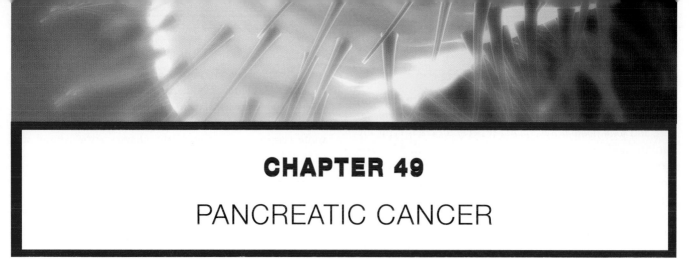

CHAPTER 49

PANCREATIC CANCER

Yu Jo Chua ■ David Cunningham

Over 90% of pancreatic cancers are ductal adenocarcinomas of the exocrine pancreas. These tumors occur twice as frequently in the pancreatic head compared to the rest of the organ, and tend to be aggressive, often presenting when locally inoperable or after distal metastases have occurred. Patients with pancreatic cancer have a poor prognosis, with a 5-year survival of only 5%. The discussion of pancreatic cancer here will be limited to ductal adenocarcinomas. Other types of pancreatic neoplasms include islet cell tumors and neuroendocrine tumors (Chap. 50).

INCIDENCE AND ETIOLOGY

Epidemiology

The lifetime risk of being diagnosed with pancreatic cancer in the United States is 1.27%. In the United States, it is estimated that approximately 37,170 people will be diagnosed with pancreatic cancer in 2007. Consistent with its associated poor prognosis, 33,370 are expected to die from this disease in the same year, making it the fourth leading cause of cancer-related death. The median age of diagnosis of pancreatic cancer is 72 years, with the peak incidence of diagnosis between the ages of 65 and 84; it is rarely diagnosed in those below the age of 50. The incidence is slightly higher in men than women, and it is also higher in African Americans than in Caucasians.

Etiology

Cigarette smoking, obesity, and nonhereditary chronic pancreatitis appear to be risk factors for the development of pancreatic cancer. With smoking, the risk seems to increase with the number of cigarettes consumed and decreases with smoking cessation. Less clear, and sometimes conflicting associations, have been observed for other environmental factors such as diet, coffee and alcohol consumption, previous partial gastrectomy or cholecystectomy, and *Helicobacter pylori*. An epidemiologic association between diabetes mellitus and pancreatic cancer has also been demonstrated; however, it is uncertain if diabetes is a precedent of, or consequence of, pancreatic cancer.

GENETIC CONSIDERATIONS

Five to 10% of patients with pancreatic cancer also have an affected first-degree relative, suggesting that in some cases genetic factors are involved. These patients seem to present earlier than sporadic cases. The risk of pancreatic cancer is increased in certain syndromes, whether directly or indirectly, such as hereditary chronic pancreatitis, Peutz-Jeghers syndrome, Von Hippel-Lindau syndrome, familial atypical multiple-mole melanoma syndrome, ataxia-telangiectasia, Gardner's syndrome [a variant of familial adenomatous polyposis (FAP)] and Lynch syndrome II, a subtype of hereditary nonpolyposis colorectal cancer (HNPCC). Heavy smokers who also have homozygous deletions of the gene for glutathione-S transferase T1 (GSTT1), a carcinogen metabolizing enzyme, may be at particular risk. Activating mutations in the K-*ras* oncogene are found in nearly all pancreatic cancer. Loss-of-function mutations in several tumor suppressor genes occur in this disease, including p53, *CDKN2A* gene (also called multiple tumor suppressor-1 gene, leading in many cases to loss of function of p16), *DPC4,* and *BRCA2*. A feature almost unique to pancreatic cancer is the combination of K-*ras* and *CDKN2A* mutations.

CLINICAL FEATURES

Presenting Features

Common presenting features of pancreatic cancer include pain (present in >80% of patients with locally advanced or metastatic disease), obstructive jaundice, weight loss, and anorexia. Patients with jaundice may also have pruritus, pale stools, and dark urine; they often have tumors in the pancreatic head, and tend to be diagnosed earlier and with earlier stage disease. Other symptoms tend to be more insidious, so that in the absence of jaundice, the interval between onset and diagnosis can be prolonged. Pain, for example, is often more of a problem in patients with lesions in the body or tail of the pancreas where the primary tumor is more likely to become quite large or to invade adjacent structures (such as the splanchnic nerves) before becoming manifest; these patients frequently have inoperable disease. When present, pain is often felt as a dull ache in the upper abdomen and may radiate to the back, and characteristically may improve upon leaning forward. It may initially be intermittent, and may worsen with meals. These patients may suffer from marked weight loss, which may result from a combination of anorexia, early satiety, malabsorption or diarrhea/steatorrhea. Other less common presenting features include the diagnosis of glucose intolerance (particularly within 2 years of cancer diagnosis), previous pancreatitis, migratory superficial thrombophlebitis (Trousseau's syndrome), gastrointestinal hemorrhage from varices, and splenomegaly.

Physical Findings

Patients with early disease may not have any significant abnormalities detectable on physical examination. Jaundice may be a presenting feature in some; in these patients a palpable, nontender gallbladder (Courvoisier's sign) may be palpated under the right costal margin. Patients with more advanced disease may have an abdominal mass, hepatomegaly, splenomegaly, or ascites. The left supraclavicular lymph node (Virchow's node) may be involved with tumor, or widespread peritoneal disease may be palpable on rectal examination in the pouch of Douglas.

DIAGNOSTIC PROCEDURES

Imaging Studies

(Fig. 49-1) Ultrasound is often used as an initial investigation for patients with jaundice, or with less-specific symptoms such as upper abdominal discomfort, and is able to assess the biliary tract, gall bladder, pancreas, and liver. Computed tomography (CT) scanning is preferable to ultrasound even though it is more costly, as it is less operator-dependent, more reproducible, and less susceptible to interference from intestinal gas. The sensitivity and specificity of CT is markedly improved by the use of pancreatic protocol scanning on modern multislice scanners. CT may show a pancreatic mass, dilatation of the biliary system or pancreatic duct, or distal spread to the liver, regional lymph nodes, or peritoneum (and/or associated ascites). When helical CT is combined with the use of intravenous contrast, it may also help determine resectability by providing information on the involvement of important vascular structures such as the celiac axis, superior mesenteric or portal vessels. Endoscopic retrograde cholangiopancreatography (ERCP) is also widely used in the diagnosis of pancreatic cancer, particularly when CT and ultrasound fail to show a mass lesion, and may reveal either stricture or obstruction in either the pancreatic or common bile duct. ERCP can also be used to obtain brushings of a stricture for cytology or for placing stents in order to relieve obstructive jaundice. Endoscopic ultrasound (EUS) may be useful in the diagnosis of small lesions (<2–3 cm in diameter) and, in some cases, for local staging as well as evaluating invasion of major vascular structures. EUS-guided fine-needle aspiration may also be used to obtain cytology for confirming the diagnosis, particularly in patients with potentially operable disease (see later). While magnetic resonance imaging (MRI) does not offer any advantages over CT in the routine evaluation of patients with possible pancreatic cancer, magnetic resonance cholangiopancreatography (MRCP) may be better than CT for defining the anatomy of the pancreatic duct and biliary tree, being able to image the ducts both above and below a stricture. The sensitivity of MRCP is comparable to ERCP, but does not require contrast administration to the ductal system, so that there is less associated morbidity. MRCP may be useful when cannulation of the pancreatic duct by ERCP has been unsuccessful or may be difficult, such as when normal anatomy is changed by surgery. Positron-emission tomography with ^{18}F-fluoro-2deoxyglucose (FDG-PET) may be useful for excluding occult distal metastasis in patients with localized disease who are being worked up for surgery or in patients with unresectable localized disease being considered for chemoradiotherapy.

Tissue Diagnosis and Cytology

Patients with disease that is potentially curable by surgery, and in whom a highly suspicious lesion is seen on imaging, are often taken directly to surgery without prior tissue confirmation of cancer. This is because of theoretical concerns that a percutaneous fine-needle aspiration may result in dissemination of cancer

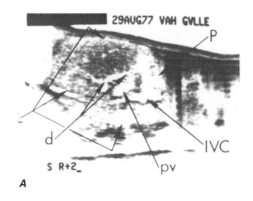

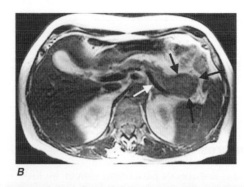

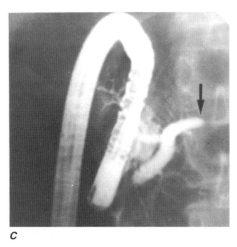

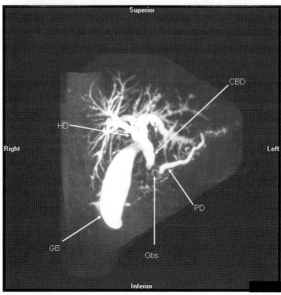

FIGURE 49-1

Carcinoma of the pancreas. _A._ Sonogram showing pancreatic carcinoma (P), dilated intrahepatic bile ducts (d), dilated portal vein (pv), and inferior vena cava (IVC). **_B._** Computed tomography scan showing pancreatic carcinoma (_dark arrows_). **_C._** Endoscopic retrograde showing abrupt cutoff of the duct of Wirsung (_arrow_). **_D._** Magnetic resonance cholangiopancreatography showing obstruction (Obs) in the pancreatic duct (PD). The gallbladder (GB), hepatic duct (HD), and common bile duct (CBD) are labeled.

intraperitoneally or along the track of the biopsy needle. In addition, negative cytology may not be sufficient evidence to avoid surgery, particularly with small lesions. EUS-guided fine-needle aspiration is increasingly being used, even in patients with potentially resectable disease, as there is less risk of intraperitoneal spread of cancer. Other methods of obtaining specimens for cytological analysis include sampling of pancreatic juices or brushings of ductal lesions obtained by ERCP.

Serum Markers

The most widely used serum marker in pancreatic cancer is cancer-associated antigen 19-9 (CA 19-9). It has a reported sensitivity and specificity of about 80–90%, and is suggestive, rather than confirmatory, of the diagnosis of pancreatic cancer. Serum levels of CA 19-9 can be elevated in patients with jaundice without pancreatic cancer present. The level of CA 19-9 may have prognostic implications, with very high levels sometimes found in patients with inoperable disease. In advanced disease, patients treated with chemotherapy who had high pretreatment levels of CA 19-9 have also been found to have a worse survival, whereas those patients whose levels of marker fell with treatment had a better outcome. In patients with cancers with elevated CA 19-9, serial evaluation of this marker is useful for monitoring responses to treatment. In patients with completely resected tumors, follow-up with CA 19-9 is useful for detecting recurrence.

Staging

In pancreatic cancer, which has a poor prognosis, the value of detailed clinical staging is limited. The most clinically relevant distinction to make is between patients with disease that may be resected with curative intent, and those with advanced disease in whom treatment is palliative (Table 49-1).

TABLE 49-1

STAGING OF PANCREATIC CARCINOMA

	STAGE GROUPING	TNM STAGING[a]
Localized resectable	I	T1–2 N0 M0
	II	T3 N0 M0 or T1–3 N1 M0
Locally advanced	III	T4 N(any) M0
Metastatic	IV	T(any) N(any) M1

[a]TNM, tumor, nodes, metastasis.

Note: T1, tumor limited to pancreas, ≤2 cm; T2, tumor limited to pancreas, >2 cm; T3, tumor extends beyond the pancreas but without involvement of celiac axis or superior mesenteric artery; T4, tumor involves celiac axis or the superior mesenteric artery (unresectable primary tumor); N0, no regional lymph node metastasis (regional lymph nodes are the peripancreatic lymph nodes, including the lymph nodes along the hepatic artery, celiac axis and pyloric/splenic regions); N1, regional lymph node metastasis; M0, no distal metastasis; M1, distal metastasis.

Source: Modified from Greene, Page; with permission.

Surveillance in High-Risk Individuals

Routine screening for pancreatic cancer is not recommended due to a high false-positive rate of the available tests. However, screening may be reasonable in certain high-risk individuals, such as those with strong family histories, although the optimal timing, frequency, and method of screening is unknown. One recommendation is to commence screening at the age of 35 in patients with hereditary pancreatitis, or 10 years before the age of the youngest diagnosis of pancreatic cancer in those with a significant family history using spiral CT, followed by EUS when CT results have been indeterminate.

℞ **Treatment: PANCREATIC CANCER**

Symptoms and the associated impaired performance status are significant issues in the management of patients with pancreatic cancer, as they can have a marked negative impact on the ability to safely deliver chemotherapy or perform curative surgery. For example, patients with malabsorption secondary to pancreatic insufficiency may be treated with pancreatic enzyme supplementation. Indeed effective symptom management is as important a therapeutic goal as survival prolongation.

ADVANCED PANCREATIC CANCER These patients have metastatic or locally advanced inoperable disease and are the majority with newly diagnosed disease. Debulking surgery or partial resections have no role, as these procedures are associated with the same risks as a curative resection but are unlikely to improve survival. Many patients may, however, benefit from endoscopic biliary or duodenal stenting, and some patients from nerve plexus blocks or ablation. Less frequently, intestinal bypass surgery is required.

The deoxycytidine analogue gemcitabine, given as a single agent (gemcitabine 1000 mg/m^2 weekly for 7 weeks followed by 1 week rest, then weekly for 3 weeks every 4 weeks thereafter), has been the preferred treatment for these patients since it was shown to yield clinical benefit (a composite parameter for evaluating symptomatic benefit of treatment used in some trials of this disease) and improved survival compared to 5-fluorouracil. The median survival observed with single-agent gemcitabine in randomized trials is about 6 months, with a 12-month survival of approximately 18%. Furthermore, two randomized trials have shown improved survival from the addition of either the oral fluoropyrimidine, capecitabine (gemcitabine 1000 mg/m^2 days 1, 8, and 15 plus capecitabine 1660 mg/m^2 days 1–21, repeated every 28 days), or the tyrosine kinase inhibitor of the epidermal growth factor receptor (EGFR), erlotinib (standard gemcitabine plus erlotinib 100 mg daily). The survival improvement observed with both of these combinations appears similar, and the addition of capecitabine to gemcitabine in this regimen does not appear to increase the toxicity above single-agent gemcitabine. Either combination should, therefore, be considered as options for treating these patients. Second-line treatment options in pancreatic cancer are limited although there may be an emerging role for oxaliplatin-based chemotherapy; fit patients who have failed first-line treatment should be offered entry into clinical trials. On-going clinical trials are evaluating the potential benefits of incorporating other novel targeted agents into the treatment of pancreatic cancer, usually together with gemcitabine.

In patients with locally advanced unresectable disease, external beam chemoradiotherapy may be useful, either as initial treatment or as consolidation after induction chemotherapy.

OPERABLE DISEASE Complete surgical resection in patients with localized disease (stage I or II disease), with distal metastases excluded by prior CT scan of the abdomen and pelvis, and CT of the chest or chest x-ray, is potentially curative. However, such surgery is only possible in 10–15% of patients, many of whom will suffer from recurrences of their disease. Indeed, the 5-year survival reported in randomized trials with surgery alone is approximately 10%, although modern series have improved on these results. Outcomes tend to be more favorable in patients with lymph node–negative disease, smaller tumors (less than 3 cm), negative resection margins and well-differentiated tumors. Despite a

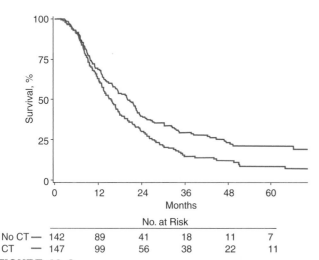

FIGURE 49-2

Survival by adjuvant chemotherapy. Kaplan-Meier estimates of survival from the European Study Group for Pancreatic Cancer 1 (ESPAC1) trial for the comparison of adjuvant chemotherapy versus no adjuvant chemotherapy (CT) in patients with resected pancreatic cancer (hazard ratio for death, 0.71; 95% confidence interval, 0.55 to 0.92; p = .009). *(Reprinted with permission from JP Neoptolemos, DD Stocken, H Friess, et al: A randomized trial of chemoradiotherapy and chemotherapy after resection of pancreatic cancer. N Engl J Med 350:1200–1210, 2004. Copyright 2004, Massachusetts Medical Society.)*

dismal long term outcome, these patients still have a better survival with surgery than with other palliative measures.

Surgery is usually preceded by laparoscopy in order to exclude peritoneal metastases not seen on other staging investigations. Pancreaticoduodenectomy, also known as the Whipple procedure, is the standard operation for cancers of the head or uncinate process of the pancreas. The procedure involves resection of the pancreatic head, duodenum, first 15 cm of the jejunum, common bile duct, and gallbladder, and a partial gastrectomy, with the pancreatic and biliary anastomosis placed 45–60 cm proximal to the gastrojejunostomy. Perioperative mortality rates have fallen to less than 5%, reflecting greater experience with the surgery and perioperative management of these patients. However, this type of surgery is highly specialized and should ideally only occur in dedicated centers with a high volume of these cases and specialized surgeons.

Adjuvant treatment for patients with curatively resected pancreatic cancer is controversial, with divergent treatment approaches preferred in the United States and in Europe, based on the results of different randomized trials conducted on both sides of the Atlantic. In the United States, fluoropyrimidine-based postoperative chemoradiotherapy followed by adjuvant chemotherapy is preferred. In Europe, because a large randomized trial (the European Study Group for Pancreatic Cancer 1 or ESPAC1 trial) showed a survival benefit for adjuvant chemotherapy with 5-fluorouracil (5FU) (**Fig. 49-2**), this approach is more common practice.

FURTHER READINGS

ALEXAKIS N et al: Current standards of surgery for pancreatic cancer. Br J Surg 91:1410, 2004

BARUGOLA G et al: The determinant factors of recurrence following resection for ductal pancreatic cancer. JOP 8(Suppl 1):132, 2007

CHANG DK et al: Role of endoscopic ultrasound in pancreatic cancer. Expert Rev Gastroenterol Hepatol 3:293, 2009

CHUA YJ, CUNNINGHAM D: Chemotherapy for advanced pancreatic cancer. Best Pract Res Clin Gastroenterol 20:327, 2006

DIMAGNO EP et al: AGA technical review on the epidemiology, diagnosis, and treatment of pancreatic ductal adenocarcinomas. American Gastroenterological Association. Gastroenterology 117:1464, 1999

GREENE FL, PAGE DL (eds): *Exocrine Pancreas, AJCC Cancer Staging Manual*, 6th ed, New York, Springer, pp 157–164, 2002

HRUBAN RH, ADSAY NV: Molecular classification of neoplasms of the pancreas. Hum Pathol 40:612, 2009

HUSER N et al: Systematic review and meta-analysis of prophylactic gastroenterostomy for unresectable advanced pancreatic cancer. Br J Surg 96:711, 2009

NEOPTOLEMOS JP et al: A randomized trial of chemoradiotherapy and chemotherapy after resection of pancreatic cancer. N Engl J Med 350:1200, 2004

WILLETT CG et al: Locally advanced pancreatic cancer. J Clin Oncol 23:4538, 2005

YEH JJ: Prognostic signature for pancreatic cancer: are we close? Future Oncol 5:313, 2009

CHAPTER 50

ENDOCRINE TUMORS OF THE GASTROINTESTINAL TRACT AND PANCREAS

Robert T. Jensen

GENERAL FEATURES OF GASTROINTESTINAL (GI) NEUROENDOCRINE TUMORS

Gastrointestinal neuroendocrine tumors (NETs) are derived from the diffuse neuroendocrine system of the GI tract, which is composed of amine- and acid-producing cells with different hormonal profiles, depending on the site of origin. The tumors can be divided into carcinoid tumors and pancreatic endocrine tumors (PETs). These tumors were originally classified as APUDomas (for *amine precursor uptake and decarboxylation*), as were pheochromocytomas, melanomas, and medullary thyroid carcinomas because they share certain cytochemical features as well as various pathologic, biologic, and molecular features (Table 50-1). It was originally proposed that APUDomas had a similar embryonic origin from neural crest cells, but it is now known the peptide-secreting cells are not of neuroectodermal origin. Nevertheless, the concept is useful because the tumors have important similarities as well as some differences (Table 50-1).

CLASSIFICATION/PATHOLOGY/TUMOR BIOLOGY OF NETs

NETs are generally composed of monotonous sheets of small round cells with uniform nuclei; mitoses are uncommon. They can be tentatively identified on routine histology; however, these tumors are now principally recognized by their histologic staining patterns due to shared cellular proteins. Historically, silver staining was used and tumors were classified as showing an argentaffin reaction if they took up and reduced silver, or as being argyrophilic if they did not reduce it. More recently immunocytochemical localization of chromogranins (A, B, C), neuron-specific enolase, or synaptophysin, which are all neuroendocrine cell markers, are used (Table 50-1). Chromogranin A is currently the most widely used.

Ultrastructurally, these tumors possess electron-dense neurosecretory granules and frequently contain small clear vesicles that correspond to synaptic vesicles of neurons. NETs synthesize numerous peptides, growth factors, and bioactive amines that may be ectopically secreted, giving rise to a specific clinical syndrome (Table 50-2).

TABLE 50-1

GENERAL CHARACTERISTICS OF GI NEUROENDOCRINE TUMORS [CARCINOIDS, PANCREATIC ENDOCRINE TUMORS (PETs)]

I. Share general neuroendocrine cell markers
   A. Chromogranins (A, B, C) are acidic monomeric soluble proteins found in the large secretory granules; chromogranin A is most widely used.
   B. Neuron-specific enolase (NSE) is the γ-γ dimer of the enzyme enolase and is a cytosolic marker of neuroendocrine differentiation.
   C. Synaptophysin is an integral membrane glycoprotein of 38,000 molecular weight found in small vesicles of neurons and neuroendocrine tumors.

II. Pathologic similarities
   A. All are APUDomas showing amine precursor uptake and decarboxylation
   B. Ultrastructurally they have dense-core secretory granules (>80 nm).
   C. Histologically appear similar with few mitoses and uniform nuclei
   D. Frequently synthesize multiple peptides/amines, which can be detected immunocytochemically but may not be secreted
   E. Presence or absence of clinical syndrome or type cannot be predicted by immunocytochemical studies.
   F. Histologic classifications do not predict biologic behavior; only invasion or metastases establishes malignancy.

III. Similarities of biologic behavior
   A. Generally slow growing, but a proportion is aggressive.
   B. Secrete biologically active peptides/amines, which can cause clinical symptoms.
   C. Generally have high densities of somatostatin receptors, which are used for both localization and treatment.

IV. Similarities/differences in molecular abnormalities
   A. Similarities
      1. Uncommon—alterations in common oncogenes (ras, jun, fos, etc.).
      2. Uncommon—alterations in common tumor-suppressor genes (p53, retinoblastoma).
      3. Alterations at MEN-1 locus (11q13) and p16^{INK4a} (9p21) occur in a proportion (10–30%).
      4. Methylation of various genes occurs in 40–87% (ras-associated domain family I, p14, p16, O^6 methyl guanosine methyltransferase, retinoic acid receptor β)
   B. Differences
      1. PETs—loss of 3p (8–47%), 3q (8–41%), 11q (21–62%), 6q (18–68%). Gains at 17q (10–55%), 7q (16–68%).
      2. Carcinoids—loss of 18q (38–67%) > 18p (33–43%) > 9p, 16q21 (21–23%). Gains at 17q, 19p (57%).

The diagnosis of the specific syndrome requires the clinical features of the disease and cannot be made from the immunocytochemistry results alone. Furthermore, pathologists cannot distinguish between benign and malignant NETs unless metastases or invasion are present.

Carcinoid tumors are frequently classified according to their anatomic area of origin (i.e., foregut, midgut, hindgut) because tumors with similar embryonic origin share functional manifestations, histochemistry, and secretory products (Table 50-3). Foregut tumors generally have a low serotonin (5HT) content, are argentaffin-negative but argyrophilic, occasionally secrete adrenocorticotropic hormone (ACTH) or 5-hydroytryptophan (5HTP) causing an atypical carcinoid syndrome (Fig. 50-1), are often multihormonal, and may metastasize to bone. They uncommonly produce a clinical syndrome due to the secreted products. Midgut carcinoids are argentaffin-positive, have a high 5HT content, most frequently cause the typical carcinoid syndrome when they metastasize (Table 50-3, Fig. 50-1), release 5HT and tachykinins (substance P, neuropeptide K, substance K), rarely secrete 5HTP or ACTH, and uncommonly metastasize to bone. Hindgut carcinoids (rectum, transverse and descending colon) are argentaffin-negative, often argyrophilic, rarely contain 5HT or cause the carcinoid syndrome (Fig. 50-1, Table 50-3), rarely secrete 5HTP or ACTH, contain numerous peptides, and may metastasize to bone.

PETs can be classified into nine well-established specific functional syndromes (Table 50-2), four possible specific functional syndromes (PETs secreting calcitonin, renin, luteinizing hormone, or erythropoietin), and nonfunctional PETs [pancreatic polypeptide (PP)–secreting tumors; PPomas]. Each of the functional syndromes is associated with symptoms due to the specific hormone released. In contrast, nonfunctional PETs release no products that cause a specific clinical syndrome. "Nonfunctional" is a misnomer in the strict sense because they frequently ectopically secrete a number of peptides (PP, chromogranin A, ghrelin, neurotensin, α subunits of human chorionic gonadotropin (hCG), neuron-specific enolase); however, they cause no specific clinical syndrome. The symptoms caused by nonfunctional PETs are entirely due to the tumor per se.

Carcinoid tumors can occur in almost any GI tissue (Table 50-3); however, at present most (70%) take origin from one of three sites: bronchus, jejunoileum, or colon/rectum. In the past, carcinoid tumors most frequently were reported in the appendix (i.e., 40%); however, the bronchus/lung and small intestine are now the most common sites. Overall, GI carcinoids are the most common site for these tumors, comprising 64%, with the respiratory tract second at 28%.

The term *pancreatic endocrine tumor*, although widely used and therefore retained here, is also a misnomer, strictly speaking, because these tumors can occur either almost entirely in the pancreas (insulinomas, glucagonomas, nonfunctional PETs, PETs causing hypercalcemia) or at both pancreatic and extrapancreatic sites [gastrinomas, VIPomas (VIP, vasoactive intestinal peptide),

TABLE 50-2

GI NEUROENDOCRINE TUMOR SYNDROMES

NAME	BIOLOGICALLY ACTIVE PEPTIDE(S) SECRETED	INCIDENCE (NEW CASES/10^6 POPULATION/ YEAR)	TUMOR LOCATION	MALIGNANT, %	ASSOCIATED WITH MEN-1, %	MAIN SYMPTOMS/ SIGNS
Established Specific Functional Syndrome						
Carcinoid tumor						
Carcinoid syndrome	Serotonin, possibly tachykinins, motilin, prostaglandins	0.5–2	Midgut (75–87%) Foregut (2–33%) Hindgut (1–8%) Unknown (2–15%)	95–100	Rare	Diarrhea (32–84%) Flushing (63–75%) Pain (10–34%) Asthma (4–18%) Heart disease (11–41%)
Pancreatic endocrine tumor						
Zollinger-Ellison syndrome	Gastrin	0.5–1.5	Duodenum (70%) Pancreas (25%) Other sites (5%)	60–90	20–25	Pain (79–100%) Diarrhea (30–75%) Esophageal symptoms (31–56%)
Insulinoma	Insulin	1–2	Pancreas (>99%)	<10	4–5	Hypoglycemic symptoms (100%)
VIPoma (Verner-Morrison syndrome, pancreatic cholera, WDHA)	Vasoactive intestinal peptide	0.05–0.2	Pancreas (90%, adult) Other (10%, neural, adrenal, periganglionic)	40–70	6	Diarrhea (90–100%) Hypokalemia (80–100%) Dehydration (83%)
Glucagonoma	Glucagon	0.01–0.1	Pancreas (100%)	50–80	1–20	Rash (67–90%) Glucose intolerance (38–87%) Weight loss (66–96%)
Somatostatinoma	Somatostatin	Rare	Pancreas (55%) Duodenum/ jejunum (44%)	>70	45	Diabetes mellitus (63–90%) Cholelithiases (65–90%) Diarrhea (35–90%)
GRFoma	Growth hormone-releasing hormone	Unknown	Pancreas (30%) Lung (54%) Jejunum (7%) Other (13%)	>60	16	Acromegaly (100%)
ACTHoma	ACTH	Rare	Pancreas (4–16% all ectopic Cushing's)	>95	Rare	Cushing's syndrome (100%)
PET causing carcinoid syndrome	Serotonin, ? tachykinins	Rare (43 cases)	Pancreas (<1% all carcinoids)	60–88	Rare	Same as carcinoid syndrome, above
PET causing hypercalcemia	PTHrP, others unknown	Rare	Pancreas (rare cause of hypercalcemia)	84	Rare	Abdominal pain due to hepatic metastases

(Continued)

TABLE 50-2 (*CONTINUED*)

GI NEUROENDOCRINE TUMOR SYNDROMES

NAME	BIOLOGICALLY ACTIVE PEPTIDE(S) SECRETED	INCIDENCE (NEW CASES/10^6 POPULATION/ YEAR)	TUMOR LOCATION	MALIGNANT, %	ASSOCIATED WITH MEN-1, %	MAIN SYMPTOMS/ SIGNS
Possible Specific Functional Syndrome						
PET secreting calcitonin	Calcitonin	Rare	Pancreas (rare) cause of hyper-calcitoninemia	>80	16	Diarrhea (50%)
PET secreting renin	Renin	Rare	Pancreas	Unknown	No	Hypertension
PET secreting luteinizing hormone	Luteinizing hormone	Rare	Pancreas	Unknown	No	Anovulation, virili-zation (female); reduced libido (male)
PET secreting erythropoietin	Erythropoietin	Rare	Pancreas	100	No	Polycythemia
No Functional Syndrome						
PPoma/ nonfunctional	None	1–2	Pancreas (100%)	>60	18–44	Weight loss (30–90%) Abdominal mass (10–30%) Pain (30–95%)

Note: MEN, multiple endocrine neoplasia; VIPoma, tumor secreting vasoactive intestinal peptide; WDHA, watery diarrhea, hypokalemia, and achlorhydria syndrome; ACTH, adrenocorticotropic hormone; PET, pancreatic endocrine tumor; PTHrP, parathyroid hormone–related peptide; PPoma, tumor secreting pancreatic polypeptide.

TABLE 50-3

CARCINOID TUMOR LOCATION, FREQUENCY OF METASTASES, AND ASSOCIATION WITH THE CARCINOID SYNDROME

	LOCATION (% OF TOTAL)	INCIDENCE OF METASTASES	INCIDENCE OF CARCINOID SYNDROME
Foregut			
Esophagus	<0.1	—	—
Stomach	4.6	10	9.5
Duodenum	2.0	—	3.4
Pancreas	0.7	71.9	20
Gallbladder	0.3	17.8	5
Bronchus, lung, trachea	27.9	5.7	13
Midgut			
Jejunum	1.8	⎰58.4	9
Ileum	14.9	⎱	9
Meckel's diverticulum	0.5	—	13
Appendix	4.8	38.8	<1
Colon	8.6	51	5
Liver	0.4	32.2	—
Ovary	1.0	32	50
Testis	<0.1	—	50
Hindgut			
Rectum	13.6	3.9	—

Source: Location is from the PAN-SEER data (1973–1999), and incidence of metastases from the SEER data (1992–1999), reported by IM Modlin et al: Cancer 97:934, 2003. Incidence of carcinoid syndrome is from 4349 cases studied from 1950–1971, reported by JD Godwin, Cancer 36:560, 1975.

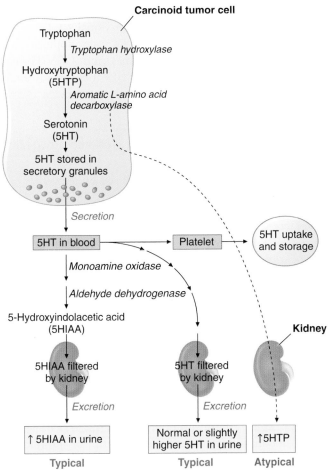

FIGURE 50-1

Synthesis, secretion, and metabolism of serotonin (5HT) in patients with typical and atypical carcinoid syndromes. Abbreviations: 5HIAA, 5-hydroxyindolacetic acid.

somatostatinomas, GRFomas (GRF, growth hormone-releasing factor)]. PETs are also called *islet cell tumors*; however, this term is discouraged because it is not established that they originate from the islets, and many can occur at extrapancreatic sites.

A uniform World Health Organization (WHO) classification for all GI NETs (including carcinoids and PETs) divides them into three general categories: (1a) well-differentiated NETs, (1b) well-differentiated neuroendocrine carcinomas of low-grade malignancy, and (2) poorly differentiated neuroendocrine carcinomas that are usually small cell neuroendocrine carcinomas of high-grade malignancy. The term *carcinoid* is synonymous with *well-differentiated NETs* (1a). This classification is further divided on the basis of tumor location and biology. Furthermore, for the first time a standard TNM classification has been proposed for the GI foregut NETs. The availability of this WHO classification and the TNM classification should greatly facilitate the comparison of clinical, pathological and prognostic features and results of treatment in GI NETs from different studies.

The exact incidence of carcinoid tumors or PETs varies according to whether only symptomatic or all tumors are considered. The incidence of clinically significant carcinoids is 7–13 cases/million population per year, whereas any malignant carcinoids at autopsy are reported in 21–84 cases/million population per year. Clinically significant PETs have a prevalence of 10 cases per million population with insulinomas, gastrinomas, and nonfunctional PETs having an incidence of 0.5–2 cases per million population per year (Table 50-2). VIPomas are 2- to 8-fold less common, glucagonomas are 17- to 30-fold less common, and somatostatinomas the least common. In autopsy studies 0.5–1.5% of all cases have a PET; however, in <1 in 1000 cases was a functional tumor thought to occur.

Both carcinoid tumors and PETs commonly show malignant behavior (Tables 50-2, 50-3). With PETs, except for insulinomas in which <10% are malignant, 50–100% in different series are malignant. With carcinoid tumors, the percentage showing malignant behavior varies in different locations. For the three most common sites of occurrence, the incidence of metastases varies greatly from jejunoileum (58%) > lung/bronchus (6%) > rectum (4%). With both carcinoid tumors and PETs, a number of factors influence survival and the aggressiveness of the tumor (Table 50-4). The presence of liver metastases is the single most important prognostic factor in single and multivariate analyses for both carcinoid tumors and PETs. Particularly important in the development of liver metastases is the size of the primary tumor. For example, with small-intestinal carcinoids, the most frequent cause of the carcinoid syndrome due to metastatic disease in the liver (Table 50-2), metastases occur in 15–25% if the tumor diameter is <1 cm, 58–80% if it is 1–2 cm, and >75% if >2 cm. Similar data exist for gastrinomas and other PETs, where the size of the primary tumor has been shown to be an independent predictor of the development of liver metastases. The presence of lymph node metastases, the depth of invasion, various histologic features [differentiation, mitotic rates, growth indices, vessel density, vascular endothelial growth factor (VEGF), and CD10 metalloproteinase expression], elevated serum alkaline phosphatase levels, and flow cytometric results (such as the presence of aneuploidy) are all important prognostic factors for the development of metastatic disease (Table 50-4). For patients with carcinoid tumors, additional poor prognostic factors include the development of the carcinoid syndrome, older age, male sex, the presence of a symptomatic tumor, or higher levels of a number of tumor markers [5-hydroxyindolacetic acid (5HIAA), neuropeptide K, chromogranin A]. With PETs or gastrinomas, the best studied PET, a worse prognosis is associated with female sex, overexpression of the *ha-ras* oncogene or p53, the absence of multiple endocrine neoplasia–type 1 (MEN-1), and higher levels of various tumor markers (i.e., chromogranin A, gastrin).

TABLE 50-4

PROGNOSTIC FACTORS IN NEUROENDOCRINE TUMORS

Both carcinoid tumors and PETs
  Presence of liver metastases ($p < .001$)
  Extent of liver metastases ($p < .001$)
  Presence of lymph node metastases ($p < .001$)
  Depth of invasion ($p < .001$)
  Elevated serum alkaline phosphatase levels ($p = .003$)
  Primary tumor site ($p < .001$)
  Primary tumor size ($p < .005$)
  Various histologic features
    Tumor differentiation ($p < .001$)
    High growth indices (high Ki-67 index, PCNA expression)
    High mitotic counts ($p < .001$)
    Vascular or perineural invasion
    Vessel density (low microvessel density, increased lymphatic density)
    Low VEGF, high CD10 metalloproteinase expression)
    Flow cytometric features (i.e., aneuploidy)
Carcinoid tumors
  Presence of carcinoid syndrome
  Laboratory results [urinary 5-HIAA level ($p < .01$), plasma neuropeptide K ($p < .05$), serum chromogranin A ($p < .01$)]
  Presence of a second malignancy
  Male sex ($p < .001$)
  Older age ($p < .01$)
  Mode of discovery (incidental > symptomatic)
  Molecular findings [TGF-α expression ($p < .05$), chr 16q LOH or gain chr 4p ($p < .05$)]
PETs
  Ha-Ras oncogene or p53 overexpression
  Female sex
  MEN-1 syndrome absent
  Laboratory findings (increased chromogranin A in some studies; gastrinomas—increased gastrin level)
  Molecular findings [increased HER2/*neu* expression ($p = .032$), chr 1q, 3p, 3q, or 6q LOH ($p = .0004$), EGF receptor overexpression ($p = .034$), gains in chr 7q, 17q, 17p, 20q]

Note: PET, pancreatic endocrine tumor; Ki-67, proliferation-associated nuclear antigen recognized by Ki-67 monoclonal antibody; PCNA, proliferating cell nuclear antigen; 5HIAA, 5-hydroxyindoleacetic acid; TGF-α, transforming growth factor α; chr, chromosome; LOH, loss of heterozygosity; MEN, multiple endocrine neoplasia; EGF, epidermal growth factor.

A number of genetic disorders are associated with an increased incidence of NETs (Table 50-5). Each one is caused by a loss of a possible tumor-suppressor gene. The most important is MEN-1, an autosomal dominant disorder due to a defect in a 10-exon gene on 11q13, which encodes for a 610-amino acid nuclear protein, menin. Patients with MEN-1 develop hyperparathyroidism due to parathyroid hyperplasia in 95–100%, PETs in 80–100%, pituitary adenomas in 54–80%, bronchial carcinoids in 8%, thymic carcinoids in 8%, and gastric carcinoids in 13–30% of the patients with Zollinger-Ellison syndrome (ZES). In patients with MEN-1, 80–100% develop nonfunctional PETs; functional PETs occur in 80%, with 54% developing ZES, 21% insulinomas, 3% glucagonomas, and 1% VIPomas. MEN-1 is present in 20–25% of all patients with ZES, in 4% with insulinomas, and in a low percentage (<5%) of the other PETs.

Three phacomatoses associated with NETs are von Hippel–Lindau disease (VHL), von Recklinghausen's disease [neurofibromatosis (NF) type 1], and tuberous sclerosis (Bourneville's disease). VHL is an autosomal dominant disorder due to defects in a gene on chromosome 3p25, which encodes a 213-amino-acid protein that interacts with the elongin family of proteins as a transcriptional regulator. In addition to cerebellar hemangioblastomas, renal cancer, and pheochromocytomas, 10–17% of these patients develop a PET. Most are nonfunctional although insulinomas and VIPomas are reported. Patients with NF-1 have defects in a gene on chromosome 17q11.2 encoding for a 2845-amino-acid protein, neurofibromin, which functions in normal cells as a suppressor of the *ras* signaling cascade. Up to 12% of these patients develop an upper GI carcinoid tumor, characteristically in the periampullary region (54%). Many are classified as somatostatinomas because they contain somatostatin immunocytochemically; however, they uncommonly secrete somatostatin or produce a clinical somatostatinoma syndrome. NF-1 has rarely been associated with insulinomas and ZES. Tuberous sclerosis is caused by mutations that alter either the 1164-amino-acid protein, hamartin (TSC1), or the 1807-amino-acid protein, tuberin (TSC2). Both hamartin and tuberin interact in a pathway related to cytosolic G protein regulation. A few cases including nonfunctional and functional PETs (insulinomas and gastrinomas) have been reported in these patients (Table 50-5).

In contrast to most common nonendocrine tumors such as carcinoma of the breast, colon, lung, or stomach, alterations in common oncogenes (*ras, myc, fos, src, jun*) or tumor-suppressor genes (p53, retinoblastoma susceptibility gene) have not been found in PETs or carcinoid tumors. Alterations that may be important in their pathogenesis include changes in the *MEN-1* gene, p16/MTS1 tumor-suppressor gene, and DPC 4/*Smad* 4 gene; amplification of the HER-2/*neu* protooncogene and growth factors and their receptors; methylation of a number of genes likely resulting in their inactivation; and deletions of unknown tumor-suppressor genes as well as gains in other unknown genes (Table 50-1). Comparative genomic hybridization and genome-wide allelotyping studies have shown differences in chromosomal losses and gains between PETs and carcinoids, some of which have prognostic significance (Table 50-4). Mutations in the *MEN-1* gene are likely particularly important. Loss of heterozygosity at the MEN-1 locus on chromosome 11q13 is seen in 93% of sporadic PETs

TABLE 50-5

GENETIC SYNDROMES ASSOCIATED WITH AN INCREASED INCIDENCE OF NEUROENDOCRINE TUMORS [NETs (CARCINOIDS OR PANCREATIC ENDOCRINE TUMORS) (PETs)]		
SYNDROME	LOCATION OF GENE MUTATION AND GENE PRODUCT	NETs SEEN/FREQUENCY
Multiple endocrine neoplasia type 1 (MEN-1)	11q13 (encodes 610-amino-acid protein, menin)	80–100% develop PETs: (nonfunctional > gastrinoma > insulinoma) Carcinoids: gastric (13–30%), bronchial/thymic (8%)
von Hippel–Lindau disease	3q25 (encodes 213-amino-acid protein)	12–17% develop PETs (almost always nonfunctional)
von Recklinghausen's disease [neurofibromatosis 1 (NF-1)]	17q11.2 (encodes 2485-amino-acid protein, neurofibromin)	Duodenal somatostatinomas (usually nonfunctional) Rarely insulinoma, gastrinoma
Tuberous sclerosis	9q34 (TSCI) encodes 1164-amino-acid protein, hamartin) 16p13 (TSC2) (encodes 1807-amino-acid protein, tuberin)	Uncommonly develop PETs [nonfunctional and functional (insulinoma, gastrinoma)]

(i.e., in patients without MEN-1) and in 26–75% of sporadic carcinoid tumors. Mutations in the *MEN-1* gene are reported in 31–34% of sporadic gastrinomas. The presence of a number of these molecular alterations (PET or carcinoid) correlates with tumor growth, tumor size, disease extent or invasiveness and may have prognostic significance.

CARCINOID TUMORS AND CARCINOID SYNDROME

CHARACTERISTICS OF THE MOST COMMON GI CARCINOID TUMORS

Appendiceal Carcinoids

These occur in 1 in every 200–300 appendectomies, usually in the appendiceal tip. In older studies, most (>90%) are reported as <1 cm in diameter without metastases, but more recent reports find that 2–35% have metastases (Table 50-3). In the SEER data of 1570 appendiceal carcinoids, 62% were localized and 27% had regional and 8% had distant metastases; half of those between 1 and 2 cm metastasized to lymph nodes. Their percentage of the total number of carcinoids has decreased from 43.9% (1950–1969) to 2.4% (1992–1999).

Small Intestinal Carcinoids

These are frequently multiple; 70–80% are present in the ileum and 70% within 6 cm (24 in.) of the ileocecal valve. Some 40% are <1 cm in diameter, 32% are 1–2 cm, and 29% are >2 cm. Between 35 and 70% are associated with metastases (Table 50-3). They characteristically cause a marked fibrotic reaction, which can lead to intestinal obstruction. Distant metastases occur to the liver in 36–60%, to bone in 3%, and to lung in 4%. Tumor size affects the frequency of metastases. However, even small carcinoid tumors of the small intestine (<1 cm) have metastases in 15–25%, whereas it increases to 58–100% for tumors 1–2 cm in diameter. Carcinoids also occur in the duodenum, with 31% having metastases. No duodenal tumor <1 cm in two series metastasized, whereas 33% of those >2 cm had metastases. Small-intestinal carcinoids are the most common cause (60–87%) of the carcinoid syndrome and are discussed below.

Rectal Carcinoids

Rectal carcinoids are found in ~1 of every 2500 proctoscopies. Nearly all occur between 4 and 13 cm above the dentate line. Most are small, with 66–80% being <1 cm in diameter, and they rarely metastasize (5%). Tumors between 1 and 2 cm can metastasize in 5–30% and tumors >2 cm, which are uncommon, in >70%.

Bronchial Carcinoids

The frequency of bronchial carcinoids is not related to smoking. A number of different classifications of bronchial carcinoid tumors are proposed. In some studies, lung NETs are classified into four categories: typical carcinoid [also called bronchial carcinoid tumor, Kulchitsky cell carcinoma (KCC)-I]; atypical carcinoid (also called well-differentiated neuroendocrine carcinoma, KCC-II); intermediate small cell neuroendocrine carcinoma; and small cell neuroendocarcinoma (KCC-III). Another proposed classification includes three categories of lung NETs: benign or low-grade malignant (typical carcinoid), low-grade malignant (atypical carcinoid), and high-grade malignant (poorly differentiated carcinoma of the large cell or small cell type). These different categories of lung NETs have different prognoses, varying from excellent for typical carcinoid to poor for small cell neuroendocrine carcinomas.

Gastric Carcinoids

These account for 3 of every 1000 gastric neoplasms. It is thought that three different subtypes of gastric carcinoids occur. Each originates from gastric enterochromaffin-like (ECL) cells in the gastric mucosa. Two subtypes are associated with hypergastrinemic states, either chronic atrophic gastritis (type I) (80% of all gastric carcinoids) or ZES, almost always as part of the MEN-1 syndrome (type II) (6% of all cases). These tumors generally pursue a benign course, with 9–30% associated with metastases. They are usually multiple, small, and infiltrate only to the submucosa. The third subtype of gastric carcinoid (type III) (sporadic) occurs without hypergastrinemia (14% of all carcinoids) and pursues an aggressive course, with 54–66% developing metastases. Sporadic carcinoids are usually single, large tumors, 50% have atypical histology, and they can be a cause of the carcinoid syndrome. Gastric carcinoids as a percentage of all carcinoids are increasing in frequency [1.96% (1969–71), 3.6% (1973–91), 5.8% (1991–99)].

CARCINOID TUMORS WITHOUT THE CARCINOID SYNDROME

The age of patients at diagnosis ranges from 10–93 years with a mean of 63 years for small intestine and 66 years for the rectum. The presentation is diverse and related to the site of origin and extent of malignant spread. In the appendix, carcinoid tumors are usually found incidentally during surgery for suspected appendicitis. Small-intestinal carcinoids in the jejunoileum present with periodic abdominal pain (51%), intestinal obstruction with ileus/invagination (31%), an abdominal tumor (17%), or GI bleeding (11%). Because of the vagueness of the symptoms, the diagnosis is usually delayed ~2 years from onset of the symptoms, ranging up to 20 years. Duodenal, gastric, and rectal carcinoids are most frequently found by chance at endoscopy. The most common symptoms of rectal carcinoids are melena/bleeding (39%), constipation (17%), and diarrhea (12%). Bronchial carcinoids are frequently discovered as a lesion on a chest radiograph, and 31% of the patients are asymptomatic. Thymic carcinoids present as anterior mediastinal masses on chest radiograph or CT scan. Ovarian and testicular carcinoids usually present as masses discovered on physical examination or ultrasound. Metastatic carcinoid tumor in the liver frequently presents as hepatomegaly in a patient who may have minimal symptoms and near-normal liver function tests.

CARCINOID TUMORS WITH SYSTEMIC SYMPTOMS DUE TO SECRETED PRODUCTS

Carcinoid tumors can contain numerous GI peptides: gastrin, insulin, somatostatin, motilin, neurotensin, tachykinins (substance K, substance P, neuropeptide K), glucagon, gastrin-releasing peptide, VIP, PP, other biologically active peptides (ACTH, calcitonin, growth hormone), prostaglandins and bioactive amines (5HT). These substances may or may not be released in sufficient amounts to cause symptoms. In various studies of patients with carcinoid tumors, elevated serum levels of PP were found in 43%, motilin in 14%, gastrin in 15%, and VIP in 6%. Foregut carcinoids are more likely to produce various GI peptides than midgut carcinoids. Ectopic ACTH production causing Cushing's syndrome is increasingly seen with foregut carcinoids (respiratory tract primarily) and in some series was the most common cause of the ectopic ACTH syndrome, accounting for 64% of all cases. Acromegaly due to GRF release occurs with foregut carcinoids, as does the somatostatinoma syndrome, but rarely occurs with duodenal carcinoids. The most common systemic syndrome with carcinoid tumors is the carcinoid syndrome.

CARCINOID SYNDROME

Clinical Features

The cardinal features at presentation as well as during the disease course are shown in Table 50-6. Flushing and diarrhea are the two most common symptoms,

TABLE 50-6

CLINICAL CHARACTERISTICS IN PATIENTS WITH CARCINOID SYNDROME		
	AT PRESENTATION	DURING COURSE OF DISEASE
Symptoms/signs		
Diarrhea	32–73%	68–84%
Flushing	23–65%	63–74%
Pain	10%	34%
Asthma/wheezing	4–8%	3–18%
Pellagra	2%	5%
None	12%	22%
Carcinoid heart disease present	11%	14–41%
Demographics		
Male	46–59%	46–61%
Age		
Mean	57 y	52–54 y
Range	25–79 y	9–91 y
Tumor location		
Foregut	5–9%	2–33%
Midgut	78–87%	60–87%
Hindgut	1–5%	1–8%
Unknown	2–11%	2–15%

occurring in up to 73% initially and in up to 89% during the course of the disease. The characteristic flush is of sudden onset; it is a deep red or violaceous erythema of the upper body, especially the neck and face, often associated with a feeling of warmth, and occasionally associated with pruritus, lacrimation, diarrhea, or facial edema. Flushes may be precipitated by stress, alcohol, exercise, certain foods such as cheese, or by certain agents such as catecholamines, pentagastrin, and serotonin reuptake inhibitors. Flushing episodes may be brief, lasting 2–5 min, especially initially, or may last hours, especially later in the disease course. Flushing is usually seen with midgut carcinoids but can also occur with foregut carcinoids. With bronchial carcinoids the flushes are frequently prolonged for hours to days, reddish in color, and associated with salivation, lacrimation, diaphoresis, diarrhea, and hypotension. The flush associated with gastric carcinoids is also reddish in color but patchy in distribution over the face and neck. It may be provoked by food and have accompanying pruritus.

Diarrhea is present in 32–73% initially and 68–84% at some time in their disease course. Diarrhea usually occurs with flushing (85% of cases). The diarrhea is usually described as watery with 60% having <1 L/day of diarrhea. Steatorrhea is present in 67%, and in 46% it is >15 g/d (normal <7 g). Abdominal pain may be present with the diarrhea or independently in 10–34% of cases.

Cardiac manifestations occur in 11% initially and in 14–41% at some time in the disease course. The cardiac disease is due to fibrosis involving the endocardium, primarily on the right side, although left side lesions can occur also. The dense fibrous deposits are most commonly on the ventricular aspect of the tricuspid valve and less commonly on the pulmonary valve cusps. They can result in constriction of the valves and pulmonic stenosis is usually predominant, whereas the tricuspid valve is often fixed open, resulting in regurgitation predominating. Up to 80% of patients with cardiac lesions develop heart failure. Lesions on the left side are much less extensive, occur in 30% at autopsy, and most frequently affect the mitral valve.

Other clinical manifestations include wheezing or asthma-like symptoms (8–18%) and pellagra-like skin lesions (2–25%). A variety of noncardiac problems due to increased fibrous tissue have been reported including retroperitoneal fibrosis causing urethral obstruction, Peyronie's disease of the penis, intraabdominal fibrosis, and occlusion of the mesenteric arteries or veins.

Pathobiology

In different studies, carcinoid syndrome occurred in 8% of 8876 patients with carcinoid tumors with a rate of 1.4–18.4%. It only occurs when sufficient concentrations of secreted products by the tumor reach the systemic circulation. In 91% of cases this occurs after distant metastases to the liver. Rarely primary gut carcinoids with

nodal metastases with extensive retroperitoneal invasion, pancreatic carcinoids with retroperitoneal lymph nodes, or carcinoids of the lung or ovary with direct access to the systemic circulation can cause the carcinoid syndrome without hepatic metastases. All carcinoid tumors do not have the same propensity to metastasize and cause the carcinoid syndrome. Midgut carcinoids account for 60–67% of the cases of carcinoid syndrome, foregut tumors for 2–33%, hindgut for 1–8%, and an unknown primary location for 2–15% (Tables 50-2, 50-3).

One of the main secretory products of carcinoid tumors involved in the carcinoid syndrome is 5HT (Fig. 50-1), which is synthesized from tryptophan. Up to 50% of dietary tryptophan can be used in this synthetic pathway by tumor cells, which can result in inadequate supplies for conversion to niacin; hence, some patients (2.5%) develop pellagra-like lesions. 5HT has numerous biologic effects including stimulating intestinal secretion with inhibition of absorption, stimulating increases in intestinal motility, and stimulating fibrogenesis. In various studies 56–88% of all carcinoid tumors were associated with 5HT overproduction; however, 12–26% of patients did not have the carcinoid syndrome. In one study, platelet 5HT was elevated in 96% of patients with midgut carcinoids, in 43% with foregut tumors, and in 0% with hindgut tumors. In 90–100% of patients with the carcinoid syndrome, evidence of 5HT overproduction is noted. 5HT is thought to be predominantly responsible for the diarrhea by its effects on gut motility and intestinal secretion, primarily through $5HT_3$ and, to a lesser degree, $5HT_4$ receptors. Serotonin receptor antagonists (especially $5HT_3$ antagonists) relieve the diarrhea in most patients. Additional studies suggest prostaglandin E_2 and tachykinins may be important mediators of the diarrhea in some patients. 5HT does not appear to be involved in the flushing because flushing is not relieved by serotonin receptor antagonists. In patients with gastric carcinoids the red, patchy pruritic flush is likely due to histamine release, because it can be prevented by H_1 and H_2 receptor antagonists. Numerous studies show tachykinins are stored in carcinoid tumors and released during flushing. However, octreotide can relieve the flushing induced by pentagastrin in these patients without altering the stimulated increase in plasma substance P, suggesting that other mediators must be involved in the flushing. Both histamine and 5HT may be responsible for the wheezing as well as the fibrotic reactions involving the heart, causing Peyronie's disease and intraabdominal fibrosis. The exact mechanism of the heart disease is unclear. The valvular heart disease caused by the appetite-suppressant drug dexfenfluramine is histologically indistinguishable from that observed in carcinoid disease. Furthermore, ergot-containing dopamine receptor agonists used for Parkinson's disease (pergolide, cabergoline) cause valvular heart disease that closely resembles that seen in the carcinoid syndrome. Metabolites of fenfluramine, as well as the dopamine receptor agonists, have high affinity for $5HT_{2B}$ receptors, activation of which is known to cause fibroblast mitogenesis. High levels of $5HT_{2B}$ receptors are known to occur in heart valves. Studies on cultured interstitial cells from human cardiac valves demonstrate that these valvulopathic drugs induce mitogenesis by activating $5HT_{2B}$ receptors and stimulating upregulation of transforming growth factor β and collagen biosynthesis. These observations support the conclusion that 5HT overproduction by carcinoid tumors is important in mediating the valvular changes, possibly by activating $5HT_{2B}$ receptors in the endocardium. Both the magnitude of serotonin overproduction and prior chemotherapy are important predictors of progression of the heart disease. Atrial natriuretic peptide overproduction is also reported in patients with cardiac disease, but its role in the pathogenesis is unknown.

Patients may develop either a typical or atypical carcinoid syndrome. In patients with the typical form, characteristically caused by a midgut carcinoid tumor, the conversion of tryptophan to 5HTP is the rate-limiting step (Fig. 50-1). Once 5HTP is formed it is rapidly converted to 5HT and stored in secretory granules of the tumor or in platelets. A small amount remains in plasma that is converted to 5HIAA, which appears in large amounts in the urine. These patients have an expanded 5HT pool size, increased blood and platelet 5HT, and increased urinary 5HIAA. Some carcinoid tumors cause an atypical carcinoid syndrome thought due to a deficiency in the enzyme dopa decarboxylase, and thus, 5HTP cannot be converted to 5HT and instead is secreted into the bloodstream. In these patients, plasma 5HT levels are normal but urinary levels may be increased because some 5HTP is converted to 5HT in the kidney. Characteristically, urinary 5HTP and 5HT are increased, but urinary 5HIAA levels are only slightly elevated. Foregut carcinoids are the most likely to cause an atypical carcinoid syndrome.

One of the most immediate life-threatening complications of the carcinoid syndrome is the development of a carcinoid crisis. This is more frequent in patients who have intense symptoms or have greatly increased urinary 5HIAA levels (i.e., >200 mg/d). The crises may occur spontaneously or be provoked by stress, anesthesia, chemotherapy, or a biopsy. Patients develop intense flushing, diarrhea, abdominal pain, cardiac abnormalities including tachycardia, hypertension, or hypotension. If not adequately treated, it can be a terminal event.

DIAGNOSIS OF THE CARCINOID SYNDROME AND CARCINOID TUMORS

The diagnosis of carcinoid syndrome relies on measurement of urinary or plasma serotonin or its metabolites in the urine. The measurement of 5HIAA is most frequently used. False-positive elevations may occur if the patient is eating serotonin-rich foods such as bananas, pineapple, walnuts, pecans, avocados, or hickory nuts or is taking certain medications (cough syrup containing guaifenesin, acetaminophen, salicylates, or L-dopa). The normal range in daily urinary 5HIAA excretion is 2–8 mg/d. In one study, 92% of patients with carcinoid syndrome had 5HT overproduction; in another, 5HIAA had a 73% sensitivity and 100% specificity for carcinoid syndrome.

Most physicians use only the urinary 5HIAA excretion rate; however, plasma and platelet serotonin levels, if available, may give additional information. Platelet serotonin levels are more sensitive than urinary 5HIAA but are not generally available. Because patients with foregut carcinoids may produce an atypical carcinoid syndrome, if this syndrome is suspected and urinary 5HIAA is minimally elevated or normal, other urinary metabolites of tryptophan, such as 5HTP or 5HT, should be measured.

Flushing occurs in a number of other conditions, such as systemic mastocytosis, chronic myeloid leukemia with increased histamine release, and menopause; as a reaction to alcohol or glutamate; and as a side effect of chlorpropamide, calcium channel blockers, and nicotinic acid. None of these conditions cause an increased urinary 5HIAA.

The diagnosis of carcinoid tumor can be suggested by the carcinoid syndrome, by recurrent abdominal symptoms in a healthy-appearing individual, or by discovering hepatomegaly or hepatic metastases associated with minimal symptoms. Ileal carcinoids, which are 25% of all clinically detected carcinoids, should be suspected in patients with bowel obstruction, abdominal pain, flushing, or diarrhea.

Serum chromogranin A levels are elevated in 56–100% of patients with carcinoid tumors, and the level correlates with tumor bulk. Serum chromogranin A levels are not specific for carcinoid tumors because they are also elevated in patients with PETs and other NETs. Plasma neuron-specific enolase levels are also used as a marker of carcinoid tumors but are less sensitive than chromogranin A, being increased in only 17–47% of patients.

Treatment: ℞ CARCINOID SYNDROME AND NON-METASTATIC CARCINOID TUMORS

CARCINOID SYNDROME Treatment includes avoiding conditions that precipitate flushing, dietary supplementation with nicotinamide, treatment of heart failure with diuretics, treatment of wheezing with oral bronchodilators, and controlling the diarrhea with antidiarrheal agents such as loperamide or diphenoxylate. If patients still have symptoms, serotonin receptor antagonists or somatostatin analogues are the drugs of choice.

There are 14 subclasses of 5HT receptors, and antagonists for most are not available. The $5HT_1$ and

5HT$_2$ receptor antagonists methysergide, cyprohepta-dine, and ketanserin have all been used to control the diarrhea but usually do not decrease flushing. Methy-sergide use is limited because it can cause retroperi-toneal fibrosis. Ketanserin diminishes diarrhea in 30–100% of patients. 5HT$_3$ receptor antagonists (ondansetron, tropisetron, alosetron) can control diar-rhea and nausea in up to 100% of patients and occa-sionally ameliorate the flushing. A combination of histamine H$_1$ and H$_2$ receptor antagonists (i.e., diphen-hydramine and cimetidine or ranitidine) may control flushing in patients with foregut carcinoids.

Synthetic analogues of somatostatin (octreotide, lan-reotide) are the most widely used agents to control the symptoms of patients with carcinoid syndrome (Fig. 50-2). These drugs are effective at relieving symptoms and decreasing urinary 5HIAA levels in patients with carcinoid

syndrome. Octreotide controls symptoms in >80% of patients, including the diarrhea and flushing, and 70% of patients have a >50% decrease in urinary 5HIAA excre-tion. Patients with mild to moderate symptoms should initially be treated with 100 µg SC every 8 h. Individual responses vary, and some patients have received as much as 3000 µg/d. Some 40% of patients escape control after a median of 4 months, and the dose may need to be increased. Similar results are reported with lanreotide.

In patients with carcinoid crises, somatostatin ana-logues are effective at both treating the condition as well as preventing symptoms during known precipitat-ing events such as surgery, anesthesia, chemotherapy, or stress. It is recommended that octreotide, 150–250 µg SC every 6–8 h, be used 24–48 h before anesthesia and then continued throughout the procedure.

Sustained-release preparations of both octreotide [octreotide-LAR (long-acting release)] and lanreotide [lan-reotide-PR (prolonged release, lanreotide autogel)] permit infrequent injections. Octreotide-LAR (30 mg/month) gives a plasma level ≥ 1 ng/mL for 25 days, whereas this requires 3–6 injections per day of the non-sustained-release form. Lanreotide-PR is given IM every 10–14 days, and the lan-reotide autogel every 4–6 weeks. Each of the sustained-release forms is highly effective at controlling the symptoms of the carcinoid syndrome (61–85% of patients).

Short-term side effects occur in 40–60% of patients receiving SC somatostatin analogues. Pain at the injec-tion site and side effects related to the GI tract (59% dis-comfort, 15% nausea, diarrhea) are the most common. They are usually short-lived and do not interrupt treat-ment. Important long-term side effects include gallstone formation, steatorrhea, and deterioration in glucose tol-erance. The overall incidence of gallstones/biliary sludge in one study was 52%, with 7% having symptomatic dis-ease requiring surgical treatment.

Interferon α(IFN-α) is effective in controlling symp-toms of the carcinoid syndrome, either alone or com-bined with hepatic artery embolization. With IFN-α alone the response rate is 42%, and with IFN-α with hepatic artery embolization, diarrhea was controlled for 1 year in 43% and flushing in 86%.

Hepatic artery embolization alone or with chemother-apy (chemoembolization) has been used to control the symptoms of carcinoid syndrome. Embolization alone is reported to control symptoms in up to 76% of patients and chemoembolization (5-fluorouracil, doxorubicin, cis-platin, mitomycin) in 60–75% of patients. Hepatic artery embolization can have major side effects including nau-sea, vomiting, pain, and fever. In two studies, 5–7% of patients died from complications of hepatic artery occlusion.

Other drugs have been used successfully in small num-bers of patients to control the symptoms of carcinoid

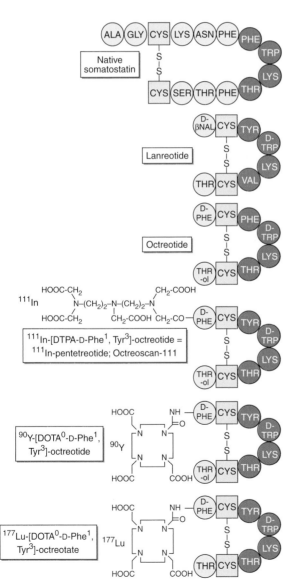

FIGURE 50-2

Structure of somatostatin and synthetic analogues used for diagnostic or therapeutic indications.

syndrome. Parachlorophenylalanine can inhibit tryptophan hydroxylase and the conversion of tryptophan to 5HTP. However, its severe side effects, including psychiatric disturbances, make it intolerable for long-term use. α-Methyldopa inhibits the conversion of 5HTP to 5HT; however, its effects are only partial.

CARCINOID TUMORS (NONMETASTATIC)

Surgery is the only potentially curative therapy. The extent of surgical resection is determined by the size of the primary. With appendiceal carcinoids, appendectomy was curative in 103 patients followed for up to 35 years. With rectal carcinoids <1 cm, local resection is curative. With small-intestinal carcinoids <1 cm, consensus had not been reached. Because 15–69% of small-intestinal carcinoids this size have metastases, some recommend a wide resection with en bloc resection of the adjacent lymph-bearing mesentery. If the carcinoid tumor is >2 cm in rectal, appendiceal, or small-intestinal sites, a full cancer operation should be done. This includes a right hemicolectomy for appendiceal carcinoid, an abdominoperineal resection or low anterior resection for rectal carcinoids and an en bloc resection of adjacent lymph nodes for small-intestinal carcinoids. For carcinoids 1–2 cm in diameter, a simple appendectomy is proposed by some for appendiceal tumors, whereas others favor a formal right hemicolectomy. For 1- to 2-cm rectal carcinoids, a wide local full-thickness excision is performed.

With type I or II gastric carcinoids, which are usually <1 cm, endoscopic removal is recommended. In type I or II gastric carcinoids >2 cm or if there is local invasion, some recommend total gastrectomy, whereas others recommend antrectomy in type 1 to reduce the hypergastrinemia; antrectomy produced regression of the carcinoids in a number of studies. For types I and III gastric carcinoids of 1–2 cm, there is no agreement, with some recommending endoscopic treatment, others surgical treatment. With type III gastric carcinoids >2 cm, excision and regional lymph node clearance is recommended. Most tumors <1 cm are treated endoscopically.

Resection of isolated or limited hepatic metastases may be beneficial (see later).

PANCREATIC ENDOCRINE TUMORS

Functional PETs usually present clinically with symptoms due to the hormone–excess state. Only late in the course of the disease does the tumor per se cause prominent symptoms such as abdominal pain. In contrast, all of the symptoms due to nonfunctional PETs are due to the tumor per se. The overall result of this is that some functional PETs may present with severe symptoms with a small or undetectable primary tumor, whereas nonfunctional tumors almost always present late in their disease course with large tumors, which are usually metastatic. The mean delay between onset of continuous symptoms and diagnosis of a functional PET syndrome is 4–7 years. Therefore, the diagnoses are frequently missed for extended periods of time.

℞ Treatment:
PANCREATIC ENDOCRINE TUMORS

Treatment of PETs requires two different strategies. (1) Treatment must be directed at the hormone excess state, such as the gastric acid hypersecretion in gastrinomas or hypoglycemia in insulinomas. Ectopic hormone secretion usually causes the presenting symptoms and can cause life-threatening complications. (2) With all of the tumors except insulinomas, >50% are malignant (Table 50-2); therefore, treatment must also be directed against the tumor itself. Because these tumors are frequently widespread, surgical resection for cure, which addresses both treatment aspects, is not possible.

GASTRINOMAS (ZOLLINGER-ELLISON SYNDROME)

A gastrinoma is a NET that secretes gastrin; the resultant hypergastrinemia causes gastric acid hypersecretion (ZES). The chronic gastric acid hypersecretion leads to growth of the gastric mucosa with increased numbers of parietal cells and proliferation of gastric ECL cells. The gastric acid hypersecretion characteristically causes peptic ulcer disease (PUD), often refractory and severe, as well as diarrhea. The most common presenting symptoms are abdominal pain (70–100%), diarrhea (37–73%), and gastroesophageal reflux disease (GERD) (30–35%); 10–20% have diarrhea only. Although peptic ulcers may occur in unusual locations, most patients have a typical duodenal ulcer. Important observations that should suggest this diagnosis include PUD with diarrhea; PUD in an unusual location or with multiple ulcers; and PUD refractory to treatment, associated with prominent gastric folds, associated with findings suggestive of MEN-1 (endocrinopathy, family history of ulcer or endocrinopathy, nephrolithiases), or without *Helicobacter pylori* present. *H. pylori* is present in >90% of idiopathic peptic ulcers but is present in <50% of patients with gastrinomas. Chronic unexplained diarrhea should also suggest gastrinoma.

About 20–25% of patients have MEN-1, and in most cases hyperparathyroidism is present prior to the gastrinoma. These patients are treated differently from those without MEN-1; therefore, MEN-1 should be sought in all patients by family history, by measuring plasma ionized calcium and prolactin levels and plasma hormone levels (parathormone, growth hormone).

Most gastrinomas (50–70%) are present in the duodenum, followed by the pancreas (20–40%) and other intraabdominal sites (mesentery, lymph nodes, biliary tract, liver, stomach, ovary). Three cases with two extraabdominal sites have been described: gastrinomas of the left ventricular septum of the heart and non-small cell lung cancer. In MEN-1, the gastrinomas are also usually in the duodenum (70–90%) or the pancreas (10–30%), and they are almost always multiple. About 60–90% of gastrinomas are malignant (Table 50-2) with metastatic spread to lymph nodes and liver. Distant metastases to bone occur in 12–30% of patients with liver metastases.

Diagnosis

The diagnosis of gastrinoma requires the demonstration of fasting hypergastrinemia and an increased basal gastric acid output (BAO) (hyperchlorhydria). Greater than 98% of patients with gastrinomas have fasting hypergastrinemia, although in 40–60% the level may be less than tenfold elevated. Therefore, when the diagnosis is suspected, a fasting gastrin level should be determined first. Potent gastric acid–suppressant drugs such as proton pump inhibitors (e.g., omeprazole, esomeprazole) can suppress acid secretion sufficiently to cause hypergastrinemia; because of their prolonged duration of action, the drugs need to be discontinued for a week before the gastrin determination. If the gastrin level is elevated, it is important to show it is increased when gastric pH ≤ 2.0; physiologic hypergastrinemia secondary to achlorhydria (atrophic gastritis, pernicious anemia) is one of the most common causes of hypergastrinemia. Nearly all gastrinoma patients have a fasting pH ≤ 2 when off antisecretory drugs. If the fasting gastrin >1000 ng/L (10 times increased) and the pH ≤ 2.0, which occurs in 40–60% of patients with gastrinoma, the diagnosis is established after ruling out the possibility of retained antrum syndrome by history. In patients with hypergastrinemia with fasting gastrin < 1000 ng/L and gastric pH ≤ 2.0, other conditions such as *H. pylori* infections, antral G cell hyperplasia/hyperfunction, gastric outlet obstruction, or rarely, renal failure can masquerade as a gastrinoma. To establish the diagnosis in this group, a determination of BAO and a secretin stimulation test should be done. In patients with gastrinomas without previous gastric acid–reducing surgery, the BAO is usually (>90%) elevated (i.e., >15 meq/h). The secretin stimulation test is usually positive, with the criterion of >120 ng/L increase over the basal level having the highest sensitivity (94%) and specificity (100%).

℞ **Treatment:**
GASTRINOMAS

Gastric acid hypersecretion in patients with gastrinomas can be controlled in almost every case by oral gastric antisecretory drugs. Because of their long duration of action and potency, allowing once or twice a day dosing, the proton pump inhibitors are the drugs of choice.

Histamine H_2-receptor antagonists are also effective, although more frequent dosing (q 4–8 h) and high doses are frequently required. In patients with MEN-1 with hyperparathyroidism, correction of the hyperparathyroidism increases the sensitivity to gastric antisecretory drugs and decreases the basal acid output.

With the increased ability to control acid hypersecretion, >50% of the patients who are not cured (>60% of patients) will die from tumor-related causes. At presentation careful imaging studies are essential to localize the extent of the tumor. A third of patients present with hepatic metastases, and in <15% of those with hepatic metastases the disease is limited, so that surgical resection may be possible. Surgical cure is possible in 30% of patients without MEN-1 or liver metastases (40% of all patients). In patients with MEN-1, long-term surgical cure is rare because the tumors are multiple, frequently with lymph node metastases. Therefore, all patients with gastrinomas without MEN-1 or a medical condition limiting life expectancy should undergo surgery by an experienced surgeon.

INSULINOMAS

An insulinoma is an endocrine tumor of the pancreas derived from beta cells that ectopically secretes insulin, which results in hypoglycemia. The average age of occurrence is 40–50 years. The most common clinical symptoms are due to the effect of the hypoglycemia on the central nervous system (neuroglycemic symptoms) and include confusion, headache, disorientation, visual difficulties, irrational behavior, or even coma. Also, most patients have symptoms due to excess catecholamine release secondary to the hypoglycemia including sweating, tremor, and palpitations. Characteristically these attacks are associated with fasting.

Insulinomas are generally small (>90% <2 cm), usually not multiple (90%), and only 5–15% are malignant; they almost invariably occur only in the pancreas, distributed equally in the pancreatic head, body, and tail.

Insulinomas should be suspected in all patients with hypoglycemia, especially with a history suggesting attacks provoked by fasting or with a family history of MEN-1. Insulin is synthesized as proinsulin, a 21-amino-acid α-chain and a 30-amino-acid β-chain connected by a 33-amino-acid connecting peptide (C peptide). In insulinomas, in addition to elevated plasma insulin levels, elevated plasma proinsulin levels are found and C-peptide levels can be elevated.

Diagnosis

The diagnosis of insulinoma requires the demonstration of an elevated plasma insulin level at the time of hypoglycemia. A number of other conditions may cause fasting hypoglycemia, such as the inadvertent or surreptitious use of insulin or oral hypoglycemic agents, severe liver disease, alcoholism, poor nutrition, or other extrapancreatic tumors. The most reliable test to diagnose insulinoma is a fast up to 72 h with serum glucose, C-peptide, and insulin measurements every 4–8 h. If at any point the patient becomes symptomatic or glucose levels are persistently <2.2 mmol/L (40 mg/dL), the test should be terminated and repeat samples for the above studies obtained before glucose is given. Some 70–80% of patients will develop hypoglycemia during the first 24 h and 98% by 48 h. In nonobese normal subjects, serum insulin levels should decrease to <43 pmol/L (<6 μU/mL) when blood glucose decreases to ≤2.2 mmol/L (≤40 mg/dL) and the ratio of insulin to glucose is <0.3 (in mg/dL). In addition to having an insulin level >6 μU/mL when blood glucose is ≤40 mg/dL, some investigators also require an elevated C-peptide and serum proinsulin level, an insulin/glucose ratio >0.3, and a decreased plasma β-hydroxybutyrate level for the diagnosis of insulinomas. Surreptitious use of insulin or hypoglycemic agents may be difficult to distinguish from insulinomas. The combination of proinsulin levels (normal in exogenous insulin/hypoglycemic agent users), C-peptide levels (low in exogenous insulin users), antibodies to insulin (positive in exogenous insulin users), and measurement of sulfonylurea levels in serum or plasma will allow the correct diagnosis to be made. The diagnosis of insulinoma has been complicated by the introduction of specific insulin assays that do not also interact with proinsulin, as do many of the older radioimmunoassays (RIAs), and therefore give lower plasma insulin levels. The increased use of these specific insulin assays has resulted in increased numbers of patients with insulinomas having lower plasma insulin values than the 43 pmol/L (6 μU/mL) levels proposed to be characteristic of insulinomas by RIA. In these patients the assessment of proinsulin and C-peptide levels at the time of hypoglycemia are particularly helpful for establishing the correct diagnosis.

℞ Treatment:
INSULINOMAS

Only 5–15% of insulinomas are malignant; therefore, after appropriate imaging (see later), surgery should be performed. In different studies, 75–95% of patients are cured by surgery. Before surgery, the hypoglycemia can be controlled by frequent small meals and the use of diazoxide (150–800 mg/d). Diazoxide is a benzothiadiazide whose hyperglycemic effect is attributed to inhibition of insulin release. Its side effects are sodium retention and GI symptoms such as nausea. Approximately 50–60% of patients respond to diazoxide. Other agents effective in some patients to control the hypoglycemia include verapamil and diphenylhydantoin. Long-acting somatostatin analogues such as octreotide are acutely effective in 40% of patients. However, octreotide needs to be used with care because it inhibits growth hormone secretion and can alter plasma glucagon levels; therefore, in some patients it can worsen the hypoglycemia.

For the 5–15% of patients with malignant insulinomas, the above drugs or somatostatin analogues are used initially. If they are not effective, various anti-tumor treatments such as hepatic arterial embolization, chemoembolization, or chemotherapy have been used (see later).

GLUCAGONOMAS

A glucagonoma is an endocrine tumor of the pancreas that secretes excessive amounts of glucagon, which causes a distinct syndrome characterized by dermatitis, glucose intolerance or diabetes, and weight loss. Glucagonomas principally occur between 45 and 70 years of age. The tumor is clinically heralded by a characteristic dermatitis (migratory necrolytic erythema) (67–90%), accompanied by glucose intolerance (40–90%), weight loss (66–96%), anemia (33–85%), diarrhea (15–29%), and thromboembolism (11–24%). The rash starts usually as an annular erythema at intertriginous and periorificial sites, especially in the groin or buttock. It subsequently becomes raised and bullae form; when the bullae rupture, eroded areas form. The lesions can wax and wane. A characteristic laboratory finding is hypoaminoacidemia, which occurs in 26–100% of patients.

Glucagonomas are generally large tumors (5–10 cm) at diagnosis. Some 50–80% occur in the pancreatic tail. From 50–82% have evidence of metastatic spread at presentation, usually to the liver. Glucagonomas are rarely extrapancreatic and usually occur singly.

Diagnosis

The diagnosis is confirmed by demonstrating an increased plasma glucagon level (normal is <150 ng/L). Plasma glucagon levels are >1000 ng/L in 90%, between 500 and 1000 ng/L in 7%, and <500 ng/L in 3%. A plasma glucagon level >1000 ng/L is considered diagnostic of glucagonoma. Other diseases causing increased plasma glucagon levels include renal insufficiency, acute pancreatitis, hypercorticism, hepatic insufficiency, prolonged fasting, or familial hyperglucagonemia. With the exception of cirrhosis, these disorders do not increase plasma glucagon to >500 ng/L.

R☓ Treatment: GLUCAGONOMAS

In 50–80% of patients, metastases are present, so curative surgical resection is not possible. Surgical debulking in patients with advanced disease or other anti-tumor treatments may be beneficial (see later). Long-acting somatostatin analogues such as octreotide or lanreotide improve the skin rash in 75% of patients and may improve the weight loss, pain, and diarrhea but usually do not improve the glucose intolerance.

SOMATOSTATINOMA SYNDROME

The somatostatinoma syndrome is due to a NET that secretes excessive amounts of somatostatin, which causes a distinct syndrome characterized by diabetes mellitus, gallbladder disease, diarrhea, and steatorrhea. There is no general distinction in the literature between a tumor that contains somatostatin-like immunoreactivity (somatostatinoma) and does (11–45%), or does not (55–89%) produce a clinical syndrome (somatostatinoma syndrome) by secreting somatostatin. In one review of 173 cases of somatostatinomas, only 11% were associated with the somatostatinoma syndrome. The mean age of patients is 51 years. Somatostatinomas occur primarily in the pancreas and small intestine, and the frequency of the symptoms differs in each. Each of the usual symptoms is more frequent in pancreatic than intestinal somatostatinomas: diabetes mellitus (95% vs 21%), gallbladder disease (94% vs 43%), diarrhea (92% vs 38%), steatorrhea (83% vs 12%), hypochlorhydria (86% vs 12%), and weight loss (90% vs 69%). Somatostatinomas occur in the pancreas in 56–74% of cases, with the primary location being in the pancreatic head. The tumors are usually solitary (90%) and large, with a mean size of 4.5 cm. Liver metastases are frequent, being present in 69–84% of patients.

Somatostatin is a tetradecapeptide that is widely distributed in the central nervous system and GI tract, where it functions as a neurotransmitter or has paracrine and autocrine actions. It is a potent inhibitor of many processes including release of almost all hormones, acid secretion, intestinal and pancreatic secretion, and intestinal absorption. Most of the clinical manifestations are directly related to these inhibitory actions.

Diagnosis

In most cases somatostatinomas have been found by accident either at the time of cholecystectomy or during endoscopy. The presence of psammoma bodies in a duodenal tumor should particularly raise suspicion. Duodenal somatostatin-containing tumors are increasingly associated with von Recklinghausen's disease. Most of these do not cause the somatostatinoma syndrome. The diagnosis of the somatostatinoma syndrome requires the demonstration of elevated plasma somatostatin levels.

R☓ Treatment: SOMATOSTATINOMAS

Pancreatic tumors are frequently (70–92%) metastatic at presentation, whereas 30–69% of small-intestinal somatostatinomas have metastases. Surgery is the treatment of choice for those without widespread hepatic metastases. Symptoms in patients with the somatostatinoma syndrome are improved by octreotide treatment.

VIPOMAS

VIPomas are endocrine tumors that secrete excessive amounts of VIP, which causes a distinct syndrome characterized by large-volume diarrhea, hypokalemia, and dehydration. This syndrome is also called Verner-Morrison syndrome, pancreatic cholera, and WDHA syndrome for *w*atery *d*iarrhea, *h*ypokalemia, and *a*chlorhydria, which some patients develop. The mean age of patients with this syndrome is 49 years; however, it can occur in children and when it does, it is usually caused by a ganglioneuroma or ganglioneuroblastoma.

The principal symptoms are large-volume diarrhea (100%) severe enough to cause hypokalemia (80–100%), dehydration (83%), hypochlorhydria (54–76%), and flushing (20%). The diarrhea is secretory in nature, persisting during fasting, is almost always >1 L/d and >3 L/d in 70%. Most patients do not have accompanying steatorrhea (16%), and the increased stool volume is due to increased excretion of sodium and potassium, which, with the anions, account for the osmolality of the stool. Patients frequently have hyperglycemia (25–50%) and hypercalcemia (25–50%).

VIP is a 28-amino-acid peptide important as a neurotransmitter, ubiquitously present in the central nervous system and GI tract. Its known actions include stimulation of small-intestinal chloride secretion, effects on smooth-muscle contractility, inhibition of acid secretion, and vasodilatory effects, which explain most features of the clinical syndrome.

In adults 80–90% of VIPomas are pancreatic in location, with the rest due to VIP-secreting pheochromocytomas, intestinal carcinoids, and, rarely, ganglioneuromas. These tumors are usually solitary, 50–75% are in the pancreatic tail, and 37–68% have hepatic metastases at diagnosis. In children <10 years old, the syndrome is usually due to ganglioneuromas or ganglioblastomas and is less often malignant (10%).

Diagnosis

The diagnosis requires the demonstration of an elevated plasma VIP level and the presence of large-volume diarrhea. A stool volume of <700 mL/day is proposed to exclude the diagnosis of VIPoma. By fasting the patient, a number of causes can be excluded that cause marked diarrhea. Other diseases that can give a secretory large-volume diarrhea include gastrinomas, chronic laxative abuse, carcinoid syndrome, systemic mastocytosis, rarely medullary thyroid cancer, diabetes, and AIDS. Of these conditions, only VIPomas cause a marked increase in plasma VIP.

℞ **Treatment:**
VASOACTIVE INTESTINAL PEPTIDOMAS

The most important initial treatment in these patients is to correct their dehydration, hypokalemia, and electrolyte losses with fluid and electrolyte replacement. These patients may require 5 L/d of fluid and >350 meq/day of potassium. Because 37–68% of adults with VIPomas have metastatic disease in the liver at presentation, a significant number of patients cannot be cured surgically. In these patients long-acting somatostatin analogues such as octreotide or lanreotide are the drugs of choice.

Octreotide will control the diarrhea in 87% of patients. In nonresponsive patients the combination of glucocorticoids and octreotide has proved helpful in a small number of patients. Other drugs reported to be helpful in small numbers of patients include prednisone (60–100 mg/d), clonidine, indomethacin, phenothiazines, loperamide, lidamidine, lithium, propanolol, and metoclopramide. Treatment of advanced disease with embolization, chemoembolization, and chemotherapy may also be helpful (see later).

NONFUNCTIONAL PANCREATIC ENDOCRINE TUMORS

Nonfunctional PETs are endocrine tumors that originate in the pancreas and either secrete no products or their products do not cause a specific clinical syndrome. The symptoms are due entirely to the tumor per se. Nonfunctional PETs secrete chromogranin A (90–100%), chromogranin B (90–100%), PP (58%), α-hCG (40%), and β-hCG (20%). Because the symptoms are due to the tumor alone, patients with nonfunctional PETs usually present late in their disease course with invasive tumors and hepatic metastases (64–92%), and the tumors are usually large (72% > 5 cm). The tumors are usually solitary except in patients with MEN-1, where they are multiple. They occur primarily in the pancreatic head. Even though these tumors do not cause a functional syndrome, immunocytochemical studies show they synthesize numerous peptides and cannot be distinguished from functional tumors by immunocytochemistry.

The most common symptoms are abdominal pain (30–80%); jaundice (20–35%); weight loss, fatigue, or bleeding; and 10–15% are found incidentally. The average time from the beginning of symptoms to diagnosis is 5 years.

Diagnosis

The diagnosis is established by histologic confirmation in a patient without either clinical symptoms or elevated plasma hormone levels. Even though chromogranin A levels are elevated in almost every patient, this is not specific for this disease as it can be found in functional PETs, carcinoids, and other neuroendocrine disorders. Plasma PP is increased in 22–71% of patients and should strongly suggest the diagnosis in a patient with a pancreatic mass because it is usually normal in patients with pancreatic adenocarcinomas. Elevated plasma PP is not diagnostic of this tumor because it is elevated in a number of other conditions such as chronic renal failure, old age, inflammatory conditions, and diabetes.

℞ **Treatment:**
NONFUNCTIONAL PANCREATIC ENDOCRINE TUMORS

Unfortunately, surgical curative resection can be considered only in the minority of the patients because 64–92% present with metastatic disease. Treatment is directed against the tumor per se using chemotherapy, embolization, chemoembolization, or hormonal therapy (see later).

GRFOMAS

GRFomas are endocrine tumors that secrete excessive amounts of GRF that causes acromegaly. The true frequency of this syndrome is not known. GRF is a 44-amino-acid peptide, and 25–44% of PETs have GRF immunoreactivity, although it is uncommonly secreted. GRFomas are lung tumors in 47–54% of cases, PETs in 29–30%, and small-intestinal carcinoids in 8–10%; up to 12% occur at other sites. Patients have a mean age of 38 years, and the symptoms are usually due to either acromegaly or the tumor itself. The acromegaly caused by GRFomas is indistinguishable from classic acromegaly. The pancreatic tumors are usually large (>6 cm), and liver metastases are present in 39%. They should be suspected in any patient with acromegaly and an abdominal tumor, in a patient with MEN-1 with acromegaly, or in a patient without a pituitary adenoma with acromegaly or associated with hyperprolactinemia, which occurs in 70% of GRFomas. GRFomas are an uncommon cause of acromegaly. The diagnosis is established by performing plasma assays for GRF and growth hormone. The normal level for GRF is <5 μg/L in men and <10 μg/L in women. Most GRFomas have a plasma GRF level ≥ 300 μg/L. Patients with GRFomas also have increased plasma insulin-like growth factor 1 levels similar to those in classic acromegaly. Surgery is the treatment of choice if diffuse metastases are not present. Long-acting somatostatin analogues such as octreotide or lanreotide are the agents of choice, with 75–100% of patients responding.

OTHER RARE PANCREATIC ENDOCRINE TUMOR SYNDROMES

Cushing's syndrome (ACTHoma) due to a PET occurs in 4–16% of all ectopic Cushing's syndrome cases. It occurs in 5% of cases of sporadic gastrinomas, almost invariably in patients with hepatic metastases, and is an independent poor prognostic factor. Paraneoplastic hypercalcemia due to PETs releasing parathyroid hormone–related peptide (PTHrP), a PTH-like material, or unknown factor, is rarely reported. The tumors are usually large, and liver metastases are usually present. Most (88%) appear to be due to release of PTHrP. PETs can occasionally cause the carcinoid syndrome. PETs secreting calcitonin have been proposed as a specific clinical syndrome. Half of the patients have diarrhea, which disappears with resection of the tumor. The proposal that this could be a discrete syndrome is supported by finding that 25–42% of patients with medullary thyroid cancer with hypercalcitoninemia develop diarrhea, likely secondary to a motility disorder. A renin-producing PET has been described in a patient presenting with hypertension; PETs secreting luteinizing hormone, resulting in masculinization or decreased libido, and a PET secreting erythropoietin, resulting in polycythemia have also been reported (Table 50-2). Ghrelin is a 28-amino-acid peptide with a number of metabolic and immunologic functions. Although it is detectable immunohistochemically in most PETs, only 1 in 24 patients (4%) with a PET had elevated plasma ghrelin levels in one study and the patient was asymptomatic. Release of ghrelin by a PET may be clinically silent.

TUMOR LOCALIZATION

Localization of the primary tumor and defining the extent of disease are essential to the proper management of all carcinoids and PETs. Numerous tumor localization methods are used in both types of NETs, including conventional imaging studies (CT, MRI, transabdominal ultrasound, selective angiography), somatostatin receptor scintigraphy (SRS), and positron emission tomographic scanning. In PETs, endoscopic ultrasound (EUS) and functional localization by measuring venous hormonal gradients are also reported useful. Bronchial carcinoids are usually detected by a standard chest radiography and assessed by CT. Rectal, duodenal, colonic, and gastric carcinoids are usually detected by GI endoscopy.

PETs, as well as carcinoid tumors, frequently overexpress high-affinity somatostatin receptors in both their primary tumors and their metastases. Of the five types of somatostatin receptors (sst_{1-5}), radiolabeled octreotide binds with high affinity to sst_2 and sst_5, lower for sst_3, and has a very low affinity for sst_1 and sst_4. Between 90 and 100% of carcinoid tumors and PETs possess sst_2, and many also have the other four sst subtypes. Interaction with these receptors can be used to localize NETs using [^{111}In-DTPA-D-Phe^1]octreotide and radionuclide scanning (SRS) as well as for treatment of the hormone excess state with octreotide or lanreotide, as discussed earlier. Because of its sensitivity and ability to localize tumor throughout the body, SRS is now the initial imaging modality of choice for localizing both primary and metastatic NETs. SRS localizes tumor in 73–89% of patients with carcinoids and in 56–100% of patients with PETs, except for insulinomas. Insulinomas are usually small and have low densities of sst receptors, resulting in SRS being positive in only 12–50% of patients with insulinomas. Figure 50-3 shows an example of the increased sensitivity of SRS in a patient with a carcinoid

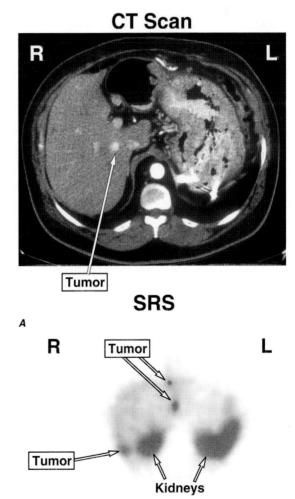

FIGURE 50-3

Ability of CT scanning (A) or somatostatin receptor scintigraphy (SRS) (B) to localize metastatic carcinoid in the liver.

tumor. The CT scan (Fig. 50-3*A*) shows a single liver metastasis, whereas the SRS demonstrates three metastases in the liver in multiple locations (Fig. 50-3*B*). Occasional false-positive responses with SRS can occur (12% in one study) because numerous other normal tissues and diseases can have high densities of sst receptors, including granulomas (sarcoid, TB, etc.), thyroid diseases (goiter, thyroiditis), and activated lymphocytes (lymphomas, wound infections). For PETs located in the pancreas, EUS is highly sensitive, localizing 77–93% of insulinomas, which occur almost exclusively within the pancreas. EUS is less sensitive for extrapancreatic tumors. If liver metastases are identified by SRS, either a CT or MRI is then recommended to assess the size and exact location of the metastases because SRS does not give information on tumor size. Functional localization measuring hormone gradients after intraarterial calcium injections in insulinomas (insulin) or gastrin gradients after secretin injections in gastrinoma is a sensitive method, being positive in 80–100% of patients. However, this method gives only regional localization and therefore is reserved for cases where other imaging modalities are negative. Positron emission tomographic scanning with ^{18}F-fluoro-DOPA in patients with carcinoids or with ^{11}C-5HTP in patients with PETs or carcinoids has greater sensitivity than conventional imaging studies or SRS and will likely be used increasingly in the future.

Treatment:
R_X **ADVANCED DISEASE (DIFFUSE METASTATIC DISEASE)**

The single most important prognostic factor for survival is the presence of liver metastases (**Fig. 50-4**). For patients with foregut carcinoids without hepatic metastases, the 5-year survival in one study was 95% and with distant metastases, 20%. With gastrinomas, the 5-year survival without liver metastases is 98%, with limited metastases in one hepatic lobe it is 78%, and with diffuse metastases, 16%. A number of different modalities are reported to be effective in advanced disease including cytoreductive surgery (removal of all visible tumor), treatment with chemotherapy, somatostatin analogues, IFN-α, hepatic embolization alone or with chemotherapy (chemoembolization), radiotherapy, and liver transplantation.

SPECIFIC ANTITUMOR TREATMENTS Cytoreductive surgery, unfortunately, is only possible in the 9–22% of patients who have limited hepatic metastases. Although no randomized studies have proven that hepatic resection extends life, results from a number of studies suggest it likely increases survival and therefore is recommended, if possible.

Chemotherapy for metastatic carcinoid tumors has generally been disappointing, with response rates of

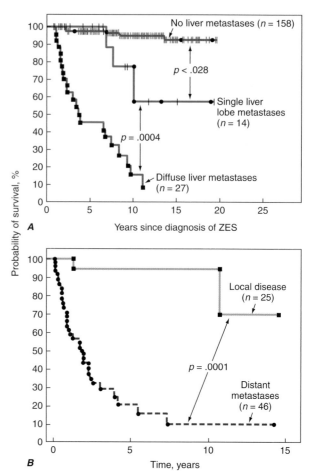

FIGURE 50-4

Effect of the presence and extent of liver metastases on survival in patients with gastrinomas (**A**) or carcinoid tumors (**B**). ZES, Zollinger-Ellison syndrome. (*A is drawn from data from 199 patients with gastrinomas modified from F Yu et al: J Clin Oncol 17:615, 1999. B is drawn from data from 71 patients with foregut carcinoid tumors from EW McDermott et al: Br J Surg 81:1007, 1994.*)

0–40% with various two- or three-drug combinations. Chemotherapy for PETs has been more successful with tumor shrinkage reported in 30–70% of patients. The current regimen of choice is streptozotocin and doxorubicin.

Long-acting somatostatin analogues such as octreotide, lanreotide, and IFN-α rarely decrease tumor size (i.e., 0–17%); however, these drugs have tumoristatic effects, stopping additional growth in 26–95% of patients with NETs. How long tumor stabilization lasts or whether it prolongs survival has not been established.

Hepatic embolization and chemoembolization (with dacarbazine, cisplatin, doxorubicin, 5-fluorouracil, or streptozotocin) have been reported to decrease tumor bulk and to help control the symptoms of the hormone-excess state. These modalities are generally reserved for cases in which treatment with somatostatin analogues, IFN-α (carcinoids), or chemotherapy (PETs) fails.

Embolization, when combined with treatment with octreotide and IFN-α, significantly reduces tumor progression (*p* = .008) over treatment with embolization and octreotide alone in patients with advanced midgut carcinoids.

Radiotherapy with radiolabeled somatostatin analogues that are internalized by the tumors is an approach under investigation. Three different radionuclides are being used: (1) high doses of [^{111}In-DTPA-D-Phe^1]octreotide (Fig. 50-2), which emits γ-rays, internal conversion, and Auger electrons; yttrium-90, which emits high-energy β-particles coupled by a DOTA chelating group to octreotide or octreotate; and (3) ^{177}lutetium-coupled analogues, which emit both β- and γ-rays. All are being tested. Tumor stabilization is reported in 41–81%, 44–88%, and 23–40%, respectively, and a decrease in tumor size in 8–30%, 6–37%, and 38%, respectively, of patients with advanced metastatic NETs. These results suggest this novel therapy may be helpful, especially in patients with advanced metastatic disease.

The use of liver transplantation has been abandoned for treatment of most metastatic tumors to the liver. However, for metastatic NETs it is still a consideration. In a review of 103 cases of malignant NETs (48 PETs, 43 carcinoids), the 2- and 5-year survival rates were 60% and 47%, respectively. However, recurrence-free survival was low (<24%). It was concluded that for younger patients with metastatic NETs limited to the liver, liver transplantation may be justified.

FURTHER READINGS

DAVIES K, CONLON KC: Neuroendocrine tumors of the pancreas. Curr Gastroenterol Rep 11:119, 2009

EHEHALT F et al: Neuroendocrine tumors of the pancreas. Oncologist 14:456, 2009

FORRER F et al: Peptide receptor radiotherapy. Best Practice Res Clin Endocrinol Metab 21:111, 2007

JENSEN RT, DOHERTY GM: Carcinoid tumors and the carcinoid syndrome, in *Cancer: Principles and Practice of Oncology*, 7th ed, VT DeVita Jr, S Hellman, SA Rosenberg (eds). Philadelphia, Lippincott Williams and Wilkins, 2005, pp 1559–1574

MODLIN IM et al: Therapeutic options for gastrointestinal carcinoids. Clin Gastrointest Hepatol 4:526, 2006

OBERG K: Somatostatin analog octreotide LAR in gastro-entero-pancreatic tumors. Expert Rev Anticancer Ther 9:557, 2009

———, ERIKSSON B: Neuroendocrine tumors. Best Pract Res Clin Endocrinol Metabol 21:1, 2007

RINDI G, BORDI C: Aetiology, molecular pathogenesis and genetics. Best Pract Res Clin Gastroenterol 19:519, 2005

——— et al (ed): Consensus guidelines on the management of patients with digestive neuroendocrine tumors. Neuroendocrinology 84:151, 2006

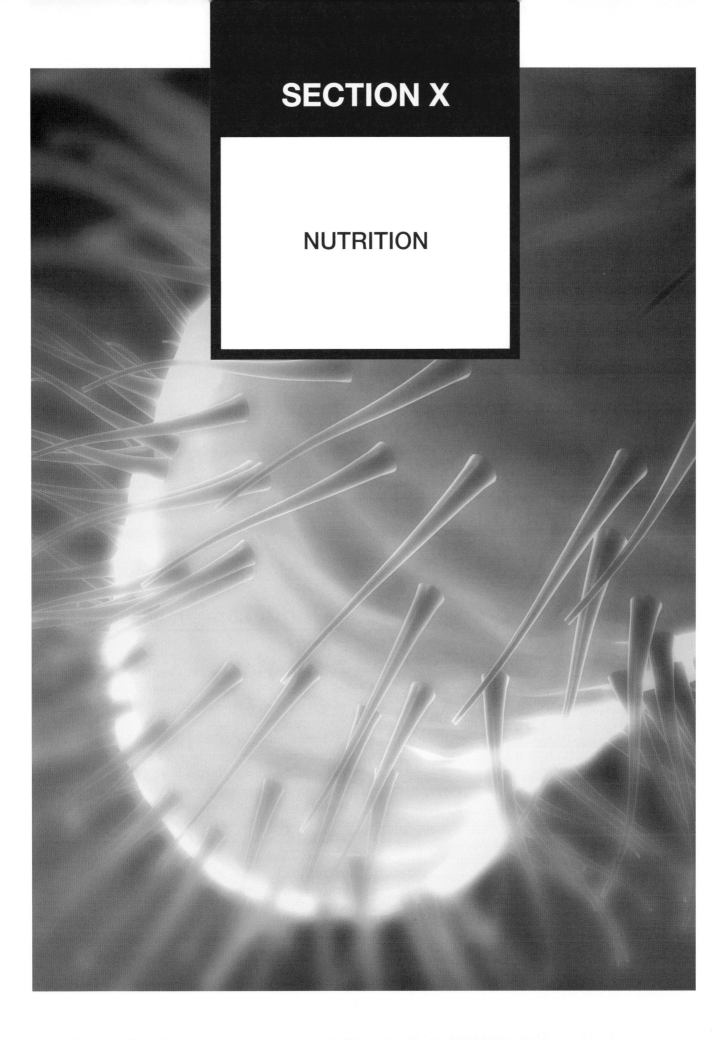

SECTION X

NUTRITION

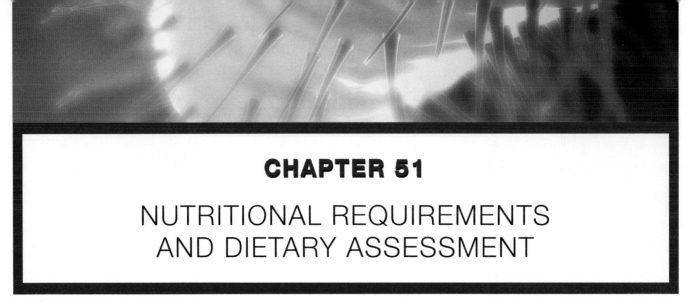

CHAPTER 51

NUTRITIONAL REQUIREMENTS AND DIETARY ASSESSMENT

Johanna Dwyer

Nutrients are substances that must be supplied by the diet because they are not synthesized in the body in sufficient amounts. Nutrient requirements for groups of healthy persons have been determined experimentally. For good health we require energy-providing nutrients (protein, fat, and carbohydrate), vitamins, minerals, and water. Specific nutrient requirements include nine essential amino acids, several fatty acids, four fat-soluble vitamins, ten water-soluble vitamins, and choline. Several inorganic substances, including four minerals, seven trace minerals, three electrolytes, and the ultratrace elements, also must be supplied in the diet.

The required amounts of the essential nutrients differ by age and physiologic state. Conditionally essential nutrients are not required in the diet but must be supplied to individuals who do not synthesize them in adequate amounts, such as those with genetic defects, those having pathologic states with nutritional implications, and developmentally immature infants. Many organic phytochemicals and zoochemicals present in foods have health effects. For example, dietary fiber has beneficial effects on gastrointestinal function. Other bioactive food constituents or contaminants such as lead may have negative health effects.

ESSENTIAL NUTRIENT REQUIREMENTS

ENERGY

For weight to remain stable, energy intake must match energy output. The major components of energy output are resting energy expenditure (REE) and physical activity; minor sources include the energy cost of metabolizing food (thermic effect of food or specific dynamic action) and shivering thermogenesis (e.g., cold-induced thermogenesis). The average energy intake is about 2800 kcal/d for American men and about 1800 kcal/d for American women, although these estimates vary with body size and activity level. Formulas for estimating REE are useful for assessing the energy needs of an individual whose weight is stable. Thus, for males, REE = $900 + 10w$, and for females, REE = $700 + 7w$, where w is weight in kilograms. The calculated REE is then adjusted for physical activity level by multiplying by 1.2 for sedentary, 1.4 for moderately active, or 1.8 for very active individuals. The final figure provides a rough estimate of total caloric needs in a state of energy balance. Formulas to provide more precise estimates of energy requirements are provided by the Food and Nutrition Board, Institute of Medicine, National Academy of Sciences in recent reports on dietary reference intakes. For further discussion of energy balance in health and disease, see Chap. 53.

PROTEIN

Dietary protein consists of both essential and other amino acids that are required for protein synthesis. The nine essential amino acids are histidine, isoleucine, leucine, lysine, methionine/cystine, phenylalanine/tyrosine, threonine, tryptophan, and valine. All amino acids can be used for energy, and certain amino acids (e.g., alanine) can also be used for gluconeogenesis. When energy intake is inadequate, protein intake must be increased, since ingested amino acids are diverted into pathways of glucose synthesis and oxidation. In extreme energy deprivation, protein-calorie malnutrition may ensue (Chap. 53).

For adults, the recommended dietary allowance (RDA) for protein is about 0.6 g/kg desirable body weight per day, assuming that energy needs are met and that the protein is of relatively high biologic value. Current recommendations for a healthy diet call for at least 10–14% of calories from protein. Biologic value tends to be highest for animal proteins, followed by proteins from legumes (beans), cereals (rice, wheat, corn), and roots. Combinations of plant proteins that complement one another in biologic value or combinations of animal and plant proteins can increase biologic value and lower total protein requirements.

Protein needs increase during growth, pregnancy, lactation, and rehabilitation after malnutrition. Tolerance to normal amounts of dietary protein is decreased in renal insufficiency and liver failure, precipitating encephalopathy in patients with cirrhosis of the liver.

FAT AND CARBOHYDRATE

Fats are a concentrated source of energy and constitute on average 34% of calories in U.S. diets. For optimal health, saturated fat and trans-fat should be limited to <10% of calories, and polyunsaturated fats to <10% of calories, with monounsaturated fats constituting the remainder of fat intake. At least 55% of total calories should be derived from carbohydrates. The brain requires about 100 g/d of glucose for fuel; other tissues use about 50 g/d. Some tissues (e.g., brain and red blood cells) rely on glucose supplied either exogenously or from muscle proteolysis. Over time, some adaptations in carbohydrate needs are possible in other tissues during hypocaloric states.

WATER

For adults, 1.0–1.5 mL water per kcal of energy expenditure is sufficient under usual conditions to allow for normal variations in physical activity, sweating, and solute load

of the diet. Water losses include 50–100 mL/d in the feces, 500–1000 mL/d by evaporation or exhalation, and, depending on the renal solute load, ≥1000 mL/d in the urine. If external losses increase, intakes must increase accordingly to avoid underhydration. Fever increases water losses by approximately 200 mL/d per °C; diarrheal losses vary but may be as great as 5 L/d with severe diarrhea. Heavy sweating and vomiting also increase water losses. When renal function is normal and solute intakes are adequate, the kidneys can adjust to increased water intake by excreting up to 18 L/d of excess water. However, obligatory urine outputs can compromise hydration status when there is inadequate intake or when losses increase in disease or kidney damage.

Infants have high requirements for water because of their large ratio of surface area to volume, the limited capacity of the immature kidney to handle high renal solute loads, and their inability to communicate their thirst. During pregnancy, 30 mL/d additional water is needed. During lactation, milk production increases water requirements by approximately 1000 mL/d, or 1 mL for each mL of milk produced. Special attention must be paid to the water needs of the elderly, who have reduced total body water and blunted thirst sensation, and may be taking diuretics.

OTHER NUTRIENTS

See Chap. 52 for a detailed description of vitamins and trace minerals.

DIETARY REFERENCE INTAKES AND RECOMMENDED DIETARY ALLOWANCES

Fortunately, human life and well-being can be maintained within a fairly wide range for most nutrients. However, the capacity for adaptation is not infinite—too much of a nutrient, as well as too little, may have adverse effects on health. Therefore, quantitative benchmark recommendations on nutrient intakes have been developed to guide clinical practice. These estimates are collectively referred to as the *dietary reference intakes* (DRIs). The DRIs supplant but include the *recommended dietary allowances* (RDAs), the single reference values used in the United States since 1989. DRIs include the *estimated average requirement* (EAR) of a nutrient, as well as three other reference values used for dietary planning for individuals: the RDA, or, if it cannot be established, the *adequate intake* (AI), and the tolerable *upper level* (UL). The current DRIs for vitamins and elements are provided in Tables 51-1 and 51-2, respectively.

ESTIMATED AVERAGE REQUIREMENT

When florid manifestations of the classic dietary deficiency diseases such as rickets, scurvy, xerophthalmia,

TABLE 51-1

DIETARY REFERENCE INTAKES: RECOMMENDED INTAKES FOR INDIVIDUALS—VITAMINS

LIFE-STAGE GROUP	VITAMIN, μg/d A[a]	C	D[b,c]	E[d]	K	THIAMINE, mg/d	RIBOFLAVIN, mg/d	NIACIN, mg/d[e]	VITAMIN B$_6$, mg/d	FOLATE, μg/d[f]	VITAMIN B$_{12}$, μg/d	PANTOTHENIC ACID, mg/d	BIOTIN, μg/d	CHOLINE, mg/d[g]
Infants														
0–6 mo	400	40	5	4	2.0	0.2	0.3	2	0.1	65	0.4	1.7	5	125
7–12 mo	500	50	5	5	2.5	0.3	0.4	4	0.3	80	0.5	1.8	6	150
Children														
1–3 y	**300**	**15**	5	**6**	30	**0.5**	**0.5**	**6**	**0.5**	**150**	**0.9**	2	8	200
4–8 y	**400**	**25**	5	**7**	55	**0.6**	**0.6**	**8**	**0.6**	**200**	**1.2**	3	12	250
Males														
9–13 y	**600**	**45**	5	**11**	60	**0.9**	**0.9**	**12**	**1.0**	**300**	**1.8**	4	20	375
14–18 y	**900**	**75**	5	**15**	75	**1.2**	**1.3**	**16**	**1.3**	**400**	**2.4**	5	25	550
19–30 y	**900**	**90**	5	**15**	120	**1.2**	**1.3**	**16**	**1.3**	**400**	**2.4**	5	30	550
31–50 y	**900**	**90**	5	**15**	120	**1.2**	**1.3**	**16**	**1.3**	**400**	**2.4**	5	30	550
51–70 y	**900**	**90**	10	**15**	120	**1.2**	**1.3**	**16**	**1.7**	**400**	**2.4**[h]	5	30	550
>70 y	**900**	**90**	15	**15**	120	**1.2**	**1.3**	**16**	**1.7**	**400**	**2.4**[h]	5	30	550
Females														
9–13 y	**600**	**45**	5	**11**	60	**0.9**	**0.9**	**12**	**1.0**	**300**	**1.8**	4	20	375
14–18 y	**700**	**65**	5	**15**	75	**1.0**	**1.0**	**14**	**1.2**	**400**[i]	**2.4**	5	25	400
19–30 y	**700**	**75**	5	**15**	90	**1.1**	**1.1**	**14**	**1.3**	**400**[i]	**2.4**	5	30	425
31–50 y	**700**	**75**	5	**15**	90	**1.1**	**1.1**	**14**	**1.3**	**400**[i]	**2.4**	5	30	425
51–70 y	**700**	**75**	10	**15**	90	**1.1**	**1.1**	**14**	**1.5**	**400**	**2.4**[h]	5	30	425
>70 y	**700**	**75**	15	**15**	90	**1.1**	**1.1**	**14**	**1.5**	**400**	**2.4**[h]	5	30	425
Pregnancy														
≤18 y	**750**	**80**	5	**15**	75	**1.4**	**1.4**	**18**	**1.6**	**600**[j]	**2.6**	6	30	450
19–30 y	**770**	**85**	5	**15**	90	**1.4**	**1.4**	**18**	**1.9**	**600**[j]	**2.6**	6	30	450
31–50 y	**770**	**85**	5	**15**	90	**1.4**	**1.4**	**18**	**1.9**	**600**[j]	**2.6**	6	30	450
Lactation														
≤18 y	**1200**	**115**	5	**19**	75	**1.4**	**1.6**	**17**	**2.0**	**500**	**2.8**	7	35	550
19–30 y	**1300**	**120**	5	**19**	90	**1.4**	**1.6**	**17**	**2.0**	**500**	**2.8**	7	35	550
31–50 y	**1300**	**120**	5	**19**	90	**1.4**	**1.6**	**17**	**2.0**	**500**	**2.8**	7	35	550

Note: This table presents recommended dietary allowances (RDAs) in **bold type** and adequate intakes (AIs) in ordinary type. RDAs and AIs may both be used as goals for individual intake. RDAs are set to meet the needs of almost all individuals (97 to 98%) in a group. For healthy breastfed infants, the AI is the mean intake. The AI for other life stage and gender groups is believed to cover needs of all individuals in the group, but lack of data or uncertainty in the data prevent being able to specify with confidence the percentage of individuals covered by this intake.

[a]As retinol activity equivalents (RAEs). 1 RAE = 1 μg retinol, 12 μg β-carotene, 24 μg α-carotene, or 24 μg β-cryptoxanthin. To calculate RAEs from retinol equivalents (REs) of provitamin A carotenoids in foods, divide the REs by 2. For preformed vitamin A in foods or supplements and for provitamin A carotenoids in supplements, 1 RE = 1 RAE.

[b]As calciferol. 1 μg calciferol = 40 IU vitamin D.

[c]In the absence of adequate exposure to sunlight.

[d]As α-tocopherol. α-Tocopherol includes *RRR*-α-tocopherol, the only form of α-tocopherol that occurs naturally in foods, and the 2*R*-stereoisomeric forms of α-tocopherol (*RRR*-, *RSR*-, *RRS*-, and *RSS*-α-tocopherol) that occur in fortified foods and supplements. It does not include the 2*S*-stereoisomeric forms of α-tocopherol (*SRR*-, *SSR*-, *SRS*-, and *SSS*-α-tocopherol), also found in fortified foods and supplements.

[e]As niacin equivalents (NE). 1 mg of niacin = 60 mg of tryptophan; 0–6 months = preformed niacin (not NE).

[f]As dietary folate equivalents (DFEs). 1 DFE = 1 μg food folate = 0.6 μg of folic acid from fortified food or as a supplement consumed with food = 0.5 μg of a supplement taken on an empty stomach.

[g]Although AIs have been set for choline, there are few data to assess whether a dietary supply of choline is needed at all stages of the life cycle, and it may be that the choline requirement can be met by endogenous synthesis at some of these stages.

[h]Because 10 to 30% of older people may malabsorb food-bound B$_{12}$, it is advisable for those >50 years to meet their RDA mainly by consuming foods fortified with B$_{12}$ or a supplement containing B$_{12}$.

[i]In view of evidence linking inadequate folate intake with neural tube defects in the fetus, it is recommended that all women capable of becoming pregnant consume 400 μg from supplements or fortified foods in addition to intake of food folate from a varied diet.

[j]It is assumed that women will continue consuming 400 μg from supplements or fortified food until their pregnancy is confirmed and they enter prenatal care, which ordinarily occurs after the end of the periconceptional period—the critical time forformation of the neural tube.

Source: Food and Nutrition Board, Institute of Medicine—National Academy of Sciences Dietary Reference Intakes, 2000, 2002, reprinted with permission. Courtesy of the Na-tional Academy Press, Washington, DC. http://www.nap.edu

TABLE 51-2

DIETARY REFERENCE INTAKES: RECOMMENDED INTAKES FOR INDIVIDUALS—ELEMENTS

LIFE-STAGE GROUP	CALCIUM, mg/d	CHROMIUM, µg/d	COPPER, µg/d	FLUORIDE, mg/d	IODINE, µg/d	IRON, mg/d	MAGNESIUM, mg/d	MANGANESE, mg/d	MOLYBDENUM, µg/d	PHOSPHORUS, mg/d	SELENIUM, µg/d	ZINC, mg/d
Infants												
0–6 mo	210	0.2	200	0.01	110	0.27	30	0.003	2	100	15	2
7–12 mo	270	5.5	220	0.5	130	11	75	0.6	3	275	20	3
Children												
1–3 y	500	11	340	0.7	90	7	80	1.2	17	460	20	3
4–8 y	800	15	440	1	90	10	130	1.5	22	500	30	5
Males												
9–13 y	1300	25	700	2	120	8	240	1.9	34	1250	40	8
14–18 y	1300	35	890	3	150	11	410	2.2	43	1250	55	11
19–30 y	1000	35	900	4	150	8	400	2.3	45	700	55	11
31–50 y	1000	35	900	4	150	8	420	2.3	45	700	55	11
51–70 y	1200	30	900	4	150	8	420	2.3	45	700	55	11
>70 y	1200	30	900	4	150	8	420	2.3	45	700	55	11
Females												
9–13 y	1300	21	700	2	120	8	240	1.6	34	1250	40	8
14–18 y	1300	24	890	3	150	15	360	1.6	43	1250	55	9
19–30 y	1000	25	900	3	150	18	310	1.8	45	700	55	8
31–50 y	1000	25	900	3	150	18	320	1.8	45	700	55	8
51–70 y	1200	20	900	3	150	8	320	1.8	45	700	55	8
>70 y	1200	20	900	3	150	8	320	1.8	45	700	55	8
Pregnancy												
≤18 y	1300	29	1000	3	220	27	400	2.0	50	1250	60	12
19–30 y	1000	30	1000	3	220	27	350	2.0	50	700	60	11
31–50 y	1000	30	1000	3	220	27	360	2.0	50	700	60	11
Lactation												
≤18 y	1300	44	1300	3	290	10	360	2.6	50	1250	70	13
19–30 y	1000	45	1300	3	290	9	310	2.6	50	700	70	12
31–50 y	1000	45	1300	3	290	9	320	2.6	50	700	70	12

Note: This table presents recommended dietary allowances (RDAs) in **bold type** and adequate intakes (AIs) in ordinary type. RDAs and AIs may both be used as goals for individual intake. RDAs are set to meet the needs of almost all individuals (97 to 98%) in a group. For healthy breastfed infants, the AI is the mean intake. The AI for other life stage and gender groups is believed to cover needs of all individuals in the group, but lack of data or uncertainty in the data prevent being able to specify with confidence the percentage of individuals covered by this intake.

Source: Food and Nutrition Board, Institute of Medicine—National Academy of Sciences Dietary Reference Intakes, 2000, 2002, reprinted with permission. Courtesy of the National Academy Press, Washington, DC. *http://www.nap.edu*

and protein-calorie malnutrition were common, nutrient adequacy was inferred from the absence of their clinical signs. Later, it was determined that biochemical and other changes were evident long before the clinical deficiency became apparent. Consequently, criteria of nutrient adequacy are now based on biologic markers when they are available. Priority is given to sensitive biochemical, physiologic, or behavioral tests that reflect early changes in regulatory processes or maintenance of body stores of nutrients. Current definitions focus on the amount of a nutrient that minimizes the risk of chronic degenerative diseases.

The EAR is the amount of a nutrient estimated to be adequate for half of the healthy individuals of a specific age and sex. The types of evidence and criteria used to establish nutrient requirements vary by nutrient, age, and physiologic group. The EAR is not useful clinically for estimating nutrient adequacy in individuals because it is a median requirement for a group; 50% of individuals in a group fall below the requirement and 50% fall above it. Thus, a person with a usual intake at the EAR has a 50% risk of an inadequate intake. For these reasons, other standards, described below, are more useful for clinical purposes.

RECOMMENDED DIETARY ALLOWANCES

The RDA is the nutrient-intake goal for planning diets of individuals; it is used in the MyPyramid food guide of the U.S. Department of Agriculture (USDA), therapeutic diets, and descriptions of the nutritional content of processed foods and dietary supplements. The nutrient content in a food is stated by weight or as a percentage of the daily value (DV), a variant of the RDA that, for an adult, represents the highest RDA for an adult consuming 2000 kcal/d.

The RDA is the average daily dietary intake level that meets the nutrient requirements of nearly all healthy persons of a specific sex, age, life stage, or physiologic condition (such as pregnancy or lactation).

The RDA is defined statistically as 2 standard deviations (SD) above the EAR to ensure that the needs of most individuals are met.

The risk of dietary inadequacy increases as intake falls further below the RDA. However, the RDA is an overly generous criterion for evaluating nutrient adequacy. For example, by definition the RDA exceeds the actual requirements of all but about 2 to 3% of the population. Therefore, many people whose intake falls below the RDA may still be getting enough of the nutrient.

ADEQUATE INTAKE

It is not possible to set an RDA for some nutrients that do not have an established EAR. In this circumstance, the AI is based on observed, or experimentally determined, approximations of nutrient intakes in healthy people. In the DRIs established to date, AIs rather than RDAs are proposed for infants up to age 1 year, as well as for calcium, chromium, vitamin D, fluoride, manganese, pantothenic acid, biotin, choline, sodium, chloride, potassium, and water for persons of all ages.

TOLERABLE UPPER LEVELS OF NUTRIENT INTAKE

Healthy individuals derive no established benefit from consuming nutrient levels above the RDA or AI. Excessive nutrient intake can disturb body functions and cause acute, progressive, or permanent disabilities. The tolerable UL is the highest level of chronic nutrient intake (usually daily) that is unlikely to pose a risk of adverse health effects for most of the population. Data on the adverse effects of large amounts of many nutrients are unavailable or too limited to establish a UL. Therefore, the lack of a UL does *not* mean that the risk of adverse effects from high intake is nonexistent. Individual nutrients in foods that most people eat rarely reach levels that exceed the UL. However, nutritional supplements provide more concentrated amounts of nutrients per dose and, as a result, pose a greater potential risk of toxicity. Nutrient supplements are labeled with "Supplement Facts" that express the amount of nutrient in absolute units or as the percent of the DV provided per recommended serving size. Total nutrient consumption, including both food and supplements, should not exceed RDA levels.

FACTORS ALTERING NUTRIENT NEEDS

The DRIs are affected by age, sex, rate of growth, pregnancy, lactation, physical activity, composition of diet, coexisting diseases, and drugs. When only slight differences exist between the requirements for nutrient sufficiency and excess, dietary planning becomes more difficult.

PHYSIOLOGIC FACTORS

Growth, strenuous physical activity, pregnancy, and lactation increase needs for energy and several essential nutrients, including water. Energy needs rise during pregnancy, due to the demands of fetal growth, and during lactation, because of the increased energy required for milk production. Energy needs decrease with loss of lean body mass, the major determinant of REE. Because both health and physical activity tend to decline with age, energy needs in older persons, especially those over 70, tend to be less than those of younger persons.

DIETARY COMPOSITION

Dietary composition affects the biologic availability and utilization of nutrients. For example, the absorption of iron may be impaired by high amounts of calcium or lead; non-heme iron uptake may be impaired by the lack of ascorbic acid and amino acids in the meal. Protein utilization by the body may be decreased when essential amino acids are not present in sufficient amounts. Animal foods, such as milk, eggs, and meat, have high biologic values with most of the needed amino acids present in adequate amounts. Plant proteins in corn (maize), soy, and wheat have lower biologic values and must be combined with other plant or animal proteins to achieve optimal utilization by the body.

ROUTE OF ADMINISTRATION

The RDAs apply only to oral intakes. When nutrients are administered parenterally, similar values can sometimes be used for amino acids, carbohydrates, fats, sodium, chloride, potassium, and most of the vitamins, since their intestinal absorption is nearly 100%. However, the oral bioavailability of most mineral elements may be only half that obtained by parenteral administration. For some nutrients that are not readily stored in the body, or cannot be stored in large amounts, timing of administration may also be important. For example, amino acids cannot be used for protein synthesis if they are not supplied together; instead they will be used for energy production.

DISEASE

Specific dietary deficiency diseases include protein-calorie malnutrition; iron, iodine, and vitamin A deficiency; megaloblastic anemia due to vitamin B_{12} or folic acid deficiency; vitamin D–deficiency rickets; scurvy due to lack of ascorbic acid; beriberi due to lack of thiamine; and pellagra due to lack of niacin and protein (Chaps. 52 and 53). Each deficiency disease is characterized by imbalances at the cellular level between the supply of nutrients or energy and the body's nutritional needs for growth, maintenance, and other functions. Imbalances in nutrient intakes are recognized as risk factors for certain chronic degenerative diseases, such as saturated and transfat and cholesterol in coronary artery disease; sodium in hypertension; obesity in hormone-dependent endometrial and breast cancers; and ethanol in alcoholism. However, the etiology and pathogenesis of these disorders are multifactorial, and diet is only one of many risk factors. Osteoporosis, for example, is associated with calcium deficiency as well as risk factors related to environment (e.g., smoking, sedentary lifestyle), physiology (e.g., estrogen deficiency), genetic determinants (e.g., defects in collagen metabolism), and drug use (chronic steroids).

DIETARY ASSESSMENT

In clinical situations, nutritional assessment is an iterative process that involves (1) screening for malnutrition; (2)

assessing food and dietary supplement intake, and establishing the absence or presence of malnutrition and its possible causes; and (3) planning for the most appropriate nutritional therapy. Some disease states affect the bioavailability, requirements, utilization, or excretion of specific nutrients. In these circumstances, specific measurements of various nutrients may be required to ensure adequate replacement (Chap. 53).

Most health care facilities have a nutrition screening process in place for identifying possible malnutrition after hospital admission. Nutritional screening is required by the Joint Commission on Accreditation of Healthcare Organizations (JCAHO), but there are no universally recognized or validated standards. The factors that are usually assessed include abnormal weight for height or body mass index (e.g., BMI <18.5 or >25); reported weight change (involuntary loss or gain of >5 kg in the past 6 months) (Chap. 7); diagnoses with known nutritional implications (metabolic disease, any disease affecting the gastrointestinal tract, alcoholism, and others); present therapeutic dietary prescription; chronic poor appetite; presence of chewing and swallowing problems or major food intolerances; need for assistance with preparing or shopping for food, eating, or other aspects of self care; and social isolation. Reassessment of nutrition status should occur periodically in hospitalized patients—at least once every week.

A more complete dietary assessment is indicated for patients who exhibit a high risk of malnutrition based on nutrition screening. The type of assessment varies with the clinical setting, severity of the patient's illness, and stability of his or her condition.

ACUTE CARE SETTINGS

Acute care settings, anorexia, various diseases, test procedures, and medications can compromise dietary intake. Under such circumstances, the goal is to identify and avoid inadequate intake and ensure appropriate alimentation. Dietary assessment focuses on what patients are currently eating, whether they are able and willing to eat, and whether they experience any problems with eating. Dietary intake assessment is based on information from observed intakes; medical record; history; clinical examination; and anthropometric, biochemical, and functional status. The objective is to gather enough information to establish the likelihood of malnutrition due to poor dietary intake or other causes and to assess whether nutritional therapy is indicated.

Simple observations may suffice to suggest inadequate oral intake. These include dietitians' and nurses' notes, the amount of food eaten on trays, frequent tests and procedures that are likely to cause meals to be skipped, nutritionally inadequate diet orders such as clear liquids or full liquids for more than a few days, fever, gastrointestinal distress, vomiting, diarrhea, a comatose state, and diseases or treatments that involve any part of the alimentary tract.

Acutely ill patients with diet-related diseases such as diabetes require assessment because an inappropriate diet may exacerbate these conditions and adversely affect other therapies. Abnormal biochemical values [serum albumin levels <35 g/L (<3.5 mg/dL); serum cholesterol levels <3.9 mmol/L (<150 mg/dL)] are nonspecific but may also indicate a need for further nutritional assessment.

Most therapeutic diets offered in hospitals are calculated to meet individual nutrient requirements and the RDA. However, there are exceptions including clear liquids, some full liquid diets, and test diets, which are inadequate for several nutrients and should not be used, if possible, for more than 24 h. As much as half of the food served to hospitalized patients is not eaten, so it cannot be assumed that the intakes of hospitalized patients are adequate. Dietary assessment should compare how much and what food the patient has consumed with the diet that has been provided. Major deviations in intakes of energy, protein, fluids, or other nutrients of special concern for the patient's illness should be noted and corrected.

Nutritional monitoring is especially important for patients who are very ill and who have extended lengths of stay. Patients who are fed by special enteral and parenteral routes also require special nutritional assessment and monitoring by physicians with training in nutrition support and/or dietitians with certification in nutrition support (Chap. 54).

AMBULATORY SETTINGS

The aim of dietary assessment in the outpatient setting is to determine whether the patient's usual diet is a health risk in itself or if it contributes to existing chronic disease-related problems. Dietary assessment also provides the basis for planning a diet that fulfills therapeutic goals while ensuring patient adherence. The outpatient dietary assessment should review the adequacy of present and usual food intakes, including vitamin and mineral supplements, medications, and alcohol, as all of these may affect the patient's nutritional status. The assessment should focus on the dietary constituents that are most likely to be involved or compromised by a specific diagnosis, as well as any comorbidities that are present. More than one day's intake should be reviewed to provide a better representation of the usual diet.

There are many ways to assess the adequacy of the patient's habitual diet. These include a food guide, a food exchange list, a diet history, or a food frequency questionnaire. A commonly used food guide for healthy persons is the USDA's food pyramid, which is useful as a basis for identifying inadequate intakes of essential nutrients, as well as likely excesses in fat, saturated fat, sodium, sugar, and alcohol (Table 51-3). The guide is available online (www.MyPyramid.gov) and can be tailored to the needs of persons of different ages and life

TABLE 51-3

MY PYRAMID: THE USDA FOOD GUIDE PYRAMID FOR HEALTHY PERSONS

SERVINGS AND EXAMPLES OF STANDARD PORTION SIZES	LOWER: 1600 kcal	MODERATE: 2200 kcal	HIGHER: 2800 kcal
Fruits, cups	1.5	2	2.5
Vegetables, cups	2	3	3.5
Grains, oz eq (1 slice bread, 1 cup ready to eat cereal, 0.5 cup cooked rice, pasta, cooked cereal)	5	7	10
Meat and beans, oz eq (1 oz lean meat, poultry, or fish; 1 egg, 1 Tbsp. peanut butter, 0.25 cup cooked dry beans, or 0.5 oz nuts or seeds)	5	6	7
Milk, cups (1 cup milk or yogurt, 1.5 oz natural or 2 oz processed cheese)	3	3	3
Oils, tsp	5	6	8
Discretionary calorie allowance, kcal (remaining calories after accounting for all of the above)	132	290	426

Note: oz eq, ounce equivalent.
Source: Data from United States Department of Agriculture. http://www.MyPyramid.com.

stages by varying the number of servings. The process of reviewing the guide with patients helps to identify food groups eaten in excess of recommendations or in insufficient quantities and helps them to transition to healthier dietary patterns. For those prescribed therapeutic diets, assessment against prescriptions stated as food exchange lists may be useful. These include, for example, the American Diabetes Association food exchange lists for diabetes, or the American Dietetic Association food exchange lists for renal disease.

NUTRITIONAL STATUS ASSESSMENT

Full nutritional status assessment is reserved for seriously ill patients and those at very high nutritional risk when the cause of malnutrition is still uncertain after initial clinical evaluation and dietary assessment. It involves multiple dimensions, including documentation of dietary intake, anthropometric measurements, biochemical measurements of blood and urine, clinical examination, health history, and functional status. For further discussion of nutritional assessment, see Chap. 53.

GLOBAL CONSIDERATIONS

New nutrient-based terminologies with dietary reference intakes have been developed not only in North America, but in the United Kingdom and Europe, and by the World Health Organization/ Food and Agricultural Organization of the United Nations (WHO/FAO). These different standards have many similarities in their basic concepts, definitions, and levels of nutrients recommended, but there are some differences, owing to assumptions made, functional criteria chosen, the timeliness of the evidence reviewed, and expert judgment.

FURTHER READINGS

Ashton K et al: Methods of assessment of selenium status in humans: a systematic review. Am J Clin Nutr 89:2025S, 2009

Fekete K et al: Methods of assessment of n-3 long-chain polyunsaturated fatty acid status in humans: a systematic review. Am J Clin Nutr 89:2070S, 2009

Gibson RS: *Principles of Nutritional Assessment*, 2d ed. Oxford University Press, London, 2005

Harvey LJ et al: Methods of assessment of copper status in humans: a systematic review. Am J Clin Nutr 89:2009S, 2009

Lowe NM et al: Methods of assessment of zinc status in humans: A systematic review. Am J Clin Nutr 89:2040S, 2009

Murphy SP et al: Multivitamin-multimineral supplements' effect on total nutrient intake. Am J Clin Nutr 85:280S, 2007

Shils ME et al (eds): *Modern Nutrition in Health and Disease*, 10th ed. Philadelphia, Lippincott Williams and Wilkins, 2005

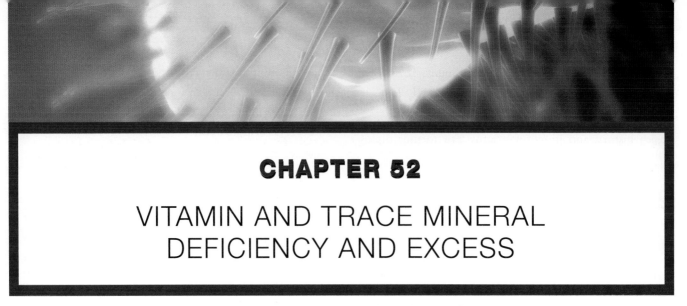

CHAPTER 52

VITAMIN AND TRACE MINERAL DEFICIENCY AND EXCESS

Robert M. Russell ■ Paolo M. Suter

Vitamins and trace minerals are required constituents of the human diet since they are either inadequately synthesized or not synthesized in the human body. Only small amounts of these substances are needed for carrying out essential biochemical reactions (e.g., acting as coenzymes or prosthetic groups). Overt vitamin or trace mineral deficiencies are rare in Western countries due to a plentiful, varied, and inexpensive food supply; however, multiple nutrient deficiencies may appear together in persons who are chronically ill or alcoholic. Moreover, subclinical vitamin and trace mineral deficiencies, as diagnosed by laboratory testing, are quite common in the normal population—especially in the geriatric age group.

Famine, emergency-affected and displaced populations, and refugees are at increased risk for protein-energy malnutrition and classic micronutrient deficiencies (vitamin A, iron, iodine), as well as for thiamine (beriberi), riboflavin, vitamin C (scurvy), and niacin (pellagra) overt deficiencies.

Body stores of vitamins and minerals vary tremendously. For example, vitamin B₁₂ and vitamin A stores are large, and an adult may not become deficient for one or more years after being on a depleted diet. However, folate and thiamine may become depleted within weeks when eating a deficient diet. Therapeutic modalities can deplete essential nutrients from the body; for example, hemodialysis removes water-soluble vitamins, which must be replaced by supplementation.

There are several roles for vitamins and trace minerals in diseases: (1) deficiencies of vitamins and minerals may be caused by disease states such as malabsorption; (2) both deficiency and excess of vitamins and minerals can cause disease in and of themselves (e.g., vitamin A intoxication and liver disease); and (3) vitamins and minerals in high doses may be used as drugs (e.g., niacin for hypercholesterolemia). The hematologic-related vitamins and minerals are considered only briefly in this chapter, as are the bone-related vitamins and minerals (vitamin D, calcium, phosphorus), since they are covered elsewhere (**Tables 52-1, 52-2,** and **Fig. 52-1**).

VITAMINS

THIAMINE (VITAMIN B₁)

Thiamine was the first B vitamin to be identified and is therefore also referred to as vitamin B₁. Thiamine functions in the decarboxylation of α-ketoacids, such as

TABLE 52-1 563

PRINCIPAL CLINICAL FINDINGS OF VITAMIN MALNUTRITION

NUTRIENT	CLINICAL FINDING	DIETARY LEVEL PER DAY ASSOCIATED WITH OVERT DEFICIENCY IN ADULTS	CONTRIBUTING FACTORS TO DEFICIENCY
Thiamine	Beriberi: neuropathy, muscle weakness and wasting, cardiomegaly, edema, ophthalmoplegia, confabulation	<0.3 mg/1000 kcal	Alcoholism, chronic diuretic use, hyperemesis
Riboflavin	Magenta tongue, angular stomatitis, seborrhea, cheilosis	<0.6 mg	—
Niacin	Pellagra: pigmented rash of sun-exposed areas, bright red tongue, diarrhea, apathy, memory loss, disorientation	<9.0 niacin equivalents	Alcoholism, vitamin B_6 deficiency, riboflavin deficiency, tryptophan deficiency
Vitamin B_6	Seborrhea, glossitis convulsions, neuropathy, depression, confusion, microcytic anemia	<0.2 mg	Alcoholism, isoniazid
Folate	Megaloblastic anemia, atrophic glossitis, depression, ↑ homocysteine	<100 µg/d	Alcoholism, sulfasalazine, pyrimethamine, triamterene
Vitamin B_{12}	Megaloblastic anemia, loss of vibratory and position sense, abnormal gait, dementia, impotence, loss of bladder and bowel control, ↑ homocysteine, ↑ methylmalonic acid	<1.0 µg/d	Gastric atrophy (pernicious anemia), terminal ileal disease, strict vegetarianism, acid reducing drugs (e.g., H_2 blockers)
Vitamin C	Scurvy: petechiae, ecchymosis, coiled hairs, inflamed and bleeding gums, joint effusion, poor wound healing, fatigue	<10 mg/d	Smoking, alcoholism
Vitamin A	Xerophthalmia, nightblindness, Bitot's spots, follicular hyperkeratosis, impaired embryonic development, immune dysfunction	<300 µg/d	Fat malabsorption, infection, measles, alcoholism, protein-energy malnutrition
Vitamin D	Rickets: skeletal deformation, rachitic rosary, bowed legs; osteomalacia	<2.0 µg/d	Aging, lack of sunlight exposure, fat malabsorption, deeply pigmented skin
Vitamin E	Peripheral neuropathy, spinocerebellar ataxia, skeletal muscle atrophy, retinopathy	Not described unless underlying contributing factor is present	Occurs only with fat malabsorption, or genetic abnormalities of vitamin E metabolism/transport
Vitamin K	Elevated prothrombin time, bleeding	<10 µg/d	Fat malabsorption, liver disease, antibiotic use

pyruvate α-ketoglutarate, and branched-chain amino acids and thus is a source of energy generation. In addition, thiamine pyrophosphate acts as a coenzyme for a transketolase reaction that mediates the conversion of hexose and pentose phosphates. It has also been postulated that thiamine plays a role in peripheral nerve conduction, although the exact chemical reactions underlying this function are unknown.

Food Sources

The median intake of thiamine in the United States from food alone is 2 mg/d. Primary food sources for thiamine include yeast, organ meat, pork, legumes, beef, whole grains, and nuts. Milled rice or grains contain little thiamine, if any. Thiamine deficiency is therefore more common in cultures that rely heavily on a rice-based diet. Tea, coffee (regular and decaffeinated), raw fish, and shellfish contain thiaminases, which can destroy the vitamin. Thus, drinking large amounts of tea or coffee can theoretically lower thiamine body stores.

Deficiency

Most dietary deficiency of thiamine worldwide is the result of poor dietary intake. In Western countries, the primary causes of thiamine deficiency are alcoholism and chronic illness, such as cancer. Alcohol interferes directly with the absorption of thiamine and with the synthesis of thiamine pyrophosphate. Thiamine should

TABLE 52-2

DEFICIENCIES AND TOXICITIES OF METALS

ELEMENT	DEFICIENCY	TOXICITY	TOLERABLE UPPER (DIETARY) INTAKE LEVEL
Boron	No biologic function determined	Developmental defects, male sterility, testicular atrophy	20 mg/d (extrapolated from animal data)
Calcium	Reduced bone mass, osteoporosis	Renal insufficiency (milk-alkali syndrome), nephrolithiasis, impaired iron absorption	2500 mg/d (milk-alkali)
Copper	Anemia, growth retardation, defective keratinization and pigmentation of hair, hypothermia, degenerative changes in aortic elastin, osteopenia, mental deterioration	Nausea, vomiting, diarrhea, hepatic failure, tremor, mental deterioration, hemolytic anemia, renal dysfunction	10 mg/d (liver toxicity)
Chromium	Impaired glucose tolerance	Occupational: renal failure, dermatitis, pulmonary cancer	ND
Fluoride	↑ Dental caries	Dental and skeletal fluorosis, osteosclerosis	10 mg/d (fluorosis)
Iodine	Thyroid enlargement, ↓ T_4, cretinism	Thyroid dysfunction, acne-like eruptions	1100 µg/d (thyroid dysfunction)
Iron	Muscle abnormalities, koilonychia, pica, anemia, ↓ work performance, impaired cognitive development, premature labor, ↑ perinatal maternal mortality	Gastrointestinal effects (nausea, vomiting, diarrhea, constipation), iron overload with organ damage, acute systemic toxicity	45 mg/d of elemental iron (GI side effects)
Manganese	Impaired growth and skeletal development, reproduction, lipid and carbohydrate metabolism; upper body rash	General: Neurotoxicity, Parkinson-like symptoms. Occupational: Encephalitis-like syndrome, Parkinson-like syndrome, psychosis, pneumoconiosis	11 mg/d (neurotoxicity)
Molybdenum	Severe neurologic abnormalities	Reproductive and fetal abnormalities	2 mg/d extrapolated from animal data
Selenium	Cardiomyopathy, heart failure, striated muscle degeneration	General: Alopecia, nausea, vomiting, abnormal nails, emotional lability, peripheral neuropathy, lassitude, garlic odor to breath, dermatitis. Occupational: Lung and nasal carcinomas, liver necrosis, pulmonary inflammation	400 µg/d (hair, nail changes)
Phosphorous	Rickets (osteomalacia), proximal muscle weakness, rhabdomyolysis, paresthesia, ataxia, seizure, confusion, heart failure, hemolysis, acidosis	Hyperphosphatemia	4000 mg/d
Zinc	Growth retardation, ↓ taste and smell, alopecia, dermatitis, diarrhea, immune dysfunction, failure to thrive, gonadal atrophy, congenital malformations	General: Reduced copper absorption, gastritis, sweating, fever, nausea, vomiting. Occupational: Respiratory distress, pulmonary fibrosis	40 mg/d (impaired copper metabolism)

Note: ND, not determined; GI, gastrointestinal.

always be replenished when refeeding a patient with alcoholism, as carbohydrate repletion without adequate thiamine can precipitate acute thiamine deficiency. Other at-risk populations are women with prolonged hyperemesis gravidarum and anorexia, patients with an overall poor nutritional status on parenteral glucose, and patients on chronic diuretic therapy due to increased urinary thiamine losses. Maternal thiamine deficiency can lead to infantile beriberi in breast-fed children. Thiamine deficiency should also be considered in the setting of motor vehicle accidents associated with head injury.

Thiamine deficiency in its early stage induces anorexia and nonspecific symptoms (e.g., irritability,

Vitamin	Active derivative or cofactor form	Principal function
Thiamine (B$_1$) 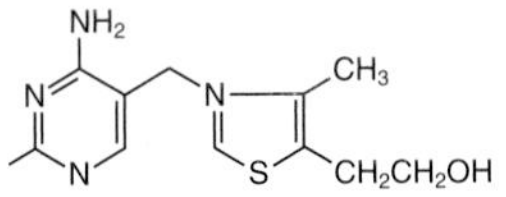	Thiamine pyrophosphate	Coenzyme for cleavage of carbon-carbon bonds; amino acid and carbohydrate metabolism
Riboflavin (B$_2$) 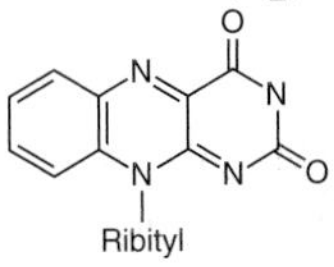	Flavin mononucleotide (FMN) and flavin adenine dinucleotide (FAD)	Cofactor for oxidation, reduction reactions, and covalently attached prosthetic groups for some enzymes
Niacin 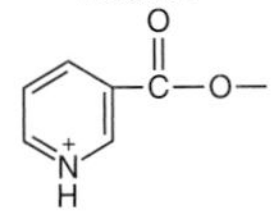	Nicotinamide adenine dinucleotide phosphate (NADP) and nicotinamide adenine dinucleotide (NAD)	Coenzymes for oxidation and reduction reactions
Vitamin B$_6$ 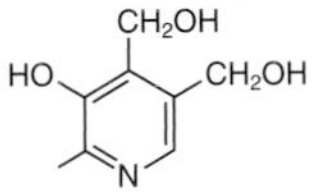	Pyridoxal phosphate	Cofactor for enzymes of amino acid metabolism
Folate 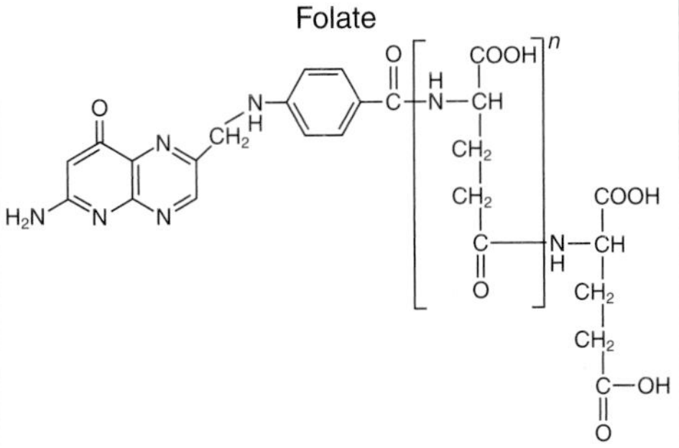	Polyglutamate forms of (5, 6, 7, 8) tetrahydrofolate with carbon unit attachments	Coenzyme for one carbon transfer in nucleic acid and amino acid metabolism
Vitamin B$_{12}$ 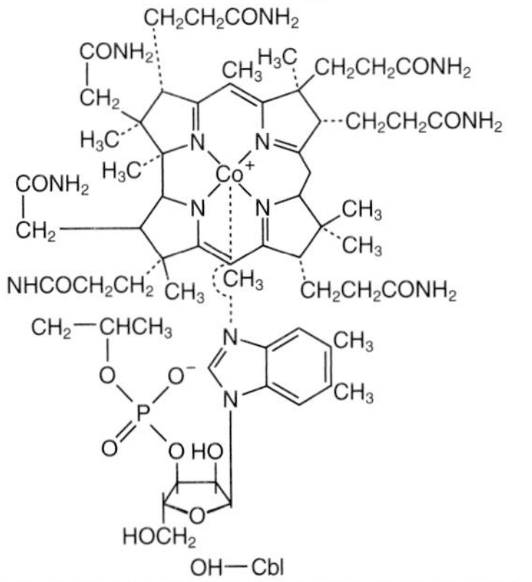	Methylcobalamine Adenosylcobalamin	Coenzyme for methionine synthase and L-methylmalonyl-CoA mutase

FIGURE 52-1

The structures and principal functions of vitamins associated with human disorders.

decrease in short-term memory). Prolonged thiamine deficiency causes beriberi, which is classically categorized as wet or dry, although there is considerable overlap. In either form of beriberi, patients may complain of pain and paresthesia. *Wet beriberi* presents primarily with cardiovascular symptoms, due to impaired myocardial energy metabolism and dysautonomia, and can occur after 3 months of a thiamine-deficient diet. Patients

Vitamin	Active derivative or cofactor form	Principal function
Vitamin C 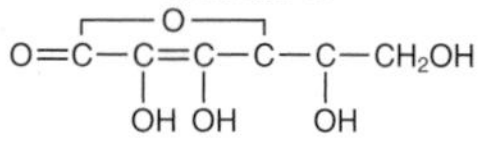	Ascorbic acid and dehydrascorbic acid	Participation as a redox ion in many biological oxidation and hydrogen transfer reactions
Vitamin A 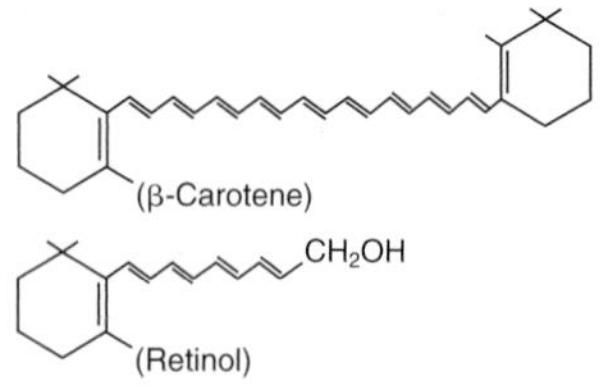 (β-Carotene) (Retinol)	Retinol, retinaldehyde, and retinoic acid	Formation of rhodopsin (vision) and glycoproteins (epithelial cell function); also regulates gene transcription
Vitamin D 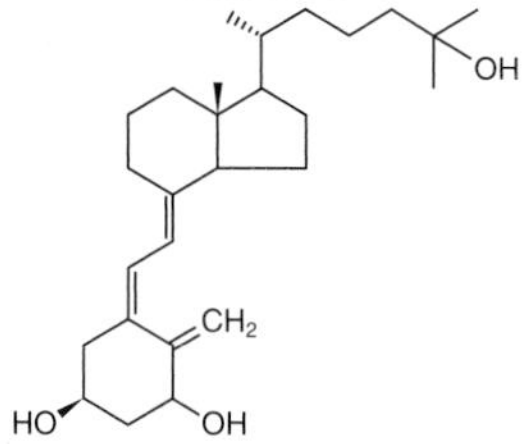	1, 25-Dihydroxyvitamin D	Maintenance of blood calcium and phosphorous levels; antiproliferative hormone
Vitamin E 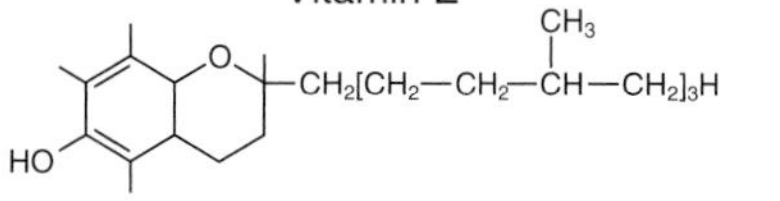	Tocopherols and tocotrienols	Antioxidants
Vitamin K 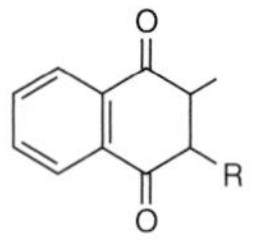	Vitamin K hydroquinone	Cofactor for posttranslation carboxylation of many proteins including essential clotting factors

FIGURE 52-1 (continued)

present with an enlarged heart, tachycardia, high-output congestive heart failure, peripheral edema, and peripheral neuritis. Patients with *dry beriberi* present with a symmetric peripheral neuropathy of the motor and sensory systems with diminished reflexes. The neuropathy affects the legs most markedly, and patients have difficulty rising from a squatting position.

Alcoholic patients with chronic thiamine deficiency may also have central nervous system (CNS) manifestations known as *Wernicke's encephalopathy*, consisting of horizontal nystagmus, ophthalmoplegia (due to weakness of one or more extraocular muscles), cerebellar ataxia, and mental impairment. When there is an additional loss of memory and a confabulatory psychosis, the syndrome is known as *Wernicke-Korsakoff syndrome*. Despite the typical clinical picture and history, Wernicke-Korsakoff syndrome is underdiagnosed.

The laboratory diagnosis of thiamine deficiency is usually made by a functional enzymatic assay of transketolase activity measured before and after the addition of thiamine pyrophosphate. A >25% stimulation by the addition of thiamine pyrophosphate (an activity coefficient of 1.25) is taken as abnormal. Thiamine or the phosphorylated esters of thiamine in serum or blood can also be measured by high-performance liquid chromatography (HPLC) to detect deficiency.

℞ **Treatment:**
THIAMINE DEFICIENCY

In acute thiamine deficiency with either cardiovascular or neurologic signs, 100 mg/d of thiamine should be given parenterally for 7 days, followed by 10 mg/d orally until there is complete recovery. Cardiovascular improvement occurs within 24 h, and ophthalmoplegic improvement occurs within 24 h. Other manifestations gradually clear, although psychosis in Wernicke-Korsakoff syndrome may be permanent or persist for several months.

Toxicity

Although anaphylaxis has been reported after high doses of thiamine, no adverse effects have been recorded from either food or supplements at high doses. Thiamine supplements may be bought over the counter in doses of up to 50 mg/d.

RIBOFLAVIN (VITAMIN B$_2$)

Riboflavin is important for the metabolism of fat, carbohydrate, and protein, reflecting its role as a respiratory coenzyme and an electron donor. Enzymes that contain flavin adenine dinucleotide (FAD) or flavin-mononucleotide (FMN) as prosthetic groups are known as *flavoenzymes* (e.g., succinic acid dehydrogenase, monoamine oxidase, glutathione reductase). FAD is a cofactor for methyltetrahydrofolate reductase and therefore modulates homocysteine metabolism. The vitamin also plays a role in drug and steroid metabolism, including detoxification reactions.

Although much is known about the chemical and enzymatic reactions of riboflavin, the clinical manifestations of riboflavin deficiency are nonspecific and similar to those of other vitamin B deficiencies. Riboflavin deficiency is manifested principally by lesions of the mucocutaneous surfaces of the mouth and skin (Table 52-1). In addition to the mucocutaneous lesions, corneal vascularization, anemia, and personality changes have been described with riboflavin deficiency.

Deficiency and Excess

Riboflavin deficiency is almost always due to dietary deficiency. Milk, other dairy products, and enriched breads and cereals are the most important dietary sources of riboflavin in the United States, although lean meat, fish, eggs, broccoli, and legumes are also good sources. Riboflavin is extremely sensitive to light, and milk should be stored in containers that protect against photodegradation. Laboratory diagnosis of riboflavin deficiency can be made by measurement of red blood cell or urinary riboflavin concentrations or by measurement of erythrocyte glutathione reductase activity, with and without added FAD. Because the capacity of the gastrointestinal tract to absorb riboflavin is limited (~20 mg if given in one oral dose), riboflavin toxicity has not been described.

NIACIN (VITAMIN B$_3$)

The term *niacin* refers to nicotinic acid and nicotinamide and their biologically active derivatives. Nicotinic acid and nicotinamide serve as precursors of two coenzymes, nicotinamide adenine dinucleotide (NAD) and NAD phosphate (NADP), which are important in numerous oxidation and reduction reactions in the body. In addition, NAD and NADP are active in adenine diphosphate–ribose transfer reactions involved in DNA repair and calcium mobilization.

Nicotinic acid and nicotinamide are absorbed well from the stomach and small intestine. Niacin bioavailability is high from beans, milk, meat, and eggs; bioavailability from cereal grains is lower. Since flour is enriched with the "free" niacin (i.e., non-coenzyme form), bioavailability is excellent. Median intakes of niacin in the United States considerably exceed the recommended dietary allowance (RDA).

The amino acid tryptophan can be converted to niacin with an efficiency of 60:1 by weight. Thus, the RDA for niacin is expressed in niacin equivalents. A lower conversion of tryptophan to niacin occurs in vitamin B$_6$ and/or riboflavin deficiencies, or in the presence of isoniazid. The urinary excretion products of niacin include 2-pyridone and 2-methyl nicotinamide, measurements of which are used in diagnosis of niacin deficiency.

Deficiency

Niacin deficiency causes *pellagra*, which is mostly found among people eating corn-based diets in parts of China, Africa, and India. Pellagra in North America is found mainly among alcoholics; in patients with congenital defects of intestinal and kidney absorption of tryptophan (Hartnup disease); and in patients with carcinoid syndrome (Chap. 50), where there is increased conversion of tryptophan to serotonin. In the setting of famine or population displacement, the occurrence of pellagra results from the absolute lack of niacin but also the deficiency of micronutrients required for the conversion of tryptophan to niacin (e.g., iron, riboflavin, and pyridoxine). The early symptoms of pellagra include loss of appetite, generalized weakness and irritability, abdominal pain, and vomiting. Bright red glossitis then ensues, followed by a characteristic skin rash that is pigmented and scaling, particularly in skin areas exposed to sunlight. This rash is known as *Casal's necklace* because it forms a ring around the neck; it is seen in advanced cases. Vaginitis and esophagitis may also occur. Diarrhea (in part due to proctitis and in part due to malabsorption), depression, seizures, and dementia are also part of the pellagra syndrome—the four *D*s: *d*ermatitis, *d*iarrhea, and *d*ementia leading to *d*eath.

R$_X$ Treatment: PELLAGRA

Treatment of pellagra consists of oral supplementation of 100–200 mg of nicotinamide or nicotinic acid three times daily for 5 days. High doses of nicotinic acid (2 g/d in a time-release form) are used for the treatment of elevated cholesterol and triglyceride levels and/or low high-density lipoprotein (HDL) cholesterol level.

Prostaglandin-mediated flushing due to binding of the vitamin to a G protein–coupled receptor has been observed at daily doses as low as 50 mg of niacin when taken as a supplement or as therapy for dyslipidemia. There is no evidence of toxicity from niacin derived from food sources. Flushing always starts in the face and may be accompanied by skin dryness, itching, paresthesia, and headache. Premedication with aspirin may alleviate these symptoms. Flushing is subject to tachyphylaxis and often improves with time. Nausea, vomiting, and abdominal pain also occur at similar doses of niacin. Hepatic toxicity is the most serious toxic reaction due to niacin and may present as jaundice with elevated aspartate aminotransferase (AST) and alanine aminotransferase (ALT) levels. A few cases of fulminant hepatitis requiring liver transplantation have been reported at doses of 3–9 g/d. Other toxic reactions include glucose intolerance, hyperuricemia, macular edema, and macular cysts. The upper limit for daily niacin intake has been set at 35 mg. However, this upper limit does not pertain to the therapeutic use of niacin.

PYRIDOXINE (VITAMIN B₆)

Vitamin B₆ refers to a family of compounds including pyridoxine, pyridoxal, pyridoxamine, and their 5′-phosphate derivatives. 5′-Pyridoxal phosphate (PLP) is a cofactor for more than 100 enzymes involved in amino acid metabolism. Vitamin B₆ is also involved in heme and neurotransmitter synthesis and in the metabolism of glycogen, lipids, steroids, sphingoid bases, and several vitamins, including the conversion of tryptophan to niacin.

Dietary Sources

Plants contain vitamin B₆ in the form of pyridoxine, whereas animal tissues contain PLP and pyridoxamine phosphate. The vitamin B₆ contained in plants is less bioavailable than that from animal tissues. Rich food sources of vitamin B₆ include legumes, nuts, wheat bran, and meat, although it is present in all food groups.

Deficiency

Symptoms of vitamin B₆ deficiency include epithelial changes, as seen frequently with other B vitamin deficiencies. In addition, severe vitamin B₆ deficiency can lead to peripheral neuropathy, abnormal electroencephalograms, and personality changes including depression and confusion. In infants, diarrhea, seizures, and anemia have been reported. Microcytic, hypochromic anemia is due to diminished hemoglobin synthesis, since the first enzyme involved in heme biosynthesis (aminolevulinate synthase) requires PLP as a cofactor.

In some case reports, platelet dysfunction has also been reported. Since vitamin B₆ is necessary for the conversion of homocysteine to cystathionine, it is possible that chronic low-grade vitamin B₆ deficiency may result in hyperhomocysteinemia and increased risk of cardiovascular disease. Independent of homocysteine, low levels of circulating vitamin B₆ have also been associated with inflammation and elevated C-reactive protein levels.

Certain medications such as isoniazid, L-dopa, penicillamine, and cycloserine interact with PLP due to a reaction with carbonyl groups. Pyridoxine should be given concurrently with isoniazid to avoid neuropathy. The increased ratio of AST (or SGOT) to ALT (or SGPT) seen in alcoholic liver disease reflects the relative vitamin B₆ dependence of ALT. Vitamin B₆ dependency syndromes that require pharmacologic doses of vitamin B₆ are rare; they include cystathionine β-synthase deficiency, pyridoxine-responsive (primarily sideroblastic) anemias, and gyrate atrophy with chorioretinal degeneration due to decreased activity of the mitochondrial enzyme ornithine aminotransferase. In these situations, 100–200 mg/d of oral vitamin B₆ is required for treatment.

High doses of vitamin B₆ have been used to treat carpal tunnel syndrome, premenstrual syndrome, schizophrenia, autism, and diabetic neuropathy but have not been found to be effective.

The laboratory diagnosis of vitamin B₆ deficiency is generally made on the basis of low plasma PLP values (20 nmol/L). Treatment of vitamin B₆ deficiency is 50 mg/d; higher doses of 100–200 mg/d are given if vitamin B₆ deficiency is related to medication use. Vitamin B₆ should not be given with L-dopa, since the vitamin interferes with the action of this drug.

Toxicity

The safe upper limit for vitamin B₆ has been set at 100 mg/d, although no adverse effects have been associated with high intakes of vitamin B₆ from food sources only. When toxicity occurs, it causes a severe sensory neuropathy, leaving patients unable to walk. Some cases of photosensitivity and dermatitis have also been reported.

VITAMIN C

Both ascorbic acid and its oxidized product dehydroascorbic acid are biologically active. Actions of vitamin C include antioxidant activity, promotion of nonheme iron absorption, carnitine biosynthesis, the conversion of dopamine to norepinephrine, and the synthesis of many peptide hormones. Vitamin C is also important for connective tissue metabolism and cross-linking (proline hydroxylation), and it is a component of many drug-metabolizing enzyme systems, particularly the mixed-function oxidase systems.

Absorption and Dietary Sources

Almost complete absorption of vitamin C occurs if <100 mg is administered in a single dose; however, only 50% or less is absorbed at doses >1 g. Enhanced degradation and fecal and urinary excretion of vitamin C occur at higher intake levels.

Good dietary sources of vitamin C include citrus fruits, green vegetables (especially broccoli), tomatoes, and potatoes. Consumption of five servings of fruits and vegetables a day provides vitamin C in excess of the RDA, 90 mg/d for males and 75 mg/d for females. In addition, approximately 40% of the U.S. population consumes vitamin C as a dietary supplement in which "natural forms" of vitamin C are no more bioavailable than synthetic forms. Smoking, hemodialysis, pregnancy, and stress (e.g., infection, trauma) appear to increase vitamin C requirements.

Deficiency

Vitamin C deficiency causes scurvy. In the United States, this is seen primarily among the poor and elderly, in alcoholics who consume <10 mg/d of vitamin C, and also in individuals consuming macrobiotic diets. In addition to generalized fatigue, symptoms of scurvy primarily reflect impaired formation of mature connective tissue and include bleeding into skin (petechiae, ecchymoses, perifollicular hemorrhages); inflamed and bleeding gums; and manifestations of bleeding into joints, the peritoneal cavity, pericardium, and the adrenal glands. In children, vitamin C deficiency may cause impaired bone growth. Laboratory diagnosis of vitamin C deficiency is made on the basis of low plasma or leukocyte levels.

Administration of vitamin C (200 mg/d) improves the symptoms of scurvy within a matter of several days. High-dose vitamin C supplementation (e.g., 1–2 g/d) might slightly decrease the symptoms and duration of upper respiratory tract infections. Vitamin C supplementation has also been reported to be useful in Chédiak-Higashi syndrome and osteogenesis imperfecta. Diets high in vitamin C have been claimed to lower the incidence of certain cancers, particularly esophageal and gastric cancers. If proved, this effect may be due to the fact that vitamin C can prevent the conversion of nitrites and secondary amines to carcinogenic nitrosamines. However, one intervention study from China did not show vitamin C to be protective.

Toxicity

Taking >2 g of vitamin C in a single dose may result in abdominal pain, diarrhea, and nausea. Since vitamin C may be metabolized to oxalate, it is feared that chronic, high-dose vitamin C supplementation could result in an increased prevalence of kidney stones. However, this has not been borne out in several trials, except in patients with preexisting renal disease. Thus, it is reasonable to advise patients with a past history of kidney stones to not take large doses of vitamin C. There is also an unproven but possible risk that chronic high doses of vitamin C could promote iron overload in patients taking supplemental iron. High doses of vitamin C can induce hemolysis in patients with glucose-6-phosphate dehydrogenase deficiency, and doses >1 g/d can cause false-negative guaiac reactions as well as interfere with tests for urinary glucose.

BIOTIN

Biotin is a water-soluble vitamin that plays a role in gene expression, gluconeogenesis, and fatty acid synthesis and serves as a CO_2 carrier on the surface of both cytosolic and mitochondrial carboxylase enzymes. The vitamin also functions in the catabolism of specific amino acids (e.g., leucine). Excellent food sources of biotin include organ meat such as liver or kidney, soy, beans, yeast, and egg yolks; however, egg white contains the protein avidin, which strongly binds the vitamin and reduces its bioavailability.

Biotin deficiency due to low dietary intake is rare; rather, deficiency is due to inborn errors of metabolism. Biotin deficiency has been induced by experimental feeding of egg white diets and in patients with short bowels who received biotin-free parenteral nutrition. In the adult, biotin deficiency results in mental changes (depression, hallucinations), paresthesia, anorexia, and nausea. A scaling, seborrheic, and erythematous rash may occur around the eyes, nose, and mouth as well as on the extremities. In infants, biotin deficiency presents as hypotonia, lethargy, and apathy. In addition, the infant may develop alopecia and a characteristic rash that includes the ears. The laboratory diagnosis of biotin deficiency can be established based on a decreased urinary concentration or an increased urinary excretion of 3-hydroxyisovaleric acid after a leucine challenge. Treatment requires pharmacologic doses of biotin, using up to 10 mg/d. No toxicity is known.

PANTOTHENIC ACID (VITAMIN B₅)

Pantothenic acid is a component of coenzyme A and phosphopantetheine, which are involved in fatty acid metabolism and the synthesis of cholesterol, steroid hormones, and all compounds formed from isoprenoid units. In addition, pantothenic acid is involved in the acetylation of proteins. The vitamin is excreted in the urine, and the laboratory diagnosis of deficiency is made on the basis of low urinary vitamin levels.

The vitamin is ubiquitous in the food supply. Liver, yeast, egg yolks, whole grains, and vegetables are particularly good sources. Human pantothenic acid deficiency has been demonstrated only in experimental feeding of diets low in pantothenic acid or by giving a specific pantothenic acid antagonist. The symptoms of pantothenic acid deficiency are nonspecific and include gastrointestinal disturbance, depression, muscle cramps, paresthesia, ataxia, and hypoglycemia. Pantothenic acid deficiency is believed to have caused the burning feet syndrome seen in prisoners of war during World War II. No toxicity of this vitamin has been reported.

CHOLINE

Choline is a precursor for acetylcholine, phospholipids, and betaine. Choline is necessary for the structural integrity of cell membranes, cholinergic neurotransmission, lipid and cholesterol metabolism, methyl-group metabolism, and transmembrane signaling. Recently, a recommended adequate intake was set at 550 mg/d for adult males and 425 mg/d for adult females, although certain genetic polymorphisms can increase an individual's requirement for choline. Choline is thought to be a "conditionally essential" nutrient, in that de novo synthesis occurs in the liver and is less than the vitamin's utilization only under certain stress conditions (e.g., alcoholic liver disease). The dietary requirement of choline depends on the status of other methyl-group donors (folate, vitamin B_{12}, and methionine) and thus varies widely. Choline is widely distributed in food (e.g., egg yolk, wheat germ, organ meat, milk) in the form of lecithin (phosphatidylcholine). Choline deficiency has occurred in patients receiving parenteral nutrition devoid of choline. Deficiency results in fatty liver, elevated transaminase levels, and skeletal muscle damage with high creatine phosphokinase values. The diagnosis of choline deficiency is currently made on the basis of low plasma levels, although nonspecific conditions (e.g., heavy exercise) may suppress plasma levels.

Toxicity from choline results in hypotension, cholinergic sweating, diarrhea, salivation, and a fishy body odor. The upper limit for choline has been set at 3.5 g/d. Therapeutically, choline has been suggested for patients with dementia and for patients at high risk of cardiovascular disease, due to its ability to lower cholesterol and homocysteine levels. However, such benefits have yet to be documented. Choline- and betaine-restricted diets are of therapeutic value in trimethylaminuria (fish odor syndrome).

FLAVONOIDS

Flavonoids constitute a large family of polyphenols that contribute to the aroma, taste, and color of fruits and vegetables. Major groups of dietary flavonoids include anthocyanidins in berries; catechins in green tea and chocolate; flavonols (e.g., quercetin) in broccoli, kale, leeks, onion, and the skins of grapes and apples; and isoflavones (e.g., genistein) in legumes. Isoflavones have a low bioavailability and are partially metabolized by the intestinal flora. The dietary intake of flavonoids is estimated to be between 10 and 100 mg/d, although this is almost certainly an underestimate due to the lack of knowledge of their concentrations in many foods. Several flavonoids have been shown to have antioxidant activity and to affect cell signaling. From observational epidemiologic studies and from limited clinical human and animal studies, flavonoids have been postulated to play a role in the prevention of several chronic diseases, including neurodegenerative disease, diabetes, and osteoporosis. The ultimate importance and usefulness of their compounds against human disease have yet to be demonstrated.

VITAMIN A

Vitamin A, in the strictest sense, refers to retinol. However, the oxidized metabolites, retinaldehyde and retinoic acid, are also biologically active compounds. The term *retinoids* includes all molecules (including synthetic molecules) that are chemically related to retinol. Retinaldehyde (11-*cis*) is the essential form of vitamin A that is required for normal vision, whereas retinoic acid is necessary for normal morphogenesis, growth, and cell differentiation. Retinoic acid does not function in vision and, in contrast to retinol, is not involved in reproduction. Vitamin A also plays a role in iron utilization, humoral immunity, T cell–mediated immunity, natural killer cell activity, and phagocytosis. Vitamin A is commercially available in esterified forms (e.g., acetate, palmitate) since it is more stable as an ester.

There are more than 600 carotenoids in nature, and approximately 50 of these can be metabolized to vitamin A. β-Carotene is the most prevalent carotenoid in the food supply that has provitamin A activity. In humans, significant fractions of carotenoids are absorbed intact and are stored in liver and fat. It is now estimated that 12 μg or greater of dietary β-carotene is equivalent to 1 μg of retinol, whereas 24 μg or greater of other dietary provitamin A carotenoids (e.g., cryptoxanthin, α-carotene) is equivalent to 1 μg of retinol.

Metabolism

The liver contains approximately 90% of the vitamin A reserves and secretes vitamin A in the form of retinol, which is bound to retinol-binding protein. Once this has occurred, the retinol-binding protein complex interacts with a second protein, transthyretin. This trimolecular complex functions to prevent vitamin A from being filtered by the kidney glomerulus, to protect the body against the toxicity of retinol and to allow retinol to be taken up by specific cell-surface receptors that recognize retinol-binding protein. A certain amount of vitamin A enters peripheral cells even if it is not bound to retinol-binding protein. After retinol is internalized by the cell, it becomes bound to a series of cellular retinol-binding proteins, which function as sequestering and transporting agents as well as co-ligands for enzymatic reactions. Certain cells also contain retinoic acid–binding proteins, which have sequestering functions but also shuttle retinoic acid to the nucleus and enable its metabolism.

Retinoic acid is a ligand for certain nuclear receptors that act as transcription factors. Two families of receptors (RAR and RXR receptors) are active in retinoid-mediated gene transcription. Retinoid receptors regulate transcription by binding as dimeric complexes to specific DNA sites, the retinoic acid response elements, in target genes. The receptors can either stimulate or repress gene expression in response to their ligands. RAR binds all-*trans* retinoic acid and 9-*cis* retinoic acid, whereas RXR binds only 9-*cis* retinoic acid.

The retinoid receptors play an important role in controlling cell proliferation and differentiation. Retinoic acid is useful in the treatment of promyelocytic leukemia and is also used in the treatment of cystic acne because it inhibits keratinization, decreases sebum secretion, and possibly alters the inflammatory reaction. RXRs dimerize with other nuclear receptors to function as coregulators of genes responsive to retinoids, thyroid hormone, and calcitriol. RXR agonists induce insulin sensitivity experimentally, perhaps because RXR is a cofactor for the peroxisome-proliferator-activated receptors (PPARs), which are targets for the thiazolidinedione drugs such as rosiglitazone and troglitazone.

Dietary Sources

The retinol activity equivalent (RAE) is used to express the vitamin A value of food. One RAE is defined as 1 μg of retinol (0.003491 mmol), 12 μg of β-carotene, and 24 μg of other provitamin A carotenoids. In older literature, vitamin A was often expressed in international units (IU), with 1 RAE being equal to 3.33 IU of retinol and 20 IU of β-carotene, but these units are no longer in current scientific use.

Liver, fish, and eggs are excellent food sources for preformed vitamin A; vegetable sources of provitamin A carotenoids include dark green and deeply colored fruits and vegetables. Moderate cooking of vegetables enhances carotenoid release for uptake in the gut. Carotenoid absorption is also aided by some fat in a meal. Infants are particularly susceptible to vitamin A deficiency because neither breast nor cow's milk supplies enough vitamin A to prevent deficiency. In developing countries, chronic dietary deficit is the main cause of vitamin A deficiency and is exacerbated by infection. In early childhood, low vitamin A status results from inadequate intakes of animal food sources and edible oils, both of which are expensive, coupled with seasonal unavailability of vegetables and fruits, and lack of marketed fortified food products. Concurrent zinc deficiency can interfere with the mobilization of vitamin A from liver stores. Alcohol interferes with the conversion of retinol to retinaldehyde in the eye by competing for alcohol (retinol) dehydrogenase. Drugs that interfere with the absorption of vitamin A include mineral oil, neomycin, and cholestyramine.

Deficiency

Vitamin A deficiency is endemic where diets are chronically poor, especially in Southern Asia, Sub-Saharan Africa, some areas of Latin America, and the Western Pacific, including parts of China. Vitamin A status is usually assessed by measuring serum retinol [normal range, 1.05–3.50 μmol/L (30–100 μg/dL)] or blood spot retinol or by tests of dark adaptation. Stable isotopic or invasive liver biopsy methods exist to estimate total body stores of vitamin A. Based on deficient serum retinol [<0.70 μmol/L (20 μg/dL)], there are more than 125 million preschool-age children with vitamin A deficiency, among whom ~4 million have an ocular manifestation of deficiency termed *xerophthalmia*. This condition includes milder stages of night blindness and conjunctival xerosis (dryness) with Bitot's spots (white patches of keratinized epithelium appearing on the sclera) as well as rare, potentially blinding corneal ulceration and necrosis. Keratomalacia (softening of the cornea) leads to corneal scarring that blinds at least a quarter of a million children each year and is associated with a fatality rate of 4–25%. However, vitamin A deficiency at any stage poses an increased risk of mortality from diarrhea, dysentery, measles, malaria, and respiratory disease. Vitamin A deficiency can compromise barrier and innate and acquired immune defenses to infection. Vitamin A supplementation can markedly reduce risk of child mortality (23–34%, on average) where deficiency is widely prevalent. About 10% of pregnant women in undernourished settings also develop night blindness, assessed by history, during the latter half of pregnancy and this moderate vitamin A deficiency is associated with an increased risk of maternal infection and mortality.

Treatment:
VITAMIN A DEFICIENCY

Any stage of xerophthalmia should be treated with 60 mg of vitamin A in oily solution, usually contained in a soft-gel capsule. The same dose is repeated 1 and 14 days later. Doses should be reduced by half for patients 6–11 months of age. Mothers with night blindness or Bitot's spots should be given vitamin A orally, either 3 mg daily or 7.5 mg twice a week for 3 months. These regimens are efficacious, and they are less expensive and more widely available than injectable water-miscible vitamin A. A common approach to prevention is to supplement young children living in high-risk areas with 60 mg every 4–6 months, with a half-dose given to infants 6–11 months of age.

Uncomplicated vitamin A deficiency rarely occurs in industrialized countries. One high-risk group, extremely low-birth-weight infants (<1000 g), is likely to be vitamin A–deficient and should be supplemented with 1500 µg (or RAE) of vitamin A, three times a week for 4 weeks. Severe measles in any society can lead to secondary vitamin A deficiency. Children hospitalized with measles should receive two 60-mg doses of vitamin A on two consecutive days. Vitamin A deficiency most often occurs in patients with malabsorptive diseases (e.g., celiac sprue, short-bowel syndrome), who have abnormal dark adaptation or symptoms of night blindness without other ocular changes. Typically, such patients are treated for 1 month with 15 mg/d of a water-miscible preparation of vitamin A. This is followed by a lower maintenance dose with the exact amount determined by monitoring serum retinol.

There are no specific deficiency signs or symptoms that result from carotenoid deficiency. It was postulated that β-carotene would be an effective chemopreventive agent for cancer because numerous epidemiologic studies had shown that diets high in β-carotene were associated with lower incidences of cancers of the respiratory and digestive systems. However, intervention studies in smokers found that treatment with high doses of β-carotene actually resulted in more lung cancers than did treatment with placebo. Non–provitamin A carotenoids, such as lutein and zeaxanthin, have been suggested to protect against macular degeneration. The non–provitamin A carotenoid lycopene has been proposed to protect against prostate cancer. However, the effectiveness of these agents has not been proven by intervention studies, and the mechanisms underlying these purported biologic actions are unknown.

Toxicity

Acute toxicity of vitamin A was first noted in Arctic explorers who ate polar bear liver and has also been seen after administration of 150 mg in adults or 100 mg in children. Acute toxicity is manifested by increased intracranial pressure, vertigo, diplopia, bulging fontanels in children, seizures, and exfoliative dermatitis; it may result in death. In children being treated for vitamin A deficiency according to the protocols outlined above, transient bulging of fontanels occurs in 2% of infants, and transient nausea, vomiting, and headache occur in 5% of preschoolers. Chronic vitamin A intoxication is largely a concern in industrialized countries and has been seen in normal adults who ingest 15 mg/d and

children who ingest 6 mg/d of vitamin A over a period of several months. Manifestations include dry skin, cheilosis, glossitis, vomiting, alopecia, bone demineralization and pain, hypercalcemia, lymph node enlargement, hyperlipidemia, amenorrhea, and features of pseudotumor cerebri with increased intracranial pressure and papilledema. Liver fibrosis with portal hypertension and bone demineralization may result from chronic vitamin A intoxication. When vitamin A is provided in excess to pregnant women, congenital malformations have included spontaneous abortions, craniofacial abnormalities, and valvular heart disease. In pregnancy, the daily dose of vitamin A should not exceed 3 mg. Commercially available retinoid derivatives are also toxic, including 13-cis-retinoic acid, which has been associated with birth defects. As a result, contraception should be continued for a least 1 year, and possibly longer, in women who have taken 13-cis retinoic acid.

High doses of carotenoids do not result in toxic symptoms but should be avoided in smokers due to an increased risk of lung cancer. Carotenemia, which is characterized by a yellowing of the skin (creases of the palms and soles) but not the sclerae, may be present after ingestion of >30 mg of β-carotene daily. Hypothyroid patients are particularly susceptible to the development of carotenemia due to impaired breakdown of carotene to vitamin A. Reduction of carotenes from the diet results in the disappearance of skin yellowing and carotenemia over a period of 30–60 days.

VITAMIN D

See Fig. 52-1, and Table 52-1.

VITAMIN E

Vitamin E is a collective name for all stereoisomers of tocopherols and tocotrienols, although only the 2R tocopherols meet human requirements. Vitamin E acts as a chain-breaking antioxidant and is an efficient pyroxyl radical scavenger, which protects low-density lipoproteins (LDLs) and polyunsaturated fats in membranes from oxidation. A network of other antioxidants (e.g., vitamin C, glutathione) and enzymes maintains vitamin E in a reduced state. Vitamin E also inhibits prostaglandin synthesis and the activities of protein kinase C and phospholipase A_2.

Absorption and Metabolism

After absorption, vitamin E is taken up from chylomicrons by the liver, and a hepatic α tocopherol transport protein mediates intracellular vitamin E transport and incorporation into very low–density lipoprotein (VLDL). The transport protein has particular affinity for the RRR isomeric form of α tocopherol; thus this natural isomer has the most biologic activity.

Requirement

Vitamin E is widely distributed in the food supply and is particularly high in sunflower oil, safflower oil, and wheat germ oil; γ tocotrienols are notably present in soybean and corn oils. Vitamin E is also found in meats, nuts, and cereal grains, and small amounts are present in fruits and vegetables. Vitamin E pills containing doses of 50–1000 mg are ingested by a large fraction of the U.S. population. The RDA for vitamin E is 15 mg/d (34.9 μmol or 22.5 IU) for all adults. Diets high in polyunsaturated fats may necessitate a slightly higher requirement for vitamin E.

Dietary deficiency of vitamin E does not exist. Vitamin E deficiency is seen in only severe and prolonged malabsorptive diseases, such as celiac disease, or after small-intestinal resection. Children with cystic fibrosis or prolonged cholestasis may develop vitamin E deficiency characterized by areflexia and hemolytic anemia. Children with abetalipoproteinemia cannot absorb or transport vitamin E and become deficient quite rapidly. A familial form of isolated vitamin E deficiency also exists; it is due to a defect in the α tocopherol transport protein. Vitamin E deficiency causes axonal degeneration of the large myelinated axons and results in posterior column and spinocerebellar symptoms. Peripheral neuropathy is initially characterized by areflexia, with progression to an ataxic gait, and by decreased vibration and position sensations. Ophthalmoplegia, skeletal myopathy, and pigmented retinopathy may also be features of vitamin E deficiency. Either vitamin E or selenium deficiency in the host has been shown to increase certain viral mutations and, therefore, virulence. The laboratory diagnosis of vitamin E deficiency is made on the basis of low blood levels of α tocopherol (<5 μg/mL, or <0.8 mg of α tocopherol per gram of total lipids).

℞ Treatment:
VITAMIN E DEFICIENCY

Symptomatic vitamin E deficiency should be treated with 800–1200 mg of α tocopherol per day. Patients with abetalipoproteinemia may need as much as 5000–7000 mg/d. Children with symptomatic vitamin E deficiency should be treated with 400 mg/d orally of water-miscible esters; alternatively, 2 mg/kg per d may be administered intramuscularly. Vitamin E in high doses may protect against oxygen-induced retrolental fibroplasia and bronchopulmonary dysplasia, as well as intraventricular hemorrhage of prematurity. Vitamin E has been suggested to increase sexual performance, to treat intermittent claudication, and to slow the aging process, but evidence for these properties is lacking. When given in combination with other antioxidants, vitamin E may help to prevent macular degeneration. High doses (60–800 mg/d) of vitamin E have been shown in controlled trials to improve parameters of immune function and to reduce colds in nursing home residents, but intervention studies using vitamin E to prevent cardiovascular disease or cancer have not shown efficacy and, at doses >400 mg/d, may even increase all-cause mortality.

Toxicity

All forms of vitamin E are absorbed and could contribute to toxicity. High doses of vitamin E (>800 mg/d) may reduce platelet aggregation and interfere with vitamin K metabolism and are therefore contraindicated in patients taking warfarin. Nausea, flatulence, and diarrhea have been reported at doses >1 g/d.

VITAMIN K

There are two natural forms of vitamin K: vitamin K₁, also known as *phylloquinone*, from vegetable and animal sources, and vitamin K₂, or *menaquinone*, which is synthesized by bacterial flora and found in hepatic tissue. Phylloquinone can be converted to menaquinone in some organs.

Vitamin K is required for the posttranslational carboxylation of glutamic acid, which is necessary for calcium binding to γ-carboxylated proteins such as prothrombin (factor II); factors VII, IX, and X; protein C; protein S; and proteins found in bone (osteocalcin) and vascular smooth muscle (e.g., matrix Gla protein). However, the importance of vitamin K for bone mineralization and prevention of vascular calcification is not known. Warfarin-type drugs inhibit γ-carboxylation by preventing the conversion of vitamin K to its active hydroquinone form.

Dietary Sources

Vitamin K is found in green leafy vegetables such as kale and spinach, and appreciable amounts are also present in margarine and liver. Vitamin K is present in vegetable oils and is particularly rich in olive, canola, and soybean oils. The average daily intake by Americans is estimated to be approximately 100 μg/d.

Deficiency

The symptoms of vitamin K deficiency are due to hemorrhage, and newborns are particularly susceptible because of low fat stores, low breast milk levels of vitamin K, sterility of the infantile intestinal tract, liver immaturity, and poor placental transport. Intracranial bleeding, as well as gastrointestinal and skin bleeding, can occur in vitamin K–deficient infants 1–7 days after birth. Thus, vitamin K (1 mg IM) is given prophylactically at the time of delivery.

Vitamin K deficiency in adults may be seen in patients with chronic small-intestinal disease (e.g., celiac disease, Crohn's disease), in those with obstructed biliary tracts, or after small-bowel resection. Broad-spectrum antibiotic treatment can precipitate vitamin K deficiency by reducing gut bacteria, which synthesize menaquinones, and by inhibiting the metabolism of vitamin K. In patients with warfarin therapy, the antiobesity drug orlistat can lead to INR changes due to vitamin K malabsorption. The diagnosis of vitamin K deficiency is usually made on the basis of an elevated prothrombin time or reduced clotting factors, although vitamin K may also be measured directly by HPLC. Vitamin K deficiency is treated using a parenteral dose of 10 mg. For patients with chronic malabsorption, 1–2 mg/d of vitamin K should be given orally, or 1–2 mg/week can be taken parenterally. Patients with liver disease may have an elevated prothrombin time because of liver cell destruction as well as vitamin K deficiency. If an elevated prothrombin time does not improve on vitamin K therapy, it can be deduced that it is not the result of vitamin K deficiency.

Toxicity

Toxicity from dietary phylloquinones and menaquinones has not been described. High doses of vitamin K can impair the actions of oral anticoagulants.

MINERALS

See Table 52-2.

ZINC

Zinc is an integral component of many metalloenzymes in the body; it is involved in the synthesis and stabilization of proteins, DNA, and RNA and plays a structural role in ribosomes and membranes. Zinc is necessary for the binding of steroid hormone receptors and several other transcription factors to DNA. Zinc is absolutely required for normal spermatogenesis, fetal growth, and embryonic development.

Absorption

The absorption of zinc from the diet is inhibited by dietary phytate, fiber, oxalate, iron, and copper, as well as by certain drugs including penicillamine, sodium valproate, and ethambutol. Meat, shellfish, nuts, and legumes are good sources of bioavailable zinc, whereas zinc in grains and legumes is less available for absorption.

Deficiency

Mild zinc deficiency has been described in many diseases, including diabetes mellitus, HIV/AIDS, cirrhosis, alcoholism, inflammatory bowel disease, malab-sorption syndromes, and sickle cell disease. In these diseases, mild chronic zinc deficiency can cause stunted growth in children, decreased taste sensation (hypogeusia), and impaired immune function. Severe chronic zinc deficiency has been described as a cause of hypogonadism and dwarfism in several Middle Eastern countries. In these children, hypopigmented hair is also part of the syndrome. Acrodermatitis enteropathica is a rare autosomal recessive disorder characterized by abnormalities in zinc absorption. Clinical manifestations include diarrhea, alopecia, muscle wasting, depression, irritability, and a rash involving the extremities, face, and perineum. The rash is characterized by vesicular and pustular crusting with scaling and erythema. Occasional patients with Wilson's disease have developed zinc deficiency as a consequence of penicillamine therapy.

The diagnosis of zinc deficiency is usually made by a serum zinc level of <12 μmol/L (<70 μg/dL). Pregnancy and birth control pills may cause a slight depression in serum zinc levels, and hypoalbuminemia from any cause can result in hypozincemia. In acute stress situations, zinc may be redistributed from serum into tissues. Zinc deficiency may be treated with 60 mg elemental zinc, orally twice a day. Zinc gluconate lozenges (13 mg elemental zinc every 2 h while awake) have been reported to reduce the duration and symptoms of the common cold in adults, but studies are conflicting.

Zinc deficiency is prevalent in many developing countries and usually coexists with other micronutrient deficiencies (especially iron). Zinc (20 mg/d) may be an effective adjunctive therapeutic strategy for diarrheal disease in children.

Toxicity

Acute zinc toxicity after oral ingestion causes nausea, vomiting, and fever. Zinc fumes from welding may also be toxic and cause fever, respiratory distress, excessive salivation, sweating, and headache. Chronic large doses of zinc may depress immune function and cause hypochromic anemia as a result of copper deficiency.

COPPER

Copper is an integral part of numerous enzyme systems including amine oxidases, ferroxidase (ceruloplasmin), cytochrome-c oxidase, superoxide dismutase, and dopamine hydroxylase. Copper is also a component of ferroprotein, a transport protein involved in the basolateral transfer of iron during absorption from the enterocyte. As such, copper plays a role in iron metabolism, melanin synthesis, energy production, neurotransmitter synthesis, and CNS function; the synthesis and cross-linking of elastin and collagen; and the scavenging of superoxide radicals. Dietary sources of copper include shellfish, liver, nuts, legumes, bran, and organ meats.

Deficiency

Dietary copper deficiency is relatively rare, although it has been described in premature infants who are fed milk diets and in infants with malabsorption (Table 52-2). Copper-deficiency anemia has been reported in patients with malabsorptive diseases and nephrotic syndrome and in patients treated for Wilson's disease with chronic high doses of oral zinc, which can interfere with copper absorption. Menkes kinky hair syndrome is an X-linked metabolic disturbance of copper metabolism characterized by mental retardation, hypocupremia, and decreased circulating ceruloplasmin. It is caused by mutations in the copper-transporting *ATP7A* gene. Children with this disease often die within 5 years because of dissecting aneurysms or cardiac rupture. Aceruloplasminemia is a rare autosomal recessive disease characterized by tissue iron overload, mental deterioration, microcytic anemia, and low serum iron and copper concentrations.

The diagnosis of copper deficiency is usually made on the basis of low serum levels of copper (<65 μg/dL) and low ceruloplasmin levels (<20 mg/dL). Serum levels of copper may be elevated in pregnancy or stress conditions since ceruloplasmin is an acute-phase reactant and 90% of circulating copper is bound to ceruloplasmin.

Toxicity

Copper toxicity is usually accidental (Table 52-2). In severe cases, kidney failure, liver failure, and coma may ensue. In Wilson's disease, mutations in the copper-transporting *ATP7B* gene lead to accumulation of copper in the liver and brain, with low blood levels due to decreased ceruloplasmin.

SELENIUM

Selenium, in the form of selenocysteine, is a component of the enzyme glutathione peroxidase, which serves to protect proteins, cell membranes, lipids, and nucleic acids from oxidant molecules. As such, selenium is being actively studied as a chemopreventive agent against certain cancers, such as prostate. Selenocysteine is also found in the deiodinase enzymes, which mediate the deiodination of thyroxine to triiodothyronine. Rich dietary sources of selenium include seafood, muscle meat, and cereals, although the selenium content of cereal is determined by the soil concentration. Countries with low soil concentrations include parts of Scandinavia, China, and New Zealand. *Keshan disease* is an endemic cardiomyopathy found in children and young women residing in regions of China where dietary intake of selenium is low (<20 μg/d). Concomitant deficiencies of iodine and selenium may worsen the clinical manifestations of cretinism. Chronic ingestion of high amounts of selenium leads to selenosis characterized by hair and nail brittleness and loss, garlic breath odor, skin rash, myopathy, irritability, and other abnormalities of the nervous system.

CHROMIUM

Chromium potentiates the action of insulin in patients with impaired glucose tolerance, presumably by increasing insulin receptor–mediated signaling, although its usefulness in treating type 2 diabetes is uncertain. In addition, improvement in blood lipid profiles has been reported in some patients. The usefulness of chromium supplements in muscle building is not substantiated. Rich food sources of chromium include yeast, meat, and grain products. Chromium in the trivalent state is found in supplements and is largely nontoxic; however, chromium-6 is a product of stainless steel welding and is a known pulmonary carcinogen, as well as a cause of liver, kidney, and CNS damage.

FLUORIDE, MANGANESE, AND ULTRATRACE ELEMENTS

An essential function for fluoride in humans has not been described, although it is useful for the maintenance of structure in teeth and bone. Adult fluorosis results in mottled and pitted defects in tooth enamel as well as brittle bone (skeletal fluorosis).

Manganese and molybdenum deficiencies have been reported in patients with rare genetic abnormalities and in a few patients receiving prolonged total parenteral nutrition. Several manganese-specific enzymes have been identified (e.g., manganese superoxide dismutase). Deficiencies of manganese have been reported to result in bone demineralization, poor growth, ataxia, disturbances in carbohydrate and lipid metabolism, and convulsions.

Ultratrace elements are defined as those needed in amounts <1 mg/d. Essentiality has not been established for most ultratrace elements, although selenium, chromium, and iodine are clearly essential. *Molybdenum* is necessary for the activity of sulfite and xanthine oxidase, and molybdenum deficiency may result in skeletal and brain lesions.

FURTHER READINGS

BONAA KH et al: Homocysteine lowering and cardiovascular events after acute myocardial infarction. N Engl J Med 354:1578, 2006

COLLINS N, SPAULDING-ALBRIGHT N: Vitamin D deficiency: shining new light on the sun nutrient. Ostomy Wound Manage 55:15, 2009

DAY E et al: Thiamine for Wernicke-Korsakoff Syndrome in people at risk from alcohol abuse. Cochrane Database Syst Rev CD004033, 2004

LICHTENSTEIN AH, RUSSELL RM: Essential nutrients in a healthy diet: Food or supplements? JAMA 294:1, 2005

MILLER ER et al: Meta-analysis: High-dosage vitamin E supplementation may increase all-cause mortality. Ann Intern Med 142:37, 2005

576 MORRIS MC et al: Dietary folate and vitamin B12 intake and cognitive decline among community-dwelling older persons. Arch Neurol 62:641, 2005

MURPHY SP et al: Multivitamin-multimineral supplements' effect on total nutrient intake. Am J Clin Nutr 85:280S, 2007

NEMEROVSKI CW et al: Vitamin D and cardiovascular disease. Pharmacotherapy 29:691, 2009

PENNISTON KL, TANUMIHARDJO: The acute and chronic toxic effects of vitamin A. Am J Clin Nutr 83:191, 2006

PRENTICE RL: Clinical trials and observational studies to assess the chronic disease benefits and risks of multivitamin-multimineral supplements. Am J Clin Nutr 85:308S, 2007

TOUVIER M et al: Dual association of beta-carotene with risk of tobacco-related cancers in a cohort of French women. J Natl Cancer Inst 97:1338, 2005

VAN DER PUTTEN GJ et al: Association of some specific nutrient deficiencies with periodontal disease in elderly people: A systemic literature review. Nutrition 25:717, 2009

VERMEER C et al: Beyond deficiency: Potential benefits of increased intakes of vitamin K for bone and vascular health. Eur J Nutr 43:325, 2004ZX

WOLFF T et al: Folic acid supplementation for the prevention of neural tube defects: An update of the evidence for the U.S. Preventive Services Task Force. Ann Intern Med 150:632, 2009

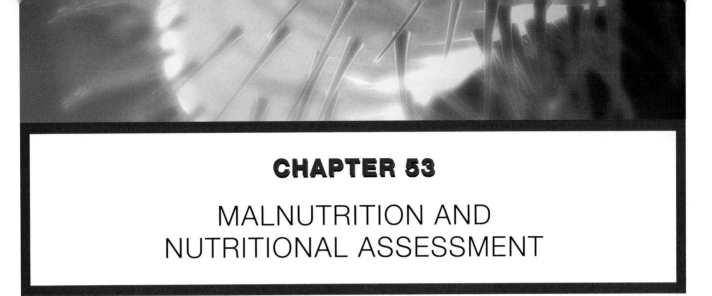

CHAPTER 53

MALNUTRITION AND NUTRITIONAL ASSESSMENT

Douglas C. Heimburger

Malnutrition can arise from primary or secondary causes, with the former resulting from inadequate or poor-quality food intake and the latter from diseases that alter food intake or nutrient requirements, metabolism, or absorption. Primary malnutrition occurs mainly in developing countries and under conditions of war or famine. Secondary malnutrition, the main form encountered in industrialized countries, was largely unrecognized until the early 1970s, when it became appreciated that persons with adequate food supplies can become malnourished as a result of acute or chronic diseases that alter nutrient intake or metabolism. Various studies have shown that protein-energy malnutrition (PEM) affects one-third to one-half of patients on general medical and surgical wards in teaching hospitals. The consistent finding that nutritional status influences patient prognosis underscores the importance of preventing, detecting, and treating malnutrition.

PROTEIN-ENERGY MALNUTRITION

The two major types of PEM are *marasmus* and *kwashiorkor*. These conditions are compared in **Table 53–1**. Marasmus and kwashiorkor can occur singly or in combination, as *marasmic kwashiorkor*. Kwashiorkor can occur

rapidly, whereas marasmus is the end result of a gradual wasting process that passes through stages of underweight, then mild, moderate, and severe cachexia.

MARASMUS

The end stage of cachexia, marasmus is a state in which virtually all available body fat stores have been exhausted due to starvation. Conditions that produce marasmus in developed countries tend to be chronic and indolent, such as cancer, chronic pulmonary disease, and anorexia nervosa. Marasmus is easy to detect because of the patient's starved appearance. The diagnosis is based on severe fat and muscle wastage resulting from prolonged calorie deficiency. Diminished skin-fold thickness reflects the loss of fat reserves; reduced arm muscle circumference with temporal and interosseous muscle wasting reflects the catabolism of protein throughout the body, including vital organs such as the heart, liver, and kidneys.

The laboratory findings in marasmus are relatively unremarkable. The creatinine-height index (the 24-h urinary creatinine excretion compared with normal values based on height) is low, reflecting the loss of muscle mass. Occasionally, the serum albumin level is reduced,

TABLE 53-1

COMPARISON OF MARASMUS AND KWASHIORKOR

	MARASMUS	KWASHIORKOR[a]
Clinical setting	↓ Energy intake	↓ Protein intake during stress state
Time course to develop	Months or years	Weeks
Clinical features	Starved appearance	Well-nourished appearance
	Weight <80% standard for height	Easy hair pluckability[b]
	Triceps skinfold <3 mm	Edema
	Mid-arm muscle circumference <15 cm	
Laboratory findings	Creatinine-height index <60% standard	Serum albumin <2.8 g/dL
		Total iron-binding capacity <200 µg/dL
		Lymphocytes <1500/µL
		Anergy
Clinical course	Reasonably preserved respon-	Infections
	siveness to short-term stress	Poor wound healing, decubitus
		ulcers, skin breakdown
Mortality	Low unless related to underlying	High
	disease	
Diagnostic criteria	Triceps skinfold <3 mm	Serum albumin <2.8 g/dL
	Mid-arm muscle circumference <15 cm	At least one of the following:
		Poor wound healing, decubitus
		ulcers, or skin breakdown
		Easy hair pluckability[b]
		Edema

[a]The findings used to diagnose kwashiorkor must be unexplained by other causes.
[b]Tested by *firmly* pulling a lock of hair from the top (not the sides or back), grasping with the thumb and forefinger. An average of three or more hairs removed easily and painlessly is considered abnormal hair pluckability.

but it stays above 2.8 g/dL in uncomplicated cases. Despite a morbid appearance, immunocompetence, wound healing, and the ability to handle short-term stress are reasonably well preserved in most patients with marasmus.

Marasmus is a chronic, fairly well-adapted form of starvation rather than an acute illness; it should be treated cautiously, in an attempt to reverse the downward trend gradually. Although nutritional support is necessary, overly aggressive repletion can result in severe, even life-threatening metabolic imbalances such as hypophosphatemia and cardiorespiratory failure. When possible, oral or enteral nutritional support is preferred; treatment started slowly allows readaptation of metabolic and intestinal functions (Chap. 54).

KWASHIORKOR

In contrast to marasmus, kwashiorkor in developed countries occurs mainly in connection with acute, life-threatening illnesses such as trauma and sepsis, and chronic illnesses that involve acute-phase inflammatory responses. The physiologic stress produced by these illnesses increases protein and energy requirements at a time when intake is often limited. A classic scenario for kwashiorkor is the acutely stressed patient who receives only 5% dextrose solutions for periods as brief as 2 weeks. Although the etiologic mechanisms are not clear, the protein-sparing response normally seen in starvation is blocked by the stressed state and by carbohydrate infusion.

In its early stages, the physical findings of kwashiorkor are few and subtle. Fat reserves and muscle mass are initially unaffected, giving the deceptive appearance of adequate nutrition. Signs that support the diagnosis of kwashiorkor include easy hair pluckability, edema, skin breakdown, and poor wound healing. The major *sine qua non* is severe reduction of levels of serum proteins such as albumin (<2.8 g/dL) and transferrin (<150 mg/dL) or iron-binding capacity (<200 µg/dL). Cellular immune function is depressed, reflected by lymphopenia (<1500 lymphocytes/µL in adults and older children) and lack of response to skin test antigens (anergy).

The prognosis of adult patients with full-blown kwashiorkor is not good, even with aggressive nutritional support. Surgical wounds often dehisce (fail to heal), pressure sores develop, gastroparesis and diarrhea can occur with enteral feeding, the risk of gastrointestinal bleeding from stress ulcers is increased, host defenses are compromised, and death from overwhelming infection

TABLE 53-2

PHYSIOLOGIC CHARACTERISTICS OF HYPOMETABOLIC AND HYPERMETABOLIC STATES

PHYSIOLOGIC CHARACTERISTICS	HYPOMETABOLIC, NONSTRESSED PATIENT (CACHECTIC, MARASMIC)	HYPERMETABOLIC, STRESSED PATIENT (KWASHIORKOR RISK[a])
Cytokines, catecholamines, glucagon, cortisol, insulin	↓	↑
Metabolic rate, O$_2$ consumption	↓	↑
Proteolysis, gluconeogenesis	↓	↑
Ureagenesis, urea excretion	↓	↑
Fat catabolism, fatty acid utilization	↑	↑
Adaptation to starvation	Normal	Abnormal

[a]These changes characterize the stressed, kwashiorkor-risk patient seen in developed countries; they differ in some respects from the characteristics of primary kwashiorkor seen in developing countries.

CHAPTER 53

Malnutrition and Nutritional Assessment

may occur despite antibiotic therapy. Unlike treatment in marasmus, aggressive nutritional support is indicated to restore better metabolic balance rapidly (Chap. 54). Although kwashiorkor in children is less foreboding, perhaps because a lesser degree of stress is required to precipitate the disorder, it is still a serious condition.

MARASMIC KWASHIORKOR

Marasmic kwashiorkor, the combined form of PEM, develops when the cachectic or marasmic patient experiences acute stress such as surgery, trauma, or sepsis, superimposing kwashiorkor onto chronic starvation. An extremely serious, life-threatening situation can occur because of the high risk of infection and other complications. It is important to determine the major component of PEM so that the appropriate nutritional plan can be developed. If kwashiorkor predominates, the need for vigorous nutritional therapy is urgent; if marasmus predominates, feeding should be more cautious.

PHYSIOLOGIC CHARACTERISTICS OF HYPOMETABOLIC AND HYPERMETABOLIC STATES

The metabolic characteristics and nutritional needs of hypermetabolic patients who are stressed from injury, infection, or chronic inflammatory illness differ from those of hypometabolic patients who are unstressed but chronically starved. In both cases, nutritional support is important, but misjudgments in selecting the appropriate approach may have disastrous consequences.

The hypometabolic patient is typified by the relatively unstressed but mildly catabolic and chronically

starved individual who, with time, will develop marasmus. The hypermetabolic patient stressed from injury or infection is catabolic (experiencing rapid breakdown of body mass) and is at high risk for developing kwashiorkor, if nutritional needs are not met and/or the illness does not resolve quickly. As summarized in Table 53-2, the two states are distinguished by differing perturbations of metabolic rate, rates of protein breakdown (proteolysis), and rates of gluconeogenesis. These differences are mediated by proinflammatory cytokines and counterregulatory hormones—tumor necrosis factor, interleukins 1 and 6, C-reactive protein, catecholamines (epinephrine and norepinephrine), glucagon, and cortisol—that are relatively reduced in hypometabolic patients and increased in hypermetabolic patients. Although insulin levels are also elevated in stressed patients, insulin resistance in the target tissues prevents insulin-mediated anabolic actions.

METABOLIC RATE

In starvation and semistarvation, the resting metabolic rate falls between 10% and 30% as an adaptive response to energy restriction, slowing the rate of weight loss. By contrast, resting metabolic rate rises in the presence of physiologic stress in proportion to the degree of the insult. It may increase by about 10% after elective surgery, 20–30% after bone fractures, 30–60% with severe infections such as peritonitis or gram-negative septicemia, and as much as 110% after major burns.

If the metabolic rate (energy requirement) is not matched by energy intake, weight loss results—slowly in hypometabolism and quickly in hypermetabolism. Losses of up to 10% of body weight are unlikely to be detrimental; however, losses greater than this in acutely ill hypermetabolic patients may be associated with rapid deterioration in body function.

PROTEIN CATABOLISM

The rate of endogenous protein breakdown (catabolism) to supply energy needs normally falls during uncomplicated energy deprivation. After about 10 days of total starvation, the unstressed individual loses about 12–18 g/d protein (equivalent to approximately 2 oz of muscle tissue or 2–3 g of nitrogen). By contrast, in injury and sepsis, protein breakdown accelerates in proportion to the degree of stress, to 30–60 g/d after elective surgery, 60–90 g/d with infection, 100–130 g/d with severe sepsis or skeletal trauma, and >175 g/d with major burns or head injuries. These losses are reflected by proportional increases in the excretion of urea nitrogen, the major byproduct of protein breakdown.

GLUCONEOGENESIS

The major aim of protein catabolism during a state of starvation is to provide the glucogenic amino acids (especially alanine and glutamine) that serve as substrates for endogenous glucose production (gluconeogenesis) in the liver. In the hypometabolic/starved state, protein breakdown for gluconeogenesis is minimized, especially as ketones derived from fatty acids become the substrate preferred by certain tissues. In the hypermetabolic/stress state, gluconeogenesis increases dramatically and in proportion to the degree of the insult, to increase the supply of glucose (the major fuel of reparation). Glucose is the only fuel that can be utilized by hypoxic tissues (anaerobic glycolysis), white blood cells, and newly generated fibroblasts. Infusions of glucose partially offset a negative energy balance but do not significantly suppress the high rates of gluconeogenesis in the catabolic patient. Hence, adequate supplies of protein are needed to replace the amino acids utilized for this metabolic response.

In summary, the hypometabolic patient is adapted to starvation and conserves body mass by reducing the metabolic rate and using fat as the primary fuel (rather than glucose and its precursor amino acids). The hypermetabolic patient also uses fat as a fuel but rapidly breaks down body protein to produce glucose, causing loss of muscle and organ tissue and endangering vital body functions.

MICRONUTRIENT MALNUTRITION

The same illnesses and reductions in nutrient intake that lead to PEM often produce deficiencies of vitamins and minerals as well (Chap. 52). Deficiencies of nutrients that are stored in small amounts (such as the water-soluble vitamins) are lost through external secretions, such as zinc in diarrhea fluid or burn exudate, and are probably more common than generally recognized.

Deficiencies of vitamin C, folic acid, and zinc are reasonably common in sick patients. Signs of scurvy such as corkscrew hairs on the lower extremities are frequently found in chronically ill and/or alcoholic patients. The diagnosis can be confirmed with plasma vitamin C levels. Folic acid intakes and blood levels are often less than optimal, even among healthy persons; when illness, alcoholism, poverty, or poor dentition is present, deficiencies are common. Low blood zinc levels are prevalent in patients with malabsorption syndromes such as inflammatory bowel disease. Patients with zinc deficiency often exhibit poor wound healing, pressure ulcer formation, and impaired immunity. Thiamine deficiency is a common complication of alcoholism, but its manifestations are often prevented by therapeutic doses of thiamine in patients treated for alcohol abuse.

Patients with low plasma vitamin C levels usually respond to the doses found in multivitamin preparations, but patients with deficiencies should be supplemented with 250–500 mg/d. Folic acid is absent from some oral multivitamin preparations; patients with deficiencies should be supplemented with about 1 mg/d. Patients with zinc deficiencies resulting from large external losses sometimes require oral daily supplementation with 220 mg of zinc sulfate one to three times daily. For these reasons, laboratory assessments of the micronutrient status of patients at high risk are desirable.

Hypophosphatemia develops in hospitalized patients with remarkable frequency and generally results from rapid intracellular shifts of phosphate in cachectic or alcoholic patients receiving intravenous glucose. The adverse clinical sequelae are numerous; some, such as acute cardiopulmonary failure, can be life-threatening.

NUTRITIONAL ASSESSMENT

Because interactions between illness and nutrition are complex, many physical and laboratory findings reflect both underlying disease and nutritional status. Therefore, the nutritional evaluation of a patient requires an integration of the history, physical examination, anthropometrics, and laboratory studies. This approach helps both to detect nutritional problems and to avoid concluding that isolated findings indicate nutritional problems when they do not. For example, hypoalbuminemia caused by an underlying illness does not necessarily indicate malnutrition.

NUTRITIONAL HISTORY

A nutritional history is directed toward identifying underlying mechanisms that put patients at risk for nutritional

TABLE 53-3

THE HIGH-RISK PATIENT

Underweight (body mass index <18.5) and/or recent loss of ≥10% of usual body weight
Poor intake: anorexia, food avoidance (e.g., psychiatric condition), or NPO status for more than about 5 days
Protracted nutrient losses: malabsorption, enteric fistulae, draining abscesses or wounds, renal dialysis
Hypermetabolic states: sepsis, protracted fever, extensive trauma or burns
Alcohol abuse or use of drugs with antinutrient or catabolic properties: steroids, antimetabolites (e.g., methotrexate),
  immunosuppressants, antitumor agents
Impoverishment, isolation, advanced age

depletion or excess. These mechanisms include inadequate intake, impaired absorption, decreased utilization, increased losses, and increased requirements of nutrients.

Individuals with the characteristics listed in Table 53-3 are at particular risk for nutritional deficiencies.

PHYSICAL EXAMINATION

Physical findings that suggest vitamin, mineral, and protein-energy deficiencies and excesses are outlined in Table 53-4. Most of the physical findings are not specific for individual nutrient deficiencies, and they must be integrated with the historic, anthropometric, and laboratory findings. For example, the finding of follicular hyperkeratosis on the back of the arms is a fairly common, normal finding. On the other hand, if it is widespread in a person who consumes little fruit and vegetables and smokes regularly (increasing ascorbic acid requirements), vitamin C deficiency is likely. Similarly, easily pluckable hair may be a consequence of chemotherapy, but in a hospitalized patient who has poorly healing surgical wounds and hypoalbuminemia, it suggests kwashiorkor.

ANTHROPOMETRICS

Anthropometric measurements provide information on body muscle mass and fat reserves. The most practical and commonly used measurements are body weight, height, triceps skinfold (TSF), and mid-arm muscle circumference (MAMC). Body weight is one of the most useful nutritional parameters to follow in patients who are acutely or chronically ill. Unintentional weight loss during illness often reflects loss of lean body mass (muscle and organ tissue), especially if it is rapid and not caused by diuresis. This can be an ominous sign since it indicates use of vital body protein stores as a metabolic fuel. The reference standard for normal body weight, body mass index (BMI, or weight in kilograms divided by height, in meters, squared), is discussed in Chap 56. BMIs <18.5 are considered underweight, 18.5–24.9 are normal, 25–29.9 are overweight, and ≥30 are obese.

Measurement of skinfold thickness is useful for estimating body fat stores, because about 50% of body fat is normally located in the subcutaneous region. Skinfold thicknesses can also permit discrimination of fat mass from muscle mass. The TSF is a convenient site that is generally representative of the body's overall fat level. A thickness of <3 mm suggests virtually complete exhaustion of fat stores. The MAMC, often used to estimate skeletal muscle mass, is calculated as follows:

$$\text{MAMC (cm)} = \text{upper arm circumference (cm)} - [0.314 \times \text{TSF (mm)}]$$

LABORATORY STUDIES

A number of laboratory tests used routinely in clinical medicine can yield valuable information about a patient's nutritional status if a slightly different approach to their interpretation is used. For example, abnormally low serum albumin levels, total iron-binding capacity, and anergy may have a distinct explanation, but collectively they may represent kwashiorkor. In the clinical setting of a hypermetabolic, acutely ill patient who is edematous and has easily pluckable hair and inadequate protein intake, the diagnosis of kwashiorkor is clear-cut. Commonly used laboratory tests for assessing nutritional status are outlined in Table 53-5. The table also provides tips to help avoid assigning nutritional significance to tests that may be abnormal for nonnutritional reasons.

Assessment of Circulating (Visceral) Proteins

The serum proteins most used to assess nutritional status include albumin, total iron-binding capacity (or transferrin), thyroxine-binding prealbumin (or transthyretin), and retinol-binding protein. Because they have differing synthesis rates and half-lives—the half-life of serum albumin is about 21 days whereas those of prealbumin and retinol-binding protein are about 2 days and 12 h, respectively—some of these proteins reflect changes in

TABLE 53-4

PHYSICAL FINDINGS OF NUTRITIONAL DEFICIENCIES

CLINICAL FINDINGS	POSSIBLE DEFICIENCY[a]	POSSIBLE EXCESS
Hair, Nails		
Corkscrew hairs and unemerged coiled hairs	Vitamin C	
Easily pluckable hair	Protein	
Flag sign (transverse depigmentation of hair)	Protein	
Sparse hair	Protein, biotin, zinc	Vitamin A
Transverse ridging of nails	Protein	
Skin		
Cellophane appearance	Protein	
Cracking (flaky paint or crazy pavement dermatosis)	Protein	
Follicular hyperkeratosis	Vitamins A, C	
Petechiae (especially perifollicular)	Vitamin C	
Purpura	Vitamins C, K	
Pigmentation, scaling of sun-exposed areas	Niacin	
Poor wound healing, decubitus ulcers	Protein, vitamin C, zinc	
Scaling	Vitamin A, essential fatty acids, biotin	Vitamin A
Yellow pigmentation sparing sclerae (benign)	Zinc (hyperpigmented)	Carotene
Eyes		
Night blindness	Vitamin A	
Papilledema		Vitamin A
Perioral		
Angular stomatitis	Riboflavin, pyridoxine, niacin	
Cheilosis (dry, cracking, ulcerated lips)	Riboflavin, pyridoxine, niacin	
Oral		
Atrophic lingual papillae (slick tongue)	Riboflavin, niacin, folate, vitamin B_{12}, protein, iron	
Glossitis (scarlet, raw tongue)	Riboflavin, niacin, pyridoxine, folate,	
Hypogeusesthesia, hyposmia	Zinc	
Swollen, retracted, bleeding gums (if teeth present)	Vitamin C	
Bones, Joints		
Beading of ribs, epiphyseal swelling, bowlegs	Vitamin D	
Tenderness, subperiosteal hemorrhage in children	Vitamin C	
Neurologic		
Confabulation, disorientation	Thiamine (Korsakoff psychosis)	
Drowsiness, lethargy, vomiting		Vitamin A
Dementia	Niacin, vitamin B_{12}, folate	
Headache		Vitamin A
Ophthalmoplegia	Thiamine, phosphorus	
Peripheral neuropathy (e.g., weakness, paresthesias, ataxia, foot drop, and decreased tendon reflexes, fine tactile sense, vibratory sense, and position sense)	Thiamine, pyridoxine, vitamin B_{12}	Pyridoxine
Tetany	Calcium, magnesium	
Other		
Edema	Protein, thiamine	
Heart failure	Thiamine ("wet" beriberi), phosphorus	
Hepatomegaly	Protein	Vitamin A
Parotid enlargement	Protein (consider also bulimia)	
Sudden heart failure, death	Vitamin C	

[a]In this table, "protein deficiency" is used to signify kwashiorkor.

TABLE 53-5

583

LABORATORY TESTS FOR NUTRITIONAL ASSESSMENT

TEST (NORMAL VALUES)	NUTRITIONAL USE	CAUSES OF NORMAL VALUE DESPITE MALNUTRITION	OTHER CAUSES OF ABNORMAL VALUE
Serum albumin (3.5–5.5 g/dL)	2.8–3.5: Compromised protein status <2.8: Possible kwashiorkor Increasing value reflects positive protein balance	Dehydration Infusion of albumin, fresh frozen plasma, or whole blood	**Low** Common: Infection and other stress, especially with poor protein intake Burns, trauma Congestive heart failure Fluid overload Severe liver disease Uncommon: Nephrotic syndrome Zinc deficiency Bacterial stasis/overgrowth of small intestine
Serum prealbumin, also called transthyretin (20–40 mg/dL; lower in prepubertal children)	10–15 mg/dL: Mild protein depletion 5–10 mg/dL: Moderate protein depletion <5 mg/dL: Severe protein depletion Increasing value reflects positive protein balance	Chronic renal failure	Similar to serum albumin
Serum total iron binding capacity (TIBC) 240–450 µg/dL	<200: Compromised protein status, possible kwashiorkor Increasing value reflects positive protein balance More labile than albumin	Iron deficiency	**Low** Similar to serum albumin **High** Iron deficiency
Prothrombin time 12.0–15.5 sec	Prolongation: vitamin K deficiency		**Prolonged** Anticoagulant therapy (warfarin) Severe liver disease
Serum creatinine 0.6–1.6 mg/dL	<0.6: Muscle wasting due to prolonged energy deficit Reflects muscle mass		**High** Despite muscle wasting: Renal failure Severe dehydration
24-h urinary creatinine 500–1200 mg/d (standardized for height and sex)	Low value: muscle wasting due to prolonged energy deficit	>24-h collection Decreasing serum creatinine	**Low** Incomplete urine collection Increasing serum creatinine Neuromuscular wasting
24-h urinary urea nitrogen (UUN) <5 g/d (depends on level of protein intake)	Determine level of catabolism (as long as protein intake is ≥10 g below calculated protein loss or <20 g total, but at least 100 g carbohydrate is provided) 5–10 g/d = mild catabolism or normal fed state 10–15 g/d = moderate catabolism >15 g/d = severe catabolism Estimate protein balance Protein balance = protein intake – protein loss where protein loss (protein catabolic rate) = [24-h UUN (g) + 4] × 6.25 Adjustments required in burn patients and others with large nonurinary nitrogen losses and in patients with fluctuating BUN levels (e.g., renal failure)		

(Continued)

TABLE 53-5 (*CONTINUED*)

LABORATORY TESTS FOR NUTRITIONAL ASSESSMENT			
TEST (NORMAL VALUES)	**NUTRITIONAL USE**	**CAUSES OF NORMAL VALUE DESPITE MALNUTRITION**	**OTHER CAUSES OF ABNORMAL VALUE**
Blood urea nitrogen (BUN) 8–23 mg/dL	<8: Possibly inadequate protein intake 12–23: Possibly adequate protein intake >23: Possibly excessive protein intake If serum creatinine is normal, use BUN If serum creatinine is elevated, use BUN/creatinine ratio (normal range is essentially the same as for BUN)		**Low** Severe liver disease Anabolic state Syndrome of inappropriate antidiuretic hormone **High** Despite poor protein intake: Renal failure (use BUN/creatinine ratio) Congestive heart failure Gastrointestinal hemorrhage

nutritional status more quickly than others. However, rapid fluctuations can also make shorter-half-life proteins less reliable.

Levels of circulating proteins are influenced by their rates of synthesis and catabolism, "third spacing" (loss into interstitial spaces), and, in some cases, external loss. Although an adequate intake of calories and protein is necessary to achieve optimal circulating protein levels, serum protein levels generally do not reflect protein intake. For example, a drop in the serum level of albumin or transferrin often accompanies significant physiologic stress (e.g., from infection or injury) and is not necessarily an indication of malnutrition or poor intake. A low serum albumin level in a burned patient with both hypermetabolism and increased dermal losses of protein may not indicate malnutrition. On the other hand, adequate nutritional support of the patient's calorie and protein needs is critical for returning circulating proteins to normal levels as stress resolves. Thus low values by themselves do not define malnutrition, but they often point to increased risk of malnutrition because of the hypermetabolic stress state. As long as significant physiologic stress persists, serum protein levels remain low, even with aggressive nutritional support. However, if the levels do not rise after the underlying illness improves, the patient's protein and calorie needs should be reassessed to ensure that intake is sufficient.

Assessment of Vitamin and Mineral Status

The use of laboratory tests to confirm suspected micronutrient deficiencies is desirable because the physical findings for these are often equivocal or nonspecific. Low blood micronutrient levels can predate more serious clinical manifestations and may also indicate drug-nutrient interactions.

ESTIMATING ENERGY AND PROTEIN REQUIREMENTS

A patient's basal energy expenditures (BEE, measured in kilocalories per day) can be estimated from height, weight, age, and gender using the Harris-Benedict equations:

Men: BEE = 66.47 + 13.75W + 5.00H − 6.76A
Women: BEE = 655.10 + 9.56W + 1.85H − 4.68A

where W is weight in kg; H is height in cm, and A is age in years. After solving these equations, total energy requirements are estimated by multiplying the BEE by a factor that accounts for the stress of illness. Multiplying by 1.1–1.4 yields a range 10–40% above basal that estimates the 24-h energy expenditure of the majority of patients. The lower value (1.1) is used for patients without evidence of significant physiologic stress; the higher value (1.4) is appropriate for patients with marked stress such as sepsis or trauma. The result is used as a 24-h energy goal for feeding.

When it is important to have a more accurate assessment of energy expenditure, it can be measured at the bedside using indirect calorimetry. This technique is useful in patients who are believed to be hypermetabolic from sepsis or trauma and whose body weights cannot be obtained accurately. Indirect calorimetry can also be useful in patients having difficulty weaning from a ventilator, as their energy needs should not be exceeded to avoid excessive CO_2 production. Patients at the extremes of weight (e.g., obese persons) and/or age are good candidates as well, because the Harris-Benedict equations were developed from measurements in adults with roughly normal body weights.

Because urea is a major byproduct of protein catabolism, the amount of urea nitrogen excreted each day can be used to estimate the rate of protein catabolism and to determine if protein intake is adequate to offset it. Total protein loss and protein balance can be calculated from the urinary urea nitrogen (UUN) as follows:

$$\text{Protein catabolic rate (g/d)} = [\text{24-h UUN (g)} + 4]$$
$$\times 6.25 \text{ (g protein/g nitrogen)}$$

The value of 4 g added to the UUN represents a liberal estimate of the unmeasured nitrogen lost in the urine (e.g., creatinine and uric acid), sweat, hair, skin, and feces. When protein intake is low (e.g., less than about 20 g/d), the equation indicates both the patient's protein requirement and the severity of the catabolic state (Table 53-5). More substantial protein intakes can raise the UUN because some of the ingested (or infused) protein is catabolized and converted to UUN. Thus at lower protein intakes the equation is useful for estimating *requirements*, and at higher protein intakes it is useful for assessing protein *balance*.

$$\text{Protein balance (g/d)} = \text{Protein intake}$$
$$- \text{Protein catabolic rate}$$

FURTHER READINGS

AMERICAN SOCIETY FOR PARENTERAL AND ENTERAL NUTRITION: *The science and practice of nutrition support: A case-based core curriculum.* Dubuque, Kendall/Hunt, 2001. Available online at: *www.nutritioncare.org*

ATINMO T et al: Breaking the poverty/malnutrition cycle in Africa and the Middle East. Nutr Rev 67 (suppl 1):S40, 2009

BAKER H: Nutrition in the elderly: Hypovitaminosis and its implications. Geriatrics 62:22, 2007

BHUTTA ZA: Addressing severe acute malnutrition where it matters. Lancet 374:94, 2009

CHAPMAN IM: Nutritional disorders in the elderly. Med Clin North Am 90:887, 2006

HEIMBURGER DC, ARD JD (eds): *Handbook of Clinical Nutrition,* 4th ed. Philadelphia, Mosby Elsevier, 2006

PEPERSACK T: Nutritional problems in the elderly. Acta Clin Belg 64:85, 2009

SHILS ME et al (eds): *Modern Nutrition in Health and Disease,* 10th ed. Baltimore, Lippincott Williams & Wilkins, 2005

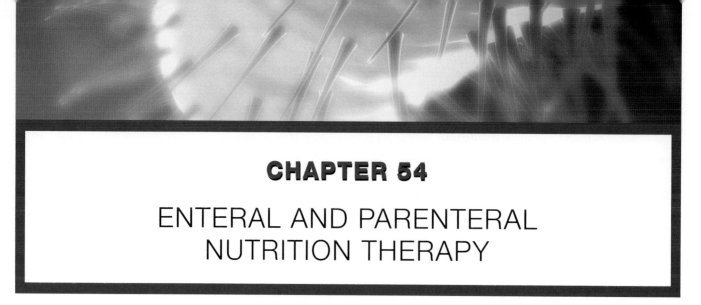

CHAPTER 54

ENTERAL AND PARENTERAL NUTRITION THERAPY

Bruce R. Bistrian ■ David F. Driscoll

The ability to provide specialized nutritional support (SNS) represents a major advance in medical therapy. Nutritional support, via either enteral or parenteral routes, is used in two main settings: (1) to provide adequate nutritional intake during the recuperative phase of illness or injury, when the patient's ability to ingest or absorb nutrients is impaired, and (2) to support the patient during the systemic response to inflammation, injury, or infection during an extended critical illness. SNS is also used in patients with permanent loss of intestinal length or function. In addition, an increasing number of elderly patients living in nursing homes and chronic care facilities receive enteral feeding, usually as a consequence of inadequate nutritional intake.

Enteral refers to feeding via a tube placed into the gut to deliver liquid formulas containing all essential nutrients. *Parenteral* refers to the infusion of complete nutrient solutions into the bloodstream via a peripheral vein or, more commonly, by central venous access to meet nutritional needs. Enteral feeding is generally the preferred route because of benefits derived from maintaining the digestive, absorptive, and immunologic barrier functions of the gastrointestinal tract. Small-bore pliable tubes have largely replaced large-bore rubber tubes, making placement easier and more acceptable to patients. Infusion pumps have also improved the delivery of nutrient solutions.

For short-term use, enteral tubes can be placed via the nose into the stomach, duodenum, or jejunum. For long-term use, these sites can be accessed through the abdominal wall using endoscopic, radiologic, or surgical procedures. Intestinal tolerance of tube feeding may be limited during acute illness by gastric retention or diarrhea. Parenteral feeding has greater risk of infection, reflecting the need for venous access, and a greater propensity for inducing hyperglycemia. However, these risks can generally be managed successfully by SNS teams. For the postoperative patient with preexisting malnutrition, or in trauma patients who were previously well nourished, SNS is strikingly cost-effective. In the most critically ill patient in the intensive care unit, SNS can dramatically enhance survival. Although enteral nutrition (EN) can be provided by most health care teams caring for hospitalized patients, safe and effective parenteral nutrition (PN) usually requires specialized teams.

Approach to the Patient:
REQUIREMENTS FOR SPECIALIZED NUTRITIONAL SUPPORT

Indications for Specialized Nutritional Support Although at least 15–20% of patients in acute care hospitals have evidence of significant malnutrition, only a small fraction will benefit from SNS. For others, wasting is an inevitable component of a terminal disease and the course of the disease will not be altered by SNS. The decision to use SNS should be based on the likelihood that preventing protein-calorie malnutrition (PCM) will increase the likelihood of recovery, reduce infection rates, improve healing, or otherwise shorten the hospital stay. In the case of the elderly or chronically ill patient for whom full recovery is not anticipated, the decision to feed is usually based on whether SNS will extend the duration and quality of life. The decision-making process used to decide when to use SNS is depicted in **Fig. 54-1**.

The first step in deciding to administer SNS is to consider the nutritional implications of the disease process. Is the condition or its treatment likely to impair food intake and absorption for a prolonged period of time? For example, a well-nourished individual can tolerate approximately 7 days of starvation while experiencing a systemic response to inflammation (SRI). The second step is to determine if the patient is already significantly malnourished to the degree that critical functions such as wound healing, immune function, or ventilatory function are impaired

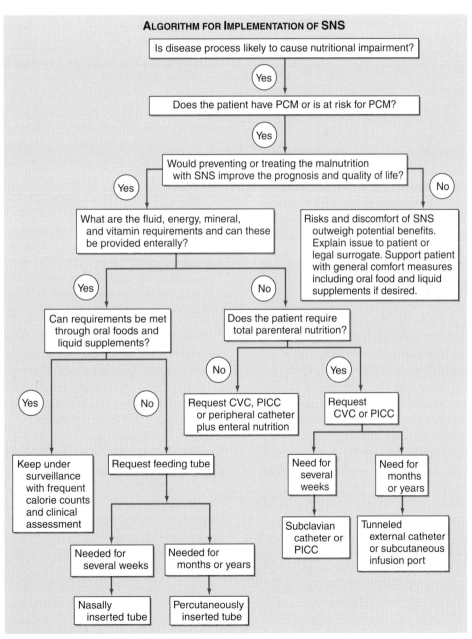

FIGURE 54-1

Decision-making for the implementation of specialized nutrition support (SNS). CVC, central venous catheter; PICC, peripherally inserted central catheter. *(Adapted from previous chapter by Lyn Howard, MD.)*

(Chap. 72). An unintentional weight loss of >10% during the previous 6 months or a weight/height <90% of standard, when associated with physiologic impairment, represents significant PCM. Weight loss >20% of usual or <80% of standard reflects severe PCM. The presence or absence of SRI should be noted, since inflammation, injury, and infection increase the rate of lean tissue loss. SRI also has pathophysiologic effects that influence nutritional responses such as fluid retention and hyperglycemia, as well as impairment of anabolic responses to nutritional support.

Once it is determined that a patient is already or at risk of becoming malnourished, the next step is to decide whether SNS will impact positively on the patient's response to disease. In the end stages of many chronic illnesses with accompanying PCM, particularly those due to cancer or terminal neurologic disorders, nutrition may not reverse the PCM or improve quality of life. While the provision of food and water is part of basic medical care, nutrition delivered by tube or catheter, either enterally or parenterally, is associated with risk and discomfort. Thus, SNS should be recommended only when potential benefits exceed risks, and should be undertaken with the consent of the patient. Like other life support measures, enteral or parenteral therapy is difficult to withdraw once started. Initiating nutrition support may be appropriate before a final prognosis can be determined, but this should not preclude its subsequent withdrawal. If preventing or treating PCM with SNS is appropriate, nutritional requirements and the method of delivery should be determined. The optimal route depends on the degree of gut function and somewhat on the available technical resources.

The timing of nutritional support is based on evaluation of the preexisting nutritional status, the presence and extent of SRI, and the anticipated clinical course. SRI is identified by the standard clinical signs of leukocytosis, tachycardia, tachypnea, and/or temperature elevation or depression. Although the degree of hypoalbuminemia provides an estimate of SRI severity, normal serum albumin levels will not be restored by adequate nutritional support until the SRI remits, even though nutritional benefits can be achieved by adequate feeding.

The SRI can be graded as severe, moderate, or mild. Examples of severe SRI include sepsis or other inflammatory conditions like pancreatitis requiring ICU care, multiple trauma with an Injury Severity Score >20–25 or APACHE II >25, closed head injury with a Glasgow Coma Scale <8, or major third-degree burns of >40% of body surface area. Moderate SRI includes less severe infections, injuries, or inflammatory conditions like pneumonia, major surgery, acute hepatic or renal insufficiency, and exacerbations of

TABLE 54-1

BODY MASS INDEX (BMI) AND NUTRITIONAL STATUS

BMI	NUTRITIONAL STATUS
>30 kg/m^2	Obese
>25–30 kg/m^2	Overweight
20–25 kg/m^2	Normal
<18.5 kg/m^2	Moderate malnutrition
<16 kg/m^2	Severe malnutrition
<13 kg/m^2	Lethal in males
<11 kg/m^2	Lethal in females

From D Driscoll, B Bistrian: Parenteral and enteral nutrition in the intensive care unit, in *Intensive Care Medicine*, R Irwin, J Rippe (eds). Lippincott Williams & Wilkins, Philadelphia, 2003.

ulcerative colitis or regional enteritis requiring hospitalization. PCM should also be defined as severe, moderate, or minimal as assessed by weight/height, percent recent weight loss, and body mass index. The body mass index in relation to nutritional status is listed in **Table 54-1.** A patient with a severe SRI requires early feeding within the first several days of care because the condition is likely to produce inadequate spontaneous intake over the next 7 days. A moderate SRI, as commonly seen during a postoperative period without oral intake that exceeds 5 days, benefits from adequate feeding by day 5–7 if the patient was initially well nourished. If severely malnourished, candidates for elective major surgery benefit from preoperative nutritional repletion for 5–7 days. However, this is not often possible. Thus, early postoperative feeding is indicated. Patients with a moderate SRI and moderate PCM also benefit from earlier feeding within the first several days.

Efficacy of SNS in Different Disease States Efficacy studies have shown that malnourished patients undergoing major thoracoabdominal surgery benefit from SNS. Critical illness requiring ICU care including major burns, major trauma, severe sepsis, closed head injury, and severe pancreatitis [positive CT scan and Acute Physiology and Chronic Health Evaluation II (APACHE II) >10] all benefit by early SNS, as indicated by reduced mortality and morbidity. In critical illness, initiation of SNS within 24 h of injury or ICU admission is associated with a ~50% reduction in mortality. Patients with nitrogen accumulation disorders of renal and hepatic failure have a likelihood of PCM of >50% and at least a moderate SRI. Improvements in morbidity, including infection rates, encephalopathy, liver or renal function, and length of hospital stay have been found with SNS. Inflammatory bowel disease—including Crohn's disease particularly, and, to a lesser degree, ulcerative colitis—often produce PCM. In the outpatient setting, SNS in Crohn's disease can improve nutritional status, quality of life, and the likelihood of remission. With pulmonary disease in the critically ill, SNS improves ventilatory status, and in acute lung injury the use of omega 3 fats as a component of SNS improves gas exchange and respiratory dynamics and reduces the need for mechanical ventilation. Low body weight in chronic obstructive pulmonary disease is associated with diminished pulmonary status and exercise capacity and higher mortality rates. However, there is little convincing evidence that SNS as caloric supplementation improves nutrition or pulmonary function. PCM is also common in the course of cancer and HIV disease, although less so in the latter with the advent of highly active antiretroviral therapy. When PCM develops as a consequence of SRI in these conditions, there is limited likelihood of substantial efficacy or benefit from SNS. However, when PCM develops as a consequence of gastrointestinal dysfunction, SNS can be effective. Although no randomized trials have been performed for SNS provided for hyperemesis gravidarum, there is considerable clinical evidence that it improves pregnancy outcomes.

Risks and Benefits of Specialized Nutrition Support The risks are determined primarily by patient factors such as state of alertness, swallowing competence, the route of delivery, underlying conditions, and the experience of the supervising clinical team. The safest and least costly approach is to avoid SNS by close attention to oral food intake, by adding an oral liquid supplement, or in certain chronic conditions by using medications to stimulate appetite. Nutrient intake monitoring by frequent calorie counts or oral formula selection is best performed by a nutritionist.

Enteral tube feeding is often required in patients with anorexia, impaired swallowing, or bowel disease. The bowel and its associated digestive organs derive 70% of their required nutrients directly from food in the lumen. Arginine, glutamine, short-chain fatty acids, long-chain omega 3 fatty acids, and nucleotides available in some specialty enteral formulas are particularly important for maintaining immunity. Enteral feeding also supports gut function by stimulating splanchnic blood flow, neuronal activity, IgA antibody release, and secretion of gastrointestinal hormones that stimulate gut trophic activity. These factors support the gut as an immunologic barrier against enteric pathogens. For these reasons, some luminal nutrition should be provided, even when PN is required to provide most of the nutritional support. The combination of some enteral feeding either by mouth or by enteral tube with parenteral feeding often shortens the transition to full enteral feeding, which can generally be used when >50% of requirements can be met enterally. Substantial nutritional benefit can be achieved by providing ~50% of energy needs for periods of up to 10 days, if protein and other essential nutrient requirements are met. For longer periods of time, it may be preferable to provide 75–80% of energy needs, rather than full feeding, if this improves gastrointestinal tolerance, glycemic control, and avoidance of excess fluid administration.

In the past, bowel rest through PN was the cornerstone of treatment for many severe gastrointestinal disorders. However, the value of providing even minimal amounts of EN is now widely accepted. The development of protocols to facilitate more widespread use of EN include initiation within 24 h of ICU admission; aggressive use of the head-upright position; postpyloric and nasojejunal feeding tubes; prokinetic agents; more rapid increases in feeding rates; tolerance of higher gastric residuals; and nurse-administered algorithms. PN alone is generally necessary only for severe gut dysfunction due to prolonged ileus, obstruction, or severe hemorrhagic pancreatitis. In the critically ill, feeding adequately by PN beginning within the first 24 h of care improves mortality and is more effective than delayed EN. Early feeding of the critically ill in the ICU is associated with a 50% reduction in mortality, but there is also a 50% increase in infection risk. Much of the increase in morbidity related to PN and EN is due to hyperglycemia, which can be significantly reduced by insulin therapy. The level of glycemia necessary to accomplish this goal, whether <110 mg/dL or only <150 mg/dL, is not yet defined.

Although PN was initially relatively expensive, its components are often less expensive than specialty enteral formulas. Percutaneous placement of a central venous catheter into the subclavian or internal jugular vein with advancement into the superior vena cava can be accomplished at the bedside by trained personnel using sterile techniques. Peripherally inserted central catheters can also be placed within the lumen in the central vein, but this technique is usually more appropriate for non-ICU patients. The subclavian or internal jugular lines can be changed over a wire, but this carries a greater risk of pneumothorax or serious vascular damage. The peripherally inserted catheters are subject to position-related flow, and the catheter cannot be changed over a wire. Inserting a nasogastric tube is a bedside procedure, but many critically ill patients have impaired gastric emptying that increases the risk of aspiration pneumonia. This risk can be reduced by feeding directly into the jejunum beyond the ligament of Treitz. This usually requires fluoroscopic guidance or endoscopic placement. In patients who have planned laparotomies or other conditions likely to require a prolonged need for SNS, it is advantageous to place a jejunal feeding tube at the time of surgery.

Although most SNS is delivered in hospitals, some patients require it on a long-term basis. If they have a safe environment and a willingness to learn the self-care techniques, SNS can be administered at home. The clinical outcomes of patients with severe intestinal disorders treated with home PN or EN are summarized in Table 54-2. PN infused at home is usually cycled overnight to give greater daytime freedom. Other important considerations in determining the appropriateness of home PN or EN are that the patient's prognosis is longer than several months and that the therapy benefits quality of life.

Disease-Specific Nutritional Support SNS is basically a support therapy and is primary therapy only for the treatment or prevention of malnutrition. Certain conditions require modification of nutritional support because of organ or system impairment. For instance, in nitrogen accumulation disorders, protein intake may need to be reduced. However, in renal disease, except for brief periods of several days, protein intakes should approach requirement levels of at least 0.8 g/kg or higher up to 1.2 g/kg as long as the blood urea nitrogen does not exceed 100 mg/dL. If this is not possible, then dialysis or hemofiltration should be considered to allow better feeding. In hepatic failure, intakes of 1.2–1.4 g/kg up to the optimal 1.5 g/kg should be attempted, as long as encephalopathy due to protein intolerance is not encountered. In the presence of protein intolerance, formulas containing 33–50% branched-chain amino

TABLE 54-2

SUMMARY OF OUTCOMES FOR PATIENTS ON HOME PARENTERAL AND ENTERAL NUTRITION (HPEN)

DIAGNOSIS	NUMBER IN GROUP	AGE IN YEARS	% SURVIVAL[a] ON THERAPY	THERAPY STATUS, % AT 1 YEAR[b] FULL ORAL NUTRITION	CONTINUED ON HPEN RX	DIED	REHABILITATION[c] STATUS, % IN 1ST YEAR C	P	M	COMPLICATIONS[d] PER PATIENT-YEAR HPEN	NONHPEN
Home Parenteral Nutrition											
Crohn's disease	562	36	96	70	25	2	60	38	2	0.9	1.1
Ischemic bowel disease	331	49	87	27	48	19	53	41	6	1.4	1.1
Motility disorder	299	45	87	31	44	21	49	39	12	1.3	1.1
Congenital bowel defect	172	5	94	42	47	9	63	27	11	2.1	1.0
Hyperemesis gravidarum	112	28	100	100	0	0	83	16	1	1.5	3.5
Chronic pancreatitis	156	42	90	82	10	5	60	38	2	1.2	2.5
Radiation enteritis	145	58	87	28	49	22	42	49	9	0.8	1.1
Chronic adhesive obstructions	120	53	83	47	34	13	23	68	10	1.7	1.4
Cystic fibrosis	51	17	50	38	13	36	24	66	16	0.8	3.7
Cancer	2122	44	20	26	8	63	29	57	14	1.1	3.3
AIDS	280	33	10	13	6	73	8	63	29	1.6	3.3
Home Enteral Nutrition											
Neurologic disorders of swallowing	1134	65	55	19	25	48	5	24	71	0.3	0.9
Cancer	1644	61	30	30	6	59	21	59	21	0.4	2.7

[a]Survival rates on therapy are values at 1 year, calculated by the life table method. This will differ from the percentage listed as died under Therapy Status, since all patients with known end points are considered in this latter measure. The ratio of observed versus expected deaths is equivalent to a Standard Mortality Ratio.
[b]Not shown are those patients who were back in hospital or who had changed therapy type by 12 months.
[c]Rehabilitation is designated complete (C), partial (P), or minimal (M), relative to the patient's ability to sustain normal age-related activity.
[d]Complications refer only to those complications that resulted in rehospitalization.
Source: Derived from North American HPEN Registry.
Table taken from previous chapter by Lyn Howard, MD.

acids are available at the 1.2–1.4-g/kg level. Cardiac patients, and many severely stressed patients, often benefit from fluid and sodium restriction to levels of 1000 mL of total parenteral nutrition (TPN) formula and 5–20 meq of sodium per day. In patients with severe chronic PCM characterized by severe weight loss and tissue wasting, TPN must be instituted gradually because of the profound antinatriuresis, antidiuresis, and intracellular accumulation of potassium, magnesium, and phosphorus. This is usually accomplished by limiting fluid intakes initially to about 1000 mL containing modest carbohydrate content of 10–20% dextrose, low sodium, and ample potassium, magnesium, and phosphorus, with careful assessment of fluid and electrolyte status. Protein need not be restricted.

THE DESIGN OF INDIVIDUAL REGIMENS

FLUID REQUIREMENTS

The normal daily requirement for fluid is 30 mL/kg of body weight from all sources (IV infusions, per tube, or oral intake), plus any replacement of abnormal losses such as an osmotic diuresis, nasogastric drainage, wound output, or diarrheal/ostomy losses. Electrolyte and mineral losses can be estimated or measured and also need to be replaced (Table 54-3). Fluid restriction may be necessary in patients with fluid overload, and fluid inputs can be limited to 1200 mL/d if urine is the only significant fluid output. When severe fluid overload occurs, the optimal PN solution for central venous administration is a concentrated 1-L solution of 7% crystalline amino acids (70 g) and 21% dextrose (210 g), which provides an amount of nitrogen and glucose that is effective at protein-sparing.

Patients requiring PN or EN in the acute care setting generally have some element of associated hormonal adaptations (e.g., increased secretion of antidiuretic hormone, aldosterone, insulin, glucagon, or cortisol) that cause fluid retention and hyperglycemia. Weight gain in the critically ill, whether receiving SNS or not, is invariably the consequence of fluid retention, since lean tissue accretion is minimal in the acute phase of illness. Because excess fluid removal can be difficult, limiting fluid intake to allow for balanced intake and output is more effective.

ENERGY REQUIREMENTS

Total energy expenditure comprises resting energy expenditure (two-thirds) plus activity energy expenditure (one-third) (Chap. 72). Resting energy expenditure includes the calories necessary for basal metabolism at bed rest. Activity energy expenditure represents one-fourth to one-third of the total, and the thermal effect of feeding is about 10% of the total energy expenditure. For normally nourished healthy individuals, the total energy expenditure is about 30–35 kcal/kg. Although critical illness increases resting energy expenditure, only in initially well-nourished individuals with the highest systemic inflammatory response, such as that from severe multiple trauma, burns, closed head injury, or sepsis, do total energy expenditures reach 40–45 kcal/kg. The chronically ill patient with lean tissue loss has reduced basal energy expenditure, and inactivity which results in a total energy expenditure of about 20–25 kcal/kg. About 95% of such patients need <30 kcal/kg to achieve energy balance. Because providing about 50% of measured energy expenditure as SNS is at least equally efficacious for the first 10 days of critical illness, actual measurement of energy expenditure is not generally necessary in the early period of SNS. However, in patients who remain critically ill beyond several weeks, in the severely malnourished for whom estimates of energy expenditure are unreliable, or in those who are difficult to wean from ventilators, it is reasonable to actually measure energy expenditure and to aim for energy balance with SNS.

TABLE 54-3

ENTERIC FLUID VOLUMES AND THEIR ELECTROLYTE CONTENT[a]						
	L/d	Na	K	Cl	HCO$_3$	H
Oral intake	2–3					
Enteric secretions						
Saliva	1–2	15	30	15	50	—
Gastric juice	1.5–2	50–70	5–15	90–120	0	70–100
Bile	0.5–1.5	120–150	5–15	80–120	30–50	—
Pancreatic	0.5–1	100–140	10	70–100	60–110	—
Small intestine	1–2	80–140	10–20	80–120	20–40	—

[a]All in mEq/L.
Source: Adapted from previous chapter by Lyn Howard, MD, in *Harrison's Principles of Internal Medicine.*

Insulin resistance is associated with increased gluconeogenesis and reduced glucose utilization, predisposing a patient to hyperglycemia. This is aggravated in patients receiving exogenous carbohydrate from SNS. Normalization of blood glucose levels by insulin infusion in critically ill patients receiving SNS reduces morbidity and mortality. In mild or moderately malnourished patients, a reasonable goal is to provide metabolic support to improve protein synthesis and maintain metabolic homeostasis. Hypocaloric nutrition providing only about 1000 kcal/d and 70 g protein for up to 10 days requires less fluid and reduces the likelihood of poor glycemic control. Energy content can be advanced to 20–25 kcal/kg with 1.5 g protein/kg as conditions permit and definitely during the second week of SNS. Patients with multiple trauma, closed head injury, and severe burns often have much higher energy expenditures, but there is little evidence that providing more than 30 kcal/kg has additional benefit, and it risks hyperglycemia.

Generally, because glucose is an essential tissue fuel, glucose and amino acids are provided parenterally until the level of resting energy expenditure is reached. At this point, adding fat becomes beneficial, since more parenteral glucose stimulates de novo lipogenesis by the liver—an energy-inefficient process. Polyunsaturated long-chain triglycerides are the chief ingredient in most parenteral fat emulsions and the majority of the fat in enteral feeding formulas. These vegetable oil–based emulsions provide essential fatty acids. Enteral feeding formulas have fat content that ranges from 3% of calories up to as much as 50% of calories, while parenteral fat comes in separate containers as 10, 20, and 30% emulsions that can be infused separately or mixed by the pharmacy under controlled conditions as all-in-one or total nutrient admixture with glucose, amino acids, lipid, electrolytes, vitamins, and minerals. Although parenteral fat is required at only about 3% of energy requirements to meet essential fatty acid requirements, when provided as an all-in-one mixture of carbohydrate, fat, and protein, 2–3% fat in the TPN mixtures, representing about 20–30% of calories as fat, is provided to ensure emulsion stability. If given separately, parenteral fat should not be provided at rates exceeding 0.11 g/kg body weight per h or about 100 g over 12 h—equivalent to 1 L of 10% parenteral fat and 500 mL of 20% parenteral fat.

Medium-chain triglycerides, which contain saturated fatty acids with chain lengths of 6, 8, 10, or 12 carbons, are provided in a number of enteral feeding formulas because they are absorbed preferentially. Fish oil contains polyunsaturated fatty acids of the omega 3 family, which have been shown to improve immune function and reduce the inflammatory response. Parenteral emulsions containing medium-chain triglycerides, olive oil, and fish oil are available in Europe and Japan but not yet in the United States.

Carbohydrates are provided as hydrous glucose providing 3.4 kcal/g in PN formulas. In enteral formulas, glucose is the carbohydrate source in so-called monomeric diets. These diets provide protein as amino acids and fat in minimal amounts (3%) to meet essential fatty acid requirements. Monomeric formulas are designed to optimize absorption in the seriously compromised gut. These formulas, like the immune-enhancing diets, are quite expensive. In polymeric diets, the carbohydrate source is usually an osmotically less active polysaccharide, protein is usually soy or casein protein, and fat is present in amounts from 25 to 50%. Such formulas are usually well tolerated by patients with normal intestinal length, and some are acceptable for oral consumption.

PROTEIN OR AMINO ACID REQUIREMENTS

Although the recommended dietary allowance for protein is 0.8 g/kg per d, maximal rates of repletion occur with 1.5 g/kg in the malnourished. In the severely catabolic patient, this higher level minimizes protein loss. In patients requiring SNS in the acute care setting, at least 1 g/kg is recommended, with greater amounts up to 1.5 g/kg as volume, renal, and hepatic tolerances allow. The standard parenteral and enteral formulas contain protein of high biologic value and meet the requirements for the eight essential amino acids. In protein-intolerant conditions such as renal and hepatic failure, modified amino acid formulas should be considered. In hepatic failure, higher branched-chain amino acid–enriched formulas appear to improve outcomes. Conditionally essential amino acids like arginine and glutamine may also have some benefit in supplemental amounts.

Protein (nitrogen) balance provides a measure of feeding efficacy of PN or EN. It is calculated as protein intake/6.25 because proteins are on average 16% nitrogen (N), minus the 24-h urine urea N (UUN) plus 4 g N, which reflects other N losses. In the critically ill, a mild negative balance of 2–4 g N/d is usually achievable with a similarly mild positive balance in the recuperating patient. Each g N represents approximately 30 g lean tissue.

MINERAL AND VITAMIN REQUIREMENTS

Parenteral electrolyte, vitamin, and trace mineral requirements are summarized in **Tables 54-4** to **54-6**. Electrolyte modifications are necessary with substantial gastrointestinal losses from nasogastric drainage or intestinal losses from fistulas, diarrhea or ostomy outputs. Such losses also imply extra calcium, magnesium, and zinc losses. Excessive urine or potassium losses with amphotericin, or magnesium losses with cisplatin or in renal failure, necessitate adjustments in sodium, potassium, magnesium, phosphorus, and acid-base balance. Vitamin and trace element requirements are met by the daily provision of a complete parenteral vitamin supple-

TABLE 54-4

USUAL DAILY ELECTROLYTE ADDITIONS TO PARENTERAL NUTRITION

ELECTROLYTE	PARENTERAL EQUIVALENT OF RDA	USUAL INTAKE
Sodium		1–2 meq/kg + replacement, but can be as low as 5–40 meq/d
Potassium		40–100 meq/d + replacement of unusual losses
Chloride		As needed for acid-base balance, but usually 2:1 to 1:1 with acetate
Acetate		As needed for acid-base balance
Calcium	10 meq	10–20 meq/d
Magnesium	10 meq	8–16 meq/d
Phosphorus	30 mmol	20–40 mmol

ment and trace elements for PN, and with the provision of adequate amounts of enteral feeding formulas that contain these micronutrients.

PARENTERAL NUTRITION

INFUSION TECHNIQUE AND PATIENT MONITORING

Parenteral feeding through a peripheral vein is limited by osmolality and volume constraints. Solutions that contain more than 3% amino acids and 5% glucose (290 kcal/L) are poorly tolerated peripherally. Parenteral fat (20%) can be given to increase the calories delivered. The total

TABLE 54-5

PARENTERAL MULTIVITAMIN REQUIREMENTS FOR ADULTS

VITAMIN	RECENTLY REVISED VALUE
Vitamin A	3300 IU
Thiamin (B_1)	6 mg
Riboflavin (B_2)	3.6 mg
Niacin (B_3)	40 mg
Folic acid	600 µg
Pantothenic acid	15 mg
Pyridoxine (B_6)	6 mg
Cyanocobalamin (B_{12})	5 µg
Biotin	60 µg
Ascorbic acid (C)	200 mg
Vitamin D	200 IU
Vitamin E	10 IU
Vitamin K[a]	150 µg

[a]A product is available that does not contain vitamin K. Vitamin K supplementation is recommended at 2–4 mg/week in patients not receiving oral anticoagulation therapy if using this product.

TABLE 54-6

PARENTERAL TRACE METAL SUPPLEMENTATION FOR ADULTS[a]

TRACE MINERAL	INTAKE
Zinc	2.5–4 mg/d, an additional 10–15 mg/d per L of stool or ileostomy output
Copper	0.5–1.5 mg/d, possibility of retention in biliary tract obstruction
Manganese	0.1–0.3 mg/d, possibility of retention in biliary tract obstruction
Chromium	10–15 µg/d
Selenium	20–100 µg/d, necessary for long-term PN, optional for short-term TPN
Molybdenum	20–120 µg/d, necessary for long-term PN, optional for short-term PN
Iodine	75–150 µg/d, necessary for long-term PN, optional for short-term PN

[a]Commercial products are available that have the first four, first five, and all seven of these metals in recommended amounts.
Note: PN, parenteral nutrition; TPN, total parenteral nutrition.

volume required to provide a marginal protein intake of 60 g and 1680 total kcal is 2.5 L. However, the risk of significant morbidity and mortality from incompatibilities of calcium and phosphate salts is greatest in these low-osmolality, low-glucose regimens. Parenteral feeding via a peripheral vein is generally intended as a supplement to oral feeding and is not optimal for the critically ill. Peripheral parenteral nutrition may benefit from small amounts of heparin at 1000 U/L and co-infusion with parenteral fat to reduce osmolality, but volume constraints still limit the value of this therapy. Peripherally inserted central catheters (PICCs) can be used for the short term to provide concentrated glucose parenteral solutions of 20–25% dextrose and 4–7% amino acids, while avoiding some of the complications of catheter placement via a large central vein. With PICC lines, however, flow can be position-related, and the lines cannot be exchanged over a wire for infection monitoring. For these reasons, in the critically ill, centrally placed catheters are preferred. The subclavian approach is best tolerated by the patient and is the easiest to dress. The jugular approach is less likely to lead to a pneumothorax. The femoral approach is discouraged because of the greater risk of catheter infection. For long-term feeding in the home, tunneled catheters and implanted ports reduce infection risk and are more acceptable to patients. However, tunneled catheters require placement in the operating room.

Catheters are made of silastic, polyurethane, or polyvinyl chloride. Silastic catheters are less thrombogenic

TABLE 54-7

MONITORING THE PATIENT ON PARENTERAL NUTRITION

Clinical Data Monitored Daily

General sense of well-being

Strength as evidenced in getting out of bed, walking, resistance exercise as appropriate

Vital signs including temperature, blood pressure, pulse, and respiratory rate

Fluid balance: weight at least several times weekly, fluid intake (parenteral and enteral) vs fluid output (urine, stool, gastric drainage, wound, ostomy)

Parenteral nutrition delivery equipment: tubing, pump, filter, catheter, dressing

Nutrient solution composition

Laboratory Daily

Finger-stick glucose	Three times daily until stable
Blood glucose, Na, K, Cl, HCO$_3$, BUN	Daily until stable and fully advanced, then twice weekly
Serum creatinine, albumin, PO$_4$, Ca, Mg, Hb/Hct, WBC	Baseline, then twice weekly
INR	Baseline, then weekly
Micronutrient tests	As indicated

Note: Hb, hemoglobin; Hct, hematocrit; INR, international normalized ratio; WBC, white blood cell count.
Source: Adapted from chapter by Lyn Howard, MD, in HPIM, 16e.

and are best for tunneled catheters. Polyurethane is best for temporary catheters. Dressing changes with dry gauze at regular intervals should be performed by nurses skilled in catheter care to avoid infection. Chlorhexidine solution is more effective than alcohol or iodine compounds. Appropriate monitoring for patients receiving PN is summarized in Table 54-7.

COMPLICATIONS

Mechanical

The insertion of a central venous catheter should be performed by trained and experienced personnel using aseptic techniques to limit the major common complications of pneumothorax and inadvertent arterial puncture or injury. Catheter position should be radiographically confirmed to be in the superior vena cava distal to the junction with the jugular or subclavian vein and not directly against the vessel wall. Thrombosis related to the catheter may occur at the site of entry into the vein and extend to encase the catheter. Catheter infection predisposes to thrombosis, as does the systemic inflammatory response. The addition of 6000 U of heparin in the daily parenteral formula in hospitalized patients with temporary catheters reduces the risk of fibrin sheath formation and catheter infection. Temporary catheters that develop a thrombus should be removed and, based on clinical

findings, treated with anticoagulants. Thrombolytic therapy can be considered for patients with permanent catheters depending on the ease of replacement and presence of alternate, reasonably acceptable venous access sites. Low-dose warfarin therapy of 1 mg/d reduces the risk of thrombosis in permanent catheters used for home PN, but full anticoagulation may be required in patients who have recurrent thrombosis related to permanent catheters. A recent U.S. Food and Drug Administration mandate to reformulate parenteral multivitamins to include vitamin K at a dose of 150 μg daily may affect the efficacy of low-dose warfarin therapy. There is a "no vitamin K" version available for patients receiving this therapy. Catheters can become mechanically occluded and may also become occluded by fibrin at the tip, or by fat, minerals, or drugs intraluminally. These occlusions can be managed with low-dose alteplase for fibrin, with indwelling 70% alcohol for fat, with 0.1 N hydrochloric acid for mineral precipitates, and with either 0.1 N hydrochloric acid or 0.1 N sodium hydroxide for drugs, depending on their pH.

Metabolic

The most common problems related to PN are fluid overload and hyperglycemia (Table 54-8). Hypertonic dextrose stimulates a much higher insulin level than meal feeding. Because insulin is a potent antinatriuretic and antidiuretic hormone, hyperinsulinemia leads to sodium and fluid retention. In the absence of gastrointestinal losses or renal dysfunction, net fluid retention is likely when total fluid intake exceeds 2000 mL/d. Close monitoring of body weight, as well as fluid intake and output, is necessary to prevent this complication. In the absence of significant renal impairment, the sodium content of the urine is likely to be <10 meq/L. Providing sodium in limited amounts of 40 meq/d and the use of both glucose and fat in the PN mixture to lower total glucose and sodium will help reduce fluid retention. The elevated insulin also increases the intracellular transport of potassium, magnesium, and phosphorus, which can precipitate a dangerous refeeding syndrome if the total glucose content of the PN solution is advanced too quickly in severely malnourished patients. It is generally best to start PN with <200 g glucose/d to assess glucose tolerance. Regular insulin can be added to the PN formula to establish glycemic control, and the insulin doses can be increased proportionately as the glucose is advanced. As a general rule, patients with insulin-dependent diabetes require about twice their usual home insulin doses when they are receiving TPN at 20–25 kcal/kg, largely as a consequence of parenteral glucose administration and some loss of insulin to the TPN container. As a rough estimate, the amount of insulin can be provided in a similar proportion to the amount of calories provided as TPN relative to full

TABLE 54-8

595

SELECTED METABOLIC DISTURBANCES AND THEIR CORRECTION

DISTURBANCE	CAUSE	CORRECTIVE ACTION WITH PN
Hyponatremia	Increased total body water or decreased total body sodium	Decrease free water or increase sodium
Hypernatremia	Occurs commonly with excessive isotonic or hypertonic fluid followed by diuretic administration with free water clearance; can also occur with dehydration and normal total body sodium	Increase free water to produce net positive fluid balance maintaining sodium and chloride balance
Hypokalemia	Inadequate intake relative to need	Use supplements
	Excessive diuresis, tubular dysfunction	Use supplements
	Magnesium deficiency	Increase PN magnesium
	Metabolic alkalosis	Correct alkalosis
	Hyperinsulinemia	Maintain constant PN, increase potassium
Hyperkalemia	Excessive provision	Reduce supplements
	Metabolic acidosis	Evaluate alkalosis, treat with PN acetate salt and decrease potassium
	Renal deterioration	Evaluate patient and adjust PN as indicated
Hypocalcemia	Reciprocal response to phosphorus repletion	Increase calcium
	Critical illness effect	Increase calcium
	Severe malabsorption	Supplement calcium
Hypercalcemia	Excessive administration or pathologic (cancer, hyperparathyroidism)	Reduce or eliminate calcium
Hypomagnesemia	Increased requirements due to diuretic use, alcoholism, malabsorption, malnutrition	Supplement magnesium
	Critical illness	Supplement magnesium
Hypophosphatemia	Inadequate intake relative to needs related to malnutrition, alcohol use	Supplement phosphorus
	Increased calcium intake	Use supplements
Hyperphosphatemia	Excessive administration or worsening renal function	Reduce phosphorus
Azotemia	Excessive amino acid infusion or worsening renal function	Reduce amino acid level but consider renal replacement therapy if cannot provide 1 g protein per kg for prolonged periods

Note: PN, parenteral nutrition.

feeding, and the insulin can be placed in the TPN formula. Subcutaneous regular insulin can be provided to improve glucose control as assessed by measurements of blood glucose every 6 h. About two-thirds of the total 24-h amount can be added to the next day's order, with subcutaneous insulin supplements as needed. Advances in TPN concentration should be made when reasonable glucose control is established, and the insulin dose adjusted proportionately to the calories added as glucose and amino acids. These are general rules, and they are conservative. Given the adverse clinical impact of hyperglycemia, it may be necessary to use continuous insulin therapy as a separate infusion with a standard protocol to initially establish control. Once established, this insulin dose can be added to the PN formula. Acid-base imbalance is also common during PN therapy. Amino acid formulas are buffered, but critically ill patients are prone to metabolic acidosis, often due to renal tubular impairment. The use of sodium and potassium acetate salts in the PN formula may address this problem. Bicarbonate salts should not be used because they are incompatible with TPN formulations. Nasogastric drainage produces a hypochloremic alkalosis

that can be managed by attention to chloride balance. Occasionally, hydrochloric acid may be required for a more rapid response or when diuretic therapy limits the ability to provide substantial sodium chloride. Up to 100 meq/L and up to 150 meq of hydrochloric acid per day may be placed in a fat-free PN formula.

Infectious

Infections of the central access catheter rarely occur in the first 72 h. Fever during this period is usually from infection elsewhere or another cause. Fever that develops during PN can be addressed by checking the catheter site and, if the site looks clean, exchanging the catheter over a wire with cultures taken through the catheter and at the catheter tip. If these cultures are negative, as they are most of the time, the new catheter can continue to be used. If a culture is positive for a relatively nonpathogenic bacteria like *Staphylococcus epidermidis*, consider a second exchange over a wire with repeat cultures or replace the catheter depending on the clinical circumstances. If cultures are positive for more pathogenic bacteria, or for fungi like *Candida albicans*, it is generally best to replace the catheter at a new site. Whether antibiotic treatment is required is a clinical decision, but *C. albicans* grown from the blood culture in a patient receiving PN should always be treated because the consequences of failure to treat can be dire.

Catheter infections can be minimized by dedicating the feeding catheter to PN, without blood sampling or medication administration. Central catheter infections are a serious complication with an attributed mortality of 12–25%. Infections in central venous catheters dedicated to feeding should occur less frequently than 3 per 1000 catheter-days. Home PN catheters that become infected may be treated through the catheter without removal of the catheter, particularly if the offending organism is *S. epidermidis*. Clearing of the biofilm and fibrin sheath by local treatment of the catheter with indwelling alteplase may increase the likelihood of eradication. Antibiotic lock therapy with high concentrations of antibiotic, with or without heparin in addition to systemic therapy, may improve efficacy. Sepsis with hypotension should precipitate catheter removal in either the temporary or permanent PN setting.

ENTERAL NUTRITION

TUBE PLACEMENT AND PATIENT MONITORING

The types of enteral feeding tubes, methods of insertion, their clinical uses, and potential complications are outlined in **Table 54-9**. The different types of enteral formulas are listed in **Table 54-10**. Patients receiving EN are at risk for many of the same metabolic complications

TABLE 54-9

ENTERAL FEEDING TUBES		
TYPE/INSERTION TECHNIQUE	**CLINICAL USES**	**POTENTIAL COMPLICATIONS**
Nasogastric Tube		
External measurement: nostril, ear, xiphisternum; tube stiffened by ice water or stylet; position verified by injecting air and auscultating, or by x-ray	Short-term clinical situation (weeks) or longer periods with intermittent insertion; bolus feeding simpler, but continuous drip with pump better tolerated	Aspiration; ulceration of nasal and esophageal tissues, leading to stricture
Nasoduodenal Tube		
External measurement: nostril, ear, anterior superior iliac spine; tube stiffened by stylet and passed through pylorus under fluoroscopy or with endoscopic loop	Short-term clinical situations where gastric emptying impaired or proximal leak suspected; requires continuous drip with pump	Spontaneous pulling back into stomach (position verified by aspirating content, pH > 6); diarrhea common, fiber-containing formulas may help
Gastrostomy Tube		
Percutaneous placement endoscopically, radiologically, or surgically; after tract established, can be converted to a gastric "button"	Long-term clinical situations, swallowing disorders, or impaired small-bowel absorption requiring continuous drip	Aspiration; irritation around tube exit site; peritoneal leak; balloon migration and obstruction of pylorus
Jejunostomy Tube		
Percutaneous placement endoscopically or radiologically via pylorus or endoscopically or surgically directly into the jejunum	Long-term clinical situations where gastric emptying impaired; requires continuous drip with pump; direct endoscopic placement (PEJ) is the most comfortable for patient	Clogging or displacement of tube; jejunal fistula if large-bore tube used; diarrhea from dumping; irritation of surgical anchoring suture
Combined Gastrojejunostomy Tube		
Percutaneous placement endoscopically, radiologically, or surgically; intragastric arm for continuous or intermittent gastric suction; jejunal arm for enteral feeding	Used for patients with impaired gastric emptying and at high risk for aspiration or patients with acute pancreatitis or proximal leaks	Clogging: especially of small bore jejunal tube

Note: All small tubes are at risk for clogging, especially if used for crushed medications. In long-term enteral patients, gastrostomy and jejunostomy tubes can be exchanged for a low-profile "button" once the tract is established.
Source: Adapted from chapter in *Harrison's Principles of Internal Medicine,* 16e, by Lyn Howard, MD.

as those who receive PN and should be monitored in the same manner. EN can be a source of similar problems, but not to the same degree, because the insulin response to EN is about half of that seen with PN. Enteral feeding formulas have fixed electrolyte compositions that are generally modest in sodium and somewhat higher in potassium content. Acid-base disturbances can be addressed to a more limited extent with EN. Acetate salts can be added to the formula to treat chronic metabolic acidosis. Calcium chloride can be added to treat mild chronic metabolic alkalosis. Medications and other additives to enteral feeding formulas can clog the tubes (e.g., calcium chloride may interact with casein-based formulas to produce insoluble calcium caseinate products) and may reduce the efficacy of some drugs (e.g., phenytoin). Since small-bore tubes are easily displaced, tube position should be checked at intervals by aspirating and measuring the pH of the gut fluid (<4 in the stomach, >6 in the jejunum).

COMPLICATIONS

Aspiration

The debilitated patient with poor gastric emptying and impairment of swallowing and cough is at risk for aspiration; this is particularly true for those who are mechanically ventilated. Tracheal suctioning induces coughing and gastric regurgitation, and cuffs on endotracheal or tracheostomy tubes seldom protect against aspiration. Preventive measures include elevating the head of the bed to 30 degrees, using nurse-directed algorithms for formula advancement, combining enteral with parenteral feeding, and using post–ligament of Treitz feeding. Tube feeding should not be discontinued for gastric residuals of <300 mL unless there are other signs of gastrointestinal intolerance such as nausea, vomiting, or abdominal distention. Continuous feeding using pumps is better tolerated intragastrically and is essential for feeding into the jejunum. For small-bowel feeding, residuals are not assessed but abdominal pain and distention should be monitored.

Diarrhea

Enteral feeding often leads to diarrhea, especially if bowel function is compromised by disease or drugs, particularly broad-spectrum antibiotics. Diarrhea may be controlled by the use of a continuous drip, with a fiber-containing formula, or by adding an antidiarrheal agent to the formula. However, *Clostridium difficile*,

TABLE 54-10

ENTERAL FORMULAS

COMPOSITION CHARACTERISTICS	CLINICAL INDICATIONS
Standard Enteral Formula	

1. Complete dietary products (+)
   a. Caloric density 1 kcal/mL
   b. Protein ~14% cals, caseinates, soy, lactalbumin
   c. CHO ~60% cals, hydrolyzed corn starch, maltodextrin, sucrose
   d. Fat ~30% cals, corn, soy, safflower oils
   e. Recommended daily intake of all minerals and vitamins in >1500 kcal/d
   f. Osmolality (mosmol/kg): ~300
	Suitable for most patients requiring tube feeding; some can be used orally

Modified Enteral Formulas	

1. Caloric density 1.5–2 kcal/mL (+)
 2. a. High protein ~20–25% protein (+)
   b. Hydrolyzed protein to small peptides (+)
   c. ↑ Arginine, glutamine, nucleotides, ω3 fat (+++)
   d. ↑ Branched-chain amino acids, ↓ aromatic amino acids (+++)
   e. Low protein of high biologic value
 3. a. Low fat, partial MCT substitution (+)
   b. ↑ Fat >40% cals (++)
 	
   c. ↑ Fat from MUFA (++)
   d. ↑ Fat from ω3 and ↓ ω6 linoleic acid (+++)
 4. Fiber provided as soy polysaccharide (+)
	Fluid-restricted patients
	 Critically ill patients
	 Impaired absorption
	 Immune-enhancing diets
	 Liver failure patients intolerant of 0.8 g/kg protein
	 Renal failure patient for brief periods if critically ill
	 Fat malabsorption
	 Pulmonary failure with CO_2 retention on standard formula, limited utility
	 Improvement in glycemic index control in diabetes
	 Improved ventilation in ARDS
	 Improved laxation

Cost: + inexpensive; ++ moderately expensive; +++ very expensive.
Note: ARDS, acute respiratory distress syndrome; CHO, carbohydrate; MCT, medium-chain triglyceride; MUFA, monounsaturated fatty acids; ω3 or ω6, polyunsaturated fat with first double bond at carbon 3 (fish oils) or carbon 6 (vegetable oils).
Source: Adapted from chapter in *Harrison's Principles of Internal Medicine,* 16e, by Lyn Howard, MD.

which is a common cause of diarrhea in patients being tube fed, should be ruled out before using antidiarrheal agents. H2 blockers may also assist in reducing the net fluid presented to the colon. Diarrhea associated with enteral feeding does not necessarily imply inadequate absorption of nutrients other than water and electrolytes. Amino acids and glucose are particularly well absorbed in the upper small bowel except in the most diseased or shortest bowel. Since luminal nutrients exert trophic effects on the gut mucosa, it is often appropriate to persist with tube feeding, despite the diarrhea, even when this necessitates supplemental parenteral fluid support.

ACKNOWLEDGMENT

The authors acknowledge the contributions of Lyn Howard, MD, the author in earlier editions of Harrison's Principles of Internal Medicine, to material in this chapter.

FURTHER READINGS

AUGUST D et al: Evidence-based approach to optimal management of HPEN access. J Parenter Enteral Nutr 30:S5, 2006

BISTRIAN B, MCCOWEN K: Nutritional support in the adult intensive care unit: Key controversies. Crit Care Med 34:1525, 2006

CENTERS FOR DISEASE CONTROL AND PREVENTION: Reduction in central line–associated bloodstream infections among patients in intensive care units—Pennsylvania, April 2001–March 2005. MMWR 54:1013, 2005

CHEN Y, PETERSON SJ: Enteral nutrition formulas: Which formula is right for your adult patient? Nutr Clin Pract 24:344, 2009

DEBAVEYE Y, VAN DEN BERGHE G: Risks and benefits of nutritional support during critical illness. Annu Rev Nutr 26:513, 2006

KORETZ RL: Enteral nutrition: a hard look at some soft evidence. Nutr Clin Pract 24:316, 2009

——— et al: Does enteral nutrition affect clinical outcome? A systematic review of the randomized trials. Am J Gastroenterol 102:412, 2007

MILNE A et al: Meta-analysis: Protein and energy supplementation in older people. Ann Intern Med 144:37, 2006

——— et al: Protein and energy supplementation in elderly people at risk from malnutrition. Cochrane Database Syst Rev Apri 15;(2):CD003288, 2009

PLANK LD, HILL GL: Energy balance in critical illness. Proc Nutr Soc 62:545, 2003

SIMPSON F, DOIG GS: Parenteral vs. enteral nutrition in the critically ill patient: A meta-analysis of trials using the intention to treat principle. Intensive Care Med 31:12, 2005

VAN DEN BERGHE G et al: Intensive insulin therapy in the critically ill patients. N Engl J Med 345:1359, 2001

SECTION X

Nutrition

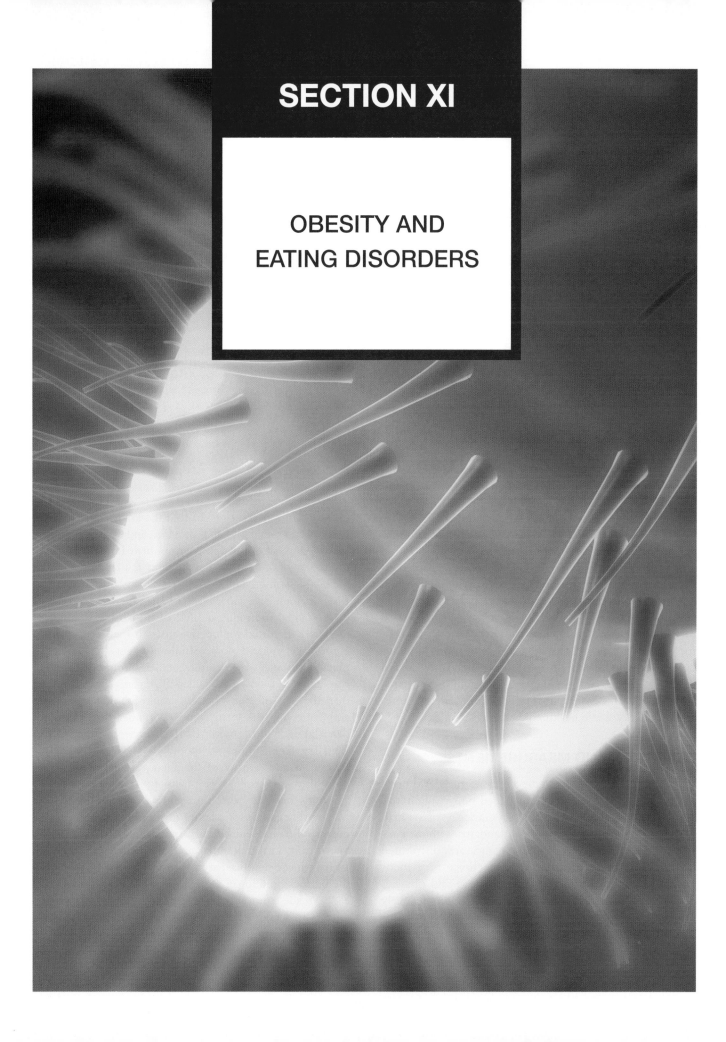

SECTION XI

OBESITY AND EATING DISORDERS

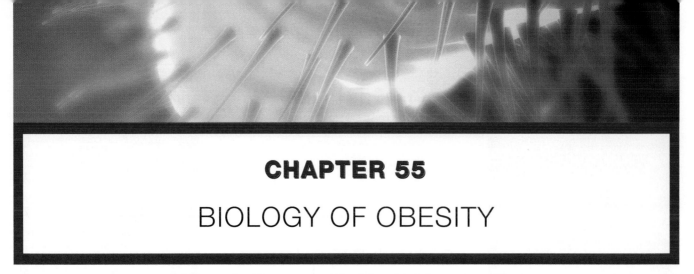

CHAPTER 55

BIOLOGY OF OBESITY

Jeffrey S. Flier ■ Eleftheria Maratos-Flier

In a world where food supplies are intermittent, the ability to store energy in excess of what is required for immediate use is essential for survival. Fat cells, residing within widely distributed adipose tissue depots, are adapted to store excess energy efficiently as triglyceride and, when needed, to release stored energy as free fatty acids for use at other sites. This physiologic system, orchestrated through endocrine and neural pathways, permits humans to survive starvation for as long as several months. However, in the presence of nutritional abundance and a sedentary lifestyle, and influenced importantly by genetic endowment, this system increases adipose energy stores and produces adverse health consequences.

DEFINITION AND MEASUREMENT

Obesity is a state of excess adipose tissue mass. Although often viewed as equivalent to increased body weight, this need not be the case—lean but very muscular individuals may be overweight by numerical standards without having increased adiposity. Body weights are distributed continuously in populations, so that choice of a medically meaningful distinction between lean and obese is somewhat arbitrary. Obesity is therefore more effectively defined by assessing its linkage to morbidity or mortality.

Although not a direct measure of adiposity, the most widely used method to gauge obesity is the *body mass index* (BMI), which is equal to weight/height^2 (in kg/m^2) (**Fig. 55-1**). Other approaches to quantifying obesity include anthropometry (skin-fold thickness), densitometry (underwater weighing), CT or MRI, and electrical impedance. Using data from the Metropolitan Life Tables, BMIs for the midpoint of all heights and frames among both men and women range from 19–26 kg/m^2; at a similar BMI, women have more body fat than men. Based on data of substantial morbidity, a BMI of 30 is most commonly used as a threshold for obesity in both men and women. Large-scale epidemiologic studies suggest that all-cause, metabolic, cancer, and cardiovascular morbidity begin to rise (albeit at a slow rate) when BMIs are ≥25, suggesting that the cut-off for obesity should be lowered. Most authorities use the term *overweight* (rather than obese) to describe individuals with BMIs between 25 and 30. A BMI between 25 and 30 should be viewed as medically significant and worthy of therapeutic intervention, especially in the presence of risk factors that are influenced by adiposity, such as hypertension and glucose intolerance.

The distribution of adipose tissue in different anatomic depots also has substantial implications for morbidity. Specifically, intraabdominal and abdominal subcutaneous fat have more significance than subcutaneous fat present in the buttocks and lower extremities. This distinction is most easily made clinically by determining the waist-to-hip ratio, with a ratio >0.9 in women and >1.0 in men being abnormal. Many of the most important complications of obesity, such as insulin resistance, diabetes, hypertension, hyperlipidemia, and hyperandrogenism in women, are linked more strongly to intraabdominal and/or upper

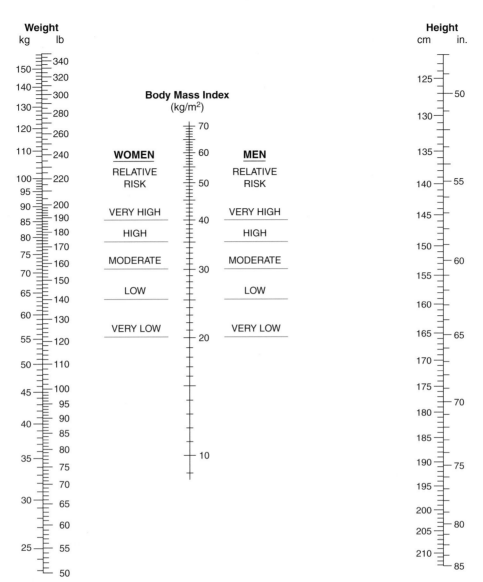

FIGURE 55-1

Nomogram for determining body mass index. To use this nomogram, place a ruler or other straight edge between the body weight (without clothes) in kilograms or pounds located on the left-hand line and the height (without shoes) in centimeters or inches located on the right-hand line. The body mass index is read from the middle of the scale and is in metric units. (*Copyright 1979, George A. Bray, M.D.; used with permission.*)

body fat than to overall adiposity (Chap. 58). The mechanism underlying this association is unknown but may relate to the fact that intraabdominal adipocytes are more lipolytically active than those from other depots. Release of free fatty acids into the portal circulation has adverse metabolic actions, especially on the liver. Whether adipokines and cytokines secreted by visceral adipocytes play an additional role in systemic complications of obesity is an area of active investigation.

PREVALENCE

Data from the National Health and Nutrition Examination Surveys (NHANES) show that the percent of the American adult population with obesity (BMI >30) has

increased from 14.5% (between 1976 and 1980) to 30.5% (between 1999 and 2000). As many as 64% of U.S. adults ≥20 years of age were overweight (defined as BMI >25) between the years of 1999 and 2000. Extreme obesity (BMI ≥40) has also increased and affects 4.7% of the population. The increasing prevalence of medically significant obesity raises great concern. Obesity is more common among women and in the poor; the prevalence in children is also rising at a worrisome rate.

PHYSIOLOGIC REGULATION OF ENERGY BALANCE

Substantial evidence suggests that body weight is regulated by both endocrine and neural components that ultimately influence the effector arms of energy intake and expenditure. This complex regulatory system is necessary because even small imbalances between energy intake and expenditure will ultimately have large effects on body weight. For example, a 0.3% positive imbalance over 30 years would result in a 9-kg (20-lb) weight gain. This exquisite regulation of energy balance cannot be monitored easily by calorie-counting in relation to physical activity. Rather, body weight regulation or dysregulation depends on a complex interplay of hormonal and neural signals. Alterations in stable weight by forced overfeeding or food deprivation induce physiologic changes that resist these perturbations: with weight loss, appetite increases and energy expenditure falls; with overfeeding, appetite falls and energy expenditure increases. This latter compensatory mechanism frequently fails, however, permitting obesity to develop when food is abundant and physical activity is limited. A major regulator of these adaptive responses is the adipocyte-derived hormone leptin, which acts through brain circuits (predominantly in the hypothalamus) to influence appetite, energy expenditure, and neuroendocrine function (see later).

Appetite is influenced by many factors that are integrated by the brain, most importantly within the hypothalamus (**Fig. 55-2**). Signals that impinge on the hypothalamic center include neural afferents, hormones, and metabolites. Vagal inputs are particularly important, bringing information from viscera, such as gut distention. Hormonal signals include leptin, insulin, cortisol, and gut peptides. Among the latter are ghrelin, which is made in the stomach and stimulates feeding, and peptide YY (PYY) and cholecystokinin, which are made in the small intestine and signal to the brain through direct action on hypothalamic control centers and/or via the vagus nerve. Metabolites, including glucose, can influence appetite, as seen by the effect of hypoglycemia to induce hunger; however, glucose is not normally a major regulator of appetite. These diverse hormonal, metabolic, and neural signals act by influencing the expression and release of various hypothalamic peptides [e.g., neuropeptide Y (NPY), Agouti-related peptide (AgRP), α-melanocyte-stimulating hormone (α-MSH), and melanin-concentrating hormone (MCH)] that are integrated with serotonergic, catecholaminergic, endocannabinoid, and opioid signaling pathways (see later). Psychological and cultural factors also play a role in the final expression of appetite. Apart from rare genetic syndromes involving leptin, its receptor, and the melanocortin system, specific defects in this complex appetite control network that influence common cases of obesity are not well defined.

Energy expenditure includes the following components: (1) resting or basal metabolic rate; (2) the energy cost of metabolizing and storing food; (3) the thermic effect of exercise; and (4) adaptive thermogenesis, which varies in response to chronic caloric intake (rising with increased intake). Basal metabolic rate accounts for ~70% of daily energy expenditure, whereas active physical activity contributes 5–10%. Thus, a significant component of daily energy consumption is fixed.

Genetic models in mice indicate that mutations in certain genes (e.g., targeted deletion of the insulin receptor in adipose tissue) protect against obesity, apparently by increasing energy expenditure. Adaptive thermogenesis occurs in *brown adipose tissue* (BAT), which plays an important role in energy metabolism in many mammals. In contrast to white adipose tissue, which is used to store energy in the form of lipids, BAT expends stored energy as heat. A mitochondrial *uncoupling protein* (UCP-1) in BAT dissipates the hydrogen ion gradient in the oxidative respiration chain and releases energy as heat. The metabolic activity of BAT is increased by a central action of leptin, acting through the sympathetic nervous system, which heavily innervates this tissue. In rodents, BAT deficiency causes obesity and diabetes; stimulation of BAT with a specific adrenergic agonist β_3 agonist) protects against diabetes and obesity. Although BAT exists in humans (especially neonates), its physiologic role is not yet established. Homologues of UCP-1 (UCP-2 and -3) may mediate uncoupled mitochondrial respiration in other tissues.

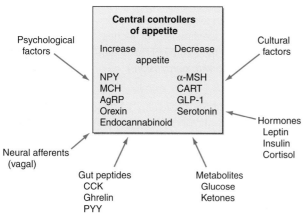

FIGURE 55-2

The factors that regulate appetite through effects on central neural circuits. Some factors that increase or decrease appetite are listed. NPY, neuropeptide Y; MCH, melanin-concentrating hormone; AgRP, Agouti-related peptide; MSH, melanocyte-stimulating hormone; CART, cocaine- and amphetamine-related transcript; GLP-1, glucagon-related peptide-1; CCK, cholecystokinin.

THE ADIPOCYTE AND ADIPOSE TISSUE

Adipose tissue is composed of the lipid-storing adipose cell and a stromal/vascular compartment in which cells including preadipocytes and macrophages reside. Adipose

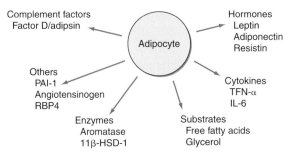

FIGURE 55-3

Factors released by the adipocyte that can affect peripheral tissues. PAI, plasminogen activator inhibitor; TNF, tumor necrosis factor; RBP4, retinal binding protein 4.

mass increases by enlargement of adipose cells through lipid deposition, as well as by an increase in the number of adipocytes. Obese adipose tissue is also characterized by increased numbers of infiltrating macrophages. The process by which adipose cells are derived from a mesenchymal preadipocyte involves an orchestrated series of differentiation steps mediated by a cascade of specific transcription factors. One of the key transcription factors is *peroxisome proliferator-activated receptor* γ (PPAR-γ), a nuclear receptor that binds the thiazolidinedione class of insulin-sensitizing drugs used in the treatment of type 2 diabetes.

Although the adipocyte has generally been regarded as a storage depot for fat, it is also an endocrine cell that releases numerous molecules in a regulated fashion (**Fig. 55-3**). These include the energy balance-regulating hormone leptin, cytokines such as tumor necrosis factor (TNF) α and interleukin (IL)-6, complement factors such as factor D (also known as *adipsin*), prothrombotic agents such as plasminogen activator inhibitor I, and a component of the blood pressure regulating system, angiotensinogen. Adiponectin, an abundant adipose-derived protein whose levels are reduced in obesity, enhances insulin sensitivity and lipid oxidation and it has vascular protective effects, whereas resistin and RBP4, whose levels are increased in obesity, may induce insulin resistance. These factors, and others not yet identified, play a role in the physiology of lipid homeostasis, insulin sensitivity, blood pressure control, coagulation, and vascular health, and are likely to contribute to obesity-related pathologies.

ETIOLOGY OF OBESITY

Though the molecular pathways regulating energy balance are beginning to be illuminated, the causes of obesity remain elusive. In part, this reflects the fact that obesity is a heterogeneous group of disorders. At one level, the pathophysiology of obesity seems simple: a chronic excess of nutrient intake relative to the level of energy expenditure. However, due to the complexity of the neuroendocrine and metabolic systems that regulate

energy intake, storage, and expenditure, it has been difficult to quantitate all the relevant parameters (e.g., food intake and energy expenditure) over time in human subjects.

Role of Genes versus Environment

Obesity is commonly seen in families, and the heritability of body weight is similar to that for height. Inheritance is usually not Mendelian, however, and it is difficult to distinguish the role of genes and environmental factors. Adoptees more closely resemble their biologic than adoptive parents with respect to obesity, providing strong support for genetic influences. Likewise, identical twins have very similar BMIs whether reared together or apart, and their BMIs are much more strongly correlated than those of dizygotic twins. These genetic effects appear to relate to both energy intake and expenditure.

Whatever the role of genes, it is clear that the environment plays a key role in obesity, as evidenced by the fact that famine prevents obesity in even the most obesity-prone individual. In addition, the recent increase in the prevalence of obesity in the United States is far too rapid to be due to changes in the gene pool. Undoubtedly, genes influence the susceptibility to obesity in response to specific diets and availability of nutrition. Cultural factors are also important—these relate to both availability and composition of the diet and to changes in the level of physical activity. In industrial societies, obesity is more common among poor women, whereas in underdeveloped countries, wealthier women are more often obese. In children, obesity correlates to some degree with time spent watching television. Although the role of diet composition in obesity continues to generate controversy, it appears that high-fat diets may promote obesity, especially when combined with diets rich in simple (as opposed to complex) carbohydrates.

Additional environmental factors may contribute to the increasing obesity prevalence. Both epidemiologic correlations and experimental data suggest that sleep deprivation leads to increased obesity. Less well supported in humans are potential changes in gut flora with capacity to alter energy balance and a possible role for obesogenic viral infections.

Specific Genetic Syndromes

For many years obesity in rodents has been known to be caused by a number of distinct mutations distributed through the genome. Most of these single-gene mutations cause both hyperphagia and diminished energy expenditure, suggesting a physiologic link between these two parameters of energy homeostasis. Identification of the *ob* gene mutation in genetically obese (ob/ob) mice represented a major breakthrough in the field. The ob/ob mouse develops severe obesity, insulin resistance, and hyperphagia, as

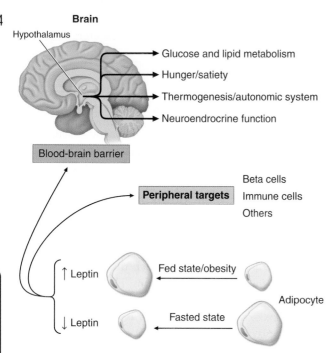

FIGURE 55-4

The physiologic system regulated by leptin. Rising or falling leptin levels act through the hypothalamus to influence appetite, energy expenditure, and neuroendocrine function and through peripheral sites to influence systems such as the immune system.

well as efficient metabolism (e.g., it gets fat even when ingesting the same number of calories as lean litter mates). The product of the *ob* gene is the peptide leptin, a name derived from the Greek root *leptos*, meaning thin. Leptin is secreted by adipose cells and acts primarily through the hypothalamus. Its level of production provides an index of adipose energy stores (**Fig. 55-4**). High leptin levels decrease food intake and increase energy expenditure. Another mouse mutant, db/db, which is resistant to leptin, has a mutation in the leptin receptor and develops a similar syndrome. The *OB* gene is present in humans and expressed in fat. Several families with morbid, early-onset obesity caused by inactivating mutations in either leptin or the leptin receptor have been described, thus demonstrating the biologic relevance of leptin in humans. The obesity in these individuals begins shortly after birth, is severe, and is accompanied by neuroendocrine abnormalities. The most prominent of these is hypogonadotropic hypogonadism, which is reversed by leptin replacement. Central hypothyroidism and growth retardation are seen in the mouse model, but their occurrence in leptin-deficient humans is less clear. To date, there is no evidence to suggest that mutations or polymorphisms in the leptin or leptin receptor genes play a prominent role in common forms of obesity.

Mutations in several other genes cause severe obesity in humans (**Table 55-1**); each of these syndromes is

TABLE 55-1

SOME OBESITY GENES IN HUMANS AND MICE

GENE	GENE PRODUCT	MECHANISM OF OBESITY	IN HUMAN	IN RODENT
Lep (ob)	Leptin, a fat-derived hormone	Mutation prevents leptin from delivering satiety signal; brain perceives starvation	Yes	Yes
LepR (db)	Leptin receptor	Same as above	Yes	Yes
POMC	Proopiomelanocortin, a precursor of several hormones and neuropeptides	Mutation prevents synthesis of melanocyte-stimulating hormone (MSH), a satiety signal	Yes	Yes
MC4R	Type 4 receptor for MSH	Mutation prevents reception of satiety signal from MSH	Yes	Yes
AgRP	Agouti-related peptide, a neuropeptide expressed in the hypothalamus	Overexpression inhibits signal through MC4R	No	Yes
PC-1	Prohormone convertase 1, a processing enzyme	Mutation prevents synthesis of neuropeptide, probably MSH	Yes	No
Fat	Carboxypeptidase E, a processing enzyme	Same as above	No	Yes
Tub	Tub, a hypothalamic protein of unknown function	Hypothalamic dysfunction	No	Yes
TrkB	TrkB, a neurotrophin receptor	Hyperphagia due to uncharacterized hypothalamic defect	Yes	Yes

rare. Mutations in the gene encoding proopiomelanocortin (POMC) cause severe obesity through failure to synthesize α-MSH, a key neuropeptide that inhibits appetite in the hypothalamus. The absence of POMC also causes secondary adrenal insufficiency due to absence of adrenocorticotropic hormone (ACTH), as well as pale skin and red hair due to absence of α-MSH. Proenzyme convertase 1 (PC-1) mutations are thought to cause obesity by preventing synthesis of α-MSH from its precursor peptide, POMC. α-MSH binds to the type 4 melanocortin receptor (MC4R), a key hypothalamic receptor that inhibits eating. Heterozygous loss-of-function mutations of this receptor account for as much as 5% of severe obesity. These five genetic defects define a pathway through which leptin (by stimulating POMC and increasing α-MSH) restricts food intake and limits weight (Fig. 55-5).

In addition to these human obesity genes, studies in rodents reveal several other molecular candidates for hypothalamic mediators of human obesity or leanness. The *tub* gene encodes a hypothalamic peptide of unknown function; mutation of this gene causes late-onset obesity. The *fat* gene encodes carboxypeptidase E, a peptide-processing enzyme; mutation of this gene is thought to cause obesity by disrupting production of one or more neuropeptides. AgRP is coexpressed with NPY in arcuate nucleus neurons. AgRP antagonizes α-MSH action at MC4 receptors, and its overexpression induces obesity. In contrast, a mouse deficient in the peptide MCH, whose administration causes feeding, is lean.

A number of complex human syndromes with defined inheritance are associated with obesity (Table 55-2). Although specific genes are undefined at present, their identification will likely enhance our understanding of more common forms of human obesity. In the Prader-Willi syndrome, obesity coexists with short stature, mental retardation, hypogonadotropic hypogonadism, hypotonia, small hands and feet, fish-shaped mouth, and hyperphagia. Most patients have a chromosome 15 deletion, and reduced expression of the signaling protein necdin may be an important cause of defective hypothalamic neural development in this disorder. Bardet-Biedl syndrome (BBS) is a genetically heterogeneous disorder characterized by obesity, mental retardation, retinitis pigmentosa, renal and cardiac malformations, polydactyly, and hypogonadotropic hypogonadism. At least eight genetic loci have been identified, and BBS may involve defects in ciliary function.

Other Specific Syndromes Associated with Obesity

Cushing's Syndrome

Although obese patients commonly have central obesity, hypertension, and glucose intolerance, they lack other specific stigmata of Cushing's syndrome. Nonetheless, a potential diagnosis of Cushing's syndrome is often entertained. Cortisol production and urinary metabolites (17OH steroids) may be increased in simple obesity. Unlike in Cushing's syndrome, however, cortisol levels in blood and urine in the basal state and in response to corticotropin-releasing hormone (CRH) or ACTH are normal; the overnight 1-mg dexamethasone suppression test is normal in 90%, with the remainder being normal on a standard 2-day low-dose dexamethasone suppression test. Obesity may be associated with excessive local reactivation of cortisol in fat by 11β-hydroxysteroid dehydrogenase 1, an enzyme that converts inactive cortisone to cortisol.

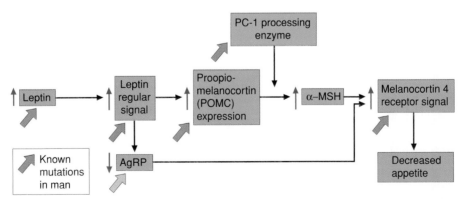

FIGURE 55-5

A central pathway through which leptin acts to regulate appetite and body weight. Leptin signals through proopiomelanocortin (POMC) neurons in the hypothalamus to induce increased production of α-melanocyte-stimulating hormone (α-MSH), requiring the processing enzyme PC-1 (proenzyme convertase 1). α-MSH acts as an agonist on melanocortin-4 receptors to inhibit appetite, and the neuropeptide AgRp (Agouti-related peptide) acts as an antagonist of this receptor. Mutations that cause obesity in humans are indicated by the solid purple arrows.

TABLE 55-2

A COMPARISON OF SYNDROMES OF OBESITY—HYPOGONADISM AND MENTAL RETARDATION

SYNDROME

FEATURE	PRADER-WILLI	LAURENCE-MOON-BIEDL	AHLSTROM	COHEN	CARPENTER
Inheritance	Sporadic; two-thirds have defect	Autosomal recessive	Autosomal recessive	Probably autosomal recessive	Autosomal recessive
Stature	Short	Normal; infrequently short	Normal; infrequently short	Short or tall	Normal
Obesity	Generalized Moderate to severe Onset 1–3 yrs	Generalized Early onset, 1–2 y	Truncal Early onset, 2–5 y	Truncal Mid-childhood, age 5	Truncal, gluteal
Craniofacies	Narrow bifrontal diameter Almond-shaped eyes Strabismus V-shaped mouth High-arched palate	Not distinctive	Not distinctive	High nasal bridge Arched palate Open mouth Short philtrum	Acrocephaly Flat nasal bridge High-arched palate
Limbs	Small hands and feet Hypotonia	Polydactyly	No abnormalities	Hypotonia Narrow hands and feet	Polydactyly Syndactyly Genu valgum
Reproductive status	1° Hypogonadism	1° Hypogonadism	Hypogonadism in males but not in females	Normal gonadal function or hypogonadotrophic hypogonadism	2° Hypogonadism
Other features	Enamel hypoplasia Hyperphagia Temper tantrums Nasal speech			Dysplastic ears Delayed puberty	
Mental retardation	Mild to moderate		Normal intelligence	Mild	Slight

606

Hypothyroidism

The possibility of hypothyroidism should be considered, but it is an uncommon cause of obesity; hypothyroidism is easily ruled out by measuring thyroid-stimulating hormone (TSH). Much of the weight gain that occurs in hypothyroidism is due to myxedema.

Insulinoma

Patients with insulinoma often gain weight as a result of overeating to avoid hypoglycemic symptoms. The increased substrate plus high insulin levels promote energy storage in fat. This can be marked in some individuals but is modest in most.

Craniopharyngioma and Other Disorders Involving the Hypothalamus

Whether through tumors, trauma, or inflammation, hypothalamic dysfunction of systems controlling satiety, hunger, and energy expenditure can cause varying degrees of obesity. It is uncommon to identify a discrete anatomic basis for these disorders. Subtle hypothalamic dysfunction is probably a more common cause of obesity than can be documented using currently available imaging techniques. Growth hormone (GH), which exerts lipolytic activity, is diminished in obesity and is increased with weight loss. Despite low GH levels, insulin-like growth factor (IGF) I (somatomedin) production is normal, suggesting that GH suppression is a compensatory response to increased nutritional supply.

Pathogenesis of Common Obesity

Obesity can result from increased energy intake, decreased energy expenditure, or a combination of the two. Thus, identifying the etiology of obesity should involve measurements of both parameters. However, it is nearly impossible to perform direct and accurate measurements of energy intake in free-living individuals, and the obese, in particular, often underreport intake. Measurements of chronic energy expenditure have only recently become available using doubly labeled water or metabolic chamber/rooms. In subjects at stable weight and body composition, energy intake equals expenditure. Consequently, these techniques allow assessment of energy intake in free-living individuals. The level of energy expenditure differs in established obesity, during periods of weight gain or loss, and in the pre- or postobese state. Studies that fail to take note of this phenomenon are not easily interpreted.

There is continued interest in the concept of a body weight "set point." This idea is supported by physiologic mechanisms centered around a sensing system in adipose tissue that reflects fat stores and a receptor, or "adipostat," that is in the hypothalamic centers. When fat stores are depleted, the adipostat signal is low, and the hypothalamus responds by stimulating hunger and decreasing energy expenditure to conserve energy. Conversely, when fat stores are abundant, the signal is increased, and the hypothalamus responds by decreasing hunger and increasing energy expenditure. The recent discovery of the *ob* gene, and its product leptin, and the *db* gene, whose product is the leptin receptor, provides important elements of a molecular basis for this physiologic concept (see earlier).

What Is the Status of Food Intake in Obesity? (Do the Obese Eat More Than the Lean?)

This question has stimulated much debate, due in part to the methodologic difficulties inherent in determining food intake. Many obese individuals believe that they eat small quantities of food, and this claim has often been supported by the results of food intake questionnaires. However, it is now established that average energy expenditure increases as individuals get more obese, due primarily to the fact that metabolically active lean tissue mass increases with obesity. Given the laws of thermodynamics, the obese person must therefore eat more than the average lean person to maintain their increased weight. It may be the case, however, that a subset of individuals who are predisposed to obesity have the capacity to become obese initially without an absolute increase in caloric consumption.

What Is the State of Energy Expenditure in Obesity?

The average total daily energy expenditure is higher in obese than lean individuals when measured at stable weight. However, energy expenditure falls as weight is lost, due in part to loss of lean body mass and to decreased sympathetic nerve activity. When reduced to near-normal weight and maintained there for a while, (some) obese individuals have lower energy expenditure than (some) lean individuals. There is also a tendency for those who will develop obesity as infants or children to have lower resting energy expenditure rates than those who remain lean.

The physiologic basis for variable rates of energy expenditure (at a given body weight and level of energy intake) is essentially unknown. A mutation in the human β_3-adrenergic receptor may be associated with increased risk of obesity and/or insulin resistance in certain (but not all) populations. Homologues of the BAT uncoupling protein, named UCP-2 and UCP-3, have been identified in both rodents and humans. UCP-2 is expressed widely, whereas UCP-3 is primarily expressed in skeletal muscle. These proteins may play a role in disordered energy balance.

One newly described component of thermogenesis, called *nonexercise activity thermogenesis* (NEAT), has been linked to obesity. It is the thermogenesis that accompanies physical activities other than volitional exercise, such as the activities of daily living, fidgeting, spontaneous muscle contraction, and maintaining posture. NEAT accounts for about two-thirds of the increased daily energy expenditure induced by overfeeding. The wide variation in fat storage seen in overfed individuals is predicted by the degree to which NEAT is induced. The molecular basis for NEAT and its regulation is unknown.

Leptin in Typical Obesity

The vast majority of obese persons have increased leptin levels but do not have mutations of either leptin or its receptor. They appear, therefore, to have a form of functional "leptin resistance." Data suggesting that some individuals produce less leptin per unit fat mass than others or have a form of relative leptin deficiency that predisposes to obesity are at present contradictory and unsettled. The mechanism for leptin resistance, and whether it can be overcome by raising leptin levels, is not yet established. Some data suggest that leptin may not effectively cross the blood-brain barrier as levels rise. It is also apparent from animal studies that leptin signaling inhibitors, such as SOCS3 and PTP1b, are involved in the leptin-resistant state.

PATHOLOGIC CONSEQUENCES OF OBESITY

(See also Chap. 56) Obesity has major adverse effects on health. Obesity is associated with an increase in mortality, with a 50–100% increased risk of death from all causes compared to normal-weight individuals, mostly due to cardiovascular causes. Obesity and overweight together are the second leading cause of preventable death in the United States, accounting for 300,000 deaths per year. Mortality rates rise as obesity increases, particularly when obesity is associated with increased intraabdominal fat (see earlier). Life expectancy of a moderately obese individual could be shortened by 2–5 years, and a 20- to 30-year-old male with a BMI >45 may lose 13 years of life. It is also apparent that the degree to which obesity affects particular organ systems is influenced by susceptibility genes that vary in the population.

Insulin Resistance and Type 2 Diabetes Mellitus

Hyperinsulinemia and insulin resistance are pervasive features of obesity, increasing with weight gain and diminishing with weight loss (Chap. 58). Insulin resistance is more strongly linked to intraabdominal fat than to fat in other depots. The molecular link between obesity and insulin resistance in tissues such as fat, muscle, and liver has been sought for many years. Major factors under investigation include: (1) insulin itself, by inducing receptor downregulation; (2) free fatty acids, known to be increased and capable of impairing insulin action;

(3) intracellular lipid accumulation; and (4) various circulating peptides produced by adipocytes, including the cytokines TNF-α and IL-6, RBP4, and the "adipokines" adiponectin and resistin, which are produced by adipocytes, have altered expression in obese adipocytes, and are capable of modifying insulin action. Despite nearly universal insulin resistance, most obese individuals do not develop diabetes, suggesting that the onset of diabetes requires an interaction between obesity-induced insulin resistance and other factors that predispose to diabetes, such as impaired insulin secretion. Obesity, however, is a major risk factor for diabetes, and as many as 80% of patients with type 2 diabetes mellitus are obese. Weight loss and exercise, even of modest degree, are associated with increased insulin sensitivity and often improve glucose control in diabetes.

Reproductive Disorders

Disorders that affect the reproductive axis are associated with obesity in both men and women. Male hypogonadism is associated with increased adipose tissue, often distributed in a pattern more typical of females. In men >160% ideal body weight, plasma testosterone and sex hormone-binding globulin (SHBG) are often reduced, and estrogen levels (derived from conversion of adrenal androgens in adipose tissue) are increased. Gynecomastia may be seen. However, masculinization, libido, potency, and spermatogenesis are preserved in most of these individuals. Free testosterone may be decreased in morbidly obese men whose weight is >200% ideal body weight.

Obesity has long been associated with menstrual abnormalities in women, particularly in women with upper body obesity. Common findings are increased androgen production, decreased SHBG, and increased peripheral conversion of androgen to estrogen. Most obese women with oligomenorrhea have the polycystic ovarian syndrome (PCOS), with its associated anovulation and ovarian hyperandrogenism; 40% of women with PCOS are obese. Most nonobese women with PCOS are also insulin-resistant, suggesting that insulin resistance, hyperinsulinemia, or the combination of the two are causative or contribute to the ovarian pathophysiology in PCOS in both obese and lean individuals. In obese women with PCOS, weight loss or treatment with insulin-sensitizing drugs often restores normal menses. The increased conversion of androstenedione to estrogen, which occurs to a greater degree in women with lower body obesity, may contribute to the increased incidence of uterine cancer in postmenopausal women with obesity.

Cardiovascular Disease

The Framingham Study revealed that obesity was an independent risk factor for the 26-year incidence of cardiovascular disease in men and women [including coronary disease, stroke, and congestive heart failure (CHF)]. The waist/hip ratio may be the best predictor of these risks. When the additional effects of hypertension and glucose intolerance associated with obesity are included, the adverse impact of obesity is even more evident. The effect of obesity on cardiovascular mortality in women may be seen at BMIs as low as 25. Obesity, especially abdominal obesity, is associated with an atherogenic lipid profile; with increased low-density lipoprotein (LDL) cholesterol, very low density lipoprotein, and triglyceride; and with decreased high-density lipoprotein cholesterol and decreased levels of the vascular protective adipokine adiponectin. Obesity is also associated with hypertension. Measurement of blood pressure in the obese requires use of a larger cuff size to avoid artifactual increases. Obesity-induced hypertension is associated with increased peripheral resistance and cardiac output, increased sympathetic nervous system tone, increased salt sensitivity, and insulin-mediated salt retention; it is often responsive to modest weight loss.

Pulmonary Disease

Obesity may be associated with a number of pulmonary abnormalities. These include reduced chest wall compliance, increased work of breathing, increased minute ventilation due to increased metabolic rate, and decreased functional residual capacity and expiratory reserve volume. Severe obesity may be associated with obstructive sleep apnea and the "obesity hypoventilation syndrome" with attenuated hypoxic and hypercapnic ventilatory responses. Sleep apnea can be obstructive (most common), central, or mixed and is associated with hypertension. Weight loss (10–20 kg) can bring substantial improvement, as can major weight loss following gastric bypass or restrictive surgery. Continuous positive airway pressure has been used with some success.

Gallstones

Obesity is associated with enhanced biliary secretion of cholesterol, supersaturation of bile, and a higher incidence of gallstones, particularly cholesterol gallstones (Chap. 43). A person 50% above ideal body weight has about a sixfold increased incidence of symptomatic gallstones. Paradoxically, fasting increases supersaturation of bile by decreasing the phospholipid component. Fasting-induced cholecystitis is a complication of extreme diets.

Cancer

Obesity in males is associated with higher mortality from cancer, including cancer of the esophagus, colon, rectum, pancreas, liver, and prostate; obesity in females is associated with higher mortality from cancer of the gallbladder, bile ducts, breasts, endometrium, cervix, and ovaries. Some of the latter may be due to increased rates of conversion of androstenedione to estrone in adipose tissue of obese individuals. It was recently estimated that obesity accounts for 14% of cancer deaths in men and 20% in women in the United States.

Bone, Joint, and Cutaneous Disease

Obesity is associated with an increased risk of osteoarthritis, no doubt partly due to the trauma of added weight bearing and joint malalignment. The prevalence of gout may also be increased. Among the skin problems associated with obesity is acanthosis nigricans, manifested by darkening and thickening of the skin folds on the neck, elbows, and dorsal interphalangeal spaces. Acanthosis reflects the severity of underlying insulin resistance and diminishes with weight loss. Friability of skin may be increased, especially in skin folds, enhancing the risk of fungal and yeast infections. Finally, venous stasis is increased in the obese.

FURTHER READINGS

EDER K et al: The major inflammatory mediator interleukin-6 and obesity. Inflamm Res Jun 19 2009 [epub ahead of print]

FAROOQI IS, O'RAHILLY S: Genetics of obesity. Philos Trans R Soc Lond B Biol Sci 361:1095, 2006

FLIER JS: Obesity wars: Molecular progress confronts an expanding epidemic. Cell 116:337, 2004

JIA JJ et al: The polymorphisms of UCP2 and UCP3 genes associated with fat metabolism, obesity and diabetes. Obes Rev Apr 1 2009 [epub ahead of print]

KERSHAW EE, FLIER JS: Adipose tissue as an endocrine organ. J Clin Endocrinol Metab 89:2548, 2004

MORTON GJ et al: Central nervous system control of food intake and body weight. Nature 443:289, 2006

MURPHY KG et al: Gut peptides in the regulation of food intake and energy homeostasis. Endocr Rev 27:719, 2006

OGDEN CL et al: Prevalence of overweight and obesity in the United States, 1999-2004. JAMA 295:1549, 2006

———et al: The epidemiology of obesity. Gastroenterology 132(6):2087, 2007

VAN BAAK MA, ASTRUP A: Consumption of sugars and body weight. Obes Rev 10 (suppl 1): 9, 1009

WELLS JC: Ethnic variability in adiposity and cardiovascular risk: the variable disease selection hypothesis. Int J Epidemiol 38:63, 2009

CHAPTER 56

EVALUATION AND MANAGEMENT OF OBESITY

Robert F. Kushner

Over 66% of U.S. adults are currently categorized as overweight or obese, and the prevalence of obesity is increasing rapidly throughout most of the industrialized world. Based on statistics from the World Health Organization, overweight and obesity may soon replace more traditional public health concerns such as undernutrition and infectious diseases as the most significant contributors to ill health. Children and adolescents are also becoming more obese, indicating that the current trends will accelerate over time. Obesity is associated with an increased risk of multiple health problems, including hypertension, type 2 diabetes, dyslipidemia, degenerative joint disease, and some malignancies. Thus, it is important for physicians to routinely identify, evaluate, and treat patients for obesity and associated comorbid conditions.

EVALUATION

The U.S. Preventive Services Task Force recommends that physicians screen all adult patients for obesity and offer intensive counseling and behavioral interventions to promote sustained weight loss. This recommendation is consistent with previously released guidelines from the National Heart, Lung, and Blood Institute (NHLBI) and a number of medical societies. The five main steps in the evaluation of obesity are described in the next sections and include (1) focused obesity-related history, (2) physical examination to determine the degree and type of obesity, (3) comorbid conditions, (4) fitness level, and (5) the patient's readiness to adopt lifestyle changes.

The Obesity-Focused History

Information from the history should address the following six questions:

- What factors contribute to the patient's obesity?
- How is the obesity affecting the patient's health?
- What is the patient's level of risk from obesity?
- What are the patient's goals and expectations?
- Is the patient motivated to begin a weight management program?
- What kind of help does the patient need?

Although the vast majority of obesity can be attributed to behavioral features that affect diet and physical activity patterns, the history may suggest secondary causes that merit further evaluation. Disorders to consider include polycystic ovarian syndrome, hypothyroidism, Cushing's syndrome, and hypothalamic disease. Drug-induced weight gain should also to be considered. Common causes include antidiabetes agents (insulin, sulfonylureas, thiazolidine-diones); steroid hormones; psychotropic agents; mood stabilizers (lithium); antidepressants (tricyclics, monoamine oxidase inhibitors, paroxetine, mirtazapine); and antiepileptic drugs (valproate, gabapentin, carbamazepine). Other medications such as nonsteroidal anti-inflammatory drugs and calcium-channel blockers may cause peripheral edema, but they do not increase body fat.

The patient's current diet and physical activity patterns may reveal factors that contribute to the development of obesity in addition to identifying behaviors to target for treatment. This type of historical information is best obtained by using a questionnaire in combination with an interview.

TABLE 56-1

BODY MASS INDEX (BMI) TABLE

HEIGHT,
INCHES
                                        BODY WEIGHT, POUNDS

BMI	19	20	21	22	23	24	25	26	27	28	29	30	31	32	33	34	35
58	91	96	100	105	110	115	119	124	129	134	138	143	148	153	158	162	167
59	94	99	104	109	114	119	124	128	133	138	143	148	153	158	163	168	173
60	97	102	107	112	118	123	128	133	138	143	148	153	158	163	168	174	179
61	100	106	111	116	122	127	132	137	143	148	153	158	164	169	174	180	185
62	104	109	115	120	126	131	136	142	147	153	158	164	169	175	180	186	191
63	107	113	118	124	130	135	141	146	152	158	163	169	175	180	186	191	197
64	110	116	122	128	134	140	145	151	157	163	169	174	180	186	192	197	204
65	114	120	126	132	138	144	150	156	162	168	174	180	186	192	198	204	210
66	118	124	130	136	142	148	155	161	167	173	179	186	192	198	204	210	216
67	121	127	134	140	146	153	159	166	172	178	185	191	198	204	211	217	223
68	125	131	138	144	151	158	164	171	177	184	190	197	203	210	216	223	230
69	128	135	142	149	155	162	169	176	182	189	196	203	209	216	223	230	236
70	132	139	146	153	160	167	174	181	188	195	202	209	216	222	229	236	243
71	136	143	150	157	165	172	179	186	193	200	208	215	222	229	236	243	250
72	140	147	154	162	169	177	184	191	199	206	213	221	228	235	242	250	258
73	144	151	159	166	174	182	189	197	204	212	219	227	235	242	250	257	265
74	148	155	163	171	179	186	194	202	210	218	225	233	241	249	256	264	272
75	152	160	168	176	184	192	200	208	216	224	232	240	248	256	264	272	279
76	156	164	172	180	189	197	205	213	221	230	238	246	254	263	271	279	287

BMI	36	37	38	39	40	41	42	43	44	45	46	47	48	49	50	51	52	53	54
58	172	177	181	186	191	196	201	205	210	215	220	224	229	234	239	244	248	253	258
59	178	183	188	193	198	203	208	212	217	222	227	232	237	242	247	252	257	262	267
60	184	189	194	199	204	209	215	220	225	230	235	240	245	250	255	261	266	271	276
61	190	195	201	206	211	217	222	227	232	238	243	248	254	259	264	269	275	280	285
62	196	202	207	213	218	224	229	235	240	246	251	256	262	267	273	278	284	289	295
63	203	208	214	220	225	231	237	242	248	254	259	265	270	278	282	287	293	299	304
64	209	215	221	227	232	238	244	250	256	262	267	273	279	285	291	296	302	308	314
65	216	222	228	234	240	246	252	258	264	270	276	282	288	294	300	306	312	318	324
66	223	229	235	241	247	253	260	266	272	278	284	291	297	303	309	315	322	328	334
67	230	236	242	249	255	261	268	274	280	287	293	299	306	312	319	325	331	338	344
68	236	243	249	256	262	269	276	282	289	295	302	308	315	322	328	335	341	348	354
69	243	250	257	263	270	277	284	291	297	304	311	318	324	331	338	345	351	358	365
70	250	257	264	271	278	285	292	299	306	313	320	327	334	341	348	355	362	369	376
71	257	265	272	279	286	293	301	308	315	322	329	338	343	351	358	365	372	379	386
72	265	272	279	287	294	302	309	316	324	331	338	346	353	361	368	375	383	390	397
73	272	280	288	295	302	310	318	325	333	340	348	355	363	371	378	386	393	401	408
74	280	287	295	303	311	319	326	334	342	350	358	365	373	381	389	396	404	412	420
75	287	295	303	311	319	327	335	343	351	359	367	375	383	391	399	407	415	423	431
76	295	304	312	320	328	336	344	353	361	369	377	385	394	402	410	418	426	435	443

CHAPTER 56 Evaluation and Management of Obesity

BMI and Waist Circumference

Three key anthropometric measurements are important to evaluate the degree of obesity-weight, height, and waist circumference. The body mass index (BMI), calculated as weight (kg)/height (m)^2, or as weight (lbs)/height (inches)^2 × 703, is used to classify weight status and risk of disease (Tables 56-1 and 56-2). BMI is used since it provides an estimate of body fat and is related to risk of disease. Lower BMI thresholds for overweight and obesity have been proposed for the Asia-Pacific region since this population appears to be at-risk at lower body weights for glucose and lipid abnormalities.

Excess abdominal fat, assessed by measurement of waist circumference or waist-to-hip ratio, is independently associated with higher risk for diabetes mellitus and cardiovascular disease. Measurement of the waist circumference is a surrogate for visceral adipose tissue and should be performed in the horizontal plane above the

TABLE 56-2

	BMI (kg/m²)	OBESITY CLASS	RISK OF DISEASE
CLASSIFICATION OF WEIGHT STATUS AND RISK OF DISEASE			
Underweight	<18.5		
Healthy weight	18.5–24.9		
Overweight	25.0–29.9		Increased
Obesity	30.0–34.9	I	High
Obesity	35.0–39.9	II	Very high
Extreme obesity	≥40	III	Extremely high

Source: Adapted from National Institutes of Health, National Heart, Lung, and Blood Institute: *Clinical Guidelines on the Identification, Evaluation, and Treatment of Overweight and Obesity in Adults.* U.S. Department of Health and Human Services, Public Health Service, 1998.

iliac crest. Cut points that define higher risk for men and women based on ethnicity have been proposed by the International Diabetes Federation (Table 56-3).

Physical Fitness

Several prospective studies have demonstrated that physical fitness, reported by questionnaire or measured by a maximal treadmill exercise test, is an important predictor of all-cause mortality independent of BMI and body composition. These observations highlight the importance of taking an exercise history during examination as well as emphasizing physical activity as a treatment approach.

Obesity-Associated Comorbid Conditions

The evaluation of comorbid conditions should be based on presentation of symptoms, risk factors, and index of suspicion. All patients should have a fasting lipid panel (total, LDL, and HDL cholesterol and triglyceride levels) and blood glucose measured at presentation along with blood pressure determination. Symptoms and diseases that are directly or indirectly related to obesity are listed in Table 56-4. Although individuals vary, the number and severity of organ-specific comorbid conditions usually rise with increasing levels of obesity. Patients at very high absolute risk include the following: established coronary heart disease; presence of other atherosclerotic diseases such as peripheral arterial disease, abdominal aortic aneurysm, and symptomatic carotid artery disease; type 2 diabetes; and sleep apnea.

Assessing the Patient's Readiness to Change

An attempt to initiate lifestyle changes when the patient is not ready usually leads to frustration and may hamper future weight-loss efforts. Assessment includes patient motivation and support, stressful life events, psychiatric status, time availability and constraints, and appropriateness of goals and expectations. Readiness can be viewed as the balance of two opposing forces: (1) motivation, or the patient's desire to change; and (2) resistance, or the patient's resistance to change.

A helpful method to begin a readiness assessment is to "anchor" the patient's interest and confidence to change on a numerical scale. Using this technique, the patient is asked to rate his or her level of interest and confidence on a scale from 0 to 10, with 0 being not so important (or confident) and 10 being very important (or confident) to lose weight at this time. This exercise helps to establish readiness to change and also serves as a basis for further dialogue.

TABLE 56-3

ETHNIC-SPECIFIC VALUES FOR WAIST CIRCUMFERENCE	
ETHNIC GROUP	**WAIST CIRCUMFERENCE**
Europeans	
Men	>94 cm (37 in)
Women	>80 cm (31.5 in)
South Asians and Chinese	
Men	>90 cm (35 in)
Women	>80 cm (31.5 in)
Japanese	
Men	>85 cm (33.5 in)
Women	>90 cm (35 in)
Ethnic South and Central Americans	Use south Asian recommendations until more specific data are available.
Sub-Saharan Africans	Use European data until more specific data are available.
Eastern Mediterranean and Middle East (Arab) populations	Use European data until more specific data are available.

Source: From KGMM Alberti et al for the IDF Epidemiology Task Force Consensus Group: The metabolic syndrome—a new worldwide definition. Lancet 366:1059, 2005.

TABLE 56-4

OBESITY-RELATED ORGAN SYSTEMS REVIEW

Cardiovascular
  Hypertension
  Congestive heart failure
  Cor pulmonale
  Varicose veins
  Pulmonary embolism
  Coronary artery disease
Endocrine
  Metabolic syndrome
  Type 2 diabetes
  Dyslipidemia
  Polycystic ovarian syndrome
Musculoskeletal
  Hyperuricemia and gout
  Immobility
  Osteoarthritis (knees and hips)
  Low back pain
  Carpal tunnel syndrome
Psychological
  Depression/low self-esteem
  Body image disturbance
  Social stigmatization
Integument
  Striae distensae
  Stasis pigmentation of legs
  Lymphedema
  Cellulitis
  Intertrigo, carbuncles
  Acanthosis nigricans
  Acrochordon (skin tags)
  Hidradenitis suppurativa

Respiratory
  Dyspnea
  Obstructive sleep apnea
  Hypoventilation syndrome
  Pickwickian syndrome
  Asthma
Gastrointestinal
  Gastroesophageal reflux disease
  Nonalcoholic fatty liver disease
  Cholelithiasis
  Hernias
  Colon cancer
Genitourinary
  Urinary stress incontinence
  Obesity-related glomerulopathy
  Hypogonadism (male)
  Breast and uterine cancer
  Pregnancy complications
Neurologic
  Stroke
  Idiopathic intracranial hypertension
  Meralgia paresthetica
  Dementia

℞ Treatment: OBESITY

THE GOAL OF THERAPY The primary goal of treatment is to improve obesity-related comorbid conditions and reduce the risk of developing future comorbidities. Information obtained from the history, physical examination, and diagnostic tests is used to determine risk and develop a treatment plan (Fig. 56-1). The decision of how aggressively to treat the patient, and which modalities to use, is determined by the patient's risk status, expectations, and available resources. Therapy for obesity always begins with lifestyle management and may include pharmacotherapy or surgery, depending on BMI risk category (Table 56-5). Setting an initial weight-loss goal of 10% over 6 months is a realistic target.

LIFESTYLE MANAGEMENT Obesity care involves attention to three essential elements of lifestyle: dietary habits, physical activity, and behavior modification. Because obesity is fundamentally a disease of energy imbalance, all patients must learn how and when energy is consumed (diet), how and when energy is expended (physical activity), and how to incorporate this information into their daily life (behavior therapy). Lifestyle management has been shown to result in a modest (typically 3–5 kg) weight loss compared to no treatment or usual care.

DIET THERAPY The primary focus of diet therapy is to reduce overall calorie consumption. The NHLBI guidelines recommend initiating treatment with a calorie deficit of 500–1000 kcal/d compared to the patient's habitual diet. This reduction is consistent with a goal of losing approximately 1–2 lb per week. This calorie deficit can be accomplished by suggesting substitutions or alternatives to the diet. Examples include choosing smaller portion sizes, eating more fruits and vegetables, consuming more whole-grain cereals, selecting leaner cuts of meat and skimmed dairy products, reducing fried foods and other added fats and oils, and drinking water instead of caloric beverages. It is important that the dietary counseling remains patient-centered and that the goals are practical, realistic, and achievable.

ALGORITHM FOR TREATMENT OF OBESITY

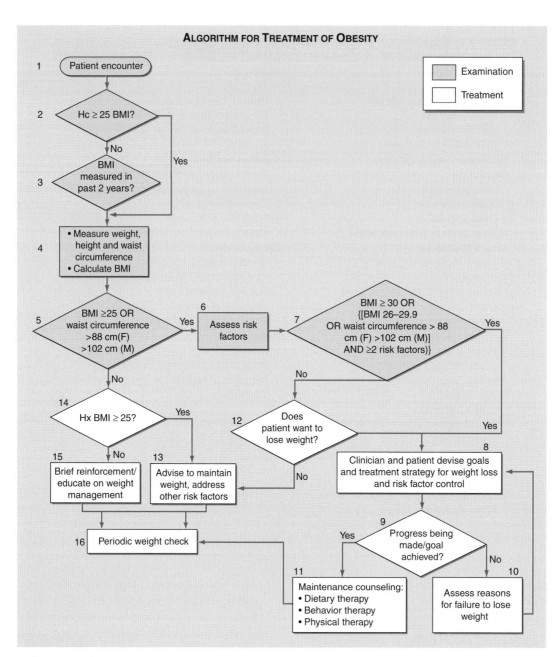

FIGURE 56-1

Treatment algorithm. This algorithm applies only to the assessment for overweight and obesity and subsequent decisions on that assessment. It does not reflect any initial overall assessment for other conditions that the physician may wish to perform. Ht, height; Hx, history; Wt, weight. *(From National, Heart, Lung, and Blood Institute: Clinical guidelines on the identification, evaluation, and treatment of overweight and obesity in adults: The evidence report. Washington, DC, US Department of Health and Human Services, 1998.)*

The macronutrient composition of the diet will vary depending on the patient's preference and medical condition. The 2005 U.S. Department of Agriculture Dietary Guidelines for Americans (Chap. 51), which focus on health promotion and risk reduction, can be applied to treatment of the overweight or obese patient. The recommendations include maintaining a diet rich in whole grains, fruits, vegetables, and dietary fiber; consuming

two servings (8 oz) of fish high in omega 3 fatty acids per week; decreasing sodium to <2300 mg/d; consuming 3 cups of milk (or equivalent low-fat or fat-free dairy products) per day; limiting cholesterol to <300 mg/d; and keeping total fat between 20 and 35% of daily calories and saturated fats to <10% of daily calories. Application of these guidelines to specific calorie goals can be found on the website *www.mypyramid.gov*. The revised Dietary

TABLE 56-5

615

A GUIDE TO SELECTING TREATMENT

TREATMENT	BMI CATEGORY				
	25–26.9	27–29.9	30–35	35–39.9	≥40
Diet, exercise, behavior therapy	With comorbidities	With comorbidities	+	+	+
Pharmacotherapy		With comorbidities	+	+	+
Surgery				With comorbidities	+

Source: From National Heart, Lung, and Blood Institute, North American Association for the Study of Obesity (2000).

Reference Intakes for Macronutrients released by the Institute of Medicine recommends 45–65% of calories from carbohydrates, 20–35% from fat, and 10–35% from protein. The guidelines also recommend daily fiber intake of 38 g (men) and 25 g (women) for persons over 50 years of age and 30 g (men) and 21 g (women) for those under 50.

Since portion control is one of the most difficult strategies for patients to manage, the use of pre-prepared products, such as meal replacements, is a simple and convenient suggestion. Examples include frozen entrees, canned beverages, and bars. Use of meal replacements in the diet has been shown to result in a 7–8% weight loss.

A current area of controversy is the use of low-carbohydrate, high-protein diets for weight loss. These diets are based on the concept that carbohydrates are the primary cause of obesity and lead to insulin resistance. Most low-carbohydrate diets (e.g., South Beach, Zone, and Sugar Busters!) recommend a carbohydrate level of approximately 40–46% of energy. The Atkins diet contains 5–15% carbohydrate, depending on the phase of the diet. Several randomized, controlled trials of these low-carbohydrate diets have demonstrated greater weight loss at 6 months with improvement in coronary heart disease risk factors, including an increase in HDL cholesterol and a decrease in triglyceride levels. Weight loss between groups did not remain statistically significant at 1 year; however, low-carbohydrate diets appear to be at least as effective as low-fat diets in inducing weight loss for up to 1 year.

Another dietary approach to consider is the concept of energy density, which refers to the number of calories (energy) a food contains per unit of weight. People tend to ingest a constant volume of food, regardless of caloric or macronutrient content. Adding water or fiber to a food decreases its energy density by increasing weight without affecting caloric content. Examples of foods with low-energy density include soups, fruits, vegetables, oatmeal, and lean meats. Dry foods and high-fat foods such as pretzels, cheese, egg yolks, potato chips, and red meat have a high-energy density. Diets containing low-energy dense foods have been shown to control hunger and result in decreased caloric intake and weight loss.

Occasionally, very-low-calorie diets (VLCDs) are prescribed as a form of aggressive dietary therapy. The primary purpose of a VLCD is to promote a rapid and significant (13–23 kg) short-term weight loss over a 3–6 month period. These propriety formulas typically supply ≤800 kcal, 50–80 g protein, and 100% of the recommended daily intake for vitamins and minerals. According to a review by the National Task Force on the Prevention and Treatment of Obesity, indications for initiating a VLCD include well-motivated individuals who are moderately to severely obese (BMI >30), have failed at more conservative approaches to weight loss, and have a medical condition that would be immediately improved with rapid weight loss. These conditions include poorly controlled type 2 diabetes, hypertriglyceridemia, obstructive sleep apnea, and symptomatic peripheral edema. The risk for gallstone formation increases exponentially at rates of weight loss >1.5 kg/week (3.3 lb/week). Prophylaxis against gallstone formation with ursodeoxycholic acid, 600 mg/d, is effective in reducing this risk. Because of the need for close metabolic monitoring, these diets are usually prescribed by physicians specializing in obesity care.

PHYSICAL ACTIVITY THERAPY Although exercise alone is only moderately effective for weight loss, the combination of dietary modification and exercise is the most effective behavioral approach for the treatment of obesity. The most important role of exercise appears to be in the maintenance of the weight loss. Currently, the *minimum* public health recommendation for physical activity is 30 min of moderate intensity physical activity on most, and preferably all, days of the week. Focusing on simple ways to add physical activity into the normal daily routine through leisure activities,

CHAPTER 56 Evaluation and Management of Obesity

travel, and domestic work should be suggested. Examples include walking, using the stairs, doing home and yard work, and engaging in sport activities. Asking the patient to wear a pedometer to monitor total accumulation of steps as part of the activities of daily living is a useful strategy. Step counts are highly correlated with activity level. Studies have demonstrated that lifestyle activities are as effective as structured exercise programs for improving cardiorespiratory fitness and weight loss. The Dietary Guidelines for Americans 2005 summarizes compelling evidence that at least 60–90 min of daily moderate-intensity physical activity (420–630 min per week) is needed to sustain weight loss (*http://www.health.gov/dietaryguidelines/dga2005/*). The American College of Sports Medicine recommends that overweight and obese individuals progressively increase to a minimum of 150 min of moderate intensity physical activity per week as a first goal. However, for long-term weight loss, a higher level of exercise (e.g., 200–300 min or ≥2000 kcal per week) is needed. These recommendations are daunting to most patients and need to be implemented gradually. Consultation with an exercise physiologist or personal trainer may be helpful.

BEHAVIORAL THERAPY Cognitive behavioral therapy is used to help change and reinforce new dietary and physical activity behaviors. Strategies include self-monitoring techniques (e.g., journaling, weighing, and measuring food and activity); stress management; stimulus control (e.g., using smaller plates, not eating in front of the television or in the car); social support; problem solving; and cognitive restructuring to help patients develop more positive and realistic thoughts about themselves. When recommending any behavioral lifestyle change, have the patient identify what, when, where, and how the behavioral change will be performed. The patient should keep a record of the anticipated behavioral change so that progress can be reviewed at the next office visit. Because these techniques are time-consuming to implement, they are often provided by ancillary office staff such as a nurse clinician or registered dietitian.

PHARMACOTHERAPY Adjuvant pharmacologic treatments should be considered for patients with a BMI >30 kg/m² or with a BMI >27 kg/m² who also have concomitant obesity-related diseases and for whom dietary and physical activity therapy has not been successful. When prescribing an antiobesity medication, patients should be actively engaged in a lifestyle program that provides the strategies and skills needed to effectively use the drug since this support increases total weight loss.

There are several potential targets of pharmacologic therapy for obesity. The most thoroughly explored treatment is suppression of appetite via centrally active medications that alter monoamine neurotransmitters.

A second strategy is to reduce the absorption of selective macronutrients from the gastrointestinal (GI) tract, such as fat. These two mechanisms form the basis for all currently prescribed antiobesity agents. A third target, selective blocking of the endocannabinoid system, has recently been identified.

Centrally Acting Anorexiant Medications
Appetite-suppressing drugs, or anorexiants, affect satiety-the absence of hunger after eating—and hunger—a biologic sensation that initiates eating. By increasing satiety and decreasing hunger, these agents help patients reduce caloric intake without a sense of deprivation. The target site for the actions of anorexiants is the ventromedial and lateral hypothalamic regions in the central nervous system (Chap. 55). Their biological effect on appetite regulation is produced by augmenting the neurotransmission of three monoamines: norepinephrine; serotonin [5-hydroxytryptamine (5-HT)]; and, to a lesser degree, dopamine. The classic sympathomimetic adrenergic agents (benzphetamine, phendimetrazine, diethylpropion, mazindol, and phentermine) function by stimulating norepinephrine release or by blocking its reuptake. In contrast, sibutramine (Meridia) functions as a serotonin and norepinephrine reuptake inhibitor. Unlike other previously used anorexiants, sibutramine is not pharmacologically related to amphetamine and has no addictive potential.

Sibutramine is the only anorexiant that is currently approved by the Food and Drug Administration (FDA) for long-term use. It produces an average loss of about 5–9% of initial body weight at 12 months. Sibutramine has been demonstrated to maintain weight loss for up to 2 years. The most commonly reported adverse events of sibutramine are headache, dry mouth, insomnia, and constipation. These are generally mild and well-tolerated. The principal concern is a dose-related increase in blood pressure and heart rate that may require discontinuation of the medication. A dose of 10–15 mg/d causes an average increase in systolic and diastolic blood pressure of 2–4 mmHg and an increase in heart rate of 4–6 beats/min. For this reason, all patients should be monitored closely and evaluated within 1 month after initiating therapy. The risk of adverse effects on blood pressure are no greater in patients with controlled hypertension than in those who do not have hypertension, and the drug does not appear to cause cardiac valve dysfunction. Contraindications to sibutramine use include uncontrolled hypertension, congestive heart failure, symptomatic coronary heart disease, arrhythmias, or history of stroke. Similar to other antiobesity medications, weight reduction is enhanced when the drug is used along with behavioral therapy, and body weight increases when the medication is discontinued.

Peripherally Acting Medications Orlistat (Xenical) is a synthetic hydrogenated derivative of a naturally occurring lipase inhibitor, lipostatin, produced by the mold *Streptomyces toxytricini*. Orlistat is a potent, slowly reversible inhibitor of pancreatic, gastric, and carboxylester lipases and phospholipase A2, which are required for the hydrolysis of dietary fat into fatty acids and monoacylglycerols. The drug acts in the lumen of the stomach and small intestine by forming a covalent bond with the active site of these lipases. Taken at a therapeutic dose of 120 mg tid, orlistat blocks the digestion and absorption of about 30% of dietary fat. After discontinuation of the drug, fecal fat usually returns to normal concentrations within 48–72 h.

Multiple randomized, 1–2 year double-blind, placebo-controlled studies have shown that after one year, orlistat produces a weight loss of about 9–10%, compared with a 4–6% weight loss in the placebo-treated groups. Because orlistat is minimally (<1%) absorbed from the GI tract, it has no systemic side effects. Tolerability to the drug is related to the malabsorption of dietary fat and subsequent passage of fat in the feces. GI tract adverse effects are reported in at least 10% of orlistat-treated patients. These include flatus with discharge, fecal urgency, fatty/oily stool, and increased defecation. These side effects are generally experienced early, diminish as patients control their dietary fat intake, and infrequently cause patients to withdraw from clinical trials. Psyllium mucilloid is helpful in controlling the orlistat-induced GI side effects when taken concomitantly with the medication. Serum concentrations of the fat-soluble vitamins D and E and β-carotene may be reduced, and vitamin supplements are recommended to prevent potential deficiencies. Orlistat was approved for other-the-counter use in 2007.

The Endocannabinoid System Cannabinoid receptors and their endogenous ligands have been implicated in a variety of physiologic functions, including feeding, modulation of pain, emotional behavior, and peripheral lipid metabolism. Cannabis and its main ingredient, Δ^9-tetrahydrocannabinol (THC), is an exogenous cannabinoid compound. Two endocannabinoids have been identified, anandamide and 2-arachidonyl glyceride. Two cannabinoid receptors have been identified: CB_1 (abundant in the brain) and CB_2 (present in immune cells). The brain endocannabinoid system is thought to control food intake through reinforcing motivation to find and consume foods with high incentive value and to regulate actions of other mediators of appetite. The first selective cannabinoid CB_1 receptor antagonist, rimonabant, was discovered in 1994. The medication antagonizes the orexigenic effect of THC and suppresses appetite when given alone in animal models. Several large prospective, randomized controlled trials have demonstrated the effectiveness of rimonabant as a weight-loss agent. Taken as a 20 mg dose, subjects lost an average of 6.5 kg (14.32 lb) compared to 1.5 kg (3.3 lb) for placebo at 1 year. Concomitant improvements were seen in waist circumference and cardiovascular risk factors. The most common reported side effects include depression, anxiety, and nausea. FDA approval of Rimonabant is still pending.

SURGERY Bariatric surgery can be considered for patients with severe obesity (BMI ≥40 kg/m²) or those with moderate obesity (BMI ≥35 kg/m²) associated with a serious medical condition. Surgical weight loss functions by reducing caloric intake and, depending on the procedure, macronutrient absorption.

Weight-loss surgeries fall into one of two categories: restrictive and restrictive-malabsorptive (**Fig. 56-2**). Restrictive surgeries limit the amount of food the stomach can hold and slow the rate of gastric emptying. The

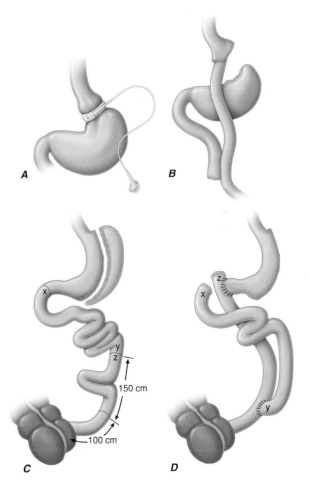

FIGURE 56-2

Bariatric surgical procedures. Examples of operative interventions used for surgical manipulation of the gastrointestinal tract. *A.* Laparoscopic gastric band (LAGB). *B.* The Roux-en-Y gastric bypass. *C.* Biliopancreatic diversion with duodenal switch. *D.* Biliopancreatic diversion. *(From ML Kendrick, GF Dakin. Surgical approaches to obesity. Mayo Clin Proc 815:518, 2006; with permission.)*

vertical banded gastroplasty (VBG) is the prototype of this category but is currently performed on a very limited basis due to lack of effectiveness in long-term trials. Laparoscopic adjustable silicone gastric banding (LASGB) has replaced the VBG as the most commonly performed restrictive operation. The first banding device, the lap-band, was approved for use in the United States in 2001. In contrast to previous devices, the diameter of this band is adjustable by way of its connection to a reservoir that is implanted under the skin. Injection or removal of saline into the reservoir tightens or loosens the band's internal diameter, thus changing the size of the gastric opening.

The three restrictive-malabsorptive bypass procedures combine the elements of gastric restriction and selective malabsorption. These procedures include Roux-en-Y gastric bypass (RYGB), biliopancreatic diversion (BPD), and biliopancreatic diversion with duodenal switch (BPDDS) (Fig. 56-2). RYGB is the most commonly performed and accepted bypass procedure. It may be performed with an open incision or laparoscopically.

Although no recent randomized controlled trials compare weight loss after surgical and nonsurgical interventions, data from meta-analyses and large databases, primarily obtained from observational studies, suggest that bariatric surgery is the most effective weight-loss therapy for those with clinically severe obesity. These procedures generally produce a 30–35% average total body weight loss that is maintained in nearly 60% of patients at 5 years. In general, mean weight loss is greater after the combined restrictive-malabsorptive procedures compared to the restrictive procedures. An abundance of data supports the positive impact of bariatric surgery on obesity-related morbid conditions, including diabetes mellitus, hypertension, obstructive sleep apnea, dyslipidemia, and nonalcoholic fatty liver disease.

Surgical mortality from bariatric surgery is generally <1% but varies with the procedure, patient's age and comorbid conditions, and experience of the surgical team. The most common surgical complications include stomal stenosis or marginal ulcers (occurring in 5–15% of patients) that present as prolonged nausea and vomiting after eating or inability to advance the diet to solid foods. These complications are typically treated by endoscopic balloon dilatation and acid suppression therapy, respectively. For patients who undergo LASGB, there are no intestinal absorptive abnormalities other than mechanical reduction in gastric size and outflow. Therefore, selective deficiencies occur uncommonly unless eating habits become unbalanced. In contrast, the restrictive-malabsorptive procedures increase risk for micronutrient deficiencies of vitamin B_{12}, iron, folate, calcium, and vitamin D. Patients with restrictive-malabsorptive procedures require lifelong supplementation with these micronutrients.

FURTHER READINGS

Bray GA, Greenway FL: Pharmacologic treatment of the overweight patient. Pharmacol Rev 59:151, 2007

———, Ryan DH: Drug treatment of the overweight patient. Gastroenterology 132:2239, 2007

Buchwald H et al: Bariatric surgery: A systematic review and meta-analysis. JAMA 292:1724, 2004

Colquitt JL et al: Surgery for obesity. Cochrane Database Syste Rev Apr 15;(2):CD003641, 2009

DeMaria EJ: Bariatric surgery for morbid obesity. N Engl J Med 356:2176, 2007

Hasani-Ranjbar S et al: A systematic review of the efficacy and safety of herbal medicines used in the treatment of obesity. World J Gastroenterol 15:3073, 2009

Haslam DW, James WPT: Obesity. Lancet 366:1197, 2005

Kendall DM et al: Clinical application of incretin-based therapy: Therapeutic potential, patient selection and clinical use. Am J Med 122 (Suppl 6):S37, 2009

Korner J et al: Regulation of energy homeostasis and health consequences in obesity. Am J Med 122 (Suppl 1):S12, 2009

Kushner RF: Roadmaps for clinical practice: Case studies in disease prevention and health promotion—assessment and management of adult obesity: A primer for physicians. Chicago, American Medical Association, 2003. (Available online at *www.ama-assn.org/ama/pub/category/10931.html*)

McTigue KM et al: Screening and interventions for obesity in adults: Summary of the evidence for the U.S. Preventive Services Task Force. Ann Intern Med 139:933, 2003. (Appendix tables available at *www.annals.org*)

National Heart, Lung, and Blood Institute, North American Association for the Study of Obesity: Practical guide: Identification, evaluation, and treatment of overweight and obesity in adults. Bethesda, MD, National Institutes of Health pub number 00-4084, Oct. 2000. Available online: *http://www.nhlbi.nih.gov/guidelines/obesity/practgde.htm*

Padwal R et al: Long-term pharmacotherapy for overweight and obesity: A systematic review and meta-analysis of randomized controlled trials. Int J Obesity 27:1437, 2003

Wadden TA et al: Lifestyle modification for the management of obesity. Gastroenterology 132:2226, 2007

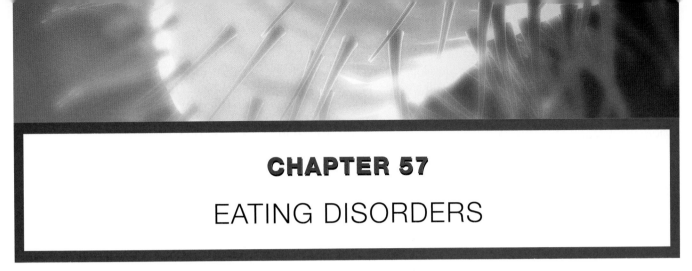

CHAPTER 57

EATING DISORDERS

B. Timothy Walsh

Anorexia nervosa and bulimia nervosa are characterized by severe disturbances of eating behavior. The salient feature of *anorexia nervosa* (AN) is a refusal to maintain a minimally normal body weight. *Bulimia nervosa* (BN) is characterized by recurrent episodes of binge eating followed by abnormal compensatory behaviors, such as self-induced vomiting. AN and BN are distinct clinical syndromes but share certain features in common. Both disorders occur primarily among previously healthy young women who become overly concerned with body shape and weight. Many patients with BN have past histories of anorexia nervosa, and many patients with AN engage in binge eating and purging behavior. In the current diagnostic system, the critical distinction between AN and BN depends on body weight: patients with AN are, by definition, significantly underweight, whereas patients with BN have body weights in the normal range or above.

Binge eating disorder (BED) is a more recently described syndrome characterized by repeated episodes of binge eating, similar to those of BN, in the absence of inappropriate compensatory behavior. Patients with BED are typically middle-aged men or women with significant obesity. They have an increased frequency of anxiety and depression compared to similarly obese patients without BED. It is not established that patients with BED are at increased risk for medical complications or that they require specific treatment interventions.

ANOREXIA NERVOSA

EPIDEMIOLOGY

Among women, the lifetime prevalence of the full syndrome of AN is approximately 1%. AN is much less common in males. AN is more prevalent in cultures where food is plentiful and in which being thin is associated with attractiveness. Individuals who pursue interests that place a premium on thinness, such as ballet and modeling, are at greater risk. The incidence of AN has increased in recent decades.

ETIOLOGY

The etiology of AN is unknown but appears to involve a combination of psychological, biologic, and cultural risk factors. Risk factors, such as sexual or physical abuse and a family history of mood disturbance, are best viewed as nonspecific risk factors that increase vulnerability to a range of psychiatric disorders, including AN.

Patients who develop AN are inclined to be more obsessional and perfectionist than their peers. The disorder often begins as a diet not distinguishable at the outset from those undertaken by many adolescents and young women. As weight loss progresses, the fear of gaining weight grows; dieting becomes stricter; and psychological, behavioral, and medical aberrations increase.

Eating disorders, including AN, may develop among individuals with type 1 diabetes mellitus and are associated with poorer glycemic control and an increased frequency of complications.

Numerous physiologic disturbances, including abnormalities in a variety of neurotransmitter systems, have been described in AN (see later). It is difficult to distinguish neurochemical, metabolic, and hormonal changes that may have a role in the initiation or perpetuation of the syndrome from those that are secondary to the disorder. The resolution of most of these abnormalities with weight restoration argues against an etiologic role.

Genetic factors contribute to the risk of development of AN, as its incidence is greater in families with one affected member and the concordance in monozygotic twins is greater than in dizygotic twins. However, specific genes have not been identified.

CLINICAL FEATURES

AN typically begins in mid to late adolescence, sometimes in association with a stressful life event such as leaving home for school (Table 57-1). The disorder occasionally develops in early puberty, before menarche, but seldom begins after age 40. Despite being underweight, patients with AN are irrationally afraid of gaining weight, often out of a concern that weight gain will get "out of control." They also exhibit a distortion of body image, which may express itself in several ways. For example, despite being emaciated, patients with AN

TABLE 57-1

COMMON CHARACTERISTICS OF ANOREXIA NERVOSA AND BULIMIA NERVOSA

	ANOREXIA NERVOSA[a]	BULIMIA NERVOSA
Clinical Characteristics		
Onset	Mid-adolescence	Late adolescence/early adulthood
Female:male	10:1	10:1
Lifetime prevalence in women	1%	1–3%
Weight	Markedly decreased	Usually normal
Menstruation	Absent	Usually normal
Binge eating	25–50%	Required for diagnosis
Mortality	~5% per decade	Low
Physical and Laboratory Findings[a]		
Skin/extremities	Lanugo Acrocyanosis Edema	
Cardiovascular	Bradycardia Hypotension	
Gastrointestinal	Salivary gland enlargement Slow gastric emptying Constipation Elevated liver enzymes	Salivary gland enlargement Dental erosion
Hematopoietic	Normochromic, normocytic anemia Leukopenia	
Fluid/Electrolyte	Increased BUN, creatinine Hypokalemia	Hypokalemia Hypochloremia Alkalosis
Endocrine	Hypoglycemia Low estrogen or testosterone Low LH and FSH Low-normal thyroxine Normal TSH Increased cortisol	
Bone	Osteopenia	

[a]Patients with the binge-eating/purging subtype of anorexia nervosa may also exhibit the physical and laboratory findings associated with bulimia nervosa.
Note: BUN, blood urea nitrogen; LH, luteinizing hormone; FSH, follicle stimulating hormone; TSH, thyroid stimulating hormone.

may believe that their body as a whole, or some part of their body, is too fat. Further weight loss is viewed by the patient as a fulfilling accomplishment, while weight gain is seen as a personal failure. Patients with AN rarely complain of hunger or fatigue and often exercise extensively. Despite the denial of hunger, one-quarter to one-half of patients with AN engage in eating binges. Patients tend to become socially withdrawn and increasingly committed to work or study, dieting, and exercise. As weight loss progresses, thoughts of food dominate mental life and idiosyncratic rules develop around eating. Patients with AN may obsessively collect cookbooks and recipes and be drawn to food-related occupations.

Physical Features

Patients with AN typically have few physical complaints but may note cold intolerance. Gastrointestinal motility is diminished, leading to reduced gastric emptying and constipation. Some women who develop AN after menarche report that their menses ceased before significant weight loss occurred. Weight and height should be measured to allow calculation of body mass index (BMI; kg/m^2). Vital signs may reveal bradycardia, hypotension, and mild hypothermia. Soft, downy hair growth (lanugo) sometimes occurs, and alopecia may be seen. Salivary gland enlargement, which is associated with starvation as well as with binge eating and vomiting, may make the face appear surprisingly full in contrast to the marked general wasting. Acrocyanosis of the digits is common, and peripheral edema can be seen in the absence of hypoalbuminemia, particularly when the patient begins to regain weight. Consumption of large amounts of vegetables containing vitamin A can result in a yellow tint to the skin (*hypercarotenemia*), which is especially notable on the palms.

Laboratory Abnormalities

Mild normochromic, normocytic anemia is frequent, as is mild to moderate leukopenia, with a disproportionate reduction of polymorphonuclear leukocytes. Dehydration may result in slightly increased levels of blood urea nitrogen and creatinine. Serum transaminase levels may increase, especially during the early phases of refeeding. The level of serum proteins is usually normal. Blood sugar is often low and serum cholesterol may be moderately elevated. Hypokalemic alkalosis suggests self-induced vomiting or the use of diuretics. Hyponatremia is common and may result from excess fluid intake and disturbances in the secretion of antidiuretic hormone.

Endocrine Abnormalities

The regulation of virtually every endocrine system is altered in AN, but the most striking changes occur in the reproductive system. Amenorrhea is hypothalamic in origin and reflects diminished production of gonadotropin-releasing hormone (GnRH). When exogenous GnRH is administered in a pulsatile manner, pituitary responses of luteinizing hormone (LH) and follicle-stimulating hormone (FSH) are normalized, indicating the absence of a primary pituitary abnormality. The resulting gonadotropin deficiency causes low plasma estrogen in women and reduced testosterone in men. The hypothalamic GnRH pulse generator is exquisitely sensitive, particularly in women, to body weight, stress, and exercise, each of which may contribute to *hypothalamic amenorrhea* in AN.

Serum leptin levels are markedly reduced in AN as a result of undernutrition and decreased body fat mass. The reduction in leptin appears to be the primary factor responsible for the disturbances of the hypothalamic-pituitary-gonadal axis, and to be an important mediator of the other neuroendocrine abnormalities characteristic of AN (Chap. 55).

Serum cortisol and 24-h urine free cortisol levels are generally elevated but without characteristic clinical signs of cortisol excess. Thyroid function tests resemble the pattern seen in euthyroid sick syndrome. Thyroxine (T_4) and free T_4 levels are usually in the low-normal range, triiodothyronine (T_3) levels are reduced, and reverse T_3 (rT_3) is elevated. The level of thyroid-stimulating hormone (TSH) is normal or partially suppressed. Growth hormone is increased, but insulin-like growth factor 1 (IGF-1), which is produced mainly by the liver, is reduced, as in other conditions of starvation. Diminished bone density is routinely observed in AN and reflects the effects of multiple nutritional deficiencies, reduced gonadal steroids, and increased cortisol. The degree of bone density reduction is proportional to the length of the illness, and patients are at risk for the development of symptomatic fractures. The occurrence of AN during adolescence may lead to the premature cessation of linear bone growth and a failure to achieve expected adult height.

Cardiac Abnormalities

Cardiac output is reduced, and congestive heart failure occurs rarely during rapid refeeding. The electrocardiogram usually shows sinus bradycardia, reduced QRS voltage, and nonspecific ST-T-wave abnormalities. Some patients develop a prolonged QT_c interval, which may predispose to serious arrhythmias, particularly when electrolyte abnormalities also are present.

DIAGNOSIS

The diagnosis of AN is based on the presence of characteristic behavioral, psychological, and physical attributes (Table 57-2). Widely accepted diagnostic criteria are provided by the American Psychiatric Association's

TABLE 57-2

DIAGNOSTIC FEATURES OF ANOREXIA NERVOSA
Refusal to maintain body weight at or above a minimally normal weight for age and height. (This includes a failure to achieve weight gain expected during a period of growth leading to an abnormally low body weight.)
Intense fear of weight gain or becoming fat.
Distortion of body image (e.g., feeling fat despite an objectively low weight or minimizing the seriousness of low weight).
Amenorrhea. (This criterion is met if menstrual periods occur only following hormone—e.g., estrogen— administration.)

Diagnostic and Statistical Manual of Mental Disorders (DSM-IV). These criteria include weight <85% of that expected for age and height, which is roughly equivalent to a BMI of 18.5 kg/m^2 for adult women. This weight criterion is somewhat arbitrary, so that a patient who meets all other diagnostic criteria but weighs between 85 and 90% of expected would still merit the diagnosis of AN. The current diagnostic criteria require that women with AN not have spontaneous menses, but occasional patients with the characteristics and complications of AN describe regular menstruation. Two mutually exclusive subtypes of AN are specified in DSM-IV. Patients whose weight loss is maintained primarily by caloric restriction, perhaps augmented by excessive exercise, are considered to have the "restricting" subtype of AN. The "binge eating/purging" subtype is characterized by binge eating and self-induced vomiting and/or laxative abuse. Patients with the binge/purge subtype are more prone to develop electrolyte imbalances, are more emotionally labile, and are more likely to have other problems with impulse control, such as drug abuse.

The diagnosis of AN can usually be made confidently in a patient with a history of weight loss accomplished by restrictive dieting and excessive exercise, accompanied by a marked reluctance to gain weight. Patients with AN often deny that they have a serious problem and may be brought to medical attention by concerned family or friends. In atypical presentations, other causes of significant weight loss in previously healthy young people should be considered, including inflammatory bowel disease, gastric outlet obstruction, diabetes mellitus, central nervous system (CNS) tumors, or neoplasm (Chap. 7).

PROGNOSIS

The course and outcome of AN are highly variable. One-quarter to one-half of patients eventually recover fully, with few psychological or physical sequelae. However, many patients have persistent difficulties with weight maintenance, depression, and eating disturbances, including BN. The development of obesity following AN is rare. The long-term mortality of AN is among the highest associated with any psychiatric disorder. Approximately 5% of patients die per decade of follow-up, primarily due to the physical effects of chronic starvation or by suicide.

Virtually all of the physiologic abnormalities associated with AN are observed in other forms of starvation and markedly improve or disappear with weight gain. A worrisome exception is the reduction in bone mass, which may not recover fully, particularly when AN occurs during adolescence when peak bone mass is normally achieved.

℞ Treatment: ANOREXIA NERVOSA

Because of the profound physiologic and psychological effects of starvation, there is a broad consensus that weight restoration to at least 90% of predicted weight is the primary goal in the treatment of AN. Unfortunately, because most patients resist this goal, the management of AN is often accompanied by frustration for the patient, the family, and the physician. Patients typically exaggerate their food intake and minimize their symptoms. Some patients resort to subterfuge to make their weights appear higher, for example, by water-loading before they are weighed. In attempting to engage the patient in treatment, it may be useful for the physician to elicit the patient's physical concerns (e.g., about osteoporosis, weakness, or fertility) and, provide education about the importance of normalizing nutritional status in order to address those concerns. The physician should reassure the patient that weight gain will not be permitted to get "out of control" but simultaneously emphasize that weight restoration is medically and psychologically imperative.

The intensity of the initial treatment, including the need for hospitalization, is determined by the patient's current weight, the rapidity of recent weight loss, and the severity of medical and psychological complications (**Fig. 57-1**). Hospitalization should be strongly considered for patients weighing <75% of expected, even if the results of routine blood studies are within normal limits. Acute medical problems, such as severe electrolyte imbalances, should be identified and addressed. Nutritional restoration can almost always be successfully accomplished by oral feeding, and parenteral methods are rarely required. For severely underweight patients, sufficient calories (approximately 1200–1800 kcal/d) should be provided initially in divided meals as food or liquid supplements to maintain weight and to permit stabilization of fluid and electrolyte balance. Calories can then be gradually increased to achieve a

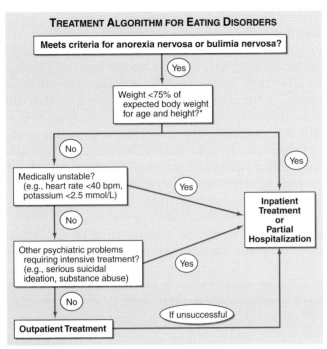

TREATMENT ALGORITHM FOR EATING DISORDERS

Meets criteria for anorexia nervosa or bulimia nervosa?

Yes

Weight <75% of expected body weight for age and height?*

No — Yes

Medically unstable? (e.g., heart rate <40 bpm, potassium <2.5 mmol/L)

Yes

No

Other psychiatric problems requiring intensive treatment? (e.g., serious suicidal ideation, substance abuse)

Yes

No

Inpatient Treatment or Partial Hospitalization

Outpatient Treatment

If unsuccessful

FIGURE 57-1

An algorithm for basic treatment decisions regarding patients with anorexia nervosa or bulimia nervosa. Based on the American Psychiatric Association's practice guidelines for the treatment of patients with eating disorders. *Although outpatient management may be considered for patients with anorexia nervosa weighing more than 75% of expected, there should be a low threshold for using more intensive interventions if the weight loss has been rapid or if current weight is <80% of expected.

weight gain of 1–2 kg (2–4 lb) per week, typically requiring an intake of 3000–4000 kcal/d. Meals must be supervised, ideally by personnel who are firm regarding the necessity of food consumption, empathic regarding the challenges entailed, and reassuring about the patient's eventual recovery. Patients have great psychological difficulty complying with the need for increased caloric consumption, and the assistance of psychiatrists or psychologists experienced in the treatment of AN is usually necessary.

Less severely affected patients may be treated in a partial hospitalization program where medical and psychiatric supervision is available and several meals can be monitored each day. Outpatient treatment may suffice for mildly ill patients. Weight must be monitored at frequent intervals, and explicit goals agreed on for weight gain, with the understanding that more intensive treatment will be required if the level of care initially employed is not successful. For younger patients, the active involvement of the family in treatment is crucial regardless of the treatment venue.

Psychiatric treatment focuses primarily on two issues. First, patients require much emotional support during the period of weight gain. Patients often intellectually agree with the need to gain weight, but strenuously resist increases in caloric intake, and often surreptitiously discard food that is provided. Second, patients must learn to base their self-esteem not on the achievement of an inappropriately low weight, but on the development of satisfying personal relationships and the attainment of reasonable academic and occupational goals. While this is often possible, some patients with AN develop other serious emotional and behavioral symptoms such as depression, self-mutilation, obsessive-compulsive behavior, and suicidal ideation. These symptoms may require additional therapeutic interventions, in the form of psychotherapy, medication, or hospitalization.

Medical complications occasionally occur during refeeding. Especially in the early stages of treatment, severely malnourished patients may develop a "refeeding syndrome" characterized by hypophosphatemia, hypomagnesemia, and cardiovascular instability. Acute gastric dilatation has been described when refeeding is rapid. As in other forms of malnutrition, fluid retention and peripheral edema may occur, but they generally do not require specific treatment in the absence of cardiac, renal, or hepatic dysfunction. Transient modest elevations in serum liver enzyme levels occasionally occur. Multivitamins should be given, and an adequate intake of vitamin D (400 IU/d) and calcium (1500 mg/d) should be provided to minimize bone loss.

No psychotropic medications are of established value in the treatment of AN; tricyclic antidepressants are contraindicated when there is prolongation of the QT_c interval. The alterations of cortisol and thyroid hormone metabolism do not require specific treatment and are corrected by weight gain. Estrogen treatment appears to have minimal impact on bone density in underweight patients, and the small benefit of bisphosphonate treatment appears to be outweighed by the potential risks of such agents in young women.

BULIMIA NERVOSA

EPIDEMIOLOGY

In women, the full syndrome of BN occurs with a lifetime prevalence of 1–3%. Variants of the disorder, such as occasional binge eating or purging, are much more common and occur in 5–10% of young women. The frequency of BN among men is less than one-tenth of that among women. The prevalence of BN increased dramatically in the early 1970s and 1980s but may have leveled off or declined somewhat in recent years.

As with AN, the etiology of BN is likely to be multifactorial. Patients who develop BN describe a higher-than-expected prevalence of childhood and parental obesity, suggesting that a predisposition toward obesity may increase vulnerability to this eating disorder. The marked increase in the number of cases of BN during the past 25 years and the rarity of BN in underdeveloped countries suggest that cultural factors are important. Several biologic abnormalities in patients with BN may perpetuate this disorder once it has begun. These include abnormalities of CNS serotonergic function, which is involved in eating behavior, and disruption of peripheral satiety mechanisms, including the release of cholecystokinin (CCK) from the small intestine.

CLINICAL FEATURES

The typical patient presenting for treatment of BN is a woman of normal weight in her mid-twenties who reports binge eating and purging 5–10 times a week for 5–10 years (Table 57-3). The disorder usually begins in late adolescence or early adulthood during or following a diet, often in association with depressed mood. The self-imposed caloric restriction leads to increased hunger and to overeating. In an attempt to avoid weight gain, the patient induces vomiting, takes laxatives or diuretics, or engages in some other form of compensatory behavior. During binges, patients with this disorder tend to consume large amounts of sweet foods with a high fat content, such as dessert items. The most frequent compensatory behaviors are self-induced vomiting and laxative abuse, but a wide variety of techniques have been described, including the omission of insulin injections by individuals with type 1 diabetes mellitus. Initially, patients may experience a sense of satisfaction that appealing food can be eaten without weight gain. However, as the disorder progresses, patients perceive diminished control over eating. Binges increase in size and frequency and are provoked by a variety of stimuli, such as transient depression, anxiety, or a sense that too much food has been consumed in a normal meal. Between binges, patients restrict caloric intake, which increases hunger and sets the stage for the next binge. Typically, patients with BN are ashamed of their behavior and endeavor to keep their disorder hidden from family and friends. Like patients with AN, those with BN place an unusual emphasis on weight and shape as a basis for their self-esteem. Many patients with BN have mild symptoms of depression. Some patients exhibit serious mood and behavioral disturbances, such as suicide attempts, sexual promiscuity, and drug and alcohol abuse. Although vomiting may be triggered initially by manual stimulation of the gag reflex, most patients with BN develop the ability to induce vomiting at will. Rarely, patients resort to the regular use of syrup of ipecac. Laxatives and diuretics are frequently taken in impressive quantities, such as 30 or 60 laxative pills on a single occasion. The resulting fluid loss produces dehydration and a feeling of emptiness but has little impact on caloric balance.

The physical abnormalities associated with BN primarily result from the purging behavior. Painless bilateral salivary gland hypertrophy (sialadenosis) may be noted. A scar or callus on the dorsum of the hand may develop due to repeated trauma from the teeth among patients who manually stimulate the gag reflex. Recurrent vomiting and the exposure of the lingual surfaces of the teeth to stomach acid lead to loss of dental enamel and eventually to chipping and erosion of the front teeth. Laboratory abnormalities are surprisingly infrequent, but hypokalemia, hypochloremia, and hyponatremia are observed occasionally. Repeated vomiting may lead to alkalosis, whereas repeated laxative abuse may produce a mild metabolic acidosis. Serum amylase may be slightly elevated due to an increase in the salivary isoenzyme.

Serious physical complications resulting from BN are rare. Oligomenorrhea and amenorrhea are more frequent than among women without eating disorders. Arrhythmias occasionally occur secondary to electrolyte disturbances. Tearing of the esophagus and rupture of the stomach have been reported and constitute life-threatening events. Some patients who chronically abuse laxatives or diuretics develop transient peripheral edema when this behavior ceases, presumably due to high levels of aldosterone secondary to persistent fluid and electrolyte depletion.

DIAGNOSIS

The critical diagnostic features of BN are repeated episodes of binge eating followed by inappropriate and abnormal behaviors aimed at avoiding weight gain (Table 57-3). The diagnosis of BN requires a candid history from the patient detailing frequent, large eating binges followed by the purposeful use of inappropriate

TABLE 57-3

DIAGNOSTIC FEATURES OF BULIMIA NERVOSA
Recurrent episodes of binge eating, which is characterized by the consumption of a large amount of food in a short period of time and a feeling that the eating is out of control.
Recurrent inappropriate behavior to compensate for the binge eating, such as self-induced vomiting.
The occurrence of both the binge eating and the inappropriate compensatory behavior at least twice weekly, on average, for 3 months.
Overconcern with body shape and weight.

Note: If the diagnostic criteria for anorexia nervosa are simultaneously met, only the diagnosis of anorexia nervosa is given.

mechanisms to avoid weight gain. Most patients with BN who present for treatment are distressed by their inability to control their eating behavior but are able to provide such details if queried in a supportive and non-judgmental fashion.

As in AN, there are two subtypes of BN. Patients with the "purging" subtype utilize compensatory behaviors that directly rid the body of calories or fluids (e.g., self-induced vomiting, laxative, or diuretic abuse), whereas those with the "nonpurging" subtype attempt to compensate for binges by fasting or by excessive exercise. Patients with the nonpurging subtype tend to be heavier and are less prone to fluid and electrolyte disturbances.

PROGNOSIS

The prognosis of BN is much more favorable than that of AN. Mortality is low, and full recovery occurs in approximately 50% of patients within 10 years. Approximately 25% of patients have persistent symptoms of BN over many years. Few patients progress from BN to AN.

℞ **Treatment:**
BULIMIA NERVOSA

BN can usually be treated on an outpatient basis (Fig. 57-1). Cognitive behavioral therapy (CBT) is a short-term (4–6 months) psychological treatment that focuses on the intense concern with shape and weight, the persistent dieting, and the binge eating and purging that characterize this disorder. Patients are directed to monitor the circumstances, thoughts, and emotions associated with binge/purge episodes, to eat regularly, and to challenge their assumptions linking weight to self-esteem. CBT produces symptomatic remission in 25–50% of patients.

Numerous double-blind, placebo-controlled trials have documented that antidepressant medications are useful in the treatment of BN but are probably somewhat less effective than CBT. Although efficacy has been established for virtually all chemical classes of antidepressants, only the selective serotonin reuptake inhibitor fluoxetine (Prozac) has been approved for use in BN by the U.S. Food

and Drug Administration. Antidepressant medications are helpful even for patients with BN who are not depressed, and the dose of fluoxetine recommended for BN (60 mg/d) is higher than that typically used to treat depression. These observations suggest that different mechanisms may underlie the utility of these medications in BN and in depression.

A subset of patients does not respond to CBT, antidepressant medication, or their combination. More intensive forms of treatment, including hospitalization, may be required.

FURTHER READINGS

AMERICAN PSYCHIATRIC ASSOCIATION: Practice guidelines for the treatment of patients with eating disorders, third edition. Am J Psychiatry, 2006

ATTIA E, WALSH BT: Behavioral management for anorexia nervosa. N Engl J Med 360:500, 2009

BECKER AE et al: Clarifying criteria for cognitive signs and symptoms for eating disorders in DSM-V. Int J Eat Disord Jul 31, 2009 [epub ahead of print]

CHAN JL, MANTZOROS CS: Role of leptin in energy-deprivation states: Normal human physiology and clinical implications for hypothalamic amenorrhoea and anorexia nervosa. Lancet 366:74, 2005

KATZMAN DK: Medical complications in adolescents with anorexia: A review of the literature. Int J Eat Disord 37(Suppl):S52, 2005

KAYE WH et al: New insights into symptoms and neurocircuit function of anorexia nervosa. Nat Rev Neurosci 10:573, 2009

KESKI-RAHKONEN A et al: Epidemiology and course of anorexia nervosa in the community. Am J Psychiatry 164:1259, 2007

KLEIN DA, WALSH BT: Eating disorders: Clinical features and pathophysiology. Physiol Behav 81:359, 2004

MEHLER PS: Clinical practice. Bulimia nervosa. N Engl J Med 349:875, 2003

SYSKO R, WALSH BT: A critical evaluation of the efficacy of self-help interventions for the treatment of bulimia nervosa and binge-eating disorder. Int J Eat Disord Oct 5 2007, epub ahead of print

THOMAS JJ et al: The relationship between eating disorder not otherwise specified (EDNOS) and officially recognized eating disorders: meta-analysis and implications for DSM. Psychol Bull 135:407, 2009

YAGER J, ANDERSEN AE: Clinical practice. Anorexia nervosa. N Engl J Med 353:1481, 2005

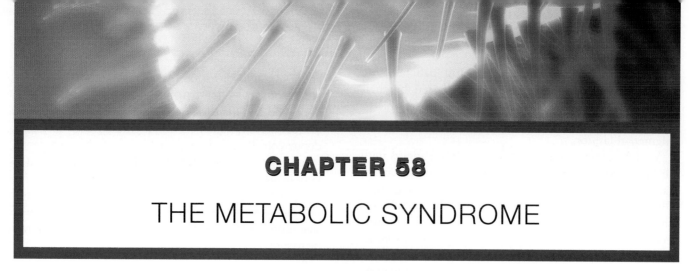

CHAPTER 58

THE METABOLIC SYNDROME

Robert H. Eckel

The metabolic syndrome (syndrome X, insulin resistance syndrome) consists of a constellation of metabolic abnormalities that confer increased risk of cardiovascular disease (CVD) and diabetes mellitus (DM). The criteria for the metabolic syndrome have evolved since the original definition by the World Health Organization in 1998, reflecting growing clinical evidence and analysis by a variety of consensus conferences and professional organizations. The major features of the metabolic syndrome include central obesity, hypertriglyceridemia, low HDL cholesterol, hyperglycemia, and hypertension (Table 58-1).

EPIDEMIOLOGY

Prevalence of the metabolic syndrome varies across the globe, in part reflecting the age and ethnicity of the populations studied and the diagnostic criteria applied. In general, the prevalence of metabolic syndrome increases with age. The highest recorded prevalence worldwide is in Native Americans, with nearly 60% of women ages 45–49 and 45% of men ages 45–49 meeting National Cholesterol Education Program, Adult Treatment Panel III (NCEP:ATPIII) criteria. In the United States, metabolic syndrome is less common in African-American men but more common in Mexican-American women. Based on data from the National Health and Nutrition Examination Survey (NHANES) III, the age-adjusted prevalence of the metabolic syndrome in the United States is 34% for men and 35% for women. In France, a 30–64–year-old cohort shows a <10% prevalence for each gender, although 17.5% are affected in the 60–64 age range. Greater industrialization worldwide is associated with rising rates of obesity, which is anticipated to dramatically increase prevalence of the metabolic syndrome, especially as the population ages. Moreover, the rising prevalence and severity of obesity in children is initiating features of the metabolic syndrome in a younger population.

The frequency distribution of the five components of the syndrome for the U.S. population (NHANES III) is summarized in Fig. 58-1. Increases in waist circumference predominate in women whereas fasting triglycerides >150 mg/dL and hypertension are more likely in men.

RISK FACTORS

Overweight/Obesity

Although the first description of the metabolic syndrome occurred in the early twentieth century, the worldwide overweight/obesity epidemic has been the driving force for more recent recognition of the syndrome. Central adiposity is a key feature of the syndrome, reflecting the fact that the syndrome's prevalence is driven by the strong relationship between waist circumference and increasing adiposity. However, despite the importance of obesity, patients who are normal weight may also be insulin-resistant and have the syndrome.

TABLE 58-1 627

NCEP:ATPIII 2001 AND IDF CRITERIA FOR THE METABOLIC SYNDROME	

NCEP:ATPIII 2001	IDF CRITERIA FOR CENTRAL ADIPOSITY[a]		
Three or More of the Following:	**Waist Circumference**		
Central obesity: Waist circumference >102 cm (M), >88 cm (F)	**Men**	**Women**	**Ethnicity**
Hypertriglyceridemia: Triglycerides ≥150 mg/dL or specific medication	≥94 cm	≥80 cm	Europid, Sub-Saharan African, Eastern & Middle Eastern
Low HDL cholesterol: <40 mg/dL and <50 mg/dL, respectively, or specific medication	≥90 cm	≥80 cm	South Asian, Chinese, and ethnic South & Central American
Hypertension: Blood pressure ≥130 mm systolic or ≥85 mm diastolic or specific medication	≥85 cm	≥90 cm	Japanese
Fasting plasma glucose ≥100 mg/dL or specific medication or previously diagnosed type 2 diabetes	**Two or More of the Following:**		
	Fasting triglycerides >150 mg/dL or specific medication		
	HDL cholesterol <40 mg/dL and <50 mg/dL for men and women, respectively, or specific medication		
	Blood pressure >130 systolic or >85 mm diastolic or previous diagnosis or specific medication		
	Fasting plasma glucose ≥100 mg/dL or previously diagnosed type 2 diabetes		

[a]In this analysis, the following thresholds for waist circumference were used: White men, ≥94 cm; African-American men, ≥94 cm; Mexican-American men, ≥90 cm; white women, ≥80 cm; African-American women, ≥80 cm; Mexican-American women, ≥80 cm. For participants whose designation was "other race—including multiracial," thresholds that were once based on Europid cut points (≥94 cm for men and ≥80 cm for women) and once based on South Asian cut points (≥90 cm for men and ≥80 cm for women) were used. For participants who were considered "other Hispanic," the IDF thresholds for ethnic South and Central Americans were used.

Note: NCEP:ATPIII, National Cholesterol Education Program, Adult Treatment Panel III; IDF, International Diabetes Foundation HDL, high-density lipoprotein.

Sedentary Lifestyle

Physical inactivity is a predictor of CVD events and related mortality. Many components of the metabolic syndrome are associated with a sedentary lifestyle, including increased adipose tissue (predominantly central); reduced HDL cholesterol; and a trend toward increased triglycerides, blood pressure, and glucose in the genetically susceptible. Compared with individuals who watched television or videos or used their computer <1 h daily, those who carried out these behaviors for >4 h daily have a twofold increased risk of the metabolic syndrome.

Aging

The metabolic syndrome affects 44% of the U.S. population older than age 50. A greater percentage of women older than age 50 have the syndrome than men. The age dependency of the syndrome's prevalence is seen in most populations around the world.

Diabetes Mellitus

DM is included in both the NCEP and International Diabetes Foundation (IDF) definitions of the metabolic syndrome. It is estimated that the large majority (~75%) of patients with type 2 diabetes or impaired glucose tolerance (IGT) have the metabolic syndrome. The presence of the metabolic syndrome in these populations relates to a higher prevalence of CVD compared to patients with type 2 diabetes or IGT without the syndrome.

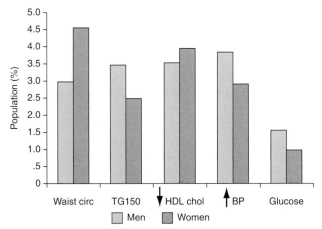

FIGURE 58-1

Prevalence of the metabolic syndrome components, from NHANES III. NHANES, National Health and Nutrition Examination Survey; TG, triglyceride; HDL, high-density lipoprotein; BP, blood pressure. *(From ES Ford et al: JAMA 287:356, 2002; with permission.)*

Coronary Heart Disease

The approximate prevalence of the metabolic syndrome in patients with coronary heart disease (CHD) is 50%, with a prevalence of 37% in patients with premature coronary artery disease (≤ age 45), particularly in women. With appropriate cardiac rehabilitation and changes in lifestyle (e.g., nutrition, physical activity, weight reduction, and, in some cases, pharmacologic agents), the prevalence of the syndrome can be reduced.

Lipodystrophy

Lipodystrophic disorders in general are associated with the metabolic syndrome. Both genetic (e.g., Berardinelli-Seip congenital lipodystrophy, Dunnigan familial partial lipodystrophy) and acquired (e.g., HIV-related lipodystrophy in patients treated with highly active antiretroviral therapy) forms of lipodystrophy may give rise to severe insulin resistance and many of the metabolic syndrome's components.

ETIOLOGY

Insulin Resistance

The most accepted and unifying hypothesis to describe the pathophysiology of the metabolic syndrome is insulin resistance, caused by an incompletely understood defect in insulin action. The onset of insulin resistance is heralded by postprandial hyperinsulinemia, followed by fasting hyperinsulinemia and, ultimately, hyperglycemia.

An early major contributor to the development of insulin resistance is an overabundance of circulating fatty acids (Fig. 58–2). Plasma albumin-bound free fatty acids (FFAs) are derived predominantly from adipose tissue triglyceride stores released by hormone-sensitive lipase. Fatty acids are also derived through the lipolysis of triglyceride-rich lipoproteins in tissues by lipoprotein lipase (LPL). Insulin mediates both antilipolysis and the

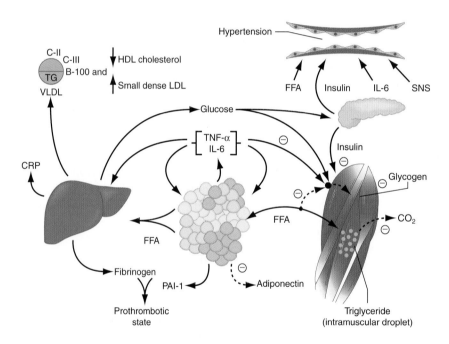

FIGURE 58-2

Pathophysiology of the metabolic syndrome. Free fatty acids (FFAs) are released in abundance from an expanded adipose tissue mass. In the liver, FFAs result in an increased production of glucose, triglycerides and secretion of very low density lipoproteins (VLDLs). Associated lipid/lipoprotein abnormalities include reductions in high-density lipoprotein (HDL) cholesterol and an increased density of low-density lipoproteins (LDLs). FFAs also reduce insulin sensitivity in muscle by inhibiting insulin-mediated glucose uptake. Associated defects include a reduction in glucose partitioning to glycogen and increased lipid accumulation in triglyceride (TG). Increases in circulating glucose, and to some extent FFA, increase pancreatic insulin secretion, resulting in hyperinsulinemia. Hyperinsulinemia may result in enhanced sodium reabsorption and increased sympathetic nervous system (SNS) activity and contribute to the hypertension, as might increased levels of circulating FFAs. The proinflammatory state is superimposed and contributory to the insulin resistance produced by excessive FFAs. The enhanced secretion of interleukin 6 (IL-6) and tumor necrosis factor α (TNF-α) produced by adipocytes and monocyte-derived macrophages results in more insulin resistance and lipolysis of adipose tissue triglyceride stores to circulating FFAs. IL-6 and other cytokines also enhance hepatic glucose production, VLDL production by the liver, and insulin resistance in muscle. Cytokines and FFAs also increase the hepatic production of fibrinogen and adipocyte production of plasminogen activator inhibitor 1 (PAI-1), resulting in a prothrombotic state. Higher levels of circulating cytokines also stimulate the hepatic production of C-reactive protein (CRP). Reduced production of the anti-inflammatory and insulin sensitizing cytokine adiponectin are also associated with the metabolic syndrome. (*Reprinted from Eckel et al., with permission from Elsevier.*)

stimulation of LPL in adipose tissue. Of note, the inhibition of lipolysis in adipose tissue is the most sensitive pathway of insulin action. Thus, when insulin resistance develops, increased lipolysis produces more fatty acids, which further decrease the antilipolytic effect of insulin. Excessive fatty acids enhance substrate availability and create insulin resistance by modifying downstream signaling. Fatty acids impair insulin-mediated glucose uptake and accumulate as triglycerides in both skeletal and cardiac muscle, whereas increased glucose production and triglyceride accumulation are seen in liver.

The oxidative stress hypothesis provides unifying theory for aging and the predisposition to the metabolic syndrome. In studies carried out in insulin-resistant subjects with obesity or type 2 diabetes, in the offspring of patients with type 2 diabetes, and in the elderly, a defect has been identified in mitochondrial oxidative phosphorylation, leading to the accumulation of triglycerides and related lipid molecules in muscle. The accumulation of lipids in muscle is associated with insulin resistance.

Increased Waist Circumference

Waist circumference is an important component of the most recent and frequently applied diagnostic criteria for the metabolic syndrome. However, measuring waist circumference does not reliably distinguish between a large waist due to increases in subcutaneous adipose tissue versus visceral fat; this distinction requires CT or MRI. With increases in visceral adipose tissue, adipose tissue-derived FFAs are directed to the liver. On the other hand, increases in abdominal subcutaneous fat release lipolysis products into the systemic circulation and avoid more direct effects on hepatic metabolism. Relative increases in visceral versus subcutaneous adipose tissue with increasing waist circumference in Asians and Asian Indians may explain the greater prevalence of the syndrome in these populations compared to African-American men in whom subcutaneous fat predominates. It is also possible that visceral fat is a marker for, but not the source of, excess postprandial FFAs in obesity.

Dyslipidemia

In general, FFA flux to the liver is associated with increased production of apoB–containing, triglyceride-rich very low density lipoproteins (VLDLs). The effect of insulin on this process is complex, but *hypertriglyceridemia* is an excellent marker of the insulin-resistant condition.

The other major lipoprotein disturbance in the metabolic syndrome is a *reduction in HDL cholesterol*. This reduction is a consequence of changes in HDL composition and metabolism. In the presence of hypertriglyceridemia, a decrease in the cholesterol content of HDL is a consequence of reduced cholesteryl ester content of the lipoprotein core in combination with cholesteryl ester

transfer protein–mediated alterations in triglyceride making the particle small and dense. This change in lipoprotein composition also results in an increased clearance of HDL from the circulation. The relationships of these changes in HDL to insulin resistance are likely indirect, occurring in concert with the changes in triglyceride-rich lipoprotein metabolism.

In addition to HDL, LDLs are also modified in composition. With fasting serum triglycerides >2.0 mM (~180 mg/dL), there is almost always a predominance of small dense LDLs. Small dense LDLs are thought to be more atherogenic. They may be toxic to the endothelium, and they are able to transit through the endothelial basement membrane and adhere to glycosaminoglycans. They also have increased susceptibility to oxidation and are selectively bound to scavenger receptors on monocyte-derived macrophages. Subjects with increased small dense LDL particles and hypertriglyceridemia also have increased cholesterol content of both VLDL1 and VLDL2 subfractions. This relatively cholesterol-rich VLDL particle may also contribute to the atherogenic risk in patients with metabolic syndrome.

Glucose Intolerance

The defects in insulin action lead to impaired suppression of glucose production by the liver and kidney and reduced glucose uptake and metabolism in insulin-sensitive tissues, i.e., muscle and adipose tissue. The relationship between impaired fasting glucose (IFG) or impaired glucose tolerance (IGT) and insulin resistance is well supported by human, nonhuman primate, and rodent studies. To compensate for defects in insulin action, insulin secretion and/or clearance must be modified to sustain euglycemia. Ultimately, this compensatory mechanism fails, usually because of defects in insulin secretion, resulting in progress from IFG and/or IGT to DM.

Hypertension

The relationship between insulin resistance and hypertension is well established. Paradoxically, under normal physiologic conditions, insulin is a vasodilator with secondary effects on sodium reabsorption in the kidney. However, in the setting of insulin resistance, the vasodilatory effect of insulin is lost, but the renal effect on sodium reabsorption is preserved. Sodium reabsorption is increased in Caucasians with the metabolic syndrome but not in Africans or Asians. Insulin also increases the activity of the sympathetic nervous system, an effect that may also be preserved in the setting of the insulin resistance. Finally, insulin resistance is characterized by pathway-specific impairment in phosphatidylinositol 3-kinase signaling. In the endothelium, this may cause an imbalance between the production of nitric oxide and secretion of endothelin-1, leading to decreased blood flow. Although these mechanisms are provocative, when insulin action is assessed by levels of fasting insulin or by the Homeostasis Model Assessment (HOMA), insulin resistance contributes only modestly to the increased prevalence of hypertension in the metabolic syndrome.

Proinflammatory Cytokines

The increases in proinflammatory cytokines, including interleukin (IL) 1, IL-6, IL-18, resistin, tumor necrosis factor (TNF) α, and C-reactive protein (CRP), reflect overproduction by the expanded adipose tissue mass (Fig. 58-2). Adipose tissue-derived macrophages may be the primary source of pro-inflammatory cytokines locally and in the systemic circulation. It remains unclear, however, how much of the insulin resistance is caused by the paracrine versus endocrine effects of these cytokines.

Adiponectin

Adiponectin is an anti-inflammatory cytokine produced exclusively by adipocytes. Adiponectin enhances insulin sensitivity and inhibits many steps in the inflammatory process. In the liver, adiponectin inhibits the expression of gluconeogenic enzymes and the rate of glucose production. In muscle, adiponectin increases glucose transport and enhances fatty acid oxidation, partially due to activation of AMP kinase. Adiponectin is reduced in the metabolic syndrome. The relative contribution of adiponectin deficiency versus overabundance of the proinflammatory cytokines remains unclear.

CLINICAL FEATURES

Symptoms and Signs

The metabolic syndrome is typically unassociated with symptoms. On physical examination, waist circumference may be expanded and blood pressure elevated. The presence of one or either of these signs should alert the clinician to search for other biochemical abnormalities that may be associated with the metabolic syndrome. Less frequently, lipoatrophy or acanthosis nigricans is found on examination. Because these physical findings are typically associated with severe insulin resistance, other components of the metabolic syndrome should be expected.

Associated Diseases

Cardiovascular Disease

The relative risk for new-onset CVD in patients with the metabolic syndrome, in the absence of diabetes, averages between 1.5- and threefold. In an 8-year follow-up of middle-aged men and women in the Framingham Offspring Study (FOS), the population attributable risk for patients with the metabolic syndrome to develop CVD was 34% in men and 16% in women. In the same

study, both the metabolic syndrome and diabetes predicted ischemic stroke with greater risk for patients with the metabolic syndrome than for diabetes alone (19% vs 7%), particularly in women (27% vs 5%). Patients with metabolic syndrome are also at increased risk for peripheral vascular disease.

Type 2 Diabetes

Overall, the risk for type 2 diabetes in patients with the metabolic syndrome is increased three- to fivefold. In the FOS's 8-year follow-up of middle-aged men and women, the population-attributable risk for developing type 2 diabetes was 62% in men and 47% in women.

Other Associated Conditions

In addition to the features specifically associated with metabolic syndrome, insulin resistance is accompanied by other metabolic alterations. These included increases in apoB and C III, uric acid, prothrombotic factors (fibrinogen, plasminogen activator inhibitor 1), serum viscosity, asymmetric dimethylarginine, homocysteine, white blood cell count, pro-inflammatory cytokines, CRP, microalbuminuria, nonalcoholic fatty liver disease (NAFLD) and/or nonalcoholic steatohepatitis (NASH), polycystic ovarian disease (PCOS), and obstructive sleep apnea (OSA).

Nonalcoholic Fatty Liver Disease

(See also Chap. 42) Fatty liver is relatively common. However, in NASH, both triglyceride accumulation and inflammation coexist. NASH is now present in 2–3% of the population in the United States and other Western countries. As the prevalence of overweight/obesity and the metabolic syndrome increases, NASH may become one of the more frequent causes of end-stage liver disease and hepatocellular carcinoma.

Hyperuricemia

Hyperuricemia reflects defects in insulin action on the renal tubular reabsorption of uric acid, whereas the increase in asymmetric dimethylarginine, an endogenous inhibitor of nitric oxide synthase, relates to endothelial dysfunction. Microalbuminuria may also be caused by altered endothelial pathophysiology in the insulin-resistant state.

Polycystic Ovary Syndrome

PCOS is highly associated with the metabolic syndrome, with a prevalence between 40 and 50%. Women with PCOS are 2–4 times more likely to have the metabolic syndrome compared to women without PCOS.

Obstructive Sleep Apnea

OSA is commonly associated with obesity, hypertension, increased circulating cytokines, IGT, and insulin resistance. With these associations, it is not surprising that the metabolic syndrome is frequently present. Moreover, when biomarkers of insulin resistance are compared between patients with OSA and weight-matched controls, insulin resistance is more severe in patients with OSA. Continuous positive airway pressure (CPAP) treatment in OSA patients improves insulin sensitivity.

DIAGNOSIS

The diagnosis of the metabolic syndrome relies on satisfying the criteria listed in Table 58-1 using tools at the bedside and in the laboratory. Because the NCEP:ATPIII and IDF criteria are similar, either can be used. The medical history should include evaluation of symptoms for OSA in all patients and PCOS in premenopausal women. Family history will help determine risk for CVD and DM. Blood pressure and waist circumference measurements provide information necessary for the diagnosis.

Laboratory Tests

Fasting lipids and glucose are needed to determine if the metabolic syndrome is present. The measurement of additional biomarkers associated with insulin resistance must be individualized. Such tests might include apo B, high-sensitivity CRP, fibrinogen, uric acid, urinary microalbumin, and liver function tests. A sleep study should be performed if symptoms of OSA are present. If PCOS is suspected based on clinical features and anovulation, testosterone, luteinizing hormone, and follicle-stimulating hormone should be measured.

℞ Treatment:
THE METABOLIC SYNDROME

LIFESTYLE (See also Chap. 56) Obesity is the driving force behind the metabolic syndrome. Thus, weight reduction is the primary approach to the disorder. With weight reduction, the improvement in insulin sensitivity is often accompanied by favorable modifications in many components of the metabolic syndrome. In general, recommendations for weight loss include a combination of caloric restriction, increased physical activity, and behavior modification. For weight reduction, caloric restriction is the most important component, whereas increases in physical activity are important for maintenance of weight loss. Some, but not all, evidence suggests that the addition of exercise to caloric restriction may promote relatively greater weight loss from the visceral depot. The tendency for weight regain after successful weight reduction underscores the need for long-lasting behavioral changes.

DIET Before prescribing a weight-loss diet, it is important to emphasize that it takes a long time for a patient to achieve an expanded fat mass; thus, the correction need not occur quickly. On the basis of ~3500 kcal = one lb of fat, ~500 kcal restriction daily equates to a weight reduction of 1 lb per week. Diets restricted in carbohydrate typically provide a rapid initial weight loss. However, after one year, the amount of weight reduction is usually unchanged. Thus, adherence to the diet is more important than which diet is chosen. Moreover, there is concern about diets enriched in saturated fat, particularly for patients at risk for CVD. Therefore, a high quality of the diet—i.e., enriched in fruits, vegetables, whole grains, lean poultry, and fish—should be encouraged to provide the maximum overall health benefit.

PHYSICAL ACTIVITY Before a physical activity recommendation is provided to patients with the metabolic syndrome, it is important to ensure that this increased activity does not incur risk. Some high-risk patients should undergo formal cardiovascular evaluation before initiating an exercise program. For the inactive participant, gradual increases in physical activity should be encouraged to enhance adherence and to avoid injury. Although increases in physical activity can lead to modest weight reduction, 60–90 min of daily activity is required to achieve this goal. Even if an overweight or obese adult is unable to achieve this level of activity, they still derive a significant health benefit from at least 30 min of moderate intensity daily activity. The caloric value of 30 min of a variety of activities can be found at *http://www.americanheart.org/presenter.jhtml?identifier=3040364*. Of note, a variety of routine activities—such as gardening, walking, and housecleaning—require moderate caloric expenditure. Thus, physical activity need not be defined solely in terms of formal exercise such as jogging, swimming, or tennis.

OBESITY (See also Chap. 56) In some patients with the metabolic syndrome, treatment options need to extend beyond lifestyle intervention. Weight-loss drugs come in two major classes: appetite suppressants and absorption inhibitors. Appetite suppressants approved by the Food and Drug Administration include phentermine (for short-term use only; 3 months) and sibutramine. Orlistat inhibits fat absorption by ~30% and is moderately effective compared to placebo (~5% weight loss). Orlistat has been shown to reduce the incidence of type 2 diabetes, an effect that was especially evident in patients with baseline IGT.

Bariatric surgery is an option for patients with the metabolic syndrome who have a body mass index (BMI) of >40 kg/m^2 or >35 kg/m^2 with comorbidities. Gastric bypass results in a dramatic weight reduction and improvement in the features of metabolic syndrome. At present, however, a survival benefit has yet to be realized.

LDL CHOLESTEROL The rationale for the NCEP: ATPIII panel to develop criteria for the metabolic syndrome was to go beyond LDL cholesterol in identifying and reducing risk for CVD. The working assumption by the panel was that LDL cholesterol goals had already been achieved, and increasing evidence supports a linear reduction in CVD events with progressive lowering of LDL cholesterol. For patients with the metabolic syndrome and diabetes, LDL cholesterol should be reduced to <100 mg/dL and perhaps further in patients with a history of CVD events. For patients with the metabolic syndrome without diabetes, the Framingham risk score may predict a 10-year CVD risk that exceeds 20%. In these subjects, LDL cholesterol should also be reduced to <100 mg/dL. With a 10-year risk of <20%, however, the targeted LDL cholesterol goal is <130 mg/dL.

Diets restricted in saturated fats (<7% of calories), trans fat (as few as possible), and cholesterol (<200 mg daily) should be applied aggressively. If LDL cholesterol remains above goal, then pharmacologic intervention is needed. Statins (HMG-CoA reductase inhibitors), which produce a 20–60% lowering of LDL cholesterol, are generally the first choice for medication intervention. Of note, for each doubling of the statin dose, there is only ~6% additional lowering of LDL cholesterol. Side effects are rare and include an increase in hepatic transaminases and/or myopathy. The cholesterol absorption inhibitor ezetimibe is well tolerated and should be the second choice. Ezetimibe typically reduces LDL cholesterol by 15–20%. The bile acid sequestrants cholestyramine and colestipol are more effective than ezetimibe but must be used with caution in patients with the metabolic syndrome because they often increase triglycerides. In general, bile sequestrants should not be administered when fasting triglycerides are >200 mg/dL. Side effects include gastrointestinal symptoms (palatability, bloating, belching, constipation, anal irritation). Nicotinic acid has modest LDL cholesterol–lowering capabilities (<20%). Fibrates are best employed to lower LDL cholesterol when both LDL cholesterol and non-triglycerides are elevated. Fenofibrate may be more effective than gemfibrozil in this group.

TRIGLYCERIDES The NCEP:ATPIII has focused on non-HDL cholesterol rather than triglycerides. However, a fasting triglyceride value of <150 mg/dL is recommended. In general, the response of fasting triglycerides relates to the amount of weight reduction achieved. A weight reduction of >10% is necessary to lower fasting triglycerides.

A fibrate (gemfibrozil or fenofibrate) is the drug of choice to lower fasting triglycerides and typically achieve a 35–50% reduction. Concomitant administration with drugs metabolized by the 3A4 cytochrome P450 system (including some statins) greatly increases the risk of myopathy. In these cases, fenofibrate may be preferable

to gemfibrozil. In the Veterans Affairs HDL Intervention Trial (VA-HIT), gemfibrozil was administered to men with known CHD and levels of HDL cholesterol <40 mg/dL. A coronary disease event and mortality benefit was experienced predominantly in men with hyperinsulinemia and/or diabetes, many of whom retrospectively had the metabolic syndrome. Of note, the amount of triglyceride lowering in the VA-HIT did not predict benefit. Although levels of LDL cholesterol did not change, a decrease in LDL particle number related to benefit. Although several additional clinical trials have been performed, these have not shown clear evidence that fibrates reduce CVD risk as a consequence of triglyceride lowering.

Other drugs that lower triglycerides include statins, nicotinic acid, and high doses of omega-3 fatty acids. When choosing a statin for this purpose, the dose must be high for the "less potent" statins (lovastatin, pravastatin, fluvastatin) or intermediate for the "more potent" statins (simvastatin, atorvastatin, rosuvastatin). The effect of nicotinic acid on fasting triglycerides is dose-related and less than fibrates (~20–40%). In patients with the metabolic syndrome and diabetes, nicotinic acid may increase fasting glucose. Omega-3 fatty acid preparations that include high doses of docosahexaenoic acid and eicosapentaenoic acid (~3.0–4.5 g daily) lower fasting triglycerides by ~40%. No interactions with fibrates or statins occur, and the main side effect is eructation with a fishy taste. This can be partially blocked by ingesting the nutraceutical after freezing. Clinical trials of nicotinic acid or high-dose omega-3 fatty acids in patients with the metabolic syndrome have not been reported.

HDL CHOLESTEROL Beyond weight reduction, there are very few lipid-modifying compounds that increase HDL cholesterol. Statins, fibrates, and bile acid sequestrants have modest effects (5–10%), and there is no effect on HDL cholesterol with ezetimibe or omega-3 fatty acids. Nicotinic acid is the only currently available drug with predictable HDL cholesterol-raising properties. The response is dose-related and can increase HDL cholesterol ~30% above baseline. There is little evidence at present that raising HDL has a benefit on CVD events independent of lowering LDL cholesterol, particularly in patients with the metabolic syndrome.

BLOOD PRESSURE The direct relationship between blood pressure and all-cause mortality has been well established, including patients with hypertension (>140/90) versus prehypertension (>120/80 but <140/90) versus individuals with normal blood pressure (<120/80). In patients with the metabolic syndrome without diabetes, the best choice for the first antihypertensive should usually be an ACE inhibitor or an angiotensin II receptor blocker, as these two classes of drugs appear to reduce the incidence of new-onset type 2 diabetes. In all patients with hypertension, a sodium-restricted diet enriched in fruits and vegetables and low-fat dairy products should be advocated. Home monitoring of blood pressure may assist in maintaining good blood pressure control.

IMPAIRED FASTING GLUCOSE In patients with the metabolic syndrome and type 2 diabetes, aggressive glycemic control may favorably modify fasting triglycerides and/or HDL cholesterol. In those patients with IFG without a diagnosis of diabetes, a lifestyle intervention that includes weight reduction, dietary fat restriction, and increased physical activity has been shown to reduce the incidence of type 2 diabetes. Metformin has also been shown to reduce the incidence of diabetes, although the effect was less than that seen with lifestyle intervention.

INSULIN RESISTANCE Several drug classes [biguanides, thiazolidinediones (TZDs)] increase insulin sensitivity. If insulin resistance is the primary pathophysiologic mechanism for the metabolic syndrome, then representative drugs in these classes should reduce its prevalence. Both metformin and TZDs enhance insulin action in the liver and suppress endogenous glucose production. TZDs, but not metformin, also improve insulin-mediated glucose uptake in muscle and adipose tissue. Benefits of both drugs have also been seen in patients with NAFLD and PCOS, and they have been shown to reduce markers of inflammation and small dense LDL. In general, the beneficial effects of TZDs appear superior to those of metformin.

FURTHER READINGS

ALBERTI KG et al: The IDF Epidemiology Task Force Consensus Group. The metabolic syndrome—a new worldwide definition. Lancet 366:1059, 2005

DUAN SZ et al: PPARs: the vasculature inflammation and hypertension. Curr Opin Nephrol Hypertens 18:128, 2009

ECKEL RH et al: The metabolic syndrome. Lancet 365:1415, 2005

EXPERT PANEL ON DETECTION EVALUATION, AND TREATMENT OF HIGH BLOOD CHOLESTEROL IN ADULTS: Executive summary of the third report of the National Cholesterol Education Program (NCEP) expert panel on detection, evaluation, and treatment of high blood cholesterol in adults (Adult Treatment Panel III). JAMA 285:2486, 2001

FORD ES: Prevalence of the metabolic syndrome defined by the International Diabetes Federation among adults in the U.S. Diabetes Care 28:2745, 2005

GRUNDY SM: Metabolic syndrome: Connecting and reconciling cardiovascular and diabetes worlds. J Am Coll Cardiol 47:1093, 2006

——— et al: Diagnosis and management of the metabolic syndrome. An American Heart Association/National Heart, Lung, and Blood Institute Scientific statement. Circulation 112:2735, 2005

KAHN R et al: The metabolic syndrome: Time for a critical appraisal. Joint statement from the American Diabetes Association and the European Association for the Study of Diabetes. Diabetes Care 28:2289, 2005

MAKYRUS AN: Treatment of hypertension in metabolic syndrome: implications of recent clinical trials. Curr Diab Rep 9:229, 2009

SAAD F, GOOREN L: The role of testosterone in the metabolic syndrome: a review. J Steroid Biochem Mol Biol 114:40, 2009

SOWERS JR et al: Narrative review: The emerging clinical implications of the role of aldosterone in the metabolic syndrome and resistant hypertension. Ann Intern Med 150:776, 2009

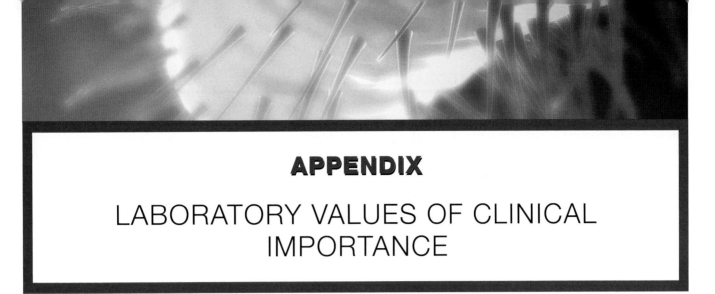

APPENDIX

LABORATORY VALUES OF CLINICAL IMPORTANCE

Alexander Kratz ■ Michael A. Pesce ■ Daniel J. Fink[†]

INTRODUCTORY COMMENTS

The following are tables of reference values for laboratory tests, special analytes, and special function tests. A variety of factors can influence reference values. Such variables include the population studied, the duration and means of specimen transport, laboratory methods and instrumentation, and even the type of container used for the collection of the specimen. The reference or "normal" ranges given in this appendix may therefore not be appropriate for all laboratories, and these values should only be used as general guidelines. Whenever possible, reference values provided by the laboratory performing the testing should be utilized in the interpretation of laboratory data. Values supplied in this Appendix reflect typical reference ranges in adults. Pediatric reference ranges may vary significantly from adult values.

In preparing the Appendix, the authors have taken into account the fact that the system of international units (SI, système international d'unités) is used in most countries and in some medical journals. However, clinical laboratories may continue to report values in "conventional" units. Therefore, both systems are provided in the Appendix. The dual system is also used in the text except for (1) those instances in which the numbers remain the same but only the terminology is changed (mmol/L for meq/L or IU/L for mIU/mL), when only the SI units are given; and (2) most pressure measurements (e.g., blood and cerebrospinal fluid pressures), when the conventional units (mmHg, mmH$_2$O) are used. In all other instances in the text the SI unit is followed by the traditional unit in parentheses.

[†]Deceased.

REFERENCE VALUES FOR LABORATORY TESTS

TABLE A-1

HEMATOLOGY AND COAGULATION

ANALYTE	SPECIMEN[a]	SI UNITS	CONVENTIONAL UNITS
Activated clotting time	WB	70–180 s	70–180 seconds
Activated protein C resistance (Factor V Leiden)	P	Not applicable	Ratio >2.1
Alpha$_2$ antiplasmin	P	0.87–1.55	87–155%
Antiphospholipid antibody panel			
PTT-LA (Lupus anticoagulant screen)	P	Negative	Negative
Platelet neutralization procedure	P	Negative	Negative
Dilute viper venom screen	P	Negative	Negative
Anticardiolipin antibody	S		
IgG		0–15 arbitrary units	0–15 GPL
IgM		0–15 arbitrary units	0–15 MPL
Antithrombin III	P		
Antigenic		220–390 mg/L	22–39 mg/dL
Functional		0.7–1.30 U/L	70–130%
Anti-Xa assay (heparin assay)	P		
Unfractionated heparin		0.3–0.7 kIU/L	0.3–0.7 IU/mL
Low-molecular-weight heparin		0.5–1.0 kIU/L	0.5–1.0 IU/mL
Danaparoid (Orgaran)		0.5–0.8 kIU/L	0.5–0.8 IU/mL
Autohemolysis test	WB	0.004–0.045	0.4%–4.50%
Autohemolysis test with glucose	WB	0.003–0.007	0.3%–0.7%
Bleeding time (adult)		<7.1 min	<7.1 min
Bone marrow: see **Table A-8**			
Clot retraction	WB	0.50–1.00/2 h	50–100%/2 h
Cryofibrinogen	P	Negative	Negative
D-Dimer	P	0.22–0.74 µg/mL	0.22–0.74 µg/mL
Differential blood count	WB		
Neutrophils		0.40–0.70	40–70%
Bands		0.0–0.05	0–5%
Lymphocytes		0.20–0.50	20–50%
Monocytes		0.04–0.08	4–8%
Eosinophils		0.0–0.06	0–6%
Basophils		0.0–0.02	0–2%
Eosinophil count	WB	150–300/µL	150–300/mm^3
Erythrocyte count	WB		
Adult males		4.30–5.60 × 10^{12}/L	4.30–5.60 × 10^6/mm^3
Adult females		4.00–5.20 × 10^{12}/L	4.00–5.20 × 10^6/mm^3
Erythrocyte life span	WB		
Normal survival		120 days	120 days
Chromium labeled, half life ($t_{1/2}$)		25–35 days	25–35 days
Erythrocyte sedimentation rate	WB		
Females		0–20 mm/h	0–20 mm/h
Males		0–15 mm/h	0–15 mm/h
Euglobulin lysis time	P	7200–14400 s	120–240 min
Factor II, prothrombin	P	0.50–1.50	50–150%
Factor V	P	0.50–1.50	50–150%
Factor VII	P	0.50–1.50	50–150%
Factor VIII	P	0.50–1.50	50–150%
Factor IX	P	0.50–1.50	50–150%
Factor X	P	0.50–1.50	50–150%
Factor XI	P	0.50–1.50	50–150%
Factor XII	P	0.50–1.50	50–150%
Factor XIII screen	P	Not applicable	Present
Factor inhibitor assay	P	<0.5 Bethesda Units	<0.5 Bethesda Units
Fibrin(ogen) degradation products	P	0–1 mg/L	0–1µg/mL

(Continued)

HEMATOLOGY AND COAGULATION

ANALYTE	SPECIMEN[a]	SI UNITS	CONVENTIONAL UNITS
Fibrinogen	P	2.33–4.96 g/L	233–496 mg/dL
Glucose-6-phosphate dehydrogenase (erythrocyte)	WB	<2400 s	<40 min
Ham's test (acid serum)	WB	Negative	Negative
Hematocrit	WB		
Adult males		0.388–0.464	38.8–46.4
Adult females		0.354–0.444	35.4–44.4
Hemoglobin			
Plasma	P	6–50 mg/L	0.6–5.0 mg/dL
Whole blood	WB		
Adult males		133–162 g/L	13.3–16.2 g/dL
Adult females		120–158 g/L	12.0–15.8 g/dL
Hemoglobin electrophoresis	WB		
Hemoglobin A		0.95–0.98	95–98%
Hemoglobin A_2		0.015–0.031	1.5–3.1%
Hemoglobin F		0–0.02	0–2.0%
Hemoglobins other than A, A_2, or F		Absent	Absent
Heparin-induced thrombocytopenia antibody	P	Negative	Negative
Joint fluid crystal	JF	Not applicable	No crystals seen
Joint fluid mucin	JF	Not applicable	Only type I mucin present
Leukocytes			
Alkaline phosphatase (LAP)	WB	0.2–1.6 μkat/L	13–100 μ/L
Count (WBC)	WB	$3.54–9.06 \times 10^9$/L	$3.54–9.06 \times 10^3$/mm^3
Mean corpuscular hemoglobin (MCH)	WB	26.7–31.9 pg/cell	26.7–31.9 pg/cell
Mean corpuscular hemoglobin concentration (MCHC)	WB	323–359 g/L	32.3–35.9 g/dL
Mean corpuscular hemoglobin of reticulocytes (CH)	WB	24–36 pg	24–36 pg
Mean corpuscular volume (MCV)	WB	79–93.3 fL	79–93.3 μm^3
Mean platelet volume (MPV)	WB	9.00–12.95 fL	9.00–12.95 μm^3
Osmotic fragility of erythrocytes	WB		
Direct		0.0035–0.0045	0.35–0.45%
Index		0.0030–0.0065	0.30–0.65%
Partial thromboplastin time, activated	P	26.3–39.4 s	26.3–39.4 s
Plasminogen	P		
Antigen		84–140 mg/L	8.4–14.0 mg/dL
Functional		0.70–1.30	70–130%
Plasminogen activator inhibitor 1	P	4–43 μg/L	4–43 ng/mL
Platelet aggregation	PRP	Not applicable	> 65% aggregation in response to adenosine diphosphate, epinephrine, collagen, ristocetin, and arachidonic acid
Platelet count	WB	$165–415 \times 10^9$/L	$165–415 \times 10^3$/mm^3
Platelet, mean volume	WB	6.4–11 fL	6.4–11.0 μm^3
Prekallikrein assay	P	0.50–1.5	50–150%
Prekallikrein screen	P		No deficiency detected
Protein C	P		
Total antigen		0.70–1.40	70–140%
Functional		0.70–1.30	70–130%
Protein S	P		
Total antigen		0.70–1.40	70–140%
Functional		0.65–1.40	65–140%
Free antigen		0.70–1.40	70–140%
Prothrombin gene mutation G20210A	WB	Not applicable	Not present
Prothrombin time	P	12.7–15.4 s	12.7–15.4 s
Protoporphyrin, free erythrocyte	WB	0.28–0.64 μmol/L of red blood cells	16–36 μg/dL of red blood cells
Red cell distribution width	WB	<0.145	<14.5%
Reptilase time	P	16–23.6 s	16–23.6 s

(Continued)

TABLE A-1 (CONTINUED)

HEMATOLOGY AND COAGULATION

ANALYTE	SPECIMEN[a]	SI UNITS	CONVENTIONAL UNITS
Reticulocyte count	WB		
Adult males		0.008–0.023 red cells	0.8–2.3% red cells
Adult females		0.008–0.020 red cells	0.8–2.0% red cells
Reticulocyte hemoglobin content	WB	>26 pg/cell	>26 pg/cell
Ristocetin cofactor (functional von Willebrand factor)	P		
Blood group O		0.75 mean of normal	75% mean of normal
Blood group A		1.05 mean of normal	105% mean of normal
Blood group B		1.15 mean of normal	115% mean of normal
Blood group AB		1.25 mean of normal	125% mean of normal
Sickle cell test	WB	Negative	Negative
Sucrose hemolysis	WB	<0.1	<10% hemolysis
Thrombin time	P	15.3–18.5 s	15.3–18.5 s
Total eosinophils	WB	150–300 × 10⁶/L	150–300/mm³
Transferrin receptor	S, P	9.6–29.6 nmol/L	9.6–29.6 nmol/L
Viscosity			
Plasma	P	1.7–2.1	1.7–2.1
Serum	S	1.4–1.8	1.4–1.8
Von Willebrand factor (vWF) antigen (factor VIII:R antigen)	P		
Blood group O		0.75 mean of normal	75% mean of normal
Blood group A		1.05 mean of normal	105% mean of normal
Blood group B		1.15 mean of normal	115% mean of normal
Blood group AB		1.25 mean of normal	125% mean of normal
Von Willebrand factor multimers	P	Normal distribution	Normal distribution
White blood cells: see "leukocytes"			

[a]P, plasma; JF, joint fluid; PRP, platelet-rich plasma; S, serum; WB, whole blood.

TABLE A-2

CLINICAL CHEMISTRY AND IMMUNOLOGY

ANALYTE	SPECIMEN[a]	SI UNITS	CONVENTIONAL UNITS
Acetoacetate	P	20–99 μmol/L	0.2–1.0 mg/dL
Adrenocorticotropin (ACTH)	P	1.3–16.7 pmol/L	6.0–76.0 pg/mL
Alanine aminotransferase (AST, SGPT)	S	0.12–0.70 μkat/L	7–41 U/L
Albumin	S		
Female		41–53 g/L	4.1–5.3 g/dL
Male		40–50 g/L	4.0–5.0 g/dL
Aldolase	S	26–138 nkat/L	1.5–8.1 U/L
Aldosterone (adult)			
Supine, normal sodium diet	S, P	55–250 pmol/L	2–9 ng/dL
Upright, normal sodium diet	S, P		2–5-fold increase over supine value
Supine, low-sodium diet	S, P		2–5-fold increase over normal sodium diet level
	U	6.38–58.25 nmol/d	2.3–21.0 μg/24 h
Alpha fetoprotein (adult)	S	0–8.5 μg/L	0–8.5 ng/mL
Alpha₁ antitrypsin	S	1.0–2.0 g/L	100–200 mg/dL
Ammonia, as NH₃	P	11–35 μmol/L	19–60 μg/dL
Amylase (method dependent)	S	0.34–1.6 μkat/L	20–96 U/L
Androstenedione (adult)	S	1.75–8.73 nmol/L	50–250 ng/dL
Angiotensin-converting enzyme (ACE)	S	0.15–1.1 μkat/L	9–67 U/L
Anion gap	S	7–16 mmol/L	7–16 mmol/L
Apo B/Apo A-1 ratio		0.35–0.98	0.35–0.98
Apolipoprotein A-1	S	1.19–2.40 g/L	119–240 mg/dL
Apolipoprotein B	S	0.52–1.63 g/L	52–163 mg/dL

(Continued)

CLINICAL CHEMISTRY AND IMMUNOLOGY

ANALYTE	SPECIMEN[a]	SI UNITS	CONVENTIONAL UNITS
Arterial blood gases			
[HCO_3^-]		22–30 mmol/L	22–30 meq/L
P_{CO_2}		4.3–6.0 kPa	32–45 mmHg
pH		7.35–7.45	7.35–7.45
P_{O_2}		9.6–13.8 kPa	72–104 mmHg
Aspartate aminotransferase (AST, SGOT)	S	0.20–0.65 μkat/L	12–38 U/L
Autoantibodies			
Anti-adrenal antibody	S	Not applicable	Negative at 1:10 dilution
Anti-double-strand (native) DNA	S	Not applicable	Negative at 1:10 dilution
Anti–glomerular basement membrane antibodies	S		
Qualitative		Negative	Negative
Quantitative		<5 kU/mL	<5 U/mL
Anti-granulocyte antibody	S	Not applicable	Negative
Anti-Jo-1 antibody	S	Not applicable	Negative
Anti-La antibody	S	Not applicable	Negative
Anti-mitochondrial antibody	S	Not applicable	Negative
Antineutrophil cytoplasmic autoantibodies, cytoplasmic (C-ANCA)	S		
Qualitative		Negative	Negative
Quantitative (antibodies to proteinase 3)		<2.8 kU/L	<2.8 kU/L
Antineutrophil cytoplasmic autoantibodies, perinuclear (P-ANCA)	S		
Qualitative		Negative	Negative
Quantitative (antibodies to myeloperoxidase)		<1.4 U/mL	<1.4 U/mL
Antinuclear antibody	S	Not applicable	Negative at 1:40
Anti–parietal cell antibody	S	Not applicable	Negative at 1:20
Anti-Ro antibody	S	Not applicable	Negative
Anti-platelet antibody	S	Not applicable	Negative
Anti-RNP antibody	S	Not applicable	Negative
Anti-Scl 70 antibody	S	Not applicable	Negative
Anti-Smith antibody	S	Not applicable	Negative
Anti-smooth-muscle antibody	S	Not applicable	Negative at 1:20
Anti-thyroglobulin	S	Not applicable	Negative
Anti-thyroid antibody	S	<0.3 kIU/L	<0.3 IU/mL
B type natriuretic peptide (BNP)	P	Age and gender specific: <167 ng/L	Age and gender specific: <167 pg/mL
Bence Jones protein, serum	S	Not applicable	None detected
Bence Jones protein, urine, qualitative	U	Not applicable	None detected in 50 × concentrated urine
Bence Jones Protein, urine, quantitative	U		
Kappa		<2.5 mg/L	<2.5 mg/dL
Lambda		<5.0 mg/L	<5.0 mg/dL
β_2-Microglobulin			
	S	<2.7 mg/L	<0.27 mg/dL
	U	<120 μg/d	<120 μg/day
Bilirubin	S		
Total		5.1–22 μmol/L	0.3–1.3 mg/dL
Direct		1.7–6.8 μmol/L	0.1–0.4 mg/dL
Indirect		3.4–15.2 μmol/L	0.2–0.9 mg/dL
C peptide (adult)	S, P	0.17–0.66 nmol/L	0.5–2.0 ng/mL
C1-esterase-inhibitor protein	S		
Antigenic		124–250 mg/L	12.4–24.5 mg/dL
Functional		Present	Present
CA 125	S	0–35 kU/L	0–35 U/mL
CA 19-9	S	0–37 kU/L	0–37 U/mL
CA 15-3	S	0–34 kU/L	0–34 U/mL
CA 27-29	S	0–40 kU/L	0–40 U/mL

(Continued)

CLINICAL CHEMISTRY AND IMMUNOLOGY

ANALYTE	SPECIMEN[a]	SI UNITS	CONVENTIONAL UNITS
Calcitonin	S		
Male		3–26 ng/L	3–26 pg/mL
Female		2–17 ng/L	2–17 pg/mL
Calcium	S	2.2–2.6 mmol/L	8.7–10.2 mg/dL
Calcium, ionized	WB	1.12–1.32 mmol/L	4.5–5.3 mg/dL
Carbon dioxide content (TCO$_2$)	P (sea level)	22–30 mmol/L	22–30 meq/L
Carboxyhemoglobin (carbon monoxide content)	WB		
Nonsmokers		0–0.04	0–4%
Smokers		0.04–0.09	4–9%
Onset of symptoms		0.15–0.20	15–20%
Loss of consciousness and death		>0.50	>50%
Carcinoembryonic antigen (CEA)	S		
Nonsmokers		0.0–3.0 µg/L	0.0–3.0 ng/mL
Smokers	S	0.0–5.0 µg/L	0.0–5.0 ng/mL
Ceruloplasmin	S	250–630 mg/L	25–63 mg/dL
Chloride	S	102–109 mmol/L	102–109 meq/L
Cholesterol: see **Table A-5**			
Cholinesterase	S	5–12 kU/L	5–12 U/mL
Complement			
C3	S	0.83–1.77 g/L	83–177 mg/dL
C4	S	0.16–0.47 g/L	16–47 mg/dL
Total hemolytic complement (CH50)	S	50–150%	50–150%
Factor B	S	0.17–0.42 g/L	17–42 mg/dL
Coproporphyrins (types I and III)	U	150–470 µmol/d	100–300 µg/d
Cortisol			
Fasting, 8 A.M.–12 noon	S	138–690 nmol/L	5–25µg/dL
12 noon–8 P.M.		138–414 nmol/L	5–15 µg/dL
8 P.M.–8 A.M.		0–276 nmol/L	0–10 µg/dL
Cortisol, free	U	55–193 nmol/24 h	20–70 µg/24 h
C-reactive protein	S	0.2–3.0 mg/L	0.2–3.0 mg/L
Creatine kinase (total)	S		
Females		0.66–4.0 µkat/L	39–238 U/L
Males		0.87–5.0 µkat/L	51–294 U/L
Creatine kinase-MB	S		
Mass		0.0–5.5 µg/L	0.0–5.5 ng/mL
Fraction of total activity (by electrophoresis)		0–0.04	0–4.0%
Creatinine	S		
Female		44–80 µmol/L	0.5–0.9 ng/mL
Male		53–106 µmol/L	0.6–1.2 ng/mL
Cryoproteins	S	Not applicable	None detected
Dehydroepiandrosterone (DHEA) (adult)			
Male	S	6.2–43.4 nmol/L	180–1250 ng/dL
Female		4.5–34.0 nmol/L	130–980 ng/dL
Dehydroepiandrosterone (DHEA) sulfate	S		
Male (adult)		100–6190 µg/L	10–619 µg/dL
Female (adult, premenopausal)		120–5350 µg/L	12–535 µg/dL
Female (adult, postmenopausal)		300–2600 µg/L	30–260 µg/dL
Deoxycorticosterone (DOC) (adult)	S	61–576 nmol/L	2–19 ng/dL
11-Deoxycortisol (adult) (compound S) (8:00 A.M.)	S	0.34–4.56 nmol/L	12–158 ng/dL
Dihydrotestosterone			
Male	S, P	1.03–2.92 nmol/L	30–85 ng/dL
Female		0.14–0.76 nmol/L	4–22 ng/dL
Dopamine	P	<475 pmol/L	<87 pg/mL
Dopamine	U	425–2610 nmol/d	65–400 µg/d
Epinephrine	P		
Supine (30 min)		<273 pmol/L	<50 pg/mL
Sitting		<328 pmol/L	<60 pg/mL
Standing (30 min)		<491 pmol/L	<90 pg/mL

CLINICAL CHEMISTRY AND IMMUNOLOGY

ANALYTE	SPECIMEN[a]	SI UNITS	CONVENTIONAL UNITS
Epinephrine	U	0–109 nmol/d	0–20 µg/d
Erythropoietin	S	4–27 U/L	4–27 U/L
Estradiol	S, P		
Female			
Menstruating:			
Follicular phase		74–532 pmol/L	<20–145 pg/mL
Mid-cycle peak		411–1626 pmol/L	112–443 pg/mL
Luteal phase		74–885 pmol/L	<20–241 pg/mL
Postmenopausal		217 pmol/L	<59 pg/mL
Male		74 pmol/L	<20 pg/mL
Estrone	S, P		
Female			
Menstruating:			
Follicular phase		55–555 pmol/L	15–150 pg/mL
Luteal phase		55–740 pmol/L	15–200 pg/mL
Postmenopausal		55–204 pmol/L	15–55 pg/mL
Male		55–240 pmol/L	15–65 pg/mL
Fatty acids, free (nonesterified)	P	<0.28–0.89 mmol/L	<8–25 mg/dL
Ferritin	S		
Female		10–150 µg/L	10–150 ng/mL
Male		29–248 µg/L	29–248 ng/mL
Follicle stimulating hormone (FSH)	S, P		
Female			
Menstruating:			
Follicular phase		3.0–20.0 IU/L	3.0–20.0 mIU/mL
Ovulatory phase		9.0–26.0 IU/L	9.0–26.0 mIU/mL
Luteal phase		1.0–12.0 IU/L	1.0–12.0 mIU/mL
Postmenopausal		18.0–153.0 IU/L	18.0–153.0 mIU/mL
Male		1.0–12.0 IU/L	1.0–12.0 mIU/mL
Free testosterone, adult			
Female	S	2.1–23.6 pmol/L	0.6–6.8 pg/mL
Male		163–847 pmol/L	47–244 pg/mL
Fructosamine	S	<285 µmol/L	<285 µmol/L
Gamma glutamyltransferase	S	0.15–0.99 µkat/L	9–58 U/L
Gastrin	S	<100 ng/L	<100 pg/mL
Glucagon	P	20–100 ng/L	20–100 pg/mL
Glucose (fasting)	P		
Normal		4.2–6.1 mmol/L	75–110 mg/dL
Impaired glucose tolerance		6.2–6.9 mmol/L	111–125 mg/dL
Diabetes mellitus		>7.0 mmol/L	>125 mg/dL
Glucose, 2 h postprandial	P	3.9–6.7 mmol/L	70–120 mg/dL
Growth hormone (resting)	S	0.5–17.0 µg/L	0.5–17.0 ng/mL
Hemoglobin A_{1c}	WB	0.04–0.06 Hb fraction	4.0–6.0%
High-density lipoprotein (HDL) (see **Table A-5**)			
Homocysteine	P	4.4–10.8 µmol/L	4.4–10.8 µmol/L
Human chorionic gonadotropin (hCG)	S		
Non-pregnant female		<5 IU/L	<5 mIU/mL
1–2 weeks postconception		9–130 IU/L	9–130 mIU/mL
2–3 weeks postconception		75–2600 IU/L	75–2600 mIU/mL
3–4 weeks postconception		850–20,800 IU/L	850–20,800 mIU/mL
4–5 weeks postconception		4000–100,200 IU/L	4000–100,200 mIU/mL
5–10 weeks postconception		11,500–289,000 IU/L	11,500–289,000 mIU/mL
10–14 weeks postconception		18,300–137,000 IU/L	18,300–137,000 mIU/mL
Second trimester		1400–53,000 IU/L	1400–53,000 mIU/mL
Third trimester		940–60,000 IU/L	940–60,000 mIU/mL
β-Hydroxybutyrate	P	0–290 µmol/L	0–3 mg/dL
5-Hydroindoleacetic acid [5-HIAA]	U	10.5–36.6 µmol/d	2–7 mg/d

(Continued)

TABLE A-2 (*CONTINUED*)

CLINICAL CHEMISTRY AND IMMUNOLOGY

ANALYTE	SPECIMEN[a]	SI UNITS	CONVENTIONAL UNITS
17-Hydroxyprogesterone (adult)	S		
Male		0.15–7.5 nmol/L	5–250 ng/dL
Female			
Follicular phase		0.6–3.0 nmol/L	20–100 ng/dL
Midcycle peak		3–7.5 nmol/L	100–250 ng/dL
Luteal phase		3–15 nmol/L	100–500 ng/dL
Postmenopausal		≤2.1 nmol/L	≤70 ng/dL
Hydroxyproline	U, 24 hour	38–500 μmol/d	38–500 μmol/d
Immunofixation	S	Not applicable	No bands detected
Immunoglobulin, quantitation (adult)			
IgA	S	0.70–3.50 g/L	70–350 mg/dL
IgD	S	0–140 mg/L	0–14 mg/dL
IgE	S	24–430 μg/L	10–179 IU/mL
IgG	S	7.0–17.0 g/L	700–1700 mg/dL
IgG_1	S	2.7–17.4 g/L	270–1740 mg/dL
IgG_2	S	0.3–6.3 g/L	30–630 mg/dL
IgG_3	S	0.13–3.2 g/L	13–320 mg/dL
IgG_4	S	0.11–6.2 g/L	11–620 mg/dL
IgM	S	0.50–3.0 g/L	50–300 mg/dL
Insulin	S, P	14.35–143.5 pmol/L	2–20 μU/mL
Iron	S	7–25 μmol/L	41–141 μg/dL
Iron-binding capacity	S	45–73 μmol/L	251–406 μg/dL
Iron-binding capacity saturation	S	0.16–0.35	16–35%
Joint fluid crystal	JF	Not applicable	No crystals seen
Joint fluid mucin	JF	Not applicable	Only type I mucin present
Ketone (acetone)	S, U	Negative	Negative
17 Ketosteroids	U	0.003–0.012 g/d	3–12 mg/d
Lactate	P, arterial	0.5–1.6 mmol/L	4.5–14.4 mg/dL
	P, venous	0.5–2.2 mmol/L	4.5–19.8 mg/dL
Lactate dehydrogenase	S	2.0–3.8 μkat/L	115–221 U/L
Lactate dehydrogenase isoenzymes	S		
Fraction 1 (of total)		0.14–0.26	14–26%
Fraction 2		0.29–0.39	29–39%
Fraction 3		0.20–0.25	20–25%
Fraction 4		0.08–0.16	8–16%
Fraction 5		0.06–0.16	6–16%
Lipase (method dependent)	S	0.51–0.73 μkat/L	3–43 U/L
Lipids: see **Table A-5**			
Lipoprotein (a)	S	0–300 mg/L	0–30 mg/dL
Low-density lipoprotein (LDL) (see **Table A-5**)			
Luteinizing hormone (LH)	S, P		
Female			
Menstruating:			
Follicular phase		2.0–15.0 U/L	2.0–15.0 U/L
Ovulatory phase		22.0–105.0 U/L	22.0–105.0 U/L
Luteal phase		0.6–19.0 U/L	0.6–19.0 U/L
Postmenopausal		16.0–64.0 U/L	16.0–64.0 U/L
Male		2.0–12.0 U/L	2.0–12.0 U/L
Magnesium	S	0.62–0.95 mmol/L	1.5–2.3 mg/dL
Metanephrine	P	<0.5 nmol/L	<100 pg/mL
Metanephrine	U	30–211 mmol/mol creatinine	53–367 μg/g creatinine
Methemoglobin	WB	0.0–0.01	0–1%
Microalbumin urine	U		
24-h urine		0.0–0.03 g/d	0–30 mg/24 h
Spot urine		0.0–0.03 g/g creatinine	0–30 μg/mg creatinine

(Continued)

CLINICAL CHEMISTRY AND IMMUNOLOGY

ANALYTE	SPECIMEN[a]	SI UNITS	CONVENTIONAL UNITS
Myoglobin	S		
Male		19–92 µg/L	19–92 µg/L
Female		12–76 µg/L	12–76 µg/L
Norepinephrine	U	89–473 nmol/d	15–80 µg/d
Norepinephrine	P		
Supine (30 min)		650–2423 pmol/L	110–410 pg/mL
Sitting		709–4019 pmol/L	120–680 pg/mL
Standing (30 min)		739–4137 pmol/L	125–700 pg/mL
N-telopeptide (cross linked), NTx	S		
Female, premenopausal		6.2–19.0 nmol BCE	6.2–19.0 nmol BCE
Male		5.4–24.2 nmol BCE	5.4–24.2 nmol BCE
Bone collagen equivalent (BCE)			
N-telopeptide (cross linked), NTx	U		
Female, premenopausal		17–94 nmol BCE/ mmol creatinine	17–94 nmol BCE/mmol creatinine
Female, postmenopausal		26–124 nmol BCE/ mmol creatinine	26–124 nmol BCE/mmol creatinine
Male		21–83 nmol BCE/ mmol creatinine	21–83 nmol BCE/mmol creatinine
Bone collagen equivalent (BCE)			
5' Nucleotidase	S	0.02–0.19 µkat/L	0–11 U/L
Osmolality	P	275–295 mOsmol/ kg serum water	275–295 mOsmol/kg serum water
	U	500–800 mOsmol/ kg water	500–800 mOsmol/kg water
Osteocalcin	S	11–50 µg/L	11–50 ng/mL
Oxygen content	WB		
Arterial (sea level)		17–21	17–21 vol%
Venous (sea level)		10–16	10–16 vol%
Oxygen percent saturation (sea level)	WB		
Arterial		0.97	94–100%
Venous, arm		0.60–0.85	60–85%
Parathyroid hormone (intact)	S	8–51 ng/L	8–51 pg/mL
Phosphatase, alkaline	S	0.56–1.63 µkat/L	33–96 U/L
Phosphorus, inorganic	S	0.81–1.4 mmol/L	2.5–4.3 mg/dL
Porphobilinogen	U	None	None
Potassium	S	3.5–5.0 mmol/L	3.5–5.0 meq/L
Prealbumin	S	170–340 mg/L	17–34 mg/dL
Progesterone	S, P		
Female			
Follicular		<3.18 nmol/mL	<1.0 ng/mL
Midluteal		9.54–63.6 nmol/L	3–20 ng/mL
Male			
Prolactin	S	0–20 µg/L	0–20 ng/mL
Prostate-specific antigen (PSA)	S		
Male			
<40 years		0.0–2.0 µg/L	0.0–2.0 ng/mL
>40 years		0.0–4.0 µg/L	0.0–4.0 ng/mL
PSA, free; in males 45–75 years, with PSA values between 4 and 20 µg/mL	S	>0.25 associated with benign prostatic hyperplasia	>25% associated with benign prostatic hyperplasia
Protein fractions	S		
Albumin		35–55 g/L	3.5–5.5 g/dL (50–60%)
Globulin		20–35 g/L	2.0–3.5 g/dL (40–50%)
Alpha$_1$		2–4 g/L	0.2–0.4 g/dL (4.2–7.2%)
Alpha$_2$		5–9 g/L	0.5–0.9 g/dL (6.8–12%)
Beta		6–11 g/L	0.6–1.1 g/dL (9.3–15%)
Gamma		7–17 g/L	0.7–1.7 g/dL (13–23%)

(Continued)

TABLE A-2 (*CONTINUED*)

CLINICAL CHEMISTRY AND IMMUNOLOGY

ANALYTE	SPECIMEN[a]	SI UNITS	CONVENTIONAL UNITS
Protein, total	S	67–86 g/L	6.7–8.6 g/dL
Pyruvate	P, arterial	40–130 μmol/L	0.35–1.14 mg/dL
	P, venous	40–130 μmol/L	0.35–1.14 mg/dL
Rheumatoid factor	S, JF	<30 kIU/L	<30 IU/mL
Serotonin	WB	0.28–1.14 μmol/L	50–200 ng/mL
Serum protein electrophoresis	S	Not applicable	Normal pattern
Sex hormone binding globulin (adult)	S		
Male		13–71 nmol/L	13–71 nmol/L
Female		18–114 nmol/L	18–114 nmol/L
Sodium	S	136–146 mmol/L	136–146 meq/L
Somatomedin-C (IGF-1) (adult)	S		
16–24 years		182–780 μg/L	182–780 ng/mL
25–39 years		114–492 μg/L	114–492 ng/mL
40–54 years		90–360 μg/L	90–360 ng/mL
>54 years		71–290 μg/L	71–290 ng/mL
Somatostatin	P	<25 ng/L	<25 pg/mL
Testosterone, total, morning sample	S		
Female		0.21–2.98 nmol/L	6–86 ng/dL
Male		9.36–37.10 nmol/L	270–1070 ng/dL
Thyroglobulin	S	0.5–53 μg/L	0.5–53 ng/mL
Thyroid-binding globulin	S	13–30 mg/L	1.3–3.0 mg/dL
Thyroid-stimulating hormone	S	0.34–4.25 mIU/L	0.34–4.25 μIU/mL
Thyroxine, free (fT_4)	S	10.3–21.9 pmol/L	0.8–1.7 ng/dL
Thyroxine, total (T_4)	S	70–151 nmol/L	5.4–11.7 μg/dL
(Free) thyroxine index	S	6.7–10.9	6.7–10.9
Transferrin	S	2.0–4.0 g/L	200–400 mg/dL
Triglycerides (see **Table A-5**)	S	0.34–2.26 mmol/L	30–200 mg/dL
Triiodothyronine, free (fT_3)	S	3.7–6.5 pmol/L	2.4–4.2 pg/mL
Triiodothyronine, total (T_3)	S	1.2–2.1 nmol/L	77–135 ng/dL
Troponin I	S		
Normal population, 99% tile		0–0.08 μg/L	0–0.08 ng/mL
Cut-off for MI		>0.4 μg/L	>0.4 ng/mL
Troponin T	S		
Normal population, 99% tile		0–0.1 μg/L	0–0.01 ng/mL
Cut-off for MI		0–0.1 μg/L	0–0.1 ng/mL
Urea nitrogen	S	2.5–7.1 mmol/L	7–20 mg/dL
Uric acid	S		
Females		0.15–0.33 μmol/L	2.5–5.6 mg/dL
Males		0.18–0.41 μmol/L	3.1–7.0 mg/dL
Urobilinogen	U	0.09–4.2 μmol/d	0.05–25 mg/24 h
Vanillylmandelic acid (VMA)	U, 24h	<30 μmol/d	<6 mg/d
Vasoactive intestinal polypeptide	P	0–60 ng/L	0–60 pg/mL

[a]P, plasma; S, serum; U, urine; WB, whole blood; JF, joint fluid.

TABLE A-3

TOXICOLOGY AND THERAPEUTIC DRUG MONITORING

DRUG	THERAPEUTIC RANGE		TOXIC LEVEL	
	SI UNITS	CONVENTIONAL UNITS	SI UNITS	CONVENTIONAL UNITS
Acetaminophen	66–199 μmol/L	10–30 μg/mL	>1320 μmol/L	>200 μg/mL
Amikacin				
Peak	34–51 μmol/L	20–30 μg/mL	>60 μmol/L	>35 μg/mL
Trough	0–17 μmol/L	0–10 μg/mL	>17 μmol/L	>10 μg/mL
Amitriptyline/Nortriptyline (Total Drug)	430–900 nmol/L	120–250 ng/mL	>1800 nmol/L	>500 ng/mL

(Continued)

TOXICOLOGY AND THERAPEUTIC DRUG MONITORING

DRUG	THERAPEUTIC RANGE		TOXIC LEVEL	
	SI UNITS	CONVENTIONAL UNITS	SI UNITS	CONVENTIONAL UNITS
Amphetamine	150–220 nmol/L	20–30 ng/mL	>1500 nmol/L	>200 ng/mL
Bromide	1.3–6.3 mmol/L	Sedation:	6.4–18.8 mmol/L	51–150 mg/dL: mild
	9.4–18.8 mmol/L	10–50 mg/dL	>18.8 mmol/L	toxicity
		Epilepsy:	>37.5 mmol/L	>150 mg/dL: Severe
		75–150 mg/dL		toxicity
				>300 mg/dL: Lethal
Carbamazepine	17–42 µmol/L	4–10 µg/mL	85 µmol/L	>20 µg/mL
Chloramphenicol				
Peak	31–62 µmol/L	10–20 µg/mL	>77 µmol/L	>25 µg/mL
Trough	15–31 µmol/L	5–10 µg/mL	>46 µmol/L	>15 µg/mL
Chlordiazepoxide	1.7–10 µmol/L	0.5–3.0 µg/mL	>17 µmol/L	>5.0 µg/mL
Clonazepam	32–240 nmol/L	10–75 ng/mL	>320 nmol/L	>100 ng/mL
Clozapine	0.6–2.1 µmol/L	200–700 ng/mL	>3.7 µmol/L	>1200 ng/mL
Cocaine			>3.3 µmol/L	>1.0 µg/mL
Codeine	43–110 nmol/mL	13–33 ng/mL	>3700 nmol/mL	>1100 ng/mL (lethal)
Cyclosporine				
Renal Transplant				
0–6 months	208–312 nmol/L	250–375 ng/mL	>312 nmol/L	>375 ng/mL
6–12 months after transplant	166–250 nmol/L	200–300 ng/mL	>250 nmol/L	>300 ng/mL
>12 months	83–125 nmol/L	100–150 ng/mL	>125 nmol/L	>150 ng/mL
Cardiac Transplant				
0–6 months	208–291 nmol/L	250–350 ng/mL	>291 nmol/L	>350 ng/mL
6–12 months after transplant	125–208 nmol/L	150–250 ng/mL	>208 nmol/L	>250 ng/mL
>12 months	83–125 nmol/L	100–150 ng/mL	>125 nmol/L	150 ng/mL
Lung Transplant				
0–6 months	250–374 nmol/L	300–450 ng/mL	>374 nmol/L	>450 ng/mL
Liver Transplant				
0–7 days	249–333 nmol/L	300–400 ng/mL	>333 nmol/L	>400 ng/mL
2–4 weeks	208–291 nmol/L	250–350 ng/mL	>291 nmol/L	>350 ng/mL
5–8 weeks	166–249 nmol/L	200–300 ng/mL	>249 nmol/L	>300 ng/mL
9–52 weeks	125–208 nmol/L	150–250 ng/mL	>208 nmol/L	>250 ng/mL
>1 year	83–166 nmol/L	100–200 ng/mL	>166 nmol/L	>200 ng/mL
Desipramine	375–1130 nmol/L	100–300 ng/mL	>1880 nmol/L	>500 ng/mL
Diazepam (and Metabolite)				
Diazepam	0.7–3.5 µmol/L	0.2–1.0 µg/mL	>7.0 µmol/L	>2.0 µg/mL
Nordazepam	0.4–6.6 µmol/L	0.1–1.8 µg/mL	>9.2 µmol/L	>2.5 µg/mL
Digoxin	0.64–2.6 nmol/L	0.5–2.0 ng/mL	>3.1 nmol/L	>2.4 ng/mL
Disopyramide	>7.4 µmol/L	2.5 µg/mL	20.6 µmol/L	>7 µg/mL
Doxepin and Nordoxepin				
Doxepin	0.36–0.98 µmol/L	101–274 ng/mL	>1.8 µmol/L	>503 ng/mL
Nordoxepin	0.38–1.04 µmol/L	106–291 ng/mL	>1.9 µmol/L	>531 ng/mL
Ethanol				
Behavioral changes			>4.3 mmol/L	>20 mg/dL
Legal limit			17 mmol/L	80 mg/dL
Critical with acute exposure			>54 mmol/L	>250 mg/dL
Ethylene Glycol				
Toxic			>2 mmol/L	>12 mg/dL
Lethal			>20 mmol/L	>120 mg/dL
Ethosuximide	280–700 µmol/L	40–100 µg/mL	>700 µmol/L	>100 µg/mL
Flecainide	0.5–2.4 µmol/L	0.2–1.0 µg/mL	>3.6 µmol/L	>1.5 µg/mL
Gentamicin				
Peak	10–21 µmol/mL	5–10 µg/mL	>25 µmol/mL	>12 µg/mL
Trough	0–4.2 µmol/mL	0–2 µg/mL	>4.2 µmol/mL	>2 µg/mL

(Continued)

TABLE A-3 (CONTINUED)

TOXICOLOGY AND THERAPEUTIC DRUG MONITORING

DRUG	THERAPEUTIC RANGE		TOXIC LEVEL	
	SI UNITS	CONVENTIONAL UNITS	SI UNITS	CONVENTIONAL UNITS
Heroin (Diacetyl Morphine)			>700 µmol/L	>200 ng/mL (as morphine)
Ibuprofen	49–243 µmol/L	10–50 µg/mL	>97 µmol/L	>200 µg/mL
Imipramine (and metabolite)				
Desimipramine	375–1130 nmol/L	100–300 ng/mL	>1880 nmol/L	>500 ng/mL
Total Imipramine+Desimipramine	563–1130 nmol/L	150–300 ng/mL	>1880 nmol/L	>500 ng/mL
Lidocaine	5.1–21.3 µmol/L	1.2–5.0 µg/mL	>38.4 µmol/L	>9.0 µg/mL
Lithium	0.5–1.3 meq/L	0.5–1.3 meq/L	>2 mmol/L	>2 meq/L
Methadone	1.3–3.2 µmol/L	0.4–1.0 µg/mL	>6.5 µmol/L	>2 µg/mL
Methamphetamine		20–30 ng/mL		0.1–1.0 µg/mL
Methanol			>6 mmol/L	>20 mg/dL
			>16 mmol/L	>50 mg/dL Severe Toxicity
			>28 mmol/L	>89 mg/dL Lethal
Methotrexate				
Low-dose	0.01–0.1 µmol/L	0.01–0.1 µmol/L	>0.1 mmol/L	>0.1 mmol/L
High-dose (24h)	<5.0 µmol/L	<5.0 µmol/L	>5.0 µmol/L	>5.0 µmol/L
High-dose (48h)	<0.50 µmol/L	<0.50 µmol/L	>0.5 µmol/L	>0.5 µmol/L
High-dose (72h)	<0.10 µmol/L	<0.10 µmol/L	>0.1 µmol/L	>0.1 µmol/L
Morphine	35–250 µmol/L	10–70 ng/mL	180–14000 µmol/L	50–4000 ng/mL
Nitroprusside (as thiocyanate)	103–499 µmol/L	6–29 µg/mL	860 µmol/L	>50 µg/mL
Nortriptyline	190–569 nmol/L	50–150 ng/mL	>1900 nmol/L	>500 ng/mL
Phenobarbital	65–172 µmol/L	15–40 µg/mL	>215 µmol/L	>50 µg/mL
Phenytoin	40–79 µmol/L	10–20 µg/mL	>118 µmol/L	>30 µg/mL
Phenytoin, Free	4.0–7.9 µg/mL	1–2 µg/mL	>13.9 µg/mL	>3.5 µg/mL
% Free	.08–.14	8–14%		
Primidone and Metabolite				
Primidone	23–55 µmol/L	5–12 µg/mL	>69 µmol/L	>15 µg/mL
Phenobarbital	65–172 µmol/L	15–40 µg/mL	>215 µmol/L	>50 µg/mL
Procainamide				
Procainamide	17–42 µmol/L	4–10 µg/mL	>51 µmol/L	>12 µg/mL
NAPA (N-acetylprocainamide)	22–72 µmol/L	6–20 µg/mL	>126 µmol/L	>35 µg/mL
Quinidine	>6.2–15.4 µmol/L	2.0–5.0 µg/mL	>31 µmol/L	>10 µg/mL
Salicylates	145–2100 µmol/L	2–29 mg/dL	>2172 µmol/L	>30 mg/dL
Sirolimus (Trough Level)				
Kidney Transplant	4.4–13.1 nmol/L	4–12 ng/mL	>16 nmol/L	>15 ng/mL
Tacrolimus (FK506) (trough)				
Kidney and Liver				
0–2 months post transplant	12–19 nmol/L	10–15 ng/mL	>25 nmol/L	>20 ng/mL
>2 months post transplant	6–12 nmol/L	5–10 ng/mL		
Heart				
0–2 months post transplant	19–25 nmol/L	15–20 ng/mL	>25 nmol/L	>20 ng/mL
3–6 months post transplant	12–19 nmol/L	10–15 ng/mL		
>6 months post transplant	10–12 nmol/L	8–10 ng/mL		
Theophylline	56–111 µg/mL	10–20 µg/mL	>140 µg/mL	>25 µg/mL
Thiocyanate				
After nitroprusside infusion	103–499 µmol/L	6–29 µg/mL	860 µmol/L	>50 µg/mL
Nonsmoker	17–69 µmol/L	1–4 µg/mL		
Smoker	52–206 µmol/L	3–12 µg/mL		
Tobramycin				
Peak	11–22 µg/L	5–10 µg/mL	>26 µg/L	>12 µg/mL
Trough	0–4.3 µg/L	0–2 µg/mL	>4.3 µg/L	>2 µg/mL
Valproic acid	350–700 µmol/L	50–100 µg/mL	>1000 µmol/L	>150 µg/mL
Vancomycin				
Peak	14–28 µmol/L	20–40 µg/mL	>55 µmol/L	>80 µg/mL
Trough	3.5–10.4 µmol/L	5–15 µg/mL	>14 µmol/L	>20 µg/mL

TABLE A-4

VITAMINS AND SELECTED TRACE MINERALS

SPECIMEN	ANALYTE[a]	REFERENCE RANGE	
		SI UNITS	CONVENTIONAL UNITS
Aluminum	S	<0.2 µmol/L	<5.41 µg/L
	U, random	0.19–1.11 µmol/L	5–30 µg/L
Arsenic	WB	0.03–0.31 µmol/L	2–23 µg/L
	U, 24 h	0.07–0.67 µmol/d	5–50 µg/d
Cadmium	WB	<44.5 nmol/L	<5.0 µg/L
Coenzyme Q10 (ubiquinone)	P	433–1532 µg/L	433–1532 µg/L
B carotene	S	0.07–1.43 µmol/L	4–77 µg/dL
Copper			
	S	11–22 µmol/L	70–140 µg/dL
	U, 24 h	<0.95 µmol/d	<60 µg/d
Folic acid	RC	340–1020 nmol/L cells	150–450 ng/mL cells
Folic acid	S	12.2–40.8 nmol/L	5.4–18.0 ng/mL
Lead (adult)	S	<0.5 µmol/L	<10 µg/dL
Mercury			
	WB	3.0–294 nmol/L	0.6–59 µg/L
	U, 24 h	<99.8 nmol/L	<20 µg/L
Selenium	S	0.8–2.0 µmol/L	63–160 µg/L
Vitamin A	S	0.7–3.5 µmol/L	20–100 µg/dL
Vitamin B$_1$ (thiamine)	S	0–75 nmol/L	0–2 µg/dL
Vitamin B$_2$ (riboflavin)	S	106–638 nmol/L	4–24 µg/dL
Vitamin B$_6$	P	20–121 nmol/L	5–30 ng/mL
Vitamin B$_{12}$	S	206–735 pmol/L	279–996 pg/mL
Vitamin C (ascorbic acid)	S	23–57 µmol/L	0.4–1.0 mg/dL
Vitamin D$_3$, 1,25-dihydroxy	S	60–108 pmol/L	25–45 pg/mL
Vitamin D$_3$, 25-hydroxy	P		
Summer		37.4–200 nmol/L	15–80 ng/mL
Winter		34.9–105 nmol/L	14–42 ng/mL
Vitamin E	S	12–42 µmol/L	5–18 µg/mL
Vitamin K	S	0.29–2.64 nmol/L	0.13–1.19 ng/mL
Zinc	S	11.5–18.4 µmol/L	75–120 µg/dL

[a]P, plasma; RC, red cells; S, serum; WB, whole blood; U, urine.

TABLE A-5

CLASSIFICATION OF LDL, TOTAL, AND HDL CHOLESTEROL

LDL Cholesterol, mg/dL (mmol/L)

<70 (<1.81)	Therapeutic option for very high risk patients
<100 (<2.59)	Optimal
100–129 (2.59–3.34)	Near optimal/above optimal
130–159 (3.36–4.11)	Borderline high
160–189 (4.14–4.89)	High
≥190 (≥4.91)	Very high

Total Cholesterol, mg/dL (mmol/L)

<200 (<5.17)	Desirable
200–239 (5.17–6.18)	Borderline high
≥240 (≥6.21)	High

HDL Cholesterol, mg/dL (mmol/L)

<40 (<1.03)	Low
≥60 (≥1.55)	High

Note: LDL, low-density lipoprotein; HDL, high-density lipoprotein

Source: Executive summary of the third report of the National Cholesterol Education Program (NCEP) expert panel on detection, evaluation, and treatment of high blood cholesterol in adults (adult treatment panel III). JAMA 285:2486, 2001; and Implications of recent clinical trials for the National Cholesterol Education Program Adult Treatment Panel III Guidelines: SM Grundy et al for the Coordinating Committee of the National Cholesterol Education Program. Circulation 110:227, 2004.

APPENDIX

Laboratory Values of Clinical Importance

TABLE A-6

CEREBROSPINAL FLUID (CSF)[a]

CONSTITUENT	REFERENCE RANGE SI UNITS	REFERENCE RANGE CONVENTIONAL UNITS
Osmolarity	292–297 mmol/kg water	292–297 mosmol/L
Electrolytes		
Sodium	137–145 mmol/L	137–145 meq/L
Potassium	2.7–3.9 mmol/L	2.7–3.9 meq/L
Calcium	1.0–1.5 mmol/L	2.1–3.0 meq/L
Magnesium	1.0–1.2 mmol/L	2.0–2.5 meq/L
Chloride	116–122 mmol/L	116–122 meq/L
CO_2 content	20–24 mmol/L	20–24 meq/L
P_{CO_2}	6–7 kPa	45–49 mmHg
pH	7.31–7.34	
Glucose	2.22–3.89 mmol/L	40–70 mg/dL
Lactate	1–2 mmol/L	10–20 mg/dL
Total protein		
Lumbar	0.15–0.5 g/L	15–50 mg/dL
Cisternal	0.15–0.25 g/L	15–25 mg/dL
Ventricular	0.06–0.15 g/L	6–15 mg/dL
Albumin	0.066–0.442 g/L	6.6–44.2 mg/dL
IgG	0.009–0.057 g/L	0.9–5.7 mg/dL
IgG index[b]	0.29–0.59	
Oligoclonal bands	<2 bands not present in matched serum sample	
Ammonia	15–47 µmol/L	25–80 µg/dL
Creatinine	44–168 µmol/L	0.5–1.9 mg/dL
Myelin basic protein	<4 µg/L	
CSF pressure		50–180 mmH$_2$O
CSF volume (adult)	~150 mL	
Red blood cells	0	0
Leukocytes		
Total	0–5 mononuclear cells per µL	0–5 mononuclear cells per mm^3
Differential		
Lymphocytes	60–70%	
Monocytes	30–50%	
Neutrophils	None	

[a]Since cerebrospinal fluid concentrations are equilibrium values, measurements of the same parameters in blood plasma obtained at the same time are recommended. However, there is a time lag in attainment of equilibrium, and cerebrospinal levels of plasma constituents that can fluctuate rapidly (such as plasma glucose) may not achieve stable values until after a significant lag phase.
[b]IgG index = CSF IgG(mg/dL) × serum albumin(g/dL)/Serum IgG(g/dL) × CSF albumin(mg/dL).

TABLE A-7

URINE ANALYSIS

	REFERENCE RANGE SI UNITS	REFERENCE RANGE CONVENTIONAL UNITS
Acidity, titratable	20–40 mmol/d	20–40 meq/d
Ammonia	30–50 mmol/d	30–50 meq/d
Amylase		4–400 U/L

(Continued)

TABLE A-7 (*CONTINUED*)

URINE ANALYSIS

	REFERENCE RANGE	
	SI UNITS	CONVENTIONAL UNITS
Amylase/creatinine clearance ratio [(Cl_{am}/Cl_{cr}) × 100]	1–5	1–5
Calcium (10 meq/d or 200 mg/d dietary calcium)	<7.5 mmol/d	<300 mg/d
Creatine, as creatinine		
Female	<760 μmol/d	<100 mg/d
Male	<380 μmol/d	<50 mg/d
Creatinine	8.8–14 mmol/d	1.0–1.6 g/d
Eosinophils	<100,000 eosinophils/L	<100 eosinophils/mL
Glucose (glucose oxidase method)	0.3–1.7 mmol/d	50–300 mg/d
5-Hydroxyindoleacetic acid (5-HIAA)	10–47 μmol/d	2–9 mg/d
Iodine, spot urine		
WHO classification		
of iodine deficiency		
Not iodine deficient	>100 μg/L	>100 μg/L
Mild iodine deficiency	50–100 μg/L	50–100 μg/L
Moderate iodine deficiency	20–49 μg/L	20–49 μg/L
Severe iodine deficiency	<20 μg/L	<20 μg/L
Microalbumin		
Normal	0.0–0.03 g/d	0–30 mg/d
Microalbuminuria	0.03–0.30 g/d	30–300 mg/d
Clinical albuminuria	>0.3 g/d	>300 mg/d
Microalbumin/creatinine ratio		
Normal	0–3.4 g/mol creatinine	0–30 μg/mg creatinine
Microalbuminuria	3.4–34 g/mol creatinine	30–300 μg/mg creatinine
Clinical albuminuria	>34 g/mol creatinine	>300 μg/mg creatinine
Oxalate		
Male	80–500 μmol/d	7–44 mg/d
Female	45–350 μmol/d	4–31 mg/d
pH	5.0–9.0	5.0–9.0
Phosphate (phosphorus) (varies with intake)	12.9–42.0 mmol/d	400–1300 mg/d
Potassium (varies with intake)	25–100 mmol/d	25–100 meq/d
Protein	<0.15 g/d	<150 mg/d
Sediment		
Red blood cells	0–2/high power field	
White blood cells	0–2/high power field	
Bacteria	None	
Crystals	None	
Bladder cells	None	
Squamous cells	None	
Tubular cells	None	
Broad casts	None	
Epithelial cell casts	None	
Granular casts	None	
Hyaline casts	0–5/low power field	
Red blood cell casts	None	
Waxy casts	None	
White cell casts	None	
Sodium (varies with intake)	100–260 mmol/d	100–260 meq/d
Specific gravity	1.001–1.035	1.001–1.035
Urea nitrogen	214–607 mmol/d	6–17 g/d
Uric acid (normal diet)	1.49–4.76 mmol/d	250–800 mg/d

Note: WHO, World Health Organization.

TABLE A-8

DIFFERENTIAL NUCLEATED CELL COUNTS OF BONE MARROW ASPIRATES[a]

	OBSERVED RANGE, %	95% CONFIDENCE INTERVALS, %	MEAN, %
Blast cells	0–3.2	0–3.0	1.4
Promyelocytes	3.6–13.2	3.2–12.4	7.8
Neutrophil myelocytes	4–21.4	3.7–10.0	7.6
Eosinophil myelocytes	0–5.0	0–2.8	1.3
Metamyelocytes	1–7.0	2.3–5.9	4.1
Neutrophils			
Males	21.0–45.6	21.9–42.3	32.1
Females	29.6–46.6	28.8–45.9	37.4
Eosinophils	0.4–4.2	0.3–4.2	2.2
Eosinophils plus eosinophil myelocytes	0.9–7.4	0.7–6.3	3.5
Basophils	0–0.8	0–0.4	0.1
Erythroblasts			
Males	18.0–39.4	16.2–40.1	28.1
Females	14.0–31.8	13.0–32.0	22.5
Lymphocytes	4.6–22.6	6.0–20.0	13.1
Plasma cells	0–1.4	0–1.2	0.6
Monocytes	0–3.2	0–2.6	1.3
Macrophages	0–1.8	0–1.3	0.4
M:E ratio			
Males	1.1–4.0	1.1–4.1	2.1
Females	1.6–5.4	1.6–5.2	2.8

[a]Based on bone marrow aspirate from 50 healthy volunteers (30 men, 20 women).
Source: From BJ Bain: The bone marrow aspirate of healthy subjects. Br J Haematol 94:206, 1996.

TABLE A-9

STOOL ANALYSIS

	REFERENCE RANGE	
	SI UNITS	CONVENTIONAL UNITS
Amount	0.1–0.2 kg/d	100–200 g/24 h
Coproporphyrin	611–1832 nmol/d	400–1200 µg/24 h
Fat		
Adult		<7 g/d
Adult on fat-free diet		<4 g/d
Fatty acids	0–21 mmol/d	0–6 g/24 h
Leukocytes	None	None
Nitrogen	<178 mmol/d	<2.5 g/24 h
pH	7.0–7.5	
Occult blood	Negative	Negative
Trypsin		20–95 U/g
Urobilinogen	85–510 µmol/d	50–300 mg/24 h
Uroporphyrins	12–48 nmol/d	10–40 µg/24 h
Water	<0.75	<75%

Source: Modified from FT Fishbach, MB Dunning III: *A Manual of Laboratory and Diagnostic Tests,* 7th ed., Lippincott Williams & Wilkins, Philadelphia, 2004.

TABLE A-10

RENAL FUNCTION TESTS

	REFERENCE RANGE	
	SI UNITS	CONVENTIONAL UNITS
Clearances (corrected to 1.72 m² body surface area)		
Measures of glomerular filtration rate		
Inulin clearance (Cl)		
Males (mean ± 1 SD)	2.1 ± 0.4 mL/s	124 ± 25.8 mL/min
Females (mean ± 1 SD)	2.0 ± 0.2 mL/s	119 ± 12.8 mL/min
Endogenous creatinine clearance	1.5–2.2 mL/s	91–130 mL/min
Measures of effective renal plasma flow and tubular function		
p-Aminohippuric acid clearance (Cl_{PAH})		
Males (mean ± 1 SD)	10.9 ± 2.7 mL/s	654 ± 163 mL/min
Females (mean ± 1 SD)	9.9 ± 1.7 mL/s	594 ± 102 mL/min
Concentration and dilution test		
Specific gravity of urine		
After 12-h fluid restriction	>1.025	>1.025
After 12-h deliberate water intake	≤1.003	≤1.003
Protein excretion, urine	<0.15 g/d	<150 mg/d
Specific gravity, maximal range	1.002–1.028	1.002–1.028
Tubular reabsorption, phosphorus	0.79–0.94 of filtered load	79–94% of filtered load

TABLE A-11

CIRCULATORY FUNCTION TESTS

TEST	RESULTS: REFERENCE RANGE	
	SI UNITS (RANGE)	CONVENTIONAL UNITS (RANGE)
Arteriovenous oxygen difference	30–50 mL/L	30–50 mL/L
Cardiac output (Fick)	2.5–3.6 L/m² of body surface area per min	2.5–3.6 L/m² of body surface area per min
Contractility indexes		
Max. left ventricular $dp/dt(dp/dt)$/DP when DP = 5.3 kPa (40 mmHg) (DP, diastolic pressure)	220 kPa/s (176–250 kPa/s) (37.6 ± 12.2)/s	1650 mmHg/s (1320–1880 mmHg/s) (37.6 ± 12.2)/s
Mean normalized systolic ejection rate (angiography)	3.32 ± 0.84 end-diastolic volumes per second	3.32 ± 0.84 end-diastolic volumes per second
Mean velocity of circumferential fiber shortening (angiography)	1.83 ± 0.56 circumferences per second	1.83 ± 0.56 circumferences per second
Ejection fraction: stroke volume/end-diastolic volume (SV/EDV)	0.67 ± 0.08 (0.55–0.78)	0.67 ± 0.08 (0.55–0.78)
End-diastolic volume	70 ± 20.0 mL/m² (60–88 mL/m²)	70 ± 20.0 mL/m² (60–88 mL/m²)
End-systolic volume	25 ± 5.0 mL/m² (20–33 mL/m²)	25 ± 5.0 mL/m² (20–33 mL/m²)
Left ventricular work		
Stroke work index	50 ± 20.0 (g•m)/m² (30–110)	50 ± 20.0 (g•m)/m² (30–110)
Left ventricular minute work index	1.8–6.6 [(kg•m)/m²]/min	1.8–6.6 [(kg•m)/m²]/min
Oxygen consumption index	110–150 mL	110–150 mL
Maximum oxygen uptake	35 mL/min (20–60 mL/min)	35 mL/min (20–60 mL/min)
Pulmonary vascular resistance	2–12 (kPa•s)/L	20–130 (dyn•s)/cm⁵
Systemic vascular resistance	77–150 (kPa•s)/L	770–1600 (dyn•s)/cm⁵

Source: E Braunwald et al: *Heart Disease,* 6th ed, Philadelphia, Saunders, 2001.

TABLE A-12

GASTROINTESTINAL TESTS

	RESULTS	
TEST	**SI UNITS**	**CONVENTIONAL UNITS**
Absorption tests		
D-Xylose: after overnight fast, 25 g xylose given in oral aqueous solution		
Urine, collected for following 5 h	25% of ingested dose	25% of ingested dose
Serum, 2 h after dose	2.0–3.5 mmol/L	30–52 mg/dL
Vitamin A: a fasting blood specimen is obtained and 200,000 units of vitamin A in oil is given orally	Serum level should rise to twice fasting level in 3–5 h	Serum level should rise to twice fasting level in 3–5 h
Bentiromide test (pancreatic function): 500 mg bentiromide (chymex) orally; *p*-aminobenzoic acid (PABA) measured		
Plasma		>3.6 (±1.1) µg/mL at 90 min
Urine	>50% recovered in 6 h	>50% recovered in 6 h
Gastric juice		
Volume		
24 h	2–3 L	2–3 L
Nocturnal	600–700 mL	600–700 mL
Basal, fasting	30–70 mL/h	30–70 mL/h
Reaction		
pH	1.6–1.8	1.6–1.8
Titratable acidity of fasting juice	4–9 µmol/s	15–35 meq/h
Acid output		
Basal		
Females (mean ± 1 SD)	0.6 ± 0.5 µmol/s	2.0 ± 1.8 meq/h
Males (mean ± 1 SD)	0.8 ± 0.6 µmol/s	3.0 ± 2.0 meq/h
Maximal (after SC histamine acid phosphate, 0.004 mg/kg body weight, and preceded by 50 mg promethazine, or after betazole, 1.7 mg/kg body weight, or pentagastrin, 6 µg/kg body weight)		
Females (mean ± 1 SD)	4.4 ± 1.4 µmol/s	16 ± 5 meq/h
Males (mean ± 1 SD)	6.4 ± 1.4 µmol/s	23 ± 5 meq/h
Basal acid output/maximal acid output ratio	≤0.6	≤0.6
Gastrin, serum	0–200 µg/L	0–200 pg/mL
Secretin test (pancreatic exocrine function): 1 unit/kg body weight, IV		
Volume (pancreatic juice) in 80 min	>2.0 mL/kg	>2.0 mL/kg
Bicarbonate concentration	>80 mmol/L	>80 meq/L
Bicarbonate output in 30 min	>10 mmol	>10 meq

TABLE A-13

NORMAL VALUES OF DOPPLER ECHOCARDIOGRAPHIC MEASUREMENTS IN ADULTS

	RANGE	**MEAN**
RVD (cm), measured at the base in apical 4-chamber view	2.6–4.3	3.5 ± 0.4
LVID (cm), measured in the parasternal long axis view	3.6–5.4	4.7 ± 0.4
Posterior LV wall thickness (cm)	0.6–1.1	0.9 ± 0.4
IVS wall thickness (cm)	0.6–1.1	0.9 ± 0.4
Left atrial dimension (cm), antero-posterior dimension	2.3–3.8	3.0 ± 0.3
Aortic root dimension (cm)	2.0–3.5	2.4 ± 0.4
Aortic cusps separation (cm)	1.5–2.6	1.9 ± 0.4
Percentage of fractional shortening	34–44%	36%
Mitral flow (m/s)	0.6–1.3	0.9
Tricuspid flow (m/s)	0.3–0.7	0.5
Pulmonary artery (m/s)	0.6–0.9	0.75
Aorta (m/s)	1.0–1.7	1.35

Note: RVD, right ventricular dimension; LVID, left ventricular internal dimension; LV, left ventricle; IVS, interventricular septum.

Source: From A Weyman: *Principles and Practice of Echocardiography,* 2d ed., Philadelphia, Lea & Febiger, 1994.

SUMMARY OF VALUES USEFUL IN PULMONARY PHYSIOLOGY

		TYPICAL VALUES	
	SYMBOL	MAN, AGE 40, 75 kg, 175 cm TALL	WOMAN, AGE 40, 60 kg, 160 cm TALL
Pulmonary Mechanics			
Spirometry—volume-time curves			
Forced vital capacity	FVC	5.1 L	3.6 L
Forced expiratory volume in 1 s	FEV_1	4.1 L	2.9 L
FEV_1/FVC	$FEV_1\%$	80%	82%
Maximal midexpiratory flow	MMF (FEF 25–27)	4.8 L/s	3.6 L/s
Maximal expiratory flow rate	MEFR (FEF 200–1200)	9.4 L/s	6.1 L/s
Spirometry—flow-volume curves			
Maximal expiratory flow at 50% of expired vital capacity	V_{max} 50 (FEF 50%)	6.1 L/s	4.6 L/s
Maximal expiratory flow at 75% of expired vital capacity	V_{max} 75 (FEF 75%)	3.1 L/s	2.5 L/s
Resistance to airflow			
Pulmonary resistance	RL (R_L)	<3.0 (cmH$_2$O/s)/L	
Airway resistance	Raw	<2.5 (cmH$_2$O/s)/L	
Specific conductance	SGaw	>0.13 cmH$_2$O/s	
Pulmonary compliance			
Static recoil pressure at total lung capacity	Pst TLC	25 ± 5 cmH$_2$O	
Compliance of lungs (static)	CL	0.2 L cmH$_2$O	
Compliance of lungs and thorax	C(L + T)	0.1 L cmH$_2$O	
Dynamic compliance of 20 breaths per minute	C dyn 20	0.25 ± 0.05 L/cmH$_2$O	
Maximal static respiratory pressures			
Maximal inspiratory pressure	MIP	>90 cmH$_2$O	>50 cmH$_2$O
Maximal expiratory pressure	MEP	>150 cmH$_2$O	>120 cmH$_2$O
Lung Volumes			
Total lung capacity	TLC	6.7 L	4.9 L
Functional residual capacity	FRC	3.7 L	2.8 L
Residual volume	RV	2.0 L	1.6 L
Inspiratory capacity	IC	3.3 L	2.3 L
Expiratory reserve volume	ERV	1.7 L	1.1 L
Vital capacity	VC	5.0 L	3.4 L
Gas Exchange (Sea Level)			
Arterial O$_2$ tension	Pa$_{O_2}$	12.7 ± 0.7 kPa (95 ± 5 mmHg)	
Arterial CO$_2$ tension	Pa$_{CO_2}$	5.3 ± 0.3 kPa (40 ± 2 mmHg)	
Arterial O$_2$ saturation	Sa$_{O_2}$	0.97 ± 0.02 (97 ± 2%)	
Arterial blood pH	pH	7.40 ± 0.02	
Arterial bicarbonate	HCO$_3^-$	24 + 2 meq/L	
Base excess	BE	0 ± 2 meq/L	
Diffusing capacity for carbon monoxide (single breath)	DL$_{CO}$	0.42 mL CO/s per mmHg (25 mL CO/min per mmHg)	
Dead space volume	V$_D$	2 mL/kg body wt	
Physiologic dead space; dead space-tidal volume ratio	V$_D$/V$_T$		
Rest		≤35% V$_T$	
Exercise		≤20% V$_T$	
Alveolar-arterial difference for O$_2$	P(A – a)$_{O_2}$	≤2.7 kPa ≤20 kPa (≤20 mmHg)	

TABLE A-15

BODY FLUIDS AND OTHER MASS DATA

	REFERENCE RANGE	
	SI UNITS	**CONVENTIONAL UNITS**
Ascitic fluid: See **Table 10-1**		
Body fluid		
Total volume (lean) of body weight	50% (in obese) to 70%	
Intracellular	0.3–0.4 of body weight	
Extracellular	0.2–0.3 of body weight	
Blood		
Total volume		
Males	69 mL per kg body weight	
Females	65 mL per kg body weight	
Plasma volume		
Males	39 mL per kg body weight	
Females	40 mL per kg body weight	
Red blood cell volume		
Males	30 mL per kg body weight	1.15–1.21 L/m^2 of body surface area
Females	25 mL per kg body weight	0.95–1.00 L/m^2 of body surface area
Body mass index	18.5–24.9 kg/m^2	18.5–24.9 kg/m^2

TABLE A-16

RADIATION-DERIVED UNITS

QUANTITY	OLD UNIT	SI UNIT	NAME FOR SI UNIT (AND ABBREVIATION)	CONVERSION
Activity	Curie (Ci)	Disintegrations per second (dps)	Becquerel (Bq)	1 Ci = 3.7 × 10^{10} Bq 1 mCi = 37 mBq 1 µCi = 0.037 MBq or 37 GBq 1 Bq = 2.703 × 10^{-11} Ci
Absorbed dose	Rad	Joule per kilogram (J/kg)	Gray (Gy)	1 Gy = 100 rad 1 rad = 0.01 Gy 1 mrad = 10^{-3} cGy
Exposure	Roentgen (R)	Coulomb per kilogram (C/kg)	—	1 C/kg = 3876 R 1 R = 2.58 × 10^{-4} C/kg 1 mR = 258 pC/kg
Dose equivalent	Rem	Joule per kilogram (J/kg)	Sievert (Sv)	1 Sv = 100 rem 1 rem = 0.01 Sv 1 mrem = 10 µSv

ACKNOWLEDGMENT

The authors acknowledge the contributions of Dr. Patrick M. Sluss, Dr. James L. Januzzi, and Dr. Kent B. Lewandrowski to this chapter in previous editions of Harrison's Principles of Internal Medicine.

FURTHER READINGS

KRATZ A et al: Case records of the Massachusetts General Hospital. Weekly clinicopathological exercises. Laboratory reference values. N Engl J Med 351:1548, 2004

LEHMAN HP, HENRY JB: SI units, in *Henry's Clinical Diagnosis and Management by Laboratory Methods*, 21st ed, RC McPherson, MR Pincus (eds). Philadelphia, Elsevier Saunders, 2007, pp 1404–1418

PESCE MA: Reference ranges for laboratory tests and procedures, in *Nelson's Textbook of Pediatrics*, 18th ed, RM Klegman et al (eds). Philadelphia, Elsevier Saunders, 2007, pp 2943–2949

SOLBERG HE: Establishment and use of reference values, in *Tietz Textbook of Clinical Chemistry and Molecular Diagnostics*, 4th ed, CA Burtis et al (eds). Philadelphia, Elsevier Saunders, 2006, pp 425–448

REVIEW AND SELF-ASSESSMENT*

Charles Wiener ■ Gerald Bloomfield ■ Cynthia D. Brown ■ Joshua Schiffer ■ Adam Spivak

QUESTIONS

DIRECTIONS: Choose the **one** best response to each question.

1. A 46-year-old man is admitted to the hospital for upper gastrointestinal (GI) bleeding. He has a known history of peptic ulcer disease, for which he takes a proton-pump inhibitor. His last admission for upper GI bleeding was 4 years ago. After fluid resuscitation, he is hemodynamically stable and his hematocrit has not changed in the past 8 h. Upper endoscopy is performed. Which of the following findings at endoscopy is most reassuring that the patient will not have a significant rebleeding episode within the next 3 days?

   A. Adherent clot on ulcer
   B. Clean-based ulcer
   C. Gastric ulcer with arteriovenous malformations
   D. Visible bleeding vessel
   E. Visible nonbleeding vessel

2. All of the following necessitate sending bacterial stool cultures in patients with diarrhea for 2 days severe enough to keep them home from work *except*

   A. age >75
   B. bloody stools
   C. dehydration
   D. recent lung transplantation
   E. temperature >38.5°C

3. All the following are causes of diarrhea *except*

   A. diabetes
   B. hypercalcemia
   C. hyperthyroidism
   D. irritable bowel syndrome
   E. metoclopramide

4. A 76-year-old man complains of frequent small stools that are not abnormally liquid or hard. There is some pain with passing the stool. He has no abdominal pain, nausea, melena, vomiting, or fever.

4. *(Continued)*
   He has approximately 8–10 bowel movements per day, which interferes with his quality of life, though there is no fecal incontinence. What is a possible diagnosis to explain his complaints?

   A. Hypothyroidism
   B. Neuromuscular disorder
   C. Proctitis
   D. Ulcerative colitis
   E. Viral gastroenteritis

5. A patient with known peptic ulcer disease presents with sudden abdominal pain to the emergency department. She is thought to have peritonitis but refuses an abdominal examination due to the discomfort caused by previous examinations. Which of the following maneuvers will provide reasonably specific evidence of peritonitis without manual palpation of the abdomen?

   A. Bowel sounds are absent on auscultation.
   B. Forced cough elicits abdominal pain.
   C. Hyperactive bowel sounds are heard on auscultation.
   D. Pain is elicited with gentle pressure at the costovertebral angle.
   E. Rectal examination reveals heme-positive stools.

6. A 46-year-old woman with a past medical history of osteoporosis presents to the hospital because of hematemesis. She reports having bright-red bloody emesis for 2 h as well as seeing "coffee-grounds" in her emesis. However, you do not witness any vomiting in the emergency department. She takes calcium, vitamin D, and alendronate. Blood pressure is 108/60 mmHg, heart rate 93 beats/min, and temperature 37.6°C. Her hematocrit is 30% (baseline 37%). You request an emergent upper endoscopy and resuscitate the patient with fluids. What is the role for immediate IV proton-pump inhibitor (PPI) therapy in this patient?

*Questions and answers were taken from Wiener C et al (eds): *Harrison's Principles of Internal Medicine Self-Assessment and Board Review*, 17th ed. New York, McGraw-Hill, 2008.

6. *(Continued)*

   A. It is contraindicated given her history of osteoporosis.

   B. It should be initiated, as this will decrease further bleeding.

   C. It should be initiated only if high-risk ulcers are identified at the time of endoscopy.

   D. It will decrease her bleeding risk, length of hospitalization, likelihood to need surgery, and overall mortality.

   E. There is no indication for immediate IV PPI therapy.

7. While waiting for endoscopy, you recheck her hematocrit 2 h later and it remains 30%. Vital signs are unchanged. You perform a gastric lavage, which returns clear fluid. Test of occult blood in the lavage is negative. What is the most appropriate intervention at this time?

   A. Perform a CT scan of the abdomen.

   B. Continue current management and plan.

   C. Perform another gastric lavage.

   D. Recheck another hematocrit in 2 h.

   E. Request psychiatric consultation for factitious bleeding.

8. A 45-year-old male says that for the last year he occasionally has regurgitated particles from food eaten several days earlier. His wife complains that his breath has been foul-smelling. He has had occasional dysphagia for solid foods. The most likely diagnosis is

   A. gastric outlet obstruction

   B. scleroderma

   C. achalasia

   D. Zenker's diverticulum

   E. diabetic gastroparesis

9. A 61-year-old male is admitted to your service for swelling of the abdomen. You detect ascites on clinical examination and perform a paracentesis. The results show a white blood cell count of 300 leukocytes/μL with 35% polymorphonuclear cells. The peritoneal albumin level is 1.2 g/dL, protein is 2.0 g/dL, and triglycerides are 320 mg/dL. Peritoneal cultures are pending. Serum albumin is 2.6 g/dL. Which of the following is the most likely diagnosis?

   A. Congestive heart failure

   B. Peritoneal tuberculosis

   C. Peritoneal carcinomatosis

   D. Chylous ascites

   E. Bacterial peritonitis

10. A 78-year-old female nursing home resident complains of rectal pain and profuse watery diarrhea for 2 days. Her nurse reports 2 weeks of constipation prior to this. A physician sent a *Clostridium difficile*

10. *(Continued)*

    stool antigen test that returned negative. What is the next step in establishing a diagnosis?

    A. Colonoscopy

    B. Digital rectal examination

    C. Repeat *C. difficile* stool antigen test

    D. Rotavirus stool antigen

    E. Stool culture

11. Which of the following is potentially associated with constipation?

    A. Colon cancer

    B. Depression

    C. Eating disorder

    D. Hypothyroidism

    E. Irritable bowel syndrome

    F. Pharmaceutical agents

    G. All of the above

12. A 62-year-old male is evaluated in the emergency department for a complaint of vomiting and inability to tolerate oral intake. These symptoms have gradually progressed from occasional episodes of emesis after meals to an extent where the patient has not been able to tolerate solid foods for the last week. He notes no significant sensation of nausea before the emesis. Instead, the patient describes vomiting partially digested foods within a half hour of eating. The patient notes no abdominal pain. He has experienced an unintentional 30-lb weight loss over 6 months. The patient has a history of diabetes mellitus that is poorly controlled, with a glycosylated hemoglobin level of 8.9%. The patient underwent partial gastrectomy for peptic ulcer disease at age 52. His only medication is insulin therapy. On physical examination the patient is cachectic with a body mass index (BMI) of 17. He has temporal wasting. The abdominal examination reveals no masses and is nontender. The bowel sounds are normoactive, and the patient's stool is hemoccult-negative. An abdominal film shows an enlarged gastric bubble with decompressed small intestinal loops. What is the most likely diagnosis?

    A. Small bowel obstruction

    B. Gastroparesis

    C. Esophageal stricture

    D. Gastric outlet obstruction

    E. Cholelithiasis

13. The patient in Question 12 undergoes upper endoscopy for further evaluation, and a large mass is seen in the fundus of the stomach. Biopsy shows gastric adenocarcinoma. All the following are risk factors for the development of this disease *except*

13. *(Continued)*
  A. atrophic gastritis
  B. alcoholism
  C. *Helicobacter pylori* infection
  D. high consumption of salted and smoked food
  E. juvenile hamartomatous polyps

14. All of the following statements regarding fat malabsorption are true *except*

  A. 90% of pancreatic exocrine function must be lost before malabsorption ensues.
  B. Celiac disease is a commonly overlooked cause of nonspecific, gastrointestinal symptoms and fat malabsorption.
  C. Nutritional deficiencies are uncommon.
  D. Steatorrhea is formally established with >7 g of fat in stool over 24 h.
  E. Symptoms include greasy, foul-smelling stools that are difficult to flush.

15. What is the most common cause of chronic secretory diarrhea in the United States?

  A. Carcinoid tumor
  B. Crohn's disease with ileitis
  C. Lactose intolerance
  D. Lymphocytic colitis
  E. Medications

16. All the following are causes of bloody diarrhea *except*

  A. *Campylobacter*
  B. *Cryptosporidia*
  C. *Escherichia coli*
  D. *Entamoeba*
  E. *Shigella*

17. One week after removal of a biliary mass, a patient still has an elevated total bilirubin. The patient is recovering well and imaging of the hepatobiliary system shows no remaining pathology. The conjugated bilirubin is decreasing but remains elevated out of proportion to the patient's recovery. What is the best explanation for this finding?

  A. Bilirubin bound to albumin
  B. Gilbert's syndrome
  C. Hibernating hepatocytes
  D. Incomplete resection
  E. Occult hemolysis

18. Which of the following statements regarding bilirubin metabolism is true?

18. *(Continued)*
  A. Bacterial β-glucuronidases unconjugate the conjugated bilirubin that reaches the distal ileum.
  B. Bilirubin solubilizes in the serum after conversion from biliverdin in the reticuloendothelial system.
  C. Conjugated bilirubin is passively transported into the bile canalicular system.
  D. Glutathione S-transferase B facilitates conjugated bilirubin's transport into the bile canalicular system.
  E. Most bilirubin that reaches the terminal ileum is reabsorbed as urobilinogen.

19. A patient with alcoholic cirrhosis has increasing ascites despite dietary sodium control and diuretics. A paracentesis shows clear, turbid fluid. There are 2300 white blood cells (WBCs) and 150 red blood cells per microliter. The WBC differential shows 75% lymphocytes. Fluid protein is 3.2 g/dL and the serum-ascites albumin gradient (SAAG) is 1.0 g/dL. What is the most appropriate next study in this patient's management?

  A. Adenosine deaminase activity of the ascitic fluid
  B. CT scan of the liver
  C. Peritoneal biopsy
  D. None; consider transplant evaluation

20. A 24-year-old patient is admitted to the intensive care unit with obtundation and jaundice over 1–2 days. No further history is available. The following laboratory findings are obtained:

Total bilirubin 7.2 mg/dL
Direct bilirubin 4.0 mg/dL
AST: 1478 U/L
ALT: 1056 U/L
Alkaline phosphatase: 132 U/L
INR: 3.1
Albumin: 3.6 g/dL

All of the following tests are indicated *except*

  A. antinuclear antibody (ANA)
  B. ceruloplasmin
  C. endoscopic retrograde cholangiopancreatography (ERCP)
  D. hepatitis B surface antigen
  E. toxicology screen

21. A defect in which of the following bilirubin metabolic processes will give rise to bilirubinuria?

  A. Conjugation of bilirubin to glucuronic acid
  B. Conversion of biliverdin to bilirubin
  C. Transport of conjugated bilirubin into bile canaliculi
  D. Transport of unconjugated bilirubin into hepatocytes

22. The differential diagnosis of an isolated unconjugated (indirect) hyperbilirubinemia is limited. In a patient with isolated unconjugated hyperbilirubinemia, which of these historic findings would be unlikely?

    A. Calcium bilirubinate gallstones
    B. Cryoglobulinemia
    C. History of gout
    D. Spherocytosis
    E. Recurrent long-bone pain crises

23. In a patient with ascites, which of the following physical examination findings suggests a superior vena cava obstruction instead of intrinsic hepatic cirrhosis?

    A. Bulging flanks
    B. Collateral venous flow downward toward the umbilicus
    C. Everted umbilicus
    D. Pulsatile liver
    E. Venous hum at the umbilicus

24. All of the following physical examination clues are helpful for differentiating jaundice caused by hyperbilirubinemia from other causes *except*

    A. greenish discoloration of the skin
    B. involvement of the nasolabial folds
    C. predominant involvement of palms, soles, and forehead
    D. sparing of non-sun-exposed areas of the body
    E. sparing of the sclera

25. When evaluating a patient with chronic ascites, a high (>1.1 g/dL) serum–ascites albumin gradient (SAAG) is consistent with all of the following diagnoses *except*

    A. cirrhosis
    B. congestive heart failure
    C. constrictive pericarditis
    D. hepatic vein thrombosis
    E. nephrosis

26. A 42-year-old man with a history of end-stage renal disease is on hemodialysis and has been taking a medication chronically for nausea and vomiting. Over the past week he has developed new-onset involuntary lip smacking, grimacing, and tongue protrusion. This side effect is most likely due to which of the following antiemetics?

    A. Erythromycin
    B. Methylprednisolone
    C. Ondansetron
    D. Prochlorperazine
    E. Scopolamine

27. A 54-year-old male patient of yours presents to your clinic complaining of unexplained weight loss. On review of his chart, you do notice that he has lost 8% of his total body weight in the past year. He has well-treated hypertension for which he takes a thiazide diuretic. Other than recently being widowed, he has no pertinent social history. He is a lifelong nonsmoker and worked as a hospital administrator. An extensive review of systems is unrevealing. Your physical examination reveals no masses or other pathology. A brief psychiatric examination shows no signs of depression. You perform initial testing with a complete blood count; electrolytes, renal function, liver function, urinalysis, thyroid-stimulating hormone, and a chest x-ray, which are unrevealing. He is up to date on his routine cancer screening. What is the next step in the workup of this patient?

    A. Chest CT scan
    B. Close follow-up
    C. Positron emission tomography (PET) scan
    D. Total-body CT scan
    E. Upper endoscopy

28. A 22-year old woman presents to the emergency department with abdominal pain and malaise. Her symptoms began about 8 h prior to presentation, and she has no diarrhea. The pain is mostly in the right flank currently but began in the periumbilical area. She has nausea and vomiting. Temperature is 100.3°C, blood pressure 129/90 mmHg, heart rate 101 beats/min. Physical examination shows only mild diffuse abdominal tenderness. The abdomen is soft and bowel sounds are diminished. She is tender in the right flank without costovertebral angle tenderness. The genitourinary and pelvic examinations are normal. White blood cell count is 10,000/μL. Urine analysis shows 2 white blood cells per high powered field, no epithelial cells, and 1 red blood cell per high powered field. A serum pregnancy test is negative. She has no past medical history and has never had similar symptoms. She is not sexually active. Which of the following is the most likely diagnosis?

    A. Abdominal aortic aneurysm rupture
    B. Acute appendicitis
    C. Pyelonephritis
    D. Mesenteric lymphadenitis
    E. Pelvic inflammatory disease

29. While doing rounds in the intensive care unit, you see a 70-year-old male patient with multisystem organ failure who is postoperative day 3. Review of his history reveals that he had a perforated appendix

29. *(Continued)*

due to a delay in the diagnosis of acute appendicitis. Prior to his surgical intervention, he was noted to be delirious. His preoperative laboratory results showed: sodium, 133 meq/dL, potassium, 5.2 meq/dL, chloride, 98 meq/dL, bicarbonate, 14 meq/dL, blood urea nitrogen 85 mg/dL, creatinine, 3.2 mg/dL. Urine analysis had no red cells, white cells, and trace protein. An electrocardiogram showed ST-segment depression in an area of an old myocardial infarct. Preoperative troponin I level was 0.09 mg/dL. He had no history of chronic renal insufficiency. What is the most likely etiology of this patient's renal failure?

A. Acute interstitial nephritis
B. Congestive heart failure
C. Glomerulonephritis
D. Ureteral injury
E. Volume depletion

30. A 28-year-old man is admitted to the hospital with a large perianal abscess. He is taken to the operating room for incision and drainage, which he tolerates well, and he is discharged home with a 2-week course of antibiotics. He returns to the hospital 2 months later for a rash on his shins. On examination, he has discrete red swollen nodules on both of his shins without fluctuance. They measure ~2 cm in diameter. He has no respiratory complaints, and the rest of his skin examination is normal. Laboratory data show a white blood cell count of 12,000 with a normal differential. Erythrocyte sedimentation rate is 64 mm/h. A chest radiograph is normal. Thyroid-stimulating hormone is 3.27 mU/L, and a glycosylated hemoglobin is 5.3%. Which of the following conditions is he also likely to have?

A. Giant cell arteritis
B. *Pneumocystis jirovecii* pneumonia
C. Sarcoidosis
D. Type 1 diabetes
E. Uveitis

31. A male patient with inflammatory bowel disease (IBD) comes to your office as a new patient. Reviewing the medical records, you note that he has had primarily rectal disease. Macroscopic photographs from his most recent colonoscopy show a lumpy, bumpy, hemorrhagic mucosa with ulcerations. Histology shows a process that is limited to the mucosa, with the deep layers unaffected. There are crypt abscesses. Which historic feature would be surprising in a patient with this form of IBD?

31. *(Continued)*

A. Age 15–30
B. Current smoker
C. Fraternal twin sister does not have IBD
D. Identical twin brother does not have IBD
E. Intact appendix

32. A 26-year-old male presents with persistent perianal pain for 2 months that is worse with defecation. The patient notes that he occasionally sees small amounts of red blood on the toilet tissue. He never has had blood staining the toilet bowl. He reports persistent constipation but has not had any incontinence. He denies anal trauma. On physical examination there is a linear ulceration with raised edges with a skin tag at the distal end. Circular fibers of the hypertrophied internal sphincter are visible. What is the most appropriate treatment of this disease?

A. Sitz baths
B. Placement of a mechanical loop followed by surgical resection
C. Steroid enemas
D. Nitroglycerin ointment
E. Mesalamine enemas

33. Which of the following proteins does not cause secretion of gastric acid?

A. Acetylcholine
B. Caffeine
C. Gastrin
D. Histamine
E. Somatostatin

34. A 62-year-old female has a 3-month history of diffuse crampy abdominal pain and watery diarrhea and has lost 14 lb over this period. There is no prior history of abdominal or gynecologic disease. She is on no regular medications, is a nonsmoker, and does not consume alcohol. Colonoscopy reveals normal colonic mucosa. Biopsies of the colon reveal inflammation with extensive subepithelial collagen deposition and lymphocytic infiltration of the epithelium. Which of the following is the most likely diagnosis?

A. Collagenous colitis
B. Crohn's disease
C. Ischemic colitis
D. Lymphocytic colitis
E. Ulcerative colitis

35. A 57-year-old man with peptic ulcer disease experiences transient improvement with *Helicobacter*

35. *(Continued)*

pylori eradication. However, 3 months later, symptoms recur despite acid-suppressing therapy. He does not take nonsteroidal anti-inflammatory agents. Stool analysis for *H. pylori* antigen is negative. Upper GI endoscopy reveals prominent gastric folds together with the persistent ulceration in the duodenal bulb previously detected and the beginning of a new ulceration 4 cm proximal to the initial ulcer. Fasting gastrin levels are elevated and basal acid secretion is 15 meq/h. What is the best test to perform to make the diagnosis?

A. No additional testing is necessary.
B. Blood sampling for gastrin levels following a meal.
C. Blood sampling for gastrin levels following secretin administration.
D. Endoscopic ultrasonography of the pancreas.
E. Genetic testing for mutations in the MEN1 gene.

36. A 29-year-old woman comes to see you in clinic because of abdominal discomfort. She feels abdominal discomfort on most days of the week, and the pain varies in location and intensity. She notes constipation as well as diarrhea, but diarrhea predominates. In comparison to 6 months ago, she has more bloating and flatulence than she has had before. She identifies eating and stress as aggravating factors, and her pain is relieved by defecation. You suspect irritable bowel syndrome (IBS). Laboratory data include white blood cell (WBC) count 8000/μL, hematocrit 32%, platelets 210,000/μL, and erythrocyte sedimentation rate (ESR) of 44 mm/h. Stool studies show the presence of lactoferrin but no blood. Which intervention is appropriate at this time?

A. Antidepressants
B. Ciprofloxacin
C. Colonoscopy
D. Reassurance and patient counseling
E. Stool bulking agents

37. After a careful history and physical and a cost-effective workup, you have diagnosed your patient with IBS. What other condition would you expect to find in this patient?

A. Abnormal brain anatomy
B. Autoimmune disease
C. History of sexually transmitted diseases
D. Hypersensitivity to peripheral stimuli
E. Psychiatric diagnosis

38. A 42-year-old male presents for evaluation of recurrent sharp substernal chest pain that occurs primarily at rest and radiates to both arms and the

38. *(Continued)*

sides of the chest. He notes that the pain is worse with eating and emotional stress. The pain lasts approximately 10 min before resolving entirely. He has undergone a full cardiac evaluation, including negative exercise echocardiography for inducible ischemia. You suspect diffuse esophageal spasm and order a barium swallow for further evaluation. Which of the following findings would best correlate with your suspected diagnosis?

A. Proximal esophageal dilatation with tapered beak-like appearance distally near the gastroesophageal junction
B. Uncoordinated distal esophageal contractions resulting in a corkscrew appearance of the esophagus
C. Dilation of the esophagus with loss of peristaltic contractions in the middle and distal portions of the esophagus
D. Reflux of barium back into the distal portion of the esophagus
E. A tapered narrowing in the distal esophagus with an apple core–like lesion

39. A 38-year-old male presents to his physician with 4–6 months of weight loss and joint complaints. He reports that his appetite is good, but he has had diarrhea with six to eight loose, foul-smelling stools each day. He has also had migratory pain in the knees and shoulders. Stool studies demonstrate steatorrhea. Which of the following diagnostic tests is most likely to be positive in this patient?

A. Serum IgA antiendomysial antibodies
B. Serum IgA antigliadin antibodies
C. Serum PCR for *Tropheryma whippelii*
D. Small bowel biopsy showing reduced villous height and crypt hyperplasia
E. Stool *Clostridium difficile* toxin

40. Inflammatory bowel disease (IBD) may be caused by exogenous factors. Gastrointestinal flora may promote an inflammatory response or may inhibit inflammation. Probiotics have been used to treat IBD. Which of the following organisms has been used in the treatment of IBD?

A. *Campylobacter* spp.
B. *Clostridium difficile*
C. *Escherichia* spp.
D. *Lactobacillus* spp.
E. *Shigella* spp.

41. A 24-year-old woman with a history of irritable bowel syndrome (IBS) has been treated with loperamide, psyllium, and imipramine. Because of

41. *(Continued)*

continued abdominal pain, bloating, and alternating constipation/diarrhea, she is started on alosetron, 0.5 mg bid. Five days later she is brought to the emergency department with severe abdominal pain. On examination she is in severe discomfort. Her temperature is 39°C, blood pressure 90/55 mmHg, heart rate 115 beats/min, respiratory rate 22 breaths/min, and oxygen saturation normal. Abdominal examination is notable for hypoactive bowel sounds, diffuse tenderness, and guarding without rebound tenderness. Her stool is heme positive. Laboratory studies are notable for a white blood cell count of 15,800 with a left shift and a slight anion gap metabolic acidosis. Which of the following is the most likely diagnosis?

A. Appendicitis
B. *Clostridium difficile* colitis
C. Crohn's disease
D. Ischemic colitis
E. Perforated duodenal ulcer

42. An 88-year-old woman is brought to your clinic by her family because she has become increasingly socially withdrawn. The patient lives alone and has been reluctant to visit or be visited by her family. Family members, including seven children, also note a foul odor in her apartment and on her person. She has not had any weight loss. Alone in the examining room, she only complains of hemorrhoids. On mental status examination, she does have signs of depression. Which of the following interventions is most appropriate at this time?

A. Head CT scan
B. Initiate treatment with an antidepressant medication
C. Physical examination including genitourinary and rectal examination
D. Screening for occult malignancy
E. Serum thyroid-stimulating hormone

43. Your 33-year-old patient with Crohn's disease (CD) has had a disappointing disease response to glucocorticoids and 5-ASA agents. He is interested in steroid-sparing agents. He has no liver or renal disease. You prescribe once-weekly methotrexate injections. In addition to monitoring hepatic function and complete blood count, what other complication of methotrexate therapy do you advise the patient of?

A. Disseminated histoplasmosis
B. Lymphoma
C. Pancreatitis
D. Pneumonitis
E. Primary sclerosing cholangitis

44. A 23-year-old Turkish female presents to the emergency department for evaluation of acute abdominal pain. She reports that she has had multiple episodes of severe abdominal pain since age 15. These episodes have been very severe, once prompting exploratory laparotomy at age 18 with removal of the appendix, which was histologically benign. She reports that the pain lasts approximately 2 or 3 days and then resolves entirely without intervention. There are no clear triggers for the pain. Past evaluation has included normal upper and lower endoscopy, normal small bowel series, and multiple CT scans that have shown only small amounts of free fluid in the abdominal cavity. In addition, the patient recently developed a migratory arthritis affecting her knees and ankles. The patient is currently on no medications. Multiple other family members have similar complaints. On physical examination the patient appears in moderate distress, lying very still. Temperature is 39.8°C (103.6°F), heart rate is 130, and blood pressure is 112/66. She has evidence of a pleural effusion on the right with decreased breath sounds and dullness to percussion of half the lung field. She has a regular tachycardia without murmurs. Bowel sounds are hypoactive, and there is moderate diffuse abdominal tenderness. There is mild rebound tenderness diffusely throughout the abdomen without guarding. Her left knee is swollen and erythematous with an effusion. Laboratory studies show a white blood cell count of 15,300/mm^3 (90% neutrophils). Erythrocyte sedimentation rate is 110 s. Arthrocentesis reveals a white blood cell count of 68,000 with 98% neutrophils. Culture is negative at 1 week. The patient's symptoms resolve over the course of 72 h. What is the best therapy for prevention of the patient's symptoms?

A. Azathioprine
B. Colchicine
C. Hemin
D. Indomethacin
E. Prednisone

45. A 22-year-old pregnant woman presents to the emergency department with abdominal pain and malaise. Her symptoms began about 8 h prior to presentation and she has no diarrhea. Her pain is mostly in the right flank currently but began in the periumbilical area. She has nausea and vomiting. She has had an uncomplicated pregnancy and she is at 24 weeks' gestation. She receives regular obstetric care, and her last examination, including an echo, was normal 1 week ago. Temperature is 100.3°C,

45. *(Continued)*
blood pressure 129/90 mmHg, and heart rate 105 beats/min. Physical examination shows only mild abdominal tenderness. The abdomen is soft and bowel sounds are diminished. She is tender in the right lower quadrant without costovertebral angle tenderness. The genitourinary examination is normal, and she has a closed os. Fetal monitoring shows a normal fetal heart rate. White blood cell count is 10,000/µL. Urine analysis shows 2 white blood cells per high powered field, no epithelial cells, and 1 red blood cell per high powered field. What is the most likely diagnosis?

    A. Acute appendicitis
    B. Fitz-Hugh–Curtis syndrome
    C. Mittelschmerz
    D. Nephrolithiasis
    E. Pyelonephritis

46. A 54-year-old male presents with 1 month of diarrhea. He states that he has 8–10 loose bowel movements a day. He has lost 8 lb during this time. Vital signs and physical examination are normal. Serum laboratory studies are normal. A 24-h stool collection reveals 500 g of stool with a measured stool osmolality of 200 mosmol/L and a calculated stool osmolality of 210 mosmol/L. Based on these findings, what is the most likely cause of this patient's diarrhea?

    A. Celiac sprue
    B. Chronic pancreatitis
    C. Lactase deficiency
    D. Vasoactive intestinal peptide tumor
    E. Whipple's disease

47. A 38-year-old male is seen in the urgent care center with several hours of severe abdominal pain. His symptoms began suddenly, but he reports several months of pain in the epigastrium after eating, with a resultant 10-lb weight loss. He takes no medications besides over-the-counter antacids and has no other medical problems or habits. On physical examination temperature is 38.0°C (100.4°F), pulse 130/min, respiratory rate 24/min, and blood pressure 110/50 mmHg. His abdomen has absent bowel sounds and is rigid with involuntary guarding diffusely. A plain film of the abdomen is obtained and shows free air under the diaphragm. Which of the following is most likely to be found in the operating room?

    A. Necrotic bowel
    B. Necrotic pancreas
    C. Perforated duodenal ulcer
    D. Perforated gallbladder
    E. Perforated gastric ulcer

48. Which of the following is the source of this patient's peritonitis?

    A. Blood
    B. Bile
    C. Foreign body
    D. Gastric contents
    E. Pancreatic enzymes

49. A 37-year-old female presents with a chief complaint of difficulty swallowing. She reports that she feels as if food gets stuck in her midchest. She notices no difference between liquids or solids but does note that the symptoms worsen when she eats hurriedly. She has had a 15-lb weight loss and reports regurgitation of undigested food after eating. The patient undergoes barium swallow. What is the most likely diagnosis? (See Fig. 13-1, Part 4)

    A. Esophageal stricture
    B. Esophageal spasm
    C. Achalasia
    D. Esophageal cancer
    E. CREST syndrome

50. Which of the following extraintestinal manifestations of inflammatory bowel disease typically worsens with exacerbations of disease activity?

    A. Ankylosing spondylitis
    B. Arthritis
    C. Nephrolithiasis
    D. Primary sclerosing cholangitis
    E. Uveitis

51. A 37-year-old woman presents with abdominal pain, anorexia, and fever of 4 days' duration. The abdominal pain is mostly in the left lower quadrant. Her past medical history is significant for irritable bowel syndrome, diverticulitis treated 6 months ago, and status post-appendectomy. Since her last bout of diverticulitis she has increased her fiber intake and avoids nuts and popcorn. Review of systems is positive for weight loss, daily chills and sweats, and "bubbles" in her urinary stream. Her temperature is 39.6°C. A limited CT scan shows thickened colonic wall (5 mm) and inflammation with pericolic fat stranding. She is admitted with a presumptive diagnosis of diverticulitis. What is the most appropriate management for this patient?

    A. A trial of rifaximin and a high-fiber diet
    B. Bowel rest, ciprofloxacin, metronidazole, and ampicillin
    C. Examination of the urine sediment
    D. Measurement of 24-h urine protein
    E. Surgical removal of the affected colon and exploration

52. A 69-year-old patient presents to the emergency department with hematochezia of 4 h duration. The patient is pale but alert and oriented. Blood pressure is 107/82 mmHg, respiratory rate is 24 breaths/min and heart rate is 96 beats/min. The hematocrit is 24%, with a baseline of 32%. Which of the following represents the best approach for localization of this patient's intestinal bleeding?

    A. Angiography is most appropriate for this massive gastrointestinal (GI) bleed.
    B. Angiography is of little utility since the patient is not stable.
    C. Colonoscopy is better suited to localize bleeding, if it is massive.
    D. Colonoscopy can be diagnostic and therapeutic in this mild GI bleed.
    E. Immediate surgery with intraoperative localization is appropriate.

53. A 36-year-old female with AIDS and a CD4 count of $35/mm^3$ presents with odynophagia and progressive dysphagia. The patient reports daily fevers and a 20-lb weight loss. The patient has been treated with clotrimazole troches without relief. On physical examination the patient is cachectic with a body mass index (BMI) of 16 and a weight of 86 lb. The patient has a temperature of 38.2°C (100.8°F). She is noted to be orthostatic by blood pressure and pulse. Examination of the oropharynx reveals no evidence of thrush. The patient undergoes EGD, which reveals serpiginous ulcers in the distal esophagus without vesicles. No yellow plaques are noted. Multiple biopsies are taken that show intranuclear and intracytoplasmic inclusions in large endothelial cells and fibro-blasts. What is the best treatment for this patient's esophagitis?

    A. Ganciclovir
    B. Thalidomide
    C. Glucocorticoids
    D. Fluconazole
    E. Foscarnet

54. A 48-year-old male seeks evaluation for diarrhea and malabsorptive symptoms. Approximately 5 years ago the patient underwent partial gastrectomy with gastrojejunostomy for a perforated duodenal ulcer. He had done well since that time until 5 months ago, when he developed abdominal pain and bloating after eating. In addition, the patient has had profound diarrhea that occurs after eating and is worse after he eats fatty foods. He notes that the diarrhea is foul-smelling and often leaves a greasy film in the toilet. On physical examination

54. (Continued)
the patient is thin with a body mass index of 19. The examination is unremarkable. His stool is hemoccult-negative. Laboratory studies are remarkable except for an albumin of 3.1 g/dL. He is noted to have a hemoglobin of 9.6 mg/dL and a mean corpuscular volume (MCV) of 106. What is the most likely diagnosis?

    A. Dumping syndrome
    B. Bile reflux gastropathy
    C. Afferent loop syndrome
    D. Postvagotomy diarrhea
    E. Zollinger-Ellison syndrome

55. A 17-year-old Asian student complains of abdominal bloating and diarrhea, particularly after eating ice cream and other milk products. Her parents have similar symptoms. The patient denies any weight loss or systemic symptoms. The physical examination is normal. Treatment with which of the following medications is most likely to reduce her symptoms?

    A. Cholestyramine
    B. Metoclopramide
    C. Omeprazole
    D. Viokase
    E. None of the above

56. An 85-year-old woman is brought to a local emergency room by her family. She has been complaining of abdominal pain off and on for several days, but this morning states that this is the worst pain of her life. She is able to describe a sharp, stabbing pain in her abdomen. Her family reports that she has not been eating and seems to have no appetite. She has a past medical history of atrial fibrillation and hypercholesterolemia. She has had two episodes of vomiting and in the ER experiences diarrhea that is hemoccult positive. On examination she is afebrile, with a heart rate of 105 beats/min and blood pressure of 111/69 mmHg. Her abdomen is mildly distended and she has hypoactive bowel sounds. She does not exhibit rebound tenderness or guarding. She is admitted for further management. Several hours after admission she becomes unresponsive. Blood pressure is difficult to obtain and at best approximation is 60/40 mmHg. She has a rigid abdomen. Surgery is called and the patient is taken for emergent laparotomy. She is found to have acute mesenteric ischemia. Which of the following is true regarding this diagnosis?

    A. Mortality for this condition is >50%.
    B. Risk factors include low-fiber diet and obesity.
    C. The "gold standard" for diagnosis is CT scan of the abdomen.

56. *(Continued)*

   D. The lack of acute abdominal signs in this case is unusual for mesenteric ischemia.

   E. The splanchnic circulation is poorly collateralized.

57. A 17-year-old woman presents to the clinic complaining of vaginal itchiness and malodorous discharge. She is sexually active with multiple partners, and she is interested in getting tested for sexually transmitted diseases. A wet-mount microscopic examination is performed, and trichomonal parasites are identified. Which of the following statements regarding trichomoniasis is true?

   A. A majority of women are asymptomatic.

   B. No treatment is necessary as disease is self-limited.

   C. The patient's sexual partner need not be treated.

   D. Trichomoniasis can only be spread sexually.

   E. Trichomoniasis is 100% sensitive to metronidazole.

58. While attending the University of Georgia, a group of friends go on a 5-day canoeing and camping trip in rural southern Georgia. A few weeks later, one of the campers develops a serpiginous, raised, pruritic, erythematous eruption on the buttocks. Strongyloides larvae are found in his stool. Three of his companions, who are asymptomatic, are also found to have strongyloides larvae in their stool. Which of the following is indicated in the asymptomatic carriers?

   A. Fluconazole

   B. Ivermectin

   C. Mebendazole

   D. Mefloquine

   E. Treatment only for symptomatic illness

59. You are a physician working on a cruise ship traveling from Miami to the Yucatán Peninsula. In the course of 24 h, 32 people are seen with acute gastrointestinal illness that is marked by vomiting and watery diarrhea. The most likely causative agent of the illness is

   A. enterohemorrhagic *Escherichia coli*

   B. norovirus

   C. rotavirus

   D. *Shigella*

   E. *Salmonella*

60. What is the best method for diagnosis?

   A. Acute and convalescent antibody titers

   B. Demonstration of Norwalk toxin in the stool

   C. Electron microscopy

   D. Isolation in cell culture

   E. Polymerase chain reaction (PCR) to identify the Norwalk-associated calcivirus

61. The most common cause of traveler's diarrhea in Mexico is

   A. *Campylobacter jejuni*

   B. *Entamoeba histolytica*

   C. enterotoxigenic *Escherichia coli*

   D. *Giardia lamblia*

   E. *Vibrio cholerae*

62. *Helicobacter pylori* colonization is implicated in all of the following conditions *except*

   A. duodenal ulcer disease

   B. gastric adenocarcinoma

   C. gastric mucosa-associated lymphoid tissue (MALT) lymphoma

   D. gastroesophageal reflux disease

   E. peptic ulcer disease

63. Which of the following statements regarding *Clostridium difficile*–associated disease relapses is true?

   A. A first recurrence does not imply greater risk of further recurrences.

   B. Most recurrences are due to antibiotic resistance.

   C. Recurrent *C. difficile*–associated disease has been associated with a higher risk of colon cancer.

   D. Recurrent disease is associated with serious complications.

   E. Testing for clearance of *C. difficile* is warranted after treating recurrences.

64. A patient presents to the clinic complaining of nausea, vomiting, crampy abdominal pain, and markedly increased flatus. The patient has not experienced any diarrhea or vomiting but notes that he has been belching more than usual and he describes a "sulfur-like" odor when he does so. He returned from a 3-week trip to Peru and Ecuador several days ago and notes that his symptoms began about a week ago. Giardiasis is considered in the differential. Which of the following is true regarding *Giardia*?

   A. Boiling water prior to ingestion will not kill *Giardia* cysts.

   B. *Giardia* is a disease of developing nations; if this patient had not travelled, there would be no likelihood of giardiasis.

   C. Hematogenous dissemination and eosinophilia are common.

   D. Ingestion of as few as 10 cysts can cause human disease.

   E. Lack of diarrhea makes the diagnosis of *Giardia* very unlikely.

65. One month after receiving a 14-day course of omeprazole, clarithromycin, and amoxicillin for *Helicobacter pylori*–associated gastric ulcer disease, a 44-year-old woman still has mild dyspepsia and pain after meals. What is the appropriate next step in management?

    A. Empirical long-term proton pump inhibitor therapy
    B. Endoscopy with biopsy to rule out gastric adenocarcinoma
    C. *H. pylori* serology testing
    D. Reassurance
    E. Second-line therapy for *H. pylori* with omeprazole, bismuth subsalicylate, tetracycline, and metronidazole
    F. Urea breath test

66. All of the following are clinical manifestations of *Ascaris lumbricoides* infection *except*

    A. asymptomatic carriage
    B. fever, headache, photophobia, nuchal rigidity, and eosinophilia
    C. nonproductive cough and pleurisy with eosinophilia
    D. right upper quadrant pain and fever
    E. small-bowel obstruction

67. In the developed world, seroprevalence of *Helicobacter pylori* infection is currently

    A. decreasing
    B. increasing
    C. staying the same
    D. unknown

68. Which of the following antibiotics has the weakest association with the development of *Clostridium difficile*–associated disease?

    A. Ceftriaxone
    B. Ciprofloxacin
    C. Clindamycin
    D. Moxifloxacin
    E. Piperacillin/tazobactam

69. All of the following factors increase the risk for *Clostridium difficile*–associated disease *except*

    A. antacids
    B. antecedent antibiotics
    C. *C. difficile* colonization
    D. enteral tube feeds
    E. increasing length of hospital stay
    F. older age

70. A 38-year-old woman presents to the emergency department with severe abdominal pain. She has no

70. *(Continued)*
    past medical or surgical history. She recalls no recent history of abdominal discomfort, diarrhea, melena, bright red blood per rectum, nausea, or vomiting prior to this acute episode. She ate ceviche (lime-marinated raw fish) at a Peruvian restaurant 3 h prior to presentation. On examination, she is in terrible distress and has dry heaves. Temperature is 37.6°C; heart rate is 128 beats per minute; blood pressure is 174/92 mmHg. Examination is notable for an extremely tender abdomen with guarding and rebound tenderness. Bowel sounds are present and hyperactive. Rectal examination is normal and guaiac test is negative. Pelvic examination is unremarkable. White blood cell count is 6738/μL; hematocrit is 42%. A complete metabolic panel and lipase and amylase levels are all within normal limits. CT of the abdomen shows no abnormality. What is the next step in her management?

    A. CT angiogram of the abdomen
    B. Pelvic ultrasonography
    C. Proton pump inhibitor therapy and observation
    D. Right upper quadrant ultrasonography
    E. Upper endoscopy

71. Which of the following statements regarding liver abscesses is true?

    A. Amebic liver abscess should be ruled out only by direct sampling and culture of pus.
    B. Alkaline phosphatase is the most likely liver function test to be abnormal in the presence of a liver abscess.
    C. *Candida* species are most commonly isolated from patients with abscesses that develop as a result of peritoneal or pelvic pathology.
    D. Patients with liver abscesses nearly always have right upper quadrant pain.
    E. All of the above are true.

72. A 52-year-old woman with alcoholic cirrhosis, portal hypertension, esophageal varices, and history of hepatic encephalopathy presents to the hospital with confusion over several days. Her husband remarks that the patient has been adherent to her medicines. These medicines include labetalol, furosemide, aldactone, and lactulose. Physical examination is notable for temperature of 38.3°C, heart rate of 115 bpm, blood pressure of 105/62 mmHg, respiratory rate of 12 breaths per minute, and oxygen saturation of 96% on room air. The patient is extremely drowsy, only intermittently able to answer questions, and disoriented. She has slight asterixis. Lungs are clear. Cardiac examination is unremarkable. Her abdomen is distended and tense

72. *(Continued)*

but non-tender. She has 3+ lower extremity edema extending to her thighs. She is guaiac negative. Her cranial nerves and extremity strength are symmetric and normal. Laboratory studies reveal a leukocyte count of 4830/μL, hematocrit = 33% (baseline = 30%), and platelet count of 94,000/μL. Basic metabolic panel is unremarkable. What is an essential component of the diagnostic workup?

A. CT scan of the head
B. Esophagastroduodenoscopy
C. Paracentesis
D. Therapeutic trial of lactulose
E. Serum ammonia level

73. You are the on-call physician practicing in a suburban community. You receive a call from a 28-year-old female with a past medical history significant for sarcoidosis who is currently on no medications. She is complaining of the acute onset of crampy diffuse abdominal pain and multiple episodes of emesis that are nonbloody. She has not had any light-headedness with standing or loss of consciousness. When questioned further, the patient states that her last meal was 5 h previously, when she joined her friends for lunch at a local Chinese restaurant. She ate from the buffet, which included multiple poultry dishes and fried rice. What should you do for this patient?

A. Ask the patient to go to the nearest emergency department for resuscitation with IV fluids.
B. Initiate antibiotic therapy with azithromycin.
C. Reassure the patient that her illness is self-limited and no further treatment is necessary if she can maintain adequate hydration.
D. Refer the patient for CT to assess for appendicitis.
E. Refer the patient for admission for IV vancomycin and ceftriaxone because of her immunocompromised state resulting from sarcoidosis.

74. A previously healthy 28-year-old male describes several episodes of fever, myalgia, and headache that have been followed by abdominal pain and diarrhea. He has experienced up to 10 bowel movements per day. Physical examination is unremarkable. Laboratory findings are notable only for a slightly elevated leukocyte count and an elevated erythrocyte sedimentation rate. Wright's stain of a fecal sample reveals the presence of neutrophils. Colonoscopy reveals inflamed mucosa. Biopsy of an affected area discloses mucosal infiltration with neutrophils, monocytes, and eosinophils; epithelial damage, including loss of mucus; glandular degeneration;

74. *(Continued)*

and crypt abscesses. The patient notes that several months ago he was at a church barbecue where several people contracted a diarrheal illness. Although this patient could have inflammatory bowel disease, which of the following pathogens is most likely to be responsible for his illness?

A. *Campylobacter*
B. *Escherichia coli*
C. Norwalk agent
D. *Staphylococcus aureus*
E. *Salmonella*

75. A 68-year-old woman has been in the medical intensive care unit for 10 days with a chronic obstructive pulmonary disease flare and pneumonia, including the initial 6 days on a mechanical ventilator. She just finished a course of moxifloxacin and glucocorticoid taper when she develops abdominal discomfort over 2 days. Vital signs reveal a temperature of 38.2°C, heart rate of 94 beats per minute, blood pressure of 162/94 mmHg, respiratory rate of 18 per minute, and oxygen saturation of 90%. On examination, she is in moderate distress. She is not using accessory muscles but is tachypneic. She has a slight bilateral wheeze with good air movement. Heart sounds are distant and unchanged. Her abdomen is moderately distended and tense, with scant bowel sounds present. There is no guarding or rebound, but she is tender throughout. Review of her records reveals no bowel movement over the past 72 h and no stool is palpable in the rectal vault. White blood cell count has increased from 7100/μL to 38,000/μL over the past 2 days. Abdominal plain film shows what is read as a probable ileus in the right lower quadrant. Aside from nasogastric (NG) tube placement with suction and NPO status, which of the following should your management also include?

A. Intravenous immunoglobulin (IVIg)
B. Metronidazole, 500 mg IV tid
C. Piperacillin/tazobactam, 3.37 g IV q6h
D. Restart moxifloxacin, 400 PO qd
E. Vancomycin, 500 mg PO qid

76. Empirical antibiotic therapy for continuous ambulatory peritoneal dialysis (CAPD) patients with peritonitis should be directed towards which organisms?

A. Enteric gram-negative rods
B. Enteric gram-negative rods and yeast
C. Gram-positive cocci
D. Gram-positive cocci plus enteric gram-negative rods
E. Gram-positive cocci plus enteric gram-negative rods plus yeast

77. A 19-year-old college student presents to the emergency room with crampy abdominal pain and watery diarrhea that has worsened over 3 days. He recently returned from a volunteer trip to Mexico. He has no past medical history and felt well throughout the trip. Stool examination shows small cysts containing four nuclei, and stool antigen immunoassay is positive for *Giardia*. Which of the following is an effective treatment regimen?

A. Albendazole
B. Clindamycin
C. Giardiasis is self-limited and requires no antibiotic therapy
D. Metronidazole
E. Paromomycin
F. Tinidazole

78. A 41-year-old man with hepatitis C–associated ascites presents with acute abdominal pain. Physical examination is notable for temperature of 38.3°C, heart rate of 115 beats per minute, blood pressure of 88/48 mmHg, respiratory rate of 16 breaths per minute, and oxygen saturation of 99% on room air. The patient is in moderate discomfort and is lying still. He is alert and oriented. Lungs are clear. Cardiac examination is unremarkable. His abdomen is diffusely tender with distant bowel sounds, mild guarding, and no rebound tenderness. Laboratory studies reveal a leukocyte count of 11,630/µL with 94% neutrophils, hematocrit of 29%, and platelet count of 24,000/µL. Paracentesis reveals 658 PMNs/µL, total protein 1.2 g/dL, glucose 24 mg/dL, and Gram stain showing gram-negative rods, gram-positive cocci in chains, gram-positive rods, and yeast forms. All of the following are indicated *except*

A. abdominal radiograph
B. broad-spectrum antibiotics
C. drotrecogin alfa
D. intravenous fluid
E. surgical consultation

79. A 34-year-old female presents to your clinic with 5 weeks of right upper quadrant pain. She denies nausea, changes in bowel habits, or weight loss. Her past medical history is unremarkable. Her only medications are a multivitamin and oral contraceptives. The examination is notable for a palpable liver mass 2 cm below the right costal margin. Serum α fetoprotein is normal. An abdominal CT scan shows two 3-cm hypervascular lesions in the right hepatic lobe that are suggestive of hepatocellular adenoma. What is the most appropriate next management step?

79. *(Continued)*
A. Observation
B. Discontinuation of oral contraceptives
C. Referral for surgical excision
D. Radiofrequency ablation (RFA)
E. CT-guided biopsy

80. Which of the following statements about alcoholic liver disease is *not* true?

A. Pathologically, alcoholic cirrhosis is often characterized by diffuse fine scarring with small regenerative nodules.
B. The ratio of AST to ALT is often higher than 2.
C. Serum aspartate aminotransferase levels are often greater than 1000 U/L.
D. Concomitant hepatitis C significantly accelerates the development of alcoholic cirrhosis.
E. Serum prothrombin times may be prolonged, but activated partial thromboplastin times are usually not affected.

81. All the following are associated with an increased risk for cholelithiasis *except*

A. chronic hemolytic anemia
B. obesity
C. high-protein diet
D. pregnancy
E. female sex

82. A 16-year-old woman had visited your clinic 1 month ago with jaundice, vomiting, malaise, and anorexia. Two other family members were ill with similar symptoms. Based on viral serologies, including a positive anti-hepatitis A virus (HAV) IgM, a diagnosis of hepatitis A was made. The patient was treated conservatively, and 1 week after first presenting, she appeared to have made a full recovery. She returns to your clinic today complaining of the same symptoms she had 1 month ago. She is jaundiced, and an initial panel of laboratory tests returns elevated transaminases. Which of the following offers the best explanation of what has occurred in this patient?

A. Co-infection with hepatitis C
B. Hepatitis A recurrence
C. Inappropriate treatment of initial infection
D. Incorrect initial diagnosis; this patient likely has hepatitis B
E. Relapsing hepatitis

83. A 29-year-old woman who recently immigrated to the United States from South America presents to a local emergency room with severe abdominal pain, jaundice, and fever. No one else at home is ill.

83. *(Continued)*

She is unsure how long her symptoms have been going on, but describes a sudden worsening over the past 3 days. She has been unable to get out of bed and has not been eating well over that period of time. She has had nausea and vomiting. She denies alcohol or illicit drug use. She is rapidly triaged and on initial laboratory studies is found to have an ALT and AST in the thousands. She is to be admitted for inpatient management, and viral hepatitis serologies are sent. In a patient with acute hepatitis B, which of the following would be the first indication of infection?

A. Anti-HBc (antibody to hepatitis B core antigen)
B. Clinical symptoms such as fever, jaundice, and abdominal pain
C. HBeAg (hepatitis B e antigen)
D. HBsAg (hepatitis B surface antigen)
E. Increased transaminases

84. The patient described above has the following laboratory results: HBsAg is positive, Anti-HBc IgM is positive, and HBeAg is positive. All other serologies are negative. She is diagnosed with acute hepatitis B. When interpreting hepatitis B serology results, the term "window period" refers to the time between which of the following?

A. Anti-HBs and anti-HBc positivity
B. Clinical symptoms and anti-HBs
C. HBsAg and anti-HBs positivity
D. HBsAg and HBeAg positivity
E. Increased transaminases and HBsAg

85. Which of the following statements about cardiac cirrhosis is true?

A. Prolonged passive congestion from right-sided heart failure results first in congestion and necrosis of portal triads, resulting in subsequent fibrosis.
B. AST and ALT levels may mimic the very high levels seen in acute hepatitis infection or acetaminophen toxicity.
C. Budd-Chiari syndrome cannot be distinguished clinically from cardiac cirrhosis.
D. Venoocclusive disease is a major cause of morbidity and mortality in patients undergoing liver transplantation.
E. Echocardiography is the gold standard for diagnosing constrictive pericarditis as a cause of cirrhosis.

86. In chronic hepatitis B virus (HBV) infection, presence of hepatitis B e antigen (HBeAg) signifies which of the following?

86. *(Continued)*

A. Development of liver fibrosis leading to cirrhosis
B. Dominant viral population is less virulent and less transmissible
C. Increased likelihood of an acute flare in the next 1–2 weeks
D. Ongoing viral replication
E. Resolving infection

87. A 26-year-old woman presents to your clinic and is interested in getting pregnant. She seeks your advice regarding vaccines she should obtain, and in particular asks about the hepatitis B vaccine. She works as a receptionist for a local business, denies alcohol or illicit drug use, and is in a monogamous relationship. Which of the following is true regarding hepatitis B vaccination?

A. Hepatitis B vaccine consists of two intramuscular doses 1 month apart.
B. Only patients with defined risk factors need be vaccinated.
C. Pregnancy is not a contraindication to the hepatitis B vaccine.
D. This patient's hepatitis serologies should be checked prior to vaccination.
E. Vaccination should not be administered to children under 2 years old.

88. A 41-year-old female presents to your clinic with a week of jaundice. She notes pruritus, icterus, and dark urine. She denies fever, abdominal pain, or weight loss. The examination is unremarkable except for yellow discoloration of the skin. Total bilirubin is 6.0 mg/dL, and direct bilirubin is 5.1 mg/dL. AST is 84 U/L, and ALT is 92 U/L. Alkaline phosphatase is 662 U/L. CT scan of the abdomen is unremarkable. Right upper quadrant ultrasound shows a normal gallbladder but does not visualize the common bile duct. What is the most appropriate next management step?

A. Antibiotics and observation
B. Endoscopic retrograde cholangiopancreatography (ERCP)
C. Hepatitis serologies
D. HIDA scan
E. Serologies for antimitochondrial antibodies

89. A 34-year-old male reports "yellow eyes" for the last 2 days during a routine employment examination. He states that since his early twenties he has had similar episodes of yellow eyes lasting 2–4 days. He denies nausea, abdominal pain, dark urine, light-colored stools, pruritus, or weight loss. He has

89. *(Continued)*

not sought prior medical attention because of finances, lack of symptoms, and the predictable resolution of the yellow eyes. He takes a multivitamin and some herbal medications. On examination he is mildly obese. He is icteric. There are no stigmata of chronic liver disease. The patient's abdomen is soft and nontender, and there is no organomegaly. Laboratory examinations are normal except for a total bilirubin of 3 mg/dL. Direct bilirubin is 0.2 mg/dL. AST, ALT, and alkaline phosphatase are normal. Hematocrit, lactate dehydrogenase (LDH), and haptoglobin are normal. Which of the following is the most likely diagnosis?

A. Crigler-Najjar syndrome type 1
B. Cholelithiasis
C. Dubin-Johnson syndrome
D. Gilbert's syndrome
E. Medication-induced hemolysis

90. What is the appropriate next management step for this patient?

A. Genotype studies
B. Peripheral blood smear
C. Prednisone
D. Reassurance
E. Right upper quadrant ultrasound

91. You are asked to consult on a 62-year-old white female with pruritus for 4 months. She has noted progressive fatigue and a 5-lb weight loss. She has intermittent nausea but no vomiting and denies changes in her bowel habits. There is no history of prior alcohol use, blood transfusions, or illicit drug use. The patient is widowed and had two heterosexual partners in her lifetime. Her past medical history is significant only for hypothyroidism, for which she takes levothyroxine. Her family history is unremarkable. On examination she is mildly icteric. She has spider angiomata on her torso. You palpate a nodular liver edge 2 cm below the right costal margin. The remainder of the examination is unremarkable. A right upper quadrant ultrasound confirms your suspicion of cirrhosis. You order a complete blood count and a comprehensive metabolic panel. What is the most appropriate next test?

A. 24-h urine copper
B. Antimitochondrial antibodies (AMA)
C. Endoscopic retrograde cholangiopancreatography (ERCP)
D. Hepatitis B serologies
E. Serum ferritin

92. An 18-year-old man presents to a rural clinic with nausea, vomiting, anorexia, abdominal discomfort, myalgias, and jaundice. He describes occasional alcohol use and is sexually active. He describes using heroin and cocaine "a few times in the past." He works as a short-order cook in a local restaurant. He has lost 15.5 kg (34 lb) since his last visit to clinic and appears emaciated and ill-appearing. On examination he is noted to have icteric sclerae and a palpable, tender liver below the right costal margin. In regard to acute hepatitis, which of the following is true?

A. A distinction between viral etiologies cannot be made using clinical criteria alone.
B. Based on age and risk factors, he is likely to have hepatitis B infection.
C. He does not have hepatitis E virus, as this infects only pregnant women.
D. This patient cannot have hepatitis C because his presentation is too acute.
E. This patient does not have hepatitis A because his presentation is too fulminant.

93. All the following are risk factors for developing cholangiocarcinoma *except*

A. choledochal cyst
B. cholelithiasis
C. liver flukes
D. sclerosing cholangitis
E. working in the rubber industry

94. A 52-year-old male with chronic hepatitis C presents to your clinic with worsening right upper quadrant pain. Examination shows a palpable right upper quadrant mass. CT scan shows a large 5×5 cm mass in the right lobe of the liver. Serum α fetoprotein is elevated. A CT-guided liver biopsy confirms the suspected diagnosis of hepatocellular carcinoma. All the following are appropriate management steps *except*

A. referral for surgical resection
B. referral for radiofrequency ablation
C. referral for liver transplantation
D. systemic chemotherapy
E. chemoembolization

95. A 26-year-old female presents to the emergency room after ingesting "lots of pills." Her boyfriend discovered her crying on the floor of their bedroom, found numerous open bottles of acetaminophen scattered throughout the apartment, and called 911. He does not know when she first took

95. *(Continued)*

the pills but had last seen her 4 h before finding her on the floor. She is nauseated and vomits once in the emergency room. Vital signs are stable. On examination she is alert and oriented. She has some epigastric tenderness to deep palpation. Otherwise the examination is unremarkable. Her acetaminophen level is 400 µg/mL. Liver function tests are normal. Which of the following statements regarding her clinical condition is *not* true?

A. *N*-acetylcysteine is the treatment of choice for acetaminophen toxicity.
B. Alkalinization of the urine is not effective as a treatment for acetaminophen toxicity.
C. The patient should be admitted and observed for 48–72 h as her hepatic injury may manifest days after the initial ingestion.
D. Liver transplantation is the only option for patients who develop fulminant hepatic failure from acetaminophen.
E. Normal liver function tests at presentation make significant liver injury unlikely.

96. Chronic active hepatitis is most reliably distinguished from chronic persistent hepatitis by the presence of

A. extrahepatic manifestations
B. hepatitis B surface antigen in the serum
C. antibody to hepatitis B core antigen in the serum
D. a significant titer of anti-smooth-muscle antibody
E. characteristic liver histology

97. A 32-year-old man who recently returned from a vacation in Thailand presents with the acute onset of jaundice, abdominal pain, and vomiting. He is able to tolerate small amounts of food. His vital signs are normal, and an abdominal examination reveals a nontender liver edge palpable 2 cm below the right costal margin. His transaminases are elevated in the thousands, hepatitis B surface (anti-HBs) antigen is positive, and antibody to hepatitis B surface antigen is negative. He has no previous medical history and abstains from alcohol use. He has never received a hepatitis B vaccine series. Which of the following do you recommend as first-line management?

A. Conservative management and close follow-up
B. Hepatitis B vaccine series
C. Hospital admission and initiation of a liver transplant workup
D. Immediate entecavir treatment until anti-HBs is positive
E. Immediate lamivudine treatment for a planned 6-month course

98. A 55-year-old male with cirrhosis is seen in the clinic to follow up a recent hospitalization for spontaneous bacterial peritonitis. He is doing well and finishing his course of antibiotics. He is taking propranolol and lactulose; besides complications of end-stage liver disease, he has well-controlled diabetes mellitus and had a basal cell carcinoma resected 5 years ago. The cirrhosis is thought to be due to alcohol abuse, and his last drink of alcohol was 2 weeks ago. He and his wife ask if he is a liver transplant candidate. He can be counseled in which of the following ways?

A. He is not a transplant candidate as he has a history of alcohol dependence.
B. He is not a transplant candidate now, but may be after a sustained period of proven abstinence from alcohol.
C. Because he has diabetes mellitus he is not a transplant candidate.
D. Because he had a skin cancer he is not a transplant candidate.
E. He is appropriate for liver transplantation and should be referred immediately.

99. A 36-year-old male presents with fatigue and tea-colored urine for 5 days. Physical examination reveals jaundice and tender hepatomegaly but is otherwise unremarkable. Laboratories are remarkable for an aspartate aminotransferase (AST) of 2400 U/L and an alanine aminotransferase (ALT) of 2640 U/L. Alkaline phosphatase is 210 U/L. Total bilirubin is 8.6 mg/dL. Which of the following is *least* likely to cause this clinical picture and these laboratory abnormalities?

A. Acute hepatitis A infection
B. Acute hepatitis B infection
C. Acute hepatitis C infection
D. Acetaminophen ingestion
E. Budd-Chiari syndrome

100. A 47-year-old woman presents to the emergency room with severe mid-abdominal pain radiating to her back. The pain began acutely and is sharp. She denies cramping or flatulence. She has had two episodes of emesis of bilious material since the pain began, but this has not lessened the pain. She currently rates the pain as a 10 out of 10 and feels the pain is worse in the supine position. For the past few months, she has had intermittent episodes of right upper and mid-epigastric pain that occur after eating but subside over a few hours. These are associated with a feeling of excess gas. She denies any history of alcohol abuse. She has no medical history of hypertension or hyperlipidemia. On physical

100. *(Continued)*

examination, she is writhing in distress and slightly diaphoretic. Vital signs are: heart rate 127 beats/min, blood pressure 92/50 mmHg, respiratory rate 20 breaths/min, temperature 37.9°C, Sa_{O_2} 88% on room air. Her body mass index is 29 kg/m^2. The cardiovascular examination reveals a regular tachycardia. The chest examination shows dullness to percussion at bilateral bases with a few scattered crackles. On abdominal examination, bowel sounds are hypoactive. There is no rash or bruising evident on inspection of the abdomen. There is voluntary guarding on palpation. The pain with palpation is greatest in the periumbilical and epigastric area without rebound tenderness. There is no evidence of jaundice, and the liver span is about 10 cm to percussion. Amylase level is 750 IU/L, and lipase level is 1129 IU/L. Other laboratory values include: aspartate amino transferase (AST) 168 U/L, alanine aminotransferase (ALT) 196 U/L, total bilirubin 2.3 mg/dL, alkaline phosphatase level 268 U/L, lactate dehydrogenase LDH 300 U/L, and creatinine 1.9 mg/dL. The hematocrit is 43%, and white blood cell (WBC) count is 11,500/μL with 89% neutrophils. An arterial blood gas shows a pH of 7.32, Pa_{CO_2} 32 mmHg, and a Pa_{O_2} of 56 mmHg. An ultrasound confirms a dilated common bile duct with evidence of pancreatitis manifested as an edematous and enlarged pancreatitis. A CT scan shows no evidence of necrosis. After 3 L of normal saline, her blood pressure comes up to 110/60 mmHg with a heart rate of 105 beats/min. Which of the following statements best describes the pathophysiology of this disease?

A. Intrapancreatic activation of digestive enzymes with autodigestion and acinar cell injury

B. Chemoattraction of neutrophils with subsequent infiltration and inflammation

C. Distant organ involvement and systemic inflammatory response syndrome related to release of activated pancreatic enzymes and cytokines

D. All of the above

101. In the case vignette presented above, which of the following factors at presentation predicts a poor outcome and increased risk of death in acute pancreatitis?

A. Body mass index (BMI) >25 kg/m^2

B. Hematocrit ≥40%

C. Lipase >1000 IU/L

D. Pa_{O_2} <60 mmHg

E. WBC count >10,000/μL

102. A 28-year-old male with HIV and a CD4 count of 4/μL is admitted to the hospital with several days of epigastric boring abdominal pain radiating to the back with associated nausea and bilious vomiting. He has a history of disseminated mycobacterial disease, cryptococcal pneumonia, and injection drug use. His current medications include fluconazole, trimethoprim-sulfamethoxazole, clarithromycin, ethambutol, and rifabutin. On physical examination he has normal vital signs, decreased bowel sounds, and tender epigastrium without rebound or guarding. Rectal exam is guaiac-negative. The remainder of the examination is normal. Amylase and lipase are elevated. The patient is treated conservatively with intravenous fluids and bowel rest, with resolution of symptoms. Right upper quadrant ultrasound is normal, and calcium and triglycerides are normal. Which of the following changes to his medical regimen should be recommended on discharge?

A. Discontinue rifabutin.

B. Substitute azithromycin for clarithromycin.

C. Substitute dapsone for trimethoprim-sulfamethoxazole.

D. Substitute amphotericin for fluconazole.

E. Discontinue trimethoprim-sulfamethoxazole.

103. Which of the following is the most common cause of acute pancreatitis in the United States?

A. Alcohol

B. Drugs

C. Gallstones

D. Hypercalcemia

E. Hyperlipidemia

104. A 50-year-old male without a significant past medical history or recent exposure to alcohol presents with midepigastric abdominal pain, nausea, and vomiting. The physical examination is remarkable for the absence of jaundice and any other specific physical findings. Which of the following is the best strategy for screening for acute pancreatitis?

A. Measurement of serum amylase

B. Measurement of serum lipase

C. Measurement of both serum amylase and serum lipase

D. Isoamylase level analysis

E. Magnetic resonance imaging

105. A 43-year-old man with alcohol dependence presents with a sharp epigastric pain radiating to the back. He also has had nausea with bilious emesis on three occasions in the past 24 h. He has had no bright red blood or coffee-ground material in his vomitus, nor has he had melena. His last alcohol

105. *(Continued)*

intake was yesterday, and he normally drinks a gallon of whiskey on a daily basis. He has a history of acute pancreatitis due to alcohol. On physical examination, he appears uncomfortable, writhing in bed. His vital signs are: heart rate 112 beats/min, blood pressure 156/92 mmHg, temperature 37.8°C, respiratory rate 24 breaths/min, and Sa_{O_2} 96% on room air. The abdominal examination reveals decreased bowel sounds and is tympanitic to percussion. There is diffuse tenderness to palpation in the midepigastrium without rebound. Voluntary guarding is present. The liver span is 15 cm to percussion, and a smooth liver edge is palpated 5 cm below the right costal margin. No spleen tip is palpable. The amylase is 580 U/L, and lipase is 690 U/L. Liver function testing reveals an AST of 280 U/L, ALT 184 U/L, alkaline phosphatase 89 U/L, and albumin 2.6 g/dL. Fecal occult blood testing is negative. Which of the following best reflects the current recommendations on treatment of acute pancreatitis in this patient?

A. A nasogastric tube with intermittent suctioning is necessary to prevent ongoing stimulation of pancreatic enzyme release by gastric secretions.
B. Early oral alimentation decreases the risk of infection and speeds recovery
C. Placement of a nasojejunal feeding tube will allow early institution of oral feeding and reduce hospital length of stay.
D. Total parenteral nutrition is indicated because the patient has evidence of chronic malnutrition and is expected to be unable to tolerate oral alimentation for >1 week.
E. Treatment with analgesia, IV fluid resuscitation, and avoidance of oral feeding will result in improvement in 3–7 days.

106. A 25-year-old female with cystic fibrosis is diagnosed with chronic pancreatitis. She is at risk for all of the following complications *except*

A. vitamin B_{12} deficiency
B. vitamin A deficiency
C. pancreatic carcinoma
D. niacin deficiency
E. steatorrhea

107. A 64-year-old man seeks evaluation from his primary care physician because of chronic diarrhea. He reports that he has two or three large loose bowel movements daily. He describes them as markedly foul-smelling, and they often leave an oily ring in the toilet. He also notes that the bowel

107. *(Continued)*

movements often follow heavy meals, but if he fasts or eats low-fat foods, the stools are more formed. Over the past 6 months, he has lost about 18 kg (40 lb). In this setting, he reports intermittent episodes of abdominal pain that can be quite severe. He describes the pain as sharp and in a midepigastric location. He has not sought evaluation of the pain previously, but when it occurs, he will limit his oral intake and treat the pain with nonsteroidal antiinflammatory drugs. He notes the pain has not lasted for >48 h and is not associated with meals. His past medical history is remarkable for peripheral vascular disease and tobacco use. He currently smokes one pack of cigarettes daily. In addition, he drinks two to six beers daily. He has stopped all alcohol intake for up to a week at a time in the past without withdrawal symptoms. His current medications are aspirin, 81 mg daily, and albuterol metered dose inhaler (MDI) on an as-needed basis. On physical examination, the patient is thin but appears well. His body mass index is 18.2 kg/m². Vital signs are normal. Cardiac and pulmonary examinations are normal. The abdominal examination shows mild epigastric tenderness without rebound or guarding. The liver span is 12 cm to percussion and palpable 2 cm below the right costal margin. There is no splenomegaly or ascites present. There are decreased pulses in the lower extremities bilaterally. An abdominal radiograph demonstrates calcifications in the epigastric area, and CT scan confirms that these calcifications are located within the body of the pancreas. No pancreatic ductal dilatation is noted. An amylase level is 32 U/L, and lipase level is 22 U/L. What is the next most appropriate step in diagnosing and managing this patient's primary complaint?

A. Advise the patient to stop all alcohol use and prescribe pancreatic enzymes.
B. Advise the patient to stop all alcohol use and prescribe narcotic analgesia and pancreatic enzymes.
C. Perform angiography to assess for ischemic bowel disease.
D. Prescribe prokinetic agents to improve gastric emptying.
E. Refer the patient for endoscopic retrograde cholangiopancreatography (ERCP) for sphincterotomy

108. All the following cancers commonly metastasize to the liver *except*

A. breast
B. colon
C. lung
D. melanoma
E. prostate

109. Which of the following statements regarding pancreatic cancer is true?

    A. Five-year survival is ~5%.
    B. Most cases present with locally confined disease amenable to a surgical cure.
    C. Pancreatic adenocarcinomas occur most frequently in the pancreatic tail.
    D. The median age of diagnosis is 49 years.
    E. The most common tumor type is an islet cell tumor.

110. You are managing a patient with stage IV pancreatic adenocarcinoma. The patient has been treated with gemcitabine for 16 weeks, and a recent CT scan confirms growth of the mass in the head of the pancreas over that time period. The patient has had biliary stents placed without complication for obstructive jaundice. The patient's weight is stable and he is able to perform activities of daily living independently. The patient wants to know what "the next step" is now that gemcitabine has seemed to fail. What is the most appropriate recommendation at this time?

    A. Initiate treatment with 5-fluorouracil.
    B. Make a referral to home hospice care.
    C. Refer for debulking surgery.
    D. Refer for external beam radiation as an adjunct to chemotherapy.
    E. Suggest enrolling in a clinical trial.

111. You are managing a patient who complains of abdominal pain. The pain is located in the epigastric area and radiates to the back. Leaning forward improves the pain. The rest of the physical examination is unremarkable and there is no jaundice. The total bilirubin is 0.7 mg/dL and CA 19-9 level is within the normal range. An ultrasound of the abdomen shows a 2.5-cm well-circumscribed mass in the tail of the pancreas. There is no ductal dilation. A CT scan confirms the presence of a 2.5-cm spiculated mass in the tail of the pancreas with no surrounding lymphadenopathy or local extension. What is the next most appropriate step in this patient's management?

    A. Magnetic resonance cholangiopancreatography
    B. Refer for surgical resection
    C. Serial CA 19-9 measurement
    D. Ultrasound-guided biopsy

112. A 49-year-old male is brought to the hospital by his family because of confusion and dehydration. The family reports that for the last 3 weeks he has had persistent copious watery diarrhea that has not

112. *(Continued)*
    abated with the use of over-the-counter medications. The diarrhea has been unrelated to food intake and has persisted during fasting. The stool does not appear fatty and is not malodorous. The patient works as an attorney, is a vegetarian, and has not traveled recently. No one in the household has had similar symptoms. Before the onset of diarrhea, he had mild anorexia and a 5-lb weight loss. Since the diarrhea began, he has lost at least 10 pounds. The physical examination is notable for blood pressure of 100/70, heart rate of 110/min, and temperature of 36.8°C (98.2°F). Other than poor skin turgor, confusion, and diffuse muscle weakness, the physical examination is unremarkable. Laboratory studies are notable for a normal complete blood count and the following chemistry results:

Na^+	146 meq/L
K^+	3.0 meq/L
Cl^-	96 meq/L
HCO_3^-	36 meq/L
BUN	32 mg/dL
Creatinine	1.2 mg/dL

A 24-h stool collection yields 3 L of tea-colored stool. Stool sodium is 50 meq/L, potassium is 25 meq/L, and stool osmolality is 170 mosmol/L. Which of the following diagnostic tests is most likely to yield the correct diagnosis?

    A. Serum cortisol
    B. Serum TSH
    C. Serum VIP
    D. Urinary 5-HIAA
    E. Urinary metanephrine

113. A 48-year-old female is undergoing evaluation for flushing and diarrhea. Physical examination is normal except for nodular hepatomegaly. A CT scan of the abdomen demonstrates multiple nodules in both lobes of the liver consistent with metastases in the liver and a 2-cm mass in the ileum. The 24-h urinary 5-HIAA excretion is markedly elevated. All the following treatments are appropriate *except*

    A. diphenhydramine
    B. interferon-α
    C. octreotide
    D. odansetron
    E. phenoxybenzamine

114. While undergoing a physical examination during medical student clinical skills, this patient develops

114. *(Continued)*

severe flushing, wheezing, nausea, and light-headedness. Vital signs are notable for a blood pressure of 70/30 mmHg and a heart rate of 135/min. Which of the following is the most appropriate therapy?

A. Albuterol
B. Atropine
C. Epinephrine
D. Hydrocortisone
E. Octreotide

115. In the evaluation of malnutrition, which of the following proteins has the shortest half-life and thus is most predictive of recent nutritional status?

A. Albumin
B. Fibronectin
C. Retinol-binding protein complex
D. Prealbumin
E. Transferrin

116. Why is it necessary to coadminister vitamin B_6 (pyridoxine) with isoniazid?

A. Vitamin B_6 requirements are higher in tuberculosis patients.
B. Isoniazid causes decarboxylation of γ-carboxyl groups in vitamin K–dependent enzymes.
C. Isoniazid interacts with pyridoxal phosphate.
D. Isoniazid causes malabsorption of vitamin B_6.
E. Isoniazid causes a conversion of homocysteine to cystathionine.

117. A 19-year-old woman with anorexia nervosa undergoes surgery for acute appendicitis. The postoperative course is complicated by acute respiratory distress syndrome, and she remains intubated for 10 days. She develops wound dehiscence on postoperative day 10. Laboratory data show a white blood cell count of 4000/μL, hematocrit 35%, albumin 2.1 g/dL, total protein 5.8 g/dL, transferrin 54 mg/dL, and iron-binding capacity 88 mg/dL. You are considering initiating nutritional therapy on hospital day 11. Which of the following is true regarding the etiology and treatment of malnutrition in this patient?

A. She has marasmus, and nutritional support should be started slowly.
B. She has kwashiorkor, and nutritional support should be aggressive.
C. She has marasmic kwashiorkor, kwashiorkor predominant, and nutritional support should be aggressive.
D. She has marasmic kwashiorkor, marasmus predominant, and nutritional support should be slow.

118. You are seeing a patient in follow-up 2 weeks after hospitalization. The patient is recovering from nosocomial pneumonia due to a resistant *Pseudomonas* spp. His hospital course was complicated by a deep venous thrombosis. The patient is currently on IV piperacillin/tazobactam and tobramycin via a tunneled catheter, warfarin, lisinopril, hydrochlorothiazide, and metoprolol. Laboratory data this morning show an INR of 8.2. At hospital discharge his INR was stable at 2.5. He has no history of liver disease. What is the most likely cause of the elevated INR?

A. The patient has inadvertently overdosed.
B. The patient has developed a recurrent deep venous thrombosis, which has affected the laboratory data.
C. The patient is deficient in vitamin K and needs supplementation.
D. The warfarin prescription was written incorrectly at the time of discharge.

119. A 51-year-old alcoholic man is admitted to the hospital for upper gastrointestinal bleeding. From further history and physical examination, it becomes apparent that his bleeding is from gingival membranes. He is intoxicated and complains of fatigue. Reviewing his chart you find that he had a hemarthrosis evacuated 6 months ago and has been lost to follow-up since then. He takes no medications. Laboratory data show platelets of 250,000, INR of 0.9. He has a diffuse hemorrhagic eruption on his legs (Fig. 119).

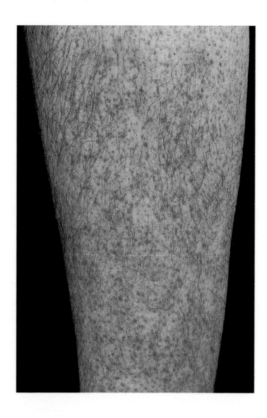

119. *(Continued)*
     What is the recommended treatment for this patient's underlying disorder?

   A. Folate
   B. Niacin
   C. Thiamine
   D. Vitamin C
   E. Vitamin K

120. While working in the intensive care unit, you admit a 57-year-old woman with acute pancreatitis and oliguric renal failure. Respiratory rate is 26 breaths/min, heart rate is 125 beats/min, and temperature is 37.2°C. Physical examination shows marked abdominal tenderness with normoactive bowel sounds. A CT scan shows an inflamed pancreas without hemorrhage. You calculate her APACHE-I score to be 28. When deciding on when to initiate nutritional replacement in this patient, which of the following statements is true?

   A. Bowel rest is the cornerstone of treatment for acute pancreatitis.
   B. Administering parenteral nutrition within 24 h will decrease the risk of infection and mortality.
   C. Enteral feeding supports gut function by secretion of gastrointestinal hormones that stimulate gut trophic activity.
   D. In severe systemic response to inflammation, feeding can be withheld initially because the patient is likely to have adequate, spontaneous oral intake in the first 7 days.

121. The resting energy expenditure is a rough estimate of total caloric needs in a state of energy balance. Of these two patients with stable weights, which person has the highest resting energy expenditure (REE): Patient A, a 40-year-old man who weighs 90 kg and is sedentary, or Patient B, a 40-year-old man who weighs 70 kg and is very active?

   A. 40-year-old man who weighs 90 kg and is sedentary
   B. 40-year-old man who weighs 70 kg and is very active
   C. REE is the same
   D. Not enough information given to calculate the REE

122. It is hospital day 16 for a 49-year-old homeless patient who is recovering from alcohol withdrawal and delirium tremens. She spent the first 9 days of this hospitalization in the intensive care unit but is now awake, alert, and conversant. She has a healing decubitus ulcer, and her body mass index is 19 kg/m². Laboratory data show an albumin of 2.9 g/dL and a prothrombin time of 18 s (normal range). Is this patient malnourished?

122. *(Continued)*
   A. Cannot be determined, need more information.
   B. No. Given her heavy alcohol intake, her prothrombin time is expected to be delayed.
   C. No. She has a low resting energy expenditure and her intact mental state argues against malnutrition.
   D. Yes, this degree of hypoalbuminemia is uncommon in cirrhosis and is likely due to malnutrition.

123. A 42-year-old male patient wants your opinion about vitamin E supplements. He has read that taking high doses of vitamin E can improve his sexual performance and slow the aging process. He is not vitamin E deficient. You explain to him that these claims are not based on good evidence. What other potential side effect should he be concerned about?

   A. Deep venous thrombosis
   B. Hemorrhage
   C. Night blindness
   D. Peripheral neuropathy
   E. Retinopathy

124. Doing rounds in the oncology center, you are see a patient with carcinoid syndrome. Due to the increased conversion of tryptophan to serotonin, this patient has developed niacin deficiency. All of the following are components of the pellagra syndrome *except*

   A. dermatitis
   B. dementia
   C. diarrhea
   D. dyslipidemia
   E. glossitis

125. An 86-year-old woman with chronic obstructive pulmonary disease (COPD), congestive heart failure, and insulin-requiring type 2 diabetes mellitus is admitted to the intensive care unit with an exacerbation of her COPD. She is intubated and treated with glucocorticoids and nebulized albuterol. She is also continued on her glargine insulin, aspirin, pravastatin, furosemide, enalapril, and metoprolol. On hospital day 8, parenteral nutrition is begun via catheter in the subclavian vein. Her insulin requirements increase on hospital day 9 due to episodes of hyperglycemia. On hospital day 10, she develops rales and an increasing oxygen requirement. A chest radiograph shows bilateral pulmonary edema. Laboratory data show hypokalemia, hypomagnesemia, and hypophosphatemia and a normal creatinine. Her weight has increased by 3 kg since admission. Urine sodium is <10 meq/dL. All of the following changes in her nutritional regimen will improve her volume status *except*

125. *(Continued)*
    A. combination of glucose and fat in the parenteral nutrition mixture
    B. decreasing the sodium content of the mixture to <40 meq per day
    C. increasing the protein content of the parenteral nutrition mixture
    D. reducing the overall glucose content

126. A new study has been published showing a benefit of 25 mg/day of vitamin X. The recommended estimated average requirement of vitamin X is 10 mg/day, 2 standard deviations below the amount published in the study. The tolerable upper limit of vitamin X is unknown. Your patient wants to know if it is safe to consume 25 mg/day of vitamin X. Which is the most appropriate answer?

    A. Two standard deviations above the estimated average requirement defines the tolerable upper limit.
    B. 25 mg/day is probably too much vitamin X in 1 day.
    C. 25 mg/day is statistically in a safe range of the estimated average requirement.
    D. The study was not designed to assess safety and therefore should not influence practice.

127. You are seeing a pediatric patient from Djibouti in consultation who was admitted with a constellation of symptoms including diarrhea, alopecia, muscle wasting, depression, and a rash involving the face, extremities, and perineum. The child has hypogonadism and dwarfism. You astutely make the diagnosis of zinc deficiency, and laboratory test confirm this (zinc level <70 µL/dL). What other clinical findings is this patient likely to manifest?

    A. Dissecting aortic aneurysm
    B. Hypochromic anemia
    C. Hypoglycemia
    D. Hypopigmented hair
    E. Macrocytosis

128. You are rotating on a medical trip to impoverished areas of China. You are examining an 8-year-old child whose mother complains of him being clumsy and sickly. He has had many episodes of diarrheal illnesses and pneumonia. His "clumsiness" is most pronounced in the evening when he has to go outside and do his chores. On examination, you notice conjunctival dryness with white patches of keratinized epithelium on the sclera. What is the cause of this child's symptoms?

    A. Autoimmune neutropenia
    B. Congenital rubella

128. *(Continued)*
    C. Spinocerebellar ataxia (SCA) type 1
    D. Vitamin A deficiency
    E. Vitamin B$_1$ deficiency

129. After being stranded alone in the mountains for 8 days, a 26-year-old hiker is brought to the hospital for evaluation of a right femoral neck fracture. He has not had anything to eat or drink for the past 6 days. Vital signs are within normal limits. Weight is 79.5 kg, which is 1.8 kg less than he weighed 6 months ago. Laboratory data show a creatinine of 2.5 mg/dL, blood urea nitrogen of 52 mg/dL, glucose 96 mg/dL, albumin 4.1 mg/dL, chloride 105 meq/L, and ferritin on 173 ng/mL. Which of the following statements is true regarding his risk of malnourishment?

    A. He has protein-calorie malnutrition due to the rate of weight loss.
    B. He has protein-calorie malnutrition due to his elevated ferritin.
    C. He is at risk, but a normal individual can tolerate 7 days of starvation.
    D. He is not malnourished because he is not hypoglycemic after 6 days of no food or water.

130. You are doing rounds in the intensive care unit on an intubated patient who is recovering from a stroke and has diabetic gastroparesis. When suctioning the patient in the morning, she coughs profusely, with thick green secretions. You are concerned about the possibility of aspiration pneumonia. All of the following measures are useful in preventing aspiration pneumonia in an intubated patient *except*

    A. combined enteral and parenteral nutrition
    B. elevating the head of the bed to 30°
    C. physician-directed methods for formula advancement
    D. post-ligament of Treitz feeding

131. Which of the following patients meets criteria for the diagnosis of the metabolic syndrome?

    A. A man with waist circumference of 110 cm, well-controlled diabetes mellitus with fasting plasma glucose of 98 mg/dL, and blood pressure of 140/75 mmHg
    B. A woman with triglycerides of 180 mg/dL, waist circumference of 75 cm, and polycystic ovary syndrome
    C. A man with nonalcoholic liver disease, obstructive sleep apnea, and blood pressure of 135/90 mmHg
    D. A woman with high-density lipoprotein (HDL) of 54 mg/dL, blood pressure of 125/80 mmHg, and fasting plasma glucose of 85 mg/dL

132. You are managing a patient with the metabolic syndrome. She is an obese woman with poorly controlled diabetes and dyslipidemia. Her Hb$_{A1C}$ is 8.8% and fasting plasma glucose is 195 mg/dL. Low-density lipoprotein (LDL) cholesterol is 98 mg/dL and triglycerides are 276 mg/dL. Her medications include insulin, atorvastatin, hydrochlorothiazide, and aspirin. What is the best option for a medication to treat this patient's hypertriglyceridemia?

    A. Cholestyramine
    B. Colestipol
    C. Ezetimibe
    D. Fenofibrate
    E. Nicotinic acid

133. Insulin resistance and fasting hyperglycemia are important when creating a treatment program for the metabolic syndrome. Often, lifestyle modifications will occur at the same time medications are prescribed. In addressing the treatment of insulin resistance and fasting hyperglycemia, which of the following statements is true?

    A. Metformin is more effective than the combination of weight reduction, dietary fat restriction, and increased physical activity for the prevention of diabetes mellitus.
    B. Metformin is superior to other drug classes for increasing insulin sensitivity.
    C. Thiazolidinediones, but not metformin, improve insulin-mediated glucose uptake in muscle.
    D. Lifestyle interventions alone are not effective in reducing the incidence of diabetes mellitus.

134. Which of the following personality traits is most likely to describe a young female with anorexia nervosa?

    A. Depressive
    B. Borderline
    C. Anxious
    D. Perfectionist
    E. Impulsive

135. All of the following clinical features are common in patients with anorexia nervosa *except*

    A. Avoid food-related occupations
    B. Distorted body image
    C. Engage in binge eating
    D. Exercise extensively
    E. Rarely complain of hunger
    F. Socially withdrawn

136. You diagnose anorexia nervosa in one of your new clinic patients. When coordinating a treatment

136. *(Continued)*
    program with the psychiatrist, what characteristics should prompt consideration for inpatient treatment instead of scheduling an outpatient assessment?

    A. Amenorrhea
    B. Exaggeration of food intake
    C. Irrational fear of gaining weight
    D. Purging behavior
    E. Weight <75% of expected body weight

137. An elevation in which of the following hormones is consistent with the effects of anorexia nervosa?

    A. Cortisol
    B. Gonadotropin-releasing hormone (GnRH)
    C. Leptin
    D. Thyroxine (T$_4$)
    E. Thyroid-stimulating hormone (TSH)

138. Which of the following statements regarding anorexia nervosa (AN) and bulimia nervosa (BN) is true?

    A. Patients with the purging subtype of BN tend to be heavier than those with the nonpurging subtype.
    B. Patients with the restricting subtype of AN are more emotionally labile than those with the purging subtype.
    C. Patients with the restricting subtype of AN are more likely to abuse illicit drugs than those with the purging subtype.
    D. The mortality of BN is lower than that of AN.

139. Which of these features represents a critical distinction between anorexia nervosa and bulimia nervosa?

    A. Binge eating
    B. Electrolyte abnormalities
    C. Self-induced vomiting
    D. Underweight

140. You are counseling a patient who is recovering from long-standing anorexia nervosa (AN). She is a 22-year-old woman who suffered the effects of AN for 8 years with a nadir body mass index of 17 kg/m^2 and many laboratory abnormalities during that time. Which of the following characteristics of AN is least likely to improve despite successful lasting treatment of the disorder?

    A. Amenorrhea
    B. Delayed gastric emptying
    C. Lanugo
    D. Low bone mass
    E. Salivary gland enlargement

ANSWERS

1. The answer is B.

(Chap. 8) Upper GI bleeding has an in-hospital mortality rate of 5–10%, with most people dying from their underlying disease rather than exsanguination. Peptic ulcers are the most common cause of upper GI bleeding requiring hospitalization, accounting for ~50% of cases. Other causes include variceal bleeding, Mallory-Weiss tears, erosive disease of the upper GI tract, malignancy, and unidentified. Characteristics of the ulcer at endoscopy provide important prognostic information. One-third of patients with an active bleeding vessel or a nonbleeding visible vessel will have rebleeding that requires surgery. Any finding other than a clean-based ulcer should prompt admission and monitoring for 3 days, as most rebleeding occurs within 3 days. Finding a clean-based ulcer is reassuring, and if the patient is stable and has no other indication for hospitalization, he may be safely discharged.

2. The answer is C.

(Chap. 6) Most causes of acute diarrhea are infectious. Dehydration is a feature of all infectious diarrheas and does not suggest bacterial etiology. Fever and bloody diarrhea are more suggestive. Immunocompromised hosts and the elderly are at greater risk for developing bacteremia and sepsis with certain pathogens, and they also may be less likely to have symptoms suggesting a bacterial pathogen. Stool cultures are typically sent in these populations unless symptoms are mild. (See Fig. 6-2.)

3. The answer is B.

(Chap. 6) Rapid transit may accompany many diarrheas as a secondary or contributing process, but primary dysmotility is an unusual cause of diarrhea. Hormonal and metabolic processes may result in increased motility. Hyperthyroidism is often clinically accompanied by complaints of diarrhea. Medications are a common cause of diarrhea either as a primary cause of motility as in the case of "prokinetic" agents such as metoclopramide and erythromycin or as a side effect of bacterial overgrowth as in the case of prolonged antibiotic administration. Diabetes results in microvascular complications of peripheral and autonomic neuropathies and may result in gastroparesis and intestinal dysmotility. Irritable bowel syndrome is extremely common. It is characterized by disturbed intestinal and colonic motor and sensory responses to various stimuli. Clinically, it is characterized by episodes of constipation and diarrhea. Although disturbances in electrolytes may cause changes in intestinal motility, hypercalcemia is typically associated with constipation, not diarrhea.

4. The answer is C.

(Chap. 6) Diarrhea is loosely defined as passage of abnormally liquid or unformed stools and an increased frequency. This patient has pseudodiarrhea, based on frequent stools, but not diarrhea as they are not loose. Rectal urgency is a common complaint in pseudodiarrhea. The differential diagnosis for pseudodiarrhea includes proctitis and irritable bowel syndrome. Neuromuscular syndromes are linked most closely with fecal incontinence, and hypothyroid most commonly leads to constipation. Ulcerative colitis presents with a broad spectrum of symptoms and cannot be entirely ruled out, but bloody diarrhea, fevers, and pain are more typical. Viral gastroenteritis is acute, self-resolving, and causes diarrhea and often nausea.

5. The answer is B.

(Chap. 1) The pain of peritoneal inflammation is steady, aching, and localized predominantly over the affected area (s). Somatic nerves supplying the parietal peritoneum transmit the pain stimulus, allowing localization. The pain of peritoneal inflammation is invariably accentuated by pressure or changes in tension of the peritoneum. Asking a patient to cough will increase the intraabdominal pressure and lead to rebound tenderness without palpating the abdomen. Another characteristic of peritoneal inflammation is the tonic reflex spasm of the abdominal musculature. Costovertebral angle tenderness, a sign suggestive of pyelonephritis, and heme-positive stools, are neither sensitive nor specific for peritonitis. The presence or quality of bowel sounds are not reliable physical examination findings to distinguish an acute abdomen from a more benign diagnosis.

6. The answer is C.

(Chap. 8) Randomized controlled trials of IV PPI therapy for upper gastrointestinal (GI) bleeding have shown that this therapy decreased further bleeding, but not mortality, for patients with high-risk ulcers (active bleeding, visible vessel, adherent clot) at the time of endoscopy. Instituting IV PPI for all patients with upper GI bleeding does not significantly improve outcomes. Studies have shown a link between long-term usage of PPIs and osteoporosis, but this does not preclude the acute use of PPI in an osteoporotic patient if there is a compelling indication.

7. The answer is B.

(Chap. 8) Hemoglobin/hematocrit levels often do not change acutely in acute GI bleeding. It may take up to 72 hours to see the hemoglobin fall. Moreover, gastric lavage can be nonbloody in 18% of cases of upper GI bleeding. This is seen when there is a duodenal source of bleeding or when the nasogastric tube does not enter the stomach. Testing nonbloody gastric aspirates for occult blood is not useful. Therefore, when there is a clinical suspicion for an upper GI bleed, endoscopy should be performed. CT scanning the abdomen will not be helpful in evaluating an upper GI bleed in the absence of other findings. Rechecking another hematocrit will not alter the indication for upper endoscopy.

8. The answer is D.

(Chaps. 5 and 13) A Zenker's diverticulum typically causes halitosis and regurgitation of saliva and particles of food consumed several days earlier. When a Zenker's diverticulum fills with food, it may produce dysphagia by compressing the esophagus. Gastric outlet obstruction can cause bloating and regurgitation of newly ingested food. Gastrointestinal disorders associated with scleroderma include esophageal reflux, the development of wide-mouthed colonic diverticula, and stasis with bacterial overgrowth. Achalasia typically presents with dysphagia for both solids and liquids. Gastric retention caused by the autonomic neuropathy of diabetes mellitus usually results in postprandial epigastric discomfort and bloating.

9. The answer is A.

(Chaps. 10 and 35) Diagnostic paracentesis is part of the routine evaluation in a patient with ascites. Fluid should be examined for its gross appearance, protein content, cell count and differential, and albumin. Cytologic and culture studies should be performed when one suspects infection or malignancy. The serum-ascites albumin gradient (SAAG) offers the best correlation with portal pressure. A high gradient (>1.1 g/dL) is characteristic of uncomplicated cirrhotic ascites and differentiates ascites caused by portal hypertension from ascites not caused by portal hypertension in more than 95% of cases. Conditions that cause a low gradient include more "exudative" processes such as infection, malignancy, and inflammatory processes. Similarly, congestive heart failure and nephrotic syndrome cause high gradients. In this patient the SAG is 1.5 g/dL, indicating a high gradient. The low number of leukocytes and polymorphonuclear cells makes bacterial or tubercular infection unlikely. Chylous ascites often is characterized by an opaque milky fluid with a triglyceride level greater than 1000 mg/dL in addition to a low SAG.

10. The answer is B.

(Chap. 6) This patient is most likely to have fecal impaction with overflow diarrhea around the impacted area. Colonoscopy is not necessary for diagnosis and may not be needed therapeutically depending on the success of manual disimpaction. C. difficile infection should always be considered in institutionalized persons, particularly the elderly, even in the absence of antecedent diarrhea. However, a negative stool antigen carries very good negative predictive value. Stool culture is indicated in the elderly with moderate to severe diarrhea, but in this case the more likely diagnosis should be ruled out before this is done. Viral gastroenteritis is also possible, but a pathogen is typically not sought as these syndromes self-resolve and there is no available antiviral agent.

11. The answer is G.

(Chap. 6) Chronic constipation occurs from inadequate fiber or fluid consumption, disordered colonic transit, disordered anorectal function due to a neurogastroenterologic

disorder, drugs, or systemic disorders that impact the gastrointestinal tract. Constipation is more often addressed from a therapeutic position by clinicians. Yet it is important not to overlook the fact that constipation can be a presenting feature of a large number of medical, surgical, and psychiatric conditions. Therefore, new or severe constipation should prompt a complete history and physical examination to ensure a key diagnosis is not being overlooked. (See Table 6-5.)

12. The answer is D.

(Chap. 5) The patient's symptoms are most consistent with an obstructive process. The progressive and gradual nature of the process is evident in worsening tolerance for solid foods over the course of months. The patient's prior partial gastrectomy predisposes him to gastric outlet obstruction as a result of stricture at the previous anastomosis. In addition, gastric ulcers often undergo malignant transformation. Although the patient has no current symptoms of peptic ulcer disease, underlying malignancy with gastric outlet obstruction must be considered as gastric ulcers may develop into cancerous lesions if left untreated. Other factors that support the diagnosis of gastric outlet obstruction are the abdominal x-ray findings of dilated gastric bubble and the lack of air in the small bowel. Small bowel obstruction presents acutely with abdominal distention, pain, and vomiting. One would expect to find dilated small bowel loops with air-fluid levels. Gastroparesis is common in poorly controlled diabetic patients, symptomatically affecting approximately 10% of those patients. Frequent vomiting of poorly digested food is reported, as in this patient. However, no abnormal findings are associated on standard radiography. Finally, cholelithiasis is most often asymptomatic but can present as biliary colic. There should be associated pain in the right upper quadrant and epigastrium with eating. Again, the abdominal radiogram is normal in this condition with the possible exception of stones seen within the gallbladder.

13. The answer is E.

(Chap. 5) Juvenile hamartomatous polyps are lesions that consist of lamina propria and dilated cystic glands. They are at increased risk of bleeding, but not malignant transformation. Other polyposis syndromes including familial adenomatous polyposis, Peutz-Jeghers syndrome, and Gardner's syndrome confer increased malignant potential throughout the GI tract. Gastric adenocarcinoma remains a prevalent malignancy worldwide despite significant decline in incidence over the last 50 years. The highest incidence of gastric cancer occurs in Japan. A major pathophysiologic risk appears to be related to bacterial conversion of ingested nitrites into carcinogens in the stomach. Risk factors for the development of gastric cancer include long-term ingestion of foods with high concentrations of nitrite (dried, smoked, salted foods) and conditions that promote bacterial colonization/infection in the stomach, such as Helicobacter infection, chronic gastritis, and achlorhydria. Duodenal ulcers are not a risk factor for gastric carcinoma.

14. The answer is C.

(Chap. 6) Greasy, foul-smelling stools that are difficult to flush are classic for fat malabsorption. The diarrhea is caused by the osmotic effects of fatty acids and neutral fats. Fat malabsorption syndromes classically lead to weight loss and many vitamin deficiencies, including iron, vitamin B_{12}, vitamin D, and vitamin K. Pancreatic insufficiency must be considered in cases of malabsorption, but destruction of the organ must be near total for this to occur, usually in the setting of long-standing alcohol abuse. Celiac disease affects 1% of Americans, often presents with symptoms similar to those of irritable bowel syndrome, and requires an endoscopy with biopsy to confirm the diagnosis. Other causes of steatorrhea include bacterial overgrowth, bariatric surgery, liver disease, and Whipple's disease. A 24-h stool collection is a formal way to confirm steatorrhea, though a consistent patient history may be adequate to begin evaluation. Small-intestinal disease typically will result in fecal fat of ~15–25 g/day, and pancreatic exocrine insufficiency may result in >30 g/day.

15. The answer is E.

(Chap. 6) Diarrhea lasting >4 weeks is considered chronic. Most causes of chronic diarrhea are noninfectious. They can be grouped into secretory, osmotic, steatorrheal, inflammatory, dysmotility, factitious, and iatrogenic causes. Secretory diarrheas are due to altered fluid or electrolyte transport across the enterocolonic mucosa. They typically are large-volume stools that persist with fasting and occur during the night. Stimulant laxatives such as bisacodyl, cascara, castor oil, and senna are very common offending agents for secretory diarrhea. Therefore, the patient's complete (not just prescribed) medication list should always be reviewed before engaging on an expensive search for causes of chronic diarrhea. Countless medications may cause diarrhea; common offenders include antibiotics and antihypertensives. Lactose intolerance is a common cause of osmotic diarrhea. Carcinoid, vasoactive intestinal polypeptide-secreting tumors, medullary thyroid carcinoma, gastrinoma, and villous adenoma are uncommon tumors that are on the differential diagnosis of secretory diarrhea. Crohn's disease can lead to bile salt–induced secretory diarrhea as a presenting feature, but this is less common than its usual presentation as an inflammatory diarrhea. Lymphocytic colitis is an inflammatory disease that causes diarrhea in the elderly.

16. The answer is B.

(Chap. 6) Campylobacter and Shigella are associated with bloody diarrhea. Fecal-oral transmission and exposure to undercooked poultry products are routes of transmission. Although bloody diarrhea is a common occurrence in amebic dysentery, patients may develop extraintestinal

manifestations in the liver, lungs, heart, and brain. Enterotoxigenic E. coli causes a watery diarrhea, but enterohemorrhagic E. coli O157:H7 (often from undercooked hamburger) may cause a severe dysentery and the development of hemolytic-uremic syndrome. Cryptosporidiosis is a common cause of diarrhea in immunodeficient individuals. It causes a profuse watery diarrhea with mucus, but blood and fecal leukocytes are extremely rare.

17. The answer is A.

(Chap. 9) The van den Bergh reaction is commonly used to identify the concentration of conjugated (direct) and total bilirubin. One shortcoming of this method is the inability to differentiate the fraction of conjugated bilirubin that is bound to albumin. Albumin-linked bilirubin (biliprotein) has a longer half-life (12–14 days) in the serum than the free form (4 h), which accounts for one of the enigmas of jaundiced patients with liver disease: the elevated serum bilirubin level declines more slowly than expected in some patients who are otherwise recovering well. Hepatobiliary function is not impaired in these patients.

18. The answer is A.

(Chap. 9) Biliverdin is converted to bilirubin in the reticuloendothelial system. Bilirubin is insoluble in serum and must be bound to albumin before it can be transported to the liver. At the hepatocyte, bilirubin is able to passively be absorbed and reach the endoplasmic reticulum. The enzyme glutathione S-transferase B appears to reduce efflux of bilirubin out of the hepatocyte. In the endoplasmic reticulum, bilirubin is conjugated to glucuronic acid yielding bilirubin mono- and diglucuronide. Conjugated bilirubin is transported into the bile canalicular system via an active process by multiple drug resistance protein 2. In the terminal ileum, bacterial glucuronidases unconjugate the conjugated bilirubin. Unconjugated bilirubin is further reduced into urobilinogen in the terminal ileum. Most (80–90%) of the urobilinogen is excreted in the feces. The remaining 10–20% are passively absorbed into the portal venous blood and either reexcreted by the liver or the kidney.

19. The answer is A.

(Chap. 10) In patients with chronic cirrhosis who develop new or worsening ascites without dietary or medication nonadherence, another occult disorder may be the reason. Common disorders that cause this phenomenon include portal vein thrombosis, hepatocellular carcinoma, portal vein thrombosis, bacterial peritonitis, alcoholic hepatitis, viral infection, and peritoneal tuberculosis. An elevated WBC count is more common when there is a neoplasm, bacterial peritonitis, or tuberculosis. The predominance of lymphocytes raises the suspicion for tuberculosis. The SAAG is classically low in cases of tuberculous peritonitis but may be high when there is concomitant cirrhosis and transudative ascites. The sensitivity of the adenosine deaminase activity is characteristically poor in patients with cirrhosis due to poor T cell–mediated response, therefore, peritoneal biopsy or visual diagnosis during laparoscopy are likely to be required for diagnosis.

20. The answer is C.

(Chap. 9) When evaluating a patient with jaundice, initial steps include determining whether the hyperbilirubinemia is predominantly unconjugated or conjugated and whether there is any other laboratory evidence of hepatobiliary dysfunction. When there are associated biochemical liver abnormalities, further discrimination into a predominantly cholestatic or hepatocellular pattern is possible. A hepatocellular pattern, as in this example characterized by ALT/AST elevated out of proportion to the alkaline phosphatase, should prompt a search for viral, autoimmune, toxicologic, and abnormal deposition disease. Acetaminophen is a common cause of mental status change, jaundice, and hepatocellular injury in the intensive care unit. Liver biopsy may ultimately become necessary. Anatomic abnormalities are more common when there is a cholestatic pattern of injury characterized by an elevated alkaline phosphatase out of proportion to the AST/ALT. In those cases, ultrasound and possible ERCP may be indicated. (See Fig. 9-1.)

21. The answer is C.

(Chap. 9) Unconjugated bilirubin is always bound to albumin in the serum, is not filtered by the kidney, and is not found in the urine. Therefore, any bilirubin found in the urine must be conjugated to glucuronic acid. The presence of bilirubinuria implies the presence of liver disease. Defects that cause elevated levels of unconjugated bilirubin will not cause bilirubinuria. A defect in bilirubin production will not cause bilirubinuria.

22. The answer is B.

(Chap. 9) Causes of isolated unconjugated (indirect) hyperbilirubinemia include inherited (sickle cell disease, spherocytosis, glucose-6-phosphate dehydrogenase deficiency) and acquired (microangiopathic hemolytic anemia, paroxysmal nocturnal hemoglobinuria, immune hemolysis) hemolytic disorders, ineffective erythropoiesis (nutritional deficiencies), inherited conditions (Gilbert's syndrome, Crigler-Najjar types I and II), and drugs (probenecid, ribavirin, rifampicin). Inherited hemolytic disorders with chronic hemolysis carry a high risk of developing calcium bilirubinate gallstones. Patients with hemolytic disorders that cause excessive heme production seldom have a serum bilirubin >5 mg/dL. Higher levels may occur during acute hemolytic conditions (sickle cell crisis) or with concomitant renal or hepatocellular disease. Probenecid (used to treat gout) and rifampicin cause unconjugated hyperbilirubinemia by diminishing hepatic uptake of bilirubin. Cryoglobulinemia is associated with hepatitis C infection which, if present, is associated with a mild hepatocellular pattern of injury and an elevated direct bilirubin.

23. The answer is B.

(Chap. 10) A carefully performed physical examination can reveal important clues concerning the etiology of abdominal swelling. Ascites and increased intraperitoneal pressure will produce stretched skin, bulging flanks, and an everted umbilicus regardless of the etiology of the ascites. Auscultating a venous hum at the umbilicus may signify portal hypertension with increased collateral blood flow around the liver but may not distinguish distal hepatic venous or superior vena cava obstruction. Prominent abdominal venous pattern with the direction of flow away from the umbilicus often reflects portal hypertension. Collateral venous flow from the lower abdomen to the umbilicus suggests inferior vena cava obstruction. Flow from the upper abdomen downward toward the umbilicus suggests superior vena cava obstruction. A pulsatile liver is classically described in severe tricuspid regurgitation.

24. The answer is D.

(Chap. 9) Jaundice that is not due to hyperbilirubinemia may be caused by excessive carotene ingestion, the use of quinacrine, and excessive exposure to phenols. In carotenoderma, the ingested pigment is predominantly deposited in the palms, soles, forehead, and nasolabial folds. The jaundice of carotenoderma, but not quinacrine usage, spares the sclera. The nasolabial folds can be involved in any cause of jaundice. When there is jaundice, skin pigment deposition does not depend on sun exposure. Over time, with bilirubin deposition, sun exposure oxidizes bilirubin to biliverdin causing a green discoloration of the skin in light-skinned patients.

25. The answer is E.

(Chap. 10) The serum-ascites albumin gradient correlates directly with portal pressure. A SAAG >1.1 g/dL is characteristic of portal hypertension with >97% accuracy. A low SAAG (<1.1 g/dL) indicates the patient does not have portal hypertension with >97% accuracy. Occult cirrhosis, intrahepatic sinusoidal destruction, massive hepatic metastases, Budd-Chiari syndrome, right-sided cardiac valve disease, right-sided heart failure, and constrictive pericarditis should be considered when evaluating new-onset ascites with a high SAAG without clear etiology. (See Table 10-1.)

26. The answer is D.

(Chap. 5) This patient has developed tardive dyskinesia that may be irreversible. Prochlorperazine is an antidopaminergic agent that suppresses emesis by acting centrally at the dopamine D_2 receptors. This class of agents is most effective for the treatment of medication-, toxin-, and metabolic-induced emesis. However, these agents freely cross the blood-brain barrier and can cause anxiety, galactorrhea, sexual dysfunction, and dystonic reactions. Tardive

dyskinesia is the most serious of these neurologic toxicities. Erythromycin is a prokinetic that may worsen nausea and vomiting. Ondansetron acts at the 5-HT$_3$ receptor and has no antidopaminergic activity. Scopolamine is an anticholinergic that may cause delirium, stupor, and other neurologic side effects, but not tardive dyskinesia. Glucocorticoids also do not cause tardive dyskinesia.

27. The answer is B.

(Chap. 7) Patients with unintentional weight loss of >5% of the total body weight over a 6- to 12-month period should prompt an evaluation. In the elderly, weight loss is an independent predictor of morbidity and mortality. Studies in the elderly have found mortality rates of 10–15%/year in patients with significant unintentional weight loss. It is important to confirm the weight loss and the duration of time over which it occurred. The causes of weight loss are protean and usually become apparent after a careful evaluation and directed testing. A thorough review of systems should be performed including constitutional, respiratory, gastrointestinal, and psychiatric. Travel history and risk factors for HIV are also important. Medications and supplements should be reviewed. The physical examination must include an examination of the skin, oropharynx, thyroid gland, lymphatic system, abdomen, rectum, prostate, neurologic system, and pelvis. A reasonable laboratory approach would include an initial phase of testing including the tests outlined in this scenario. In the absence of signs or symptoms, close follow-up rather than undirected testing is appropriate. Total-body scanning with PET or CT has not been shown to be effective as screening tests without a clinical indication.

28. The answer is B.

(Chap. 21) In acute appendicitis, tenderness is invariably present at some point in the development of the disorder. Tenderness to palpation will often occur at McBurney's point, anatomically located on a line one-third of the way between the anterior iliac spine and the umbilicus. Abdominal tenderness may be completely absent if there is a retrocecal or pelvic appendix, in which case the sole physical finding may be tenderness in the flank. This is the case with the patient in this scenario. The pain which began in the periumbilical region is pathognomonic for appendicitis. The differential diagnosis of acute appendicitis includes pelvic inflammatory disease, mesenteric lymphadenitis, ruptured ovarian follicle, nephrolithiasis, and pyelonephritis. Pelvic inflammatory disease is less likely because of the history and negative pelvic examination. The urinalysis does not suggest pyelonephritis. There is no history of chronic gastrointestinal disorder (e.g., Crohn's disease) associated with mesenteric lymphadenitis. Ruptured aortic aneurysm is not likely in a young person with no history of congenital atherosclerosis and would most likely present with shock, not inflammatory symptoms.

29. The answer is E.

(Chap. 21) This patient had acute peritonitis secondary to a ruptured appendix. Acute peritonitis is associated with decreased intestinal motor activity, resulting in distention of the intestinal lumen with gas and fluid. The accumulation of fluid in the bowel together with the lack of oral intake leads to rapid intravascular volume depletion. In the presence of systemic inflammation, there is also widespread third space loss. In the current case, this manifested as acute renal failure as well as in the cardiac and central nervous systems. Ureteral injury is a complication of abdominal surgery, but this patient's renal failure predated the procedure. Glomerulonephritis and acute interstitial nephritis are causes of acute renal failure; however, there is no evidence of red cell casts or pyuria. While not mentioned, it is likely that the urine specific gravity was elevated.

30. The answer is E.

(Chap. 18) Anorectal abscess is more prevalent in immunocompromised patients such as those with diabetes, inflammatory bowel disease (IBD), or hematologic disorders and in persons who are HIV-positive. They are more common in men than women and typically occur in young patients. The greatly elevated erythrocyte sedimentation rate (ESR) (corrected for age) suggests an inflammatory state, and the skin nodules would suggest erythema nodosum. IBD often presents with perianal abscesses and is associated with an elevated ESR, erythema nodosum, and uveitis, among other extraintestinal manifestations. Giant cell arteritis would be uncommon in a patient this young. A normal glycosylated hemoglobin makes type 1 diabetes less likely. Acute sarcoidosis may present with erythema nodosum (Löfgrens syndrome), but there is typically mediastinal adenopathy. There is no association between sarcoidosis and perianal abscess. While patients with HIV infection commonly develop anorectal abscess, *Pneumocystis* pneumonia would typically present with respiratory complaints and an abnormal radiograph, not erythema nodosum.

31. The answer is B.

(Chap. 16) The location and description of this form of IBD, without mention of other parts of the gastrointestinal tract involved and superficial involvement of the mucosa, is highly suggestive of ulcerative colitis (UC). The effects of cigarette smoking are different on UC and Crohn's disease (CD). The risk of UC in smokers is less than half that of nonsmokers. In contrast, smoking is associated with a twofold risk of CD. UC is equally common in males and females, whereas CD is more common in women. The age distribution is similar for UC and CD. Appendectomy is protective in UC. There is 0% concordance for dizygotic twins in UC and only 6% concordance for monozygotic disease. CD has a substantially higher concordance in monozygotic twins, but a 5% concordance in dizygotic twins.

32. The answer is D.

(*Chap. 18*) The patient has a chronic anal fissure. Anal fissures are often diagnosed by history alone, with severe anal pain made worse with defecation. There is often mild associated bleeding, but less than that seen with hemorrhoidal bleeding. The blood is usually described as staining the toilet paper or coating the stool. Associated conditions include constipation, trauma, Crohn's disease, and infections, including tuberculosis and syphilis. Acute anal fissures appear like a linear laceration, whereas chronic fissures show evidence of hypertrophied anal papillae at the proximal end with a skin tag at the distal end. Often the circular fibers of the internal anal sphincter can be seen at the base of the fissure. Acute anal fissures are treated conservatively with increased dietary fiber intake, topical anesthetics or glucocorticoids, and sitz baths. Treatment for chronic anal fissures is aimed at finding methods to decrease anal sphincter tone. Topical nitroglycerin or botulinum toxin injections may be used. In some cases surgical therapy becomes necessary with lateral internal sphincterotomy and dilatation.

33. The answer is E.

(*Chap. 14*) Gastric parietal cells create hydrochloric acid through a process of oxidative phosphorylation involving the H^+-K^+-ATPase pump. For each molecule of hydrochloric acid produced, a bicarbonate ion is released into the gastric venous circulation, creating the "bicarbonate tide." Control of gastric acid secretion is primarily under the control of the parasympathetic system. Postganglionic vagal fibers stimulate muscarinic receptors on parietal cells to increase acid secretion. In addition, cholinergic stimulation increases gastrin release from antral G cells as well as increasing the sensitivity of parietal cells to circulating gastrin. Gastrin is the most potent stimulus of gastric acid secretion and is released from antral G cells in response to cholinergic stimuli. Histamine is also a potent stimulus for gastric acid secretion. It is stored in enterochromaffin-like cells in the oxyntic glands of the stomach. Stimuli for histamine release include gastrin and acetylcholine. Finally, caffeine stimulates gastrin release and thus increases acid secretion.

34. The answer is A.

[*Chap. 16; Am J Gastroenterol 98 (12 Suppl): S31–S36, 2003.*] Collagenous colitis is one of the two atypical (microscopic) colitides that should be included in the differential diagnosis of inflammatory bowel disease. The other atypical colitis is lymphocytic colitis. These diseases present typically with watery diarrhea in 50-to 60-year-old patients. Collagenous colitis is markedly more common in women, whereas lymphocytic colitis has an equal sex distribution. Both have normal endoscopic appearances and require biopsy for diagnosis. Collagenous colitis features increased subepithelial collagen deposition and inflammation with increased intraepithelial lymphocytes.

In lymphocytic colitis, there is no collagen deposition and there are greater numbers of intraepithelial lymphocytes than is the case in collagenous colitis. Treatment for collagenous colitis ranges from sulfasalazine or mesalamine to glucocorticoids, depending on severity. Lymphocytic colitis is usually treated with 5-ASA or prednisone.

35. The answer is C.

(*Chap. 14*) Fasting gastrin levels can be elevated in a variety of conditions including atrophic gastritis with or without pernicious anemia, G-cell hyperplasia, and acid suppressive therapy (gastrin levels increase as a consequence of loss of negative feedback). The diagnostic concern in a patient with persistent ulcers following optimal therapy is Zollinger-Ellison syndrome (ZES). The result is not sufficient to make a diagnosis because gastrin levels may be elevated in a variety of conditions. Elevated basal acid secretion also is consistent with ZES, but up to 12% of patients with peptic ulcer disease may have basal acid secretion as high as 15 meq/h. Thus, additional testing is necessary. Gastrin levels may go up with a meal (>200%) but this test does not distinguish G-cell hyperfunction from ZES. The best test in this setting is the secretin stimulation test. An increase in gastrin levels >200 pg within 15 min of administering 2 µg/kg of secretin by intravenous bolus has a sensitivity and specificity of >90% for ZES. Endoscopic ultrasonography is useful in locating the gastrin-secreting tumor once the positive secretin test is obtained. Genetic testing for mutations in the gene that encodes the menin protein can detect the fraction of patients with gastrinomas that are a manifestation of multiple endocrine neoplasia type 1 (Wermer's syndrome). Gastrinoma is the second most common tumor in this syndrome behind parathyroid adenoma, but its peak incidence is generally in the third decade.

36. The answer is C.

(*Chap. 17*) Although this patient has signs and symptoms consistent with IBS, the differential diagnosis is large. Few tests are required for patients who have typical IBS symptoms and no alarm features. In this patient, alarm features include anemia, an elevated ESR, and evidence of WBCs in the stool. Alarm features warrant further investigation to rule out other gastrointestinal disorders such as diverticular disease or inflammatory bowel disease. Reassurance, stool bulking agents, and antidepressants are all therapies to consider if a patient does indeed have IBS

37. The answer is E.

(*Chap. 17*) Up to 80% of patients with IBS also have abnormal psychiatric features; however, no single psychiatric diagnosis predominates. The mechanism is not well understood but may involve altered pain thresholds. Although these patients are hypersensitive to colonic stimuli, this does not carry over to the peripheral nervous system. Functional brain imaging shows disparate activation in, for example, the mid-cingulate cortex, but brain anatomy does not discriminate IBS patients from those without IBS. An association between a history of sexual abuse and IBS has been reported but not with sexually transmitted diseases. Patients with IBS do not have an increased risk of autoimmunity.

38. The answer is B.

(Chap. 13) Diffuse esophageal spasm is a disorder of esophageal motility marked by disorganized nonperistaltic contractions. The contractions are due to dysfunction of the inhibitory nerves, with pain correlating with contractions of long duration and large amplitude. Clinically, patients present with sharp substernal chest pain that may mimic cardiac disease with radiation to the arms, chest, and jaw. Symptoms last for a few seconds to minutes and may be related to swallowing or emotional stress. Dysphagia with or without pain often coexists. The presence of cardiac disease needs to be evaluated before consideration of a noncardiac cause of chest pain. The diagnostic procedure of choice is barium swallow, which shows loss of normal peristaltic contractions below the level of the aortic arch. Instead, there are numerous uncoordinated simultaneous contractions that produce multiple ripples in the esophageal wall with sacculation and pseudodiverticula. This creates the characteristic appearance of a "corkscrew" esophagus. Treatment is aimed primarily at preventing these contractions with medications that cause smooth muscle relaxation, such as nitrates and calcium channel blockers. The other options listed describe other diseases of the esophagus. A beaklike appearance of the distal esophagus is characteristic of achalasia. Scleroderma causes atrophy of the smooth muscle within the lower two-thirds of the esophagus and is represented on barium swallow as dilation of the distal esophagus with loss of peristaltic contractions. Gastroesophageal reflux disease is a common disorder that affects 15% of persons at least once per week and is marked by loss of lower esophageal sphincter tone with reflux of barium back into the distal esophagus. Esophageal narrowing with apple-core lesions is typical of esophageal cancer.

39. The answer is C.

(Chap. 15) The combination of steatorrhea, weight loss, and migratory large joint arthralgias is consistent with the diagnosis of Whipple's disease. Whipple's disease may also cause cardiac and central nervous system (CNS) disease, including dementia. It is caused by chronic infection with T. whippelii. The disease occurs predominantly in middle-aged white men. Whipple's disease may also be diagnosed by a small bowel (or other involved organ) showing macrophages staining positive for PAS and containing the small Whipple's bacillus. Treatment for Whipple's disease requires prolonged (1 year) therapy with trimethoprim-sulfamethoxazole or chloramphenicol. Antiendomysial antibodies, antigliadin IgA antibodies, and the

small bowel biopsy findings described above are characteristic of celiac sprue. Antibiotic-associated colitis caused by C. difficile does not cause steatorrhea.

40. The answer is D.

[Chap. 16, Cochrane Database Syst Rev 2007 Oct 17; (4)] Despite being described as a clinical entity for over a century, the etiology of IBD remains cryptic. Current theory is related to an interplay between inflammatory stimuli in genetically predisposed individuals. Recent studies have identified a group of genes or polymorphisms that confer risk of IBD. Multiple microbiologic agents, including some that reside as "normal" flora, may initiate IBD by triggering an inflammatory response. Anaerobic organisms (e.g., Bacteroides and Clostridia spp.) may be responsible for the induction of inflammation. Other organisms, for unclear reasons, may have the opposite effect. These "probiotic" organisms include Lactobacillus spp., Bifidobacterium spp., Taenia suis, and Saccharomyces boulardii. Shigella, Escherichia, and Campylobacter spp. are known to promote inflammation. Studies of probiotic therapy in adults and children with IBD have shown potential benefit for reducing disease activity.

41. The answer is D.

(Chap. 17) Serotonin receptor antagonists enhance the sensitivity of the afferent neurons projecting from the gut. Alosetron, a 5-HT$_3$ receptor antagonist, reduces perception of painful visceral stimulation, induces rectal relaxation, and delays colonic transport in patients with IBS. Clinical studies have shown the long-term efficacy of alosetron for IBS. However, in postrelease surveillance, 84 cases of ischemic colitis were reported soon after patients were placed on alosetron. Of these, 44 cases required surgery and 4 patients died. Most cases developed within 30 days of starting the medication, and many were within 1 week. Alosetron was withdrawn voluntarily in 2000 but has been reintroduced with a strict monitoring program. Given the temporal relation and compatible clinical presentation, that is the most likely diagnosis in this case. A CT scan would likely show diffuse colitis. Therapy involves discontinuation of the drug, supportive therapy, and possible surgical resection. The other diagnoses may present with a similar clinical picture and should be on the differential diagnosis.

42. The answer is C.

(Chap. 18) This patient has symptoms (social isolation), signs (foul odor), and risk factors (multiparity) for procidentia (rectal prolapse) and fecal incontinence. Procidentia is far more common in women than men and is often associated with pelvic floor disorders. It is not uncommon for these patients to become socially withdrawn and suffer from depression because of the associated fecal incontinence. The foul odor is a result of poor perianal hygiene due to the prolapsed rectum. Although depression in the elderly is an important medical problem, it is too premature in the evaluation to initiate medical therapy for depression. Occult malignancy and thyroid abnormalities may cause fecal incontinence and depression, but a physical examination would be diagnostic and avoid costly tests. Often patients are concerned they have a rectal mass or carcinoma. Examination after an enema often makes the prolapse apparent. Medical therapy is limited to stool bulking agents or fiber. Surgical correction is the mainstay of therapy.

43. The answer is D.
(Chap. 16) Methotrexate, azathioprine, cyclosporine, tacrolimus, or anti-tumor necrosis factor (TNF) antibody are reasonable options for patients with CD, depending on the extent of macroscopic disease. Pneumonitis is a rare but serious complication of methotrexate therapy. Primary sclerosing cholangitis is an extraintestinal manifestation of inflammatory bowel disease (IBD). Pancreatitis is an uncommon complication of azathioprine, and IBD patients treated with azathioprine are at fourfold increased risk of developing a lymphoma. Anti-TNF antibody therapy is associated with an increased risk of tuberculosis, disseminated histoplasmosis, and a number of other infections.

44. The answer is B.
(Chap. 18) This is a classic presentation of familial Mediterranean fever, an inherited disease most common in Armenians, Arabs, Turks, and non-Ashkenazi Jews. Febrile episodes begin in early childhood, with more than 90% of patients experiencing the first attack by age 20. Fever is invariably a feature of an acute attack. Other common features include severe serositis presenting most frequently as peritonitis or pleuritis. The pain is often so severe that exploratory laparotomy may be performed to search for a source of peritonitis. CT imaging shows only small amounts of free fluid in the abdomen or pleural space. On laboratory testing this fluid represents sterile neutrophilia in response to the intense serosal inflammation. Other manifestations of the disease include acute monoarthritis with large sterile, neutrophilic effusions and a rash that resembles erysipelas on the lower extremity. The attacks are self-limited and resolve within 72 h, although the joint symptoms may persist. Amyloidosis as a result of chronic inflammation is a common manifestation late in the disease. Laboratory studies are nonspecific, showing changes expected with acute inflammation. Diagnosis usually can be made with clinical criteria alone, although there is gene testing available for the most common mutations that cause the disease. Treatment is targeted at preventing attacks with colchicine, a drug that inhibits microtubule formation and has been demonstrated to decrease the frequency and intensity of the attacks. In addition, it can prevent the development of amyloidosis. There are no alternative therapies available,

although investigations into the use of interferon and tumor necrosis factor inhibitors are ongoing.

45. The answer is A.
(Chap. 21) Appendicitis occurs in every 500–2000 pregnancies and tends to be most common during the second trimester. It is important to consider acute appendicitis in this population due to the frequent occurrence of mild abdominal discomfort, nausea, and vomiting during pregnancy. The unremarkable urine analysis makes pyelonephritis or nephrolithiasis less likely. Rupture of a Graafian follicle (mittelschmerz) occurs during menses, not pregnancy. Fitz-Hugh–Curtis (perihepatitis) syndrome could present with these symptoms during pregnancy; however, there is no cervicitis on examination, and the initial periumbilical pain makes appendicitis more likely.

46. The answer is D.
(Chap. 15) This patient has a stool osmolality gap (measured stool osmolality – calculated stool osmolality) of <50 mosmol/L, suggesting a secretory rather than an osmotic cause for diarrhea. Secretory causes of diarrhea include toxin-mediated diarrhea (cholera, enterotoxigenic *Escherichia coli*) and intestinal peptide–mediated diarrhea in which the major pathophysiology is a luminal or circulating secretagogue. The distinction between secretory diarrhea and osmotic diarrhea aids in forming a differential diagnosis. Secretory diarrhea will not decrease substantially during a fast and has a low osmolality gap. Osmotic diarrhea will generally decrease during a fast and has a high (>50 mosmol/L) osmolality gap. Celiac sprue, chronic pancreatitis, lactase deficiency, and Whipple's disease all cause an osmotic diarrhea.

47. and 48. The answers are C and D.
(Chap. 21) The patient presents with several months of epigastric abdominal pain that is worse after eating. His symptoms are highly suggestive of peptic ulcer disease, with the worsening pain after eating suggesting a duodenal ulcer. The current presentation with acute abdomen and free air under the diaphragm diagnoses perforated viscus. Perforated gallbladder is less likely in light of the duration of symptoms and the absence of the significant systemic symptoms that often accompany this condition. As the patient is relatively young with no risk factors for mesenteric ischemia, necrotic bowel from an infarction is highly unlikely. Pancreatitis can have a similar presentation, but a pancreas cannot perforate and liberate free air. Peritonitis is most commonly associated with bacterial infection, but it can be caused by the abnormal presence of physiologic fluids, for example, gastric contents, bile, pancreatic enzymes, blood, or urine, or by foreign bodies. In this case peritonitis most likely is due to the presence of gastric juice in the peritoneal cavity after perforation of a duodenal ulcer has allowed these juices to leave the gut lumen.

49. The answer is C.

(Chap. 13) The patient has typical symptoms of, and barium findings for, achalasia, an esophageal disease marked by abnormal motility and failure of the lower esophageal sphincter to relax normally with swallowing. The underlying abnormality is loss of the intramural neurons that control the inhibitory neurotransmitters. Other diseases that can cause secondary achalasia through destruction of these neurons include Chagas' disease, malignancy, and viral infections. Typical clinical symptoms of achalasia include dysphagia with both solids and liquids equally and worsening of symptoms with emotional stressors and rapid eating. Aspiration and regurgitation of undigested food are also common. The presence of esophageal reflux symptoms is inconsistent with the diagnosis of achalasia. The course is usually progressive, with weight loss occurring over several months. Diagnosis can be made from the classic appearance on barium swallow of esophageal dilatation with a beaklike appearance of the lower esophagus representing the failure of the lower esophageal sphincter (LES) to relax. Other diagnostic maneuvers include manometry demonstrating increased LES tone, and endoscopy should be performed to exclude coincident carcinoma. Treatment is often difficult. Nitrates and calcium channel blockers offer short-term benefits for relief of symptoms but lose efficacy over time. Endoscopic injections of botulinum toxin are also effective for short periods but may lead to fibrosis with repeated injections. Balloon dilatation is effective in approximately 85% of patients with the side effect of perforation or bleeding. Finally, some patients ultimately require surgical intervention with myotomy, which has equal success compared to balloon dilatation.

50. The answer is B.

(Chap. 16) Arthritis, typically involving the large joints of the upper and lower extremities, develops in 15–20% of patients with inflammatory bowel disease (IBD). It is more common in Crohn's disease (CD) than in ulcerative colitis (UC) and flares with disease activity. Treatment is focused on controlling bowel inflammation. Erythema nodosum and venous thromboembolism also generally correlate with intestinal disease activity. In contrast, the other extraintestinal manifestations of IBD listed above typically do not correlate with disease activity. Ankylosing spondylitis is more common in CD than in UC and may occur in up to 10% of these patients. The course is often progressive and debilitating. Nephrolithiasis occurs more frequently in CD with ileal disease resulting from calcium oxalate stones. Primary sclerosing cholangitis (PSC) occurs in 1–5% of patients with IBD. Most patients with PSC have IBD. PSC may be detected before active bowel disease and may even occur years after proctocolectomy in patients with UC. Ten percent of patients with PSC will develop cholangiocarcinoma. Uveitis is associated with UC and CD

and may occur during remission or after bowel resection. Without timely treatment with corticosteroids, vision loss may ensue.

51. The answer is E.

(Chap. 18) Surgical therapy is indicated in all low-risk surgical patients with complicated diverticular disease. Patients with at least two episodes of diverticulitis requiring hospitalization, with disease that does not respond to medical therapy, or who develop intra-abdominal complications are considered to have complicated disease. Complicating this patient's relapse of diverticulitis is probably an enterovesicular fistula causing pneumaturia. Studies indicate that younger patients (<50 years) may experience a more aggressive form of the disease than older patients, and therefore waiting for more than two attacks before considering surgery is not recommended. Rifaximin is a poorly absorbed broad-spectrum antibiotic that, when combined with a fiber-rich diet, is associated with less frequent symptoms in patients with uncomplicated diverticular disease. Pneumaturia represents a potential surgical urgency and should not be confused with proteinuria.

52. The answer is A.

(Chap. 18) Hemorrhage from a colonic diverticulum is the most common cause of hematochezia in patients >60 years of age. Patients with atherosclerosis, hypertension, and increased bleeding risk are most commonly affected. Most bleeds are intense, but are self-limited and stop spontaneously. They usually arise from the right colon. The lifetime risk of rebleeding is 25%. While colonoscopy can be both diagnostic and therapeutic in lower GI bleeding, the ability to visualize the mucosa is limited when the bleeding is brisk. Angiography can localize the bleeding and, if the patient is stable, bleeding is best managed by mesenteric angiography. If identified, the bleeding vessel may be successfully occluded with a coil in 80% of cases with <10% risk of colonic ischemia. This patient is normotensive and has a normal heart rate, suggesting that he is stable for angiography. Surgery is reserved for patients with unstable bleeding or a >6 unit/24 h bleeding episode.

53. The answer is A.

(Chap. 13) This patient has symptoms of esophagitis. In patients with HIV various infections can cause this disease, including herpes simplex virus (HSV), cytomegalovirus (CMV), varicella zoster virus (VZV), *Candida*, and HIV itself. The lack of thrush does not rule out *Candida* as a cause of esophagitis, and EGD is necessary for diagnosis. CMV classically causes serpiginous ulcers in the distal esophagus that may coalesce to form large giant ulcers. Brushings alone are insufficient for diagnosis, and biopsies must be performed. Biopsies reveal intranuclear and intracytoplasmic inclusions with

enlarged nuclei in large fibroblasts and endothelial cells. Intravenous ganciclovir is the treatment of choice, and valganciclovir is an oral preparation that has been introduced recently. Foscarnet is useful in treating ganciclovir-resistant CMV.

Herpes simplex virus manifests as vesicles and punched-out lesions in the esophagus with the characteristic finding on biopsy of ballooning degeneration with ground-glass changes in the nuclei. It can be treated with acyclovir or foscarnet in resistant cases. *Candida* esophagitis has the appearance of yellow nodular plaques with surrounding erythema. Treatment usually requires fluconazole therapy. Finally, HIV alone can cause esophagitis that can be quite resistant to therapy. On EGD these ulcers appear deep and linear. Treatment with thalidomide or oral glucocorticoids is employed, and highly active antiretroviral therapy should be considered.

54. The answer is C.

(*Chap. 15*) The patient's symptoms are consistent with bacterial overgrowth in the afferent loop. These patients complain of abdominal bloating and pain 20 min to 1 h after eating. There may be associated vomiting. In addition, malabsorptive diarrhea is common and ceases with fasting. The report of foul-smelling diarrhea that floats should prompt an evaluation for fat malabsorption. This patient also has a macrocytic anemia, which can result from vitamin B_{12} deficiency.

Many other complications have been noted after surgery for peptic ulcer disease. Dumping syndrome refers to a spectrum of vasomotor symptoms that occur after peptic ulcer surgery, including tachycardia, light-headedness, and diaphoresis. It can occur within 30 min of eating and is related to rapid delivery of hyperosmolar contents to the proximal small intestine, resulting in large fluid shifts. A late dumping syndrome can also occur, with similar symptoms developing 90 min to 3 h after eating. It is related to meals containing large amounts of simple carbohydrates and thus causes insulin surges and hypoglycemia. Bile reflux gastropathy presents after partial gastrectomy with abdominal pain, early satiety, and vomiting. Histologic examination reveals minimal inflammation but extensive epithelial injury. Treatment consists of prokinetic agents and bile acid sequestrants. Finally, postvagotomy diarrhea occurs in 10% of patients after peptic ulcer surgery. These patients usually complain of severe diarrhea that occurs 1–2 h after meals. Abdominal bloating and malabsorption are not usually part of this syndrome.

55. The answer is E.

(*Chap. 15*) This patient most likely has primary lactase deficiency. Carbohydrates in the diet are composed of starches, disaccharides (lactose, sucrose), and glucose. Only monosaccharides (glucose, galactose) are absorbed in the small intestine so that starches and disaccharides must be digested before absorption. Starches are digested by amylase (pancreatic > salivary). Lactose, the disaccharide present in milk, requires digestion by brush border lactase into glucose and galactose. Lactase is present in the intestinal brush border in all species during the postnatal period but disappears except in humans. There are marked racial differences in the persistence of lactase, with Asians having among the highest prevalence of lactase deficiency and Northern Europeans having the lowest prevalence. In primary lactase deficiency other aspects of intestinal nutrient absorption and brush border function are normal. Symptoms usually arise in adolescence or adulthood and consist of diarrhea, abdominal pain, cramps, bloating, and flatus after the consumption of milk products. The differential diagnosis includes irritable bowel syndrome. Treatment involves avoidance of foods with a high lactose content (milk, ice cream) and use of oral galactosidase ("lactase") enzyme replacement. The efficacy of the enzyme replacement treatments varies with the product, the food, and the individual. Cholestyramine is useful in cases of bile acid diarrhea. Viokase is used in patients with chronic pancreatic insufficiency (chronic pancreatitis, resection, cystic fibrosis) and contains amylase, protease, and lipase. Metoclopramide is a promotility agent and will not help symptoms of lactase deficiency. Omeprazole is a proton pump inhibitor and will decrease gastric acid secretion. (See Table 15-5.)

56. The answer is A.

(*Chap. 19*) Mesenteric ischemia is a relatively uncommon and highly morbid illness. Acute mesenteric ischemia is usually due to arterial embolus (usually from the heart) or from thrombosis in a diseased vascular bed. Major risk factors include age, atrial fibrillation, valvular disease, recent arterial catheterization, and recent myocardial infarction. Ischemia occurs when the intestines are inadequately perfused by the splanchnic circulation. This blood supply has extensive collateralization and can receive up to 30% of the cardiac output, making poor perfusion an uncommon event. Patients with acute mesenteric ischemia will frequently present with pain out of proportion to their initial physical examination. As ischemia persists, peritoneal signs and cardiovascular collapse will follow. Mortality is >50%. While radiographic imaging can suggest ischemia, the gold standard for diagnosis is laparotomy.

57. The answer is D.

(*Chap. 32*) Trichomoniasis is transmitted via sexual contact with an infected partner. Many men are asymptomatic but may have symptoms of urethritis, epididymitis, or prostatitis. Most women will have symptoms of infection that include vaginal itching, dyspareunia, and malodorous discharge. These symptoms do not distinguish *Trichomonas* infection from other forms of vaginitis, such as bacterial vaginosis. Trichomoniasis is not a self-limited infection and should be treated for symptomatic and public health reasons. Wet-mount examination for motile trichomonads has a sensitivity of 50–60% in routine examination. Direct immunofluorescent antibody staining of secretions is more sensitive and can also be performed immediately. Culture is not widely available and takes 3–7 days. Treatment should consist of metronidazole either as a single 2-g dose or 500-mg doses twice daily for 7 days; all sexual partners should be treated. Trichomoniasis resistant to metronidazole has been reported and is managed with increased doses of metronidazole or with tinidazole.

58. The answer is B.

(Chap. 33) Strongyloides is the only helminth that can replicate in the human host, allowing autoinfection. Humans acquire strongyloides when larvae in fecally contaminated soil penetrate the skin or mucus membranes. The larvae migrate to the lungs via the bloodstream, break through the alveolar spaces, ascend the respiratory airways, and are swallowed to reach the small intestine where they mature into adult worms. Adult worms may penetrate the mucosa of the small intestine. Strongyloides is endemic in Southeast Asia, Sub-Saharan Africa, Brazil, and the Southern United States. Many patients with strongyloides are asymptomatic or have mild gastrointestinal symptoms or the characteristic cutaneous eruption, larval currens, as described in this case. Small-bowel obstruction may occur with early heavy infection. Eosinophilia is common with all clinical manifestations. In patients with impaired immunity, particularly glucocorticoid therapy, hyperinfection or dissemination may occur. This may lead to colitis, enteritis, meningitis, peritonitis, and acute renal failure. Bacteremia or gram-negative sepsis may develop due to bacterial translocation through disrupted enteric mucosa. Because of the risk of hyperinfection, all patients with strongyloides, even asymptomatic carriers, should be treated with ivermectin, which is more effective than albendazole. Fluconazole is used to treat candidal infections. Mebendazole is used to treat trichuriasis, enterobiasis (pinworm), ascariasis, and hookworm. Mefloquine is used for malaria prophylaxis.

59. and 60. The answers are B and E.

(Chap. 22) Norovirus, or the so-called Norwalk-like agent, was initially described as a cause of food-borne illness in Norwalk, Ohio, in 1968. Since that time the virus responsible has been identified as a small RNA virus of the Calciviridae family. The initial detection of the Norwalk agent was poor, relying on electron microscopy or immune electron microscopy. Using these techniques, the Norwalk agent was identified as the causative agent in 19–42% of nonbacterial diarrheal outbreaks. With the development of more sensitive

molecular assays (reverse transcriptase PCR, enzyme-linked immunosorbent assay), Norwalk-like viruses are being found as increasingly frequent causes of diarrheal outbreaks. Treatment is supportive as symptoms improve within 10–51 h. Rotavirus is the most common cause of viral diarrhea in infants but is uncommon in adults. Salmonella, shigella, and *E. coli* present with more colonic and systemic manifestations.

61. The answer is C.

(Chap. 22) Enterotoxigenic *E. coli* is responsible for 50% of traveler's diarrhea in Latin America and 15% in Asia. Enterotoxigenic and enteroaggregative *E. coli* are the most common isolates from persons with classic secretory traveler's diarrhea. Treatment of frequent watery stools due to presumed *E. coli* infection may be with ciprofloxacin, or because of concerns regarding increasing ciprofloxacin resistance, azithromycin. *E. histolytica* and *V. cholerae* account for smaller percentages of traveler's diarrhea in Mexico. *Campylobacter* is more common in Asia and during the winter in subtropical areas. *Giardia* is associated with contaminated water supplies and in campers who drink from freshwater streams.

62. The answer is D.

(Chap. 25) Helicobacter pylori is thought to colonize ~50% (30% in developed countries, >80% in developing countries) of the world's population. The organism induces a direct tissue response in the stomach, with evidence of mononuclear and polymorphonuclear infiltrates in all of those with colonization, regardless of whether or not symptoms are present. Gastric ulceration and adenocarcinoma of the stomach arise in association with this gastritis. MALT is specific to *H. pylori* infection and is due to prolonged B cell activation in the stomach. Though *H. pylori* does not directly infect the intestine, it does diminish somatostatin production, indirectly contributing to the development of duodenal ulcers. Gastroesophageal reflux disease is not caused by *H. pylori*, and some early, controversial research may suggest that it is in fact protective against this condition.

63. The answer is D.

(Chap. 23) Clostridium difficile–associated disease recurrences are most often due to reinfection (because patients carry similar risk factors as they did before first infection) or relapse (due to persistence of spores in the bowel). Approximately 15–30% of patients have at least one relapse. Recurrent disease has been associated with ~10% risk of serious complications including shock, megacolon, perforation, colectomy, or death in 30 days. Metronidazole resistance occurs but is actually a very rare event. Metronidazole and vancomycin have a similar efficacy in a first episode of recurrence. Repeated courses of metronidazole should be avoided due to neurotoxicity. Unfortunately, patients who recur are

more likely to recur again, and many patients receive multiple cycles of antibiotics and are even candidates for more extreme measures such as intravenous immunoglobulin or fecal transplant via stool enema. Testing for clearance is not likely to be informative. A negative stool antigen would not change management, as symptomatic improvement is the true goal of therapy. A positive stool antigen and toxin test in a patient whose symptoms have improved after standard therapy implies colonization, not disease. It can therefore be needlessly discouraging to patients and again does not impact clinical management. There is no known association between *C. difficile*–associated disease and colon cancer.

64. The answer is D.

(Chap. 32) Giardia lamblia is one of the most common parasitic diseases, with worldwide distribution. It occurs in developed and developing countries. Infection follows ingestion of environmental cysts, which excyst in the small intestine releasing flagellated trophozoites. *Giardia* does not disseminate hematogenously; it remains in the small intestine. Cysts are excreted in stool, which accounts for person-to-person spread; however, they do not survive for prolonged periods in feces. Ingestion of contaminated water sources is another major form of infection. *Giardia* cysts can thrive in cold water for months. Filtering or boiling water will remove cysts. As few as 10 cysts can cause human disease, which has a broad spectrum of presentations. Most infected patients are asymptomatic. Symptoms in infected patients are due to small-intestinal dysfunction. Typical early symptoms include diarrhea, abdominal pain, bloating, nausea, vomiting, flatus, and belching. Diarrhea is a very common complaint, particularly early, but in some patients constipation will occur. Later, diarrhea may resolve, with malabsorption symptoms predominating. The presence of fever, eosinophilia, blood or mucus in stools, or colitis symptoms should suggest an alternative diagnosis. Diagnosis is made by demonstrating parasite antigens, cysts, or trophozoites in the stool.

65. The answer is F.

(Chap. 25, Figure 25-2) It is impossible to know whether the patient's continued dyspepsia is due to persistent *H. pylori* as a result of treatment failure or to some other cause. A quick noninvasive test to look for the presence of *H. pylori* is a urea breath test. This test can be done as an outpatient and gives a rapid, accurate response. Patients should not have received any proton pump inhibitors or antimicrobials in the meantime. Stool antigen test is another good option if urea breath testing is not available. If the urea breath test is positive >1 month after completion of first-line therapy, second-line therapy with a proton pump inhibitor, bismuth subsalicylate, tetracycline, and metronidazole may be indicated. If the urea breath test is negative, the remaining symptoms are

unlikely due to persistent *H. pylori* infection. Serology is useful only for diagnosing infection initially, but it can remain positive and therefore misleading in those who have cleared *H. pylori*. Endoscopy is a consideration to rule out ulcer or upper gastrointestinal malignancy but is generally preferred after two failed attempts to eradicate *H. pylori*.

66. The answer is B.

(Chap. 33) Ascaris lumbricoides is the longest nematode (15–40 cm) parasite of humans. It resides in tropical and subtropical regions. In the United States, it is found mostly in the rural Southeast. Transmission is through fecally contaminated soil. Most commonly the worm burden is low and it causes no symptoms. Clinical disease is related to larval migration to the lungs or to adult worms in the gastrointestinal tract. The most common complications occur due to a high gastrointestinal adult worm burden leading to small-bowel obstruction (most often in children with a narrow-caliber small-bowel lumen) or migration leading to obstructive complications such as cholangitis, pancreatitis, or appendicitis. Rarely, adult worms can migrate to the esophagus and be orally expelled. During the lung phase of larval migration (9–12 days after egg ingestion) patients may develop a nonproductive cough, fever, eosinophilia, and pleuritic chest pain. Eosinophilic pneumonia syndrome (Löffler's syndrome) is characterized by symptoms and lung infiltrates. Meningitis is not a known complication of ascariasis but can occur with disseminated strongyloidiasis in an immunocompromised host.

67. The answer is A.

(Chap. 25) H. pylori is a disease of overcrowding. Transmission has therefore decreased in the United States as the standard of living has increased. It is predicated that the percentage of duodenal ulcers due to factors other than *H. pylori* (e.g., use of nonsteroidal anti-inflammatory drugs) will increase over the upcoming decades. Controversial, but increasing, evidence suggests that *H. pylori* colonization may provide some protection from recent emerging gastrointestinal disorders, such as gastroesophageal reflux disease (and its complication, esophageal carcinoma). Therefore, the health implications of *H. pylori* eradication may not be simple.

68. The answer is E.

(Chap. 23) Clindamycin, ampicillin, and cephalosporins (including ceftriaxone) were the first antibiotics associated with *C. difficile*–associated disease, and still are. More recently, broad-spectrum fluoroquinolones, including moxifloxacin and ciprofloxacin, have been associated with outbreaks of *C. difficile*, including outbreaks in some locations of a more virulent strain that has caused severe disease among elderly outpatients. For unclear reasons, β-lactams other than the later generation

cephalosporins appear to carry a lesser risk of disease. Penicillin/β-lactamase combination antibiotics appear to have lower risk of *C. difficile*–associated disease than the other agents mentioned. Cases have even been reported associated with metronidazole and vancomycin administration. Nevertheless, all patients initiating antibiotics should be warned to seek care if they develop diarrhea that is severe or persists for more than a day, as all antibiotics carry some risk for *C. difficile*–associated disease.

69. The answer is C.
(Chap. 23) Interestingly, a number of recent studies have found that colonization is not a risk factor for disease. This may be because strains that are apt to colonize may provide some immunity to the host or are less toxigenic than disease-causing strains. In either case, this serves as a reminder that stool testing should be conducted only on symptomatic patients, as a positive test carries a totally different meaning if clinical suspicion for *C. difficile*–associated disease is low. Patients should not be considered to have *C. difficile*–associated disease based on culture results alone. Additional information to make a diagnosis in a patient with the appropriate clinical findings includes demonstrating presence of toxin A or B or demonstration of pseudomembranes at colonoscopy. Risk factors for *C. difficile*–associated disease are well defined: the most important is antecedent antibiotics, especially fluoroquinolones, cephalosporins, and clindamycin. Age, high patient acuity, enteral feedings, antacids, and length of time in a health care facility are also predictive of developing *C. difficile*–associated disease.

70. The answer is E.
(Chap. 33) This patient's most likely diagnosis is anisakiasis. This is a nematode infection where humans are an accidental host. It occurs hours to days after ingesting eggs that previously settled into the muscles of fish. The main risk factor for infection is eating raw fish. Presentation mimics an acute abdomen. History is critical as upper endoscopy is both diagnostic and curative. The implicated nematodes burrow into the mucosa of the stomach causing intense pain and must be manually removed by endoscope or, on rare occasion, surgery. There is no medical agent known to cure anisakiasis.

71. The answer is B.
(Chap. 24) Microbiologic data are critical in establishing the source of a liver abscess. Polymicrobial samples of pus or blood cultures with gram-negative rods, enterococcus, and anaerobes suggest an abdominal or pelvic source. Hepatosplenic candidiasis once commonly occurred in leukemia or stem cell transplant patients not receiving antifungal prophylaxis. Fungemia was thought to develop in the portal vasculature with poor clearance of yeast during neutropenia. The rejuvenation of neutrophils correlated with symptoms of hepatic abscess.

Hepatosplenic candidiases is now quite rare, given the widespread use of fluconazole prophylaxis in patients with prolonged neutropenia. Certain species such as *Streptococcus milleri* or *Staphylococcus aureus* likely indicate a primary bacteremia and warrant a search for the source of this, depending on the typical ecologic niche of the organism isolated. Amebic abscesses should be considered in the context of host epidemiology: those with a low to medium pretest probability based on travel history, who also have a negative amebic serology, are effectively ruled out for disease, without needing to sample the abscess percutaneously. Fever is the most common presenting sign of liver abscess. Only 50% of patients with liver abscess have right upper quadrant pain, hepatomegaly, or jaundice. Therefore, half of patients may have no signs localizing to the liver. An elevated alkaline phosphatase level is the most sensitive laboratory finding in liver abscess, present in ~70% of cases. Other liver function abnormalities are less common.

72. The answer is C.
(Chap. 24) Primary bacterial peritonitis is a complication of ascites associated with cirrhosis. Clinical presentation can be misleading as only 80% of patients have fever, and abdominal symptoms are only variably present. Therefore, when patients with known cirrhosis develop worsening encephalopathy, fever, and/or malaise, the diagnosis should strongly be considered and ruled out. In this case, a peritoneal polymorphonuclear leukocyte count of >250/μL would be diagnostic of bacterial peritonitis even if Gram's stain were negative. The paracentesis also might provide microbiologic confirmation. CT of the head would be useful for the diagnosis of cerebral edema associated with severe hepatic encephalopathy or in the presence of focal neurologic findings suggesting an epidural bleed. Cirrhotic patients are at great risk of gastrointestinal (GI) bleeding and it may worsen hepatic encephalopathy by increasing the protein load in the colon. Esophagastroduodenoscopy would be a reasonable course of action, particularly if stools were guaiac positive or there was gross evidence of hematemesis or melena. In this case, there is no evidence of GI bleeding and there is mild hemoconcentration, possibly from peritonitis. Lactulose, and possibly neomycin or rifaximin, is a logical therapeutic trial in this patient if peritonitis is not present. Serum ammonia level may suggest hepatic encephalopathy, if elevated, but does not have sufficient predictive value on its own to rule in or rule out this diagnosis.

73. The answer is C.
(Chap. 22) The patient most likely has food poisoning because of contamination of the fried rice with *Bacillus cereus*. This toxin-mediated disease occurs when heat-resistant spores germinate after boiling. Frying before serving may not destroy the preformed toxin. The

emetic form of illness occurs within 6 h of eating and is self-limited. No therapy is necessary unless the patient develops severe dehydration. This patient currently has no symptoms consistent with volume depletion; therefore, she does not need IV fluids at present. Sarcoidosis does not predispose patients to infectious diseases.

74. The answer is A.
(*Chap. 28*) Campylobacters are motile, curved gram-negative rods. The principal diarrheal pathogen is *C. jejuni*. This organism is found in the gastrointestinal tract of many animals used for food production and is usually transmitted to humans in raw or undercooked food products or through direct contact with infected animals. Over half the cases are due to insufficiently cooked contaminated poultry. *Campylobacter* is a common cause of diarrheal disease in the United States. The illness usually occurs within 2–4 days after exposure to the organism in food or water. Biopsy of an affected patient's jejunum, ileum, or colon reveals findings indistinguishable from those of Crohn's disease and ulcerative colitis. Although the diarrheal illness is usually self-limited, it may be associated with constitutional symptoms, lasts more than 1 week, and recurs in 5–10% of untreated patients. Complications include pancreatitis, cystitis, arthritis, meningitis, and Guillain-Barré syndrome. The symptoms of *Campylobacter* enteritis are similar to those resulting from infection with *Salmonella, Shigella,* and *Yersinia*; all these agents cause fever and the presence of fecal leukocytes. The diagnosis is made by isolating *Campylobacter* from the stool, which requires selective media. *E. coli* (enterotoxigenic) generally is not associated with the finding of fecal leukocytes; nor is the Norwalk agent. *Campylobacter* is a far more common cause of a recurrent relapsing diarrheal illness that could be pathologically confused with inflammatory bowel disease than are *Yersinia, Salmonella, Shigella,* and enteropathogenic *E. coli.*

75. The answer is B.
(*Chap. 23*) Severe *C. difficile*–associated disease may mimic a surgical abdomen and patients may not have diarrhea. The lack of diarrhea should not overshadow the other signs and risk factors that are suggestive of *C. difficile*–associated disease, including significant leukocytosis, long hospitalization, prior antibiotics, and probable enteral tube feeds while on the ventilator. Adynamic ileus is a serious and well-known complication of *C. difficile*–associated disease. All potentially serious manifestations that could be *C. difficile*–associated disease should be empirically treated as such until stool antigen tests are negative and an alternative clinical explanation is found. Intravenous metronidazole may be less optimal then oral vancomycin for severe cases, and this patient may fail therapy. However, oral medicines are less likely to reach the target organ in the presence of an adynamic ileus,

necessitating IV metronidazole. Some advocate combining administration of oral vancomycin by NG tube with IV metronidazole. All potentially offending antibiotics should be stopped (if possible, as is the case here with the patient having recovered from her pneumonia) rather than continued. Surgical colectomy may be necessary in fulminant cases when there is no response to medical therapy. Intravenous immunoglobulins, which may provide antibodies to *C. difficile* toxin, are reserved for severe or multiple recurrent cases of *C. difficile*–associated disease.

76. The answer is D.
(*Chap. 24*) CAPD-associated peritonitis is different from primary and secondary peritonitis in that most infections are caused by skin flora rather than gut pathogens. Therefore, antibiotics should usually ultimately be directed towards *Staphylococcus* species, especially *S. aureus.* These species, including coagulase-negative staphylococci, account for 40–50% of cases. Recently, *S. aureus* has increased in frequency. Typical signs include diffuse pain and peritoneal signs. Peritoneal fluid will be cloudy with >100 WBCs/μL with >50% neutrophils. Vancomycin is necessary in areas where methicillin-resistant *S. aureus* is common. Intraperitoneal loading doses of this drug are typically given. Though gram-negative and *Candida* infections do occur and should be covered prior to the return of culture data, they are less common. The presence of more than one species in culture should prompt an evaluation for secondary peritonitis. Once definitive culture data are returned, then antibiotics can be narrowed towards only the offending pathogen. If there is no symptomatic improvement within 48 h or the patient appears septic, then catheter removal is standard. These infections are in many ways similar to vascular catheter infections, and their management therefore has many parallels.

77. The answer is D or F.
(*Chap. 32*) Giardiasis is diagnosed by detection of parasite antigens, cysts, or trophozoites in feces. There is no reliable serum test for this disease. As a wide variety of pathogens are responsible for diarrheal illness, some degree of diagnostic testing beyond the history and physical examination is required for definitive diagnosis. Colonoscopy does not have a role in diagnosing *Giardia.* Giardiasis can persist in symptomatic patients and should be treated. Cure rates with 5 days of oral metronidazole tid are >90%. A single oral dose of tinidazole is reportedly at least as effective as metronidazole. Paromomycin, an oral poorly absorbed aminoglycoside, can be used for symptomatic patients during pregnancy, but its efficacy for eradicating infection is not known. Clindamycin and albendazole do not have a role in treatment of giardiasis. Refractory disease can be treated with longer duration of metronidazole.

78. The answer is C.

(Chap. 24) It is important to distinguish between primary (spontaneous) and secondary peritonitis. Primary peritonitis is a result of longstanding ascites, usually as a result of cirrhosis. The pathogenesis is poorly understood but may involve bacteremic spread or translocation across the gut wall of usually only a single species of pathogenic bacteria. Secondary peritonitis is due to rupture of a hollow viscous or irritation of the peritoneum due to a contiguous abscess or pyogenic infection. It typically presents with peritoneal signs and in most cases represents a surgical emergency. Secondary peritonitis in a cirrhotic patient is difficult to distinguish on clinical grounds from primary (spontaneous) peritonitis. It is often overlooked because classic peritoneal signs are almost always lacking, and it is uniformly fatal in the absence of surgery. Suspicion for this diagnosis should occur when ascites shows a protein >1g/dL, LDH greater than serum LDH, glucose <50 mg/dL, and/or a polymicrobial Gram stain. Once this diagnosis is suspected, an abdominal film is indicated to rule out free air, and prompt surgical consultation is warranted. Unlike with primary (spontaneous) bacterial peritonitis, in cases of secondary peritonitis antibiotics should include anaerobic coverage and often antifungal agents. This patient requires IV fluid as he has hypotension and tachycardia due to sepsis. Drotrecogin alfa has been shown to reduce mortality in patients with sepsis; however, patients with thrombocytopenia, cirrhosis, and ascites were excluded from inclusion in phase III trials of this agent.

79. The answer is B.

(Chaps. 48 and 34) Hepatic adenomas are benign tumors of the liver found in women in the third and fourth decades. Hormones are thought to play an essential pathophysiologic role. The risk of adenomas is increased among those taking oral contraceptives, anabolic steroids, and exogenous androgens. These adenomas typically occur in the right lobe and are often asymptomatic and are discovered incidentally. Clinical features may include pain or a palpable mass. Diagnosis is usually made by a combination of modalities, including ultrasound, CT, MRI, and nuclear medicine. The risk of malignant transformation is low. Surveillance is recommended for asymptomatic small lesions. However, since this patient has significant pain, an intervention is necessary. In light of the relationship with hormones and the low risk of malignant transformation, the first option would be discontinuation of oral contraceptive therapy and follow-up in 4–6 weeks. Tumors that do not shrink after discontinuation of oral contraceptives may require surgical excision. RFA has no established role, and biopsy is not indicated as the clinical picture is highly suggestive of a benign lesion. Advice should be given to patients with large adenomas that pregnancy may exacerbate symptoms and promote hemorrhage.

80. The answer is C.

(Chap. 41) Alcoholic cirrhosis is the most common type of cirrhosis encountered in North America. Unlike some other causes of cirrhosis, pathologically it is characterized by small, fine scarring and small regenerative nodules. Therefore, it sometimes is referred to as micronodular cirrhosis. There is clear evidence that excessive alcohol use in the setting of chronic hepatitis C strongly increases the risk of development of cirrhosis; therefore, screening and appropriate counseling are essential. Ethanol results in proportionally greater inhibition of ALT synthesis than AST synthesis. Therefore, serum AST is usually disproportionately elevated relative to ALT, resulting in a ratio greater than 2. The liver is the site of vitamin K–dependent carboxylation of coagulation factors II, VII, IX, and X. Therefore, with progressive deterioration in liver function, elevations in serum prothrombin time result, as the extrinsic pathway of coagulation is primarily dependent on tissue factor and factor II. The intrinsic pathway contains many other unaffected factors, and the activated partial thromboplastin time is often normal. Unlike the case in acute viral hepatitis, acetaminophen toxicity, and vascular congestion, alcoholic injury to the liver rarely elevates the transaminases above levels in the hundreds. Elevations in the AST above 500 to 600 U/L should prompt a search for alternative or coincident diagnoses.

81. The answer is C.

(Chap. 43) Gallstones are very common, particularly in Western countries. Cholesterol stones are responsible for 80% of cases of cholelithiasis; pigment stones account for the remaining 20%. Cholesterol is essentially water-insoluble. Stone formation occurs in the setting of factors that upset cholesterol balance. Obesity, cholesterol-rich diets, high-calorie diets, and certain medications affect biliary secretion of cholesterol. Intrinsic genetic mutations in certain populations may affect the processing and secretion of cholesterol in the liver. Pregnancy results in both an increase in cholesterol saturation during the third trimester and changes in gallbladder contractility. Pigment stones are increased in patients with chronic hemolysis, cirrhosis, Gilbert's syndrome, and disruptions in the enterohepatic circulation. Although rapid weight loss and low-calorie diets are associated with gallstones, there is no evidence that a high-protein diet confers an added risk of cholelithiasis.

82. The answer is E.

(Chap. 37) Hepatitis A is an acute, self-limited virus that is acquired almost exclusively via the fecal-oral route. It is classically a disease of poor hygiene and overcrowding. Outbreaks have been traced to contaminated water, milk, frozen raspberries and strawberries, green onions, and shellfish. Infection occurs mostly in children and young adults. It almost invariably resolves spontaneously

and results in lifelong immunity. Fulminant disease occurs in ≤0.1% of cases, and there is no chronic form (in contrast to hepatitis B and C). Diagnosis is made by demonstrating a positive IgM antibody to HAV, as described in the case above. An IgG antibody to HAV indicates immunity, obtained by previous infection or vaccination. A small proportion of patients will experience relapsing hepatitis weeks to months after a full recovery to HAV infection. This too is self-limited. There is no approved antiviral therapy for hepatitis A disease. An inactivated vaccine has decreased the incidence of the disease, and it is recommended for all U.S. children, for high-risk adults, and for travelers to endemic areas. Passive immunization with immune globulin is also available, and it is effective in preventing clinical disease before exposure or during the early incubation period.

83. and 84. The answers are D and C.
(Chap. 37) The clinical hallmarks of acute hepatitis are rarely subtle and consist of general malaise, abdominal discomfort, nausea, vomiting, anorexia, weight loss, headache, fever, and jaundice. After viral infection due to hepatitis B occurs, HBsAg begins to circulate in the blood and is the first viral marker present. HBsAg precedes elevated transaminases and clinical symptoms by several weeks. It becomes undetectable within several months of the onset of jaundice. The replicative stage of hepatitis B virus (HBV) infection is the time of maximal infectivity and liver-injury. HBeAg is a qualitative marker of this phase. HBV DNA is a quantitative marker of the infectivity and liver injury phase. Anti-HBc is typically the next detectable viral marker and precedes anti-HBs by weeks to months. As the appearance of anti-HBs is variable, some patients will experience a period of time in which the only detectable serum marker of hepatitis B infection will be anti-HBc. In other words, there is a gap, or "window period," between the disappearance of HBsAg and the appearance of anti-HBs. As more sensitive immunoassays have been developed, this window period has become less prevalent. Figure 37-2 demonstrates the time course of serum markers and clinical symptoms in acute hepatitis B.

85. The answer is B.
(Chap. 41) Severe right-sided heart failure may lead to chronic liver injury and cardiac cirrhosis. Elevated venous pressure leads to congestion of the hepatic sinusoids and of the central vein and centrilobular hepatocytes. Centrilobular fibrosis develops, and fibrosis extends outward from the central vein, not the portal triads. Gross examination of the liver shows a pattern of "nutmeg liver." Although transaminases are typically mildly elevated, severe congestion, particularly associated with hypotension, may result in dramatic elevation of AST and ALT 50- to 100-fold above normal. Budd-Chiari syndrome, or occlusion of the hepatic veins or inferior vena cava,

may be confused with congestive hepatopathy. However, the signs and symptoms of congestive heart failure are absent in patients with Budd-Chiari syndrome, and these patients can be easily distinguished clinically from those with heart failure. Venoocclusive disease may result from hepatic irradiation and high-dose chemotherapy in preparation for hematopoietic stem cell transplantation. It is not a typical complication of liver transplantation. Although echocardiography is a useful tool for assessing left and right ventricular function, findings may be unimpressive in patients with constrictive pericarditis. A high index of suspicion for constrictive pericarditis (e.g., prior episodes of pericarditis, mediastinal irradiation) should lead to a right-sided heart catheterization with demonstration of "square root sign," limitation of right heart filling pressure in diastole that is suggestive of restrictive cardiomyopathy. Cardiac magnetic resonance imaging may also be helpful in determining which patients should proceed to cardiac surgery.

86. The answer is D.
(Chap. 39) In the course of acute hepatitis B, HBeAg positivity is common and usually transient. Persistence of HBeAg in the serum for >3 months indicates an increased likelihood of development of chronic hepatitis B. In chronic hepatitis B, presence of HBeAg in the serum indicates ongoing viral replication and increased infectivity. It is also a surrogate for inflammatory liver injury but not fibrosis. The development of antibody to HBeAg (anti-HBe) is indicative of the nonreplicative phase of HBV infection. During this phase, intact virions do not circulate and infectivity is less. Currently, quantification of HBV DNA with polymerase chain reaction allows risk stratification as $<10^3$ virions/μL is the approximate threshold for liver injury and infectivity.

87. The answer is C.
(Chap. 37) The current hepatitis B vaccine is a recombinant vaccine consisting of yeast-derived hepatitis B surface antigen particles. A strategy of vaccinating only high-risk individuals in the United States has been shown to be ineffective, and universal vaccination against hepatitis B is now recommended. Pregnancy is *not* a contraindication to vaccination. Vaccination should ideally be performed in infancy. Routine evaluation of hepatitis serologies is not cost-effective and is not recommended. The vaccine is given in three divided intramuscular doses at 0, 1, and 6 months.

88. The answer is B.
(Chap. 43) The clinical presentation is consistent with a cholestatic picture. Painless jaundice always requires an extensive workup, as many of the underlying pathologies are ominous and early detection and intervention often offers the only hope for a good outcome. The gallbladder showed no evidence of stones and the patient shows

no evidence of clinical cholecystitis, and so a HIDA scan is not indicated. Similarly, antibiotics are not necessary at this point. The cholestatic picture without significant elevation of the transaminases on the liver function tests makes acute hepatitis unlikely. Antimitochondrial antibodies are elevated in cases of primary biliary cirrhosis (PBC), which may present in a similar fashion. However, PBC is far more common in women than in men, and the average age of onset is the fifth or sixth decade. The lack of an obvious lesion on CT scan does not rule out a source of the cholestasis in the biliary tree. Malignant causes such as cholangiocarcinoma and tumor of the ampulla of Vater and nonmalignant causes such as sclerosing cholangitis and Caroli's disease may be detected only by direct visualization with ERCP. ERCP is useful both diagnostically and therapeutically as stenting procedures may be done to alleviate the obstruction.

89. and 90. The answers are D and D.
(Chap. 36) Gilbert's syndrome is characterized by a mild unconjugated hyperbilirubinemia. UGT1A1 activity is typically reduced to 10–35% of normal, resulting in impaired conjugation. Diagnosis occurs during young adulthood. Exacerbations occur during times of stress, fatigue, alcohol use, or decreased caloric intake. Episodes are self-limited and benign. No treatment is required, and patient reassurance is recommended. Crigler-Najjar syndrome type 1 is a congenital disease characterized by more dramatic elevations in bilirubin that occur first in the neonatal period. Dubin-Johnson syndrome is another congenital hyperbilirubinemia. However, it is a predominantly conjugated hyperbilirubinemia. Medications and toxins may produce jaundice in the setting of cholestasis or hepatocellular injury. Similarly, medications may induce hemolysis; however, the normal hematocrit, LDH, and haptoglobin eliminate hemolysis as a possibility. Obstructive cholelithiasis is characterized by right upper quadrant pain that is often exacerbated by fatty meals. The absence of symptoms or elevation in other liver function tests also makes this diagnosis unlikely.

91. The answer is B.
(Chap. 41) The presence of cirrhosis in an elderly woman with no prior risk factors for viral or alcoholic cirrhosis should raise the possibility of primary biliary cirrhosis (PBC). It is characterized by chronic inflammation and fibrous obliteration of intrahepatic ductules. The cause is unknown, but autoimmunity is assumed as there is an association with other autoimmune disorders, such as autoimmune thyroiditis, CREST syndrome, and the sicca syndrome. The vast majority of patients with symptomatic disease are women. AMA is positive in over 90% of patients with PBC and only rarely is positive in other conditions. This makes it the most useful initial test in the diagnosis of PBC. Since there are false-positives, if AMA is positive, a liver biopsy is performed to confirm

the diagnosis. The 24-h urine copper collection is useful in the diagnosis of Wilson's disease. Hepatic failure from Wilson's disease typically occurs before age 50 years. Hemochromatosis may result in cirrhosis. It is associated with lethargy, fatigue, loss of libido, discoloration of the skin, arthralgias, diabetes, and cardiomyopathy. Ferritin levels are usually increased, and the most suggestive laboratory abnormality is an elevated transferrin saturation percentage. Although hemochromatosis is a possible diagnosis in this case, PBC is more likely in light of the clinical scenario. Although chronic hepatitis B and hepatitis C are certainly in the differential diagnosis and must be ruled out, they are unlikely because of the patient's history and lack of risk factors.

92. The answer is A.
(Chap. 37) A clear distinction between viral etiologies of acute hepatitis cannot be made on clinical or epidemiologic features alone. This patient is at risk of many forms of hepatitis due to his lifestyle. Given his occupation in food services, from a public health perspective it is important to make an accurate diagnosis. Serologies must be obtained to make a diagnosis. While hepatitis C virus typically does not present as an acute hepatitis, this is not absolute. Hepatitis E virus infects men and women equally and resembles hepatitis A virus in clinical presentation. This patient should be questioned regarding IV drug use, and in addition to hepatitis serologies, an HIV test should be performed.

93. The answer is B.
(Chaps. 48 and 43) Cholangiocarcinoma occurs most commonly in the sixth and seventh decades of life. Patients often present with symptoms and signs of biliary obstruction, including right upper quadrant pain, jaundice, and cholangitis. Unfortunately, most patients present with unresectable disease, and 5-year survival is dismal. Diagnosis is often made by cholangiography. Chronic infection with the liver flukes *Opisthorchis* and *Clonorchis* confers an added risk of cholangiocarcinoma. Similarly, exposure to toxic dyes in the automobile and rubber industries, primary sclerosing cholangitis, and congenital malformations of the biliary tree such as choledochal cysts and Caroli disease predispose to the development of cholangiocarcinoma. Cholelithiasis is not clearly a predisposing factor.

94. The answer is D.
(Chaps. 48 and 39) Hepatocellular carcinoma (HCC) is one of the most common tumors in the world. Its high prevalence in Asia and sub-Saharan Africa is related to the prevalence of chronic hepatitis B infection in those areas. The rising incidence in the United States is related to the presence of chronic hepatitis C. It is more common in men than in women and usually arises from a cirrhotic liver. The incidence peaks in the fifth and sixth

decades of life in Western countries but one to two decades earlier in regions of Asia and Africa. Chronic liver disease with other etiologies, such as hemochromatosis, primary biliary cirrhosis, and alcoholic cirrhosis, also carries an increased risk of HCC. Patients often present with an enlarging abdomen in the setting of chronic liver failure. α Feto-protein levels may be elevated. The primary treatment modality is surgery. Surgical resection offers the best hope for a cure. In cases in which there are multiple lesions or resection is technically not feasible, other options, such as radiofrequency ablation, may be tried. Liver transplantation in selected patients offers a survival that is the same as the survival after transplantation for nonmalignant liver disease. Chemoembolization may confer a survival benefit in patients with nonresectable disease. Systemic chemotherapy is generally not effective and is reserved for palliation when other, more local strategies have been tried.

95. The answer is E.
(Chap. 38) Drug-induced liver injury is common. Acetaminophen is one of the most common causes of drug-induced injury. It is often ingested in suicide attempts or accidentally by children. Acetaminophen is metabolized by a phase II reaction to innocuous sulfate and glucuronide metabolites. However, a small proportion of acetaminophen is metabolized by a phase I reaction to a hepatoxic metabolite, *N*-acetylbenzoquinoneimine (NAPQI). When excessive amounts of NAPQI are formed, glutathione levels are depleted and covalent binding of NAPQI is thought to occur, with hepatocyte macromolecules leading to hepatic injury. Patients often present with confusion, abdominal pain, and sometimes shock. Treatment includes gastric lavage, activated charcoal, and supportive measures. The risk of toxicity is derived from a nomogram plot where acetaminophen plasma levels are plotted against time after ingestion. In this patient the level was above 200 µg/mL at 4 h, indicating a risk of toxicity. Therefore, *N*-acetylcysteine, a sulfhydryl compound, is administered as a reservoir of sulfhydryl groups to support the reserves of glutathione. Normal liver function tests at the time of presentation do not indicate a benign course. Rather, patients must be observed for a period of days as the hepatic toxicity and transaminitis may manifest 4–6 days after the initial ingestion. Alkalinization plays no role. However, in patients who develop signs of hepatic failure (e.g., progressive jaundice, coagulopathy, confusion), liver transplantation is the only established option.

96. The answer is E.
(Chap. 39) Although chronic active hepatitis may be associated with extraintestinal manifestations (e.g., arthritis) and the presence in the serum of autoantibodies (e.g., anti-smooth-muscle antibody), these factors are not invariably present. The distinction between chronic active hepatitis and chronic persistent hepatitis can be established only by doing a liver biopsy. In chronic active hepatitis there is piecemeal necrosis (erosion of the limiting plate of hepatocytes surrounding the portal triads), hepatocellular regeneration, and extension of inflammation into the liver lobule; these features are not seen in chronic persistent hepatitis. Both diseases may be associated with serologic evidence of hepatitis B infection.

97. The answer is A.
(Chap. 37) In healthy adults without a previous history of liver disease, complete recovery from acute hepatitis B infection occurs in about 99% of cases. In this population, including the patient described above, antiviral treatment is unlikely to improve this excellent prognosis and should be avoided. A resolved infection will induce lifelong immunity, and a vaccine series is not necessary. Based on experience with antiviral therapy for chronic hepatitis B infection, some practitioners will treat severe cases of acute hepatitis B with antivirals such as lamivudine or entecavir, though there are no clinical trials in this patient population.

98. The answer is B.
(Chap. 44) The patient has advanced cirrhosis with a high risk of mortality as evidenced by his episode of spontaneous bacterial peritonitis. His diabetes and remote skin cancers are not absolute contraindications for liver transplantation, but active alcohol abuse is. The other absolute contraindications to transplantation are life-threatening systemic disease, uncontrolled infections, preexisting advanced cardiac or pulmonary disease, metastatic malignancy, and life-threatening congenital malignancies. Ongoing drug or alcohol abuse is an absolute contraindication, and patients who would otherwise be suitable candidates should immediately be referred to appropriate counseling centers to achieve abstinence. Once that is achieved for an acceptable period of time, transplantation can be considered. Indeed, alcoholic cirrhosis accounts for a substantial portion of the patients who undergo liver transplantation.

99. The answer is C.
(Chaps. 37 and 39) Causes of extreme elevations in serum transaminases generally fall into a few major categories, including viral infections, toxic ingestions, and vascular/hemodynamic causes. Both acute hepatitis A and hepatitis B infections may be characterized by high transaminases. Fulminant hepatic failure may occur, particularly in situations in which acute hepatitis A occurs on top of chronic hepatitis C infection or if hepatitis B and hepatitis D are cotransmitted. Most cases of acute hepatitis A or B infection in adults are self-limited. Hepatitis C is an RNA virus that does not typically cause acute hepatitis. However, it is associated with a high probability of chronic infection. Therefore, progression

to cirrhosis and hepatoma is increased in patients with chronic hepatitis C infection. Extreme transaminitis is highly unlikely with acute hepatitis C infection. Acetaminophen remains one of the major causes of fulminant hepatic failure and is managed by prompt administration of N-acetylcysteine. Budd–Chiari syndrome is characterized by posthepatic thrombus formation. It often presents with jaundice, painful hepatomegaly, ascites, and elevated transaminases.

100. **The answer is D.**

(*Chap. 46*) The pathophysiology of acute pancreatitis evolves in three phases. During the initial phase, pancreatic injury leads to intrapancreatic activation of digestive enzymes with subsequent autodigestion and acinar cell injury. Acinar injury is primarily attributed to activation of zymogens (proenzymes), particularly trypsinogen, by lysosomal hydrolases. Once trypsinogen is converted to trypsin, the activated trypsin further perpetuates the process by activating other zymogens to further autodigestion. The inflammation initiated by intrapancreatic activation of zymogens leads to the second phase of acute pancreatitis, with local production of chemokines that causes activation and sequestration of neutrophils in the pancreas. Experimental evidence suggests that neutrophilic inflammation can also cause further activation of trypsinogen, leading to a cascade of increasing acinar injury. The third phase of acute pancreatitis reflects the systemic processes that are caused by release of inflammatory cytokines and activated proenzymes into the systemic circulation. This process can lead to the systemic inflammatory response syndrome with acute respiratory distress syndrome, extensive third-spacing of fluids, and multiorgan failure.

101. **The answer is D.**

(*Chap. 46*) Several risk factors have been identified that predict an increased risk of death in acute pancreatitis. Pancreatic necrosis and evidence of multiorgan failure have been the strongest predictors of death in multiple case series. This includes the presence of shock, hypoxemia (Pa_{O_2} <60 mmHg), renal failure (creatinine >2.0 mg/dL), hemoconcentration with a hematocrit >44%, and gastrointestinal bleeding. In addition, other clinical factors including obesity (BMI >30 kg/m^2) and age >70 predict poorer outcomes. Values of amylase and lipase have not been shown to predict the course of acute pancreatitis, and amylase can be spuriously elevated in the presence of a pH <7.32. The Ranson criteria include a variety of biochemical markers at admission and at 48 h that predict outcome in acute pancreatitis. This patient does not meet any of the Ranson criteria at admission (age >55, WBC count >16,000/μL, glucose >200 mg/dL, AST >250 U/L, LDH >350 U/L). A reevaluation at 48 h would be necessary to use Ranson criteria to assess the patient's risk of death to see if any of the six additional criteria had been fulfilled.

102. **The answer is C.**

(*Chap. 46*) A diagnosis of pancreatitis is made in an appropriate clinical setting with abdominal pain radiating to the back and elevated amylase and lipase. Although there are many causes of acute pancreatitis, among the most common are medications, alcohol, and gallstones. This patient does not drink alcohol and right upper quadrant ultrasound does not show cholelithiasis, leaving medications as the likely etiology. Commonly associated drugs are sulfonamides, estrogens, 6-mercaptopurine, azathioprine, anti-HIV medications, and valproic acid. The patient was taking sulfa-methoxazole, which is a sulfonamide. He should be advised to discontinue this medication, and different *Pneumocystis carinii* pneumonia prophylaxis should be prescribed. Alternative regimens include dapsone, aerosolized pentamidine, and atovaquone. Discontinuation of all *Pneumocystis* pneumonia prophylaxis with his degree of immune suppression is unadvisable.

103. **The answer is C.**

(*Chap. 46*) All of the listed choices are causes of acute pancreatitis. Gallstone disease remains the most common cause, responsible for 30–60% of all acute pancreatitis. The second most common cause of acute pancreatitis is alcohol (15–30%). The risk of pancreatitis in alcoholics is quite low, with only 5 cases of pancreatitis per 100,000 individuals. All of the other possible answers each account for <10% of all acute pancreatitis.

104. **The answer is C.**

(*Chap. 46*) Though it is widely used as a screening test to rule out acute pancreatitis in a patient with acute abdominal or back pain, only about 85% of patients with acute pancreatitis have an elevated serum amylase level. Confounding issues include delay between symptoms and the obtaining of blood samples, the presence of chronic pancreatitis, and hypertriglyceridemia, which can falsely lower levels of both amylase and lipase. Because the serum amylase level may be elevated in other conditions, such as renal insufficiency, salivary gland lesions, tumors, burns, and diabetic ketoacidosis, as well as in other abdominal diseases, such as intestinal obstruction and peritonitis, amylase isoenzyme levels have been used to distinguish among these possibilities. Therefore, the pancreatic isoenzyme level can be used to diagnose acute pancreatitis more specifically in the setting of a confounding condition. The serum lipase assay is less subject to confounding variables. However, the sensitivity of the serum lipase level for acute pancreatitis may be as low as 70%. Therefore, recommended screening for acute pancreatitis includes both serum amylase and serum lipase.

105. **The answer is E.**

(*Chap. 46*) This patient present with acute pancreatitis related to alcohol use and has a past history of similar episodes. His presentation does not suggest severe pancreatitis. In this setting, 85–90% of patients will recover spontaneously in 3–7 days with conservative management. Analgesics should be given to control pain and will likely also aid in decreasing this patient's blood pressure. In addition, patients with pancreatitis are frequently volume-depleted due to a variety of factors, including decreased oral intake, vomiting, and third-spacing of fluid with increased vascular permeability. Intravenous volume repletion should be initially given at a high rate to replace volume loss on presentation. After initial volume resuscitation, IV fluids containing glucose should be continued until the patient is able to tolerate oral feeding. In mild pancreatitis, no oral alimentation is recommended until pain has adequately resolved, because the time period that NPO status is maintained is expected to be ≤1 week. In severe cases of pancreatitis, individuals are hypermetabolic and are frequently expected to remain NPO for extended periods. In this setting, alimentation with nasojejunal feeding is preferred over total parenteral nutrition as there appears to be less infection with use of the enteral feedings. This is thought to be due to better maintenance of the gut mucosal barrier function with enteral feeding. Use of nasogastric suctioning offers no clinical benefit in mild pancreatitis, and its use is considered elective.

106. The answer is D.

(Chap. 46) Chronic pancreatitis is a common disorder in any patient population with relapsing acute pancreatitis, especially patients with alcohol dependence, pancreas divisum, and cystic fibrosis. The disorder is notable for both endocrine and exocrine dysfunction of the pancreas. Often diabetes ensues as a result of loss of islet cell function; though insulin-dependent, it is generally not as prone to diabetic ketoacidosis or coma as are other forms of diabetes mellitus. As pancreatic enzymes are essential to fat digestion, their absence leads to fat malabsorption and steatorrhea. In addition, the fat-soluble vitamins, A, D, E, and K, are not absorbed. Vitamin A deficiency can lead to neuropathy. Vitamin B$_{12}$, or cobalamin, is often deficient. This deficiency is hypothesized to be due to excessive binding of cobalamin by cobalamin-binding proteins other than intrinsic factor that are normally digested by pancreatic enzymes. Replacement of pancreatic enzymes orally with meals will correct the vitamin deficiencies and steatorrhea. The incidence of pancreatic adenocarcinoma is increased in patients with chronic pancreatitis, with a 20-year cumulative incidence of 4%. Chronic abdominal pain is nearly ubiquitous in this disorder, and narcotic dependence is common. Niacin is a water-soluble vitamin, and absorption is not affected by pancreatic exocrine dysfunction.

107. The answer is A.

(Chap. 46) This patient likely has chronic pancreatitis related to long-standing alcohol use, which is the most common cause of chronic pancreatitis in adults in the United States. Chronic pancreatitis can develop in individuals who consume as little as 50g of alcohol daily (equivalent to ~30–40 ounces of beer). The patient's description of his loose stools is consistent with steatorrhea, and the recurrent bouts of abdominal pain are likely related to his pancreatitis. In most patients, abdominal pain is the most prominent symptom. However, up to 20% of individuals with chronic pancreatitis present with symptoms of maldigestion alone. The evaluation for chronic pancreatitis should allow one to characterize the pancreatitis as large- vs. small-duct disease. Large-duct disease is more common in men and is more likely to be associated with steatorrhea. In addition, large-duct disease is associated with the appearance of pancreatic calcifications and abnormal tests of pancreatic exocrine function. Women are more likely to have small-duct disease, with normal tests of pancreatic exocrine function and normal abdominal radiography. In small-duct disease, the progression to steatorrhea is rare, and the pain is responsive to treatment with pancreatic enzymes. The characteristic findings on CT and abdominal radiograph of this patient are characteristic of chronic pancreatitis, and no further workup should delay treatment with pancreatic enzymes. Treatment with pancreatic enzymes orally will improve maldigestion and lead to weight gain, but they are unlikely to fully resolve maldigestive symptoms. Narcotic dependence can frequently develop in individuals with chronic pancreatitis due to recurrent and severe bouts of pain. However, as this individual's pain is mild, it is not necessary to prescribe narcotics at this point in time. An ERCP or magnetic resonance cholangiopancreatography (MRCP) may be considered to evaluate for a possible stricture that is amenable to therapy. However, sphincterotomy is a procedure performed via ERCP that may be useful in treating pain related to chronic pancreatitis and is not indicated in the patient. Angiography to assess for ischemic bowel disease is not indicated as the patient's symptoms are not consistent with intestinal angina. Certainly, weight loss can occur in this setting, but the patient usually presents with complaints of abdominal pain after eating and pain that is out of proportion with the clinical examination. Prokinetic agents would likely only worsen the patient's malabsorptive symptoms and are not indicated.

108. The answer is E.

(Chaps. 48 and 34) The liver is particularly vulnerable to invasion by tumor cells because of its dual blood supply by the portal vein and the hepatic arteries. Most patients with liver metastases present with symptoms from the primary tumor. Sometimes hepatic involvement is suggested by features of active hepatic disease, including abdominal pain, hepatomegaly, and ascites. Liver biochemical tests are often the first clue to metastatic disease, but the elevations are often mild and nonspecific.

Typically, alkaline phosphatase is the most sensitive indicator of metastatic disease. Lung, breast, and colon cancer are the most common tumors that metastasize to the liver. Melanoma, particularly ocular melanoma, also commonly seeds the hepatic circulation. Prostate cancer is a much less common cause of hepatic metastases.

109. The answer is A.
(Chap. 49) Ductal adenocarcinomas of the exocrine pancreas are the most common type (>90%) of pancreatic neoplasm. The pancreatic head is the most common site. The median age of diagnosis is 72 years, with the peak incidence between 65 and 85 years. The incidence is slightly higher in men than women and in African Americans than Caucasians. Pancreatic carcinoma is uncommon below the age of 50. These tumors are aggressive and usually present with locally inoperable disease with local and distal metastases. The 5-year survival is only about 5%. It is the fourth leading cause of cancer death. Other less common types of pancreatic neoplasms include islet cell tumors and neuroendocrine tumors.

110. The answer is E.
(Chap. 49) When first-line therapy for pancreatic cancer has failed, fit patients should be referred for enrollment in clinical trials to identify novel therapeutic agents. Gemcitabine has been shown to be superior to treatment with 5-fluorouracil. Patients with little life expectancy or who have a poor functional status may benefit by incorporating palliative or hospice care into their treatment plan. External beam chemoradiotherapy may be helpful when the disease is locally advanced and causing significant morbidity. Debulking surgery has no role in the treatment of advanced pancreatic cancer since the risk of the procedure is similar to that of a curative resection and offers no survival benefit. Biliary stenting is useful for relieving obstructive jaundice.

111. The answer is B.
(Chap. 49) Patients with a suspicious pancreatic lesion seen on imaging that may be curable with local resection are often taken to surgery without further tissue characterization. Transcutaneous biopsy carries with it the theoretical risk of seeding the surrounding tissues as the needle is passed. Endoscopic ultrasound-guided fine-needle aspiration is increasing being utilized for biopsies as there is less risk of intraperitoneal spread of tumor. A negative biopsy or fine-needle aspiration may not be sufficient to rule out a neoplasm when the lesion is small. The dismal prognosis for advanced disease calls for prompt surgical referral for potentially curable lesions. An elevated CA 19-9 level is suggestive of pancreatic cancer but may also be elevated in cases of jaundice without pancreatic cancer. The reported sensitivity and specificity of the CA 19-9 assay for pancreatic cancer is

reported between 80 and 90%, but it should not be used to confirm or exclude pancreatic cancer when the clinical scenario suggests the diagnosis.

112. The answer is C.
(Chap. 50) This patient presents with the classic findings of a VIPoma, including large-volume watery diarrhea, hypokalemia, dehydration, and hypochlorhydria (WDHA, or Verner-Morrison, syndrome). Abdominal pain is unusual. The presence of a secretory diarrhea is confirmed by a stool osmolal gap [2(stool Na + stool K) – (stool osmolality)] <35 and persistence during fasting. In osmotic or laxative-induced diarrhea, the stool osmolal gap is over 100. In adults, over 80% of VIPomas are solitary pancreatic masses that usually are larger than 3 cm at diagnosis. Metastases to the liver are common and preclude curative surgical resection. The differential diagnosis includes gastrinoma, laxative abuse, carcinoid syndrome, and systemic mastocytosis. Diagnosis requires the demonstration of large-volume secretory diarrhea (over 700 mL/d) and elevated serum VIP. CT scan of the abdomen will often demonstrate the pancreatic mass and liver metastases.

113. and 114. The answers are E and E.
(Chap. 50) In patients with a nonmetastatic carcinoid, surgery is the only potentially curative therapy. The extent of surgical resection depends on the size of the primary tumor because the risk of metastasis is related to the size of the tumor. Symptomatic treatment is aimed at decreasing the amount and effect of circulating substances. Drugs that inhibit the serotonin $5-HT_1$ and $5-HT_2$ receptors (methysergide, cyproheptadine, ketanserin) may control diarrhea but not flushing. $5-HT_3$ receptor antagonists (odansetron, tropisetron, alosetron) control nausea and diarrhea in up to 100% of these patients and may alleviate flushing. A combination of histamine H_1 and H_2 receptor antagonists may control flushing, particularly in patients with foregut carcinoid tumors. Somatostatin analogues (octreotide, lanreotide) are the most effective and widely used agents to control the symptoms of carcinoid syndrome, decreasing urinary 5-HIAA excretion and symptoms in 70–80% of patients. Interferon α, alone or combined with hepatic artery embolization, controls flushing and diarrhea in 40–85% of these patients. Phenoxybenzamine is an $α_1$-adrenergic receptor blocker that is used in the treatment of pheochromocytoma.

115. The answer is B.
(Chap. 53) Albumin has a half-life of 2–3 weeks and is a sensitive but nonspecific measure of protein-calorie malnutrition. Other situations in which albumin is low include sepsis, surgery, overhydration, and increased plasma volume, including congestive heart failure, renal failure, and chronic liver disease. Among the other markers of nutritional state, transferrin has a half-life of

1 week. Prealbumin and retinol-binding protein complex have the same half-life of 2 days. Fibronectin has the shortest half-life: 1 day.

116. The answer is C.
(*Chap. 52*) Certain medications, including isoniazid used for tuberculosis, L-dopa used for Parkinson's disease, and penicillamine used for scleroderma, promote vitamin B_6 (pyridoxine) deficiency by reacting with a carbonyl group on 5-pyridoxal phosphate, which is a cofactor for a host of enzymes involved in amino acid metabolism. Foods that contain vitamin B_6 include legumes, nuts, wheat bran, and meat. Vitamin B_6 deficiency produces seborrheic dermatitis, glossitis, stomatitis, and cheilosis (also seen in other vitamin B deficiencies). A microcytic, hypochromic anemia may result from the fact that the first enzyme in heme synthesis (aminolevulinic synthetase) requires pyridoxal phosphate as a cofactor. However, vitamin B_6 is also necessary for the conversion of homocysteine to cystathionine. Consequently, a deficiency of this vitamin could produce an increased risk of cardiovascular disease caused by the resultant hyperhomocysteinemia.

117. The answer is C.
(*Chap. 53*) The two major types of protein energy malnutrition are marasmus and kwashiorkor; differentiating the two is extremely important in the malnourished patient since this directly effects your therapy. This patient has marasmic kwashiorkor due to the impact of her anorexia nervosa, the acute stressor of the surgery, and the 10 days of starvation. This patient has chronic starvation (marasmus) as well as the major sine qua non of kwashiorkor; i.e., reduction of levels of serum proteins. She is kwashiorkor predominant because of the acute starvation and the severely low levels of serum proteins. Vigorous nutritional therapy is indicated for kwashiorkor.

118. The answer is C.
(*Chap. 52*) There are two natural sources of vitamin K. Vitamin K_1 comes from vegetable and animal sources. Vitamin K_2 is synthesized by enteric bacterial flora and is found in hepatic tissue. Vitamin K deficiency in adults can be seen with chronic small-intestinal disease, in those with obstructed biliary tracts, after small-bowel resection, or in those on broad-spectrum antibiotics. As a result of reducing gut bacteria, antibiotics can precipitate vitamin K deficiency. Overdose and medication error are plausible explanations but are less likely to be the root cause given the antibiotic exposure. Acute venous thromboses can deplete levels of coagulant proteins (especially protein C and protein S), but the INR should not be affected.

119. The answer is D.
(*Chap. 52*) This patient has the classic perifollicular hemorrhagic rash of scurvy (vitamin C deficiency). In the United States, scurvy is primarily a disease of alcoholics and the elderly who consume <10 mg/d of vitamin C. In addition to nonspecific symptoms of fatigue, these patients also have impaired ability to form mature connective tissue and can bleed into various sites, including the skin and gingiva. A normal INR excludes symptomatic vitamin K deficiency. Thiamine, niacin, and folate deficiencies are also seen in patients with alcoholism. Thiamine deficiency may cause a peripheral neuropathy (beri-beri). Folate deficiency causes macrocytic anemia and thrombocytopenia. Niacin deficiency causes pellagra, which is characterized by glossitis and a pigmented, scaling rash that may be particularly noticeable in sun exposed areas.

120. The answer is C.
(*Chap. 54*) In the past, bowel rest was the cornerstone of treatment; however, the value of adding minimal amounts of enteral nutrition (EN) is widely accepted. Timing of enteral therapy is important. Although administering EN can improve mortality, there is an increased risk of infection. Patients with severe SRI are unlikely to be able to take adequate, spontaneous oral intake within the first week of their hospitalization. Therefore, enteral nutrition should be considered early for severely sick patients.

121. The answer is B.
(*Chap. 51*) For patients with stable weights, REE can be calculated if the gender, weight, and activity level are provided. For males, REE = 900 + 10w, and for females, REE = 700 + 7w, where w is weight in kilograms. The REE is then adjusted for activity level by multiplying 1.2 for sedentary, 1.4 for moderately active, and 1.8 for very active individuals. Patient A has an REE of 2160 kcal/day. Patient B has an REE of 2880 kcal/day. For a given weight, a higher level of activity increases the REE more than a 20-kg change in weight at a given level of activity.

122. The answer is A.
(*Chap. 53*) Interactions between illness and nutrition are complex, therefore many physical and laboratory findings reflect both underlying disease and nutritional status. The nutritional evaluation of a patient requires an integration of history, physical examination, anthropometrics, and laboratory studies. The finding of isolated hypoalbuminemia may be due to her underlying liver disease and does not necessarily indicate malnutrition. This patient is at high risk for malnutrition, but her current status may reflect malnutrition or sequelae of chronic alcoholism.

123. The answer is B.
(*Chap. 52*) High doses of vitamin E (>800 mg/d) may reduce platelet aggregation and interfere with vitamin K

metabolism. Doses >400 mg/d may increase mortality from any cause. Vitamin E excess is not related to increased risk of venous thrombosis. Peripheral neuropathy and a pigmented retinopathy may be seen in vitamin E deficiency. Vitamin A deficiency is a cause of night blindness.

124. The answer is D.
(Chap. 52) Pellagra (niacin deficiency) is most commonly a disorder among people eating corn-based diets but can also be seen in alcoholics. Tryptophan is converted to niacin with an efficiency of 60:1 by weight. Therefore, in a patient with congenital defects in tryptophan absorption or with increased conversion of tryptophan to serotonin, niacin deficiency can develop. The early symptoms of pellagra include anorexia, irritability, abdominal pain and vomiting, and glossitis. Vaginitis and esophagitis may also occur. The four Ds of pellagra are *d*ermatitis, *d*iarrhea, and *d*ementia leading to *d*eath. Dyslipidemia is not a part of the pellagra syndrome.

125. The answer is C.
(Chap. 54) The most common metabolic problems related to parenteral nutrition (PN) are fluid overload and hyperglycemia. Hypertonic dextrose stimulates a much higher insulin level than normal feeding, which is evident on hospital day 9 in this scenario. Hyperinsulinemia stimulates antinatriuretic and antidiuretic hormone, which leads to sodium and fluid retention as well as increased intracellular transport of potassium, magnesium, and phosphorus. It is not uncommon to see an increase in weight and a low urine sodium in patients with normal renal function. Providing sodium in limited amounts of 40 meq/day and the use of both glucose and fat in the PN mixture will help reduce fluid retention. Reducing the overall glucose content will also abate the need for higher insulin level. The fluid retention in this scenario is not mediated by low protein levels.

126. The answer is C.
(Chap. 51) The estimated average requirement (EAR) is the amount of a nutrient estimated to be adequate for half of the individuals of a specific age and sex. It is not useful clinically for estimating nutritional adequacy because it is a median requirement for a group; 50% of the individuals in a group fall below the requirement and 50% fall above it. A person taking the EAR of a vitamin has a 50% risk of inadequate intake. The recommended dietary allowance (RDA) is defined statistically as 2 standard deviations above the EAR to ensure that the needs of most individuals are met. In this case the study used a dosage of 2 standard deviations above the EAR, which would be the RDA. Data on the tolerable upper limit of a vitamin are usually inadequate to establish a value for upper limit of tolerability. The absence of a published tolerable upper limit does not imply that the risks are nonexistent.

127. The answer is D.
(Chap. 52) Hypozincemia is most commonly due to poor oral intake of zinc, although some medications can also inhibit zinc absorption (e.g., sodium valproate, penicillamine, ethambutol). Severe chronic zinc deficiency has been described among children from Middle Eastern countries as a cause of hypogonadism and dwarfism. Hypopigmented hair is also a part of this syndrome. Hypochromic anemia can be seen in a number of vitamin deficiency/excess disorders, including zinc toxicity and copper deficiency. Copper deficiency is also associated with dissecting aortic aneurysm. Hypoglycemia does not correlate with hypozincemia. Macrocytosis is associated with folate and vitamin B_{12} deficiency.

128. The answer is D.
(Chap. 52) Vitamin A deficiency remains a problem of children with chronically poor diets in parts of Asia, Africa, and China. This child has xerophthalmia with evidence of mild night blindness. He also has Bitot's spots (white patches on the sclera). Vitamin A deficiency also impairs the host's ability to fight infection. Mortality amongst vitamin A–deficient children is substantially higher when infected with diarrhea, dysentery, measles, malaria, or respiratory disease. Supplementation improves the mortality. SCA type 1 does not have any associated ophthalmologic findings. Autoimmune neutropenia may account for the repeated bouts of infection, but the constellation of Bitot's spots and recurrent infection argues against this as the cause. Congenital rubella causes congenital cataracts, not Bitot's spots. Vitamin B_1 (thiamine) deficiency causes beri-beri, which is associated with high output cardiac failure or peripheral neuropathy.

129. The answer is C.
(Chap. 53) The energy stores in a healthy 70-kg man include ~15 kg as fat, 6 kg as protein, and 500 mg as glycogen. During the first day of a fast, most energy needs are met by consumption of liver glycogen. During longer fasting, resting energy expenditure will decrease by up to 25% (provided there is no ongoing inflammation). In the presence of water intake and no inflammation, a normal individual may fast for months. A well-nourished individual can tolerate ~7 days of starvation while experiencing a systemic response to inflammation. The hiker in this scenario has starved for 6 days and, except for mild acute renal failure, he has compensated well for his starvation. Greater than 10% weight loss in 6 months represents significant protein-calorie malnutrition. This person's ferritin is only mildly elevated, although a true systemic response to inflammation (SRI) does increase the rate of lean tissue loss. Moreover, he has no other indicators that he is experiencing the systemic inflammatory response syndrome (SIRS). SRI often causes hyperglycemia, not hypoglycemia.

130. The answer is C.

(Chap. 54) Tracheal suctioning induces coughing and gastric regurgitation and cuffs on endotracheal tubes seldom protect against aspiration. Effective preventive measures include elevating the head of the bed to 30°, nurse-directed algorithms for formula advancement, combining enteral and parenteral feeding, and using post-ligament of Treitz feeding. Recent studies have suggested that constant suction above the endotracheal cuff may reduce ventilator-associated pneumonia.

131. The answer is A.

(Chap. 58) The metabolic syndrome (according to the NCET:ATP III guidelines) is defined by three or more of the following: central obesity (men >102 cm; women >88 cm), hypertriglyceridemia (≥150 mg/dL or on specific medication), low HDL cholesterol (men <40 mg/dL; women <50 mg/dL), hypertension (systolic ≥130 mmHg or diastolic ≥85 mmHg, or on specific medication), and hyperglycemia (fasting plasma glucose ≥100 mg/dL, or previous diagnosis of diabetes mellitus, or on specific medication). The International Diabetes Foundation also has criteria that further subdivide the cut-offs of waist circumference based on ethnicity. Patients with the metabolic syndrome are at greater risk than patients without the syndrome for developing conditions such as atherosclerotic cardiovascular disease, type 2 diabetes mellitus, peripheral vascular disease, sleep apnea, and polycystic ovary syndrome. The presence of one of the criteria should prompt the clinician to search for other criteria and treat the conditions as necessary.

132. The answer is D.

(Chap. 58) According to the NCEP:ATP III guidelines, treating the dyslipidemia of the metabolic syndrome should first be directed towards LDL cholesterol goals (usually <100 mg/dL, depending on the presence of risk factors). If triglyceride levels are ≥200 mg/dL after the LDL goal is reached, the clinician should set a secondary goal for non-high-density lipoprotein cholesterol 30 points higher than the LDL goal. When triglyceride levels are between 200 and 499 mg/dL, options include nicotinic acid, a fibrate, or intensifying therapy with an HMG-CoA reductase inhibitor (statin). Average efficacy of these drug classes are as follows: nicotinic acid, 20–40%; fibrate, 35–50%; statin, 7–30%). Cholestyramine and colestipol are bile acid sequestrants. They lower cholesterol but often increase triglyceride levels and should not be used in patients with triglycerides >200 mg/dL. The effects of ezetimibe on hypertriglyceridemia are not well established. Nicotinic acid is effective for treating hypertriglyceridemia but may worsen glucose control and therefore should be used cautiously in patients with the metabolic syndrome. Gemfibrozil is more likely to worsen statin myopathy than fenofibrate.

133. The answer is C.

(Chap. 58) Reversing insulin resistance and hyperglycemia can be achieved by lifestyle modifications, metformin or other biguanide medications, and/or thiazolidinedione medications. Of the medications, only the thiazolidinediones improve insulin-mediated glucose uptake in the muscle and adipose tissue. The mechanism of action of metformin is uncertain, but it appears to work by reducing hepatic gluconeogenesis and intestinal absorption of glucose. In a large trial of lifestyle modifications and metformin in the prevention of diabetes (Diabetes Prevention Program), subjects in the lifestyle arm of the trial had a more significant reduction in the incidence of diabetes than those assigned to metformin. In resource-poor settings and the developing world, lifestyle modifications have also been shown to be more cost-effective than metformin for preventing diabetes.

134. The answer is D.

(Chap. 57) The most important feature of patients with anorexia nervosa is refusal to maintain even a low-normal body weight. The full syndrome of anorexia nervosa occurs in about 1 in 200 individuals. These patients are always markedly underweight, hardly ever menstruate, and often engage in binge eating. The mortality rate is 5% per decade. The etiology of this serious eating disorder is unknown but probably involves a combination of psychological, biologic, and cultural risk factors. This illness often begins in an obsessive or perfectionist patient who starts a diet. As weight loss progresses, the patient has increasing fears of gaining weight and engages in stricter dieting practices. This disorder essentially occurs only in cultures in which thinness is valued, suggesting a strong cultural influence. Bulimia nervosa, in which patients continue to maintain a normal body weight but typically engage in overeating with binges followed by compensatory purging or purging behavior, has a higher than expected prevalence in patients with childhood or parental obesity. It is unclear whether anorexia nervosa is hereditary in nature.

135. The answer is A.

(Chap. 57) Anorexia nervosa (AN) is much less common in men than women and is more prevalent in cultures where food is plentiful and where thinness is associated with attractiveness. Individuals who pursue occupations that place a premium on thinness, such as ballet or modeling, are at greater risk of developing anorexia nervosa. In patients with AN, as weight loss increases thoughts of food dominate mental life. AN patients may obsessively collect cookbooks and recipes and tend to be drawn to food-related occupations. These patients become socially withdrawn and may also engage in binge eating, similar to bulimia nervosa patients. AN patients rarely complain of hunger or fatigue and will exercise extensively as a means to achieve weight loss.

136. The answer is E.

(Chap. 57) Based on the American Psychiatric Association's practice guidelines, inpatient treatment or partial hospitalization is indicated for patients whose weight <75% of expected for age and height, have severe metabolic disturbances (e.g., electrolyte disturbances, bradycardia, hypotension), or who have serious concomitant psychiatric problems (e.g., suicidal ideation, substance abuse). There should be a low threshold for inpatient treatment if there has been rapid weight loss or if weight <80% of expected. Amenorrhea, exaggeration of food intake, and fear of gaining weight are part of the diagnostic criteria for AN, and purging is not uncommon in this population. Weight restoration to 90% of predicted weight is the goal of nutritional therapy.

137. The answer is A.

(Chap. 57) Regulation of virtually every endocrine system is disturbed in patients with anorexia nervosa (AN). Hypothalamic amenorrhea reflects diminished production of GnRH. Serum leptin levels are reduced due to decreased mass of adipose tissue, and this is thought to be the mediator of the other neuroendocrine abnormalities associated with AN. Thyroid function tests resemble the pattern seen in euthyroid sick syndrome (low-normal or depressed TSH and T_4, depressed T_3, increased reverse T_3). Serum cortisol and 24-h urine free cortisol are generally elevated without the expected clinical consequences of hypercortisolism.

138. The answer is D.

(Chap. 57) The mortality of AN is ~5% per decade and is much lower in patients with BN. This is probably mediated by the weight loss and malnutrition associated with AN. There are two subtypes of BN: purging and nonpurging.

Patients with the nonpurging subtype tend to be heavier and are less prone to electrolyte disturbances. There are also two mutually exclusive subtypes of AN: restricting and purging. Patients with the purging subtype are more emotionally labile and tend to have other problems with impulse control such as illicit drug abuse.

139. The answer is D.

(Chap. 57) Anorexia nervosa (AN) and bulimia nervosa (BN) are distinct clinical entities but share certain features. Many patients with BN have a history of anorexia, and patients with AN engage in binge eating and abnormal compensatory behaviors such as purging. The critical distinction between AN and BN depends on body weight: patients with AN are significantly underweight, whereas patients with BN have normal weight or are overweight. The presence of electrolyte disturbances confers an increased morbidity for both disorders.

140. The answer is D.

(Chap. 57) Approximately 25–50% of patients with anorexia nervosa (AN) recover fully with few physiologic or psychological sequelae. However, many patients have persistent difficulties with weight maintenance, depression, and eating disturbances. Approximately 5% of patients die per decade, usually due to the physical effects of chronic starvation or from suicide. Virtually all of the physiologic derangements associated with anorexia nervosa will improve with weight gain. One exception is the loss of bone mass, which may not recover fully when AN occurs during adolescence (i.e., during peak bone mass formation). Psychological health also improves with successful treatment, although these patients remain at risk for depression, recurrence, and development of bulimia nervosa.

Bold number indicates the start of the main discussion of the topic; numbers with "f" and "t" refer to figure and table pages.

Derived from Harrison's Principles of Internal Medicine, 17th Edition

Editors

ANTHONY S. FAUCI, MD
Chief, Laboratory of Immunoregulation;
Director, National Institute of Allergy and Infectious Diseases,
National Institutes of Health, Bethesda

DENNIS L. KASPER, MD
William Ellery Channing Professor of Medicine,
Professor of Microbiology and Molecular Genetics,
Harvard Medical School; Director, Channing Laboratory,
Department of Medicine,
Brigham and Women's Hospital, Boston

DAN L. LONGO, MD
Scientific Director, National Institute on Aging,
National Institutes of Health, Bethesda and Baltimore

EUGENE BRAUNWALD, MD
Distinguished Hersey Professor of Medicine,
Harvard Medical School; Chairman, TIMI Study Group,
Brigham and Women's Hospital, Boston

STEPHEN L. HAUSER, MD
Robert A. Fishman Distinguished Professor and Chairman,
Department of Neurology,
University of California, San Francisco

J. LARRY JAMESON, MD, PhD
Professor of Medicine; Vice President for Medical
Affairs and Lewis Landsberg Dean,
Northwestern University Feinberg
School of Medicine, Chicago

JOSEPH LOSCALZO, MD, PhD
Hersey Professor of Theory and Practice of Medicine,
Harvard Medical School; Chairman, Department of Medicine;
Physician-in-Chief, Brigham and Women's Hospital, Boston

HARRISON'S
Gastroenterology and Hepatology